W9-CQZ-485

AMERICAN HANDBOOK OF PSYCHIATRY

Volume Eight

AMERICAN HANDBOOK OF PSYCHIATRY

Silvano Arieti, EDITOR-IN-CHIEF

Volume One
The Foundations of Psychiatry
EDITED BY SILVANO ARIETI

Volume Two
Child and Adolescent Psychiatry, Sociocultural and Community Psychiatry
EDITED BY GERALD CAPLAN

Volume Three
Adult Clinical Psychiatry
EDITED BY SILVANO ARIETI AND EUGENE B. BRODY

Volume Four
Organic Disorders and Psychosomatic Medicine
EDITED BY MORTON F. REISER

Volume Five
Treatment
EDITED BY DANIEL X. FREEDMAN AND JARL E. DYRUD

Volume Six
New Psychiatric Frontiers
EDITED BY DAVID A. HAMBURG AND H. KEITH H. BRODIE

Volume Seven
Advances and New Directions
EDITED BY SILVANO ARIETI AND H. KEITH H. BRODIE

Volume Eight
Biological Psychiatry
EDITED BY PHILIP A. BERGER AND H. KEITH H. BRODIE

AMERICAN HANDBOOK OF PSYCHIATRY

SECOND EDITION

Silvano Arieti · Editor-in-Chief

VOLUME EIGHT

Biological Psychiatry

PHILIP A. BERGER AND H. KEITH H. BRODIE · *Editors*

BASIC BOOKS, INC., PUBLISHERS · NEW YORK

Library of Congress Cataloging-in-Publication Data

Biological psychiatry.

(American handbook of psychiatry, second edition; v. 8)
Includes indexes.
1. Bilogical psychiatry.   I. Berger, Philip A.
II. Brodie, H. Keith H. (Harlow Keith Hammond),
1939-   . II. Series. [DNLM: 1. Biological
Psychiatry.   WM 100 A503 v. 8]
RC435.A562 vol. 8   616.89 s   85–48020
[RC341]   [616.89]
ISBN 0–465–00159–9

Second Edition
Copyright © 1986 by Basic Books, Inc.
Printed in the United States of America
86 87 88 MPC 9 8 7 6 5 4 3 2 1

This book is dedicated to

Meredith and Brenda

CONTRIBUTORS

Huda Akil, M.D.

Associate Professor, Director of Research, Department of Psychiatry, University of Michigan, Ann Arbor; Associate Research Scientist, Mental Health Research Institute, University of Michigan, Ann Arbor.

Ross J. Baldessarini, M.D.

Professor of Psychiatry and Neuroscience, Harvard Medical School; Psychiatrist and Interim Director, Mailman Laboratories for Psychiatric Research, McLean Hospital, Belmont, Massachusetts; Psychiatrist, Massachusetts General Hospital, Boston.

H. Thomas Ballantine, Jr., M.D.

Clinical Professor of Surgery (Neurosurgery), Emeritus, Harvard Medical School, Senior Neurosurgeon, Massachusetts General Hospital, Boston.

Jack D. Barchas, M.D.

Nancy Friend Pritzker Professor of Psychiatry and Behavioral Sciences; Director, Nancy Pritzker Laboratory of Behavioral Neurochemistry, Stanford University Medical Center, Stanford, California.

Philip A. Berger, M.D.

Director, Norris Mental Health Clinical Research Center at Stanford University and Kenneth T. Norris, Jr., Professor of Psychiatry and Behavioral Sciences, Stanford University, Stanford, California.

Garth Bissette, Ph.D.

Assistant Professor of Psychiatry, Assistant Director, Laboratory of Psychoneuroendocrinology, Duke University Medical Center, Durham, North Carolina.

John J. Bonica, M.D., D.Sc., FFARCS

Chairman Emeritus and Professor, Department of Anesthesiology, and Director Emeritus, Multidisciplinary Pain Center, University of Washington School of Medicine, Seattle.

Roger A. Boshes, Ph.D., M.D.

Research Psychiatrist, Department of Central Research, Illinois State Psychiatric Institute, Chicago; Assistant Professor, Department of Psychiatry, University of Illinois, College of Medicine, Chicago.

H.K.H. Brodie, M.D.

President and James B. Duke Professor of Psychiatry and Law, Duke University, Durham, North Carolina.

Monte S. Buchsbaum, M.D.

Professor of Psychiatry, Department of Psychiatry, University of California, Irvine.

William E. Bunney, Jr., M.D.

Professor and Chairman, Department of Psychiatry and Human Behavior, University of California School of Medicine, Irvine.

C. Richard Chapman, Ph.D.

Professor, Departments of Anesthesiology, Psychiatry, and Behavioral Sciences and Psychology, and Associate Director for Research, Multidisciplinary Pain Center, University of Washington School of Medicine, Seattle.

Roland D. Ciaranello, M.D.

Professor, Department of Psychiatry and Behavioral Sciences, and Chief, Division of Child Psychiatry and Child Development, Stanford School of Medicine, Stanford, California.

Thomas B. Cooper

Director, Analytical Psychopharmacology, Nathan Kline Institute and New York State Psychiatric Institute, New York.

Jacqueline N. Crawley, Ph.D.

Chief, Unit on Behavioral Neuropharmacology, Clinical Neuroscience Branch, National Institute of Mental Health, Bethesda, Maryland.

Michael Davidson, M.D.

Instructor, Department of Psychiatry, Mt. Sinai School of Medicine, New York; Psychiatry Service, Veterans Administration Medical Center, Bronx, New York.

John M. Davis, M.D., Ph.D.

Gillman Professor of Psychiatry, University of Illinois, Chicago; Director of Research, Illinois State Psychiatric Institute, Chicago.

Kenneth L. Davis, M.D.

Professor of Psychiatry and Pharmacology, Mt. Sinai School of Medicine, New York; Chief, Psychiatry Service, Veterans Administration Medical Center, Bronx, New York.

Susan R. Donaldson, M.D.

Staff Psychiatrist, St. Elizabeth's Hospital, Brighton, Massachusetts; Instructor in Psychiatry, Harvard Medical School, Boston.

Meredith J. Dunn, M.A., Dip. Ed.

Research Associate, Norris Mental Health Clinical Research Center at Stanford University, Stanford, California.

Burr Eichelman, M.D., Ph.D.

Professor of Psychiatry, University of Wisconsin, Madison; Chief, Psychiatry Service, William S. Middleton Memorial Veterans Administration Hospital, Madison, Wisconsin.

Glen R. Elliott, Ph.D., M.D.

Research Physician, Department of Psychiatry and Behavioral Sciences, Stanford School of Medicine, Stanford, California.

Alan J. Gelenberg, M.D.

Psychiatrist-in-Chief, The Arbour Hospital, Jamaica Plain, Massachusetts; Chief, Special Studies Clinic, Department of Psychiatry, Massachusetts General Hospital; Associate Professor of Psychiatry, Harvard Medical School, Boston.

Robert H. Gerner, M.D.

Chief, Psychiatry Research, Long Beach Veterans Administration Medical Center, Long Beach, California; Associate Professor, Department of Psychiatry, University of California, Irvine.

Alexander H. Glassman, M.D.

Chief, Department of Clinical Psychopharmacology, New York State Psychiatric Institute, New York; Professor of Psychiatry, College of Physicians and Surgeons, Columbia University, New York.

David J. Greenblatt, M.D.

Chief, Division of Clinical Pharmacology, Tufts-New England Medical Center Hospital, Boston.

Katherine A. Halmi, M.D.

Associate Professor of Psychiatry, Cornell University Medical College, New York; Associate Attending Psychiatrist, New York Hospital—Westchester Division, White Plains, New York.

Thomas B. Horvath, M.D., FRACP

Clinical Director, Psychiatry Service, Bronx Veterans Administration Medical Center, Bronx, New York: Vice-Chairman, Department of Psychiatry, Mount Sinai School of Medicine, New York.

Andrei C. Iager, M.D.

Staff Psychiatrist, National Institute of Mental Health, St. Elizabeth's Hospital, Washington, D.C.

Terry L. Jernigan, Ph.D.

Staff Psychologist, Veterans Administration Medical Center, San Diego; Assistant Professor of Psychiatry and Radiology, School of Medicine, University of California, San Diego.

Dilip V. Jeste, M.D.

Chief, Unit on Movement Disorders, National Institute of Mental Health, St. Elizabeth's Hospital, Washington, D.C.

Russell T. Joffe, M.D.

Staff Psychiatrist, Biological Psychiatry Branch, National Institutes of Health, Bethesda, Maryland.

Celeste A. Johns, M.D.

Department of Psychiatry, Mt. Sinai School of Medicine, New York; Veterans Administration Medical Center, Bronx, New York.

Seymour S. Kety, M.D.

Professor Emeritus of Neuroscience in Psychiatry, Harvard University, Boston; Senior Science Advisor to the Alcohol, Drug Abuse and Mental Health Administration, National Institutes of Health, Bethesda, Maryland.

Henry Khachaturian, Ph.D.

Research Investigator, Mental Health Research Institute, University of Michigan, Ann Arbor.

Kerry D. Kravitz, M.D., Ph.D.

Resident in Psychiatry, Stanford University Medical Center, Stanford, California.

Michael E. Lewis, Ph.D.

Research Investigator, Mental Health Research Institute, University of Michigan, Ann Arbor.

Miklos F. Losonczy, M.D., Ph.D

Instructor, Department of Psychiatry, Mt. Sinai School of Medicine, New York; Psychiatry Service, Veterans Administration Medical Center, Bronx, New York.

Martin T. Lowy, Ph.D.

Assistant Professor of Psychiatry, Department of Psychiatry, Case Western Reserve University School of Medicine, Cleveland, Ohio.

Steven Matthysse, Ph.D.

Associate Professor of Psychobiology, Harvard Medical School, Boston; Associate Psychobiologist, McLean Hospital, Belmont, Massachusetts.

Herbert Y. Meltzer, M.D.

Douglas Bond Professor of Psychiatry, Department of Psychiatry, Case Western Reserve University School of Medicine, Cleveland, Ohio.

Victor Milstein, Ph.D.

Professor of Psychology/Psychiatry, Indiana University School of Medicine, Indianapolis.

Marcelle A. Mostert, M.D.

Research Psychiatrist, University of Illinois School of Medicine, Chicago.

Charles B. Nemeroff, M.D., Ph.D.

Associate Professor of Psychiatry, Director, Laboratory of Psychoneuroendocrinology, Duke University Medical Center, Durham, North Carolina.

Paul J. Orsulak, Ph.D., M.B.A.

Research Associate Professor, Psychiatry and Pathology, University of Texas Health Science Center, Dallas; Veterans Administration Medical Center, Dallas.

Barbara L. Parry, M.D.

Clinical Psychobiology Branch, National Institute of Mental Health, Bethesda, Maryland; Department of Psychiatry, University of California at San Diego, La Jolla, California.

Steven M. Paul, M.D.

Chief, Clinical Neuroscience Branch, National Institute of Mental Health, Bethesda, Maryland.

Adolf Pfefferbaum, M.D.

Associate Professor of Psychiatry and Behavioral Sciences, Stanford University School of Medicine, Stanford; Chief, Clinical Services, Psychiatry, and Assistant Chief, Psychiatry Service, Palo Alto Veterans Administration Medical Center, Palo Alto, California.

Alfred Pope, M.D.

Professor Emeritus of Neuropathology, Harvard Medical School, Boston; Senior Neuropathologist, McLean Hospital, Belmont, Massachusetts.

Robert M. Post, M.D.

Chief, Biological Psychiatry Branch, National Institute of Mental Health, Bethesda, Maryland.

Norman E. Rosenthal, M.D.

Chief of Out-Patient Services, Psychobiology Branch, National Institute of Mental Health, Bethesda, Maryland.

Walton T. Roth, M.D.

Associate Professor of Psychiatry and Behavioral Sciences, Stanford University School of Medicine, Stanford; Chief, Psychiatric Consultation Service, Palo Alto Veterans Administration Medical Center, Palo Alto, California.

David A. Sack, M.D.

Clinical Psychobiology Branch, National Institute of Mental Health, Bethesda, Maryland.

Joseph J. Schildkraut, M.D.

Professor of Psychiatry, Harvard Medical School; Director, Neuropsychopharmacology Laboratory, Massachusetts Mental Health Center; Director, Psychiatric Chemistry Laboratory, New England Deaconess Hospital, Boston.

Marc A. Schuckit, M.D.

Professor of Psychiatry, University of California at San Diego; Director of Alcohol Treatment Program, Veterans Administration Medical Center, San Diego.

Richard I. Shader, M.D.

Professor and Chairman, Department of Psychiatry, Tufts University School of Medicine; Psychiatrist-in-Chief, New England Medical Center Hospital, Boston.

Rajiv P. Sharma, M.D.

Assistant Professor, Department of Psychiatry, University of Illinois; Research Psychiatrist, Illinois State Psychiatric Institute, Chicago.

Phil Skolnick, Ph.D.

Chief, Section on Neurobiology, Laboratory of Bio-organic Chemistry, National Institute of Arthritis and Diabetes, Bethesda, Maryland.

Iver F. Small, M.D.

Professor of Psychiatry, Indiana University School of Medicine, Indianapolis.

Joyce G. Small, M.D.

Professor of Psychiatry, Indiana University School of Medicine, Indianapolis.

Stephen M. Stahl, M.D., Ph.D.

Executive Director of Clinical Neuroscience, Merck Sharp & Dohme Research Laboratories, Neuroscience Research Centre, Harlow, Essex, United Kingdom; Associate Professor of Psychiatry and Pharmacology, University of California, Los Angeles.

Alan A. Stone, M.D.

Touroff-Glueck Professor of Law and Psychiatry, Harvard University, Cambridge.

Albert J. Stunkard, M.D.

Professor of Psychiatry, University of Pennsylvania, Philadelphia.

Stanley J. Watson, Ph.D., M.D.

Associate Professor of Psychiatry and Associate Director of the Mental Health Research Institute, University of Michigan, Ann Arbor.

Thomas A. Wehr, M.D.

Chief, Clinical Psychobiology Branch, National Institute of Mental Health, Bethesda, Maryland.

Richard Jed Wyatt, M.D.

Chief, Adult Psychiatry Branch, National Institute of Mental Health, St. Elizabeth's Hospital, Washington, D.C.

CONTENTS

Volume Eight

PART ONE: *The Neurobiology of Psychiatric Disorders*

PART TWO: *Scientific Approaches to Biological Investigation in Psychiatry*

PART THREE: *The Biology and Treatment of Specific Psychiatric Disorders*

PART FOUR: *Controversies in Biological Psychiatry*

PREFACE

PSYCHIATRY is a biomedical science. This is not a trivial statement. Nor could psychiatry have been called a science twenty years ago, when theoretical debates took place in the absence of empirical evidence. Today, a remarkable body of new knowledge relates neurobiology to psychiatric disorders. This new knowledge is being uncovered at an exponentially increasing rate by a new generation of neuroscientist-physicians. The fundamental concern of these scientist-physicians is to apply scientific investigation to the alleviation of human suffering from psychiatric disorders.

The central theme of the *American Handbook of Psychiatry,* volume VIII, Biological Psychiatry, is the search for new knowledge on the etiology, pathophysiology, and treatment of the major psychiatric disorders. Arising from a variety of scientific disciplines, this new knowledge is based on the use of innovative scientific approaches to the biological investigation of neurobiology and behavior. This text is an attempt to integrate the basic scientific and clinical advances that are revolutionizing our conceptions of the functioning human brain both in health and in illness.

The first part of the volume describes six basic science disciplines where exciting new findings are increasingly relevant to our understanding of mental illness. A major theme of this first part is the importance of chemical neuroregulators. These chemical messengers serve either as transmitters between neurons or as modulators of neuronal action. A remarkable amount has been discovered about these neuroregulators in the past two decades, and the first part is a summary of this new knowledge.

The normal and abnormal structure of the human brain as a basis for biological psychiatry is outlined in the chapters on chemical neuroanatomy and neuropathology. A chapter on behavioral neurochemistry describes our new understanding of the relationship between neuroregulators and behavior. Endocrine hormones and peptides form a new class of neuroregulators, and their relevance to mental illness is described in the chapters on neuroendocrine function and neuropeptides in psychiatric disorders. The final chapter in part one reveals the enormous potential of new knowledge in molecular genetics for an eventual understanding of the genetic bases of psychiatric illness.

The second part of the volume describes several new methods in neuroscience research that are adding to our understanding of normal and abnormal brain function and behavior. Animal models of psychiatric disorders are increasingly important in testing biological hypotheses of psychopathology and evaluating potential treatments for mental illness. The study of human brain electrical potentials and their anatomical origins is helping neuroscientists bridge the gap between neuronal activity and human cognition. Innovative neuroimaging techniques are currently producing pictures of the human brain that are unprecedented in their depiction of anatomical detail and revolutionary in their aesthetic representation of living brain activities.

The central theme of the volume, the theory and practice of biological psychiatry, is contained in part three. This section describes the major psychiatric disorders that are responsible for an enormous amount of human suffering. These disorders include the affective disorders, depression and mania; schizophrenia; anxiety disorders and phobias; agressive disorders; Alzheimer's disease; chronic pain; anorexia nervosa; obesity; childhood mental disorders; alcoholism and other substance abuse; and the psychiatric disturbances that are part of other medical diseases.

Part three is structured to begin with a summary of biological hypotheses of each psychiatric disorder. This is followed by a chapter that describes the theoretical and practical aspects of the psychopharmacological treatment of mental illness. These treatments have caused a revolution in the care of patients with mental disorders and have helped return psychiatric inquiry to biomedical science, which is the basis for innovative therapies in other areas of medicine. The treatments are far from perfect, however, and do have troublesome side effects. Thus, the volume includes a chapter on the medical side effects of psychopharmacological treatments and a chapter on the biology and experimental treatment of tardive dyskinesia—the most important side effect limiting the drug treatment of schizophrenia.

The presentation of the biological hypotheses of the etiology and pathophysiology of psychiatric diseases is powerful evidence of the significant progress in the neurobiological investigation and conceptualization of psychiatric disorders. The chapters on the biological treatment of psychiatric disorders, with their emphasis on the indications for pharmacological treatment, drug dosage and selection, and the side effects of pharmacological treatments, compose a practical manual of psychopharmacological therapeutics.

The final part of the volume discusses areas of particular controversy in biological psychiatry. Of course, the earlier chapters of the book also reflect the innumerable controversies that are an inevitable part of a rapidly expanding scientific enterprise. Currently, electroconvulsive therapy, psychosurgery, and the use of laboratory tests for the diagnosis and selection of treatment in psychiatric disorders are three areas of particularly vociferous debate. The final chapter appropriately concerns the numerous ethical dilemmas posed by the scientific investigation of human behavior and its abnormalities.

This volume is tangible evidence of the explosion of knowledge on the etiology, pathophysiology, and biological treatment of severe psychiatric diseases. Physicians attempting to reduce the enormous burden of mental illness on individuals and on society require knowledge of the scientific basis of psychiatric treatments. We believe this volume offers a comprehensive, yet practical review of biological psychiatry for the students, scientists, and clinicians who care deeply about the relief of human suffering and have learned that science can help.

PHILIP A. BERGER, M.D.
Norris Professor of Psychiatry
Stanford University
Stanford, California

H. KEITH H. BRODIE, M.D.
President
Duke University
Durham, North Carolina

ACKNOWLEDGMENTS

THE EDITORS acknowledge the contributors for their dedication to the task of summarizing scientific information. We and all of society are indebted to scientists throughout the world who have produced the new knowledge that is the heart of this volume.

We are grateful to Christie Wills Price for her enthusiasm and skill in editing and thank Pamela J. Elliott for coordinating and typing this monograph. Library research, editing, and proofreading were also shared cheerfully among Carolyn Benson, Meredith Dunn, Ken McClain, and Lisa Jordan.

We thank Jo Ann Miller and Maureen Bischoff at Basic Books, Inc., who nurtured this volume from conception to reality, and Debra Manette and Pamela Dailey for editorial and production work, respectively.

Finally, we thank the National Institute of Mental Health, the Research Service of the Veterans Administration, the MacArthur Foundation, the Kenneth T. and Eileen L. Norris Foundation, and especially Kenneth T. Norris, Jr., for invaluable support of scientific research.

PART ONE

The Neurobiology of
Psychiatric Disorders

CHAPTER 1

CHEMICAL NEUROANATOMY AS A BASIS FOR BIOLOGICAL PSYCHIATRY

Stanley J. Watson, Henry Khachaturian, Michael E. Lewis, and Huda Akil

¶ Introduction

The focus of this chapter is the interface between chemical neuroanatomy on one hand and the pharmacology/ physiology of neurotransmission on the other, particularly in relation to biological psychiatry. We will not focus on neurotransmitter or hormone biochemistry in depth; those issues are covered in other chapters. Rather, our mandate is to provide a sense of neurotransmitter-specific circuits as they relate to brain function in general and biological psychiatry in particular.

In considering the problem of brain function, one is struck by the perspectives inherent in neurotransmitter-specific anatomy, as contrasted with those found in a gross and microscopic brain anatomy. Classically, central nervous system (CNS) anatomy has focused on gross brain structure and the connectivity between brain nuclei. These classical observations are the basis for our general view of brain structure. In the first part of this chapter, we briefly summarize the gross anatomy of the limbic system, noting some of the connections between limbic nuclei as well as between limbic structures and the rest of the brain. The bulk of the chapter, however, is concerned with the anatomy/ physiology/pharmacology of several key neuronal systems. Anatomically, they are distributed only partially in the classical anatomical pathways. In fact, one of the clearest conclusions that can be drawn from pathway studies of neurotransmitter systems is that they derive from subgroups of known nuclei and have highly complex projection patterns. The neurotransmitter systems are often at variance with general patterns seen in general studies of CNS system pathways. To properly appreciate these anatomical patterns, it is important to appreciate both sets of knowledge—that is, classical CNS structure and pathways, as well as neurotransmitter anatomy.

This chapter presents two main types of biochemical anatomy important to the psychiatrist. The first is the neurotransmitter anatomy and related information (pharmacology, physiology, clinical relevance) on the monoamine, amino acid, cholinergic, and peptidergic systems in brain. Most of the text in this part of the chapter focuses on a few well-studied substances. However, it should be recognized that to date over forty neurotransmitters and neuropeptides have been isolated from the CNS (see table 1–1).

The second part of the chapter approaches a historically well-studied system, the hypothalamus-pituitary-adrenal (HPA) axis, from a relatively new perspective. The main message concerns the biochemical-anatomical links in this system, especially corticotropin-releasing factor (CRF) and vasopressin in hypothalamus as they influence pituitary function (release of adrenocorticotrophic hormone [ACTH] and beta-endorphin) and eventually the adrenal. We discuss the relationship of this system to current and future studies of affective disease.

¶ The Limbic System: An Overview

Most classical anatomical descriptions of the CNS reflect arbitrary division based largely on structure and have only a minor emphasis on function. The relatively recent discovery of neurotransmitters and neurohormones, however, have in effect revolutionized neuroanatomy into a powerful functional tool. Nevertheless, there exist in the brain distinct domains of activity that are structurally distinct from, although extensively interconnected with, other brain regions. For example, neocortical areas are clearly involved in sensory processing and integration, but also exert influence on the activity of diverse subcortical brain areas. Other regions, concentrated mainly in the reticular core of the brain stem, are more directly involved in autonomic brain function (dealing with, e.g., respiration, cardiovascular or neuroendocrine control, etc.). In-

TABLE 1–1.

Some Known Neurotransmitters and Neuropeptides in the Mammalian Central Nervous System

Acetylcholine	Glycine
ACTH (adrenocorticotrophic hormone)	Insulin
Angiotensin	LH (luteinizing hormone)
Aspartate	LHRH (luteinizing hormone-releasing hormone)
Bombesin	Motilin
Bradykinin	MSH (melanocyte-stimulating hormone)
Calcitonin	Neuropeptide Y
Carnosine	Neurotensin
CCK (cholecystokinin)	Norepinephrine
CRF (corticotropin-releasing factor)	Oxytocin
Dopamine	Prolactin
Dynorphins (multiple peptides)	Secretin
Endorphins (multiple peptides)	Serotonin
Enkephalins (multiple peptides)	Sleep peptide(s)
Epinephrine	Somatostatin
GABA (gamma-aminobutyric acid)	Substance P
Gastrin	TRH (thyrotropin-releasing hormone)
GH (growth hormone)	TSH (thyroid-stimulating hormone)
GHRH (growth hormone-releasing hormone)	Vasopressin
Glucagon	VIP (vasoactive intestinal peptide)
Glutamate	

terposed between the higher cortical and brain stem domains of activity are a number of functionally linked structures in the forebrain and midbrain that integrate information from the neocortex and reticular formation and in turn influence the function of both. These latter areas are collectively known as the *limbic system* (see figure 1–1) (for reviews, see Isaacson, [80] Kupfermann, [103] and Nieuwenhuys, Voogd, and van Huijzen [126]). The limbic system is a strong modulator of the autonomic nervous system through one of its components, the hypothalamus. The hypothalamus and other limbic areas are also reciprocally connected with the neocortex. Most important for the purpose of this chapter, the interplay between the limbic system and neocortex constitutes an anatomical-functional substrate for behavioral expression and regulation.

"Limbic system" is a term derived from the "limbic lobe" concept first defined by Paul Broca in 1878[21] to describe those phylogenetically old cortical areas that lie beneath the neocortex and that border (Latin: *limbus*) the brain stem. Broca's "limbic lobe" comprised the cingulate and hippocampal gyri and parolfactory areas. Because of their strong olfactory connections, these areas were also collectively referred to as rhinencephalon (smell brain). However, many other areas of the brain, including structures in the telencephalon, diencephalon, and mesencephalon, are integral parts of the limbic system and, by means of extensive interconnections, form a functional unit. The telencephalic components of the limbic system include the amygdala, hippocampus, septal nuclei, nucleus of the diagonal band of Broca, bed nucleus of stria terminalis, and preoptic area. In addition, several transitional cortical and neocortical areas are also involved in limbic circuitry, namely parahippocampal, periamygdaloid, entorhinal, and

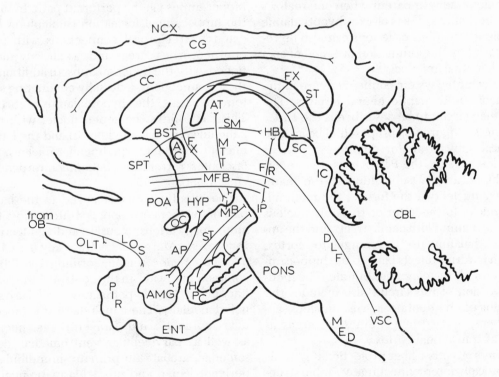

Figure 1–1. The limbic system. Parasagittal view of a schematized primate brain showing the major limbic system nuclei and their interconnections. For simplicity the fornix (FX) and stria terminalis (ST) are shown as discontinuous behind the midbrain. See Isaacson[80] for more details.

cingulate cortex, as well as the orbitofrontal part of neocortex. The olfactory system is intimately connected with some parts of the limbic telencephalon. In the diencephalon, limbic structures include the hypothalamus and parts of thalamus and "epithalamus," or habenula. The limbic midbrain areas occupy a paramedian position and include the ventral tegmental area, dorsal tegmental nucleus, and parts of the periaqueductal gray and midbrain raphe nuclei.

The structures of the limbic system can be grouped into rostral and caudal components, with the hypothalamus interposed between the two poles. An extensive array of short and long ascending and descending fiber pathways, many of which course through the hypothalamus, interconnect the various components, forming a so-called limbic system-midbrain circuit.[123,124] The hypothalamus is thus a nodal point of limbic system activity. The importance of the latter point becomes readily apparent when one realizes that most of the effects of extrahypothalamic limbic stimulations or lesions can also be reproduced by the stimulation or lesion of specific hypothalamic loci.[80]

Many limbic system connections are in the form of multisynaptic neural circuits. The first such circuit to be described is the *Papez circuit* (see figure 1–1), proposed to be an anatomical substratum for emotions.[134] In its simplest version, the Papez circuit connects the hippocampus (subiculum) to the mammillary nuclei (via the fornix), the mammillary nuclei to the anterior thalamic nucleus (via the mammillothalamic tract), and the anterior thalamus to the cingulate cortex, which in turn projects back to the hippocampus through the cingulum bundle. The modern version of this circuit also includes the presubiculum, dentate gyrus, nucleus accumbens, and certain brain stem areas as well as transitional cortex.

Numerous other fiber projectional systems reciprocally interconnect many limbic structures. One of the most prominent of these pathways is the *medial forebrain bundle,* which courses through the lateral hypothalamus to the limbic forebrain and midbrain.

The *dorsal longitudinal fasciculus* interconnects the hypothalamus with the midbrain periaqueductal gray, dorsal tegmental nucleus, as well as visceral sensory and visceral and somatic motor autonomic centers in the caudal medulla (e.g., nucleus tractus solitarius and dorsal motor nucleus of vagus). The amygdala has reciprocal connections with the thalamus, hypothalamus, hippocampus, and cingulate gyrus. Amygdaloid neurons further project (via stria terminalis) to the bed nucleus of stria terminalis, septal nuclei, and nucleus accumbens, while receiving input from the olfactory apparatus (via lateral olfactory stria). Lesions or stimulation of the amygdala produce wide-ranging alterations in emotional states, autonomic responses, and feeding.[80]

Furthermore, the neocortex can influence limbic system activity. The associational cortex projects to, among other areas, the entorhinal cortex, which in turn projects to the hippocampus via the perforant path. In turn, the hippocampal formation (subiculum) has extensive reciprocal connections with several neocortical areas and, as already mentioned, with the hypothalamus. In addition to these connections, a dorsally conducting system bypasses the hypothalamus entirely. This route links the septal nuclei with the habenula (via stria medullaris) and the latter nuclei with the interpeduncular nucleus, via fasciculus retroflexus (habenulointerpeduncular tract).

The hypothalamus, localized to the basal part of the diencephalon, is strategically situated for various neural and endocrine reflexes (see Morgane[122]). It is a key *neuroendocrine effector* region, forming the "final common pathway" in the control of the pituitary gland. Most hypothalamic nuclei are situated medially. These include the magnocellular supraoptic and paraventricular nuclei, as well as parvicellular ventromedial, dorsomedial, arcuate (in primate infundibular), periventricular, and suprachiasmatic nuclei. Many of these nuclei contain peptide-producing neurons that control the pituitary gland and additionally project to various other brain regions (see section entitled

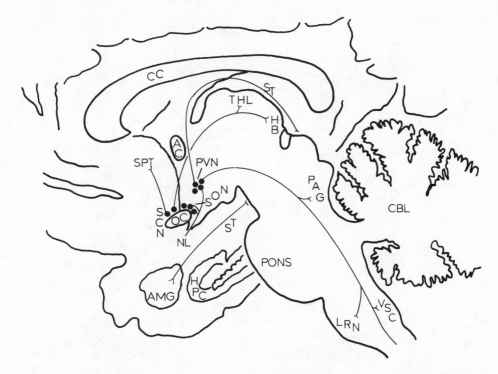

Figure 1–2. Vasopressin and oxytocin systems. Perikarya (open circles) and projections of the vasopressin and oxytocin-producing neurons are shown in this schematized parasagittal view of a primate brain.
SOURCE: M. V. Sofroniew et al., "Immunohistochemistry of Vasopressin, Oxytocin and Neurophysin in the Hypothalamus and Extrahypothalamic Regions of the Human Brain," *Acta Histochemica,* 24 (Supplement) (1981):79–95.

"Peptide-containing Neuronal Systems"). In the lateral hypothalamic area, cells form extensive multisynaptic ascending and descending connections via several fiber tracts, including, as mentioned, the medial forebrain bundle. For example, monoaminergic neurons situated in the brain stem have extensive projections to the hypothalamus and other limbic and neocortical structures through the medial forebrain bundle and the cingulum bundle (see section entitled "Monoamine-containing Neuronal Systems"). Many other fiber-projection systems interconnect the various hypothalamic regions to the brain stem, thalamus, hippocampus, and amygdala. These latter projections include fibers that course through the dorsal longitudinal fasciculus, the mammillotegmental and mammillothalamic tracts, the fornix, and stria terminalis.

A major function of the hypothalamus is to integrate various incoming neural stimuli and to translate this information into the control of the pituitary gland through its numerous peptide-producing neurons.[131] These peptidergic neurons function as "neuroendocrine transducers," receiving neural information and converting it into hormonal information. For example, the neuropeptides vasopressin and oxytocin are synthesized in the supraoptic and paraventricular nuclei. These project to the neural lobe of the pituitary (see figure 1–2), where vasopressin and oxytocin are released into general circulation.[47,158] On the other hand, various hypothalamic releasing and release-inhibiting hormones (e.g., thyrotropin-releasing hormone [TRH], luteinizing hormone-releasing hormone [LHRH], somatostatin) are synthesized in hypothalamic neurons with axons that terminate on the portal capillaries in the median eminence.[131] The peptide hormones

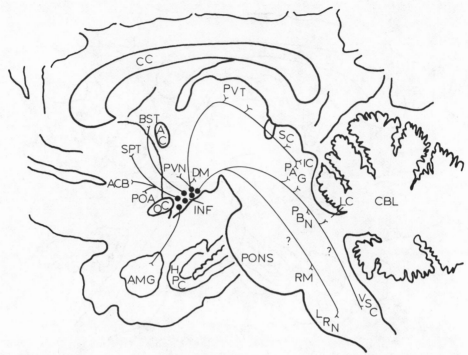

Figure 1–3. Pro-opiomelanocortin systems. Neuronal perikarya (open circles) that produce beta-endorphin, ACTH, alpha-MSH, and other end products of pro-opiomelanocortin reside in the infundibular nucleus (INF) of the hypothalamus. The projections of these neurons are shown in this schematic parasagittal view of a primate brain. While most of our knowledge of these projections comes from work done on the rodent brain,[93] many of these terminal innervation fields have been confirmed in the primate brain as well (Khachaturian, unpublished data). (See also color plate 1b)

and other factors released into the portal circulation in turn modulate the synthesis and release of specific anterior pituitary hormones into the general circulation (see section entitled "Neuroendocrine Anatomy").

In addition to regulating this neuroendocrine apparatus, the various hypothalamic peptidergic neurons also project to many other brain sites, most notably to structures in the limbic system and several autonomic centers in the brain. For example, the paraventricular nucleus has extensive vasopressinergic and oxytocinergic projections to the amygdala, locus coeruleus, parabrachial nuclei, and nucleus tactus solitarius (see figure 1–2), areas that are involved in limbic and autonomic brain function.[157,158,159] Other hypothalamic and extrahypothalamic peptidergic neurons also play important roles in the

modulation of various limbic-associated functions.[148,188] For example, the beta-endorphin-producing neurons in the infundibular (arcuate) nucleus (see figure 1–3 and color plate 1b) have extensive extrahypothalamic projections to the amygdala, bed nucleus of stria terminalis, midline thalamus, midbrain periaqueductal gray, and to brain stem catecholamine-producing regions.[93] Beta-endorphin is thought to modulate neuroendocrine, cardiovascular, respiratory, thermoregulatory, sexual, and other behaviors. Furthermore, beta-endorphin and other classes of opioid peptides, notably the enkephalins, also appear to play an important role in the modulation of nociceptive mechanisms by acting on the brain opioid receptors.[3,182]

In conclusion, the limbic system functions

to integrate endocrine, autonomic, and other neural activity. However, it is important to emphasize that while one can describe an anatomically distinct limbic system, this does not imply that the structures involved function independently of any other system of the brain. On the contrary, structures in the limbic system are connected, directly or indirectly, with all of the rest of the brain. It is ultimately this complexity with which we must deal in defining brain processes regulating behavior.

¶ Monoamine-containing Neuronal Systems

Neurons containing monoamine neurotransmitters (see chapter 2) are localized mainly within the brain stem reticular formation, an extensively, yet specifically, connected conglomeration of nerve cells situated in the core of the medulla, pons, and midbrain (see Nieuwenhuys, Voogd, and van Huijzen[126]). A typical reticular neuron has extensive dendritic arborizations ideally situated for communication with ascending and descending fibers. Each reticular neuron, in turn, possesses a unique biochemical identity and has widespread rostral and caudal connections with other parts of the brain. For example, a single locus coeruleus neuron (noradrenergic) gives rise to extensive collateral branches to the neocortex, hippocampus, cerebellum, and spinal cord.[167] In general, the monoaminergic reticular neurons do not conform to any particular nucleus in the brain stem, with a few notable exceptions (i.e., the locus coeruleus and raphe nuclei). Monoamine-producing neurons are grouped according to their neurotransmitter substance, namely dopamine (DA), norepinephrine (NE), or serotonin (5-hydroxytryptamine; 5HT). NE and DA are catecholamines derived enzymatically from the amino acid tyrosine. 5HT, on the other hand, is an indolamine, enzymatically derived from the amino acid tryptophan. In the rat brain, there are fifteen catecholaminergic and nine serotonergic cell groups.[42] Many of these

have also been described in the primate, including human, brain (see Felten and Sladek[54] and Nieuwenhuys, Voogd, and van Huijzen[126]).

Noradrenergic Systems

ANATOMY

NE-producing neurons are localized to pontine and medullary reticular formation (see color plate 1–A and figure 1–4). They were first discovered in the rodent CNS through fluorescence histochemistry.[42] Since most noradrenergic cell groups do not conform to any particular nuclear boundary, they have been designated A1 through A7.[42] Several cell groups have also been recognized in primates, including man.* The following is a brief review of some major groups. Group A1 cells in the lower medulla are partially located in the lateral reticular nucleus. Group A2 cells, also in the lower medulla, are situated beneath the fourth ventricle, mainly within the nucleus tractus solitarius. These two cell groups, along with relatively minor contributions from groups A5 and A7, give rise to an ascending fiber system, the ventral noradrenergic bundle,[167] which ascends rostrally, entering the medial forebrain bundle. The A1 and A2 groups contribute to the innervation of the mesencephalon, periaqueductal gray, the entire hypothalamus (in particular the periventricular, dorsomedial, arcuate, supraoptic, and paraventricular nuclei), preoptic area, and bed nucleus of stria terminalis.[164] Other descending bulbospinal projections of these noradrenergic cells have also been described.[42,167]

Another major noradrenergic nucleus is the locus coeruleus (group A6), a distinct, densely packed nucleus in the dorsal pons (see color plate 1) containing roughly half the number of NE-producing neurons in the brain.[64,163] The neurobiologies of this nucleus and of central noradrenergic transmission are among the most extensively studied

*See references 54, 55, 64, 78, and 127.

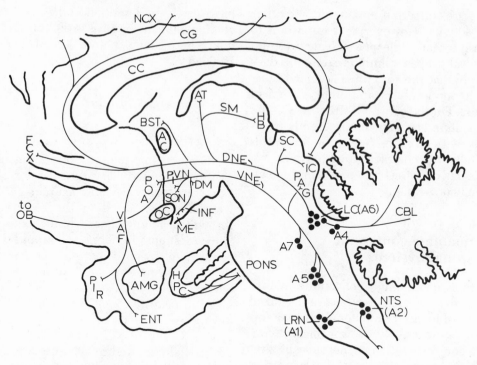

Figure 1–4. Noradrenergic systems. This schematized parasagittal view of a primate brain shows the location of major norepinephrine-producing cell bodies (open circles) and their major projections. These cell groups have been designated A1 to A7 by Dahlstrom and Fuxe.[42] (See also color plate 1a.)

SOURCE: R. Nieuwenhuys, J. Voogd, and Chr. van Huijzen, *The Human Central Nervous System* (New York: Springer-Verlag, 1981), pp. 221–230.

of any neurotransmitter system[170,171] in brain. The locus coeruleus, along with relatively minor contributions from groups A_4 and A_7, gives rise to extensively branched ascending and descending projections. A major ascending fiber system is the dorsal tegmental noradrenergic bundle,[167] which courses rostrally through the midbrain and lateral hypothalamic area to enter the telencephalon, where it then courses through the cingulum bundle in the cingulate cortex. Locus coeruleus neurons innervate the periaqueductal gray, superior and inferior colliculi, thalamic nuclei (anterior, ventral, and lateral nuclei; medial and lateral geniculate nuclei), habenular nuclei, amygdala, substantia innominata, hippocampus, cingulate and entorhinal cortex, and all of the neocortex.[164,167] The descending projections of the locus coeruleus innervate some brain stem structures as well as the spinal cord.[128]

PHYSIOLOGY AND PHARMACOLOGY

Most physiological studies of the noradrenergic systems have focused on the projections of the locus coeruleus (A6). The postsynaptic effect of activating the A6 neurons is usually a hyperpolarization and an increase in membrane resistance, which appear to be due to activation of alpha-adrenergic receptors that are positively coupled to adenylate cyclase.[170] The actions of NE may be best explained as "modulatory"—that is, as diminishing or enhancing the activity of other putative neurotransmitters.[189] Thus the physiological consequences of noradrenergic neurotransmission appear to depend on which other neurotransmitter systems are present and active. The implication of this view is that pharmacological intervention at noradrenergic synapses (e.g., with alpha-adrenoceptor blocking agents or NE reuptake–blocking tricyclic antidepressants) is likely to have complex, region-specific effects that are dependent on the activity of anatomically coextensive neural systems.

RELEVANCE TO PSYCHIATRY

The pathophysiological significance of the central noradrenergic systems is still poorly understood (see van Dongen[171] for review). Although Redmond[140] has suggested that locus coeruleus activity is involved in the production of fear or anxiety, this view is not universally accepted.[171] Nevertheless, pathological anxiety has been treated with NE uptake–blocking tricyclic antidepressants,[98] while situational anxiety is responsive to beta-blockers (e.g., propranolol hydrochloride); however, this latter effect appears to be due largely to peripheral beta-adrenoreceptor blockade.[68] Furthermore, the anxiolytic actions of benzodiazepines, which exhibit sensitization, are not pharmacologically consistent with their effects on locus coeruleus cells, which exhibit tolerance.[70]

An involvement of the central noradrenergic systems in affective disorders has been proposed on the basis of diverse findings (described elsewhere in this volume). The neuroanatomical evidence includes the finding that a group of unipolar, endogenous depressed patients exhibits a decreased content of NE in the amygdala and nucleus ruber, as well as of its metabolite, 3-methoxy-4-hydroxy-phenylglycol (MHPG), in many regions, including the hypothalamus and nucleus accumbens.[15,145] Nevertheless, the etiological significance of this apparent decline of activity in noradrenergic systems is uncertain. While acute administration of secondary tricyclic antidepressants enhances noradrenergic activity via blockade of reuptake, the chronic, therapeutically relevant effect is to diminish the postsynaptic effects of this monoamine.[109,162]

The role of noradrenergic systems in schizophrenia is similarly unclear. Postmortem assay of NE has indicated increased content in several brain regions (e.g., nucleus interstitialis, stria terminalis, and nucleus accumbens) from paranoid, but not nonparanoid, schizophrenic patients.[171] Unfortunately, neither the functional nor the etiological significance of these findings is apparent: Increased NE levels may indicate enhanced or diminished activity. Propranolol has been reported to be an effective antipsychotic, particularly in paranoid schizophrenics,[13,191,192] although mediation of this effect by central beta-adrenoceptors has not been demonstrated. Mason[115] has argued that the enhanced NE levels are due to a hypoactivity of noradrenergic systems in schizophrenia, a view[72,116,144] that has engendered lively debate. Nevertheless, this hypothesis still requires clinical evaluation. Based on the DA-NE interaction hypothesis,[6] previous findings of opposite actions of dopaminergic drugs in Parkinson's disease and schizophrenia, and the finding that clonidine hydrochloride worsened the symptoms of the former,[28] a beneficial effect of clonidine on schizophrenic symptoms was predicted[106] and later confirmed.[59]

Dopaminergic Systems

ANATOMY

Neurons that synthesize DA are confined mainly to the mesencephalon, with a few other groups in the diencephalon and telencephalon (see figure 1–5). Dahlstrom and Fuxe[42] have designated these groups A8 through A15. The substantia nigra (A9) is a major mesencephalic DA-containing nucleus.[64] Other neurons are situated in the mesencephalic reticular formation (A8) and ventral tegmental area (A10).[55,78] Substantia nigra and A8 neurons give rise to a major ascending bundle, the nigrostriatal dopaminergic system,[5,167] which traverses the lateral hypothalamic area and the internal capsule to innervate the caudate and putamen nuclear groups. From A10, neurons originate ascending fibers that comprise the mesolimbic dopaminergic system, which courses within the medial forebrain bundle to innervate various limbic and cortical structures including the bed nucleus of stria terminalis, nucleus accumbens, septal

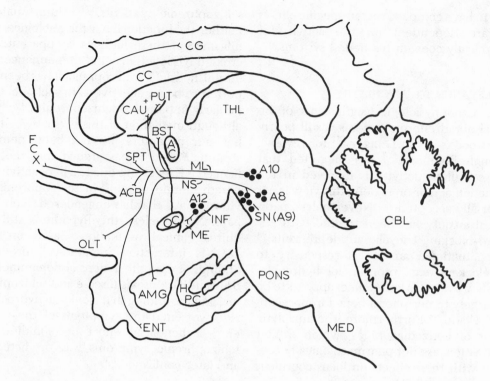

Figure 1–5. Dopaminergic systems. This schematized parasagittal view of a primate brain demonstrates the location of dopamine-containing cells (open circles) designated A8 to A10, A12,[42] and their major projections.

SOURCE: R. Nieuwenhuys, J. Voogd, and Chr. van Huijzen, *The Human Central Nervous System* (New York: Springer-Verlag, 1981), pp. 221–230.

nuclei, and frontal, cingulate, and entorhinal cortical areas.[108,167]

Dopaminergic cell groups of the diencephalon[16,55] are for the most part confined to various hypothalamic nuclei, including the caudal periventricular nucleus (A11) and the arcuate or infundibular nucleus (A12 and its rostral continuation, A14). Group A13 is situated in the zona incerta, while group A15 is localized within the olfactory bulb.[71] It is relevant here to mention that the DA-containing neurons in the hypothalamic infundibular nucleus (A12) give rise to the tubero-infundibular dopaminergic system, a major neuroendocrine link that innervates the external layer of the median eminence.

PHYSIOLOGY AND PHARMACOLOGY

The physiology of central DA neurons has developed into an increasingly complex and controversial area of study. In the striatum, iontophoretic studies have usually indicated an inhibitory response to DA, although there are persistent reports of excitation as well. Electrical stimulation of the substantia nigra and ventral tegmental area results in a bewildering mixture of excitatory and inhibitory responses of varying latencies. Superimposed upon this confusion is an unresolved debate regarding the number, locus, and function of DA receptor subtypes. According to the simplest view, these are either positively coupled (D–1) or negatively coupled (or uncoupled) (D–2) to adenylate cyclase. Within the nigrostriatal system, these receptors appear to be present at multiple loci:[104] (1) striatal presynaptic D–2 receptors controlling tyrosine hydroxylase, (2) striatal postsynaptic D–2 receptors, (3) striatal postsynaptic D–1 receptors, (4) nigral presynaptic D–1 receptors, and (5) nigral D–2 autoreceptors.

In contrast, mesocortical DA neurons do not appear to have perikaryal or terminal autoreceptors.[8]

These complexities and regional differences are reflected in the pharmacological actions of neuroleptics. Clinically effective neuroleptics all share the property of blocking D–2 DA receptors, but differ in their ability to induce extrapyramidal side effects. These side effects (parkinsonism and tardive dyskinesia) have been thought to be due to actions on the A9 neurons innervating the striatum, while the antipsychotic actions are thought to be mediated by actions on the A10 neurons innervating the cortical and limbic areas. These suppositions have been supported by recent electrophysiological studies of the differential effects of "classical" (e.g., haloperidol) and "atypical" (e.g., clozapine) neuroleptics on A9 and A10 neural activity.[29,186] The view that has emerged from these and related studies is that the antipsychotic activity of both classes of neuroleptics is due to an inactivation of A10 neurons (by depolarization block, an effect of *chronic* administration); in contrast, only the "atypical" neuroleptics, which have a low incidence of extrapyramidal side effects, do not induce depolarization block of the A9 neurons.

RELEVANCE TO PSYCHIATRY

The diverse lines of evidence for the involvement of DA systems in schizophrenia have been reviewed before[104,106,118,156] and are considered elsewhere in this volume. The neuroanatomical evidence, based on postmortem assays of dissected brain regions, has usually indicated elevated levels of DA and D–2 DA receptors in several forebrain regions (e.g., caudate nucleus, nucleus accumbens) from schizophrenic patients.* While the increase in D–2 receptors is consistent with the supersensitivity version of the DA hypothesis of schizophrenia, the increase in DA levels cannot be interpreted functionally. Crow and associates[35,36] have argued that the increase in D–2 receptors is

*See references 14, 34, 105, 114, 130, and 141.

associated with the disease process, and not neuroleptic therapy, and further that the increase may be associated with the "type I" syndrome of positive, neuroleptic-sensitive symptoms (e.g., delusions, hallucinations) rather than the "type II" syndrome of negative, neuroleptic-insensitive symptoms (e.g., affective flattening, poverty of speech). This view should be regarded as an attractive working hypothesis for guiding future investigations relating DA receptor abnormalities in different brain regions to preexisting symptoms. Such investigations must also consider laterality as a variable; Reynolds[143] has reported an abnormally and selectively high concentration of DA in the left amygdala from schizophrenic brain, a finding reminiscent of earlier studies pointing to laterality disturbances in schizophrenia.[113]

Serotonergic Systems

ANATOMY

Serotonergic neurons are distributed within midline raphe nuclei in the medulla, pons, and mesencephalon (see figure 1–6). These cell groups have been designated B1 through B9 in the rodent brain[42] and have also been described in the primate brain.[55,79] The raphe nuclei of the medulla include the nuclei raphe pallidus (B1), raphe obscurus (B2), and raphe magnus (B3). The nuclei raphe pontis (B5) and raphe medianus (B6 and B8) are situated in the pons. A rather large mesencephalic serotonergic cell group (B7) is localized in the nucleus raphe dorsalis. Other indolamine-containing neurons have also been localized to hypothalamic and habenular nuclei.[27] The projections of the serotonergic raphe neurons are extensive, encompassing the entire neuraxis,[42,61,167] particularly limbic and reticular formation structures.

A major ventral ascending serotonergic pathway originates from the nuclei raphe medianus and raphe dorsalis. This projection traverses the ventral mesencephalic tegmentum and the lateral hypothalamic area to enter the telencephalon. Along this

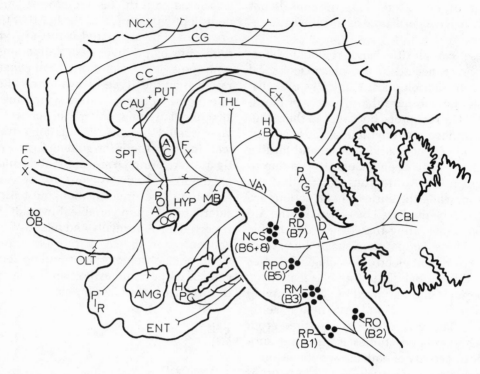

Figure 1–6. Serotonergic systems. Schematic parasagittal view of a primate brain depicting the serotonin cell groups (open circles) and their major projections. These groups were designated B1 to B9 by Dahlstrom and Fuxe.[42]

SOURCE: R. Nieuwenhuys, J. Voogd, and Chr. van Huijzen, *The Human Central Nervous System* (New York: Springer-Verlag, 1981), pp. 221–230.

course, serotonergic fibers innervate the interpeduncular nucleus, substantia nigra, and habenular nuclei, several thalamic nuclei, the lateral hypothalamic area, the nuclei caudate and putamen, amygdala, hippocampus, the entorhinal and cingulate cortex, as well as the neocortex.[61,133] The dorsal ascending serotonergic pathway is composed of fibers arising from the nuclei raphe magnus, raphe pontis, and raphe dorsalis. This periventricular bundle courses along the dorsal longitudinal fasciculus (of Schutz) to innervate the periaqueductal gray and the posterior hypothalamus.[54] Other relatively minor serotonergic pathways include projections to the cerebellum, pontine and medullary reticular formation, and spinal cord.[167]

PHYSIOLOGY AND PHARMACOLOGY

Microiontophoretic studies with 5HT have demonstrated region-dependent increases or, less commonly, decreases in the firing rate of spontaneously active neurons. In the facial motor nucleus, for example, intracellular recordings show that 5HT produces a slow depolarization together with some increase in membrane resistance; these effects enhance cellular responsivity to other excitatory inputs. Binding studies have revealed two subtypes of 5HT receptors that may be differentially coupled to adenylate cyclase and may possibly mediate the inhibitory and excitatory effects of 5HT on central neurons.[137] The hallucinogen LSD appears to bind to both sites with similarly high affinities,[136] and it is interesting to note that this drug appears to act as an agonist on neurons inhibited by 5HT, but as an antagonist on neurons excited by 5HT (see Peroutka, Lebovitz, and Snyder[137]). Clinically useful drugs affecting the serotonergic systems include the monoamine oxidase inhibitors (MAOIs;

e.g., phenelzine sulfate) and reuptake blockers (e.g., amitriptyline), the uses of which are described elsewhere in this volume.

RELEVANCE TO PSYCHIATRY

Historically, the hypothesis of a disorder of serotonergic systems in schizophrenia arose from the realization that several potential endogenous psychotogens are methylated derivatives of tryptamine or 5HT (see Lewis[106] for a review). This early version of the transmethylation hypothesis, which rewarded its investigators with countless frustrations and difficulties, has now been abandoned.[154] Other investigators have proposed an etiological role of abnormal serotonergic activity, independent of the possible formation of related psychotogens.[184] Although there is some evidence for altered 5HT turnover in several forebrain regions (e.g., the nucleus accumbens and bed nucleus of stria terminalis) from schizophrenic patients,[52] the 5HT hypothesis is plagued by pharmacological inconsistencies. First, haloperidol and promethazine hydrochloride, which differ greatly in clinical potency, are almost equipotent in displacing specific [³H]LSD binding.[10] Second, and even more unfortunately, 5HT receptor blockade with cinanserin hydrochloride or methysergide is therapeutically ineffective in schizophrenic patients (see Abrams[1] and Lewis[106] for references). Initial reports of a decline in [³H]LSD binding in frontal cortex from schizophrenic patients[11] could not be confirmed by other investigators.[185]

The possible involvement of 5HT systems in affective disorders has been explored for many years, but the direct (i.e., nonpharmacological) evidence is inconclusive.[1] While some studies found a reduced probenecid-induced accumulation of the metabolite 5-hydroxyindoleacetic acid (5-HIAA) in the cerebrospinal fluid (CSF) of depressed patients, this index of serotonergic activity was unchanged in other studies.[1,138] The usefulness of probenecid studies in measuring amine turnover now appears rather limited,[33,53] although such studies seem to have

been useful in predicting antidepressant therapeutic effects.[172] Postmortem studies have usually revealed decreased levels of 5-HIAA in brain regions (including the raphe nuclei) from suicide victims,[172] but these studies have been criticized for lack of diagnostic validity, and for the possibility that premorbid drug intake and/or the toxicity of the suicide procedures affected metabolite levels.[1] Even if the declines are not artifactual, as suggested by some CSF studies in diagnostically confirmed depressed patients, it appears that decreased CSF 5-HIAA may be related to impulsive aggression rather than to suicidal behavior per se.[22]

¶ Amino Acid–containing Neuronal Systems

ANATOMY

It is becoming increasingly clear that amino acid neurotransmitters constitute a major means of interneuronal communication in the mammalian CNS. At present, several amino acids are considered to be full-fledged or potential neurotransmitters. These include gamma-aminobutyric acid (GABA), glycine, aspartate, and glutamate. GABA and glycine are thought to be inhibitory neurotransmitters, while glutamate and aspartate probably serve excitatory functions (see Curtis and Johnston[40] and Fagg and Foster[50] for reviews).

Glutamate- and aspartate-containing neurons are distributed widely throughout the neuraxis and have equally widespread fiber projections. One of the more extensively studied systems is the hippocampal system of glutamate and aspartate neurons. Glutamate appears to be a major neurotransmitter in the perforant path, the lateral entorhinal input to hippocampal molecular layer, while aspartate may be involved in hippocampal input to the dentate gyrus (see Cotman and Nadler[32]). Additionally, hippocampal pyramidal cell projections to the septum, nucleus accumbens, bed nucleus of stria terminalis, nucleus of diagonal band, and hypothalamus may utilize glutamate or aspartate as a neurotransmitter.[175] In the cerebral cortex, glutamate has been shown to be a possible neurotransmitter in the cortical pyramidal cell projections to the neostriatum, possibly influencing striatal dopaminergic nerve terminals.[74,149] Other corticofugal pathways that may use glutamate as a neurotransmitter include projections to the nucleus accumbens, amygdala, thalamus, substantia nigra, superior colliculus, and spinal cord.[58,193] In the cerebellum, the granule cells that give rise to the parallel fibers appear to be glutamatergic,[194] while the cerebellar climbing fibers that originate from the inferior olive contain aspartate.[187] Finally, in the spinal cord, aspartate and glutamate are neurotransmitter candidates in excitatory interneurons and primary afferent fibers, respectively.[67]

GABA-containing neurons are distributed somewhat less extensively in the brain, exerting a primarily inhibitory influence over short distances. For example, in the basal ganglia, GABAergic neurons in caudate-putamen give rise to projections that terminate in the globus pallidus and the substantia nigra.[57,86] Yet another source of nigral GABA projections may be the neurons of the nucleus accumbens.[174] In the hippocampal formation, the basket cells forming interneuronal networks among pyramidal and granule cells also appear to contain GABA as a neurotransmitter.[161] Other GABAergic neuronal systems in the brain include the cerebellar Purkinje's cells, the source of innervation of deep cerebellar nuclei and vestibular nuclei in the brain stem.[111] In the spinal cord, GABA may be the neurotransmitter released by Renshaw cells, thereby inhibiting the activity of spinal motorneurons.[38] Last, glycine-producing neurons are thought to function as inhibitory interneurons in both the spinal cord (possibly in the Renshaw cells) and the brain stem.[41,67]

PHYSIOLOGY AND PHARMACOLOGY

Of the potential amino acid neurotransmitters, we have chosen to focus on GABA since the others have not as yet been explored significantly in a psychiatric context. Although GABA is generally considered to be the major inhibitory neurotransmitter in the CNS, depolarizing effects have been detected in spinal cord cells.[9] The more typical hyperpolarizing effects are reversed by the antagonist bicuculline and appear to be due to a receptor-mediated increase in chloride ion conductance.[102]

Brain GABA systems have been of particular interest to neuropharmacologists because of compelling evidence for GABA-DA interactions.[63] For example, chronic administration of classical (but not atypical) neuroleptics results in an increased number of GABA binding sites in rat substantia nigra,[62] an effect that may be related to the production of extrapyramidal side effects. GABA has also received attention for its possible role in the mechanism of action of benzodiazepines, the anxiolytic effects of which may be mediated via facilitation of GABA synaptic actions,[20,110,166] rather than inhibition of depolarization-induced cyclic guanosine monophosphate (GMP) stimulation.[153]

RELEVANCE TO PSYCHIATRY

Based on the role of GABA as a major inhibitory central neurotransmitter, Roberts proposed[147] that some aspects of schizophrenia, such as patients' reported experience of "sensory flooding," could be due to a defect in GABA-mediated neuronal inhibition. Stevens, Wilson, and Foote[160] subsequently reported behavioral evidence for dopaminergic hyperactivity (e.g., stereotypies) following bicuculline infusion near mesencephalic DA neurons. However, changes in GABA or its synthesizing enzyme, glutamic acid decarboxylase, are not realiably detected in postmortem samples of schizophrenic patients' brains, nor is administration of GABA agonists therapeutically effective. A possible role of GABA systems in affective disease has been proposed based on findings of reduced GABA levels in the CSF of depressed patients.[65,66,89] However, these findings were not obtained in one other

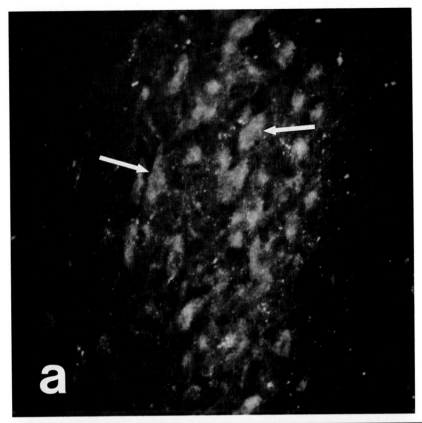

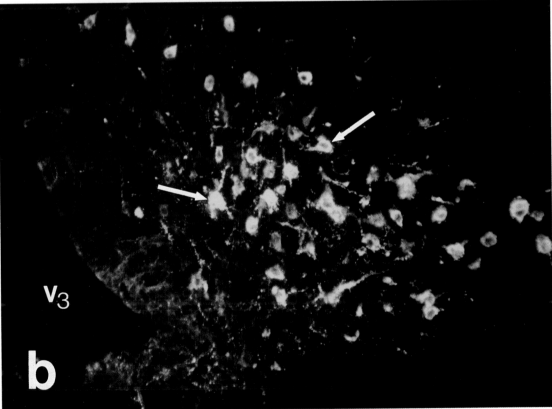

COLOR PLATE 1. Panel (a) shows formaldehyde condensation fluorescence of norepinephrine in neurons (arrows) of the rat locus coeruleus; the fluorescence was induced via ultraviolet excitation. Panel (b) shows fluorescent beta-endorphin neurons (arrows) in the rat arcuate hypothalamic nucleus. Primary rabbit antiserum against human beta-endorphin was used in this immunofluorescent histochemical technique. V_3: 3rd ventricle.

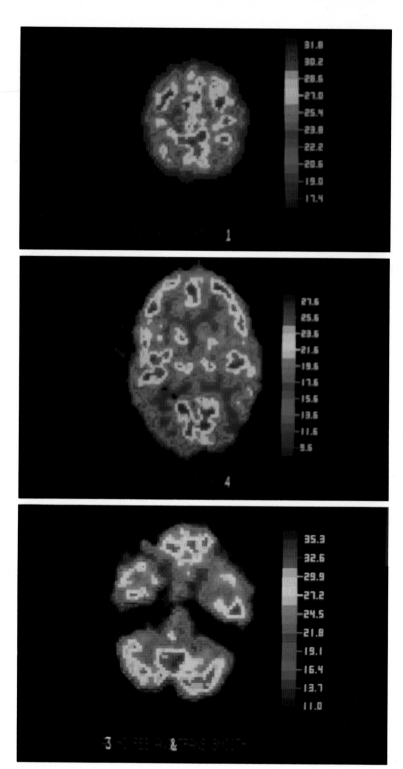

COLOR PLATE 2 (a, b, and c). Horizontal slice images of the rate of glucose metabolism in the human brain using ^{18}Fluoro-2-deoxyglucose (^{18}F-2DG) as a tracer. The color bar scale gives the rate in micromoles of glucose per 100 grams of brain tissue per minute. The subject viewed a series of blurred numbers and responded to an occasional "0" stimulus. Slices are computed parallel to the canthomeatal (CM) line —a line joining the outer canthus of the eye with the auditory meatus.

Top (95 mm above the CM line) shows the frontal and parietal cortex. Middle (55 mm) reveals the active visual regions at the occiput and frontal lobe activation. The basal ganglia and thalamus are visible in the slice center. Bottom (5 mm) shows the active frontal lobes, the circles of the temporal poles, and the cerebellum.

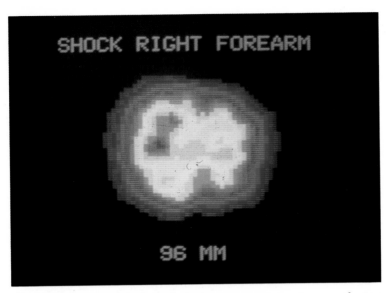

COLOR PLATE 3. Slice through the somatosensory cortex near the top of the brain of subject receiving brief electrical shocks to his right forearm reveals activation of sensory areas in the left hemisphere.

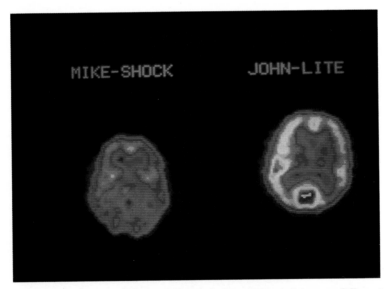

COLOR PLATE 4. Identical adult twins participated in two different tasks and have very different scans. "Mike" received the sequence of electrical stimuli to the right forearm, (see reference 7 in chapter 10) whereas John viewed a series of light flashes and counted them. Slices are at the level of thalamus and visual cortex posteriorly. Note that John, the subject doing the visual vigilance task of counting light flashes, has an area of high metabolism in his calcarine region. Mike, who sat in the dark while receiving the shocks, has an area of quite low metabolism in this area.

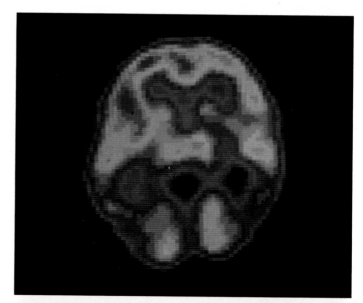

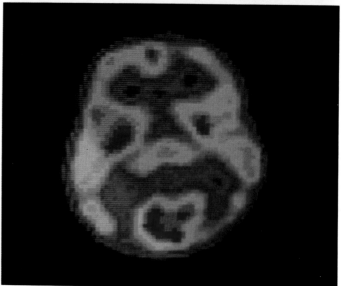

COLOR PLATE 5 (a, b, and c). PET scans at midventricular level during somatosensory stimulation in completely darkened room. (Top) Normal control (the author) shows little activity in calcarine fissure and clearly active thalamus and frontal cortex. (Middle) Patient with schizophrenia off-medication shows active visual cortex but less activity in frontal regions, especially on right side. (Bottom) Patient with bipolar affective disorder, euthymic during testing, shows low rate of frontal glucose metabolism.

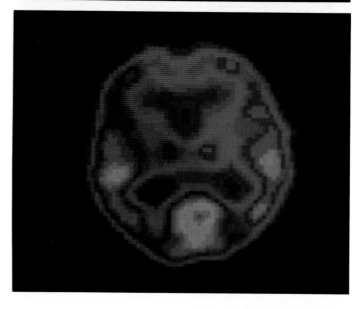

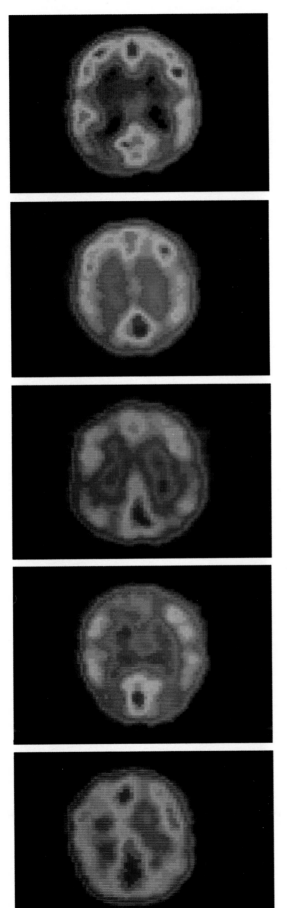

COLOR PLATE 6 (a, b, c, d, and e). Normal
control (top) and the four identical Genain
quadruplets, concordant for schizophrenia.
The slice level is above the ventricles. From
top to bottom, Nora, Iris, Myrna, and Hester.
Note that all four have relatively more activity
in posterior regions than in the anterior cortex.
No clear relationship to severity of illness or
lifetime neuroleptic dosage was seen.

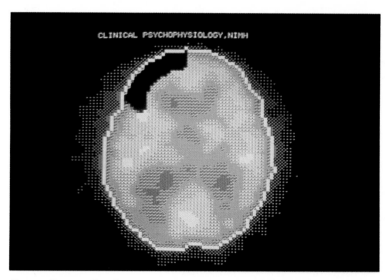

COLOR PLATE 7. Computer reconstruction of slice-images into lateral surface views for comparison with cerebral blood flow. The first step begins with the extraction of the cortical peel from each slice-image. A radial scan program selects values lying on a line joining slice center and a cortical outline.

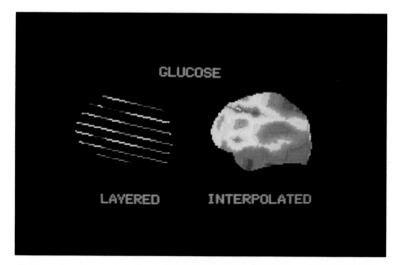

COLOR PLATE 8. Each cortical strip is placed on an approximately equal area projection of the cortical surface at the appropriate height above the canthomeatal line. Next, the spaces between slice centers are filled by interpolation, providing a continuous surface. The normal volunteer shows the visual pattern of maximal frontal glucose metabolic rate with low rates in temporal and occipital lobes. This PET lateral view comes from a set of scans of which the slice-image in color plate 5 (a) is a member.

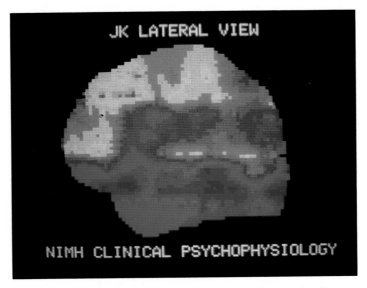

COLOR PLATE 9. Lateral cortical view of normal control subject resting with eyes closed imaged by PET with [18]F-2DG followed by cortical reconstruction. Normal hyperfrontal pattern is seen.

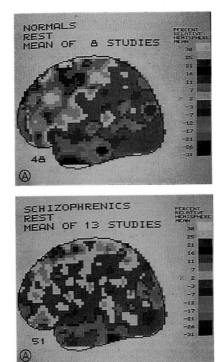

COLOR PLATE 10. Cerebral blood flow assessed with intracarotid xenon study by Ingvar and associates.[20] Top, control subjects can be compared closely with color plate 11, indicating the close parallels between the normal resting patterns of cerebral glucose use and blood flow. Bottom, patients with schizophrenia show a less pronounced frontal flow.

COLOR PLATE 11 (a, b, and c). (Top) Average lateral glucose metabolic rate across group of normal volunteers[8] and (middle) patients with schizophrenia. (Bottom) Map of statistical comparisons with t-test done on each picture element of the lateral cortical surface; red is $p < 0.05$ normals greater than schizophrenic patients and purple is $p < 0.05$ schizophrenic patients greater than normals. This exploratory technique provides a new way of visualizing diagnostic group differences or the deviation of an individual from population norms in a graphic way. Note also the similarity with cerebral blood flow data of color plate 10 (below)—with patients with schizophrenia showing less pronounced frontal glucose use.

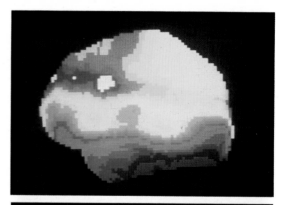

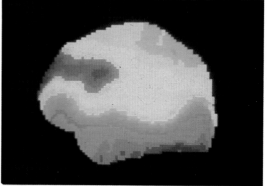

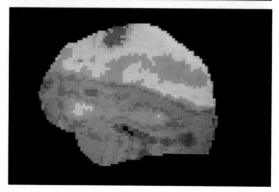

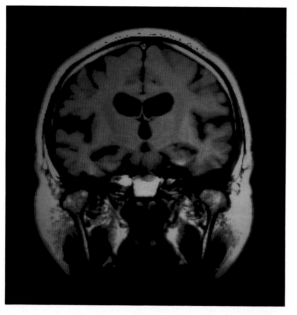

COLOR PLATE 12. A 1H magnetic resonance image of the human head. This coronal section of an elderly male with Alzheimer-type dementia illustrates several aspects of the power of MR imaging for studying the brain. First, unlike x-ray CT, images can be reconstructed from a wide range of planes, so that areas of interest are visualized optimally. Second, both ventricular and sulcal enlargement are seen clearly, without the bone artifact that interferes with CT images close to the brain surface. Also, differences in white and gray matter show plainly and can be enhanced even further with changes in the collection method.

NOTE: This picture, generated on a 1.5 Tesla General Electric Instrument at Stanford School of Medicine, was kindly supplied by Adolf Pfefferbaum, M.D.

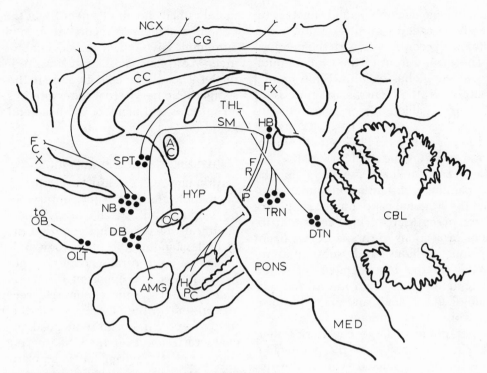

Figure 1–7. Cholinergic systems. Parasagittal view of a schematized primate brain showing the distribution of cholinergic cell bodies (open circles) and their projections. Note that while some of these systems have also been confirmed in the human brain, most of our current knowledge of cholinergic systems stems from studies in the rodent brain (see Cuello and Sofroniew[37]).

study of manic and depressed patients,[139] and, unfortunately, there have been no reports on the effects of GABA agonists on patients with affective disease. Finally, despite the apparent mechanism of action of the benzodiazepines, there is no evidence as yet for a disturbance of GABA neurotransmission in anxiety.

¶ **Acetylcholine-containing Neuronal Systems**

ANATOMY

Acetylcholine (ACh) was the first chemically identified substance to be considered as a putative neurotransmitter. Still, relatively little is known about the CNS distribution of cholinergic neurons (see figure 1–7) when compared to the monoamines or even the more recently discovered neuropeptides.

What knowledge we have of ACh localization in the brain is derived primarily from histochemical studies in the rat, cat, and monkey of acetylcholinesterase* and choline acetyltransferase,† enzymes responsible for ACh degradation and biosynthesis, respectively. Other methods for measuring ACh, enzyme concentrations, or cholinergic muscarinic receptor autoradiography have proven less useful in providing much anatomical detail of central cholinergic systems (see Armstrong et al.[7]).

Two detailed immunocytochemical mappings of choline acetyltransferase (CAT) distribution in the rat brain have recently been published.[7,37] Cholinergic perikarya are localized in several discrete brain regions. In the striatum complex, perikarya are distributed in the caudate-putamen and as-

*See references 81, 87, 107, 119, 132, 135, and 152.
†See references, 7, 94, 95, 112, and 120.

sociated nucleus accumbens and olfactory tubercle, the so-called ventral striatum, which is anatomically continuous with the neostriatum. The main output of the caudate-putamen is to the globus pallidus. Equivalently, the output of the ventral striatum is to the "ventral pallidum," or substantia innominata.

A large population of CAT-containing neurons also exists in the nucleus basalis. This includes magnocellular perikarya in the globus pallidus, substantia innominata, nucleus of the diagonal band, medial septal nucleus, and preoptic area. These areas contribute fiber projections to the neocortex (from the globus pallidus and substantia innominata), to the hippocampal formation and cingulate cortex (from the medial septum and diagonal band), and to the piriform cortex (from the preoptic area).

Another group of large cholinergic neurons is partially situated in the pedunculopontine tegmental nucleus within the nucleus cuneiformis. These neurons form a continuous band that extends from an area dorsolateral to the substantia nigra to the pontine tegmentum, near (but excluding) the parabrachial nuclei. The pedunculopontine tegmental nucleus projections ascend mainly to extrapyramidal structures, namely the substantia nigra, subthalamic nucleus, thalamus, entopeduncular nucleus, globus pallidus, striatum, and cerebral cortex. This ascending cholinergic pathway apparently corresponds to the so-called ascending reticular activating system that influences cortical activity.

The brain stem motor nuclei of the cranial nerves also contain CAT-positive neurons. These fall into three categories: somatic motor, special visceral motor, and general visceral motor. The large somatic motor cholinergic neurons are situated in the oculomotor, trochlear, abducens, and hypoglossal nuclei, which are involved in the control of eye and tongue movements. The equally large, cholinergic, special visceral motor neurons are located in trigeminal, facial, and ambiguus nuclei, which control muscles of facial expression, head and neck. In contrast, the mainly small cholinergic neurons of the general visceral motor category are found in the autonomic divisions of the oculomotor (Edinger-Westphal), facial, ambiguus, and vagus nuclei. These latter cells give rise to the parasympathetic nerves that innervate intraocular muscles and many of the head and neck glands.

Physiology and Pharmacology

Although ACh's neurotransmitter role has been known for over half a century, the slow development of specific assay and histochemical procedures has retarded progress in understanding the physiology and pharmacology of central cholinergic neurons. Nevertheless, it is apparent that both nicotinic and muscarinic cholinergic receptors are present in the CNS.[102] While the nicotinic receptor has been sequenced and well characterized outside the CNS (see, e.g., Mishina et al.[121]) and mediates depolarization via a relatively nonselective increase in small cation permeability, less is known about the receptor in brain. Muscarinic receptors, in contrast, have been extensively studied in the brain and appear to mediate a more complex range of electrophysiological responses (see, e.g., Cole and Nicoll[30]) through a variety of coupling mechanisms[73] such as phospholipid turnover.[56] Central cholinergic neurotransmission can be enhanced by administration of the reversible acetylcholinesterase inhibitor, physostigmine, or the ACh precursors, deanol acetamidobenzoate and choline.

Relevance to Psychiatry

Evidence for a possible disturbance of cholinergic neurotransmission in schizophrenia has come largely from pharmacological studies,[12] although the effects reported (e.g., the beneficial action of cholinergic agonists) tend to be ephemeral. The hypothesis that such effects are mediated by interactions with forebrain DA systems[85] is supported by animal studies showing[44,83,97] that both cholinomimetics (e.g., physostigmine) and neuroleptics block DA agonist–induced stereotypies. Although there is some evidence for altered activity of the biosynthetic enzyme, CAT, and the cholinesterases in postmortem brain samples from schizophrenic patients,[48] the direction of changes reported by different investigators is inconsistent. Furthermore, acute treatment of schizophrenic patients with physostigmine or choline chloride did not result in symptomatic improvement,[12] although the effects of chronic treatment still require evaluation. Unfortunately, the agonists currently available tend to have unpleasant side effects.

Relying wholly on pharmacological studies, several investigators have proposed an involvement of ACh systems in affective diseases; cholinergic hypoactivity has been argued to have a role in mania,[45,84] while cholinergic hyperactivity has been suggested to be associated with depression.[43,84] The cholinergic hypotheses[12,26,82] still are impressively consistent with the pharmacological effects of cholinomimetics (such as physostigmine, choline, and deanol) in psychotic patients, and are supported further by evidence that depressed patients exhibit an enhanced release of hypophyseal beta-endorphin in response to physostigmine.[146]

¶ Peptide-containing Neuronal Systems

ANATOMY

During the past fifteen years, over thirty neuroactive peptides have been characterized and shown to exist in the central nervous system (see table 1–1).* Many of these peptides, which were originally localized to the hypothalamus, are the so-called hypothalamic-releasing hormones (e.g., corticotropin-releasing factor [CRF], luteinizing hormone releasing hormone [LHRH], thyrotropin-releasing hormone [TRH], somatostatin). Other classes of peptides were first described in the pituitary gland, such as the anterior lobe hormones ACTH and beta-endorphin, or the neurohypophyseal hormones vasopressin and oxytocin. Still other peptides were initially characterized in nonneural tissue, mainly in the gastrointestinal tract (e.g., insulin, cholecystokinin [CCK], vasoactive intestinal peptide [VIP], etc.), and were subsequently shown to exist in the brain.

Peptides are localized in neuronal perikarya and projections throughout the neuraxis (see, e.g., figures 1–3, 1–8). Almost every neuropeptide identified to date has been localized to hypothalamic neurons.[99] Some are also found in extrahypothalamic neurons. The hypothalamic-releasing hormones and the neurohypophyseal hormones are synthesized in neurons located in various hypothalamic nuclei. For example, vasopressin and oxytocin are localized to the magnocellular supraoptic and paraventricular nuclei, with axonal projections to the neural lobe of the pituitary (see figure 1–2).[47,158] CRF[39,165] is found in parvocellular neurons of the paraventricular nucleus (see figure 1–8) that project to the median eminence portal capillary plexus. In addition to this neuroendocrine role, the magnocellular neurons, as well as those containing the releasing hormones, have extensive extrahypothalamic axonal projections (see figure 1–2), consistent with a possible neurotransmitter role (see Roberts et al.,[148] Sterba et al.,[159] and Woodhams et al.[188]). Other peptidergic neurons found in the hypothalamus with extensive extrahypothalamic projections include those containing beta-endorphin and ACTH, localized to the arcuate nucleus (human infudibular nucleus) with projections to limbic forebrain and brain stem structures (see figure 1–3).* Likewise, many other peptides are synthesized in neurons in a number of brain areas. For example, the enkephalins† and dynorphins‡ are found in separate neuronal perikarya in the hypothalamus, midbrain, brain stem, spinal cord, and many limbic and cortical areas. Other peptides contained in perikarya in diverse brain areas include sub-

---

*For reviews, see Hokfelt et al.,[76] Krieger,[99] Krieger and Martin,[100,101] and Snyder.[155]

*See references 17, 18, 93, 177, and 179.
†See references 49, 69, 75, 90, 92, and 178.
‡See references 91, 173, 180, 181, and 183.

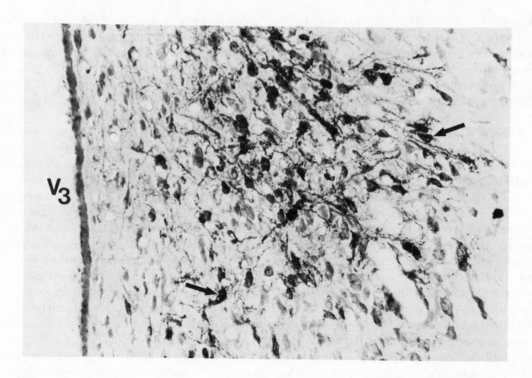

Figure 1–8. CRF immunostained neurons (arrows) are seen in the parvocellular para-ventricular nucleus of the rat hypothalamus. The method used was peroxidase-antiperoxidase immunocytochemistry using primary rabbit antiserum against ovine CRF. V_3: 3rd ventricle.

stance P, somatostatin, neurotensin, CCK, TRH, and VIP, to name a few (see Krieger[99]).

It is now well established that many peptides coexist in the same neurons with either another peptide or a "classical" neurotransmitter.[77] For example, vasopressin and dynorphin coexist in certain supraoptic and paraventricular neurons.[181] Interestingly, under certain experimental conditions (e.g., adrenalectomy) vasopressin has also been localized to parvocellular paraventricular neurons[96,151] that "normally" produce only CRF. This latter observation has profound neurobiological implications: Synthesis of a particular peptide can be induced, under certain physiological conditions, in neurons that normally do not produce that peptide. The coexistence of neuropeptides and classical neurotransmitters has also been demonstrated. These include substance P and TRH in certain medullary serotonergic neurons,

as well as gastrin in some midbrain DA-containing perikarya.[77] These observations have raised new questions regarding the synthesis, storage, release, and interactions of neuropeptides and monoamine neurotransmitters from the same neurons.

From the foregoing brief account, it is apparent that there exist in the brain many biologically active peptides that fall under one or more classifications, such as hypothalamic-releasing hormones, pituitary hormones, and so on. However, other means of classifying peptides might prove more useful in terms of functional or biosynthetic relationships. For example, those peptides that share the core amino acid sequence, Tyr-Gly-Gly-Phe-Met (or Leu) and that bind to one or more of the opioid receptor subtypes have been classified as opioid peptides. These include the enkephalins, dynorphin, beta-endorphin, and their molecular variants (see Akil et al.[3]).

Conversely, peptides can be classified according to their biosynthetic origin. Peptide synthesis in the brain, like peptide synthesis elsewhere in the body, occurs via a precursor molecule (a prohormone). The latter is then posttranslationally cleaved into smaller peptides, one or more of which may be biologically active. An example that has been the subject of most intensive investigation is the precursor pro-opiomelanocortin (POMC), which gives rise to the biologically active peptides beta-endorphin, alpha-MSH, and ACTH (see Akil and Watson[2]). For further discussion of POMC and its biologically active products, see the next section.

PHYSIOLOGY, PHARMACOLOGY, AND RELEVANCE TO PSYCHIATRY

It is impossible, within the limits of this chapter, to begin to do justice to the burgeoning literature on neuropeptide physiology and pharmacology. An excellent overview is provided by Cooper, Bloom, and Roth,[31] and current reviews on the individual peptides are plentiful.[99,125] In particular, the opioid peptides, and their possible role in psychiatric disorders, are reviewed by us elsewhere [2,3,176,182] and by others in this volume. In the following section we present some recent findings relating the HPA axis and affective disease as an example of the rich interfaces that are possible between peptide biology, neuroanatomy, endocrinology, and psychiatry.

¶ Neuroendocrine Anatomy— The Hypothalamus-Pituitary-Adrenal Axis

General Framework

We have chosen to include this section in order to focus more clearly on both a major neuroendocrine aspect of biological psychiatry as well as the intimate linkage between that endocrine system and associated brain neurotransmitter systems. A considerable amount of energy has gone into the "use" of the HPA axis (see figure 1–9) as a window into the brain.[24,182] While there have been some difficulties with such an approach, it has generally been a very rich and rewarding framework. The traditional logic of HPA studies in psychiatry has been to focus on adrenal cortisol regulation with modest attention toward pituitary function and almost none toward the hypothalamus. In effect, as a field, we have studied that most accessible part of the axis. In the last few years, the biology of both the pituitary and hypothalamic branches of this axis have been much more clearly delineated and can now be studied in

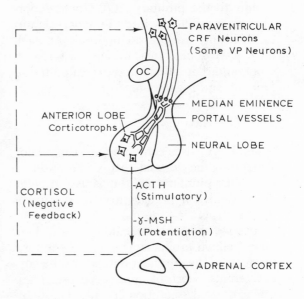

Figure 1–9. Hypothalamus-pituitary-adrenal axis. Corticotropin-releasing factor (CRF) and possibly vasopressin (VP), produced by certain paraventricular hypothalamic neurons (see also figure 1–9), are released into the median eminence portal vessels, thus stimulating the releases of ACTH and other pro-opiomelanocortin peptides from the anterior lobe corticotrophs. ACTH (and other factors) in turn stimulate corticosteroid (e.g., cortisol) secretion from the adrenal cortex. In addition to their normal metabolic regulatory functions, corticosteroids can also inhibit the synthesis and secretion of both CRF from the hypothalamus and ACTH from the anterior lobe, thus establishing a feedback loop. OC: optic chiasm.

greater depth. While our real problem is the technical limit imposed by trying to study the biochemistry of specific brain cell function in humans, fortunately we can use carefully selected indirect pharmacological tools to study a few aspects of hypothalamic cellular function—as reflected in pituitary activities.

Our discussion of the HPA axis as reflected in cortisol, ACTH/beta-endorphin, and CRF could be from either a historical or a logical perspective. We have chosen the latter approach, as it allows the reader a clearer view of the various links of regulatory control of this major system. Specifically, we will begin at the cortisol end of the circuit and move rapidly to the pituitary ACTH/beta-endorphin cells and finally into the hypothalamus to CRF and vasopressin neurons. At each level, we will note relevant clinical research observations or animal studies related to the function and regulation.

The HPA Axis

The HPA axis is composed of three major structures: the adrenal cortex, the anterior lobe of the pituitary, and the paraventricular nucleus of the hypothalamus (and possibly a fourth structure—the posterior pituitary). Figure 1–9 shows these structures and their major cellular products. The major secretory products of the adrenal medulla are the corticosteroids (cortisol and corticosterone). Corticosteroid secretion is regulated by ACTH from the anterior pituitary. In turn, the release of ACTH is under CRF and vasopressin control, both synthesized in the paraventricular nucleus (see figure 1–8).

While the corticoids are powerful and complex modifiers of general cellular metabolism, they also play a role in psychological adaptation, stress, and very likely mental illness. Within psychology, the neurosciences, and psychiatry, they are most clearly associated either with a general response to stress or for their strong correlation with severe affective disease. Salient observations on cortisol in melancholia include those from

the work of Sachar and associates [150] and Carroll and coworkers, [23,25] and a host of other laboratories. Among those observations are the hypersecretion, blunted circadian rhythm, increased frequency of secretion, and "escape" from dexamethasone suppression observed in plasma cortisol of endogenously depressed patients.

Given the general organizations of the HPA axis, it is logical to ask whether the source of the secretory and regulatory anomalies seen in depression is the adrenal. Can one imagine autonomous adrenal cortisol regulation as central to affective disease? Or is it that the adrenal is accurately reflecting its history of control from the pituitary? That is, do depressed subjects have normal adrenals (given their history of stimulation from "on high")? Can we move the level of discourse to the pituitary, especially to the corticotrophs (the cells that secrete ACTH and beta-endorphin)? Is the pituitary also "dysregulated," when compared to adrenal cortisol function?

Over the last decade, the biochemistry and biology of the ACTH/beta-endorphin–producing cells in pituitary has progressed very rapidly. In brief, there is a common 31,000 Dalton precursor for ACTH, alpha-MSH, gamma-MSH, beta-lipotropin, and beta-endorphin. This precursor, POMC, is cleaved to produce the various active peptide fragments just listed (plus a few that are not well studied at this point). The peptide of interest here is ACTH, as it is most clearly related to cortisol synthesis and release. It should be noted that measurement of any one of the several products from the POMC prohormone can probably be used to reflect ACTH release into plasma.

One can rephrase the question surrounding the HPA axis dysfunction in depression to include measurement of ACTH or beta-endorphin in plasma. There have been only a few such studies of these peptides in affective disease.* After careful logical and technical evaluation, these studies (and related

*See references 4, 46, 51, 88, 117, 142, 146, and 190.

endocrine studies) generally produce the following interpretations:

1. Both beta-endorphin and ACTH can be suppressed by dexamethasone in normal subjects and nonendogenous psychiatric controls.
2. Endogenously depressed subjects often show abnormal regulation of either plasma ACTH or beta-endorphin.
3. The same subject may or may not also be abnormal as measured by cortisol, after dexamethasone.
4. This dissociation between pituitary and adrenal dysregulation suggests different patterns of dysfunction in different patients.

Given these (and related) observations, one is forced to conclude that the pituitary is also disturbed in some endogenous patients. Yet it is another, different group of patients that is seen with cortisol measures in plasma. Again, we can ask if it is clear that the pituitary is "defective," or is it that the pituitary is actually following the messages it receives from elsewhere? What controls the pituitary corticotrophs? Is that substance (i.e., CRF) properly regulated in depression? Is it the only releaser of ACTH and beta-endorphin? What neuronal systems impact on the CRF neurons in hypothalamus? Can a case be made for "rational" adrenal and pituitary responses in depression, while the limbic system is dysfunctional?

Over the last fifteen to twenty years, a case has been made for at least two substances from nervous tissue capable of releasing peptides from the corticotrophs. These studies have identified one minor releasing factor, vasopressin (also known as antidiuretic hormone) and one major releasing factor, CRF (see Frohman and Berelowitz,[60] Vale et al.[168] and Vale et al.[169]). As noted before, both of these substances are produced in cells in the hypothalamus. Vasopressin is synthesized in the cells of the supraoptic nucleus, paraventricular nucleus, and suprachiasmatic nucleus. Cells from these nuclei project widely in the CNS and often project heavily to the posterior pituitary, where they release their peptides into plasma for distal

effect, probably including the anterior pituitary. These same vasopressin-producing cells also synthesize and release other peptides, including the opioid peptide dynorphin.[181] Of interest is the fact that both of these peptide precursors have been cloned (via recombinant DNA methods) and are known to be from totally separate genes. As an aside, it can be noted here that this type of pattern (multiple peptides from the same precursor and multiple peptide precursors in one cell) is observed with increasing frequency in brain and endocrine tissue.

The major corticotrophic-releasing factor (i.e., CRF) has cell bodies widely distributed throughout the CNS[19,39,129,165] The major hypothalamic cell group is found on the medial parvocellular subdivision of the paraventricular nucleus, with the fibers from these cells heavily represented in the external layer of the median eminence, closely apposed to the portal vascular network for the anterior pituitary. Three other peptides have been localized to CRF-secreting cells—dynorphin, oxytocin, and vasopressin. Thus the corticotrophs can receive release stimuli from vasopressin or CRF within the posterior pituitary or the median eminence portal system—or both!

The complex neuropeptide biology of these two types of cells (vasopressin and CRF producers), when considered with the substances that synapse on them, makes this a very complex and tightly regulated circuit.

In returning to the problem of affective disease and its analysis with the dexamethasone suppression test (DST), one can now consider the next steps, those regulating the release of pituitary hormones. For example, one might ask whether the corticotroph responds normally to CRF from hypothalamus. Is there any support for an abnormal CRF receptor on the corticotroph? If it is unusually super- or subsensitive, is that a sign of corticotroph dysfunction, or merely a reflection of high CRF release rate and/or unusual CRF release activity?

Let us assume a "normal" adrenal and pituitary (given their stimulation history).

What then? In one sense we are now completely in the CNS, specifically the limbic system. From the perspective of a psychiatrist and a neuroscientist, that is where we should be. It is an article of faith at this point, but depression has to be a CNS disease. What can we do to study affective disease given the road map we have discussed?

Risch and collaborators[146] have carried out a series of studies using cholinergic pharmacology in endogenous depression. They measured pituitary hormones and concluded that there is hypersecretion of beta-endorphin (and, implicitly, ACh) after physostimine. Thus they suggest that ACh regulates CRF, which in return controls ACTH and beta-endorphin release. They further hypothesize that depressed patients often escape from this cholinergic control, partially causing the "dysregulation" seen in the DST.

In concluding this excursion into endocrine anatomy and function, we need then to think of a series of neuron-neuron interactions in brain. Recent immunocytochemical studies with antisera against CAT strongly support a cholinergic impact on CRF neurons. Earlier studies with the monoamines implicate NE and epinephrine as neuronal influences on the general CRF cellular area. The anatomical intimacy within the paraventricular nucleus of CRF, dynorphin, vasopressin, somatostatin, and neurotensin (to name a few) opens the door for the study of these systems in affective disease. The long-distance linkage between the hypothalamus and brain stem nucleus tractus solitarius (part of the gut-Vagal nerve system) also implicates these systems, gut affective responses, and the sympathetic systems as a whole. Finally, the problematic observation of peptide cotransmission in the same neuron strongly suggests the need for a uniquely careful set of basic studies, prior to launching into clinical ones. In effect, as a field, biological psychiatry is increasingly asked to recognize very rapid progress in basic endocrinology and neuroscience. In return, major avenues are opening up for understanding and using the biology of neurotransmission in the study of mental illness.

¶ Acknowledgments

This work was supported by NIMH Grant #MH36168, NIDA Grant #DA02265, NIMH Training Grant #T32MH15794 (ML), and the Theophile Raphael Fund. We wish to thank Ms. Adele Henry for manuscript preparation.

¶ Bibliography

1. ABRAMS, R. "Serontonin and Affective Disorders," in W. B. Essman, ed., *Serotonin in Health and Disease*, vol. 3; *The Central Nervous System.* New York: Spectrum Publishing, 1978, pp. 203–229.

2. AKIL, H., and WATSON, S. J. "Beta-endorphin and Biosynthetically Related Peptides in the Central Nervous System," in L. Iversen, S. D. Iversen, and S. H. Snyder, eds., *Handbook of Psychopharmacology*, vol. 16. New York: Plenum Publishing Co., 1983, pp. 209–253.

3. AKIL, H., et al. "Endogenous Opioids: Biology and Function," in W. M. Cowan, ed., *Annual Review of Neuroscience.* Palo Alto: Annual Reviews Inc., 1984, pp. 223–255.

4. AMSTERDAM, J. D., et al. "Cosyntropin Stimulation Test in Depressed Patients and Healthy Subjects," *American Journal of Psychiatry,* 140 (1983):907–908.

5. ANDEN, N. E., et al. "Demonstration and Mapping Out of Nigroneostriatal Dopamine Neurons," *Life Sciences,* 3 (1964):523–530.

6. ANTELMAN, S. M., and CAGGIULA, A. R. "Norepinephrine-dopamine Interactions and Behavior," *Science* 195 (1977): 646–653.

7. ARMSTRONG, D. M., et al. "Distribution of Cholinergic Neurons in Rat Brain: Demonstrated by the Immunocytochemical Localization of Choline Acetyltransferase," *Journal of Comparative Neurology,* 216 (1983):53–68.

8. BANNON, M. J., et al. "Unique Response to Antipsychotic Drugs Is Due to Absence of Terminal Autoreceptors in Mesocor-

tical Dopamine Neurones," *Nature,* 196 (1982):444–446.

9. BARKER, J. L., MacDONALD, J. F., and MATHERS, D. A. "Three GABA Receptor Functions on Mouse Spinal Neurons," *Brain Research Bulletin,* 5 (1980): 43–49.

10. BENNETT, J. P., and SNYDER, S. H. "Stereospecific Binding of D-lysergic Acid Diethylamide (LSD) to Brain Membranes: Relationship to Serotonin Receptors," *Brain Research,* 94 (1975):523–544.

11. BENNETT, J. P., et al. "Neurotransmitter Receptors in Frontal Cortex of Schizophrenics," *Archives of General Psychiatry,* 36 (1979):927–934.

12. BERGER, P. A., DAVIS, K. L., and HOLLISTER, L. E. "Pharmacological Investigations of Cholinergic Mechanisms in Schizophrenia and Manic Psychosis," in K. L. Davis and P. A. Berger, eds., *Brain Acetylcholine and Neuropsychiatric Disease.* New York: Plenum Press, 1979, pp. 15–32.

13. BIGELOW, L. B., et al. "Propranolol Treatment of Chronic Schizophrenia: Clinical Response, Catecholamine Metabolism and Lymphocyte Beta-receptors," in E. Usdin, I. J. Kopin, and J. Barchas, eds., *Catecholamines: Basic and Clinical Features.* New York: Pergamon Press, 1979, pp. 1851–1853.

14. BIRD E. D., SPOKES, E.G.S., and IVERSEN, L. L. "Increased Dopamine Concentration in Limbic Area of Brain from Patients Dying with Schizophrenia," *Brain,* 102 (1979):347–360.

15. BIRKMAYER, W., et al. "Nucleus Ruber and L-DOPA Psychosis: Biochemical Post Mortem Findings," *Journal of Neural Transmission,* 35 (1974):93–116.

16. BJORKLUND, A., and NOBIN, A. "Histochemical and Microspectrofluormetric Mapping of Dopamine and Noradrenaline Cell Groups in the Rat Diencephalon," *Brain Research,* 51 (1973):193–205.

17. BLOCH, B., et al. "Immunocytochemical Evidence That the Same Neurons in the Human Infundibular Nucleus Are Stained with Anti-endorphins and Antisera of Other Related Peptides," *Neuroscience Letters,* 10 (1978):147–152.

18. BLOOM, F., et al. "Neurons Containing Beta-endorphin in Rat Brain Exist Separately from Those Containing Enkephalin: Immunocytochemical Studies," *Proceedings of the National Academy of Science USA,* 75 (1978):1591–1595.

19. BLOOM, F., et al. "Corticotropin Releasing Factor (CRF): Immunoreactive Neurons and Fibers in Rat Hypothalamus," *Regulatory Peptides,* 4 (1982):43–58.

20. BRAESTRUP, C., and NIELSEN, M. "Benzodiazepine Receptors," in L. L. Iversen, S. D. Iversen, and S. H. Snyder, eds., *Handbook of Psychopharmacology.* New York: Plenum Press, 1983, pp. 285–384.

21. BROCA, P. "Anatomic Comparee Circonvolutions Cerebrales. Le Grand Lobe Limbique et la Scissure Limbique dans la Serie des Mammiferes," *Revue Anthropologie* (Ser. 2), 1 (1878):384–498.

22. BROWN, G. L., et al. "Aggression, Suicide, and Serotonin: Relationship to CSF Amine Metabolites," *American Journal of Psychiatry,* 139 (1982):741–746.

23. CARROLL, B. J., CURTIS, G. C., and MENDELS, J. "Neuroendocrine Regulation in Depression: I. Limbic System-adrenocortical Dysfunction," *Archives of General Psychiatry,* 33 (1976): 1039–1044.

24. CARROLL, B. J., et al. "Neurotransmitter Studies of Neuroendocrine Pathology in Depression," *Acta Psychiatrica Scandinavica,* 280 (1980):183.

25. CARROLL, B. J., et al. "A Specific Laboratory Test for the Diagnosis of Melancholia," *Archives of General Psychiatry,* 38 (1981):15–22.

26. CASEY, D. E. "Affective Changes with Deanol," in K. L. Davis and P. A. Berger, eds., *Brain Acetylcholine and Neuropsychiatric Disease.* New York: Plenum Press, 1979, pp. 33–44.

27. CHAN-PALAY, V. "Indoleamine Neurons and Their Processes in the Normal Rat Brain and in Chronic Diet-induced Thiamine Deficiency Demonstrated by Uptake of ^{3}H-serotonin," *Journal of Comparative Neurology,* 176 (1977):467–494.

28. CHASE, T. N., and SHOULSON, I. "Dopaminergic Mechanisms in Patients with Extrapyramidal Disease," in D. B. Calne, T. N. Chase, and A. Barbeau, eds., *Advances in Neurology.* New York: Raven Press, 1975, pp. 359–366.

29. CHIODO, L. A., and BUNNEY, B. S. "Typical and Atypical Neuroleptics: Differential Effects of Chronic Administration on the Activity of A9 and A10 Midbrain Dopaminergic Neurons," *Journal of Neuroscience,* 3 (1983):1607–1619.

30. COLE, A. E., and NICOLL, R. A. "Acetylcholine Mediates a Slow Synaptic Potential in Hippocampal Pyramidal Cells," *Science,* 221 (1983):1299–1301.

31. COOPER, J. R., BLOOM, F. E., and ROTH, R. H. *The Biochemical Basis of Neuropharmacology,* 4th ed. New York: Oxford University Press, 1982.

32. COTMAN, C. W., and NADLER, J. V. "Glutamate and Aspartate as Hippocampal Transmitters: Biochemical and Pharmacological Evidence," in P. J. Roberts, J. Storm-Mathisen, and G.A.R. Johnston, eds., *Glutamate: Transmitter in the Central Nervous System.* New York: John Wiley & Sons, 1981, pp. 117–154.

33. COWDRY, R. W., et al. "Cerebrospinal Fluid Probenecid Studies: A Reinterpretation," *Biological Psychiatry,* 18 (1983):1287–1297.

34. CROSS, A. J., CROW, T. J., and OWEN, F. " ^{3}H-Flupenthixol Binding in Post-Mortem Brains of Schizophrenics: Evidence for a Selective Increase in Dopamine D2 Receptors," *Psychopharmacology,* 74 (1981):122–124.

35. CROW, T. J. "Two Syndromes in Schizophrenia?" *Trends in Neuroscience,* 5 (1982):351–354.

36. CROW, T. J., et al. "Changes in D2 Receptor Numbers in Post-mortem Brain in Schizophrenia in Relation to the Presence of the Type I Syndrome and Movement Disorder," in R. Collu et al., eds., *Brain Neurotransmitters and Hormones.* New York: Raven Press, 1982, pp. 43–53.

37. CUELLO, A., and SOFRONIEW, M. V. "The Anatomy of the CNS Cholinergic Neurons," *Trends in Neurosceinces,* 7 (1984):74–78.

38. CULLHEIM, S., and KELLERETH, J.-O. "Two Kinds of Recurrent Inhibition of Cat Spinal Alpha-motoneurones as Differentiated Pharmacologically," *Journal of Physiology* (London), 312 (1981):209–224.

39. CUMMINGS, S., et al. "Corticotropin-releasing Factor Immunoreactivity Is Widely Distributed Within the Central Nervous System of the Rat: An Immunohistochemical Study," *Journal of Neuroscience,* 3 (1983):1355–1368.

40. CURTIS, D. R., and JOHNSTON, G.A.R. "Amino Acid Transmitters in the Mammalian Central Nervous System," *Ergebnisse der Physiologie,* 69 (1974):97–188.

41. CURTIS, D. R., et al. "A Pharmacological Study of Renshaw Cell Inhibition," *Journal of Physiology* (London), 258 (1976):227–242.

42. DAHLSTROM, A., and FUXE, K. "Evidence for the Existence of Monoamine-containing Neurons in the Central Nervous System," *Acta Physiological Scandinavica,* 62 (1964):1–55.

43. DAVIS, K., and BERGER, P. "Pharmacological Investigations of the Cholinergic Imbalance Hypotheses of Movement Disorders and Psychosis," *Biological Psychiatry,* 13 (1978):23–49.

44. DAVIS, K., HOLLISTER, L. E., and TEPPER, J. "Cholinergic Inhibition of Methylphenidate-induced Stereotypy with Oxotremorine," *Psychopharmacology,* 56 (1978):1.

45. DAVIS, K., et al. "A Cholinergic Imbalance Hypothesis of Psychoses and Movement Disorders: Strategies for Evaluation," *Psychopharmacology Communications,* 1 (1975):533.

46. DEMISKAH, K., et al. "Comparison of the ACTH Suppression Test and Dexamethasone Suppression Test in Depressed Patients," *American Journal of Psychiatry,* 140 (1983):1511–1512.

47. DIERICKX, K. "Immunocytochemical Localization of the Vertebrate Cyclic Nonapeptide Neurohypophyseal Hormones and Neurophysins," *International Review of Cytology,* 62 (1980):119–185.

48. DOMINO, E. F. "Brain Cholinergic Enzymes in Schizophrenia," in K. L. Davis and P. A. Berger, eds., *Brain Acetylcholine and Neuropsychiatric Disease.* New York: Plenum Press, 1979, pp. 63–74.

49. ELDE, R., et al. "Immunohistochemical Studies Using Antibodies to Leucine-

enkephalin: Initial Observations on the Nervous System of the Rat," *Neuroscience*, 1 (1976):349–351.

50. FAGG, G. E., and FOSTER, A. C. "Amino Acid Neurotransmitters and Their Pathways in the Mammalian Central Nervous System," *Neuroscience*, 9 (1983): 701–719.

51. FANG, V. S., et al. "Plasma ACTH and Cortisol Levels in Depressed Patients: Relation to Dexamethasone Suppression Test," *Life Sciences*, 29 (1981):931–938.

52. FARLEY, I. J., SHANNAK, K. S., and HORNYKIEWICZ, O. "Brain Monoamine Changes in Chronic Paranoid Schizophrenia and Their Possible Relation to Increased Dopamine Receptor Sensitivity," in G. Pepeu, M. J. Kuhar, and S. J. Enna, eds., *Receptors for Neurotransmitters and Peptide Hormones*. New York: Raven Press, 1980, pp. 427–433.

53. FAULL, K. F., et al. "Clinical Application of the Probenecid Test for the Measurement of Monoamine Turnover in the CNS," *Biological Psychiatry*, 16 (1981):879–899.

54. FELTEN, D. L., and SLADEK, J. R., Jr. "Monoamine Distribution in Primate Brain. V. Monoaminergic Nuclei: Anatomy, Pathways and Local Organization," *Brain Research Bulletin*, 10 (1983):171–284.

55. FELTEN, D. L., LATIES, A. M., and CARPENTER, M. B. "Monoamine-containing Cell Bodies in the Squirrel Monkey Brain," *American Journal of Anatomy*, 139 (1974):153–166.

56. FISHER, S. K., KLINGER, P. D., and AGRANOFF, B. W. "Muscarinic Agonist Binding and Phospholipid Turnover in Brain," *Journal of Biological Chemistry*, 258 (1983):7358–7363.

57. FONNUM, F., GOTTESFELD, Z., and GROFOVA, I. "Distribution of Glutamate Decarboxylase, Choline Acetyltransferase and Aromatic Amino Acid Decarboxylase in the Basal Ganglia of Normal and Operated Rats. Evidence for Striatopallidal, Striatoentopeduncular and Striatonigral GABAergic Fibres," *Brain Research*, 143 (1978):125–138.

58. FONNUM, F., et al. "Glutamate in Cortical Fibers," *Advanced Biochemical Psychopharmacology*, 27 (1981):29–42.

59. FREEDMAN, R., et al. "Clonidine Treatment of Schizophrenia. Double-blind Comparison to Placebo and Neuroleptic Drugs," *Acta Psychiatrica Scandinavica*, 65 (1982):35–45.

60. FROHMAN, L. A., and BERELOWITZ, M. "The Physiological and Pharmacological Control of Anterior Pituitary Hormone Secretion," in C. B. Nemeroff and A. J. Dunn, eds., *Peptides, Hormones and Behavior*. New York: Spectrum Publications, 1984, pp. 119–172.

61. FUXE, K., and JONSSON, G. "Further Mapping of Central 5-hydroxytryptamine Neurons: Studies with the Neurotoxic Dihydroxytryptamines," in E. Costa, G. L. Gessa, and M. Sandler, eds., *Advances in Biochemical Psychopharmacology*, vol. 10. New York: Raven Press, 1974, pp. 1–12.

62. GALE, K. "Chronic Blockage of Dopamine Receptors by Antischizophrenic Drugs Enhances GABA Binding in Substantia Nigra," *Nature*, 283 (1980):569–570.

63. GALE, K., and CASU, M. "Dynamic Utilization of GABA in Substantia Nigra: Regulation by Dopamine and GABA in the Striatum, and Its Clinical and Behavioral Implications," *Molecular and Cellular Biochemistry*, 39 (1981):369–405.

64. GARVER, D. L., and SLADEK, J. R., Jr. "Monoamine Distribution in Primate Brain. I. Catecholamine-containing Perikarya in the Brain Stem of *Macaca speciosa*," *Journal of Comparative Neurology*, 159 (1975):289–304.

65. GERNER, R. H., and HARE, T. A., "CSF GABA in Normal Subjects and Patients with Depression, Schizophrenia, Mania, and Anorexia Nervosa," *American Journal of Psychiatry*, 138 (1981): 1098–1101.

66. GOLD, B. I., et al. "GABA Levels in CSF of Patients with Psychiatric Disorders," *American Journal of Psychiatry*, 137 (1980):362–364.

67. GRAHAM, L. T., et al. "Distribution of Some Synaptic Transmitter Suspects in Cat Spinal Cord: Glutamic Acid, Aspartic Acid, Gamma-aminobutyric Acid, Glycine and Glutamine," *Journal of Neurochemistry*, 14 (1967):465–472.

68. GREENBLATT, D. J., and SHADER, R. I.

"Pharmacotherapy of Anxiety with Benzodiazepines and Beta Adrenergic Blockers," in M. A. Lipton, A. DiMascio, and K. F. Killam, eds., *Psychopharmacology: A Generation of Progress.* New York: Raven Press, 1978, pp. 1381–1390.

69. HABER, S., and ELDE, R. "The Distribution of Enkephalin Immunoreactive Fibers and Terminals in the Monkey Central Nervous System: An Immunohistochemical Study," *Neuroscience,* 7 (1982):1049–1095.

70. HAEFELY, W. E. "Behavioral and Neuropharmacological Aspects of Drugs Used in Anxiety and Related States," in M. A. Lipton, A. DiMascio, and K. F. Killam, eds., *Psychopharmacology: A Generation of Progress.* New York: Raven Press, 1978, pp. 1359–1374.

71. HALASZ, N., et al. "Transmitter Histochemistry of the Rat Olfactory Bulb. I. Immunohistochemical Localization of Monoamine Synthesizing Enzymes. Support for Intrabulbar Periglomerular Dopamine Neurons," *Brain Research,* 126 (1977):455–474.

72. HARRISON-READ, P. E. "Noradrenergic and Other Strategies for Devising New Drug Treatments of Schizophrenia," *Trends in Pharmacological Science,* 5 (1984):139–141.

73. HARTZELL, H. C. "Physiological Consequences of Muscarinic Receptor Activation," *Trends in Pharmacological Science,* 3 (1982):213–214.

74. HASSLER, R., et al. "Effect of Motor and Premotor Cortex Ablation on Concentrations of Amino Acids, Monoamines, and Acetylcholine and on the Ultrastructure in Rat Striatum. A Confirmation of Glutamate as the Specific Corticostriatal Transmitter," *Journal of Neurochemistry,* 38 (1982):1087–1098.

75. HOKFELT, T., et al. "The Distribution of Enkephalin-immunoreactive Cell Bodies in the Rat Central Nervous System," *Neuroscience Letters,* 5 (1977):25–31.

76. HOKFELT, T., et al. "Peptidergic Neurones," *Nature,* 284 (1980):515–521.

77. HOKFELT, T., et al. "Coexistence of Peptides and Putative Transmitters in Neurons," *Advances in Biochemical Psychopharmacology,* 22 (1980):1–23.

78. HUBBARD, J. E., and DI CARLO, V. "Fluorescence Histochemistry of Monoamine-containing Cell Bodies in the Brain Stem of the Squirrel Monkey *(Saimiri sciureus).* II. Catecholamine-containing Groups," *Journal of Comparative Neurology,* 153 (1974):369–384.

79. ———. "Fluorescence Histochemistry of monoamine-containing Cell Bodies in the Brain Stem of the Squirrel Monkey *(Saimiri sciureus).* III. Serotonin-containing Groups," *Journal of Comparative Neurology,* 153 (1974):385–398.

80. ISAACSON, R. L. *The Limbic System,* 2d ed. New York: Plenum Press, 1982.

81. JACOBOWITZ, D. M., and PALKOVITS, M. "Topographic Atlas of Catecholamine and Acetylcholinesterase-containing Neurons in the Rat Brain. I. Forebrain (Telencephalon, Diencephalon)," *Journal of Comparative Neurology,* 157 (1974):13–28.

82. JANOWSKY, D. S. and DAVIS, J. M. "Psychological Effects of Cholinomimetic Agents," in K. L. Davis and P. A. Berger, eds., *Brain Acetylcholine and Neuropsychiatric Disease.* New York: Plenum Press, 1979, pp. 3–14.

83. JANOWSKY, D. S., et al. "Cholinergic Antagonism of Methylphenidate-induced Stereotyped Behavior," *Psychopharmacologia,* 27 (1972):295.

84. JANOWSKY, D. S., et al. "A Cholinergic Hypothesis of Mania and Depression," *Lancet* 2 (1972):632.

85. JANOWSKY, D. S., et al. "Antagonistic Effects of Physostigmine and Methylphenidate in Man," *American Journal of Psychiatry,* 130 (1973):1370.

86. JESSELL, T. M., et al. "Topographic Projections of Substance P and GABA Pathways in the Striato- and Pallido-nigral System: A Biochemical and Immunohistochemical Study," *Brain Research,* 152 (1978):487–498.

87. JOHNSTON, M. V., McKINNEY, M., and COYLE, J. T. "Evidence for a Cholinergic Projection to Neocortex from Neurons in Basal Forebrain," *Proceedings of the National Academy of Science USA,* 10 (1979):5392–5396.

88. KALIN, N. H., WEILER, S. J., and SHELTEN, S. E. "Plasma ACTH and Cortisol Concentrations Before and After Dexame-

thasone," *Psychiatry Research*, 7 (1982):87–92.

89. KASA, K., et al. "Cerebrospinal Fluid, Gamma-aminobutyric Acid and Homovanillic Acid in Depressive Disorders," *Biological Psychiatry*, 17 (1982):877–883.

90. KHACHATURIAN, H., LEWIS, M. E., and WATSON, S. J. "Enkephalin Systems in Diencephalon and Brainstem of the Rat," *Journal of Comparative Neurology*, 220 (1983):310–320.

91. KHACHATURIAN, H., et al. "Dynorphin Immunocytochemistry in the Rat Central Nervous System," *Peptides*, 3 (1982):941–954.

92. KHACHATURIAN, H., et al. "Telencephalic Enkephalinergic Systems in the Rat Brain," *Journal of Neuroscience*, 3 (1983):844–855.

93. KHACHATURIAN, H., et al. "Beta Endorphin, Alpha-MSH, ACTH, and Related Peptides," in T. Hokfelt and A. Bjorklund, eds., *Handbook of Chemical Neuroanatomy*, vol. 4, *Neuropeptides in the CNS*. Holland: Elsevier Biomedical Publishers, forthcoming.

94. KIMURA, H., et al. "Choline Acetyltransferase–containing Neurons in Rodent Brain Demonstrated by Immunohistochemistry," *Science*, 208 (1980):1057–1059.

95. KIMURA, H., et al. "The Central Cholinergic System Studied by Choline Acetyltransferase Immunohistochemistry in the Cat," *Journal of Comparative Neurology*, 200 (1981):151–201.

96. KISS, J. Z., MEZEY, E., and SKIRBOLL, L. "Corticotropin-releasing Factor-immunoreactive Neurons of the Paraventricular Nucleus Become Vasopressin Positive After Adrenalectomy," *Proceedings of the National Academy of Science USA*, 81 (1984):1854–1858.

97. KLAWANS, H. L., et al. "Cholinergic and Anticholinergic Influences on Amphetamine-induced Stereotyped Behavior," *Journal of Neurological Science*, 17 (1972):303.

98. KLEIN, D. F., ZITRIN, C. M., and WOERNER, M. "Antidepressants, Anxiety, Panic and Phobias," in M. A. Lipton, A. DiMascio, and K. F. Killam, eds., *Psychopharmacology: A Generation of Progress*. New York: Raven Press, 1978, pp. 1401–1410.

99. KRIEGER, D. T. "Brain Peptides: What, Where, and Why?" *Science*, 222 (1983):975–981.

100. KRIEGER, D. T., and MARTIN, J. B. "Brain Peptides (First of Two Parts)," *New England Journal of Medicine*, 304 (1981):876–884.

101. ———. "Brain Peptides (Second of Two Parts)," *New England Journal of Medicine*, 304 (1981):944–951.

102. KRNJEVIC, K. "Chemical Nature of Synaptic Transmission in Vertebrates," *Physiological Review*, 54 (1974):418–540.

103. KUPFERMANN, I. "Hypothalamus and Limbic System. I: Peptidergic Neurons, Homeostasis, and Emotional Behavior," in E. R. Kandel and J. H. Schwartz, eds., *Principles of Neuroscience*. Amsterdam: Elsevier-North-Holland; 1981, pp. 433–449.

104. LANGER, D. H., BROWN, G. L., and DOCHERTY, J. P. "Dopamine Receptor Supersensitivity and Schizophrenia: A Review," *Schizophrenia Bulletin*, 7 (1981):208–224.

105. LEE, T., et al. "Binding of ^{3}H-neuroleptics and ^{3}H-apomorphine in Schizophrenic Brains," *Nature*, 274 (1978):897–900.

106. LEWIS, M. E. "Biochemical Aspects of Schizophrenia," in M.B.H. Youdim, et al., eds., *Essays in Neurochemistry and Neuropharmacology*, vol. 4. New York: John Wiley & Sons, 1980, pp. 1–67.

107. LEWIS, P. R., and SHUTE, C.C.D. "The Cholinergic Limbic System: Projections to Hippocampal Formation, Medial Cortex Nuclei of the Ascending Cholinergic Reticular System and the Subfornical Organ and Supraoptic Crest," *Brain*, 90 (1967):521–542.

108. LINDVALL, O., et al. "Mesencephalic Dopamine Neurons Projecting to Neocortex," *Brain Research*, 81 (1974):325–331.

109. MAAS, J. W. "Neurotransmitters and Depression. Too Much, Too Little, or Too Unstable?" *Trends in Neuroscience*, 2 (1979):306–308.

110. MACDONALD, R. L., and BARKER, J. L. "Benzodiazepines Specifically Modulate GABA-mediated Postsynaptic Inhi-

bition in Cultured Mammalian Neurons," *Nature,* 271 (1978):563–564.

111. McGEER, P. L., HATTORI, T., and McGEER, E. G. "Chemical and Autoradiographic Analysis of Gamma-aminobutyric Acid Transport in Purkinje Cells of the Cerebellum," *Experimental Neurology,* 47 (1975):26–41.

112. McGEER, P. L., et al. "Choline Acetyltransferase Localization in the Central Nervous System by Immunohistochemistry," *Brain Research,* 81 (1974):373–379.

113. MACKAY, A.V.P. "Sinistral Findings in Schizophrenia," *Trends in Neuroscience,* 7 (1984):107–108.

114. MACKAY, A.V.P., et al. "Increased Brain Dopamine and Dopamine Receptors in Schizophrenia," *Archives of General Psychiatry,* 39 (1982):991–997.

115. MASON, S. T. "Designing a Non-Neuroleptic Antischizophrenic Drug: The Noradrenergic Strategy," *Trends in Pharmacological Science,* 4 (1983):353–356.

116. MASON, S. T. "Reply," *Trends in Pharmacological Science,* 5 (1984): 141.

117. MATTHEWS, J., et al. "Plasma Measures of Beta-endorphin-like Immunoreactivity in Depressives and Other Psychiatric Subjects," *Life Sciences,* 31 (1982):1867–1870.

118. MATTHYSSE, S. "Antipsychotic Drug Action: A Clue to the Neuropathology of Schizophrenia," *Federation Proceedings,* 32 (1973):200–205.

119. MESULAM, M. M., and van HOESEN, G. W. "Acetylcholinesterase-rich Projections from the Basal Forebrain of the Rhesus Monkey to Neocortex," *Brain Research,* 109 (1976):152–157.

120. MESULAM, M. M., et al. "Cholinergic Innervation of Cortex by the Basal Forebrain: Cytochemistry and Cortical Connections of the Septal Area, Diagonal Band Nuclei, Nucleus Basalis (Substantia Innominata), and Hypothalamus in the Rhesus Monkey," *Journal of Comparative Neurology,* 214 (1983):170–197.

121. MISHINA, M., et al. "Expression of Functional Acetylcholine Receptor from Cloned cDNAs," *Nature,* 307 (1984):604–608.

122. MORGANE, P. J. "Historical and Modern Concepts of Hypothalamic Organization and Function," in P. J. Morgane and J. Panksepp, eds., *Handbook of the Hypothalamus,* vol. 1, *Anatomy of the Hypothalamus.* New York: Marcel Dekker, 1979, pp. 1–64.

123. NAUTA, W. J. H. "The Central Visceromotor System: A General Survey," in C. C. Hockman, ed., *Limbic System Mechanics and Autonomic Function.* Springfield, Ill.: Charles C Thomas, 1972, pp. 21–38.

124. NAUTA, W. J. H., and Haymaker, W. "Hypothalamic Nuclei and Fiber Connections," in W. Haymaker, E. Anderson, and W.J.H. Nauta, eds., *The Hypothalamus.* Springfield, Ill.: Charles C Thomas, 1969, pp. 136–209.

125. NEMEROFF, C. B., and DUNN, A. J., eds., *Peptides, Hormones and Behavior.* New York: Spectrum Publications, 1984.

126. NIEUWENHUYS, R., VOOGD, J., and van HUIJZEN, CHR. *The Human Central Nervous System.* New York: Springer-Verlag, 1981.

127. NOBIN, A., and BJORKLUND, A. "Topography of the Monoamine Neuron Systems in the Human Brain as Revealed in Fetuses," *Acta Physiological Scandinavica,* 388 (Supplement) (1973): 1–40.

128. NYGREN, L.-G., and OLSON, L. "A New Major Projection from Locus Coeruleus: The Main Source of Noradrenergic Nerve Terminals in the Ventral and Dorsal Columns of the Spinal Cord," *Brain Research,* 132 (1977):85–93.

129. OLSCHOWKA, J.A., et al. "The Distribution of Corticotropin Releasing Factor–like Immuonreactive Neurons in Rat Brain," *Peptides,* 3 (1982):995–1015.

130. OWEN, F., et al. "Increased Dopamine-receptor Sensitivity in Schizophrenia," *Lancet,* 2 (1978):223–225.

131. PALKOVITS, M. "Neuropeptides in the Median Eminence: Their Sources and Destinations," *Peptides,* 3 (1982):299–303.

132. PALKOVITS, M., and JACOBOWITZ, D. M. "Topographic Atlas of Catecholamine and Acetylcholinesterase-containing Neurons in the Rat Brain. II. Hindbrain (Mesencephalon, Rhomben-

cephalon)," *Journal of Comparative Neurology,* 157 (1974):29–42.

133. PALKOVITS, M., et al. "Serotonergic Innervation of the Forebrain: Effect of Lesions on Serotonin and Tryptophan Hydroxylase Levels," *Brain Research,* 130 (1977):121–134.

134. PAPEZ, J. W. "A Proposed Mechanism of Emotion," *Archives of Neurological Psychiatry,* 38 (1937):725–743.

135. PARENT, A., and O'REILLY-FROMENTIN, J. "Distribution and Morphological Characteristics of Acetylcholinesterase-containing Neurons in the Basal Forebrain of the Cat," *Brain Research,* 8 (1982):-183–196.

136. PEROUTKA, S. J., and SNYDER, S. J. "Multiple Serotonin Receptors: Differential Binding of [³H]5-hydroxytryptamine, [³H]Lysergic Acid Diethylamide, and [³H]Spiroperidol," *Molecular Pharmacology,* 16 (1979):687–699.

137. PEROUTKA, S. J., LEBOVITZ, R. M., and SNYDER, S. H. "Two Distinct Central Serotonin Receptors with Different Physiological Functions," *Science,* 212 (1981):827–829.

138. POST, R. M., and GOODWIN, F. K. "Approaches to Brain Amines in Psychiatric Patients: A Reevaluation of Cerebrospinal Fluid Studies," in L. L. Iversen, S. D. Iversen, and S. H. Snyder, eds., *Handbook of Psychopharmacology,* vol. 13. London: Plenum Press, 1978, pp. 147–185.

139. POST, R. M., et al. "Cerebrospinal Fluid GABA in Normals and Patients with Affective Disorders," *Brain Research Bulletin,* 5 (1980):755–759.

140. REDMOND, D. E., Jr. "Alteration in the Functions of the Nucleus Locus Coeruleus: A Possible Model for Studies of Anxiety," in I. Hanin and E. Usdin, eds., *Animal Models in Psychiatry and Neurology.* New York: Pergamon Press, 1977, pp. 293–306.

141. REISINE, T. D., et al. "Opiate and Neuroleptic Receptor Alterations in Human Schizophrenic Brain Tissue," in G. Pepeu, M. J. Kuhar, and S. J. Enna, eds., *Receptors for Neurotransmitters and Peptide Hormones.* New York: Raven Press, 1980, pp. 443–450.

142. REUS, V. I., JOSEPH, M. S., and DALLMAN, M. F. "ACTH Levels After the Dexamethasone Suppression Test in Depression," *New England Journal of Medicine,* 306 (1982):238–239.

143. REYNOLDS, G. P. "Increased Concentrations and Lateral Asymmetry of Amygdala Dopamine in Schizophrenia," *Nature,* 305 (1983):527–529.

144. ———. "Noradrenaline and Schizophrenia," *Trends in Pharmacological Science,* 5 (1984): 138.

145. RIEDERER, P., and BIRKMAYER, W. "A New Concept: Brain Area Specific Imbalance of Neurotransmitters in Depression Syndrome—Human Brain Studies," in E. Usdin, T. L. Sourkes, and M.B.H. Youdim, eds., *Enzymes and Neurotransmitters in Mental Disease.* Chichester, England: John Wiley & Sons, 1980, pp. 261–280.

146. RISCH, S. C. Beta-endorphin Hypersecretion in Depression: Possible Cholinergic Mechanisms," *Biological Psychiatry,* 17 (1982):1071–1079.

147. ROBERTS, E. "An Hypothesis Suggesting that There Is a Defect in the GABA System in Schizophrenia," *Neuroscience Research Program Bulletin,* 10 (1972):-468–482.

148. ROBERTS, G. W., et al. "Distribution of Neuropeptides in the Limbic System of the Rat: The Amygdaloid Complex," *Neuroscience,* 7 (1982):99–131.

149. ROBERTS, P. J., et al. "Striatal Glutamatergic Function: Modifications Following Specific Lesions," *Brain Research,* 235 (1982):83–91.

150. SACHAR, E. J., et al. "Disrupted 24-hour Pattern of Cortisol Secretion in Psychotic Depression," *Archives of General Psychiatry,* 28 (1973):19–24.

151. SAWCHENKO, P. E., SWANSON, L. W., and VALE, W. W. "Co-expression of Corticotropin-releasing Factor and Vasopressin Immunoreactivity in Parvocellular Neurosecretory Neurons of the Adrenalectomized Rat," *Proceedings of the National Academy of Science USA,* 81 (1984):1883–1887.

152. SHUTE, C.C.D., and LEWIS, P. R. "The Ascending Cholinergic Reticular System: Neocortical, Olfactory and Subcortical Projections," *Brain,* 90 (1967):497–520.

153. SMITH, C. C., LEWIS, M. E., and TALL-

MAN, J. F. "Effect of Benzodiazepines on Cyclic GMP Formation in Rat Cerebellar Slices," *Pharmacology, Biochemistry and Behavior*, 16 (1982):29–33.

154. SMYTHIES, J. R. "The Transmethylation Hypotheses of Schizophrenia Reevaluated," *Trends in Neuroscience*, 7 (1984):45–47.

155. SNYDER, S. H. "Brain Peptides as Neurotransmitters," *Science*, 209 (1980):976–983.

156. SNYDER, S. H., et al. "Drugs, Neurotransmitters, and Schizophrenia," *Science*, 184 (1974):1243–1253.

157. SOFRONIEW, M. V. "Projections from Vasopressin, Oxytocin, and Neurophysin Neurons to Neural Targets in the Rat and Human," *Journal of Histochemistry and Cytochemistry*, 28 (1980):475–478.

158. SOFRONIEW, M. V., et al. "Immunohistochemistry of Vasopressin, Oxytocin and Neurophysin in the Hypothalamus and Extrahypothalamic Regions of the Human Brain," *Acta Histochemica*, 24 (Supplement) (1981):79–95.

159. STERBA, G., et al. "The Neurosecretory Hypothalamo-hindbrain Pathway and Its Possible Significance for the Regulation of Blood Pressure and the Milk-ejection Reflex," *Cell and Tissue Research*, 196 (1979):321–336.

160. STEVENS, J., WILSON, K., and FOOTE, W. "GABA Blockade, Dopamine and Schizophrenia: Experimental Studies in the Cat," *Psychopharmacologia*, 39 (1974):105–119.

161. STORM-MATHIESEN, J. "Localization of Transmitter Candidates in the Brain: The Hippocampal Formation as a Model," *Progress in Neurobiology*, 8 (1977):119–181.

162. SULSER, F., VETULANI, J., and MOBLEY, P. L. "Mode of Action of Antidepressant Drugs," *Biochemical Pharmacology*, 27 (1978):257–261.

163. SWANSON, L. W. "The Locus Coeruleus: A Cytoarchitectonic, Golgi and Immunohistochemical Study in the Albino Rat," *Brain Research*, 110 (1976):39–56.

164. SWANSON, L. W., and HARTMAN, B. K. "The Central Adrenergic System, an Immunofluorescence Study of the Location of Cell Bodies and Their Efferent Connections in the Rat Utilizing Dopa-

mine Beta-hydroxylase as a Marker," *Journal of Comparative Neurology*, 163 (1975):467–506.

165. SWANSON, L. W., et al. "Organization of Ovine Corticotropin-releasing Factor Immunoreactive Cells and Fibers in the Rat Brain: An Immunohistochemical Study," *Neuroendocrinology*, 36 (1983):165–186.

166. TALLMAN, J. F., et al. "Receptors for the Age of Anxiety: Pharmacology of the Benzodiazepines," *Science*, 207 (1980):274–281.

167. UNGERSTEDT, U. "Stereotaxic Mapping of the Monoamine Pathways in the Rat Brain," *Acta Physiologica Scandinavica*, 367 (1971):1–48.

168. VALE, W., et al. "Characterization of a 41 Residue Ovine Hypothalamic Peptide That Stimulates Secretions of Corticotrophin and Beta-endorphin," *Science*, 213 (1981):1394–1397.

169. VALE, W., et al. "Corticotropin Releasing Factor," in D. T. Krieger, M. J. Brownstein, and J. B. Martin, eds., *Brain Peptides*. New York: John Wiley & Sons, 1983, pp. 961–974.

170. VAN DONGEN, P.A.M. "The Central Noradrenergic Transmission and the Locus Coeruleus: A Review of the Data and Their Implications for Neurotransmission and Neuromodulation," *Progress in Neurobiology*, 16 (1981):117–143.

171. ———. "The Human Locus Coeruleus in Neurology and Psychiatry," *Progress in Neurobiology*, 17 (1981):97–139.

172. VAN PRAAG, H. M. "Significance of Biochemical Parameters in the Diagnosis, Treatment, and Prevention of Depressive Disorders," *Biological Psychiatry*, 12 (1977):101–131.

173. VINCENT, S. R., et al. "Dynorphin-immunoreactive Neurons in the Central Nervous System of the Rat," *Neuroscience Letters*, 33 (1982):185–190.

174. WALAAS, I., and FONNUM, F. "Biochemical Evidence for Gamma-aminobutyrate-containing Fibers from the Nucleus Accumbens to the Substantia Nigra and Ventral Tegmental Area in the Rat," *Neuroscience*, 5 (1980):63–72.

175. ———. "Biochemical Evidence for Glutamate as a Transmitter in Hippocampal Efferents to the Basal Forebrain and

Hypothalamus in the Rat Brain," *Neuroscience,* 5 (1980):1691–1698.

176. WATSON, S. J., ALBALA, A. A., and BERGER, P. "Peptides and Psychiatry," in D. Krieger, M. Brownstein, and J. Martin, eds., *Brain Peptides.* New York: John Wiley & Sons, 1983, pp. 349–368.

177. WATSON, S. J., RICHARD, C. W., III, and BARCHAS, J. D. "Adrenocorticotropin in Rat Brain: Immunocytochemical Localization in Cells and Axons," *Science,* 200 (1978):1180–1182.

178. WATSON, S. J., et al. "Immunocytochemical Localization of Methionine Enkephalin: Preliminary Observations," *Life Sciences,* 25 (1977):733–738.

179. WATSON, S. J., et al "Evidence for Two Separate Opiate Peptide Neuronal Systems," *Nature,* 275 (1978):226–228.

180. WATSON, S. J., et al. "Dynorphin Immunocytochemical Localization in Brain and Peripheral Nervous System: Preliminary Studies," *Proceedings of the National Academy of Science USA,* 78 (1981):1260–1263.

181. WATSON, S. J., et al. "Dynorphin and Vasopressin: Common Localization in Magnocellular Neurons," *Science,* 216 (1982):85–87.

182. WATSON, S. J., et al. "Opioid Systems: Anatomical, Physiological and Clinical Perspectives," in H.O.J. Collier, et al. *Opioids: Past, Present and Future.* London: Taylor and Francis, 1984, pp. 145–178.

183. WEBER, E., ROTH, K. A., and BARCHAS, J. D. "Immunocytochemical Distribution of Alpha-neo-endorphin/dynorphin Neuronal Systems in Rat Brain: Evidence for Colocalization," *Proceedings of the National Academy of Science USA,* 79 (1982):3062–3066.

184. WEIL-MALHERBE, H. "Serotonin and Schizophrenia," in W. B. Essman, ed., *Serotonin in Health and Disease,* vol. 3: *The Central Nervous System.* New York: Spectrum Publications, 1978, pp. 231–291.

185. WHITAKER, P. M., CROW, T. J., and FERRIER, N. "Tritiated LSD Binding in Frontal Cortex in Schizophrenia," *Archives of General Psychiatry,* 38 (1981):278–280.

186. WHITE, F. J., and WANG, R. Y. "Differential Effects of Classical and Atypical Antipsychotic Drugs on A9 and A10 Dopamine Neurons," *Science,* 221 (1983):1054–1056.

187. WIKLUND, L., TOGGENBURGER, G., and CUENOD, M. "Aspartate: Possible Neurotransmitter in Cerebellar Climbing Fibers," *Science,* 216 (1982):78–80.

188. WOODHAMS, P. L., et al. "Distribution of Neuropeptides in the Limbic System of the Rat: The Bed Nucleus of the Stria Terminalis, Septum and Preoptic Area," *Neuroscience,* 8 (1983):677–703.

189. WOODWARD, D. J., et al. "Modulatory Actions of Norepinephrine in the Central Nervous System," *Federation Proceedings,* 38 (1979):2109–2116.

190. YEREVANIAN, B. I., and WOOLF, P. D. "Plasma ACTH Levels in Primary Depression: Relationship to the 24-hour Dexamethasone Suppression Test," *Psychiatry Research,* 9 (1983):319–327.

191. YORKSTON, N. J., et al. "Propranolol as an Adjunct to the Treatment of Schizophrenia," *Lancet,* 11 (1977):575–578.

192. YORKSTON, N. J., et al. "DL-propranolol and Chlorpromazine Following Admission for Schizophrenia. A Controlled Comparison," *Acta Psychiatrica Scandinavica,* 63 (1981):13–27.

193. YOUNG, A. B., BROMBERG, M. B., and PENNEY, J. B. "Decreased Glutamate Uptake in Subcortical Areas Deafferented by Sensorimotor Cortex Ablation in the Cat," *Journal of Neuroscience,* 1 (1981):241–249.

194. YOUNG, A. B., et al. "Glutamic Acid: Selective Depletion by Viral-induced Granule Cell Loss in Hamster Cerebellum," *Brain Research,* 73 (1974):1–13.

CHAPTER 2

BEHAVIORAL NEUROCHEMISTRY: THE STUDY OF BRAIN AND BEHAVIOR

Glen R. Elliott and Jack D. Barchas

¶ Introduction

One of the truly exciting success stories of the past few decades has been the explosion of knowledge about how nerve cells communicate with each other and how such communications translate into behavior. Closely coupled with these advances have been discoveries of powerful "mind-altering" drugs and of medications that have completely changed treatment approaches for many mental disorders. This rich milieu has spawned the field of behavioral neurochemistry, which seeks to refine and expand knowledge about the intimate connections between brain neuronal function and behavior.

It seems unlikely that even the most optimistic researchers in the 1930s and 1940s would have dared to predict the rapid flowering of behavioral neurochemistry to its present robust state. Those in the field now concern themselves with levels of neuronal organization ranging from the nerve cell nucleus and cytoplasm through individual connections between nerves to neuronal networks and major brain regions. Furthermore, they seek to apply information gained from studies at each of these levels to analyses of normal and abnormal behavior in animals and human beings. Such research draws on many disciplines, including molecular genetics, analytical neurochemistry, biochemistry, neurophysiology, histology, neuroanatomy, neuropharmacology, physiological psychology, behavioral psychology, sociopharmacology, and psychiatry. The fruits of behavioral neurochemistry are also its constant motivating force—new insights into biochemical aspects of brain function that suggest exciting directions for research into normal behavior and mental disorders and should lead to improvements in methods of diagnosing, treating, and perhaps preventing severe mental disorders.

Other chapters in this volume amply attest to the power of behavioral neurochemistry in generating hypotheses about mental disorders. They also describe the rich array of pharmacological approaches now available for treating many mental disorders, as well as the limitations such treatments still have. In this chapter, we restrict ourselves mainly to a brief review of the development of behavioral neurochemistry as a field and of current thinking about brain function. We conclude by describing several exciting developments that promise to add substantially to the knowledge base over the next few years, as investigators begin to apply emerging technologies for studying brain function *in vivo* in living animals and human beings.

¶ Neuroregulators

Typically, T. R. Elliott, a Cambridge student in the early 1900s, is credited with the first formal enunciation of a hypothesis that nerve cells communicate by chemical transmission.[69,70] The concept did not develop in a vacuum but rather crystallized comments found in even earlier works. For example, in an 1877 paper, Du Bois-Reymond[63] suggested that communication between neurons could occur electrically or chemically. Also, by 1895 Oliver and Shafer[159] had shown that extracts from adrenal glands can produce physiological effects resembling those that follow sympathetic nerve stimulation. Even earlier work by Schmiedeberg and Koppe[179] had shown that muscarine can mimic many of the effects of parasympathetic nerve stimulation. Furthermore, Sherrington[186] had coined the term synapse in 1887 for the specialized regions along nerve axons where they interfaced with other neurons. Clearly, such clues to neuronal function were influential precursors to the enunciation of the chemical transmission hypothesis.

Initial experimental tests of the hypothesis of neurochemical transmission were done on acetylcholine (ACh). In 1906 Dixon[61] suggested that the physiological effects of muscarine might result from its mimicking a muscarinelike substance normally released

from parasympathetic fibers. That same year Hunt and Taveau[105] described the physiological effects of ACh, among other choline derivatives. Over the next decade Dale, Barger, and coworkers published a series of studies culminating in the conclusion that ACh was involved in transmitting signals in parasympathetic fibers.[9,54,55]

In 1921 Loewi[139] began the work that provided the first compelling evidence of chemical neurotransmission. In his classic experiment, Loewi used a perfusion medium to connect isolated frog hearts. Stimulation of the vagus nerve of the first, innervated heart released a substance—*vagusstoff*—into the perfusion medium that slowed the rate of the second, denervated heart. Later, isolation and identification of *vagusstoff* showed it to be ACh.[140]

Also in 1921, Cannon and Uridil[30] reported the isolation of "sympathin," a substance released from liver following stimulation of sympathetic nerves. They and other investigators showed that sympathin was released from all sympathetic nerves. Furthermore, it bore a strong resemblance to epinephrine, although the two compounds could be distinguished pharmacologically. Absolute identification of sympathin came slowly. Bacq[5] was one of the first to suggest that sympathin might be norepinephrine (NE), but he believed that epinephrine was the actual neurotransmitter. Proof that sympathin was NE was not available until 1946, when von Euler applied newly available fluorometric techniques to measure small amounts of NE quantitatively.[211,212]

All of the work just described was done on peripheral neuronal systems. Although there were occasional suggestions that chemical transmission also might be important in the central nervous system (CNS), the general wisdom for many years was that only electrical processes could be sufficiently rapid to satisfy the demands in the CNS for information transfer. Lively—if not always enlightening—debates on this issue gradually began to yield to experimental data in the early 1950s (see Eccles[66]). For example, researchers developed ways to record electrical activ-

TABLE 2–1
Possible CNS Neuroregulators

Dopamine (DA)	Serotonin (5-hydroxytryptamine; 5HT)
Norepinephrine (NE)	Melatonin
Epinephrine (E)	Tryptamine
Tyramine	Dimethyltryptamine (DMT)
Octopamine	5-Methoxytryptamine
Phenylethylamine (PE)	Tryptolines
Phenylethanolamine	
Tetrahydroisoquinolines (THIQ)	
Acetylcholine (ACh)	Prostaglandins
Histamine	Vasopressin
gamma-Aminobutyric acid (GABA)	Estrogens
gamma-Hydroxybutyrate (GHB)	Testosterone
Glycine	Corticosteroids
Taurine	Cholecystokinin
Purine	Oxytocin
Aspartate	Bradykinin
Glutamate	Angiotensin
Histidine	Neurophysin
Thyroid hormone	Insulin
Substance P	Vasoactive intestinal polypeptide (VIP)
Substance P (5–11)	Gastric inhibitory peptide (GIP)
Neuromedins B, C, and K	Gastrin-releasing peptide (Bombesin)
Substance K	Delta-sleep-inducing peptide
Somatostatin	Sleep-promoting substance (SPS)
Adrenocorticotropic hormone (ACTH)	Uridine
alpha-melanocyte-stimulating hormone (alpha-MSH)	Carnosine
Luteinizing hormone (LH)	Thyroid-releasing hormone (TRH)
Growth hormone-releasing hormone	Secretin
Gonadotropin-releasing hormone	FMRF amide
	Hydra head activator
Met-enkephalin (met-ENK)	Calcitonin
Met-enkephalin-Arg-Gly-Leu	Calcitonin-gene related peptide
Met-enkephalin-Arg-Phe	Cerebellin
Leu-enkephalin (leu-ENK)	BAM 12
alpha-Endorphin	BAM 18
beta-Endorphin (1–31)	BAM 22
beta-Endorphin (1–27)	Neuropeptide Y
beta-Endorphin (1–26)	Peptide E
gamma-Endorphin	Peptide F
alpha-Neo-endorphin	Peptide YY
Dynorphin A	Peptide HI
Dynorphin A(1–8)	Galanin
Dynorphin B	Motilin
Metorphamide	Neuropeptide K
beta-Lipotropin	

SOURCE: J. D. Barchas et al., "Behavioral Neurochemistry: Neuroregulators and Behavioral States," *Science*, 200 (1978):964–973. See also Krieger[126] and Krieger, Brownstein, and Martin.[127]

ity of single cells with microelectrodes[78,218] and to apply minute amounts of a substance directly onto a neuron with microiontophoresis.[53,57] The results from such studies in brain could not be reconciled with predicted characteristics of electrical neuronal junctions. Furthermore, Vogt[210] showed that NE and epinephrine were present in the CNS and changed in predictable ways with the physiological state of the animal or following administration of certain drugs.

For many years concepts of CNS neurotransmission were derived by analogy from research on peripheral neuronal systems. Even as recently as the early 1970s, fewer than ten substances were widely recognized as putative CNS neurotransmitters; the best-known of these were ACh, serotonin (5HT), dopamine (DA), NE, and gamma-aminobutyric acid (GABA). However, marked improvements in analytical methodology such as high-performance liquid chromatography, gas chromatography/mass spectrometry, radioimmunology, and radio-enzymology greatly extended the scope, sensitivity, and specificity of assays.[8,42] As a result, researchers have identified an increasingly heterogeneous and rapidly growing number of substances in brain tissues. Initially, most of the substances were small molecules like those mentioned; however, in the past decade researchers have identified an astounding array of small- and medium-sized peptides that also seem to be key components to brain function. Table 2–1 offers a sampling of substances thought to play a role in communication among nerves.

The proliferation of identified neuroactive substances has strained early concepts of chemical transmission severely.[23,160] A number of investigators have proposed nomenclatures to impose some order on the rapidly expanding range of identified substances and actions related to neuronal activity (see Dismukes[59]). We have suggested the term neuroregulators to refer to the full panoply of compounds directly involved in the regulation of interneuronal communication, with neuroregulators being divided into two broad categories—neurotransmitters and neuromodulators.[8,68] (See table 2–2).

Neurotransmitters

Light and electron microscopic studies have revealed in considerable detail the sites —synapses—at which information is con-

TABLE 2–2
A Nomenclature for Substances Involved in Communication Among Neurons

Neuroregulators: Any substances that directly contribute to the regulation of signal transmission from one neuron to another.

Neurotransmitters: Substances that carry a signal from one neuron to another unidirectionally within an identified synaptic structure.

Voltage-independent neurotransmitters produce characteristic postsynaptic effects across a wide range of postsynaptic membrane voltages.

Voltage-dependent neurotransmitters produce characteristic postsynaptic effects only in a narrow band of postsynaptic membrane voltages.

Neuromodulators: Substances that alter signal transmission between neurons or neuronal activity through mechanisms other than neurotransmission.

Synaptic neuromodulators act locally in synapses at a specific site of action to alter the activity of a neurotransmitter.

Hormonal neuromodulators affect neuronal activity at relatively great distances and numerous sites either by acting at specific receptors inside or outside synapses or by interfering with neurotransmission.

SOURCE: G. R. Elliott and J. D. Barchas, "Changing Concepts About Neuroregulation: Neurotransmitters and Neuromodulators," in D. de Wied and P. A. van Keep, eds., *Hormones and the Brain.* Lancaster, England: MTP Press, 1980, pp. 43–52.

veyed from one nerve cell to another (see Feldman and Quenzer[83]). Based on a variety of experimental data, a concept of neurotransmission has emerged that is captured in highly stylized form in figure 2–1.[8,42,167] Although accumulating evidence continually underscores its limitations, this model still illustrates some key aspects of neurotransmission that remain heuristically valuable.

The presynaptic side of the synapse contains the enzymatic machinery necessary to synthesize the neurotransmitter. The complexity of synthesis varies from one neurotransmitter to the next, as do degradative pathways. For many of the small-molecule neurotransmitters, including amino acids such as GABA and the catecholamines and 5HT, considerable information now is available about the enzymes responsible for synthesis and degradation. Many neurotransmit-

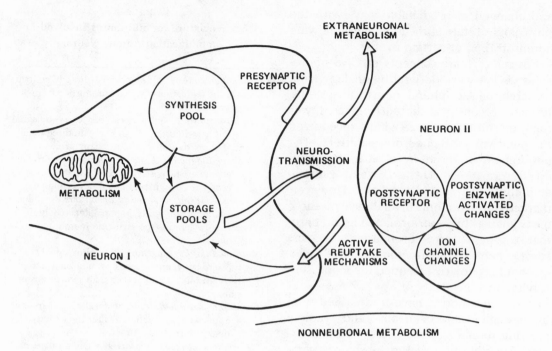

Figure 2–1. Model of neurotransmission.

ters appear to be stored in presynaptic structures called vesicles that have specialized uptake and storage mechanisms for that particular neurotransmitter.

Electrical transmission of a signal along a nerve axon has been studied extensively and is reasonably well understood.[83,98,106] Much less is known about how depolarization of the presynaptic membrane leads to release of the neurotransmitter into the synaptic cleft. Calcium is known to be involved,[17] and the predominant theory suggests that vesicles somehow begin to fuse with the membrane, releasing their contents into the extracellular space.[97,162] Whether the vesicles are the sole or even major storage site for transmitters remains controversial.[39,224] Calmodulin, a ubiquitous protein involved in a wide range of cellular functions, appears to be one piece of the puzzle of how calcium promotes neurotransmitter release with depolarization. The calcium-calmodulin complex is thought to activate an enzyme system that phosphorylates synaptic vesicles, somehow facilitating their attachment to the cellular membrane.[36,58,148]

Once in the synapse, the neurotransmitter diffuses across the small synaptic cleft, where it comes in to contact with postsynaptic receptors—proteins in the postsynaptic membrane with which it interacts in a highly specific manner.[152,191] Interaction of the neurotransmitter and its receptor has characteristic effects on the postsynaptic neuron. Any given neurotransmitter may have a number of receptors, each with different properties and effects on neuronal activity.[116,131,134] Among the common actions of receptors are changes in ion channels, creating fluxes that may either facilitate or inhibit subsequent activation of the neuron,[115] and activation of certain enzymatic systems whose functions still are poorly understood.[93,184]

Functionally, there must be a way to terminate a signal. Typically this involves disassociation of the transmitter from its receptor, followed by removal of the transmitter by, for example, passive diffusion out of the synaptic cleft or enzymatic degradation within the cleft.[8,42] Some neurons have specific reuptake mechanisms that actively return the transmitter to the presynaptic neuron, where it is either metabolized or stored for reuse.[107,130]

Within the past few years, innovative research of synapses has suggested the need for increasingly complex refinements of this idealized model. For instance, as already noted, some neurotransmitters have receptors on both the pre- and postsynaptic membranes; the former are thought to provide a mechanism of rapid feedback for turning off cell firing.[1,173,205] For several transmitters that have been studied in some detail, pre- and postsynaptic receptors are pharmacologically distinct, leading to some interesting suggestions for new treatment strategies for such mental disorders as schizophrenia.[29,174,176]

Another interesting evolution in the concept of neurotransmission is the suggestion that some transmitters may be voltage dependent.[128] At some synapses, a neurotransmitter appears to have no effect at certain postsynaptic voltages; yet at other voltages it acts as a typical neurotransmitter. Or in some instances it may inhibit postsynaptic firing at some voltages but promote it at others. The full implications of such mechanisms for understanding mental disorders remain to be determined.

Research on both peripheral and CNS neurotransmitter systems suggests certain general criteria for defining a neurotransmitter (see table 2–3). For a few substances, especially in the periphery, all of these criteria have been satisfied; for the vast majority of putative CNS neurotransmitters, many of the criteria remain untestable. For the clinician, the greatest value of such criteria may be enumeration of sites at which neurotransmission can go awry.

Neuromodulators

Even as recently as the early 1970s, the predominant focus on brain function involved studies of small groups of substances thought to be acting as neurotransmitters. For many years, a major tenet of such research was Dale's principle. First defined by Eccles,[67] who based it on early work by Dale,[55] the principle asserts that a given neuron uses the same neurotransmitter at all synapses. Synapses were thought to use only a single neurotransmitter, so Dale's principle generalized into a one-neuron/one-neurotransmitter rule.

For many years Dale's principle held up remarkably well. An especially striking example came from work with the marine snail *Aplysia*, where a single neuron was found to be excitatory to one cell and inhibitory to another.[195,199] These differential effects proved to be a result of postsynaptic interactions, with ACh being the neurotransmitter in both instances. However, in the late 1960s and early 1970s reports began to appear that suggested that neurons might contain more than one neuroactive substance.[27,118] First reported for neurons in invertebrate systems, these findings raised the possibility of much more complex neuronal regulation than the popular model of neurotransmission suggested.

Two developments in the mid-1970s further stimulated a reassessment of neuronal mechanisms. The first was the astonishing discovery of an endogenous opioid system, heralded by the identification of opioid receptors in the mammalian brain.[90,164,188,200] Subsequent research revealed that the nervous system contained opiatelike substances that acted on these receptors. The initial isolation of met-enkephalin and leu-enkephalin in 1975[104,189] led to the discovery of a whole family of previously unsuspected neuroregulators, now collectively called endorphins.[125] Furthermore, it stimulated a wider search for neuroregulator peptides, which continues to add regularly to the list of possible neuroregulators[34,45,126,127] (see table 2–1).

A second important development involved technical advances that greatly enhanced the ability of investigators to identify specific neuroregulators in cells. Especially useful has been the technique of immunohistofluorescence, in which antibodies specifically directed against a particular

TABLE 2–3

Criteria for Establishing the Identity of a Neuroregulator in the Central Nervous System

Neurotransmitter

- The substance must be present in presynaptic elements of a neuronal synapse.
- Precursors and synthetic enzymes must be present in the neuron, probably in close proximity to the site of action.
- Stimulation of neuronal afferents should cause release of the substance in physiologically significant amounts.
- Stimulation of afferents and direct application to the synapse of the substance in physiological amounts should produce identical effects.
- Specific receptors for the substance must be present on the postsynaptic membranes and may be present presynaptically.
- Interaction of the substance with its postsynaptic receptor—possibly only at certain membrane potentials—must produce changes in membrane permeability that promote either excitatory or inhibitory postsynaptic potentials.
- Specific inactivating mechanisms should exist to stop interactions of the substance with its receptor within a physiologically reasonable time.
- Stimulation of afferents and direct application of the substance should be equally responsive to and similarly affected by interventions at postsynaptic sites or on inactivating mechanisms.

Neuromodulator

- The substance must permit sensitive and specific modulation of neuronal *signals*, rather than being involved mainly in a neuronal process such as cell catabolism.
- The substance must be present in physiological fluids and must have access to the presumed modulatory site in physiologically relevant concentrations.
- Both direct application of the substance and alteration of its endogenous concentration should affect neuronal activity consistently and predictably.
- The substance should have one or more specific sites of action through which it can alter neuronal activity incrementally as a function of its concentration.
- Inactivating mechanisms should account for the time course of neuronal effects produced by endogenously or exogenously induced changes in concentrations of the substance.
- Interventions that alter the neuronal effects of increasing the endogenous concentrations of the substance also should alter the neuronal effects of its direct application to the presumed site of action.

SOURCE: G. R. Elliott and J. D. Barchas, "Changing Concepts About Neuroregulation: Neurotransmitters and Neuromodulators," in D. de Wied and P. A. van Keep, eds., *Hormones and the Brain.* Lancaster, England: MTP Press, 1980, pp. 43–52.

neuroregulator are used to identify the neurons[74,99,146,207] containing that neuroregulator. Clever applications of that technique have provided indisputable evidence that colocalization of two or more neuroregulators in the same neuron seems to be the rule, rather than the exception.* There appear to be "families" of peptides coming from the same precursor. For example, Mains, Eipper, and Ling[144] showed that a single protein, pro-opiomelanocortin, was the common precursor for beta-lipoprotein, beta-endorphin, adrenocorticotropin factor (ACTH), and several other neuronally active peptides. Stud-

*See references 34, 100, 196, 207, and 215.

ies of this and analogous precursor molecules have led to suggestions that one aspect of neuronal regulation may involve enzymatic control of the cleavage of such molecules to create differential amounts of final products.[7,222]

The proliferation of identified neuroregulators has raised questions about mechanisms other than neurotransmission that may play a role in interneuronal communication. We have proposed the term neuromodulation for such functions.[8,68] Neuromodulators may influence neuronal activity in a number of ways. In general, we conceive of their effects as involving greater numbers of cells than the transsynaptic event of neurotransmission or providing a "fine-tuning mechanism" for neurotransmitter activity (see figure 2–2).

Hormonal neuromodulators may be released from neurons, glial cells, or even distant parts of the body to alter the "tone" of synaptic activity. In contrast to neurotransmitters, neuromodulators may have prolonged effects on neurons, altering their spontaneous firing rates or sensitivity to other signals. For example, beta-endorphin, which has receptors widely distributed throughout the brain, seems likely to be a neuromodulator.[15] Many of the peripheral hormones, including the glucocorticoids, may have similar CNS modulatory roles.[8]

The coexistence of several putative neuroregulators in the same synapse, mentioned earlier, at least opens the possibility of such interactions. In some instances, two or more neurotransmitters may be released from the presynaptic site and interact with different receptors on the postsynaptic side.[10,128] Alternatively, the interactions among neuroregulators may take the form of a local perturbation of neurotransmission. As indicated in figure 2–2, such synaptic

neuromodulation may occur at many different sites, including direct effects on pre- or postsynaptic receptors and more indirect actions on neurotransmitter synthesis, release, inactivation, or receptor interactions. Although a great deal of work remains to be done to limn the possible activities of neuromodulators, table 2–3 presents some criteria.

As yet, no one has definitively demonstrated synaptic modulation through corelease of substances from the same synapse. Still, the concept offers interesting new ways to think about possible defects in neuroregulation. For instance, we have been interested for some years in the tryptolines—aldehyde condensation products of tryptamine, 5HT, and other indoleamines.[103] It is possible that these substances, some of which occur naturally in animals and human beings,[24,110] play some role in the effects of alcohol consumption. Another example of neuromodulation can be seen in the peripheral nervous system with the effects of NE on parasympathetic activity. NE released from sympathetic neurons reduces the release of ACh following electrical stimulation of parasympathetic

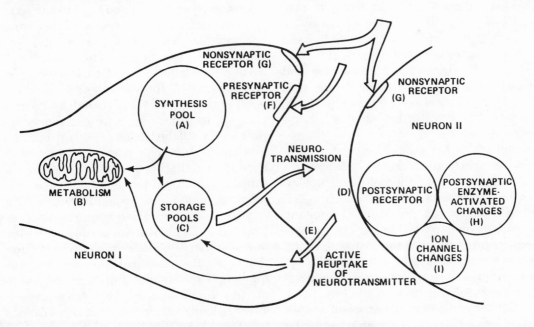

Figure 2–2. Model of neuromodulation.

neurons,[163] apparently through alpha-2 adrenergic receptors located on the presynaptic membrane of the parasympathetic neurons.[62,217] A number of other possible examples of modulation also have been suggested in recent years.[208]

¶ Techniques for Studying Neuroregulators

Much of the burgeoning knowledge about neuronal function can be attributed directly to advances in analytical methods of identifying and quantitating neuroregulators. A full review of such techniques is beyond the scope of this chapter, but a brief description of some of the analytical tools now available to researchers helps to explain the excitement that currently pervades the field of behavioral neurochemistry.

In the first half of this century, essentially all studies of neuroregulators entailed the use of bioassays, in which the presence or absence of a substance and sometimes its amount were assessed on the basis of a specific biological activity. Thus 5HT was identified—and named—from its ability to constrict blood vessels.[161] Although many of these bioassays had great sensitivity and even good specificity for a particular compound, they often were cumbersome and difficult to standardize. Also, the search for a unique physiological assay for each new substance of interest was arduous and not always successful.

As already described, the successful application of spectrophotometric and spectrophotofluorometric methods to creating assays for simple neuroregulators such as NE and 5HT confirmed the value of applying analytic techniques for behavioral neurochemical problems. For the first time rapid, reproducible measures of many samples became feasible.[204] However, it also taught another lesson that researchers continue to relearn: One can never assume that an assay is free of artifact, and all new assays must be checked and rechecked for possible sources of error. For fluorometric methods, chroma-

tographic separation methods had to be introduced for studying samples from complex biological sources to ensure that compounds with similar spectral properties did not interfere with the measures.

During the 1960s and 1970s, analytical approaches to measuring neuroregulators diverged in a number of fruitful directions. Gas chromatography became popular[31,76] and still is used in selected instances.[96] However, problems with sensitivity and specificity guaranteed the continued search for better methods. One modification of this technique that proved especially useful for behavioral neurochemists was the addition of a mass spectrometer as a detector.[109,114,124] Mass spectrometry characterizes substances by their molecular fragmentation properties. Combined with various chromatographic techniques to further isolate substances of interest, it has become established as a versatile tool[80,96,123] with a wide range of applications. One of the limitations of mass spectrometry has been its utility only for compounds of relatively low molecular weight, so that it has had few applications for studies of peptide neuroregulators.[136] However, the recent introduction of a new form of mass spectrometry using fast atom bombardment holds promise of greatly extending the potential uses of the technique.[135]

High-performance liquid chromatography also is invaluable for researchers. First developed in the 1950s for automated amino acid analyses, its other uses were not widely appreciated until the late 1960s and 1970s, when investigators discovered its utility for detecting and quantitating a wide range of biologically important substances.[117,121] The equipment is much less expensive than that required for gas chromatography/mass spectrometry, making it more readily accessible to researchers. In addition, sample preparation is relatively minimal and rapid, increasing sample throughput. Furthermore, a variety of columns and detectors have given it a remarkably diverse set of applications for both low- and high-molecular-weight neuroregulators.[26]

Augmenting the chromatographic and

mass spectrometric methods have been three other techniques using quite different approaches. Radioenzymatic assays take advantage of enzymes that are known to act only on a limited range of substances, for example, catecholamines. By cleverly picking enzymes that could attach a radioactive label to the neuroregulator of interest, researchers developed several simple, sensitive, and specific assays for substances of interest.[48,175] However, the technique was limited by the need to find just the right enzyme and largely has been replaced with radioreceptor and radioimmunoassays.

In the 1950s Berson, Yalow, and their colleagues discovered that some insulin-dependent diabetic patients had circulating antibodies against insulin.[18,19] They found that under appropriate conditions these antibodies could be used to devise an extremely sensitive assay for insulin—a technique they called radioimmunoassay (RIA),[220] for which Yalow won a Nobel Prize in 1978. Well over 10,000 RIAs probably are in use now for a broad spectrum of substances.[28,192] Briefly, an assay is devised by preparing the compound of interest in a form that will produce an antibody response in a host animal, often a rabbit. Once antibody production has been established, investigators must show that it is specific to the substance of interest, with relatively little cross-reactivity to similar compounds that also might be present in a sample. In addition to their uses for assays, such antibodies also are vital for modern neuroanatomists, who use them for specific labeling of neuronal systems containing various neuroregulators (see Chan-Palay and Palay[34] and Usdin, Hamburg, and Barchas[206]). Although RIA is versatile and relatively simple to use, issues of specificity are key. For example, such assays are used widely in studies of endogenous peptides, where careful identification of what actually is being measured and potential cross-reactivities with other, perhaps unknown, peptides may be crucial.

Radioreceptor assays grew out of efforts to characterize the sites of action of neuroregulators and psychopharmacologi-cally active drugs.[90,190] Through such considerations, criteria emerged for defining specific binding sites for a particular substance. In a manner analogous to RIA, binding can be used as an assay by defining standard curves for how much of a radioactively labeled marker is displaced from the specific binding site by various amounts of the unlabeled compound of interest.[72] Again, such assays have become ubiquitous in basic and clinical research, finding applications that range from autoradiographic determinations of receptor anatomy[73] to clinical measures of drug potency.[49,183]

¶ Approaches to Studying Neuroregulators and Behavior

Over the past decade neuroscientists have developed and employed ever more sophisticated efforts to study biochemical changes associated with behavioral states in vertebrate and mammalian systems. Powerful approaches have clarified key neuroregulatory processes in specific behavioral systems in invertebrate systems. A rapidly expanding body of evidence also has proven the feasibility of studying in animals—and to a growing degree in human beings—how behavior can influence brain function and how altered biochemistry may affect behavior.

Model Systems

For most behaviors of interest, including severe mental disorders, human beings are not suitable candidates for study by neuroscientists. On the one hand, genetic and environmental influences are so complex and intertwined that they are hard to study. On the other hand, most available tools for research are too destructive or dangerous to use in people. Therefore, basic researchers continually look for simpler models of such behaviors on which to perform their studies. Models that have provided invaluable insights into human brain function and dysfunction range from the single cell through nonhuman primates.

The ideal model would be readily reproducible, involve a relatively simple nerve system or its equivalent, and permit analysis of defined biochemical systems.[112] Perhaps the simplest yet a surprisingly rich model has emerged from the efforts of Koshland and his colleagues, who use bacterial systems to study biochemical processes underlying approach and avoidance behaviors.[122] Their research shows that these behaviors are under the control of quite basic biochemical systems. A strong advantage in using "simple" model systems is the ready ability to study controlled genetic alterations.[37]

The work of Kandel and his colleagues on a marine snail (*Aplysia*) to illuminate biochemical processes of associative learning is one of the outstanding uses of simple models.[113] Their studies have shown that certain forms of associative learning involve neuroregulator systems of several different types. For example, 5HT systems that act through a cyclic–adenosine monophosphate–dependent set of processes may be involved in both long- and short-term associative learning. Elucidation of the multiple steps involved and the ways in which they can be disrupted already is providing a rich source of information about basic neuronal processes and has implications for psychiatric disorders.[111]

Studying the Effects on Behavior of Changing Neuroregulator Activity

Until quite recently behavioral neurochemistry research on vertebrate and mammalian systems usually has involved the study either of how changes in a given neuroregulatory system alter behavior or of how the presence or absence of the behavior affects that neuroregulatory system.[101,203] Such work has been aided by the discovery of drugs that disrupt certain biochemical processes in relatively well-defined ways.[42] For example, suppose investigators wish to elucidate the role of a particular neuroregulator system in a given behavior. Typical experiments entail the administration of specific inhibitors of synthesis, metabolism, or reuptake or of agonists or antagonists to putative receptors for the neuroregulator. Predictable and consistent changes in the observed behavior with controlled increases and decreases in activity provide at least indirect evidence for a relationship between the neuroregulator and the behavior. Also useful in this regard are chemical or electrical lesions directed toward a single neuronal system.

Such techniques are powerful, if used correctly; but major problems of interpretation can arise because few of the available drugs are truly specific for only a single neuroregulatory system.[101] A classic example involves reserpine, used for many years because of its effects on the storage of a few biogenic amines. Over time investigators discovered that the drug had effects on many amines and acted on a variety of other biochemical systems as well. Nevertheless, the disruption of specific neuroregulator systems or processes remains a valuable approach to elucidating biochemical mechanisms, even as behavioral neurochemists continue to seek other more specific techniques.[2]

Studying the Effects on Neuroregulator Activity of a Behavior

An alternative to disrupting a neuroregulatory system involves the more naturalistic study of how the system changes in the presence or absence of the behavior of interest.[8] Such research can range from relatively crude measures of a neuroregulator—for example, its whole-brain concentrations—to much more sophisticated assessments of processes controlling its synthesis, storage, release, postsynaptic effects, and inactivation in specific brain regions of interest. Invariably such research presses analytic techniques to the limit, as investigators strive for increasingly refined assessments of a system.

Such biochemical studies in vertebrate behavioral systems require not only accurate, sensitive, and appropriate neurochemical measures but equally precise assessments of the behavior of interest.[101] This need mandates the use of reliable and valid behaviors within the animal's species-specific repertoire. Also critical is the degree to which other behaviors can be inactivated or suppressed to enable researchers to disentangle the specific neurochemistry of the behavior of interest.[158] The behavior under study must be carefully defined and articulated in a way that enables other researchers to reproduce it reliably.[203] For example, analyses of neurochemical processes demand careful attention to the time parameters of the behavioral state. Indeed, one common technique involves studying changes in neurochemical mechanisms over time—for example, before, during, and after a specific behavior. Such studies of time-dependent effects, combined with regional analysis of brain, provide a powerful way to probe relationships between a neuroregulatory system and a behavioral process.

Approaches to Sample Collection

Existing methods for obtaining brain tissue samples are a major limitation for most neurochemical studies in animals. The very act of killing an animal to dissect and analyze brain parts may alter brain biochemistry so greatly that no meaningful information about the normal brain can be gained. For example, GABA concentrations increase rapidly after death unless enzymes are deactivated by killing the animal with powerful microwave irradiation.[6] Even the use of intense freezing temperatures (liquid nitrogen) or rapid fixation of tissue (microwave radiation) has associated problems, for no technique is truly instantaneous. Also, there is always the possibility of unsuspected artifacts from the destructive process itself. Furthermore, techniques that require the death of the organism prevent examination of changes through the time course of a behavior in the same animal.

Several recently developed techniques enable researchers to acquire samples of brain fluids in living, awake, behaving animals.

These methods take many forms. Two especially promising approaches are *in vivo* voltammetry and perfusion of small, specific brain areas. Also exciting is the emergence of *in vivo* magnetic resonance spectrometry, described in chapter 11.

In vivo voltammetry now can be used to measure concentrations of specific neuroregulators. Recent attention has been directed to the use of specialized microelectrodes to assess concentrations of DA and related substances in highly specific areas of a brain. Exploration of these techniques is at an early phase. The basic methodology of electrochemical assays of tissue extracts, developed by Ralph Adams and his colleagues, has found widespread applications.[120,150,151] *In vivo* applications of the technique have been hampered by lack of specificity of the assays; however, these problems are being overcome with the use of carbon-based microelectrodes implanted in the brain and careful choice of parameters.[51,145] These techniques, which have been refined to the degree that most artifacts are known and can be controlled, may permit study of several different neuroregulator systems using the same electrode.

Perfusion methods also have been useful for studying biochemical processes in living animals. One method has entailed perfusion of a portion of the brain ventricular system or direct perfusion of a small brain region.[33] This "push-pull cannula" technique may create problems of specificity of site as well as artifacts resulting from tissue damage. Still, it was one of the first methods to enable investigators to monitor the neuroregulator release over time in conscious animals during a behavior of interest, such as temperature regulation, self-stimulation, or monitoring the effects of drugs.[102,154,156] More recently intracerebral dialysis has become feasible for studying neurochemical processes. In this method, a loop of dialysis tubing is implanted in the brain, with perfusion accomplished using physiological fluids.[185] Samples are collected at timed intervals and analyzed by high-performance liquid chromatography or mass spectrometry.

Such techniques as intracerebral dialysis and *in vivo* voltammetry should help researchers obtain a much more dynamic understanding of neurochemical processes associated with behavior. However, simply noting a correlation between changes in certain neurochemical processes and a specific behavior does not prove a causal link between them. For example, a change may be a key biochemical event, a secondary effect of another primary biochemical process, or even an effect of some secondary behavior. The many potential intervening factors add to the difficulty of unraveling such interconnections. Suggested criteria for establishing such links are described in table 2–4.

Levels of Study

Each step in the processing of neuroregulators offers a potentially useful area for studying their relation to behavioral states. The examples given have entailed measuring concentrations of the neuroregulator and its precursors and metabolites, but assessment of the dynamic processes that produce those final concentrations is especially important. Neuroregulator formulation, storage, uptake, release, and metabolism—all may be central to under-

TABLE 2–4

Criteria for Linking a Behavior and a Neuroregulator

The neuroregulator must be present in or have access to the brain region or regions controlling the behavior.

Occurrence of the behavior should be associated with a characteristic pattern of neuroregulator activity.

Induction of that characteristic pattern of neuroregulator activity should elicit the behavior.

Inhibition and enhancement of neuroregulator activity should have opposing behavioral effects.

Destruction of the site or sites of neuroregulator action should abolish normal control of the behavior.

Neuroregulators that affect the neuroregulator of interest also should alter the behavior in ways consistent with their effects on the neuroregulator.

SOURCE: J. D. Barchas et al., "Behavioral Neurochemistry: Neuroregulators and Behavioral States," *Science*, 200 (1978):

standing its role. It still is far too early to predict which are the "key" steps; indeed, each of the steps indicated in figure 2–1 may be vital for one or another behavioral process. Extant literature shows changes in synthesis, regulation of rate-limiting enzymes, reuptake and release. The possibility that there may be multiple changes in interacting neuroregulatory systems adds to the complexity.

Receptor mechanisms are a relatively new area of investigation generating a great deal of excitement.[133,221] Studies range from measurements of the number of various receptors to determinations of their affinities for the substances with which the receptor interacts. The degree to which receptors are mutable is an area of active investigation.[88] It is clear that receptor density and characteristics can be changed by such environmental influences as drug administration, chronic stress, and behavior.[50] Strong evidence implicates receptor dysfunction with a number of physical illnesses, and some stimulating hypotheses also have begun to link receptor changes to certain mental and addictive disorders.[176]

Autoradiography has opened one exciting approach to studying receptors by enabling researchers to create quantitative maps of their anatomical distributions in brain slices, using a variant of the RIAs.[129] Substances that interact specifically with the receptor are labeled with a radioactive tag and then incubated with a tissue slice. By applying recently developed methods of image analysis and carefully controlling for artifacts, investigators can quantitate regional densities for some receptors. Such methods may make possible studies of how receptor patterns in a specific microregion of the brain change during development and with acute and chronic environmental changes.

Genetic approaches are invaluable for studying relationships between neuroregulators and behavior.[87] Traditional genetic analyses, which utilize selective breeding, are exemplified in studies of inbred mouse strains. Such research has shown that it is possible to select for animals with markedly different behavioral traits along such dimensions as sleeping time or aggression. These selected strains then serve as interesting models for assessing associated biochemical differences. Such research clearly demonstrates that many critical .steps in neuroregulator processing are under some degree of genetic control. For example, the steady-state activity levels of the enzymes involved in formation of brain catecholamines are under genetic control.[119,168] Genetic factors also are involved in neuroregulator release, metabolism, reuptake, and receptor interactions.[7,25,41] The degree to which behavior can function within different genetically determined neurochemical capabilities is a fascinating area for future research.

Molecular neurobiology is providing astonishing new tools for research in behavioral neurochemistry. These methods[155,197,198] make it possible to discover new, previously unrecognized neuropeptide neuroregulators. Further, they permit investigation of some aspects of their regulation and processing and study of the effects of environmental and behavioral conditions and of drugs and hormones.[64,65] They also may be useful for histochemical localization of neuroregulator processing with *in situ* hybridization.[85] Most important, they may provide identifying markers of certain severe mental and neurological disorders, as already has been suggested for Huntington's disease,[94] and ultimately may allow new methods of treatment.

The Neuropeptides as a Model of Behavioral Neurochemistry Research

Consideration of the evolving concepts about the peptide neuroregulator systems are illustrative of the problems of investigating the relationships between neuroregulators and behavior.[153] As described earlier, the story of the opioid peptides has unfolded at an incredible pace since the first descriptions of opiate receptors in the early 1970s. To date, three gene families and multiple active products have been identified, with evidence of differential processing depending on the brain region and environmental factors.[214] Yet complete elucidation of the connection between one or more of these systems and a specific behavior or mental disorder remains an unfulfilled dream.

One strategy for clarifying the role of neuropeptides in brain regulation and behavior has entailed administration of a given neuropeptide and observation of a wide range of behaviors, including pain threshold, sleep, eating, thirst, motor activity, self-stimulation, learning, or effects on single neurons.* The outcomes of such studies are highly dependent on the dose of the peptide, its route of administration, and the time course during which the behavior is monitored.[16] Major unsettled issues in this type of research include what constitutes an appropriate dose for behavioral studies and whether a given dose provides useful information about real physiological actions. Furthermore, exogenously administered peptides typically have a pattern of inactivation that differs markedly from that of endogenous stores of the same substance, and they may act on brain regions where they would never occur normally.

Some of these problems can be overcome with the use of peptide neuroregulator analogues or derivatives. Such substances may be resistant to enzymatic degradation or interact only at specific receptors, either as agonists or as antagonists. For example, studies showing that certain highly specific opioid agonists will stop a form of conditioned learning provide a powerful argument for the involvement of that opioid system in such learning mechanisms.[147] Overall, despite its limitations, research on neuroregulator-induced behavioral changes is a powerful first step in defining what behavioral processes are affected. Still, it rarely is possible to demonstrate that a single substance "controls" a particular behavior.

Researchers also have altered behavior and monitored changes in opioid peptides.

---

*See references 11, 56, 60, 84, and 89 for examples of these strategies.

For example, this strategy was used to demonstrate that physiological stress causes an increase in the concentration of brain opioid peptides and that the change correlates with an increased pain threshold.[143] Even a peptide present in very small concentrations can be important in behavior, and it is impossible to assume that concentration alone indicates its relative significance. Turnover—the rapidity with which a substance is being utilized—may be more relevant. For some peptides it is possible to study turnover and rate of utilization by using tracer techniques with a radiolabeled tag; but most methods used for measuring turnover in simple monoamine neuroregulators are not applicable to peptides, so new techniques are being explored.[170] One promising approach lies in the development of ways to monitor the mechanisms involved in creating the precursor molecules for such peptides, including measures of messenger ribonucleic acid (RNA). Still, even this powerful method offers information about only one aspect of the total steps of processing and degradation that contribute to the turnover of a specific peptide.

The discovery of neuroregulator colocalization in the same neurons, which was described earlier, has further complicated efforts to understand neuronal function. Not only can two or more peptides exist in the same neuron, but they may be there together with other classes of neuroregulators, such as the biogenic amines.[23,174] These possibilities suggest that interactions between neuropeptides and behavior may require study of several different systems simultaneously. Such studies are relatively rare because of their conceptual and technical complexity; also, few investigators have the range of skills that may be needed to study quite different neuroregulator systems such as the biogenic amines and peptides (see Costa[44] and Krieger, Brownstein, and Martin[127]). Nevertheless, the research now is being carried out, frequently with the use of pharmacological agents to enhance or block one or another system.[34]

It has become clear that, even in low concentrations, peptides have potent behavioral effects. Furthermore, their actions may last for hours rather than minutes. The differential effects of two forms of the opioid peptide dynorphin highlight these features. There are multiple forms of dynorphin with strikingly different localization.[40,91,213] The effects of one form of dynorphin, dynorphin$_{1-8}$, are much briefer than dynorphin$_{1-17}$ and may reflect a transmitter function; evidence suggests that dynorphin$_{1-17}$ could be acting as a hormonal neuromodulator.[43,108]

¶ Approaches to Studying Neuroregulators and Mental Disorders

A growing body of indirect evidence strongly suggests that dysfunctions in neuroregulator systems play an important etiological role in some mental illnesses, including some forms of depression, some psychoses such as schizophrenia and mania, and certain forms of anxiety and panic disorder. Other chapters in this volume document the current state of knowledge about these interrelationships, so we will not review that evidence here. However, it is important to note that, to date, no incontrovertible causal link has yet been forged between any neuroregulator system and a particular mental or addictive disorder.[14]

Progress in the study of human disorders starts with the development of basic knowledge. Hence it is impossible to ask a question about a particular neuroregulator and its role in brain function until that substance has been discovered. No better example of the linkage of basic knowledge to clinical concerns can be given than the process that led to the use of levodopa in the treatment of Parkinson's disease. Arvid Carlsson discovered DA through research at the most basic level, without overt concern for a practical result.[32] However, its discovery was followed closely by recognition that its localization in brain was consistent with a possible role in regulating movement. A direct test of that hypothesis was possible, and the clinical use of levodopa provided the first instance of a precursor-loading approach to treating a brain disease.[46,177]

Despite the success of that example, formidable problems hamper efforts to study neuroregulator changes associated with mental disorders, primarily as a result of the remarkable degree to which the brain is protected and isolated. Several strategies have been developed for estimating key aspects of brain function in human beings with major mental and addictive disorders.[206] To date, the bulk of such research has involved measurements of the concentrations of neuroregulators and their metabolites in cerebrospinal fluid (CSF); studies of neuroregulator content, enzymes, and receptors in autopsied brain material; applications of molecular neurobiology techniques to human tissue; and the use of pharmacological probes—for example, precursors or enzyme inhibitors that change neuroregulator concentrations and agents that act on specific receptors (see chapters 12, 17, 21, and 25; see also Gottesman and Shields[92] and Post and Ballenger[166]). Although each of these methods has major drawbacks, together they have helped to suggest answers to some important questions.

Because these approaches have been used in a number of studies, we will describe in some detail their utility and limits in efforts to identify changes in neuroregulators in mental illnesses. Useful analytic methods were mentioned earlier in this chapter. Such techniques as mass spectrometry[79,80,123] and high-performance liquid chromatography[149] are essential for this research because they have the sensitivity and specificity needed to assay substances present in nanogram or picogram amounts. Many neuroregulators, including the biogenic amines and their derivatives, can be studied in this way.

Appropriate clinical research centers are essential for much of the needed research on patients with mental disorders.[13] For example, some studies can be done only with unmedicated patients who are willing to delay their own treatment so that researchers can learn more about their illness. Very few patients have been studied who have not had prior drug administration. Often, with great effort, patients can remain drug-free for several weeks; yet even that period may be too short to eliminate long-lasting effects of drugs on some neuroregulator systems. Helping such generous individuals stay off drugs and contain their illness while they participate in the research requires a skilled and dedicated staff. Furthermore, maximum utilization of this rare and valuable resource requires researchers who are thoroughly versed in the art and science of careful observation, using the best available assessment instruments.[3,193] Such centers also create an environment in which it is feasible to collect the huge amounts of data about past history, current symptoms, family history, social support systems, psychological state, and other key aspects of an individual's behavior that help to amplify and clarify any biochemical studies and ultimately may pave the way for studies of individual variation.

Studying Mental Disorders with Cerebrospinal Fluid

Biogenic amine metabolites in CSF have been studied in patients with a wide range of mental disorders, with a few promising leads.* The method, potentially quite powerful, also has difficulties. For example, CSF samples are obtained from the lumbar region of the spinal column because taps there carry minimal risk. As a result, the sample is obtained far from the brain and reflects the sum of all activity in the brain and spinal cord that adds to and subtracts from the pool of the neuroregulators of interest; even a 10 percent change, which might reflect the total absence or great enhancement of a neuroregulator in a specific brain region, would be difficult to detect. In addition, active mechanisms continually remove many neuroregulators and their metabolites from CSF. Only a relatively small fraction of the original amount makes it to the lumbar re-

*See references 4, 15, 86, 137, and 141.

gion—indeed, a gradient for certain neuroregulators and their metabolites has been demonstrated.[12,157,187,223] It may well be that safe methods need to be developed to obtain fluid samples safely from sites closer to brain.

CSF measures do not lend themselves readily to estimating turnover and utilization rates of a particular neuroregulator. There was considerable hope that such a determination could be made using probenecid, which blocks the active transport of many neuroregulator metabolites out of the CSF.[47,81,202] If preprobenecid concentrations of a neuroregulator and its metabolites are comparable, differences among subject groups in their concentrations after probenecid administration have been suggested to reflect differences in the turnover of that neuroregulator. Unfortunately, probenecid has not been as valuable as expected because of its side effects when given in required doses and because of the difficulty in obtaining adequate blockade of the transport system.

Other methods for estimating neuroregulator turnover have been suggested, including administering isotope-labeled precursors and monitoring the rate of appearance of the isotope-labeled neuroregulators or metabolites.[35] This potentially powerful method is limited by the difficulty of obtaining multiple CSF samples in the same patient and the necessity of administering substantial amounts of the isotope. Although not as sensitive as radioactive labels, stable-isotope labeling avoids concerns about ionizing radiation and is completely compatible with mass spectroscopic analytic techniques.

Another problem with the use of CSF samples stems from the need to obtain samples from normal individuals or other groups that can serve as appropriate controls; comparisons of different patient groups offer only a partial solution. Only a few institutions have been able to obtain CSF samples from physically healthy human volunteers without mental or addictive disorders.[82,95,181,182] De-

spite the inherent problems, this approach deserves more investigation.

To date, few CSF studies[71,165,178,201] have been done of neuropeptides in mental disorders. Especially given the low concentrations of neuropeptides, their assays are much less specific than are those for biogenic amines. They typically involve the use of antibodies that may react with several different peptides and classes of peptides, leaving open serious questions about what exactly is being measured. Even when the antibodies are quite specific, other nonspecific factors such as ion concentrations can change the apparent peptide concentration. Isolation and absolute identification of the peptide is essential in such studies and promises to be an important development. The difficulties created by artifacts are perhaps best reflected in the burgeoning group of reports of "opioidlike" peptides in CSF, which provides a confusing picture of increased, decreased, and unchanged concentrations of an uncharacterized peptide in some patient groups. Despite the difficulties, this clearly represents a stimulating area for research.

Studying Mental Disorders with Autopsied Brain

Brain obtained at autopsy is an important resource that has had relatively little use in research on mental disorders. Several brain banks now exist in the United States from which investigators can obtain samples of brain tissue taken at autopsy from patients whose history, diagnosis, and treatment are documented. The goals of research that has been done with such samples have been clear-cut—to determine the pattern of change in neuroregulators or their receptors in relation to specified mental illness.* Once again, such studies are feasible now because of advances in analytical neurochemistry, enzymology, receptorology, immunohistochemistry, and molecular biology. Use of autopsy material has several important

*See references 21, 22, 52, 138, 142, 169, and 180.

advantages, including the fact that it permits localized investigation and may enable scientists to detect changes involving only a limited area of the brain.

A serious problem with autopsy material is the difficulty of obtaining appropriate controls. Deaths among young people and those who have had a mental or addictive disorder for only a brief period of time are rare. Most of those with mental disorders who come to autopsy have been ill for years, have been treated for long periods with various medications, and often have had a long history of poor dietary habits. Furthermore, mental disorders themselves seldom are fatal, so death often is a result of some other type of illness. Identifying the key sources of artifact from among the large number of potential factors and then securing brain tissue from appropriate controls who are free of mental illness is impossible. Instead, researchers must constantly watch for and try to correct errors that may arise as a result of poor matches. [20,77]

Regardless of the source, brain tissue begins to deteriorate immediately after death, at least up to the time it is removed and stored at cryogenic temperatures. [75,171,209,219] Many neuroregulator systems are affected by postmortem changes, and much work remains to be done to determine the exact effects of death on neuroregulators of interest and other factors involved in their regulation. [194,216] At least equally important is a careful postmortem evaluation of the patient's diagnosis and clinical course; such evaluations are nontrivial, often having to rely on incomplete medical records.

Despite the clear problems of this type of research, it opens up otherwise inaccessible avenues for understanding what goes wrong in mental illness. No other method exists for measuring enzyme systems and receptors in individuals who have severe mental disorders that may arise because of dysfunctions at that level of neuronal regulation. Resolution of legal issues and other related problems that hamper efforts to collect samples rapidly and that complicate the acquisition of brain samples from healthy controls could markedly enhance the pace of research and knowledge.

Studying Mental Disorders with Molecular Biology

Perhaps nothing generates more excitement among neuroscientists at present than the potential uses of molecular neurobiological techniques for elucidating the causes of severe mental and addictive disorders. [38] These methods may enable researchers to use peripheral cells—for example, elements in the blood—to identify and monitor factors of genetic predisposition and expression associated with particular disorders. They also may be applied to autopsy tissue to study messenger RNA, which under some conditions is relatively resistant to postmortem changes. Recent strides toward identifying the gene responsible for Huntington's disease is a striking example of the potential of these techniques. [94] Although no gene linkage has yet been proven for any mental disorder or subtype of mental disorder, studies of genes and their regulatory mechanisms clearly are needed.

Studying Mental Disorders with Drugs

Drug probes are invaluable in research on neuroregulator processes in relation to mental illnesses and addictive disorders. Useful probes include substances that may act as precursors of specific neuroregulators and drugs with specific and well-defined actions —for example, agonists or antagonists at specific receptor sites. Chapters in this volume that deal with specific mental disorders highlight some applications of such probes, so we will focus here on their uses and limitations.

Pharmacological probes not only have helped elucidate mechanisms of disorders but also have suggested treatments. However, they also have created substantial confusion and led investigators to incorrect conclusions. A probe is only as good as the basic science that sustains its use. There are many instances of drugs thought to have only one major action that actually act on a number of neuroregulators, sometimes in ways that interfere with or augment the action of interest. Nevertheless, this cautionary note does not alter the reality: Well-defined drug probes can be key for efforts to identify subtypes of mental disorders and to facilitate the development of better therapies.

¶ Conclusion

The growing sophistication of behavioral neurochemistry is everywhere evident, and psychiatry has begun to enjoy the fruits of its efforts. This volume attests amply to advances in diagnosing mental disorders, identifying useful animal models of mental illness, and assessing behavior. In addition, advanced technologies are providing powerful tools for *in vivo* studies of brain function in living animals and human beings. Some of those methods are described in this chapter; other exciting developments highlighted elsewhere in this volume include computer-analyzed electroencephalograms (chapter 8), computed tomography (chapter 9), positron emission tomography (chapter 10), and magnetic resonance imaging and spectroscopy (chapter 11). Such techniques make it possible to pose many important questions that cannot be addressed with current methods.

Efforts to connect neuroregulator function to behavior and to mental and addictive disorders require great imagination and constant reformulations of old concepts to accommodate new facts. It is possible that a simple model such as a relative excess or a relative deficiency of a specific neuroregulatory substance may be helpful and even valid for understanding some behaviors, and such models have been the rule to date in hypotheses of mental disorders. However, given the complexity of the brain and of most normal and pathological behaviors, that level of analysis seems unlikely to provide lasting answers.

Over the past few decades, basic scientists have identified an ever-growing list of neuroregulators and elucidated their complex regulatory mechanisms with increasing precision. Given the incredible amount of observable diversity in behavior, regardless of the organism, "normal" behavior almost certainly can accommodate a wide range of activity levels for any single neuroregulator. In addition, many neuroregulators appear to be paired with or balanced against others, markedly enhancing tolerance for individual variability. Furthermore, researchers continue to find previously unsuspected mechanisms that monitor and adjust neuroregulator activity. What are needed now are conceptual frameworks that apply that level of sophisticated knowledge to the problem of understanding normal and abnormal brain function.

Particularly important for the study of mental illness and addictive disorders will be the way in which behavior interacts with neuroregulator processes. Too often, investigators have assumed a one-way effect of the neuroregulator function on behavior, without considering how behavior might, in turn, alter neuronal function. Exploration of these changes in regulatory steps, which has only begun, has yet to be extended to human disorders or behaviors. It seems likely that many mental disorders represent a spectrum of biological and behavioral influences. For some disorders—for example, phenylketonuria—the biochemical substrates may be overwhelmingly important; for others, psychosocial components may be predominant; and for many, the final outcome may be influenced markedly by both factors. Such a range of possibilities may exist even within a set of disorders that have a common final pathway underlying the clinical presentation of the disorder. If so, good research will require increasingly sophisticated measures both of neuroregulatory processes and of behavior and thought processes.

In addition to needing disease models that incorporate the growing number of putative neuroregulators and their interactions, behavioral neurochemists must consider the ways in which genetic and environmental influences may work together to produce mental and addictive disorders. Although genetic processes have a great role in determining the range within which a particular system can function, psychosocial influences also may play a key role in setting such "regulostats," at least at critical stages of development. If so, such an effect might "lock in" a particular biochemical process that subsequently could predispose an individual to developing a specific mental disorder. Such a model could be relevant, for example, to the episodes of schizophrenia that occur in relation to life stress. In those instances one could hypothesize that a neuroregulator system that is functional in the absence of major stress changes in response to the stress in a way that leads to psychosis. A similar set of mechanisms could be relevant to depressions that are induced in a subset of individuals who experience social loss.

Impressive as the advances in neurochemistry have been and will continue to be, they are only one aspect of a trend that seems to be leading toward a marked change in current concepts about mental disorders—possibly of a magnitude that Thomas Kuhn[132] would call a scientific revolution. Within that context, behavioral neurochemists are beginning to recognize the inadequacies of available conceptual frameworks in explaining the results from increasingly sophisticated studies of brain neurochemistry and behavior. At present, the field lacks even the vocabulary for expressing such interrelationships in their complexity. At least in our view, the progress being made toward creating such a vocabulary constitutes the blocks from which will arise a future psychiatry. We cannot predict the final form of that new psychiatry, but it almost certainly will be built with the skills of an enormous range of scholarly disciplines.

¶ Acknowledgments

Supported by grants from the National Institute of Mental Health and the MacArthur Foundation. We should like to thank Edward D. and Marjorie R. Gray for their encouragement.

¶ Bibliography

1. AGHAJANIAN, G. K., and WANG, R. Y. "Physiology and Pharmacology of Central Serotonergic Neurons," in M. A. Lipton, A. DiMascio, and K. F. Killam, eds., *Psychopharmacology: A Generation of Progress.* New York: Raven Press, 1978, pp. 171–183.

2. AGRANOFF, B. W. "Learning and Memory: Biochemical Approaches," in G. Siegel et al., eds., *Basic Neurochemistry.* Boston: Little, Brown, 1981, pp. 801–820.

3. ANDREASEN, N. C., et al. "Assessment of Reliability in Multicenter Collaborative Research with a Videotape Approach," *American Journal of Psychiatry,* 139 (1982):876–882.

4. ASBERG, M., et al. "Serotonin Depression—A Biochemical Subgroup Within the Affective Disorders?" *Science,* 191 (1976):478–780.

5. BACQ, Z. M. "La Pharmacologie du Système Nerveux Autonomie, et Particulièrement du Sympathique d'après la Théorie Neurohumorale," *Annales de Physiologie et de Physicochimie Biologique,* 10 (1934):467–553.

6. BALCOM, G. J., LENOX, R. H., and MEYERHOFF, J. L. "Regional Gamma-Amino-butyric Acid Levels in Rat Brain Determined After Microwave Fixation," *Journal of Neurochemistry,* 24 (1975):609–613.

7. BARCHAS, J. D., and SULLIVAN, S. "Opioid Peptides as Neuroregulators: Potential Areas for the Study of Genetic-behavioral Mechanisms," *Behavior Genetics,* 12 (1982):69–91.

8. BARCHAS, J. D., et al. "Behavioral Neurochemistry: Neuroregulators and Behavioral States," *Science,* 200 (1978):964–973.

9. BARGER, G., and DALE, H. H. "Chemical Structure and Sympathomimetic Action of Amines," *Journal of Physiology* (London), 41 (1910):19–59.

10. BARKER, J. L., and SEGAL, M. "Coexistence of Transmitter Functions in Ex-

citable Membranes of Cultured CNS Neurons," in V. Chan-Palay and S. L. Palay, eds., *Coexistence of Neuroactive Substances in Neurons.* New York: John Wiley & Sons, 1984, pp. 339–362.

11. BARKER, J. L., and SMITH, T. G., Jr. *The Role of Peptides in Neuronal Function.* New York: Marcel Dekker, 1980.

12. BECK, O., et al. "5-Hydroxytryptophol in Human Cerebrospinal Fluid: Conjugation, Concentration Gradient, Relationship to 5-Hydroxyindole-acetic acid, and Influence of Hereditary Factors," *Journal of Neurochemistry,* 43 (1984): 388–393.

13. BERGER, P. A. "Medical Treatment of Mental Illness," *Science,* 200 (1978):974–981.

14. BERGER, P. A., and BARCHAS, J. D. "Biochemical Hypotheses of Mental Disorders," in G. Siegel et al., eds., *Basic Neurochemistry,* 3rd ed. Boston: Little, Brown, 1981, pp. 759–773.

15. BERGER, P. A., et al. "CSF Monoamine Metabolites in Depression and Schizophrenia," *American Journal of Psychiatry,* 137 (1980):174–180.

16. BERGER, P. A., et al. "Behavioral Pharmacology of the Endorphins," *Annual Review of Medicine,* 33 (1982):397–415.

17. BERL, S. "The Actomyosin-like System in Nervous Tissue," in D. B. Tower, ed., *The Nervous System,* vol. 1, *The Basic Neurosciences.* New York: Raven Press, 1975, pp. 565–573.

18. BERSON, S., and YALOW, R. "Isotopic Tracers in the Study of Diabetes," *Advances in Biological Medicine and Physics,* 6 (1958):349–430.

19. BERSON, S., et al. "Insulin-I[131] Metabolism in Human Subjects: Demonstration of Insulin Binding Globulin in the Circulation of Insulin Treated Subjects," *Journal of Clinical Investigation,* 35 (1956):170–190.

20. BIRD, E. D., SPOKES, E. G., and IVERSEN, L. L. "Brain Norepinephrine and Dopamine in Schizophrenia," *Science,* 204 (1979):93–94.

21. BIRD, E. D., et al. "Increased Brain Dopamine and Reduced Glutamic Acid Decarboxylase and Choline Acetyl Transferase Activity in Schizophrenia

and Related Psychoses," *Lancet,* 2 (1977):1157–1159.

22. BIRKMAYER, W., and RIEDERER, P. "Biochemical Postmortem Findings in Depressed Patients," *Journal of Neural Transmission,* 37 (1975):95–109.

23. BLOOM, F. E. "The Functional Significance of Neurotransmitter Diversity," *American Journal of Physiology,* 246 (1984):C184–C194.

24. BLOOM, F. E., et al., eds. *Beta-Carbolines and Tetrahydroisoquinolines.* New York: Alan R. Liss, 1982.

25. BOEHME, R., and CIARANELLO, R. "Genetic Control of Dopamine and Serotonin Receptors in Brain Regions of Inbred Mice," *Brain Research,* 266 (1982):51–65.

26. BOHLEN, P., and NECKERS, L. M. "High Performance Liquid Chromatography in the Neurosciences: Methodology," in I. Hanin and S. H. Koslow, eds., *Physico-Chemical Methodologies in Psychiatric Research.* New York: Raven Press, 1980, pp. 1–22.

27. BROWNSTEIN, M. J., et al. "Coexistence of Several Putative Neurotransmitters in Single Identified Neurones of *Aplysia,*" *Proceedings of the National Academy of Science* (USA), 7 (1974): 4662–4665.

28. BRUNSWICK, D. "Principles of Radioimmunoassay," in I. Hanin and S. H. Koslow, eds., *Physico-Chemical Methodologies in Psychiatric Research.* New York: Raven Press, 1980, pp. 37–63.

29. BUNNEY, B. S., et al. "3-PPP: A Selective Dopamine Autoreceptor Agonist? Electrophysiological Studies," *Acta Pharmaceutica Suecica,* 1 (Supplement) (1983):138–144.

30. CANNON, W. B., and URIDIL, J. E. "Studies on the Conditions of Activity in Endocrine Glands. VIII. Some Effects on the Denervated Heart of Stimulating the Nerves of the Liver," *American Journal of Physiology,* 58 (1921):353–534.

31. CAPELLA, P., and HORNING, E. C. "Separation and Identification of Derivatives of Biologic Amines by Gas-liquid Chromatography," *Analytical Chemistry,* 38 (1966):316–321.

32. CARLSSON, A. "The Occurrence, Distribu-

tion and Physiological Role of Catecholamines in the Nervous System," *Pharmacological Reviews*, 11 (1959):490–493.

33. CARMICHAEL, E. A., FELDBERG, W., and FLEISCHAUER, K. "Methods for Perfusing Different Parts of the Cerebral Ventricles with Drugs," *Journal of Physiology* (London), 173 (1964):354–359.

34. CHAN-PALAY, V., and PALAY, S. L., eds. *Coexistence of Neuroactive Substances in Neurons*. New York: John Wiley & Sons, 1984.

35. CHASE, T. N., et al. "Oxygen-18 Use for Clinical Studies of Central Monoamine Metabolism," in E. Usdin and J. Barchas, eds., *Catecholamines: Basic and Clinical Frontiers*. New York: Pergamon Press, 1979, pp. 1569–1571.

36. CHEUNG, W. Y. "Calmodulin Plays a Pivotal Role in Cellular Regulation," *Science*, 207 (1980):19–27.

37. CLEGG, D. O., and KOSHLAND, D. E. "The Role of a Signaling Protein in Bacterial Sensing: Behavioral Effects of Increased Gene Expression," *Proceedings of the National Academy of Science* (USA), 81 (1984):5056–5060.

38. COLD SPRING HARBOR. *Molecular Neurobiology: Symposia on Quantitative Biology*, vol. 48. Cold Spring Harbor, N.Y.: Cold Spring Harbor Laboratory, 1983.

39. COLLIER, B. "Synaptic Vesicles and Acetylcholine Quanta," *Trends in Neurosciences*, 2 (1979):285–287.

40. CONE, R. I., et al. "Regional Distribution of Dynorphin and Neo-endorphin Peptides in Rat Brain, Spinal Cord, and Pituitary," *Journal of Neuroscience*, 3 (1983):2146–2152.

41. COOPER, D., and STOLK, J. "Differences Between Inbred Rat Strains in the Alteration of Adrenal Catecholamine Synthesizing Enzyme Activities After Immobilization Stress," *Neuroscience*, 4 (1979):1163–1172.

42. COOPER, J. R., BLOOM, F. E., and ROTH, R. H. *The Biochemical Basis of Neuropharmacology*. New York: Oxford University Press, 1978.

43. CORBETT, A. D., et al. "Dynorphin $_{1-8}$ and Dynorphin$_{1-9}$ Are Ligands for the K-subtype of Opiate Receptor," *Nature*, 299 (1982):79–81.

44. COSTA, E. "Coexistence of Neuromodulators: Biochemical and Pharmacological Consequences," *Federation Proceedings*, 42 (1983):2910–2911.

45. COSTA, E., and TRABUCCHI, M., eds. *Neural Peptides and Neuronal Communication*. New York: Raven Press, 1981.

46. COTZIAS, G. C., et al. "Treatment of Parkinson's Disease and Allied Conditions," in D. B. Tower, ed., *The Nervous System*, vol. 2, *The Clinical Neurosciences*. New York: Raven Press, 1975, pp. 323–329.

47. COWDRY, R. W., et al. "Cerebrospinal Fluid Probenecid Studies: A Reinterpretation," *Biological Psychiatry*, 18 (1983):1287–1299.

48. COYLE, J. T., and HENRY, D. "Catecholamines in Fetal and Newborn Rat Brain," *Journal of Neurochemistry*, 21 (1973):61–67.

49. CREESE, I., and SNYDER, S. H. "A Simple and Sensitive Radioreceptor Assay for Antischizophrenic Drugs in Blood," *Nature*, 270 (1977):180–182.

50. CREESE, I., BURT, D. R., and SNYDER, S. H. "Dopamine Receptor Binding Enhancement Accompanies Lesion-induced Behavioral Supersensitivity," *Science*, 197 (1977):596–598.

51. CRESPI, F., et al. "Differential Pulse Voltametry: Simultaneous *in vivo* Measurement of Ascorbic Acid, Catechols and 5-Hydroxyindoles in the Rat Striatum," *Brain Research*, 322 (1984):135–138.

52. CROW, T. J., et al. "Monoamine Mechanisms in Chronic Schizophrenia: Postmortem Neurochemical Findings," *British Journal of Psychiatry*, 134 (1979):249–256.

53. CURTIS, D. R., and ECCLES, R. M. "The Effect of Diffusional Barriers upon the Pharmacology of Cells Within the Central Nervous System," *Journal of Physiology* (London), 141 (1958):446–463.

54. DALE, H. H. "The Action of Certain Esters and Ethers of Choline, and Their Relation to Muscarine," *Journal of Pharmacology and Experimental Therapeutics*, 6 (1914):147–190.

55. ———. "Pharmacology and Nerve-

endings," *Proceedings of the Royal Society of Medicine,* Therapeutics Section, 23 (1935):319–332.

56. DELANOY, R. L., DUNN, A. J., and TINTER, R. "Behavioral Responses to Intracerebroventricularly Administered Neurohypophyseal Peptides in Mice," *Hormones and Behavior,* 11 (1978):348–362.

57. DEL CASTILLO, J., and KATZ, B. "On the Localization of Acetylcholine Receptors," *Journal of Physiology* (London), 128 (1955):157–181.

58. DELORENZO, R. J. "Calmodulin in Neurotransmitter Release and Synaptic Function," *Federation Proceedings,* 41 (1982):2265–2272.

59. DISMUKES, R. K. "New Concepts of Molecular Communication Among Neurons," *Behavior and Brain Sciences,* 2 (1979):409–448.

60. DISMUKES R. K., and LIEBESKIND, J. C. "How Much Can Psychopharmacology Tell Us About Behavior?" *Neurosciences Research Program Bulletin,* 16 (1978):493–497.

61. DIXON, W. E. "Vagus Inhibition," *British Medical Journal,* 2 (1906):1807.

62. DREW, G. M. "Presynaptic Alpha-adrenoceptors: Their Pharmacological Characterisation and Functional Significance," in S. Z. Langer, K. Starke, and M. L. Dubocovich, eds., *Presynaptic Receptors.* Oxford: Pergamon Press, 1979, pp. 59–65.

63. DU BOIS-REYMOND, E. "Gesammelte Abhandlung das Allgemeinen," *Muskel- und Nervenphysik,* 2 (1877):700.

64. EBERWINE, J., and ROBERTS, J. "Analysis of POMC Gene Structure and Function," *DNA,* 2 (1983):1–8.

65. ———. "Glucocorticoid Regulation of Pro-opiomelanocortin Gene Transcription in the Rat Pituitary," *Journal of Biological Chemistry,* 259 (1984):2166–2170.

66. ECCLES, J. C. *The Neurophysiological Basis of Mind.* Oxford: Clarendon, 1953.

67. ———. *The Physiology of Nerve Cells.* Baltimore: Johns Hopkins Press, 1957.

68. ELLIOTT, G. R., and BARCHAS, J. D. "Changing Concepts About Neuroregulation: Neurotransmitters and Neuromodulators," in D. de Wied and P. A. van Keep, eds., *Hormones and the Brain.* Lancaster, England: MTP Press, 1980, pp. 43–52.

69. ELLIOTT, T. R. "On the Action of Adrenalin," *Journal of Physiology* (London), 31 (1904):xx–xxi.

70. ———. "The Action of Adrenaline," *Journal of Physiology* (London), 32 (1905): 401–467.

71. EMRICH, H. M., et al. "Beta-endorphin-like Immunoreactivity in Cerebrospinal Fluid and Plasma of Patients with Schizophrenia and Other Neuropsychiatric Disorders," *Pharmakopsychiatrie,* 12 (1979):269–276.

72. ENNA, S. J. "Radioreceptor Assays," in I. Hanin and S. H. Koslow, eds., *Physico-Chemical Methodologies in Psychiatric Research.* New York: Raven Press, 1980, pp. 83–101.

73. ENNA, S. J., et al. "Neurotransmitter Receptor Binding: Regional Distribution in Human Brain," *Journal of Neurochemistry,* 28 (1977):233–236.

74. ERICHSEN, J. T., REINER, A. L., and KARTEN, H. J. "Co-occurrence of Substance P-like and Leu-enkephalin-like Immunoreactivities in Neurones and Fibres of Avian Nervous System," *Nature,* 295 (1982):407–410.

75. FAHN, S., and COTE, L. J. "Stability of Enzymes in Postmortem Rat Brain," *Journal of Neurochemistry,* 26 (1976):1039–1042.

76. FALES, H. M., and PISANO, J. J. "Gas Chromatography of Biologically Important Amines," *Analytical Biochemistry,* 3 (1962):337–342.

77. FARLEY, I. J., et al. "Norepinephrine in Chronic Paranoid Schizophrenia: Above Normal Levels in Limbic Forebrain," *Science,* 200 (1978):456–458.

78. FATT, P., and KATZ, B. "An Analysis of the End-plate Potential Recorded with an Intra-cellular Electrode," *Journal of Physiology* (London), 115 (1951):320–370.

79. FAULL, K. F., and BARCHAS, J. D. "Analysis of Catecholamines and Their Metabolites by Combined Gas Chromatography/Mass Spectrometry," in T. Nagatsu, ed., *Methods in Biogenic Amine Research.* Amsterdam: Elsevier/North Holland, 1983, pp. 189–236.

80. ———. "Mass Spectrometric Analysis of Neurotransmitters and Their Metabo-

lites," in D. Glick, ed., *Methods of Biochemical Analysis*, vol. 29. New York: John Wiley & Sons, 1983, pp. 325–383.

81. FAULL, K. F., et al. "A Review: Clinical Application of the Probenecid Test for Measurement of Monoamine Turnover in the CNS," *Biological Psychiatry*, 16 (1981):879–899.

82. FAULL, K. F., et al. "Systems Theory as a Tool for Integrating Functional Interactions Among Biogenic Amines," in E. Usdin, ed., *Catecholamines: Neuropharmacology and Central Nervous System —Therapeutic Aspects.* New York: Alan R. Liss, 1984, pp. 143–152.

83. FELDMAN, R. S., and QUENZER, L. F. *Fundamentals of Neuropsychopharmacology.* Sunderland, Mass.: Sinauer, 1984.

84. FREDERICKSON, R.C.A., and NORRIS, F. H. "Enkephalin-induced Depression of Single Neurons in Brain Areas with Opiate Receptors—Antagonism by Naloxone," *Science*, 194 (1976):440–442.

85. GEE, C. E., et al. "Identification of Proopiomelanocortin Neurones in Rat Hypothalamus by *in situ* cDNA-mRNA Hybridization," *Nature*, 306 (1983):374–376.

86. GERNER, R. H., et al. "CSF Neurochemistry in Depressed, Manic, and Schizophrenic Patients Compared with That of Normal Controls," *American Journal of Psychiatry*, 141 (1984):1533–1540.

87. GERSHON, E., et al., eds. *Genetic Research Strategies in Psychobiology and Psychiatry.* Pacific Grove, Calif.: Boxwood Press, 1981.

88. GNEGY, M. E., and COSTA, E. "Catecholamine Receptor Supersensitivity and Subsensitivity in the Central Nervous System," in M.B.H. Youdim et al., eds., *Essays in Neurochemistry and Neuropharmacology*, vol. 4. New York: John Wiley & Sons, 1980, pp. 249–282.

89. GOLD, P. E., and MCGAUGH, J. L. "Hormones and Memory," in L. H. Miller, C. A. Sandman, and A. J. Kastin, eds., *Neuropeptide Influences on the Brain and Behavior.* New York: Raven Press, 1977, pp. 127–143.

90. GOLDSTEIN, A., LOWNEY, L. J., and PAL, B. K. "Stereospecific and Nonspecific Interactions of the Morphine Congener Levorphanol in Subcellular Fractions of Mouse Brain," *Proceedings of the National Academy of Science* (USA), 68 (1971):1742–1747.

91. GOLDSTEIN, A., et al. "Porcine Pituitary Dynorphin: Complete Amino Acid Sequence of the Biologically Active Heptadecapeptide," *Proceedings of the National Academy of Science* (USA), 78 (1981):7219–7223.

92. GOTTESMAN, I. I., and SHIELDS, J. *Schizophrenia: The Epigenetic Puzzle* London: Cambridge University Press, 1982.

93. GREENGARD, P. "Some Chemical Aspects of Neurotransmitter Action," *Trends in Pharmacological Sciences*, 1 (1979):27–29.

94. GUSELLA, J. F., et al. "A Polymorphic DNA Marker Genetically Linked to Huntington's Disease," *Nature*, 306 (1983):234–238.

95. HAGENFELDT, L., et al. "Amino Acids in Plasma and CSF and Monoamine Metabolites in CSF: Interrelationship in Healthy Subjects," *Journal of Neurochemistry*, 42 (1984):833–837.

96. HANIN, I., and SHIH, T.-M. "Gas Chromatography, Mass Spectrometry, and Combined Gas Chromatrography-Mass Spectrometry," in I. Hanin and S. H. Koslow, eds., *Physico-Chemical Methodologies in Psychiatric Research.* New York: Raven Press, 1980, pp. 111–154.

97. HEUSER, J. E. "Synaptic Vesicle Exocytosis Revealed in Quick-frozen Frog Neuromuscular Junctions Treated with 4-Aminopyridine and Given a Single Electric Shock," in W. M. Cowan and J. A. Ferrendelli, eds., *Society for Neuroscience Symposia*, vol. 2. Bethesda, Md.: Society for Neuroscience, 1977, pp. 215–239.

98. HODGKIN, A. L. "The Ionic Basis of Nervous Conduction," *Science*, 145 (1964):1148–1153.

99. HOKFELT, T., et al. "Immunohistochemical Localization of Somatostatin (Growth Hormone Releasing Factor) in the Guinea Pig Brain," *Brain Research*, 80 (1974):165–169.

100. HOKFELT, T., et al. "Peptidergic Neurones," *Nature*, 284 (1980):515–521.

101. HOLMAN, R. B., BARCHAS, J. D., and ELLI-

OTT, G. R. "Perspectives in Behavioral Neurochemistry," in M. B. H. Youdim and W. Lovenberg, eds., *Essays in Neurochemistry and Neuropharmacology*, vol. 2. London: John Wiley & Sons, 1977, pp. 1–20.

102. HOLMAN, R. B., et al. "In vivo Release of Neurotransmitters Monitored by Continuous Cerebral Ventricular Perfusion in the Rat: Effects of Alcohol," in E. Usdin, I. Kopin, and J. D. Barchas, eds., *Catecholamines: Basic and Clinical Frontiers*. New York: Pergamon Press, 1979, pp. 1798–1800.

103. HOLMAN, R. B., et al. "Tryptolines: The Role of Indoleamine-aldehyde Condensation Products in the Effects of Alcohol," in M. Sandler, ed., *Psychopharmacology of Alcohol*. New York: Raven Press, 1980, pp. 155–169.

104. HUGHES, J., et al. "Identification of Two Related Pentapeptides from the Brain with Potent Opiate Agonist Activity," *Nature*, 258 (1975):577–579.

105. HUNT, R., and TAVEAU, R. deM. "On the Physiological Action of Certain Cholin Derivatives and New Methods of Detecting Cholin," *British Medical Journal*, 2 (1906):1788–1791.

106. HUXLEY, A. F. "Excitation and Conduction in Nerve: Quantitative Analysis," *Science*, 145 (1964):1154–1159.

107. IVERSEN, L. L. "Uptake Processes for Biogenic Amines," in L. L. Iversen, S. D. Iversen, and S.H. Snyder, eds., *Handbook of Psychopharmacology*, vol. 3. New York: Plenum Press, 1975, pp. 381–442.

108. ———. "Yet Another Opioid Peptide?" *Nature*, 299 (1982):578–579.

109. JENDEN, D. J., and CHO, A. K. "Applications of Integrated Gas Chromatography/Mass Spectrometry in Pharmacology and Toxicology," *Annual Review of Pharmacology*, 13 (1973):371–390.

110. JOHNSON, J. V., and VOST, R. A. "Tandem Mass Spectrometry for the Trace Determination of Tryptolines in Crude Brain Extracts," *Analytical Chemistry*, 56 (1984):1655–1661.

111. KANDEL, E. R. "From Metapsychology to Molecular Biology: Explorations into the Nature of Anxiety," *American Journal of Psychiatry*, 140 (1983):1277–1293.

112. KANDEL, E. R., and SCHWARTZ, J. H. *Principles of Neural Science*. New York: Elsevier, 1981.

113. ———. "Molecular Biology of Learning: Modulation of Transmitter Release," *Science*, 218 (1982):433–443.

114. KAROUM, F., et al. "Mass-fragmentography of Nanogram Quantities of Biogenic Amine Metabolites in Human Cerebrospinal Fluid and Whole Rat Brain," *Biomedical Mass Spectrometry*, 2 (1975):183–189.

115. KATZ, B., and MILEDI, R. "The Statistical Nature of the Acetylcholine Potential and Its Molecular Components," *Journal of Physiology* (London), 224 (1972): 665–699.

116. KEBABIAN, J. W. "Multiple Receptors for Dopamine," *Nature*, 277 (1979):93–96.

117. KELLER, R., et al. "Liquid Chromatographic Analysis of Catecholamines. Routine Assay for Regional Brain Mapping," *Life Sciences*, 19 (1976):995–1004.

118. KERKUT, G. A., SEDDEN, C. L., and WALKER, R. T. "Uptake of DOPA and 5-Hydroxytryptophan by Monoamine-forming Neurone in the Brain of *Helix Aspersa*," *Comparative Biochemistry and Physiology*, 23 (1967):159–162.

119. KESSLER, S., et al. "Genetic Variation in Catecholamine-synthesizing Enzyme Activity," *Proceedings of the National Academy of Science*, 69 (1972):2448–2450.

120. KISSINGER, P. T., et al. "An Electrochemical Detector for Liquid Chromatography with Picogram Sensitivity," *Analytical Letters*, 6 (1973):465–477.

121. KISSINGER, P. T., et al. "Recent Developments in the Clinical Assessment of the Metabolism of Aromatics by High Performance Reverse Phase Chromatography with Amperometric Detection," *Clinical Chemistry*, 23 (1977):1449–1455.

122. KOSHLAND, D. E., JR. *Bacterial Chemotaxis as a Model Behavioral System*. New York: Raven Press, 1980.

123. KOSLOW, S. "A Quantitative Probe for Biological Psychiatry: Selected Ion Monitoring," in I. Hanin and S. H. Koslow,

eds., *Physico-Chemical Methodologies in Psychiatric Research.* New York: Raven Press, 1980, pp. 155–170.

124. KOSLOW, S., and SCHLUMPF, M. "Quantitation of Adrenaline in Rat Brain Nuclei and Areas by Mass Fragmentography," *Nature,* 251 (1974):530–531.

125. KOSTERLITZ, H. W., ed. *Opiates and Endogenous Opioid Peptides.* Amsterdam: North Holland Publishing Co., 1976.

126. KRIEGER, D. T. "Brain Peptides: What, Where, and Why?" *Science,* 222 (1983): 975–985.

127. KRIEGER, D. T., BROWNSTEIN, M. J., and MARTIN, J. B., eds. *Brain Peptides.* New York: Wiley-Interscience, 1983.

128. KRNJEVIC, K. "Physiological Actions of Multiple Transmitters," in V. Chan-Palay and S. L. Palay, eds., *Coexistence of Neuroactive Substances in Neurons.* New York: John Wiley & Sons, 1984, pp. 363–377.

129. KUHAR, M. J. "Receptor Localization with the Microscope," in H. Yamamura, S. Enna, and M. Kuhar, eds., *Neurotransmitter Receptor Binding, 2nd Edition.* New York: Raven Press, 1984, pp. 153–176.

130. KUHAR, M. J., AGHAJANIAN, G. K., and ROTH, R. H. "Serotonin Neurons: A Synaptic Mechanism for the Reuptake of Serotonin," *Advances in Biochemical Psychopharmacology,* 10 (1974):287–295.

131. KUHAR, M. J., PERT, C. B., and SNYDER, S. H. "Regional Distribution of Opiate Receptor Binding in Monkey and Human Brain," *Nature,* 245 (1973):447–450.

132. KUHN, T. S. *The Structure of Scientific Revolutions.* Chicago: University of Chicago Press, 1962.

133. LAJTHA, A., ed. *Receptors in the Nervous System.* New York: Plenum Press, 1984.

134. LEFKOWITZ, R. J. "Identification and Regulation of Adrenergic Receptors," in M. A. Lipton, A. DiMascio, and K. F. Killam, eds., *Psychopharmacology: A Generation of Progress.* New York: Raven Press, 1978, pp. 389–396.

135. LEHMANN, W. D., KESSLER, M., and KONIG, W. A. "Investigations on Basic Aspects of Fast Atom Bombardment Mass Spectrometry: Matrix Effects, Sample Effects, Sensitivity and Quantification," *Biomedical Mass Spectrometry,* 11 (1984):217–222.

136. LEMAIRE, S., et al. "Mass Spectrometric Identification of Various Molecular Forms of Dynorphin in Bovine Adrenal Medulla," *Biochemical and Biophysical Research Communications,* 108 (1982): 51–58.

137. LINNOILA, M., et al. "Reliability of Norepinephrine and Major Monoamine Metabolite Measurements in CSF of Schizophrenic Patients," *Archives of General Psychiatry,* 40 (1983):1290–1294.

138. LLOYD, K. J., et al. "Serotonin and 5-hydroxyindoleacetic Acid in Discrete Areas of the Brainstem of Suicide Victims and Control Patients," *Advances in Biochemical Psychopharmacology,* 11 (1974):387–397.

139. LOEWI, O. "Uber Humorale Ubertragbarkeit der Herznervenwirkung," *Archiv fur die gesamte Physiologie des Menschen und der Tiere,* 189 (1921):239–242.

140. LOEWI, O., and NAVRATIL, E. "Uber Humorale Ubertragbarkeit der Herznervenwirkung. X. Mitteilung. Uber das Schicksal des Vagusstoff," *Archiv fur die gesamte Physiologie des Menschen und der Tiere,* 214 (1926):678–688.

141. MAAS, J. W., et al. "Pretreatment Neurotransmitter Metabolite Levels and Response to Tricyclic Antidepressant Drugs," *American Journal of Psychiatry,* 141 (1984):1159–1171.

142. MACKAY, A.V.P., et al. "Increased Brain Dopamine and Dopamine Receptors in Schizophrenia," *Archives of General Psychiatry,* 39 (1982):991–997.

143. MADDEN, J. IV, et al. "Stress-induced Parallel Changes in Central Opioid Levels and Pain Responsiveness in the Rat," *Nature,* 266 (1977):358–360.

144. MAINS, R. E., EIPPER, B. A., and LING, N. "Common Precursor to Corticotropins and Endorphins," *Proceedings of the National Academy of Science* (USA), 74 (1977):3014–3018.

145. MARSDEN, C. A., BRAZELL, M. P., and MAIDMENT, N. T. "An Introduction to in vivo Voltammetry," in C. A. Marsden, ed., *Measurement of Neurotrans-*

mitter Release. Chichester, U.K.: John Wiley & Son, 1984.

146. MASON, D. Y., and SAMMONS, R. E. "Alkaline Phosphatase and Peroxidase for the Double Immunoenzymatic Labelling of Cellular Constituents," *Journal of Clinical Pathology,* 31 (1978):454–462.

147. MAUK, M. D., et al. "Opiates and Classical Conditioning: Selective Abolition of Conditioned Responses by Activation of Opiate Receptors Within the Central Nervous System," *Proceedings of the National Academy of Science* (USA), 79 (1982):7598–7602.

148. MEANS, A. R., and DEDMAN, J. R. "Calmodulin—An Intracellular Calcium Recept," *Nature,* 285 (1980):73–77.

149. MEFFORD, I. N. "HPLC with Electrochemical Detection in Neurochemical Analysis: Assay for Catecholamines, Serotonin and Their Metabolites in Rat Brain," *Journal of Neuroscience Methods,* 3 (1981):207–224.

150. MEFFORD, I. N., and BARCHAS, J. D. "LCEC Analysis of Indoles in Biological Tissues," *Advances in Biochemical Psychopharmacology,* 34 (1982):107–116.

151. MEFFORD, I. N., et al. "Analysis of Catecholamines, Metabolites and Sulfate Conjugates in Brain Tissue and Plasma by High Performance Liquid Chromatography with Electrochemical Detection," in T. Nagatsu, ed., *Methods in Biogenic Amine Research.* Amsterdam: Elsevier/North Holland Biomedical Press, 1983, pp. 101–112.

152. MOLINOFF, P. B., WOLFE, B. B., and WEILAND, G. A. "Quantitative Analysis of Drug-receptor Interactions. II. Determination of the Properties of Receptor Subtypes," *Life Sciences,* 29 (1981):427–443.

153. MOSS, R. L., and DUDLEY, C. A. "The Challenge of Studying the Behavioral Effects of Neuropeptides," in L. Iversen, S. Iversen, and S. Snyder, eds., *Handbook of Psychopharmacology,* vol. 18. New York: Plenum Press, 1984, pp. 397–454.

154. MYERS, R. D. "Chronic Methods: Intraventricular Infusion, Cerebrospinal Fluid Sampling, and Push-pull Perfusion," in R. D. Myers, ed., *Methods in*

Psychobiology, vol. 3. New York: Academic Press, 1977, pp. 281–315.

155. NAKANISHI, S., et al. "Nucleotide Sequence of Cloned cDNA for Bovine Corticotropin-beta-lipotropin Precursor," *Nature,* 278 (1979):423–427.

156. NIEOULLON, A., CHERAMY, A., and GLOWINSKI, J. "Release of Dopamine *in vivo* from Cat Substantia Nigra," *Nature,* 266 (1977):375–377.

157. NORDIN, C., SIWERS, B., and BERTILSSON, L. "Site of Lumbar Puncture Influences Levels of Monoamine Metabolites," *Archives of General Psychiatry,* 39 (1982): 1445.

158. OLDS, J. *Drives and Reinforcements: Behavioral Studies of Hypothalamic Functions.* New York: Raven Press, 1977.

159. OLIVER, G., and SHAFER, E. A. "The Physiological Effects of Extracts of the Suprarenal Capsules," *Journal of Physiology* (London), 18 (1895):230–276.

160. OSBORNE, N. N., ed. *Dale's Principle and Communication Between Neurones.* Oxford: Pergamon Press, 1983.

161. PAGE, I. H. "Serotonin (5-hydroxytryptamine)," *Physiological Reviews,* 34 (1954):563–588.

162. PARSEGIAN, V. A. "Considerations in Determining the Mode of Influence of Calcium on Vesicle-membrane Interaction," in W. M. Cowan and J. A. Ferrendelli, eds., *Society for Neuroscience Symposia,* vol. 2. Bethesda, Md.: Society for Neuroscience, 1977, pp. 161–171.

163. PATON, W. D. M., and VIZI, E. S. "The Inhibitory Action of Noradrenaline and Adrenaline on Acetylcholine Output by Guinea-pig Ileum Longitudinal Muscle Strip," *British Journal of Pharmacology,* 35 (1969):10–28.

164. PERT, C. B., and SNYDER, S. H. "Properties of Opiate-receptor Binding in Rat Brain," *Proceedings of the National Academy of Science* (USA), 70 (1973): 2243–2247.

165. PICKAR, D., et al. "Endorphins in the Cerebrospinal Fluid of Psychiatric Patients," *Annals of the New York Academy of Science,* 398 (1981):399–411.

166. POST, R. M., and BALLENGER, J. C. *Neuro-*

biology of Mood Disorders. Baltimore, Md.: Williams & Wilkins, 1984.

167. REICHARDT, L. F., and KELLY, R. B. "A Molecular Description of Nerve Terminal Function," *Annual Review of Biochemistry*, 52 (1983):871–926.

168. REIS, D., et al. "A Genetic Control of the Number of Dopamine Neurons in Mouse Brain: Its Relationship to Brain Morphology, Chemistry, and Behavior," in E. Gershon et al., eds. *Genetic Research Strategies in Psychobiology and Psychiatry*. Pacific Grove, Calif.: Boxwood Press, 1981, pp. 215–229.

169. REVELEY, M. A., et al. "Brain Monoamine Oxidase Activity in Schizophrenics and Controls," *Archives of General Psychiatry*, 38 (1981):663–665.

170. ROBERTS, J. L., et al. "Effect of Glucocorticoids on the Synthesis and Processing of the Common Precursor to Adrenocorticotropin and Endorphin in Mouse Pituitary Tumor Cells," in G. H. Sato and R. Ross, eds., *Hormones and Cell Culture*, Book B. Cold Spring Harbor, N.Y.: Cold Spring Harbor Laboratory, 1979, p. 827.

171. ROBINSON, D. S., et al. "Monoamine Metabolism in Human Brain," *Archives of General Psychiatry*, 34 (1977):89–92.

172. ROTH, K. A., WEBER, E., and BARCHAS, J. D. "Immunoreactive Corticotropin Releasing Factor (CRF) and Vasopressin Are Colocalized in a Subpopulation of the Immunoreactive Vasopressin Cells in the Paraventricular Nucleus of the Hypothalamus," *Life Sciences*, 31 (1982):1857–1860.

173. ROTH, R. H. "Dopamine Autoreceptors: Pharmacology, Function, and Comparison with Postsynaptic Dopamine Receptors," *Communications in Psychopharmacology*, 3 (1979):429–445.

174. ROTH, R. H., et al. "Dopaminergic Neurons: Role of Impulse Flow and Presynaptic Receptors in the Regulation of Tyrosine Hydroxylase," in E. Usdin and W. E. Bunney, Jr., eds., *Pre- and Postsynaptic Receptors*. New York: Marcel Dekker, 1975, pp. 5–58.

175. SAAVEDRA, J. M., BROWNSTEIN, M., and AXELROD, J. "A Specific and Sensitive Enzymatic-isotopic Microassay for Serotonin in Tissues," *Journal of Pharmacology and Experimental Therapeutics*, 186 (1973):508–515.

176. SALAMA, A. I., ed. *Presynaptic Modulation of Postsynaptic Receptors in Mental Diseases*. New York: New York Academy of Sciences, 1984.

177. SCATTON, B., et al. "Neurochemistry of Monoaminergic Neurons in Parkinson's Disease," in E. Usdin et al., eds., *Catecholamines: Neuropharmacology and Central Nervous System—Therapeutic Aspects*. New York: Alan R. Liss, 1984, pp. 43–52.

178. SCHLACHTER, L. B., et al. "Persistence of Beta-endorphin in Human Cerebrospinal Fluid After Hypophysectomy," *Journal of Clinical Endocrinology and Metabolism*, 57 (1983):221–224.

179. SCHMIEDEBERG, O., and KOPPE, R. *Das Muscarin, das giftige Alkaloid des Fliegenpilzes (Agaricus muscarius, L.) seine Darstellung, chemischen Eigenschaften, physiologischen Wirkungen, toxicologische Bedeutung und sein Verhaltniss zur Pilzvergiftung im Allgemeinen*. Leipzig: Vogel, 1869.

180. SCHWARTZ, M. A., AIKENS, A. M., and WYATT, R. J. "Monoamine Oxidase Activity in Brains from Schizophrenics and Mentally Normal Individuals," *Psychopharmacologia*, 38 (1974):319–328.

181. SEDVALL, G., and WODE-HELGODT, B. "Aberrant Monoamine Metabolite Levels in CSF and Family History of Schizophrenia," *Archives of General Psychiatry*, 37 (1980):1113–1116.

182. SEDVALL, G., et al. "Genetic Studies of CSF Monoamine Metabolites," E. Usdin et al., eds., *Frontiers in Biochemical and Pharmacological Research in Depression*. New York: Raven Press, 1984, pp. 79–85.

183. SEEMAN, P., et al. "Antipsychotic Drug Doses and Neuroleptic/Dopamine Receptors," *Nature*, 261 (1976):717–719.

184. SEEMAN, P., et al. "Dopamine Receptors in the Central Nervous System," *Federation Proceedings*, 37 (1978):130–136.

185. SHARP, T., et al. "Changes in Monoamine Metabolites Measured by Simultaneous in vivo Differential Pulse Voltammetry

and Intracerebral Dialysis," *Neuroscience,* 12 (1984):1213–1221.

186. SHERRINGTON, C. S. "The Central Nervous System," in M. Foster, ed., *A Textbook of Physiology,* vol. 3. London: Macmillan, 1887.

187. SIEVER, L., et al. "Gradients of Biogenic Amine Metabolites in Cerebrospinal Fluid," *Diseases of the Nervous System,* 36 (1975):13–16.

188. SIMON, E. J., HELLER, J. M., and EDELMAN, I. "Stereospecific Binding of the Potent Narcotic Analgesic [^{3}H]etorphine to Rat Brain Homogenate," *Proceedings of the National Academy of Science* (USA), 70 (1973):1947–1949.

189. SIMONTOV, R., and SNYDER, S. H. "Isolation and Structure Identification of a Morphine-like Peptide 'Enkephalin' in Bovine Brain," *Life Sciences,* 18 (1976): 781–788.

190. SNYDER, S. H., and BENNET, J. P. "Neurotransmitter Receptors in the Brain: Biochemical Identification," *Annual Review of Physiology,* 38 (1976):153–175.

191. SNYDER, S. H., and GOODMAN, R. R. "Multiple Transmitter Receptors," *Journal of Neurochemistry,* 35 (1980):5–15.

192. SPECTOR, S. "Radioimmunoassay," *Annual Review of Pharmacology,* 13 (1973):359–370.

193. SPITZER, R. L., ENDICOTT, J., and ROBINS, E. "Research Diagnostic Criteria: Rationale and Reliability," *Archives of General Psychiatry,* 35 (1978):773–782.

194. SPOKES, E. G. "An Analysis of Factors Influencing Measurements of Dopamine, Noradrenaline, Glutamate Decarboxylase, and Choline Acetylase in Human Postmortem Brain Tissue," *Brain,* 102 (1979):333–346.

195. STRUMWASSER, F. "Post-synaptic Inhibition and Excitation Produced by Different Branches of a Single Neurone and the Common Transmitter Involved," Paper presented at the 22nd International Congress of Physiological Science, Leiden, The Netherlands, September 10–17, 1962.

196. TAKEDA, N., et al. "Immunohistochemical Evidence for the Coexistence of Histidine Decarboxylase-like and Glutamate Decarboxylase-like Immunoreactivities

in Nerve Cells of the Magnocellular Nucleus of the Posterior Hypothalamus of Rats," *Proceedings of the National Academy of Science* (USA), 81 (1984): 7647–7650.

197. TATEMOTO, K. "Isolation of New Peptides from Brain and Intestine," *Frontiers in Hormone Research,* 12 (1984):27–30.

198. TATEMOTO, K., and MUTT, V. "Chemical Determination of Polypeptide Hormones," *Proceedings of the National Academy of Science* (USA), 75 (1978): 4115–4119.

199. TAUC, L., and GERSCHENFELD, H. M. "Cholinergic Transmission Mechanisms for Both Excitation and Inhibition in Molluscan Central Synapses," *Nature,* 192 (1961):366–367.

200. TERENIUS, L. "Stereospecific Interaction Between Narcotic Analgesics and a Synaptic Plasma Membrane Fraction of Rat Cerebral Cortex," *Acta Pharmacologica et Toxicologica,* 32 (1973):317–320.

201. TERENIUS, L., et al. "Increased Levels of Endorphins in Chronic Psychosis," *Neuroscience Letters,* 3 (1976):157–162.

202. THIEMANN, S., et al. "CSF Probenecid and Biogenic Amines," *Biological Psychiatry,* 19 (1984):1357–1358.

203. THOMPSON, R. F., BERGER, T. W., and MADDEN, J., IV. "Cellular Processes of Learning and Memory in the Mammalian CNS," *Annual Review of Neuroscience,* 6 (1983):447–491.

204. UDENFRIEND, S. *Fluorescence Assay in Biology and Medicine.* New York: Academic Press, 1964.

205. U'PRICHARD, D. C. "Biochemical Characteristics and Regulation of Brain Alpha$_2$-adrenoceptors," *Annals of the New York Academy of Science,* 430 (1984):-55–75.

206. USDIN, E., HAMBURG, D. A., and BARCHAS, J. D., eds. *Neuroregulators and Psychiatric Disorders.* New York: Oxford University Press, 1977.

207. VARNDELL, I. M., and POLAK, J. M. "The Use of Immunogold Staining Procedures in the Demonstration of Neurochemical Coexistence at the Ultrastructural Level," in N. N. Osborne, ed., *Dale's Principle and Communication*

Between Neurones. Oxford: Pergamon Press, 1983, pp. 179–200.

208. VIZI, E. S. "Non-synaptic Interneuronal Communication: Physiological and Pharmacological Implication," in N. N. Osborne, ed., *Dale's Principle and Communication Between Neurones.* Oxford: Pergamon Press, 1983, pp. 83–111.

209. VOGEL, W. H., ORFEI, V., and CENTURY, B. "Activities of Enzymes Involved in the Formation and Destruction of Biogenic Amines in Various Areas of Human Brain," *Journal of Pharmacology and Experimental Therapeutics,* 165 (1969):196–203.

210. VOGT, M. "The Concentration of Sympathin in Different Parts of the Central Nervous System Under Normal Conditions and After Administration of Drugs," *Journal of Physiology* (London), 123 (1954):451–481.

211. VON EULER, U. S. "A Specific Sympathomimetic Ergone in Adrenergic Nerve Fibers (sympathin) and Its Relations to Adrenaline and Noradrenaline," *Acta Physiologica Scandanavia,* 12 (1946):73–97.

212. ———. *Noradrenalin: Chemistry, Physiology, Pharmacology, and Clinical Aspects.* Springfield, Ill: Charles C. Thomas, 1956.

213. WEBER, E., EVANS, C. J., and BARCHAS, J. D. "Opioid Peptide Dynorphin: Predominance of the Aminoterminal Octapeptide Fragment in Rat Brain Regions," *Nature,* 299 (1982):77–79.

214. ———. "Multiple endogenous ligands for opioid receptors," *Trends in Neurosciences,* 6 (1983):333–336.

215. WEBER, E., ROTH, K. A., and BARCHAS, J. D. "Colocalization of Alpha-neo-endorphin and Dynorphin Immunoreactivity in Hypothalamic Neurones," *Biochemical and Biophysical Research Communications,* 103 (1981):951–958.

216. WHITEHORSE, P. J., LYNCH, D., and KUHAR, M. J. "Effects of Postmortem Delay and Temperature on Neurotransmitter Receptor Binding in a Rat Model of the Human Autopsy Process," *Journal of Neurochemistry,* 43 (1984):553–559.

217. WIKBERG, J. "Pharmacological Classification of Adrenergic Alpha-receptors in the Guinea-pig Ileum," *Nature,* 273 (1978):164–166.

218. WOODBURY, J. W., and PATTON, H. D. "Electrical Activity of Single Spinal Cord Elements," *Cold Spring Harbor Symposium on Quantitative Biology,* 17 (1952):185–188.

219. WYATT, R. J., et al. "Difficulties in Comparing Catecholamine-related Enzymes from the Brains of Schizophrenics and Controls," *Biological Psychiatry,* 13 (1978):317–334.

220. YALOW, R. S., and BERSON, S. A. "Immunoassay of Endogenous Plasma Insulin in Man," *Journal of Clinical Investigation,* 39 (1960):1157–1175.

221. YAMAMURA, H., ENNA, S., and KUHAR, M., eds. *Neurotransmitter Receptor Binding,* 2nd ed. New York: Raven Press, 1984.

222. ZAMIR, N., et al. "Differential Processing of Prodynorphin and Proenkephalin in Specific Regions of the Rat Brain," *Proceedings of the National Academy of Science* (USA), 81 (1984):6886–6889.

223. ZIEGLER, M., et al. "Norepinephrine and MHPG Gradients in Human Cerebrospinal Fluid," *American Journal of Psychiatry,* 134 (1977):565–568.

224. ZIMMERMAN, H. "On the Vesicle Hypothesis," *Trends in Neuroscience,* 2 (1979): 282–284.

CHAPTER 3

NEUROPEPTIDES IN PSYCHIATRIC DISORDERS

Charles B. Nemeroff and Garth Bissette

¶ **Introduction: The Neurobiology of Neuropeptides**

Study of the physiological role and actions of an increasingly large number of peptides in the central and peripheral nervous system, as well as in nonneural tissue, has become a major focus of research for many neuroscientists in the last decade. More than forty peptides have thus far been isolated and sequenced (see table 3–1). They range in size from dipeptides (two amino acids joined by a single peptide bond) to large molecules such as corticotropin-releasing factor (CRF), which is comprised of forty-one amino acids. Detailed and comprehensive reviews of the neuroanatomical distribution and neurochemical, neurophysiological, neuropharmacological, and behavioral effects of a variety of neuropeptides have appeared.* In this section, we briefly

*See references 21, 47, 89, 102, 107, 132, 138, 162, 167, 169, 170, 185, 190, 191, 196, 207, 208, 232, and 249.

review these data, with special attention to the literature concerning the human central nervous system (CNS). In particular, we compare and contrast the neurobiology of neuropeptides with that of the better known monoamine neurotransmitters.

Identification of Neuropeptides

With a few notable exceptions, the pattern of peptide discovery has been as follows: first, a crude extract of brain (or some other tissue) is found to possess one or another biological activity. This activity is then found to be due to the presence of a peptide, and the peptide is eventually purified and sequenced. In 1931 substance P (sub P) was discovered by von Euler and Gaddum,[161] but forty years were to pass before its chemical identity was elucidated. A few peptides were discovered in the 1950s, such as insulin, though their presence in the CNS was not recognized until approximately twenty years later. In the 1940s and

TABLE 3–1

Neuropeptides Identified in Mammalian Brain

Thyrotropin-releasing hormone (TRH)
Gonadotrophin-releasing hormone (GnRH, LHRH)
Somatostatin (SRIF, GHIH)
Corticotropin-releasing factor (CRF)
Growth hormone-releasing factor (GRF, GHRH)
Thyroid-stimulating hormone (thyrotropin, TSH)
Adrenocorticotropin (ACTH)
Luteinizing hormone (LH)
Prolactin (PRL)
Growth hormone (GH)
Alpha-endorphin
Beta-endorphin
Gamma-endorphin
Met-enkephalin (met-ENK)
Leu-enkephalin (leu-ENK)
Dynorphin
Kytorphin
Alpha-melanocyte-stimulating hormone (alpha-MSH)
Beta-melanocyte-stimulating hormone (beta-MSH)
Neurotensin (NT)
Substance P (sub P)
Bombesin (BOM)
Gastrin
Cholecystokinin (CCK)
Secretin
Gastrin-releasing peptide
Calcitonin
Carnosine
Insulin
Glucagon
Neuromedin N
Neuropeptide Y
Vasoactive intestinal peptide (VIP)
Vasopressin
Oxytocin
Vasotocin
Delta-sleep–inducing peptide (DSIP)
Melanocyte-stimulating hormone-release inhibiting factor (MIF-I)
Angiotensin
Kallikrein
Bradykinin

1950s, the pioneering work of a few investigators spawned the "new" multidisciplinary field of neuroendocrinology.

For approximately twenty years the greatest stimulus for research in neuropeptide neurobiology was the discovery that the various endocrine axes are organized in a hierarchical fashion, with the CNS at the summit; the chemical regulators of anterior pituitary hormone secretion are now known to be neuropeptides, the release and release-inhibiting factors. The chemotransmitter-portal vessel hypothesis, expounded by Harris and his colleagues[94] and others,[210] postulated the presence of neurohormones that are released from nerve endings in the median eminence region of the hypothalamus and are transported from the primary capillary plexus to the adenohypophysis by the hypothalamo-hypophysial venous portal system. Once vascularly transported to the anterior pituitary, these hypophysiotropic hormones bind to specific membrane receptors, which results in the release (or inhibition of release) of one (or more) pituitary trophic hormones. Millions of sheep and pig hypothalami were extracted to eventually yield a few precious milligrams of the first hypothalamic releasing hormones to be discovered.[250] These include thyrotropin-releasing hormone (TRH, a tripeptide), luteinizing hormone releasing hormone (LHRH, a decapeptide), and somatostatin (SRIF, a tetradecapeptide).

These findings have not only resulted in major diagnostic and treatment breakthroughs in clinical endocrinology, but they have had considerable impact in psychiatry as well. It is now becoming more evident that particular psychiatric disorders are often associated with robust and reproducible neuroendocrine abnormalities; these findings are described in detail in chapter 4. The major purview of this chapter, then, rests on several distinct but related discoveries that have led to one inexorable conclusion—that neuropeptides are important neuroregulators in the CNS, they function there as neurotransmitters or neuromodulators and, consequently, they also modulate behavior. Moreover, some evidence is concordant with the view that alterations of specific neuropeptide-containing neurons occur in certain neuropsychiatric diseases.

Evidence That Neuropeptides Are Neurotransmitters in the CNS

Space constraints preclude a detailed discussion of the evidence that supports a neurotransmitter role for each of the more than forty neuropeptides (see table 3–1) present in the mammalian CNS. As with the monoamines, controversy still exists as to whether or not these chemical messengers fulfill all of the requisite neurotransmitter criteria.

Neuropeptides are heterogeneously distributed in the CNS. The pattern of distribution of each peptide is relatively unique. Thus in man and other mammals, neurotensin (NT) is found in high concentrations in the hypothalamus, amygdala, nucleus accumbens, and septum.[113, 158] In contrast, vasoactive intestinal peptide (VIP) and cholecystokinin (CCK) are present in high concentrations in the cerebral cortex, as well as in the hippocampus.[140,175] Other neuropeptides, like LHRH or growth hormone-releasing factor (GRF), have much more restricted patterns of distribution—they are found almost exclusively in the diencephalon.[109,125]

Because it would be impossible to discuss each of the neuropeptides in detail in this section, we have instead focused on a single one, NT. It is hoped that this will serve to acquaint the reader with the experimental approaches utilized by different investigators to determine whether a candidate neuropeptide fulfills neurotransmitter criteria, as well as with the data present in the current literature.

NT is a tridecapeptide that was discovered in 1973 by Carraway and Leeman[39] in extracts of bovine hypothalamus. It was characterized, purified, and finally sequenced by use of several bioassays—that is, the crude extract produced hypotension, hyperglycemia, and vasodilation after intravenous injection in the rat and smooth muscle contraction *in vitro*. Once sequenced (pGlu-Leu-Tyr-Glu-Asn-Lys-Pro-Arg-Arg-Pro-Tyr-Ile-Leu-OH), the synthetic peptide was synthesized, and antisera were raised against it. Such antisera were subsequently utilized for both immunohistochemical and radioimmunoassay experiments, and the results in both animal and human CNS revealed a strikingly heterogeneous distribution of NT.*

Very high concentrations of NT were found in limbic (e.g., nucleus accumbens, amygdala, habenula, septum) and hypothalamic regions (median eminence, paraventricular nucleus, preoptic area), and low concentrations were found in the hippocampus, cerebral cortex, and cerebellum. Density gradient centrifugation revealed that the majority of NT is concentrated in the synaptosomal fraction, and further subcellular fractionation indicated that the peptide is found in synaptic vesicles.[246] Immunohistochemical studies at the electron microscopic level have confirmed the presence of NT in vesicles contained within nerve terminals.[104]

NT is released from brain slices by high concentrations of potassium, and this release is calcium-dependent.[108] Enzymes (peptidases) that degrade NT have been identified in the mammalian brain. Very little is currently known about NT biosynthesis. However, if the biosynthesis of NT within neurons is similar to that described for other neuropeptides,[152] such as the opioid peptides, insulin and somatostatin, then it would be contained within the sequence of a larger prohormone that is synthesized, like most proteins, by deoxyribonucleic acid (DNA) transcription and subsequent translation. After the prohormone is formed, the active neuropeptide is thought to be liberated by the action of specific peptidase cleaving enzymes. Once released from the presynaptic terminal, peptides are believed to act on specific high-affinity postsynaptic membrane receptors. Indeed, radiolabeled NT has been used *in vitro* to identify such membrane receptors in the human and rat brain.[142,209,247]

Unlike the monoamines, neuropeptides, once released into the synaptic cleft, are inactivated primarily by enzymatic degradation and not by reuptake into the presynaptic terminal. Current knowledge about the transduction of the signal that occurs after

---

*See references 113, 123, 131, 133, 158, and 248.

neuropeptides bind to their membrane receptor(s) is also quite limited. However, electrophysiological changes in neuronal firing rates have repeatedly been observed after microiontophoretic application of neuropeptides such as NT.[31,95] Finally, behavioral changes and modifications in response to centrally acting pharmacological agents have been observed after intracerebroventricular or direct CNS administration of neuropeptides.[96,186,190] These latter findings suggest that changes in the extracellular fluid concentration of neuropeptides can produce marked physiological and pharmacobehavioral alterations.

Prior to a consideration of the role of neuropeptides in psychiatric disorders, one should carefully compare the neurobiology of neuropeptides with that of the more well-studied monoamines. These differences, highlighted by Hughes,[102] are summarized in table 3–2. One major difference between these two classes of neuroregulators is their mode of biosynthesis. As noted earlier, neuropeptides are synthesized by protein synthesis in ribosomes in the perikaryon (usually as a large prohormone) and, after packaging, are transported down the axon to the nerve terminal, where they are subsequently released in active form. In contrast, monoamines are synthesized largely in the nerve terminal region by a series of well-characterized enzymatic steps from an amino acid precursor (see chapter 2). The mode of inactivation of these two classes of neuroregulators is also quite different: Peptides are inactivated by enzymes (peptidases),[92,156] whereas monoamines are removed from the synaptic cleft largely by transmitter reuptake into the presynaptic terminal. The physiological consequences of monoamine release are brief, whereas the action of neuropeptides can be quite sustained.

It is indeed fascinating to consider the recent findings of Hokfelt and his colleagues[98] and others[103] that have convincingly demonstrated colocalization of neuropeptides and monoamines. The colocalization of sub P and serotonin (5HT) in descending spinal path-

TABLE 3–2
Comparison of Aminergic and Peptidergic Systems

Amine	Neuropeptides
Biosynthesis	
Local synthesis in terminals via specific catabolic enzymes subject to feedback control.	Ribosomal synthesis of protein precursor and enzymatic cleavage to active products in nerve axon. Posttranslational peptide modification occurs (amidation, acetylation, pulfation).
Storage	
Large and small vesicles, often granulated. Specific uptake and storage mechanisms in vesicles.	Large granular vesicles. Protein carriers.
Tissue concentrations vary from 1 to 100 nmol/g.	Tissue concentrations vary from 1 to 1000 pmol/g.
Release	
Calcium-dependent exocytosis.	Calcium-dependent.
Quantal.	
Fractional release 10^{-6} to 10^{-6}	
Inactivation	
Reuptake into nerve terminal; ester hydrolysis, methylation, and deamination.	Aminopeptidases. Endopeptidases. Carboxypeptidases.

SOURCE: J. Hughes, "Strategies for Manipulating Peptidergic Transmission," in R. J. Wurtman, S. H. Corkin, and J. H. Growden, eds., *Alzheimer's Disease: Advances in Basic Research Therapies.* Zurich: Proceedings of the 3rd Meeting of the International Study Group on Treatment of Memory Disorders Associated with Aging, 1984, pp. 259–273.

ways has been the most closely scrutinized example of colocalization. Recently compelling evidence for colocalization of CCK and dopamine (DA) has appeared.[97]

In summary, a large number of neuropeptides are now known to be present in the mammalian CNS—their unique anatomical localization and the concatenation of behavioral, electrophysiological, and pharmacological properties attributed to them make neuropeptides prime candidates for one of the classes of endogenous substances (endocoids) that modulate normal and abnormal behavior. In the remainder of this chapter, we consider three types of evidence to evaluate this hypothesis. First, studies in postmortem brain tissue and cerebrospinal fluid (CSF) have been conducted to determine whether the integrity or activity of neuropeptide-containing systems (and their receptors) are altered in neuropsychiatric disorders. Second, studies in which peptides have been administered to humans to evaluate their potential therapeutic use are reviewed. Finally, the effects of peptide receptor antagonists on the behavior and mood of normal volunteers and psychiatric patients is reviewed in detail.

There are, of course, problems with each of these approaches. The postmortem tissue and CSF studies have recently been reviewed by Edwardson and McDermott[65] and Rossor,[215] and by Post and associates,[204] respectively. In both types of studies, several potentially confounding variables must be carefully evaluated; these include patient age and sex, and drug effects. Such considerations increase the likelihood that alterations in peptide concentration (or receptor number) are related to patient diagnosis and not to these "nuisance variables." In postmortem tissue studies, stability of the peptide to be measured must be taken into consideration as well as agonal state, postmortem delay, and cause of death. In CSF and postmortem studies, the time of day (and year) the sample is obtained may be important because of possible circadian and circannual rhythms in the concentrations of certain neurotransmitters and their metabo-

lites (e.g., melatonin, endorphins).[272] In general, neuropeptides have been found to be remarkably stable in postmortem brain tissue and CSF. However, the complexity of neuropeptide neurobiology is demonstrated by the presence of multiple forms of certain neuropeptides that have been found in brain and CSF.[240]

The studies in which peptides have been administered to patients as potential therapeutic drugs have been quite problematical. It is unclear at this time whether neuropeptides penetrate the blood-brain barrier in appreciable quantities after systemic injection, and therefore, any subsequent effects observed may not be due to direct peptide actions on the CNS. Of course, studies of peptides as putative pharmacotherapeutic agents must be judged with the same rigor as any other drug trial. Ideally, there should be randomized, placebo-controlled, double-blind studies with large numbers per group conducted by clinically experienced investigators. The peptide antagonist studies, largely limited at this time to naloxone hydrochloride and naltrexone, the opiate receptor blockers, are also not without problems. The duration of action of the agonists is relatively brief, and at higher doses, they produce effects on nonopioid systems.[224]

In several places in the succeeding text, we describe, while reviewing a reported finding, the specificity of the antiserum used to measure a peptide and the method of statistical analysis employed. We recognize that many readers might consider this to be unnecessarily detailed descriptions of methodology, but we believe it to be justified. First, differences in methodology may well explain discrepant reports in the literature. Second, inclusion of methodological considerations increases their visibility, and this can only have a positive effect in psychiatry. The use of inappropriate statistical tests leads investigators to incorrect conclusions; therefore, data analysis must be carefully scrutinized. In the discussion at the end of this chapter, we list our recommendations for ideal clinical study design.

¶ Schizophrenia

Evidence That
Neuropeptide-containing Systems Are
Altered in Schizophrenia

OPIOID PEPTIDES

The neuropeptides that have clearly received the greatest attention in neurobiology are the endorphins, and this is also true in schizophrenia research. Named for the endogenous opiate receptor ligand that has been known to exist since 1975, the endorphins are now known to comprise a family of peptides.[231] A number of reviews on the biology of opioid peptides and their potential role(s) in psychiatric disorders are available.* The notion that schizophrenia is due to an endorphin deficiency is based mainly on animal studies in which centrally administered beta-endorphin produced a neurolepticlike catalepsy and also on the clinical studies in which endorphins appear to possess antipsychotic effects. The hypothesis of endorphin excess in schizophrenia is based on the increase in CSF endorphins observed by some workers and on the purported antipsychotic effects of naloxone, the opioid receptor antagonist.

Terenius and associates[242] first reported alterations in endogenous opioid peptide concentrations in CSF of schizophrenic patients. Their radioreceptor assay utilized ^{3}H-dihydromorphine as the ligand and measured total opioid activity without discrimination as to which particular opioid was present. In this original report, the CSF opioid activity of four chronic schizophrenic patients (ill for at least ten years but drug-free for four weeks) was compared before, and two and four weeks after, clozapine treatment. The diagnostic criteria used were not specified in this early report. The CSF was filtered and chromatographed on Sephadex G-10; two fractions with opiate receptor activity were

*See references 12, 13, 17, 36, 56, 136, 155, 239, 253, 255, and 260.

isolated (Fraction I and II). Methionine-enkephalin (met-ENK) co-eluted with Fraction II, but only the concentration of Fraction I was changed after neuroleptic treatment. Two of the four schizophrenic patients had elevated CSF Fraction I opioid concentrations after four weeks of neuroleptic treatment, but no statistical test was performed on this small sample. In a later study, Lindström and co-workers[147] reported that when CSF opioid activity, as defined with the same radioreceptor assay, was measured in nine chronic schizophrenic patients after a drug-free period of one to two months, six of the patients had higher Fraction I opioid concentrations than the mean Fraction I concentration of nineteen normal volunteers. In addition, the schizophrenic patients with higher CSF Fraction I levels, when retested after treatment with antipsychotic drugs (clozapine, flupenthixol, or chlorpromazine for twelve days to two months), exhibited values close to the mean of the normal controls. In another study[211] using these same methods, CSF Fraction I opioid activity was measured in eighteen drug-free acute schizophrenic patients (eleven had never received neuroleptics, seven had stopped neuroleptic treatment four to eight weeks before this study) and in twenty-four chronic schizophrenic patients who had been neuroleptic-free for at least two weeks. The schizophrenic patients fulfilled Feighner's criteria[18] for definite schizophrenia, and only the chronic patients whose symptoms worsened during the two-week drug holiday were studied (nine of twelve). Two of nine chronic schizophrenic patients, four of six relapsed patients, and six of nine acute schizophrenic patients had elevated CSF Fraction I opioid concentrations when compared to mean values for normal controls from Lindström and associates' study.[147] In another recent study, this same group[148] found that either Fraction I or II CSF opioid activity was elevated above their previously published mean normal control values[147] in 72 percent of fifty-three neuroleptic-free (for one week) schizophrenic patients (using Bleuler's criteria).[18] These elevations did not attain statistical significance when compared to normal controls, but within the schizophrenic group, the CSF Fraction I opioid activity was significantly higher in the hebephrenic (N = 23) than in the undifferentiated (N = 21) subgroup. No significant correlations were noted between CSF opioid activity of either Fraction I or II and duration of disease, length of neuroleptic treatment, or psychotic symptoms. There are, of course, many obvious problems in comparing data between diagnostic groups assayed at different times.

Dupont and associates,[63] using a radio-receptor assay employing ^{3}H-naloxone as the radioactive ligand, found decreased CSF concentrations of opioid activity in nineteen chronic schizophrenic patients when compared to nine controls. The diagnostic criteria used were not specified, and all of the schizophrenic patients were receiving neuroleptics. The CSF opioid(s) that displaced ^{3}H-naloxone binding co-eluted with met-ENK and leucine-enkephalin (leu-ENK) on Sephadex G-25, but the decreases observed in the schizophrenic patients were reported as not significant, although the method of statistical analysis was not described. After incubation of CSF for five hours at 37° C, the schizophrenic group had no measurable immunoreactivity in CSF, while the mean control CSF concentration remained at 80 percent of preincubation levels, implying higher peptide degradative (enzymatic) activity of opioids in the schizophrenic group. This latter finding has not been confirmed by Burbach and associates[37] in a study of nine schizophrenic patients and neurological controls.

The molecular nature of the opioid material in CSF is clearly an important issue. Akil and coworkers[2] measured CSF met-ENK by radioimmunoassay (RIA) and opioid activity by radioreceptor assay in ten healthy volunteers and expressed the results as pg met-ENK equivalents per ml in order to compare the two methods directly. Both assays used ^{3}H-met-ENK as the radiolabeled ligand, CSF was extracted with acid-methanol, and the peptides were separated using two liquid chromatography columns. Both assays found levels of met-ENK/opioid activity that agreed with those reported by the Swedish group for Fraction II.

In contrast, Jeffcoate and others[112] reported on the measurement of beta-endorphin by RIA in CSF of twenty "normal" patients undergoing diagnostic lumbar punctures or pneumoencephalograms; the CSF concentrations of beta-endorphin were in the same range as the opioid activity reported by Dupont and associates.[63] Because almost all antisera to beta-endorphin recognize beta-lipotropin (beta-LPH, a precursor to beta-endorphin), Jeffcoate and coworkers[112] separated the two immunoreactive forms on Sephadex G-25 and used an antiserum that was directed toward beta-LPH, but not beta-endorphin, to assess the contribution of beta-LPH to the total immunoreactivity. Beta-endorphin accounted for more than 90 percent of the immunoreactivity in all of the samples tested. These two studies[2,112] established a standard for what may be considered normal concentrations of met-ENK and beta-endorphin in CSF. Naber and Pickar[177] have comprehensively reviewed the problems of measuring endorphins in biological fluids, including CSF.

In a preliminary report, Domschke, Dickschas, and Mitznegg[62] presented data on the CSF concentration of beta-endorphin in five acute and seven chronic (greater than ten years) schizophrenic patients compared to seven normal controls and ten patients with herniated vertebral discs. No diagnostic criteria for schizophrenia were provided and all psychiatric patients were receiving neuroleptic drug therapy. The CSF was extracted in silicic acid and acetone, and beta-endorphin was estimated by RIA. Inappropriately using Student's t-test to analyze the data, this group claimed that the acute schizophrenic patients had increased, and the chronic schizophrenic patients decreased, CSF beta-endorphin concentrations, when compared to the controls.

Burbach and coworkers[37] compared CSF concentrations of beta-endorphin and met-ENK in nine neurologically diseased "controls" and nine schizophrenic patients. No diagnostic criteria were reported for the schizophrenic patients, and all were currently treated with neuroleptics. Both peptides were measured by RIA. No significant group-related differences in CSF beta-endorphin or met-ENK concentrations were observed. As just noted, after five hours of incubation at $37°$ C, there was still no significant group-related difference in CSF concentrations of either peptide. Concentrations of beta-endorphin in CSF were in agreement with other reported values, but the met-ENK concentrations were higher than those previously reported.

Naber and others[179,180] and Naber and Pickar,[177] using a radioreceptor assay for opioid activity and an RIA for beta-endorphin, studied CSF from psychiatric patients with a variety of diagnoses, including schizophrenia ($N = 27$), schizo-affective disorder ($N = 17$), depression ($N = 35$), mania ($N = 13$), as well as from normal controls. Schizophrenic patients were diagnosed by Research Diagnostic Criteria (RDC)[18] and were medication-free for two weeks prior to the study. The radioreceptor assay used a met-ENK analogue, ^{3}H-D-ala-L-Leu-enkephalinamide (D-ALA) and the RIA used 125-I-beta-endorphin as the tracer. Opiate receptor activity was significantly reduced in the schizophrenic males only ($p < 0.005$, Student's t-test, two-tailed), but beta-endorphin concentrations were much lower than those reported by others. Recently Naber and associates[178] reported that in twenty-three unmedicated acute schizophrenic patients, serum beta-endorphin concentrations were not correlated with baseline measures of psychotic behavior, nor were they associated with the therapeutic efficacy of neuroleptics.

Emrich and coworkers[69,70] and Hollt and others[100] measured the concentration of beta-endorphin-like immunoreactivity by RIA in CSF and plasma of eight "normal" controls (CSF was obtained to diagnose meningitis/encephalitis and found to be negative) compared to fifteen schizophrenic patients and a variety of other neurological patients. Schizophrenic patients were diagnosed by the International Classification of Disease (ICD) nomenclature[18] and were medication-free for four weeks. Plasma, but not CSF, beta-endorphin was extracted with a silicic acid/acetone mixture. No significant concentration differences between controls and schizophrenic patients were detected in CSF or plasma.

Van Kammen and associates[252] measured both beta-endorphin concentration and opioid activity in CSF from thirty schizophrenic patients; in addition, vasopressin and angiotensin I and II concentrations were also assayed. The results were compared to those obtained in fifty-two normal controls. Schizophrenic patients fulfilled RDC[18] and were drug-free for an average of thirty-three days before treatment. Concentrations of beta-endorphin, vasopressin, and angiotensin I and II were measured by RIA using 125-I-labeled peptides, and opioid activity was assessed by radioreceptor assay with ^{3}H-D-ALA as the radioligand. The concentration of vasopressin was found to be reduced by approximately 40 percent ($p < 0.01$) in the CSF of male schizophrenic patients; no change in the concentration of the other peptides was found.

Recently Wen, Lo, and Ho[276] measured CSF met-ENK levels in chronic schizophrenic patients ($N = 18$; duration of illness greater than ten years) and neurological controls ($N = 18$; eight stroke, ten headache). The schizophrenic patients were rated before CSF withdrawal according to the Brief Psychiatric Rating Scale (BPRS); no mention was made of medication status. The RIA employed recognized met-O-enkephalin, and therefore 125-I-met-O-enkephalin was used as the radioactive trace; all CSF samples were passed through Sep-Pak filters and oxidized with hydrogen peroxide to form met-O-enkephalin. Recovery was estimated at 70 percent and schizophrenic patients were reported to have significantly less met-ENK present in CSF than controls ($p < 0.02$, Student's t-test). No significant correlation was seen between BPRS score and met-ENK concentration. In a second study using identical biochemical methodology, this same group,[151] while investigating the purported antipsychotic effects of naloxone in schizophrenic patients, found a significant correlation between the increase in CSF met-ENK concentrations and the naloxone-induced decrease in psychotic symptoms in seven schizophrenic patients.

At the present time, we must conclude that the data provided by measuring opioids in CSF and plasma provide no compelling evidence for a significant role of these peptides in schizophrenia.

OTHER NEUROPEPTIDES

There have been several reports in which nonopioid peptides have been measured in the CSF of schizophrenic patients. Our group[277] assayed CSF NT concentrations by RIA in twenty-one schizophrenic patients (diagnosed by RDC[18]) and twelve age- and sex-matched healthy volunteers. This study was undertaken because several findings in neurochemistry, neuroanatomy, and neuropharmacology have unequivocally demonstrated NT-DA interactions in the CNS,[183,184,187] and the DA hypothesis of schizophrenia remains the most viable theory concerning pathogenesis of this disorder.

The schizophrenic patients were drug-free for at least two weeks, and psychiatric symptoms were assessed with the Comprehensive Psychopathological Rating Scale (CPRS). Group mean CSF concentrations of NT-like immunoreactivity were not significantly different, but the schizophrenic group was shown to consist of two subgroups; one of these had very low CSF concentrations of NT-like immunoreactivity. After neuroleptic treatment, this latter subgroup exhibited normalization of CSF NT concentrations. Only one of sixteen items in the CPRS was significantly correlated with the concentration of NT in CSF from the schizophrenic group: slowness of movement ($p < .01$). In this regard, it is of interest that all of the catatonic schizophrenic patients were in the low NT subgroup.

Recently, in collaboration with Widerlöv and Lindström, we have confirmed this decrease of NT-like immunoreactivity in the CSF of schizophrenic patients, but changes in NT concentration after neuroleptic treatment were not found. No such CSF NT reductions were observed in patients with major depression, anorexia-bulimia, or premenstrual syndrome.[159] Some of the patients were pretreated with probenecid, an inhibitor of acidic monoamine metabolite transport from CSF, which produced no discernible effect on the concentration of CSF NT.

Recently our group, in collaboration with Widerlöv and his coworkers,[22] measured CSF concentrations of SRIF in ten healthy volunteers, twenty-nine demented patients, twenty-three patients with major depression, and ten schizophrenic patients (DSM-III criteria[18]). The antiserum recognized $SRIF_{1-14}$ (cyclic or linear), $SRIF_{1-25}$, and $SRIF_{1-28}$. All three psychiatric diagnostic groups had significantly reduced CSF concentrations of SRIF when compared to the controls. Thus decreases in CSF SRIF appear not to be specific to a particular disease state but may reflect cognitive impairment (see discussion in "Affective Disorders" and "Alzheimer's Disease" sections).

Gerner and Yamada[83] assayed CSF concentrations of immunoreactive CCK, SRIF, and bombesin (BOM) in normal healthy volunteers ($N = 29$) and patients with anorexia nervosa ($N = 23$), mania ($N = 10$), primary depression ($N = 28$), and chronic schizophrenia ($N = 13$), all ill for more than six months. Diagnoses were made using RDC,[72] and schizophrenic patients were neuroleptic-free for fourteen days prior to CSF sampling. A small, but statistically insignificant, decrease in BOM-like immunoreactivity was observed in the schizophrenic patients when compared to the controls; no diagnostic group-related differences in CSF concentrations of SRIF- or CCK-like immunoreactivity were found.

In a more recent study,[81] BOM, SRIF, and CCK were measured by RIA in CSF obtained from thirty-one normal controls, nineteen schizophrenic patients (from California hospitals), and fifty-three schizophrenic patients (from the National Institute of Mental Health

[NIMH]). All schizophrenic patients fulfilled RDC[18] and were neuroleptic-free for at least fourteen days. Only the schizophrenic patients from NIMH exhibited significant differences—that is, elevations in CCK and SRIF concentrations and decreases in BOM—when compared to controls. CCK, SRIF, or BOM did not show any consistent change in CSF concentration after blockade of acid transport by treatment with probenecid or after treatment with the neuroleptic drug pimozide. No significant correlation was seen between CSF concentration of CCK, SRIF, or BOM and concentrations of homovanillic acid (HVA), 5-hydroxyindoleacetic acid (5-HIAA), 3-methoxy-4-hydroxy-phenylglycol (MHPG), beta-endorphin, tyrosine, tryptophan, gamma-aminobutyric acid (GABA), or cortisol. The SRIF findings are in contrast to those of Bissette and coworkers[22] in schizophrenia and in contrast to those of Rubinow and associates[220] in depression.

Verbanck and others[259] measured CSF CCK concentrations in control subjects and in patients with Parkinson's disease ($N = 13$), depression ($N = 30$), and schizophrenia ($N = 15$). Schizophrenic patients were diagnosed using Feighner's criteria.[18] Nine patients were drug-free for six weeks, and six received haloperidol prior to CSF withdrawal. The antiserum used to measure CCK also recognized gastrin and caerulein, and 125-I-gastrin was used as the radioligand in the CCK assay. The concentration of CCK in CSF was reported to be significantly decreased in the drug-free schizophrenic patients when compared to the normal controls.

Rimon and others[212] recently measured the concentration of sub P in CSF from fifteen controls (x-ray or urology patients), twelve depressed patients, and twelve schizophrenic patients. Schizophrenic patients fulfilled Feighner's criteria[18] and were drug-free for two weeks. Samples of CSF were filtered on Sep-Pak cartridges and sub P was measured by RIA. The schizophrenic patients were reported to have significantly increased CSF concentrations of this undecapeptide. Gel electrophoresis of the sub P

immunoreactivity in CSF revealed that less than 10 percent of the observed immunoreactivity was due to the presence of the intact sub P molecule; fragments co-eluting with sub P_{5-11} and sub P_{3-11} represented the bulk of the immunoreactivity.

Kaiya and associates[119] measured the concentration of sub P–like immunoreactivity in plasma of schizophrenic patients, normal controls, and patients with other psychiatric diagnoses. After more than one year of antipsychotic drug treatment, plasma sub P–like immunoreactivity was elevated when compared to controls, but this finding was observed only in the medicated schizophrenic patients.

Lindström and coworkers[149] measured the CSF concentrations of immunoreactive delta-sleep–induced peptide (DSIP) in healthy volunteers ($N = 20$), schizophrenic patients ($N = 22$), and depressed patients ($N = 10$). Schizophrenic patients fulfilled RDC[18] and were drug-free for two weeks before the first CSF sample was obtained. The DSIP antisera was directed toward the N-terminal end of the DSIP molecule and 125-I-DSIP was used as the radioactive ligand. Schizophrenic patients had significantly lower CSF DSIP concentrations than controls, both in the drug-free state and after four weeks of neuroleptic treatment.

In addition to neuropeptide measurement in CSF, investigators have also examined postmortem brain tissue from schizophrenic patients in the hope that the neurotransmitter(s) involved in the etiology and pathogenesis of schizophrenia might be elucidated. As yet, few reports have appeared concerning alterations in neuropeptide concentrations in postmortem brain regions of patients who had been, in life, diagnosed as schizophrenic. Indeed, few studies describing the concentrations of these peptides in the normal human brain have been conducted.

Recently Crow and his colleagues have measured the concentrations of several centrally active neuropeptides in brain regions from twelve controls and fourteen schizophrenic patients.[75,76,214] All schizophrenic patients fulfilled Feighner's criteria[18] and were further subclassified into type I ($N = 7$) and type II ($N = 7$) based on the presence or absence of "positive" and "negative" symptoms as described by Crow.[51] Five neuropeptides (NT, sub P, CCK, SRIF, and VIP) were assayed by RIA in temporal, frontal, parietal, and cingulate cortices and several subcortical regions including the hippocampus, amygdala, globus pallidus, putamen, dorsomedial thalamus, and lateral thalamus. Significant alterations were observed for CCK (reduced in temporal cortex) and sub P (increased in hippocampus) in the total group of schizophrenic patients compared to controls. Type II schizophrenic patients had significantly decreased mean concentrations of CCK in the amygdala and significantly decreased SRIF and CCK concentrations in the hippocampus; type I schizophrenic patients had elevated levels of VIP in the amygdala. No significant correlation was seen for any regional neuropeptide concentration with age, postmortem delay, or presence of neuroleptic medication.

Our laboratory[188] has measured the regional postmortem brain concentrations of NT, SRIF, and TRH in controls (free of neurological or psychiatric disease, $N = 50$), patients with Huntington's chorea ($N = 24$), and schizophrenic patients ($N = 46$). Schizophrenic patients were diagnosed by RDC[18] and were on various neuroleptic regimens before and, in some cases, up to the time of death. All peptides were measured by RIA, and analysis of variance was utilized to determine whether significant group-related differences in a particular regional peptide concentration were present. No significant differences in NT, SRIF, or TRH concentrations were seen between controls and schizophrenic patients in the caudate nucleus, nucleus accumbens, amygdala, or hypothalamus. A significant decrease in SRIF ($p < 0.05$) and TRH ($p < 0.004$) concentrations in Brodmann's area 12 (frontal cortex) and a significant decrease ($p < 0.05$) in TRH concentration in Brodmann's area 32 (frontal cortex) were observed in the schizophrenic patients when compared to the controls; in contrast, NT content was significantly elevated ($p <$

0.006) in Brodmann's area 32 (frontal cortex) in the schizophrenic group.

Kleinman and associates[129] measured the concentrations of four neuropeptides (met-ENK, sub P, NT, and CCK) by RIA in postmortem brain regions from normal control subjects ($N = 18$), alcoholic patients ($N = 7$), opiate users ($N = 12$), suicide victims ($N = 19$), and psychotic patients ($N = 40$). The psychotic group was subdivided by RDC[18] into chronic paranoid schizophrenics ($N = 11$), chronic undifferentiated schizophrenics ($N = 6$), and "other" psychotic disorders (unspecified functional psychoses and affective psychoses). No significant differences between normals and psychotic patients were found in met-ENK concentrations in the nucleus accumbens, hypothalamus, globus pallidus, or putamen. Similarly, no significant group-related differences in NT concentrations in the nucleus accumbens, globus pallidus, or hypothalamus were observed. Moreover, no significant differences were seen between control and psychotic patients in CCK levels in the amygdala, nucleus accumbens, caudate nucleus, frontal cortex, substantia nigra, hippocampus, or temporal cortex. Met-ENK concentrations were reported to be significantly ($p < 0.05$) decreased in the caudate nucleus of chronic paranoid schizophrenic patients compared to other diagnostic groups or controls; sub P levels were significantly increased in the caudate nucleus of patients with psychoses when compared to diagnoses other than schizophrenia.

Biggins and coworkers[20] have recently measured amygdaloid concentrations of NT and TRH by RIA in normals ($N = 7$) and patients with senile dementia of the Alzheimer's type ($N = 7$), depressive illness ($N = 7$), or schizophrenia ($N = 7$). No criteria was given for the diagnosis of schizophrenia, and no mention was made of medication status. No significant difference was seen in amygdaloid concentrations of TRH or NT between the four diagnostic groups. No correlation was seen between patient age and peptide concentration, but irrespective of diagnostic group, males had almost twice as much NT in the amygdala as females. A significant positive correlation between the concentrations of TRH and NT was noted in this brain region. Total NT and TRH immunoreactivity in the amygdala was characterized on high-performance liquid chromatography (HPLC); NT immunoreactivity co-eluted with the synthetic standard as a single peak, while TRH immunoreactivity consisted of a major peak (50 percent) and several minor peaks.

TREATMENT OF SCHIZOPHRENIA WITH NEUROPEPTIDES

Several clinical studies with beta-endorphin, enkephalin analogues, and derivatives of the endorphins (e.g., des-tyr[1]-gamma-endorphin, DTγE) have been conducted in schizophrenic patients. In an early study that stimulated considerable further research, Kline and associates[130] administered beta-endorphin (1.5 mg intravenously [IV]) to three schizophrenic patients and reported a rapid worsening of their cognitive difficulties —for example, more difficulty conceptualizing. Less than two weeks later, a second trial was conducted with higher doses of beta-endorphin. One schizophrenic patient who had not responded to the previous 1 mg dose responded to 4 mg beta-endorphin IV by looking more energetic, smiling frequently, and speaking rapidly. He spoke of plans for the future and a new lack of fear of others. However, after 7 mg beta-endorphin IV, he again looked fatigued and spoke in a halting manner. Two other schizophrenic patients who received 3 mg beta-endorphin IV showed no behavioral changes. Gerner and coworkers[84] treated eight drug-free schizophrenic patients with beta-endorphin (10 mg) in a double-blind, placebo-controlled, crossover design. No significant behavioral improvement was observed using a variety of standard rating scales. Six of the eight patients deteriorated further.

Berger, Barchas, and their colleagues[9,15,17] reported that a high dose of beta-endorphin (20 mg IV) produced small (clinically insignificant) but statistically significant improvements in the symptoms of nine unmedicated male schizophrenic patients in a double-blind, crossover-designed study. However, Petho and others[197] administered 4 mg beta-endorphin IV to six drug-free schizophrenic patients using a double-blind design and observed no salutary effects. The experiment had to be stopped in four of the patients because of increasing anxiety. Pickar and associates,[200] in a double-blind study, administered beta-endorphin (4–15 mg IV) to six unmedicated schizophrenic patients; no beneficial effects were observed using the BPRS.

The effects of a potent and stable met-ENK analogue, FK-33-824, have been studied in schizophrenia. The studies by Nedopil, Jungkunz, and their coworkers have been summarized by Klein and associates.[127] In an open study of nine paranoid schizophrenic patients, treatment with FK-33-824 (0.5 mg IV on day 1, 1.0 mg on day 2) resulted in three patients dropping out of the study because of a dramatic worsening of symptoms. However, five of the remaining six patients were improved, as evidenced by a significant decrease in BPRS scores. In contrast, in a later double-blind, two-day study,[117] the effects of FK-33-824 (3 mg intramuscularly [IM] per day) or diazepam (20 mg IM per day) in sixteen schizophrenic patients were evaluated. No clinical improvement was observed in any of the patients.

In a series of reports, DeWied, van Ree, Verhoeven, and their associates from Utrecht in the Netherlands have postulated that schizophrenia is a disorder of endorphin metabolism—an overproduction of alpha-type endorphins, which purportedly have amphetaminelike properties, and/or an underproduction of gamma-type endorphins, which purportedly possess neuroleptic properties. Such theoretical considerations and the preclinical data concordant with these hypotheses have led to clinical trials of DTγE and related peptides in schizophrenic patients. These theoretical issues and early clinical trials have been described in a series of reviews.[59,254,256,257]

The preclinical studies with gamma-endorphin fragments by the Utrecht group have been criticized on the grounds that the tests used to detect "neuroleptic activity" are atypical—for example, the pole-jumping test and the grip test[60]—when compared to standard tests such as inhibition of conditioned avoidance responding or blockade of the actions of DA agonists. Such criticisms are only partially warranted, because use of standard neuroleptic screening tests may reveal only activity of compounds with DA receptor blocking activity, and these drugs may possess unwanted side effects (extrapyramidal effects, tardive dyskinesia) that we wish to avoid in future antipsychotic drug development.

Endorphin derivatives with purported antipsychotic activity have been tested for antipsychotic efficacy in schizophrenic patients by the Utrecht group. In the first study,[263] six schizophrenic patients were withdrawn from neuroleptic drugs one week prior to the clinical trial. The patients then received daily IM treatments with 0.5 to 1.0 mg DTγE for ten days. All six patients were reported to show dramatic improvement, although three patients rapidly relapsed during treatment with the peptide.

In a second study by the same group,[257,264] schizophrenic patients were maintained on neuroleptics during treatment with DTγE. In this double-blind, crossover-designed study, sixteen patients received DTγE (1 mg IM daily for sixteen days) or placebo. The authors reported a significant improvement after combined neuroleptic and DTγE treatment when compared to the combined neuroleptic and placebo treatment. The patients became progressively less psychotic, and hallucinations and delusions were significantly reduced. Eight patients were reported to exhibit dramatic improvements.

Further impetus for the study of DTγE was provided by the report of Metz, Busch, and Meltzer,[166] who found effects of DTγE on the H-reflex in schizophrenic patients to be similar to those of neuroleptic drugs. The H-reflex is an electrically evoked monosynaptic spinal reflex.

In contrast to these findings, Emrich and his colleagues,[71] in a double-blind trial using daily IM injections of 2 mg DTγE, found no significant antipsychotic effects of the peptide in thirteen patients maintained on neuroleptic medication. (Patients were maintained on neuroleptics in an attempt to replicate the conditions used by Verhoeven and associates.[263]) Other largely negative studies have been published, including those of Fink and associates,[78] Manchandra and Hirsch,[160] Meltzer and coworkers,[164] and Tamminga and others.[238] In these studies and the recent one by Volavka and colleagues,[270] the antipsychotic effects of DTγE, when evident at all, were short-lived, barely attained statistical significance, and were not clinically robust.

DeWied[59] has stated that these negative results from other centers can be attributed to the fact that schizophrenia is a heterogeneous disorder; thus only a subgroup of patients respond to DTγE. In addition, the Utrecht group has found that duration of illness, duration of last episode, and patient age correlate negatively with response to DTγE.

Recently the Utrecht group has studied the clinical effects of des-enkephalin-gamma-endorphin (DEγE), the shortest fragment of gamma-endorphin with neurolepticlike activity in preclinical studies. Both single-blind and double-blind studies have been conducted.[265] In the single-blind study of four patients (one neuroleptic-free), two patients received 1 mg DEγE IM and two received 10 mg DEγE IM. All four patients were reported to show a marked amelioration of psychotic symptomatology, and two of these were discharged from the hospital. In the double-blind study, nineteen patients were studied and received 3 mg DEγE IM. A significant reduction in BPRS scores was associated with the peptide treatment. Two patients showed no response; four, a slight to moderate response; four, a moderate to marked response; and three, a very marked response.

In their latest review van Ree and De-Wied,[256] adding together results from several of their studies, reported that of forty-three schizophrenic patients treated with

DTγE and twenty-one with DEγE (total of sixty-four patients), thirteen showed no response (<20 percent improvement), nineteen showed a slight response (20–50 percent improvement), sixteen showed a moderate response (50–80 percent), and sixteen showed a marked response (>80 percent). In a recent study Verhoeven and coworkers[266] treated eighteen neuroleptic-free schizophrenic patients with DTγE (1 mg IM/day for ten days) in a double-blind, crossover design. Six patients showed little or no response, seven exhibited a moderate response, and five had a marked response. Paranoid and hebephrenic patients benefited most from DTγE treatment. Clearly, further clinical trials are warranted in this area to determine why, with few exceptions, only the Utrecht group has observed the dramatic and marked antipsychotic effects of DTγE.

Two other neuropeptides have been tested clinically for antipsychotic effects: CCK and TRH. Based on compelling evidence of colocalization of CCK and DA in the mesolimbic system,[97] the effects of treatment with CCK or a related homologous decapeptide, ceruletide, on the symptoms of schizophrenia have been studied. Moroji and associates[171,172] treated twenty chronic schizophrenic patients maintained on antipsychotic drugs with a single injection of ceruletide (0.3 or 0.6 μg/kg, IV), and the BPRS was used to rate symptoms in an open study. After the low dose, five of twelve patients showed improvement in mood, and one patient reported a reduction in auditory hallucinations. After the high dose of the peptide, improved mood was noted in sixteen patients, and reduction in auditory hallucinations was observed in three patients. These improvements were reported to persist for three weeks after injection.

Another group[26,181] has studied the effects of CCK-33 (0.3 μg/kg IV) in chronic schizophrenia. Six chronic paranoid schizophrenic patients maintained on neuroleptic drugs were studied in their first trial. In this open, uncontrolled study, CCK produced a significant reduction in the BPRS score that was maintained for six weeks. In a second study, a single dose of CCK-8 (0.04 μg/kg, IV) was administered to eight chronic schizophrenic patients maintained on neuroleptic drugs. A rapid improvement in psychopathology was observed, and their BPRS and Present State Examination (PSE) scores were significantly reduced. In contrast, no changes in the nurses' observation scale (NOSIE) were observed. Peak improvement was observed six days post-CCK injection.

Stimulated by these preliminary findings, three research groups have evaluated the effects of ceruletide in schizophrenia using a double-blind, placebo-controlled protocol. The results have been quite disappointing.

Hommer and others[101] treated eight neuroleptic-treated schizophrenic patients with ceruletide, increasing IM doses beginning at 0.3 μg per kg twice per day to reach a final dose of 0.6 μg per kg. The peptide produced no amelioration in schizophrenic symptoms as assessed by several rating scales, including the BPRS. Albus and associates[3] have conducted both an open study (six patients) and a double-blind study (twenty patients) with ceruletide. No antipsychotic effects of the peptide were observed. Finally, Mattes and coworkers,[163] in a double-blind study of seventeen chronic, neuroleptic-treated schizophrenic patients, administered ceruletide (0.6 μg/kg IM) or placebo (one week apart). The evaluation included ratings of twenty-nine variables related to prognosis in schizophrenia, as well as BPRS and symptom checklist (SCL)-90 scales. No beneficial effects of the peptide were observed. Recently, Tamminga and her colleagues and Itoh and his colleagues have conducted double-blind trials of CCK in schizophrenia.* No salutary effects of the peptide were observed.

The effects of TRH have been most widely studied in affective disorders; a few studies with schizophrenic patients have been conducted. This literature has been reviewed

---

*Information on the work of Tamminga and colleagues and Itoh and colleagues was gained through personal communications.

most recently by Loosen and Prange[153] in a comprehensive treatise. In general, the results are disappointing, with the exception of one research group. In a single-blind study, TRH was administered orally (4 mg/day) to sixty-two chronic, neuroleptic-treated schizophrenic patients. A beneficial effect was reported within two weeks in 75 percent of the patients. A double-blind study of 143 chronic schizophrenic patients by the same Japanese group confirmed the initial findings. Motivation and social contact were repeatedly most improved. The studies in which TRH was administered IV to schizophrenic patients have been disappointing. Moreover, several investigators have reported that TRH apparently worsened the symptoms of paranoid schizophrenic patients.

TREATMENT OF SCHIZOPHRENIA WITH PEPTIDE ANTAGONISTS

The only neuropeptide antagonists that have been evaluated as putative antipsychotic agents are the opiate/opioid receptor blockers naloxone and naltrexone. Many, but not all, of the trials that have been conducted are described in the following text and the interested reader can refer to the comprehensive reviews of Mueser and Dysken[174] and McNichols and Martin.[157] These studies are based on the hypothesis that schizophrenia is associated with excess CNS opioid activity, and therefore the opioid receptor blockade should ameliorate the symptoms of schizophrenia.

Further impetus for this work was provided by the provocative report of Gunne and associates,[93] who, in a single-blind pilot study, reported that naloxone (0.4 mg IV), but not saline, temporarily reduced or abolished auditory hallucinations in four cases of chronic schizophrenia. The beneficial effects persisted for up to seven hours. Since this initial report, the effects of naloxone in schizophrenia have been intensively studied by some of the best-known clinical neuropsychopharmacology research groups, with mixed results. For the purposes of clarity, we shall first discuss those reports describing positive results.

Lehmann, Nair, and Kline[143] conducted single- and double-blind studies of the effects of naloxone (10 mg IV) in seven chronic schizophrenic men. The diagnostic criteria used and the medication status of the patients was not described. Naloxone was reported to produce statistically significant improvement. In a single case report, Orr and Oppenheimer[194] reported that naloxone (0.4 mg IV), but not placebo, produced a marked reduction in auditory hallucinations and a mild euphoria on three separate occasions in a twenty-eight-year-old chronic schizophrenic patient maintained on antipsychotic drugs.

Watson and his coworkers[273] also used a relatively high dose of naloxone (10 mg IV) in a double-blind, crossover-designed study; all the patients fulfilled DSM-III criteria for schizophrenia (undifferentiated or paranoid). Five patients were maintained on neuroleptics throughout the study, and six were neuroleptic-free for at least two weeks. Both the BPRS and NIMH rating scales were used. Two subjects were studied in a single-blind design and nine in a double-blind paradigm. Of the latter nine patients, six reported a clear-cut improvement in hallucinations, one showed borderline improvement, and two showed no change. The improvement in clinical state reached statistical significance. In a subsequent study,[16] this same group conducted a placebo-controlled, double-blind crossover study to evaluate the effects of naloxone (10 mg IV) in fourteen male chronic schizophrenic patients. The results in this study were similar to their first one: A significantly greater reduction in hallucinations was observed following naloxone than with placebo.

An NIMH study[128] largely confirmed and extended the findings of the Stanford group. In the double-blind NIMH study, naloxone (15 mg IV) produced significant improvement in abnormal thought content in medicated, but not unmedicated, chronic schizophrenic patients. A total of seventeen patients were studied. A World Health Organization (WHO) Collaborative Study[198,202] confirmed these findings—a naloxone-induced reduction in schizophrenic symptom ratings (e.g., auditory hallucinations) in the neuroleptic-treated patients ($N = 19$), but not in the drug-free patients ($N = 13$). Finally, Cohen, Pickar, and Cohen[43] treated four chronic unmedicated schizophrenic patients (DSM-III criteria) with a high dose of naloxone (2 mg/kg IV) versus drug vehicle in a double-blind design. Three of the four patients showed improvements after naloxone, as evidenced by a decrease in BPRS scores.

In contrast to these positive findings, several experienced research groups could detect absolutely no antipsychotic effects of naloxone. In an early study Janowsky and associates[110] reported that naloxone (1.2 mg IV) produced no change in BPRS items associated with schizophrenic symptomatology in eight male schizophrenic patients. In a study with findings one could consider both negative and positive, Davis and co-workers[57] found no effect of naloxone (0.4 mg IV) on global assessment or ratings of hallucinations, psychosis, or conceptual disorganization in nineteen (mostly drug-free) schizophrenic patients. However, a single item, unusual thought content, improved significantly after naloxone.

Volavka and others,[268] using an almost identical experimental design and dose of naloxone, found no significant effects of the drug in seven chronic, neuroleptic-treated schizophrenic patients. Similarly negative findings were reported by Lipinski and colleagues[150] in seven neuroleptic-treated schizophrenic patients who received naloxone (16 mg IV). Verhoeven and associates,[261] who participated in the WHO study on naloxone in schizophrenia, found no effect of naloxone (20 mg subcutaneously [SC]) in a double-blind trial of five chronic schizophrenic patients. In a later study,[262] this same group treated ten schizophrenic patients with naloxone (20 mg SC) for four days. No effects of the opioid antagonist were detected in this double-blind study.

Naber and Leibl[176] studied the effects of repeated high-dose naloxone (20 mg SC for four days) treatment in seven schizophrenic patients (four were neuroleptic-treated). In this double-blind, crossover-designed study, no antipsychotic effects were observed at all.

The orally active opiate antagonist naltrexone has also been studied in schizophrenic patients, with largely negative results—as in the studies of Mielke and Gallant[168] and Simpson, Branchey, and Lee.[229] Mueser and Dysken[174] have reviewed these studies and summarized the current literature; of forty-two schizophrenic patients treated with naltrexone (50–800 mg orally for two to six weeks), only seven improved. The more beneficial results with naloxone compared to naltrexone may be due to the fact that at higher doses, naltrexone reportedly has opiate agonist as well as antagonist properties.

A prudent conclusion from these opiate antagonist studies is that naloxone appears to exert antipsychotic effects in a *subgroup* of *neuroleptic-treated* chronic schizophrenic patients. The magnitude of the antipsychotic effect is not, however, very robust and appears limited to a reduction in the incidence of auditory hallucinations and/or unusual thought content. In addition, naloxone increased motor activity in catatonic schizophrenic patients. The reasons for the conflicting results in the literature are probably multifactorial. These include the heterogeneous composition of any group of schizophrenic patients and the growing awareness of the existence of multiple opiate receptors —at least three (mu, kappa, and sigma) and possibly a fourth (delta)—and the fact that naloxone has differing affinities for these receptors. Further study is clearly warranted.

One of the most problematical and controversial areas in modern psychiatry has been the use of hemodialysis to treat schizophrenia. The therapeutic efficacy of this treatment has recently been refuted in several studies. These studies are, however, pertinent to the neuropeptide literature, because the improvement in schizophrenic patients after hemodialysis was reported to be associated with the appearance in the dialysate of high concentrations of beta-leu[5]-endorphin, a molecule identical to beta-endorphin except for the substitution of leucine for methionine in position 5. It was proposed that this abnormal endorphin, found in extraordinarily high concentrations in schizophrenic patients, was removed from blood by hemodialysis, and therefore, that this peptide might be involved in the pathogenesis of this psychiatric disease.

The reports of abnormally high concentrations of beta-leu[5]-endorphin in plasma or hemodialysates of schizophrenic patients have now been refuted by three research groups.[99,146,214] Lewis and associates[146] examined hemodialysates of two schizophrenic patients and two controls for the presence of beta-leu[5]-endorphin using a radioreceptor assay after gel filtration and HPLC. No beta-leu[5]-endorphin or beta-endorphin was found in the hemodialysates of either the schizophrenic patients or the controls. Ross, Berger, and Goldstein[214] measured beta-endorphin-like immunoreactivity in plasma in ninety-eight schizophrenic patients and forty-two normal controls, using an antiserum that recognized both beta-endorphin and beta-leu[5]-endorphin. No differences in plasma beta-endorphin immunoreactivity were found between the schizophrenic and control subjects. Moreover, no beta-endorphin immunoreactivity was detected in hemodialysates of eight nonpsychotic renal patients and nine schizophrenic patients. Finally, Hollt and coworkers[99] used a sensitive RIA, with equal sensitivity to beta-endorphin and beta-leu[5]-endorphin, to measure the concentration of these peptides in plasma before and after hemodialysis in three schizophrenic patients. The plasma concentrations of beta-endorphin-like immunoreactivity were not elevated in the schizophrenic patients when compared to controls, and moreover, an unexpected increase in beta-endorphin-like immunoreactivity was observed in the schizophrenic patients after hemodialysis. In addition, *in vitro* experiments revealed that neither endorphin is appreciably removed by dialysis. Taken together, the

findings of these three research groups do not support the hypothesis that schizophrenic patients have an excess of an abnormal endorphin molecule, beta-leu[5]-endorphin.

¶ Affective Disorders

Evidence That Neuropeptide-containing Systems Are Altered in Affective Disorders

OPIOID PEPTIDES

The earliest work on opioids in depression was that of Terenius and associates,[242] and we discussed this report in a previous section of this chapter. In this pilot report, the CSF concentration of opioid activity in thirteen manic-depressive patients was measured by radioreceptor assay with ^{3}H-dihydromorphine as the trace ligand during manic, euthymic, and depressed stages of their illness. No diagnostic criteria were described, and lithium treatment was continued during the study. No statistical comparison was sought, since no normal controls were included. Fraction I activity tended to be highest during the manic phase. No correlations between Fraction II concentrations and mental state were evident.

In another early study, Terenius, Wahlström, and Agren[241] presented case histories of five depressed women treated with naloxone (4.8 mg SC, three times per day). No diagnostic criteria were provided, a variety of tricyclic and anxiolytic drug treatments were continued during the trial, and no normal controls or statistical analyses were included. CSF was obtained at least twice, and up to four times, per patient over a twelve-month period, and CSF opioid activity was measured by a radioreceptor assay using ^{3}H-dihydromorphine as the radioactive ligand. No effect of naloxone on Fraction II opioid concentrations was observed, but Fraction I concentrations seemed to decrease with continued naloxone treatment.

These early uncontrolled studies are very

difficult to interpret because of the absence of controls and the inability to characterize what opioid peptide(s) comprise Fraction I. In a later study,[147] nineteen normal controls were compared to four manic-depressive patients. No data were included on the age or sex of these manic-depressive patients, the diagnostic criteria used to classify them, or their current medication status. Radioreceptor assay of the CSF fractions after Sephadex G-10 filtration revealed slightly higher levels of Fraction I opioid activity in the manic phase when compared to the "normal" or depressed phase of the illness.

Recently Terenius and coworkers[1] attempted to assess the possibility of seasonal variation in Fraction I opioid concentrations of unipolar and bipolar depressed patients. The patient population consisted of sixty-two unipolar patients and thirty-two bipolar patients (diagnosed by RDC[18]) who were medication-free, except for benzodiazepines, for at least ten days prior to lumbar puncture. The Fraction I concentrations of opioid activity were adjusted to the same sex, age, height, and weight values by analysis of covariance and plotted according to time of year. No normal controls were used for comparison, and no patient was assessed more than once, rendering interpretation of the findings difficult.

Naber and associates[179,180] and Pickar and others[201] have compared the levels of endogenous opioid activity and immunoreactive beta-endorphin concentrations in CSF of forty-one normal volunteers and thirty-five unipolar and thirteen bipolar patients (diagnosed by RDC[18]). Patients were drug-free for at least fourteen days before CSF collection. This group used ^{3}H-[D-Ala^2] enkephalin-(L-leu-amide)[5] as the competing ligand in the radioreceptor assay for opioid activity and an antiserum to beta-endorphin that exhibited significant cross-reactivity with beta-LPH. Two-way analysis of variance failed to reveal significant differences between the controls and either depressed group or any effect due to sex in either opioid activity or beta-endorphin immunoreactivity. This same group has determined whether carbamazepine alters

CSF opioid activity in a study of thirteen depressed, three manic, and one euthymic patient (diagnosed by RDC[18]). Patients were drug-free for ten days before the first sample of CSF was obtained, and they were then treated with carbamazepine (200–400 mg/day) for an average of thirty-three days before a second CSF sample was obtained. No significant carbamazepine-induced difference in CSF opioid activity was detected.

Gerner and associates[82,85] compared CSF beta-endorphin concentrations in nine normals and in nineteen unipolar and eight bipolar depressed patients (diagnosed by RDC[18]) who were free of antidepressant medication for at least seven days. The antisera used to measure beta-endorphin cross-reacted equally with beta-LPH. Column chromatography of pooled CSF fractions showed beta-LPH in a molar ratio of 1.3 to 1 with beta-endorphin. The use of analysis of variance failed to reveal statistically significant differences in the mean CSF concentrations of beta-endorphin immunoreactivity between either group of depressed patients and the controls.

Brambilla and colleagues[33] measured beta-LPH and beta-endorphin immunoreactivity in the plasma of thirty-five psychiatrically normal controls and nine unipolar primary affective disorder (diagnosed by RDC[18]) and seven secondary affective disorder patients who were drug-free for ten days. The plasma concentration of both beta-LPH and beta-endorphin immunoreactivity was significantly increased ($p < 0.001$, Student's t-test) in the secondary affective disorder patients, while only beta-LPH immunoreactivity in plasma was significantly increased ($p < 0.001$) in the primary affective disorder patients.

Alexopoulos and coworkers[4] and Inturrisi and others[106] reported the effect of the first and second electroconvulsive therapy (ECT) treatment on plasma beta-endorphin concentrations in eleven depressed patients (diagnosed by RDC[18]) and sixteen neurological controls. Patients were drug-free for at least ten days before ECT, and blood was drawn immediately before and fifteen minutes after each ECT treatment. Plasma was extracted with talc, acetone, and hydrochloric acid, and the antiserum to beta-endorphin had approximately 25 percent cross-reactivity to beta-LPH. The concentration of plasma beta-endorphin-like immunoreactivity increased approximately threefold ($p < 0.05$, two-tailed t-test) after each ECT treatment and returned to initial values within forty-eight hours.

OTHER NEUROPEPTIDES

Several other CNS neuropeptides have been measured in the CSF, plasma, and postmortem brain tissue of depressed patients. Gerner and Yamada[83] compared CSF concentrations of SRIF in twenty-eight patients with primary depression, ten patients with mania (diagnosed by RDC[18]), and twenty-nine normal, healthy volunteers. Depressed patients were drug-free for seven days. Antisera to $SRIF_{1-14}$ was directed toward the cyclic part of the $SRIF_{1-14}$ molecule and exhibited 50 percent cross-reactivity with $SRIF_{1-28}$. Depressed, but not manic, patients had significantly less ($p < 0.01$, ANOVA and t-test) SRIF-like immunoreactivity than controls.

Rubinow and associates[220] also reported decreases in CSF concentrations of SRIF-like immunoreactivity in depression. In this comprehensive study, thirty-nine normal, healthy volunteers were compared to eighteen bipolar depressed, seven unipolar depressed, and seven manic patients (diagnosed by RDC[18]). Patients were drug-free for fourteen days. The antisera to SRIF was directed toward the C-terminal, and linear $SRIF_{1-14}$ exhibited 33 percent cross-reactivity. The concentration of SRIF-like immunoreactivity was significantly decreased ($p < 0.001$, t-test) in both unipolar and bipolar patients compared to controls, while the slightly decreased concentrations in manic patients did not achieve statistical significance.

Our research group[22] has also confirmed this decrease in CSF concentrations of SRIF in depression. Healthy volunteers ($N = 10$) were compared to patients ($N = 23$) with a DSM-III diagnosis of major depression. Patients were drug-free for at least two weeks, and unextracted CSF was assayed with an antiserum to cyclic $SRIF_{1-14}$ that has equal affinity for linear $SRIF_{1-14}$ and $SRIF_{1-28}$. Depressed patients had significantly lower concentrations ($p < 0.05$, Student-Newman-Keuls test after ANOVA) of SRIF-like immunoreactivity in CSF than the normal controls.

Recently Rubinow and coworkers[221] observed drug-induced alterations of CSF SRIF-like immunoreactivity. Patients ($N = 15$) with primary affective disorder (diagnosed by RDC[18]) had lumbar CSF withdrawn before and after treatment with carbamazepine (400–1600 mg/day, plasma concentrations of 8.5–12 µg/ml, average treatment duration thirty-two days). Patients were drug-free for at least fourteen days before the first CSF sample was obtained; the CSF was collected in acetic acid. Using a paired t-test, carbamazepine was found to significantly decrease ($p < 0.01$) the CSF concentration of SRIF-like immunoreactivity, while depressed patients treated with desmethylimipramine ($N = 3$), lithium ($N = 6$), or piribedil ($N = 4$) showed no change.

Kirkegaard, Hummer, and Rogowski[126] have measured TRH-like immunoreactivity in CSF of patients ($N = 15$) with endogenous depression before and after ECT and of a variety of nonpsychiatric patients ($N = 20$) undergoing diagnostic lumbar puncture. The diagnostic criteria utilized were not provided, patients were drug-free for one week before CSF withdrawal, and the antiserum to TRH exhibited significant cross-reactivity with both urea and SRIF. Concentrations of TRH-like immunoreactivity in endogenous depression were significantly increased ($p < 0.01$, Wilcoxon test) before and after ECT when compared to the control group.

Gold and associates[88] compared CSF concentrations of arginine vasopressin (AVP) in twenty-one depressed patients, eight manic patients (diagnosed by RDC[18]), and thirty-two normal, healthy volunteers. Patients were drug-free for at least three weeks before the CSF sample was obtained. Unextracted CSF was used, and the antiserum to AVP was reported to be highly specific, with no cross-reactivity toward arginine vasoticin or oxytocin. No sex or age differences were noted. However, depressed patients exhibited CSF AVP concentrations that were significantly lower than controls. When nine bipolar depressed patients were compared to eight manic patients, the manic patients exhibited significantly higher CSF concentrations of AVP than the depressed patients.

Stein and others[237] measured urinary concentrations of AVP in nineteen women on the second to seventh postpartum days and attempted to correlate this with postpartum mood changes. Using a mood rating scale that they devised, mood, thirst, twenty-four-hour weight change, fluid intake, and urine sodium and volume were assessed. No standard errors, patient drug information, RIA methodology, or statistical analysis were presented, but there was reportedly no correlation between the variables listed and urine AVP concentrations.

CCK has been measured in the CSF of twenty-eight depressed and ten manic (diagnosed by RDC[18]) patients and twenty-nine normal, healthy volunteers by Gerner and Yamada.[83] Patients were drug-free for seven days before CSF was obtained, and CCK was assayed by an antiserum that cross-reacts with gastrin, though the latter peptide was not detected in CSF using another antiserum. No significant difference in CSF concentrations of CCK-like immunoreactivity was observed between any of the diagnostic groups, and no effect of age or sex was evident. Verbanck and colleagues[259] have also measured CCK-like immunoreactivity in thirty depressed patients (Feighner's criteria[18]) and fifty-one psychiatrically normal controls. Depressed patients were drug-free for fourteen days before CSF withdrawal, CSF was not extracted, and the CCK antisera reacted equally with $gastrin_{2-17}$ and both sulfated and nonsulfated forms of CCK. The bipolar depressed ($N = 12$), but not the unipolar depressed ($N = 18$), patients had significantly lower ($p < 0.05$) concentrations of CSF CCK-like immunoreactivity when compared to the controls.

Perry and associates[195] measured the concentration of CCK in the entorhinal cortex of nine patients with "chronic, unipolar depression" and compared them to twelve normal controls. No criteria for the diagnosis of depression or patient medication information was included, no rationale for scrutiny of this particular brain region was provided, and no statistical method was identified. No differences in the entorhinal cortex concentration of CCK was observed between the depressed patients and the controls.

Sub P has been measured in the CSF of twelve depressed patients (diagnosed by RDC[18]) and fifteen controls receiving either treatment for urologic disease or undergoing diagnostic x-ray procedures.[212] Patients were drug-free for at least two weeks prior to CSF withdrawal. The CSF was extracted with Sep-Pak cartridges, recovery was 60 to 80 percent, and the antiserum recognized sub P_{1-5}. The depressed group had significantly elevated concentrations of CSF sub P–like immunoreactivity. Electrophoresis of pooled CSF showed very little authentic sub P_{1-11}, with the 5–11 and 3–11 fragments contributing the majority of the immunoreactivity.

Kaiya and associates[119] measured sub P–like immunoreactivity in unextracted plasma obtained from thirteen normal volunteers, eight patients with bipolar affective disorder, and twenty-four patients with major depression (DSM-III criteria[18]). The medication status of the patients was not described, and no information about the specificity of the antiserum was provided. No significant group-related differences in plasma sub P concentrations were found.

Gerner and Yamada[83] compared CSF concentrations of BOM in twenty-nine normal volunteers, ten manic patients, and twenty-eight patients with major depression (diagnosed by RDC[18]). Patients were drug-free for seven days prior to CSF withdrawal, CSF was assayed unextracted, and the antiserum to BOM did not cross-react with a variety of structural homologs and other peptides. Use of ANOVA and t-test failed to reveal any statistically significant difference between either patient group and the controls.

Our research group[192] has measured CSF concentrations of CRF in ten normal volunteers and twenty-three patients with major depression (DSM-III criteria[18]). The impetus for this study was provided by the finding that approximately two-thirds of depressed patients exhibit hyperactivity of the hypothalamic-pituitary-adrenal axis. Measurement of CRF in CSF should provide information about possible CRF hypersecretion in depression. Patients were drug-free for at least fourteen days before CSF withdrawal, CSF was assayed unextracted, and the antiserum used recognizes the 33 to 41 amino acid region of CRF. Both ANOVA followed by Student-Newman-Keuls test and Mann-Whitney U-test found significant ($p < 0.05$ and $p < 0.025$, respectively) elevations in CSF concentrations of CRF-like immunoreactivity in the depressed group compared to the controls. However, post-dexamethasone plasma cortisol concentrations were not correlated with CSF concentrations of CRF-like immunoreactivity in the depressed patients. We have recently confirmed these findings in a collaborative study with Fink at Stonybrook and Banki in Hungary.[24]

Gjerris and coworkers[86] have compared CSF and plasma concentrations of VIP in sixteen neurological controls and eight manic, fourteen nonendogenously depressed, and twenty-four endogenously depressed patients (ICD criteria[18]). CSF was obtained before drug or ECT was initiated. Aprotinin, a peptidase inhibitor, was used in the collection of CSF and blood, and an RIA for VIP was used. Using the Kruskal-Wallis test and the median concentration values rather than arithmetic means, patients with nonendogenous depression were reported to exhibit CSF concentrations of VIP that were statistically ($p < 0.01$) lower than controls. After the patients received drug or ECT, CSF was again obtained from five manic patients, six nonendogenously depressed patients, and thirteen endogenously depressed patients to assess whether any alteration in CSF or

plasma VIP concentrations had occurred. However, no differences in either CSF or plasma were seen after clinical recovery, and no differences in plasma concentration were seen between patient groups.

Lindström and associates[149] have measured DSIP concentrations in the CSF of twenty normal controls and ten patients with major depression (diagnosed by RDC[18]). Patients were drug-free for at least two weeks before CSF withdrawal, CSF was centrifuged before assay, and the antiserum to DSIP was specific for the N-terminal region of the molecule. No significant difference was found between the mean depressed and control group CSF concentrations of DSIP-like immunoreactivity.

Carman and coworkers[38] measured the concentration of calcitonin in the CSF from forty-two normal volunteers, nineteen manic patients, seventeen bipolar depressed patients, and ten unipolar depressed patients (diagnosed by RDC[18]). Patients were medication-free for four weeks before CSF withdrawal, CSF was not extracted, and the antiserum was directed toward the midportion of the calcitonin molecule. Although detectable levels of calcitonin were present in only 51 percent of the normal and depressed patients and 11 percent of the manic patients, Student's t-test was used to claim a significant decrease ($p < 0.05$) in the concentration of calcitoninlike immunoreactivity of CSF in the manic patients compared to both control and depressed groups. Not unexpectedly, a positive correlation was observed between CSF concentrations of Ca^{++} and calcitonin.

Treatment of Affective Disorders with Neuropeptides

Patients with endogenous depression and mania have been treated with neuropeptides in the hope that one might prove to be an effective pharmacotherapeutic agent. The work with opioid peptides has been reviewed by Brambilla, Genazzani, and Facchinetti[32] and Berger and associates.[17] Kline and others,[130] in the same early uncontrolled study in which beta-endorphin was administered to schizophrenic patients, also administered the peptide to patients with unipolar depression. Of three patients tested (on one or two occasions), the mood of the depressed patients was reportedly improved after beta-endorphin (1.5–6.0 mg IV). It is difficult to evaluate this open study with so few patients.

Gerner and colleagues[84] administered beta-endorphin (10 mg IV) to ten depressed patients (and eight schizophrenic patients) in a double-blind, placebo-controlled, crossover design. The depressed patients were significantly improved in overall ratings. Patients were reported to show altered facial expression, reduced psychomotor retardation, increased social interaction, and a less depressed speech content after beta-endorphin. This same group found similar, though statistically insignificant, effects in another study.[41] In an uncontrolled study, Angst and associates[6] reported that three of six depressed patients became hypomanic after IV injection of 10 mg beta-endorphin. Pickar and coworkers[200] conducted a double-blind, placebo-controlled study of four depressed patients to evaluate the effects of intravenously administered beta-endorphin (0.15 mg/kg). No significant effects of the peptide were observed.

The effects of the stable met-ENK analogue FK-33-824 in depressed patients (ICD classification[18]) have been evaluated in an open study[127] using the Hamilton Rating Scale for depression. Nine depressed patients received 0.5 mg of the peptide on day 1 and 1.0 mg on day 2. No beneficial effects of FK-33-824 were found.

Other neuropeptides have been studied as potential antidepressants; these include TRH, LHRH, melanocyte-stimulating hormone-release inhibiting factor (MIF-I), and calcitonin.

The effects of TRH have been intensively studied in patients with affective disorders, and these findings have been comprehensively reviewed by Prange and his coworkers.[153,205,207,208] In 1972 Prange and Wilson[206] reported that TRH (500 μg IV) produced a prompt, partial but significant antidepressant effect in ten unipolar depressed women. The study used a placebo-controlled, double-blind, crossover design, and the behavioral responses were assessed with the Hamilton Rating Scale for depression. Similar results were obtained by Kastin and his colleagues.[122]

A large number of clinical trials with TRH have subsequently been conducted—the results have been quite disappointing. It is now clear that TRH is not a clinically efficacious antidepressant agent. However, many studies have confirmed that approximately 25 percent of depressed patients exhibit a blunted or absent TSH response after IV TRH administration. This is described in detail in chapter 4.

The only report concerning treatment with LHRH in affective disorders is the brief note by German and Stampfer.[80] In this uncontrolled study of twenty patients with major depression (unipolar or bipolar) and eight patients with "stress-associated" depression (no criteria for either diagnosis), each patient received a single IM injection of LHRH (500 mg). All twenty-seven patients reported improved sleep the following night, and the eight patients characterized with "stress-associated" depressions continued to have improved sleep for several months. No indication of concurrent medication status was provided, no controls were included, and no statistical comparison was performed.

The antidepressant effects of MIF-I were first described by Ehrensing and Kastin.[66,67] In their first double-blind study, depressed women (involutional melancholia or manic-depressive illness, depressed type) received oral MIF-I (60 or 150 mg) for six days. The lower dose was more effective than the higher one; four of five patients improved in the low-dose group. In their second study, this same group examined the effects of daily MIF-I (75 or 750 mg orally) in eight depressed patients, using a randomized double-blind design. Again the lower dose produced greater improvement than the higher one or placebo, as assessed by four depression rating scales.

Recently Levy, DeNigris, and Davis[145]

compared the effects of orally administered MIF-I (60 mg/day) with imipramine hydrochloride (75 mg/day), a clinically efficacious antidepressant, in patients fulfilling RDC[18] for major depressive disorder. Three of the six patients receiving MIF-I did very poorly and were dropped from the study. These authors concluded that this tripeptide was devoid of antidepressant properties and was certainly not superior to imipramine.

In contrast, van der Velde[251] reported a rapid and robust antidepressant effect of MIF-I. In this study, twenty psychiatric inpatients (fifteen males, five females) who fulfilled RDC[18] for major depressive disorder were assigned in a double-blind study to either daily MIF-I (60 mg orally) or imipramine (150 mg in a divided dose). The Hamilton and Zung rating scales, as well as a global assessment scale, were utilized, and the data were statistically evaluated by analysis of variance for repeated measures. The study was designed so that patients not improving after one week would be dropped—two MIF-I-treated patients and four imipramine-treated patients were removed from the trial. Both MIF-I and imipramine exerted a significant antidepressant effect, but the MIF-I effect was more rapid; on day 8 of the study, the MIF-treated group had significantly lower Hamilton Rating Scale scores than the imipramine-treated group. These findings are concordant with those of Ehrensing and Kastin and indicate that MIF-I may indeed possess antidepressant properties. Further work is clearly warranted in larger patient populations with this peptide.

Gold and his colleagues[88] have scrutinized the vasopressinergic system in affective disorders and have also studied the effects of a behaviorally active vasopressin analogue that is devoid of pressor activity, 1-desamino-8-D-arginine vasopressin (DDAVP), on cognitive function in depressed patients. The peptide was administered intranasally, 40 to 160 μg per day for two to seven weeks, to four depressed patients; controls received 60 μg DDAVP per day for two to three weeks. A statistically significant increase in learning and memory scores was observed in both the depressed patients and the control subjects after DDAVP treatment. In two of the four depressed patients, DDAVP produced an apparent antidepressant effect. Three other depressed patients exhibited improved cognitive function without any significant effect on their depressed mood. In addition, the effects of DDAVP on ECT-induced retrograde amnesia in two patients were also studied, and the peptide reversed this troublesome side effect. The effects of vasopressin have also been studied in normal volunteers and in patients with a variety of other neuropsychiatric disorders; these data are described in a later section.

Treatment of Affective Disorders with Peptide Antagonists

As in schizophrenia research, considerable attention has been directed to the potential role of endogenous opioid systems in mood disorders. As described, several investigators have hypothesized that depression is a state of opioid deficiency, and they have therefore tested beta-endorphin as a potential therapeutic agent. Others, in contrast, have used the opiate antagonists as potential drugs to treat depression or mania, with the view that one of these affective disorders is associated with hyperactivity of opioid systems. These studies have been comprehensively reviewed by Pert and associates,[196] Berger,[13] and Brambilla and others.[32]

The consensus of several studies appears clear: Naloxone either has no effect or worsens the symptoms of patients with major depression.[57,241] In a recent study Cohen and coworkers[45] studied the effects of naloxone (2 mg/kg IV) in six depressed inpatients and eight normal controls in a double-blind paradigm. The opioid antagonist produced a significant worsening in the signs and symptoms of depression in the patient group, without any noticeable effect in the normal controls.

In contrast to the null or deleterious effects observed after naloxone treatment in depressed patients are the salutary effects reported after naloxone administration in patients with mania. Davis and associates[57] observed a clear antimanic effect of naloxone (0.4–30 mg IV) in one of four patients. The following year Judd and his colleagues[116] treated eight manic patients with naloxone (20 mg IV), and four exhibited a clear reduction in symptoms. Janowsky and others[111] observed similar effects. However, in the WHO Collaborative Study,[202] naloxone (0.3 mg SC) was found to have no beneficial effect in twenty-six manic patients. One obvious difference between the different trials of naloxone in mania is the dose of the drug tested. High doses of naloxone seem necessary for it to have an antimanic effect.

Captopril is not a peptide receptor antagonist but an inhibitor of angiotensin-converting enzyme and enkephalinase. Zubenko and Nixon[283] recently reported that three depressed patients exhibited substantial mood-elevation after oral captopril treatment.

¶ Alzheimer's Disease

Evidence That Neuropeptide-containing Systems Are Altered in Alzheimer's Disease

Alzheimer's disease (AD) is now believed to be the most disabling disease of the elderly; it accounts for approximately one-half of all cases of dementia. It has been estimated to be the fourth leading cause of death of the elderly in the United States. The emotional, physical, and economic stress on the family members of patients with AD is very high. The magnitude of this problem is expected to increase as the elderly population of this country increases. First described in 1906 by Alois Alzheimer, AD is characterized by progressive loss of cognitive and other higher intellectual functions.[135] Considerable research has confirmed and extended Alzheimer's original findings of neuropathological alterations in the CNS of these patients. Neurofibrillary tangles and senile (neuritic)

plaques, particularly in the neocortex and hippocampus, are the anatomical hallmarks of the disease (see Terry and Katzman[243]).

It is now clear that there is a genetic component to AD. In the last several years, a multitude of advances in basic neuroscience, specifically neurochemistry, have resulted in a greater understanding of the function of several neurotransmitter systems in the brain. The capability of quantitating regional brain concentrations of monoamine, amino acid, and neuropeptide neurotransmitter substances (and, in some cases, their associated biosynthetic enzymes and receptors) has now been applied to research in AD. Several independent research groups have now unequivocally demonstrated a marked reduction in the activity of choline acetyltransferase (CAT), the enzyme that synthesizes acetylcholine (ACh), in several postmortem brain regions of patients with AD.[30,48,49] Immunohistochemical studies have revealed a marked loss of cholinergic perikarya in the substantia innominata (basal nucleus of Meynert), and other aspects of cholinergic function, such as ACh synthesis and choline uptake, are also reduced in AD.[48]

The integrity of neuropeptide-containing systems has also been investigated in AD. Several research groups have observed a marked reduction in the concentration of SRIF, an endogenous tetradecapeptide, in postmortem samples of cerebral cortex and hippocampus from patients with AD.* In their first study, Davies and his colleagues[55] observed a marked reduction in the concentration of SRIF, measured by RIA, in postmortem tissue (hippocampus, frontal cortex, parietal cortex, and superior temporal gyrus) of patients with AD (histologically verified) when compared to samples from twelve neurologically normal controls. In a second study, Davies and Terry[54] measured SRIF immunoreactivity in eight postmortem brain regions of twelve normal controls and twelve cases of AD. Of the eight regions examined, SRIF concentrations were reduced in seven (midfrontal cortex, inferior parietal cortex,

*See references 54, 55, 74, 189, and 216.

occipital cortex, superior temporal gyrus, midtemporal gyrus, inferior temporal gyrus, and hippocampus) and unchanged in one (anterior cingulate gyrus). Use of a Biogel P-10 chromatography column indicated that greater than 80 percent of the SRIF immunoreactivity eluted with the synthetic peptide. Crystal and Davies[52] also noted that the most profound reductions in SRIF concentrations occurred in the AD patients with an early onset of the disease.

Our group[189] has obtained somewhat similar findings in ten AD patients and ten controls. SRIF-like immunoreactivity was significantly reduced in two cortical areas, Brodmann's areas 10 and 38 (frontal and temporal cortex) and the hypothalamus, but unchanged in the caudate, substantia innominata, posterior hippocampus, nucleus accumbens, amygdala, and Brodmann's area 7 (parietal cortex). Rossor and his colleagues[216] obtained results almost identical to our own. The concentration of SRIF immunoreactivity was significantly reduced in AD in the temporal cortex (Brodmann's area 21) but not in the two other cortical areas (Brodmann's areas 10 and 21) nor in the amygdala, posterior hippocampus, or putamen. In contrast, CAT was reduced in all of the regions studied except the putamen.

Ferrier and associates[74] measured the concentration of several neuropeptides, including SRIF, in postmortem brain tissue from twelve patients with AD and thirteen controls. The concentration of SRIF was significantly reduced in the septum and three cortical areas (temporal, parietal, and frontal cortex) and increased in the substantia innominata. No change in SRIF levels was seen in the hippocampus, amygdala, putamen, globus pallidus, nucleus accumbens, dorsomedial thalamus, lateral thalamus, hypothalamus, or cingulate cortex. In the temporal cortex, a significant correlation between CAT activity and SRIF concentration was found for the total number of subjects studied (controls and AD patients); animal studies have revealed no significant colocalization of SRIF and ACh in the projections from the substantia innominata.[49]

Recently Rossor and his colleagues[219] have reviewed their nine studies of neuropeptides in AD. Of eight peptides measured, only SRIF was significantly reduced in AD. They confirmed the findings of Crystal and Davies[52]—that is, only the younger AD patients exhibit the SRIF deficit. In addition, a significant inverse correlation between neuropathological indices of severity (plaque counts and neurofibrillary tangle estimates) and SRIF reduction in temporal cortex was observed.

Recently Arai, Moroji, and Kosaka[7] measured SRIF by RIA in twenty-one regions of postmortem brain from seven histologically verified AD patients and ten controls. The concentration of SRIF was significantly reduced in the orbital cortex, hippocampus, and putamen. Finally, Joynt and McNeill[115] have utilized immunocytochemical methods to investigate SRIF-containing neural systems in AD. They studied four cases of AD and appropriate controls. SRIF-containing neuronal perikarya were distributed largely in layers III and V of the middle frontal cortex. In the AD tissue, the SRIF-containing neurons were shrunken and irregularly shaped, and the number of small-sized SRIF neurons was increased, with a concomitant decrease in the large SRIF-containing multipolar and bipolar cells.

The concentrations of other neuropeptides have been studied in AD. We found no differences in TRH concentration between controls and AD patients in a variety of subcortical and cortical areas,[189] and similar findings have been reported by Yates and others[282] and Biggins and coworkers.[20] The integrity of VIP-containing neurons has been studied in AD, largely because of its high concentration in the normal cerebral cortex. In an early study Rossor and associates[217] measured VIP by RIA in five cortical areas, as well as in the hippocampus, caudate, and globus pallidus, of seven control and seven histologically confirmed cases of AD. No AD-associated alteration in VIP content was observed in any brain region. Perry and coworkers[195] assayed VIP in the postmortem entorhinal cortex of twelve normal controls and ten patients with AD; no difference in VIP concentration was observed in the AD group when compared to the controls. Ferrier and colleagues[74] assayed VIP by RIA in fourteen brain areas from twelve patients with AD and thirteen controls. No alteration in VIP concentration in any brain area was observed in the AD group.

In contrast to all of these findings is the recent report of Arai, Moroji, and Kosaka,[7] who found a significant reduction in VIP concentration in two (insular and cingular) of twenty-one regions studied in seven postmortem AD cases when compared to the results obtained in ten normal controls.

CCK, a peptide found in very high concentration in the cerebral cortex, has been assayed in AD. All investigators agree that this peptide is not reduced in postmortem brain samples of patients with AD,[74,196,217,222] although the latter group found *increases* of CCK immunoreactivity in the white, but not gray, matter of the cortex, from patients with AD.

Crystal and Davies[52] measured the concentration of sub P in eight postmortem brain regions of thirteen normal controls and twelve patients with AD. The undecapeptide was reported to be slightly, but significantly, reduced in five of seven cortical areas but not in the hippocampus of AD patients. This finding has not been confirmed by Ferrier and his colleagues.[74]

Recently Rossor and his coworkers[219] summarized their studies of neuropeptides in AD. With the exception of the reduction of SRIF just described, they have found no alteration in the concentration of CCK, TRH, VIP, vasopressin, oxytocin, enkephalin, or NT. Our group[187] has also measured the concentrations of NT in AD. Only in the amygdala did we observe a significant (30 percent) reduction in NT. Sanders, Zahedi-Asl, and Marr[222] reported that glucagon concentrations are unchanged in the CNS of AD patients.

Bissette and associates[23] have recently discovered a marked decrease in the concentrations of CRF-like immunoreactivity in AD in the frontal cortex (Brodmann's area 10), temporal cortex (Brodmann's area 38), and caudate nucleus, with normal concentrations in the parietal cortex (Brodmann's area 7), amygdala, nucleus accumbens, posterior hippocampus, hypothalamus, and substantia innominata.

Several investigators have measured neuropeptides in CSF of AD patients in the hope that a diagnostic test might be forthcoming from such results. There is widespread agreement that CSF SRIF concentrations are indeed reduced in AD patients. However, as noted, SRIF concentrations are also reduced in patients with major depression and other diseases in which cognitive dysfunction is prominent. Thus, as a diagnostic test, measurement of SRIF in CSF has apparently reasonable sensitivity but poor specificity.

In brief, SRIF has been found to be reduced in CSF of patients with AD, "mixed dementia," Huntington's chorea, multiple sclerosis, Parkinson's disease with dementia, brain atrophy, and depression.* Of particular interest is our recent observation[121] that AD patients who are exposed to intensive environmental stimulation (increased emotional and intellectual contact) exhibit significant increases in CSF SRIF, but not CCK or CRF, concentrations.

Other neuropeptides have been measured in the CSF of dementia patients. Kaiya and associates[120] reported that the concentration of beta-endorphin is reduced in CSF of patients with AD, Huntington's chorea, and brain vascular disease, although the largest reductions were observed in the AD group. This finding has now been confirmed.[114] Facchinetti and coworkers[73] reported a small, statistically insignificant reduction in CSF beta-endorphin in AD but a marked reduction in CSF ACTH concentrations.

Two groups have measured CSF AVP concentrations in AD and have obtained opposite results. Tsuji, Takahashi, and Akazawa[245] found elevated CSF AVP concentrations in sixteen patients with AD when compared to

---

*See references 10, 22, 50, 64, 114, 134, 141, 193, 220, 228, 233, 235, 236, and 281.

eight controls. Sorensen and colleagues[235] found lower CSF AVP concentrations in sixteen AD patients when compared to twenty-eight control patients.

Treatment of Alzheimer's Disease with Neuropeptides

The rationale for the study of neuropeptides as potentially useful therapeutic drugs in the treatment of AD comes from two sources. First are the studies, described earlier, in which neuropeptides (e.g., SRIF) have been shown to be reduced in concentration in postmortem tissue of AD patients. Based on these findings, one obvious approach is to "replace" the neuropeptide loss. The second strategy is provided by preclinical studies that demonstrate cognitive improvement in animals after treatment with a neuropeptide (e.g., adrenocorticotrophic hormone [ACTH] or vasopressins). The problems and promises of this approach have recently been reviewed by Berger and Tinklenberg.[14]

Few studies of either kind have been adequately conducted. In a recent brief report, Cutler and associates[53] have evaluated the effects of a stable and potent analog of SRIF (L363,586) in AD. Ten patients with mild AD received a short IV infusion (120 μg for 30 min) followed by a longer infusion at a slower rate (40 μg/hr for 5.5 hrs). After the study, plasma and CSF concentrations of the analogue were assayed. No effect of L363, 586 on either social or paired-associate learning was found; a small, almost significant increase in arithmetic scores was observed, but this was said to be clinically irrelevant. Plasma concentrations of the SRIF analogue were increased, but CSF concentrations were undetectable.

The potent $ACTH_{4-9}$ fragment (ORG 2766) has been studied in AD patients. Ferris[77] treated fifty mildly to moderately impaired senile dementia outpatients with ORG 2766 (10–20 mg daily for two weeks). Ratings of mood appeared to improve, but cognitive improvement was minimal. Soininen and others[234] conducted a double-blind, six-month, placebo-controlled study of ORG 2766 (20 mg b.i.d.) in seventy-seven patients with AD. No beneficial effects of the peptide were evident.

Vasopressins have also been tested in AD, and these findings have been reviewed by Ferris[77] and Tinklenberg and associates.[244] The results are very disappointing. For example, Chase and coworkers[42] administered lysine-VP to seventeen AD patients in a placebo-controlled, double-blind study. No salutary effects of the peptide were evident.

¶ Neuropeptides and Other Psychiatric Disorders

Measurement of Neuropeptides in Other Psychiatric Disorders

The major focus of neuropeptide research in psychiatry has been in schizophrenia, affective disorders, and AD. In addition, the role of neuropeptides in nociception and chronic pain states is of interest. This subject has been comprehensively reviewed[154] and is discussed in chapter 26 of this book. It is therefore omitted from this chapter. Opioid peptides have been measured in other disease states. For example, Katz and associates[124] measured CSF beta-endorphin-like immunoreactivity in seventy-five children with acute leukemia, and the data were analyzed in relation to the degree of behavioral stress in these children. The results derived were all correlational in nature due to the absence of any controls. It appeared that CSF beta-endorphin increased with increasing distress. Genazzani[79] and coworkers measured the concentrations of beta-endorphin, beta-LPH, and ACTH in plasma and CSF of twenty-nine alcoholic subjects (three to ten days postwithdrawal) and eight normal volunteers. No differences in plasma concentrations of the three peptides were noted, but alcoholic subjects had markedly elevated CSF beta-endorphin levels and markedly low ACTH levels, when compared to the controls. This finding suggests alterations in pro-opiomelanocortin peptide circuits in the CNS of alcoholic subjects. Savoldi[223] has recently reviewed and updated these data. Thirty-two healthy male volunteers and thirty-four alcoholic subjects have now been studied. The latest results confirm the initial observations.

Veith and colleagues[258] studied nine normally cycling women and seven women taking oral contraceptives to determine whether any relationship existed between plasma beta-endorphin concentrations and anxiety during the menstrual cycle. A significant correlation between plasma beta-endorphin levels and anxiety was found throughout the menstrual phase. Marked variance in plasma beta-endorphin concentrations was found in the ovulatory phase.

Finally, Coid, Allolio, and Rees[46] measured plasma met-ENK, ACTH, and beta-LPH concentrations in ten drug-free patients who habitually mutilated themselves (habitual self-mutilation and DSM-III borderline personality disorder) and in healthy controls. Mean plasma met-ENK concentrations were significantly elevated in the patients who habitually mutilated themselves compared to controls.

Effects of Neuropeptides in Normal Volunteers and Patients with Other Psychiatric or Medical Disorders

The effects of opioid peptides in a variety of disease states have been evaluated. Von Graffenried and associates[271] reported that the enkephalin analogue FK-33-824 (0.1–1.2 mg IM or 0.5 mg IV) produced feelings of heaviness in the muscles of the body, pressure in the chest, and tightness in the throat (with concomitant anxiety). Most subjects exhibited an increase in bowel sounds, redness of the face, and conjunctival injection and chemosis, but none of the classical effects of morphine (e.g., changes in alertness and affective state). Electroencephalogram (EEG) recordings revealed a slowing of alpha waves and an increase in the beta band.

Recently Pickar, Dubois, and Cohen[199] re-ported that a patient with adenocarcinoma of the pancreas (with metastases) who received 3 mg beta-endorphin intrathecally noted a decrease in pain, but this was followed by progressive euphoria, confusion, fragmented thought, disorientation, agitation, and stereotyped motor behavior. Auditory and visual hallucinations were also present more than twenty-four hours after the beta-endorphin injection. By the third day postinjection, the patient's mental status returned to his baseline state.

Opioid peptides, as expected, have been shown to suppress withdrawal symptoms in heroin addicts. For example, Wen and Ho[275] reported that dynorphin$_{1-13}$ (60 μg/kg IV) suppressed withdrawal symptoms in eighteen heroin addicts. Unfortunately, no methadone group was included to compare with the dynorphin group; this would have provided direct comparison with the efficacy of a currently used and effective therapeutic modality.

Earlier in this chapter, we reviewed the data on treatment of schizophrenia with DTγE. In two studies by Casey and his colleagues,[40] this peptide has been administered to patients with tardive dyskinesia (TD). Fourteen patients with TD received DTγE (0.5–120 mg IM); no beneficial effects of the peptide were observed.

As noted, vasopressins have been administered to patients with affective disorders. These peptides have also been administered to young and old normal male volunteers to evaluate their effects on memory. Nebes, Reynolds, and Horn[182] conducted a double-blind crossover study to assess the effects of the vasopressin DDAVP (20–90 μg intranasally/day) on memory function in twenty-four young men (ages twenty to thirty years) and twenty-four older men (ages sixty to seventy years). Although the peptide did not alter semantic memory retrieval time or simple vocal reaction time, it did reduce memory comparison time and perceptual motor time of short-term memory, as well as retrieval time in long-term memory in both young and old subjects. Weingartner and associates[274] reported that DDAVP

(30–60 μg t.i.d. for 2–3 weeks) improved serial learning and recall of semantically related words and prompted free recall. Beckwith and others[11] found that DDAVP enhanced learning in a concept shift task, but not in a simple novel memory test. Anderson and coworkers[5] reported that two of three children with Lesch-Nyhan syndrome, previously unable to learn a passive avoidance task, did so after treatment with DDAVP. Stimulated by these findings, Eisenberg and others[68] treated seventeen children with learning disorders (e.g., attention deficit disorder) with DDAVP (20 μg intranasally) or placebo for ten days. There was a tendency for the peptide to exert a beneficial effect, although the changes were not statistically significant.

The putative memory-enhancing effects of ACTH and ACTH fragments in preclinical studies have led to their evaluation in man. In general, the human studies have been disappointing. For example, D'Elia and Frederiksen[58] have evaluated the effects of $ACTH_{4-10}$ on memory function in twenty depressed patients undergoing ECT and in twenty healthy normal controls using a double-blind paradigm. A single dose of $ACTH_{4-10}$ (30 mg IV) had no effect in the normal controls or in the depressed patients receiving ECT. The results from the double-blind studies are not consistent with the notion that $ACTH_{4-10}$ is useful to treat memory dysfunction in man. The behavioral effects of ACTH have been comprehensively reviewed by Branconnier.[34]

In the last few years, increasing attention has been paid to DSIP, a nonapeptide found in the CNS that induces a delta-sleep EEG pattern in experimental animals. These studies have been reviewed by Schoenenberger and Schneider-Helmert.[227] In their first double-blind study of six normal controls, slow IV infusion of DSIP (25 nmol/kg/20 min) administered in the morning resulted in the feeling of sleepiness and, consequently, increased sleep. That night, sleep onset was reduced, stage 1 sleep was relatively reduced, and sleep efficiency increased. In a study of six

middle-aged chronic insomniac patients, DSIP (25 nmol/kg) also resulted in longer sleep duration, a higher quality of sleep, and more rapid-eye-movement sleep. There was no daytime sedation and the salutary effects persisted for up to six nights. Repeated DSIP injections in four severe insomniac patients led to increasingly greater total sleep duration. These behavioral findings were confirmed by EEG recordings. Surprisingly, DSIP produced an increase of alertness two to twenty hours postinjection. In many cases, repeated DSIP injections completely normalized the disturbed sleep of chronic insomniac patients.[226] In a recent study, DSIP was administered to two patients with neurotic insomnia who were studied under double-blind, placebo-controlled conditions on a psychotherapy unit. The patients were noted to have improved ego function after DSIP by both rating psychotherapists—the patients were less rigid, confronted their problems better, and were more extroverted and self-assured. One must wonder whether these effects of DSIP on ego function are merely secondary to the improved sleep of the patients. Recently Kaeger[118] reported that in an open study, ten IV injections of DSIP (25 μmol/kg over 4 min) over fourteen days, given to seven chronic insomniac patients, normalized sleep in all but one patient for three to seven months.

Of considerable interest is the recent report of Dick and associates,[61] who studied the effect of DSIP (25 nmol/kg IV) injections (as many as six injections per day) on withdrawal syndromes from alcohol and opiates. Forty-seven patients undergoing ethanol withdrawal were studied. DSIP produced a marked reduction in physical and psychological withdrawal symptoms in both opiate and alcohol withdrawal states, although the former group required more DSIP injections to achieve clinical improvement.

CCK has, as noted earlier, been studied as a potentially novel treatment of schizophrenia. However, this peptide has also been studied as an appetite suppressant in animals and man. The satiety produced by CCK in rats has been extensively studied by Smith, Gibbs, and their colleagues, and these findings have been reviewed recently.[230] In man, CCK also reduces food consumption.

The effects of TRH in normal volunteers have been studied, and these findings have recently been reviewed by Loosen and Prange.[153] In an early study Wilson and associates,[279] using a double-blind paradigm, reported that TRH (500 μg IV) produced relaxation, mild euphoria, and a sense of increased energy in ten normal women. These findings were largely confirmed by Betts and colleagues[19] in a study of ten normal women who were treated with TRH (80 mg orally) or placebo in a double-blind paradigm. Recently Wilson, Prange, and Loosen[278] reported that thyroid hormone pretreatment (25 μg T_3 + 100 μg T_4) blocked the mild euphoric effects of TRH in normal women, and Winokur and his colleagues[280] have confirmed these findings. In a double-blind study of ten healthy women, TRH (400 μg IV) produced a significant improvement in ratings of tension using a visual analogue scale (100 mm line test).

Effects of Opioid Antagonists in Normal Controls and Patients with Other Psychiatric Disorders

Naloxone has been administered to normal volunteers in order to determine the effects of blockade of opioid receptors and therefore to investigate the physiological role of endorphins and enkephalins. Goldstein and Hansteen,[90] in an unusual double-blind case study, administered IV naloxone (3 or 10 mg) or saline to a thirty-five-year-old male staff member who proceeded to masturbate five minutes after the IV injection. Time to erection, time from erection to ejaculation, and total time from erection to ejaculation were no different after naloxone treatment than after saline treatment. The authors concluded that opioids do not mediate sexual arousal, penile erection, ejaculation, or orgasm in human males. Cohen and associ-

ates[44] have studied the effects of high dose (0.3–4.0 mg/kg IV) naloxone infusions in nine healthy volunteers (five women and four men) in a single-blind design to determine the effects of complete blockade of endogenous opioid systems. As the dose of the opioid antagonist was increased, significant dysphoria (tension-anxiety and anger-hostility), decreased performance on memory testing, and increased systolic blood pressure and respiratory rate were noted. These findings are concordant with the view that endogenous opioid systems modulate mood, memory, and certain autonomic functions. Mendelson and colleagues[165] evaluated the effects of naltrexone (50 mg orally) on mood in seven normal male volunteers in a double-blind study. All subjects correctly identified naltrexone from placebo. Like the naloxone study of Cohen and others,[44] naltrexone produced dysphoria characterized by fatigue, sleepiness, light-headedness, nausea, sweating, and occasional feelings of unreality. In contrast to the single case report of Goldstein and Hansteen[90] concerning naloxone, three of the seven subjects reported spontaneous penile erections after naltrexone.

Investigators have administered naloxone and measured pain sensitivity to determine if blockade of opioid receptors alters nociception. Levine and associates[144] reported that naloxone (9 mg IV) enhanced the pain present after surgical removal of impacted molars. Buchsbaum, Davis, and Bunney[35] reported that naloxone (2 mg IV) increased pain sensitivity in normal subjects found at baseline to be relatively pain insensitive. In contrast, Grevert and Goldstein[91] found no effect of naloxone (2 or 10 mg IV) in a double-blind study on chronic pain in twelve subjects. A significant decrease in tension and anxiety was observed. Arnsten and coworkers[8] recently reported that naloxone (2 mg IV) augments electrophysiological correlates of selective attention in normal volunteers; auditory stimuli were utilized. Ewing and McCarthy[72] have studied the effects of naloxone treatment on the intoxicating effects of ethanol. Naloxone (0.4 mg SC) did not modify the mood or physiological changes associated with ethanol intoxication. These findings do not support the hypothesis that the CNS effects of ethanol are mediated by endogenous opioids.

The pathophysiology of TD is currently poorly understood. The possibility that endogenous opioid systems may play a role in TD has been studied. Bjorndal, Casey, and Gerlach[25] treated eight psychiatric patients with TD with either naloxone (0.8 mg IM), morphine (10 mg SC), or the met-ENK analogue FK-33-824 (1–3 mg IM). The study was conducted by blind evaluation of videotapes. The opiates exerted a slight, but significant, effect in reducing the symptoms of TD in the neuroleptic-treated patients, whereas naloxone produced no significant effects. Blum and associates[29] evaluated the effects of naloxone (0.4 mg IV) in two schizophrenic women with TD in a placebo-controlled, double-blind study. In one of the two patients, naloxone significantly reduced orofacial dyskinetic movements. In a separate study, these same authors[27] reported that a thirty-six-year-old woman with diagnosed partial adrenal 21-hydroxylase deficiency, schizophreniform psychosis, and TD responded to naloxone (0.4 mg IV every four hours for four days followed by 0.8 mg IV every four hours for two and one-half days) with improvement in her psychiatric symptoms and elimination of the dyskinetic movements. Volavka, Anderson, and Goz[267] studied the effects of naloxone and naltrexone in TD and found no beneficial effects of these opioid receptor antagonists. Blum and Korczyn[27] have reviewed the evidence for the involvement of neuropeptides in the pathophysiology of TD. They concluded that data provided by animal research lent plausibility to the hypothesis that neuropeptides such as endorphins, CCK, sub P, and NT are involved in the pathogenesis of TD, but the available clinical data has yet to be generated. The finding that cyclo-leu-Gly treatment inhibits the proliferation of D-2 DA receptors after chronic haloperidol administration should serve as an impetus to determine if it could prevent the development of TD in man.

Volavka and associates[269] evaluated the effects of naloxone (10 or 20 mg IV) on short-term memory in twenty-six male volunteers. No significant effects on immediate recall, delayed recall, or delayed recognition were observed after administration of the opiate antagonist.

The involvement of endogenous opioid systems in obsessive-compulsive disorder has been studied by Insel and Pickar[105] by treating two such patients with naloxone. Both patients experienced an exacerbation of chronic obsessional doubt after naloxone in a double-blind, placebo-controlled study.

Finally, naltrexone is now routinely being used to treat opiate addicts after detoxification.[87] Once patients are withdrawn from opiates and placed on a chronic naltrexone regimen, opiate administration no longer produces rewarding euphoric effects.

¶ Discussion

In this review, we have attempted to provide an overview of neuropeptides in psychiatric disorders. This research field, in its infancy, has provided results of sufficient interest to stimulate further study. Although much remains to be elucidated, a few findings seem of particular interest. There is no doubt that much of our ignorance concerning the role of neuropeptides in the pathogenesis of neuropsychiatric disorders resides with the lack of tools sufficient to assess the functional activity of neuropeptide-containing systems in the CNS. The current situation is indeed reminiscent of our understanding of monoamine systems in the 1960s. We now have available exquisitely sensitive RIAs that can usually measure as little as 0.5 pg of a peptide. However, their specificity is often not adequately studied, and the nature of the peptide immunoreactivity has frequently not been characterized. One potential problem in measuring neuropeptides in postmortem tissue is rapid degradation after death; fortunately, neuropeptides such as SRIF and NT are remarkably stable in this regard. Of equal concern is our inability to routinely measure neuropeptide turnover or biosynthesis. However, advances in molecular biology are now being applied to neuropeptide biosynthesis and processing. Only recently have structural analogues of neuropeptides been synthesized which, when radiolabeled, result in radioligands suitable to detect high-affinity binding sites for these substances in brain membranes. Simply stated, we can determine whether neuropeptide concentrations are altered in postmortem brain tissue or CSF in a particular disease state, but what such a finding means is still unclear. Thus, a 50 percent reduction in the concentration of a neuropeptide might be due to degeneration of neuropeptide-containing neurons or, perhaps, to greatly increased utilization of neuropeptide-containing circuits in which biosynthesis cannot keep up with release. Whether CSF or tissue concentrations of neuropeptides accurately reflect extracellular fluid concentrations at relevant synaptic receptor sites in the CNS also remains to be determined.

The current literature on measurement of neuropeptides in human CSF and brain tissue is difficult to evaluate because of the existence of several potentially confounding variables. Some of these can be controlled, but others are inherent to this type of experimentation. First, we must consider the confounding effects of the use of different diagnostic criteria. This problem cannot be solved at the present time, because the validity of each currently used nosological classification (DSM-III, RDC, etc.) is undetermined, and also because application of the same diagnostic criteria within different research centers often results in poor interrater reliability. It is evident that the inclusion of a nonpsychiatric control group must be considered a requirement in all future studies.

Patient drug use in CSF and postmortem tissue studies is an obvious confounding factor; therefore, this variable must be described, and, if possible, patients should be drug-free for as long a time as is practicable and ethical prior to obtaining CSF or plasma for neuropeptide measurement. In the CSF studies, some researchers use one or another extraction method, whereas others assay the CSF without extraction (neat). Generally speaking, such an extraction step is unnecessary unless there are substances present that interfere with the assay or unless enzymes are present in the biological tissue or fluid that will degrade the neurohumor under investigation. Virtually none of the reports that use extracted CSF have presented data showing its necessity. Plasma, urine, and, of course, tissue samples must be extracted because of the variety and concentration of substances they contain. Regardless of whether or not an extraction step is performed, data on recovery of exogenously added peptide should be included in the report. Unfortunately, less than 5 percent of published studies include this essential information. When describing an RIA, it is necessary to explicitly describe the sensitivity and specificity of the assay. Specificity should include information as to which region or amino acid sequence of the molecule is recognized by the antiserum and whether structures containing homologous sequences exhibit cross-reactivity. It is, of course, important to know that a variety of other neuropeptides (with dissimilar structures) do not cross-react with your antiserum; however, this is not the most important data. The most pertinent information in evaluating a particular RIA is the concentration at which one observes 50 percent displacement of trace ligand (IC_{50}), the minimal detectable concentration (sensitivity, pg/tube), and the inter- and intraassay coefficients of variation. In reviewing the literature for this chapter, we found very few reports that supply this minimal epidemiological, drug-related, and assay information.

When working with plasma, CSF, urine, or any uncharacterized tissue source of immunoreactivity, some attempt must be made to identify the nature of the immunoreactivity. Liquid column chromatography, gel permeation chromatography, and HPLC are some of the methods that may be employed to study this problem; the method chosen usually depends on the quantity of the starting material.

It is disturbing to report that *most* of the studies we reviewed contained either no statistical analysis or used an inappropriate statistical test. The use of Student's t-test should be restricted to comparing two groups (total in the entire study) of normally distributed data. With the advent of advanced computer statistical software and, it is hoped, the appreciation that statistical analysis of data is essential, there is no longer any excuse for inappropriate or nonexistent statistical methodology. We believe that reports without appropriate statistical analysis should not be accepted for publication, with the exception, possibly, of clinical case reports.

The criticisms we have outlined in this section are not meant to belittle or demean the research performed to date, which, in many instances, is in fact pioneering work. Instead, these guidelines are intended to provide a framework for future study design so that cross-study comparison can be made with a minimum of confounding factors. In these types of human studies, it is certainly the retrospective examination of a variety of observations among different investigators and patient populations that will eventually reveal the important, diagnostically dependent, group differences.

What is left is to draw conclusions from the current literature. Our thoughts parallel our organization of the chapter. As a treatment, neuropeptides have certainly not yet been shown to be effective in any major psychiatric disorder, including schizophrenia, affective disorders, or anxiety. Beta-endorphin is clearly ineffective in schizophrenia, and the use of DTγE in schizophrenia remains quite controversial. As noted earlier, the Utrecht group has consistently observed antipsychotic effects with DTγE in schizophrenic patients. In open studies, CCK seems to possess antipsychotic effects, but this has not been confirmed in double-blind studies. The opioids seem to have no significant antidepressant activity, and of the other neuropeptides tested, the most positive studies are of those with MIF-I. In three double-blind studies, it has exhibited significant antidepressant activity. One must conclude that the neuropeptide treatment strategy is in its infancy, and considerable work in drug design and clinical neuropsychopharmacology must take place.

The peptide antagonist studies are of considerable interest. It seems clear that naloxone, in a subset of schizophrenic patients, reduces hallucinations and unusual thought content. Naloxone either has no effect or worsens depression. In contrast, a few groups have observed clear-cut antimanic effects of the opioid antagonist.

As we discussed, the peptide measurement studies (in CSF, brain tissue, plasma, and urine) are fraught with difficulties of data interpretation. Nevertheless, several promising findings have emerged. The reduction in the concentration of SRIF in brain tissue from patients with AD has now been widely confirmed. The peptide has even been observed as components of the neurofibrillary tangles and plaques that are the neuropathological hallmark of AD. Thus, along with ACh-containing neurons, SRIF-containing neurons degenerate in AD. Preliminary results from our own laboratory indicate a decrease in CRF-like immunoreactivity in two cortical brain areas in AD. Clearly, neuropeptide systems are pathophysiologically involved in AD. As the neurobiology of these neuropeptidergic systems is elucidated, appropriate treatment regimens might be devised to "normalize" the peptidergic dysfunction.

Other promising findings from the measurement studies must provoke interest. Although the CSF opioid peptide studies in schizophrenia have not been fruitful, the NT, CCK, and DSIP studies in similar patients showed differences worth additional study. The postmortem tissue measurements studies have not revealed large differences between controls and any diagnostic psychiatric group regarding peptide concentrations. Nevertheless, the data base is very small, and further peptide study is certainly warranted.

Peptide receptor studies will provide valuable data.

The therapeutic use of peptides in other psychiatric disorders is a new research area. Of the studies conducted thus far, the use of DSIP in insomnia seems the most reproducible and exciting.

We have repeatedly emphasized throughout the chapter the notion that advances in clinical neuropeptide neuropsychopharmacology must await advances in neuropeptide physiology and pharmacology. For example, basic questions relating to the passage of administered neuropeptides from the blood to the brain remain unanswered. This is, of course, a flaw of all of the peptide treatment studies; in almost no case did any of the investigators have relevant clinical or animal data on whether the peptide, in the dose used, actually entered the CNS to increase its concentrations at relevant extracellular fluid sites in the vicinity of peptidergic receptors. If peptides have difficulty penetrating the blood-brain barrier, then drug design strategies must be appreciably altered. The opioids provide a convenient example. The entry of beta-endorphin into the CNS from the vascular compartment is low, but measurable. In contrast, opiate alkaloids such as morphine and dihydromorphine are lipophilic and are, therefore, readily able to enter brain and act at opiate receptor sites. It may be imperative to identify nonpeptidergic, lipophilic compounds that act on peptidergic receptor sites and can readily enter the CNS. If we regard the last fifteen years of research as preliminary findings, then the next decade will almost certainly witness a veritable explosion in neuropeptide research, with an emphasis on molecular biology. The impact of this research in psychiatry, especially in the areas of stress and its associated disorders (e.g., anxiety), depression, and AD, will certainly be great.

¶ Acknowledgments

We are grateful to Mary Lassiter for help in preparation of this manuscript. The authors are supported by NIMH MH-39415, MH-40524, MH-40159, and a grant from the Schizophrenia Research Foundation. Charles B. Nemeroff is the recipient of a Nanaline H. Duke Fellowship from Duke University. The authors' research in schizophrenia is also supported by the Gorrell Family Psychiatric Research Fund.

¶ Bibliography

1. AGREN, H., and TERENIUS, L. "Depression and CSF Endorphin Fraction I: Seasonal Variations and Higher Levels in Unipolar Than Bipolar Patients," *Psychiatry Research*, 10 (1983):303–311.

2. AKIL, H., et al. "Enkephalin-like Material in Normal Human CSF: Measurement and Levels," *Life Sciences*, 23 (1978): 121–126.

3. ALBUS, M., et al. "Ceruletide: A New Drug for the Treatment of Schizophrenic Patients?" *Archives of General Psychiatry*, 41 (1984):528.

4. ALEXOPOULOS, G. S., et al. "Plasma Immunoreactive β-endorphin Levels in Depression," *Archives of General Psychiatry*, 40 (1983):181–183.

5. ANDERSON, L. T., et al. "Avoidance Learning in Lesch-Nyhan Disease. Effect of 1-Desamino-8-arginine-vasopressin," *Life Sciences*, 24 (1979):905–910.

6. ANGST, J., et al. "Preliminary Results of Treatment With β-endorphin in Depression," in E. Usdin, W. E. Bunney, Jr., and N. S. Kline, eds., *Endorphins in Mental Health Research*. London: Macmillan, 1979, pp. 518–528.

7. ARAI, H., MOROJI, T., and KOSAKA, K. "Somatostatin and Vasoactive Intestinal Polypeptide in Post-Mortem Brains from Patients with Alzheimer-Type Dementia," *Neuroscience Letters*, 52 (1984):73–78.

8. ARNSTEN, A.F.T., et al. "Naloxone Augments Electrophysiological Signs of Selective Attention in Man," *Nature*, 304 (1983):725–727.

9. BARCHAS, J. D., et al. "Opioid Agonists and Antagonists in Schizophrenia," in E. Costa and M. Trabucchi, eds., *Neural Peptides and Neuronal Communica-*

tion. New York: Raven Press, 1980, pp. 447–453.

10. BEAL, M. F., and MARTIN, J. B. "Somatostatin: Normal and Abnormal Observations in the Central Nervous System," in R. J. Wurtman, S. H. Corkin, and J. H. Growden, eds., *Alzheimer's Disease: Advances in Basic Research and Therapies.* Zurich: Center for Brain Sciences and Metabolism Charitable Trust, 1984, pp. 229–257.

11. BECKWITH, B. E., et al. "Vasopressin Analog (DDAVP) Facilitates Concept Learning in Human Males," *Peptides,* 3 (1982):627–630.

12. BERGER, P. A. "Biochemistry and the Schizophrenias: Old Concepts and New Hypotheses," *Journal of Nervous and Mental Disease,* 169 (1981):90–99.

13. ———. "Endorphins in Emotions, Behavior and Mental Illness," in L. Temoshok, C. Van Dike, and L. S. Vegans, eds., *Mind and Medicine: Emotions in Health and Illness.* New York: Grune & Stratton, 1983, pp. 153–166.

14. BERGER, P. A., and TINKLENBERG, J. R. "Neuropeptides and Senile Dementia," in T. Cook and S. Gershon, eds., *Strategies for the Development of an Effective Treatment for Senile Dementia.* New Haven, Conn.: Mark Powley Assoc., 1981, pp. 155–171.

15. BERGER, P. A., et al. "β-endorphin and Schizophrenia," *Archives of General Psychiatry,* 37 (1980):635–640.

16. BERGER, P. A., et al. "The Effects of Naloxone in Chronic Schizophrenia," *American Journal of Psychiatry,* 138 (1981): 913–918.

17. BERGER, P. A., et al. "Behavioral Pharmacology of the Endorphins," *Annual Review of Medicine,* 33 (1983):397–415.

18. BERNER, P., et al. *Diagnostic Criteria for Schizophrenia and Affective Psychoses.* Washington, D.C.: World Psychiatric Association, American Psychiatric Press, 1984.

19. BETTS, T. A., et al. "The Effects of Thyrotropin-releasing Hormone on Measures of Mood in Normal Women," *British Journal of Clinical Pharmacology,* 3 (1976):469–473.

20. BIGGINS, J., et al. "Post-mortem Levels of Thyrotropin-releasing Hormone and Neurotensin in the Amygdala in Alzheimer's Disease, Schizophrenia and Depression," *Journal of Neurological Sciences,* 58 (1983):117–122.

21. BISSETTE, G., and NEMEROFF, C. B. "Neuropeptides and Schizophrenia," *Progress in Brain Research,* in press.

22. BISSETTE, G., et al. "Reductions of Cerebrospinal Fluid Concentrations of Somatostatin-like Immunoreactivity in Dementia, Major Depression and Schizophrenics (Abstract)," *Society of Neuroscience,* 10 (1984):1093.

23. BISSETTE, G., et al. "Reduced Cortical and Striatal Concentrations of Corticotropin-releasing Factor (CRF)-like Immunoreactivity in Senile Dementia of the Alzheimer Type," *Journal of the American Medical Association,* in press.

24. BISSETTE, G., et al. "Further Studies of Corticotropin-releasing Factor-like Immunoreactivity in CSF of Patients with Affective Disorders (Abstract)," *Society of Neuroscience,* 11, in press.

25. BJORNDAL, N., CASEY, D. E., and GERLACH, J. "Enkephalin, Morphine, and Naloxone in Tardive Dyskinesia," *Psychopharmacology,* 69 (1980):133–136.

26. BLOOM, D. M., NAIR, N.P.V., and SCHWARTZ, G. "CCK-8 in the Treatment of Schizophrenia," *Psychopharmacology Bulletin,* 19 (1983):361–363.

27. BLUM, I., and KORCZYN, A. D. "Peptide Neurotransmitters and Their Implications for the Treatment of Tardive Dyskinesia," *Modern Problems in Pharmacopsychiatry,* 21 (1983):187–195.

28. BLUM, I., et al. "Effect of Naloxone on the Neuropsychiatric Symptoms of a Woman with Partial Adrenal 21-Hydroxylase Deficiency," *American Journal of Psychiatry,* 140 (1983):1058–1060.

29. BLUM, I., et al. "Naloxone May Be Beneficial in the Treatment of Tardive Dyskinesia," *Clinical Neuropharmacology,* 7 (1984):265–267.

30. BOWEN, D. M., et al. "Choline Acetyltransferase Activity and Histopathology of Frontal Neocortex from Biopsies of Demented Patients," *Journal of Neurological Sciences,* 57 (1982):191–202.

31. BRAITMAN, D. J., AUKER, C. R., and CAR-

PENTER, D. O. "Thyrotropin-releasing Hormone Has Multiple Actions in Cortex," *Brain Research,* 194 (1980):244–248.

32. BRAMBILLA, F., GENAZZANI, A., and FACCHINETTI, F. "Endogenous Opioid Peptides in Schizophrenia and Affective Disorders," in N. S. Shah and A. G. Donald, eds., *Psychoneuroendocrine Dysfunction.* New York: Plenum Press, 1984, pp. 309–329.

33. BRAMBILLA, F., et al. "β-Endorphin and β-Lipotropin Plasma Levels in Chronic Schizophrenia, Primary Affective Disorders and Secondary Affective Disorders," *Psychoneuroendocrinology,* 6 (1981):321–330.

34. BRANCONNIER, R. J. "The Human Behavioral Pharmacology of the Common Core Heptapeptides," *Pharmacology and Therapeutics,* 14 (1981):161–175.

35. BUCHSBAUM, M. S., DAVIS, G. C., and BUNNEY, W. E., Jr. "Naloxone Alters Pain Perception and Somatosensory Evoked Potentials in Normal Subjects," *Nature,* 270 (1977):620–622.

36. BUCHSBAUM, M. S., DAVIS, G. C., and VAN KAMMEN, D. P. "Diagnostic Classification and the Endorphin Hypothesis of Schizophrenia: Individual Differences and Psychopharmacological Strategies," in C. Baxter and T. Melnechuk, eds., *Perspectives in Schizophrenia Research.* New York: Raven Press, 1980, pp. 177–191.

37. BURBACH, J.P.H., et al. "Schizophrenia and Degradation of Endorphins in Cerebrospinal Fluid," *Lancet,* 2 (1979):480–481.

38. CARMAN, J. S., et al. "Reduced CSF Calcitonin in Mania," in C. Perris, G. Strüwe, and B. Jansson, eds., *Biological Psychiatry.* Amsterdam: Elsevier/ North Holland Biomedical Press, 1981, pp. 457–461.

39. CARRAWAY, R., and LEEMAN, S. E. "The Isolation of a New Hypotensive Peptide, Neurotensin, From Bovine Hypothalamus," *Journal of Biological Chemistry,* 248 (1973):6854–6861.

40. CASEY, D. E., et al. "Effect of Des-Tyrosine-γ-Endorphin in Tardive Dyskinesia," *Archives of General Psychiatry,* 38 (1981):158–160.

41. CATLIN, D. H., et al. "Clinical Studies with Human β-Endorphin," in R. F. Beers, Jr., and E. G. Bassett, eds., *Polypeptide Hormones.* New York: Raven Press, 1980, pp. 337–345.

42. CHASE, T. N., et al. "Vasopressin Treatment of Cognitive Deficits in Alzheimer's Disease," in S. Corkin et al., eds., *Alzheimer's Disease: A Report of Progress.* New York: Raven Press, 1982, pp. 457–461.

43. COHEN, M. R., PICKAR, D., and COHEN, R. M. "High-dose Naloxone Administration in Chronic Schizophrenia," *Biological Psychiatry,* 20 (1985):573–575.

44. COHEN, M. R., et al. "High Dose Naloxone Infusions in Normals," *Archives of General Psychiatry,* 40 (1983):613–619.

45. COHEN, M. R., et al. "High Dose Naloxone in Depression," *Biological Psychiatry,* 19 (1984):825–832.

46. COID, J., ALLOLIO, B., and REES, L. H. "Raised Plasma Met-Enkephalin in Patients Who Habitually Mutilate Themselves," *Lancet,* 2 (1983):545.

47. COSTA, E., and TRABUCCHI, M. "Regulatory Peptides: From Molecular Biology to Function," *Advances in Biochemical Psychopharmacology,* 33 (1982):1–561.

48. COYLE, J. T., PRICE, D. L., and DELONG, M. R. "Alzheimer's Disease: Disorder of Cortical Cholinergic Innervation," *Science,* 219 (1983):1184–1190.

49. COYLE, J. T., et al. "Neurotransmitter Specific Alterations in Dementing Disorders: Insights from Animal Models," *Journal of Psychiatric Research,* 18 (1984):501–512.

50. CRAMER, H., et al. "Huntington's Chorea —Measurements of Somatostatin, Substance P and Cyclic Nucleotides in the Cerebrospinal Fluid," *Journal of Neurology,* 225 (1981):183–187.

51. CROW, T. J. "Schizophrenia," in T. J. Crow, ed., *Disorders of Neurohumoural Transmission.* London: Academic Press, 1982, pp. 287–340.

52. CRYSTAL, H. A., and DAVIES, P. "Cortical Substance P-like Immunoreactivity in Cases of Alzheimer's Disease and Senile Dementia of the Alzheimer Type," *Journal of Neurochemistry,* 38 (1982): 1781–1784.

53. CUTLER, N. R., et al. "Evaluation of an

Analogue of Somatostatin (L363,586) in Alzheimer's Disease," *New England Journal of Medicine,* 312 (1985):725.

54. DAVIES, P., and TERRY, R. D. "Cortical Somatostatin-like Immunoreactivity in Cases of Alzheimer's Disease and Senile Dementia of the Alzheimer Type," *Neurobiology of Aging,* 2 (1981):9–14.

55. DAVIES, P., KATZMAN, R., and TERRY, R. D. "Reduced Somatostatin-like Immunoreactivity in Cerebral Cortex from Cases of Alzheimer's Disease and Alzheimer Senile Dementia," *Nature,* 288 (1980):279–280.

56. DAVIS, G. C., BUCHSBAUM, M. S., and BUNNEY, W. E. "Research in Endorphins and Schizophrenia," *Schizophrenia Bulletin,* 5 (1979):244–250.

57. DAVIS, G. C., et al. "Intravenous Naloxone Administration in Schizophrenia and Affective Illness," *Science,* 197 (1977): 74–77.

58. D'ELIA, G., and FREDERIKSEN, S-O. "$ACTH_{4–10}$ and Memory in ECT-Treated Patients and Untreated Controls. II. Effect on Retrieval," *Acta Psychiatria Scandinavica,* 62 (1980): 429–435.

59. DEWIED, D. "Endorphins and Psychopathology," in R. Collu et al., eds., *Brain Peptides and Hormones.* New York: Raven Press, 1982, pp. 137–147.

60. DEWIED, D., et al. "Neuroleptic-like Activity of [Des-Tyr^1]-γ-Endorphin in Rats," *Lancet,* 1 (1978):1046.

61. DICK, P., et al. "DSIP in the Treatment of Withdrawal Syndromes from Alcohol and Opiates," *European Neurology,* 23 (1984):364–371.

62. DOMSCHKE, W., DICKSCHAS, A., and MITZNEGG, P. "CSF β-Endorphin in Schizophrenia," *Lancet,* 1 (1979):1024.

63. DUPONT, A., et al. "Rapid Inactivation of Enkephalin-like Material by CSF in Chronic Schizophrenia," *Lancet,* 2 (1978):1107.

64. DUPONT, E., et al. "Low Cerebrospinal Fluid Somatostatin in Parkinson's Disease: An Irreversible Abnormality," *Neurology,* 32 (1982):312–314.

65. EDWARDSON, J. A. and McDERMOTT, J. R. "Neurochemical Pathology of Brain Peptides," *British Medical Bulletin,* 38 (1982):259–264.

66. EHRENSING, R. H., and KASTIN, A. J. "Melanocyte-Stimulating Hormone Release Inhibiting Hormone as an Antidepressant: A Pilot Study," *Archives of General Psychiatry,* 35 (1974): 63–65.

67. ———. "Dose-Related Biphasic Effect of Prolyl-leucyl-Glycinamide (MIF) in Depression," *American Journal of Psychiatry,* 135 (1978):562–566.

68. EISENBERG, J., et al. "A Controlled Trial of Vasopressin Treatment of Childhood Learning Disorder," *Biological Psychiatry,* 19 (1984):1137–1141.

69. EMRICH, H. M., et al. "A Measurement of β-Endorphin-Like Immunoreactivity in CSF and Plasma of Neuropsychiatric Patients," in Y. H. Erlich et al., eds., *Modulators, Mediators and Specifiers in Brain Function.* New York: Plenum Press, 1979, pp. 307–317.

70. EMRICH, H. M., et al. "β-Endorphin-Like Immunoreactivity in Cerebrospinal Fluid and Plasma of Patients with Schizophrenia and Neuropsychiatric Disorders," *Pharmakopsychiatria,* 12 (1979): 269–276.

71. EMRICH, H. M., et al. "Des-tyrosyl-γ-endorphin in Schizophrenia: A Double-blind Trial in 13 Patients," *Pharmakopsychiatria,* 13 (1980):290–298.

72. EWING, J. A., and McCARTHY, D. "Are the Endorphins Involved in Mediating the Mood Effects of Ethanol?" *Alcoholism: Clinical and Experimental Research,* 7 (1983):271–275.

73. FACCHINETTI, F., et al. "Central ACTH Deficit in Degenerative and Vascular Dementia," *Life Sciences,* 35 (1984): 1691–1697.

74. FERRIER, I. N., et al. "Neuropeptides in Alzheimer's Type Dementia," *Journal of Neurological Sciences,* 62 (1983):159–170.

75. FERRIER, I. N., et al. "Reduced Cholecystokinin-like and Somatostatin-like Immunoreactivity in Limbic Lobe Is Associated with Negative Symptoms in Schizophrenia," *Life Sciences,* 33 (1983):475–482.

76. FERRIER, I. N., et al. "Alterations in Neuropeptides in the Limbic Lobe in Schizophrenia," in M. R. Trimble and E. Zaritan, eds., *Psychopharmacology of*

the Limbic System. Oxford: Oxford University Press, 1984, pp. 244–254.

77. FERRIS, S. H. "Neuropeptides in the Treatment of Alzheimer's Disease," in B. Reisberg, ed., *Alzheimer's Disease: The Standard Reference.* New York: Macmillan, 1983, pp. 369–373.

78. FINK, M., et al. "Clinical Trials with Destyr-gamma Endorphin (GK-78)," in C. Perris, G. Strüwe, and B. Jansson, eds., *Biological Psychiatry.* Amsterdam: Elsevier/North Holland Biomedical Press, 1981, pp. 398–401.

79. GENAZZANI, A. R., et al. "Central Deficiency of β-Endorphin in Alcohol Addicts," *Journal of Clinical Endocrinology and Metabolism,* 55 (1982):583–586.

80. GERMAN, D., and STAMPFER, H. G. "Hypothalamic Releasing Factor for Reactive Depression," *Lancet,* 2 (1979):789.

81. GERNER, R. H. "Cerebrospinal Fluid Cholecystokinin and Bombesin in Psychiatric Disorders and Normals," in R. M. Post and J. C. Ballenger, eds., *Neurobiology of Mood Disorders,* Baltimore: Williams & Wilkins, 1984, pp. 388–392.

82. GERNER, R. H., and SHARP, B. "CSF β-Endorphin-immunoreactivity in Normal, Schizophrenic, Depressed, Manic, and Anorexic Subjects," *Brain Research,* 237 (1982):244–247.

83. GERNER, R. H., and YAMADA, T. "Altered Neuropeptide Concentrations in Cerebrospinal Fluid of Psychiatric Patients," *Brain Research,* 238 (1982):298–302.

84. GERNER, R. H., et al. "β-Endorphin: Intravenous Infusion Causes Behavioral Change in Psychiatric Inpatients," *Archives of General Psychiatry,* 37 (1980): 642–647.

85. GERNER, R. H., et al. "Endorphins: CSF Levels and Multidose Studies in Psychiatric Subjects," in C. Perris, G. Strüwe, and B. Jansson, eds., *Biological Psychiatry.* Amsterdam: Elsevier/North Holland Biomedical Press, 1981, pp. 386–389.

86. GJERRIS, A. G., et al. "Vasoactive Intestinal Polypeptide (VIP) in Cerebrospinal Fluid in Psychiatric Disorders," in C. Perris, G. Strüwe, and B. Jansson, eds., *Biological Psychiatry.* Amsterdam: Elsevier/North Holland Biomedical Press, 1981, pp. 359–362.

87. GOLD, M. S., et al. "Naltrexone, Opiate Addiction and Endorphins," *Medicinal Research Reviews,* 2 (1982):211–246.

88. GOLD, P. W., et al. "Vasopressin in Affective Illness: Direct Measurement, Clinical Trials and Response to Hypertonic Saline," in R. M. Post and J. C. Ballenger, eds., *Neurobiology of Mood Disorders.* Baltimore: William & Wilkins, 1984, pp. 323–339.

89. GOLDSTEIN, A. "Opioid Peptides (Endorphins) in Pituitary and Brain," *Science,* 193 (1976):1081–1086.

90. GOLDSTEIN, A., and HANSTEEN, R. W. "Evidence Against Involvement of Endorphins in Sexual Arousal and Orgasm in Man," *Archives of General Psychiatry,* 34 (1977):1179–1180.

91. GREVERT, P., and GOLDSTEIN, A. "Effects of Naloxone on Experimentally Induced Ischemic Pain and/or Mood in Human Subjects," *Proceedings of the National Academy of Sciences* (USA), 74 (1977):1291–1294.

92. GRIFFITHS, E. C., MCDERMOTT, J. R., and SMITH, A. I. "A Comparative Study of Neurotensin Inactivation by Brain Peptidases from Different Vertebrate Species," *Comparative and Biochemical Physiology,* 77C (1984):363–366.

93. GUNNE, L-M, LINDSTRÖM, L., and TERENIUS, L. "Naloxone-induced Reversal of Schizophrenic Hallucinations," *Journal of Neural Transmission,* 40 (1977):13–19.

94. HARRIS, G. W. "Humours and Hormones," *Journal of Endocrinology,* 53 (1972):ii–xxiii.

95. HENRY, J. L. "Electrophysiological Studies on the Neuroactive Properties of Neurotensin," *Annals of the New York Academy of Science,* 400 (1982):216–227.

96. HOEBEL, B. "Neurotransmitters in the Control of Feeding and Its Rewards: Monoamines, Opiates and Brain-gut Peptides," in A. J. Stunkard and E. Stellar, eds., *Eating and Its Disorders.* New York: Raven Press, 1984, pp. 15–38.

97. HOKFELT, T., et al. "Evidence for Coexistence of Dopamine and CCK in Mesolimbic Neurons," *Nature,* 285 (1980): 476–478.

98. HOKFELT, T., et al. "Occurrence of Neurotensin-like Immunoreactivity in Subpopulations of Hypothalamic, Mesencephalic and Medullary Catecholamine Neurons," *Journal of Comparative Neurology,* 222 (1984):543–559.

99. HOLLT, V., et al. "Endorphins in Schizophrenia: Hemodialysis/Hemoperfusion are Ineffective in Clearing β-leu⁵-Endorphin and β-endorphin from Human Plasma," *Pharmakopsychiatria,* 12 (1979):399–406.

100. HOLLT, V., et al. "β-Endorphin-like Immunoreactivity in CSF and Plasma of Neuropsychiatric Patients," in N. S. Shah and A. G. Donald, eds., *Endorphins and Opiate Antagonists in Psychiatry.* New York: Plenum Press, 1982, pp. 231–243.

101. HOMMER, D. W., et al. "The Effects of Ceruletide in Schizophrenia," *Archives of General Psychiatry,* 41 (1984):617–619.

102. HUGHES, J. "Strategies for Manipulating Peptidergic Transmission," in R. J. Wurtman, S. H. Corkin, and J. H. Growden, eds., *Alzheimer's Disease: Advances in Basic Research Therapies.* Zurich: Proceedings of the 3rd Meeting of the International Study Group on Treatment of Memory Disorders Associated with Aging, 1984, pp. 259–273.

103. IBATA, Y., et al. "Co-existence of Dopamine and Neurotensin in Hypothalamic Arcuate and Periventricular Neurons," *Brain Research,* 269 (1983):177–179.

104. IBATA, Y., et al. "Light and Electron Microscopic Immunocytochemistry of Neurotensin-like Immunoreactive Neurons in the Rat Hypothalamus," *Brain Research,* 302 (1984):221–230.

105. INSEL, T. R., and PICKAR, D. "Naloxone Administration in Obsessive-compulsive Disorder: Report of Two Cases," *American Journal of Psychiatry,* 140 (1983):1219–1220.

106. INTURRISI, C. E., et al. "β-Endorphin Immunoreactivity in the Plasma of Psychiatric Patients Receiving Electroconvulsive Treatment," *Annals of the New York Academy of Science,* 413 (1982):413–423.

107. IVERSEN, L. L., IVERSEN, S. D., and SNYDER, S. H., eds. *Neuropeptides,* vol. 16 of *Handbook of Psychopharmacology.* New York: Plenum Press, 1983, pp. 1–577.

108. IVERSEN, L. L., et al. "Calcium-dependent Release of Somatostatin and Neurotensin from Rat Brain *In Vitro,*" *Nature,* 273 (1978):161–162.

109. JACOBOWITZ, D. M., et al. "Localization of GRF-like Immunoreactive Neurons in the Rat Brain," *Peptides,* 4 (1983):521–524.

110. JANOWSKY, D. S., et al. "Lack of Effect of Naloxone on Schizophrenic Symptoms," *American Journal of Psychiatry,* 134 (1977):926–927.

111. JANOWSKY, D., et al. "Naloxone Effects on Manic Symptoms and Growth Hormone Levels," *Lancet,* 2 (1978):8084.

112. JEFFCOATE, W. J., et al. "β-Endorphin in Human Cerebrospinal Fluid," *Lancet,* 2 (1978):119–121.

113. JENNES, L., STUMPF, W. E., and KALIVAS, P. W. "Neurotensin: Topographical Distribution in Rat Brain by Immunohistochemistry," *Journal of Comparative Neurology,* 210 (1982):211–224.

114. JOLKKONEN, J. T., SOININEN, H. S., and RIEKKINEN, P. J. "Cerebrospinal Fluid Cholinesterase, β-endorphin and Somatostatin in Alzheimer's Disease," *Acta Universitatis Tamperensis,* 21 (Series B) (1984):104–109.

115. JOYNT, R. J., and McNEILL, T. H. "Neuropeptides in Aging and Dementia," *Peptides,* 5 (Supplement 1) (1984):269–274.

116. JUDD, L. L., et al. "Naloxone Related Attenuation of Manic Symptoms in Certain Bipolar Depressives," in J. M. van Ree and L. Terenius, eds., *Characteristic and Function of Opioids.* Amsterdam: Elsevier/North Holland Biomedical Press, 1978, pp. 173–174.

117. JUNGKUNZ, G., NEDOPIL, N., and RUTHER, E. "Acute Effects of the Synthetic Analogue of Methionine Enkephalin (FK-33-824) in Schizophrenic Patients: A Double Blind Trial," *Pharmacopsychiatria,* 17 (1984): 76–78.

118. KAEGER, H. E. "A Clinical Trial with DSIP," *European Neurology,* 23 (1984): 386–388.

119. KAIYA, H., et al. "Substance P-like Immunoreactivity in Plasma of Psychiatric

Patients and Effects of Neuroleptics and Electroconvulsive Therapy," *Psychiatry Research*, 5 (1981):11–21.

120. KAIYA, H., et al. "Decreased Level of β-endorphin-like Immunoreactivity in Cerebrospinal Fluid of Patients with Senile Dementia of Alzheimer Type," *Life Sciences*, 33 (1983):1039–1043.

121. KARLSSON, I., et al. "Changes of CSF Neuropeptides After Environmental Stimulation in Dementia," *Nordic Journal of Psychiatry*, 39 (Supplement 11) (1985):75–82.

122. KASTIN, A. J., et al. "Improvement in Mental Depression with Decreased Thyrotropin Response After Administration of Thyrotropin-releasing Hormone," *Lancet*, 2 (1972):740.

123. KATAOKA, K., MIZENO, N., and FROHMAN, L. A. "Regional Distribution of Immunoreactive Neurotensin in Monkey Brain," *Brain Research Bulletin*, 14 (1979):57–60.

124. KATZ, E. R., et al. "β-Endorphin Immunoreactivity with Acute Behavioral Distress in Children with Leukemia," *Journal of Nervous and Mental Disease*, 170 (1982):72–77.

125. KING, J. C., et al. "The LHRH System in Normal and Neonatally Androgenized Female Rats," *Peptides*, 1 (Supplement 1) (1980):85–100.

126. KIRKEGAARD, C. F., HUMMER, L., and ROGOWSKI, P. "Increased Levels of TRH in Cerebrospinal Fluid from Patients with Endogenous Depression," *Psychoneuroendocrinology*, 4 (1979): 227–235.

127. KLEIN, H., et al. "Clinical Effects of the Synthetic Analogue of Met-enkephalin FK-33-824," in C. Perris, G. Strüwe, and B. Jansson, eds., *Biological Psychiatry*. Amsterdam: Elsevier/North Holland Biomedical Press, 1981, pp. 390–393.

128. KLEINMAN, J. E., et al. "Naloxone in Chronic Schizophrenic Patients: Neuroendocrine and Behavioral Effects," *Psychiatry Research*, 7 (1982):1–7.

129. KLEINMAN, J. E., et al. "Postmortem Measurements of Neuropeptides in Human Brain," *Psychopharmacology Bulletin*, 19 (1983):375–377.

130. KLINE, N. S., et al. "β-Endorphin-induced Changes in Schizophrenic and De-pressed Patients," *Archives of General Psychiatry*, 34 (1977):1111–1113.

131. KOBAYASHI, R. M., BROWN, M., and VALE, W. "Regional Distribution of Neurotensin and Somatostatin in Rat Brain," *Brain Research*, 126 (1977):584–588.

132. KOCH, G., and RICHTER, D. *Biochemical and Clinical Aspects of Neuropeptides: Synthesis, Processing and Gene Function*. New York: Academic Press, 1983.

133. KOHLER, C., and ERIKSSON, L. G. "An Immunohistochemical Study of Somatostatin and Neurotensin Positive Neurons in the Septal Nuclei of the Rat Brain," *Anatomy and Embryology*, 170 (1984): 1–10.

134. KOHLER, J., SCHROTER, E., and CRAMER, H. "Somatostatin-like Immunoreactivity in the Cerebrospinal Fluid of Neurological Patients," *Archives für Psychiatrie und Nervenkranken*, 231 (1982):503–508.

135. KOKMEN, E. "Dementia-Alzheimer Type," *Mayo Clinic Proceedings*, 59 (1984):35–42.

136. KOOB, G., LEMOAL, M., and BLOOM, F. E. "The Role of Endorphins in Neurobiology, Behavior and Psychiatric Disorders," in C. B. Nemeroff and A. J. Dunn, eds., *Peptides, Hormones and Behavior*. New York: Spectrum Publications, 1984, pp. 349–384.

137. KORSGAARD, S., CASEY, D. E., and GERLACK, J. "High Dose Des-tyrosine-γ-endorphin in Tardive Dyskinesia," *Psychopharmacology*, 78 (1982):285–286.

138. KRIEGER, D. T., BROWNSTEIN, M. J., and MARTIN, J. B. *Brain Peptides*. New York: John Wiley & Sons, 1983.

139. KURLAND, A. A., et al. "The Treatment of Perceptual Disturbances in Schizophrenia with Naloxone Hydrochloride," *American Journal of Psychiatry*, 134 (1977):1408–1410.

140. LAMERS, C. B., et al. "Immunological and Biological Studies on Cholecystokinin in Rat Brain," *American Journal of Physiology*, 239 (1980):232–235.

141. LANCRANJAN, I., et al. "Decrease of Somatostatin-like Immunoreactivity in the CSF of Patients with Alzheimer's Disease," in R. J. Wurtman, S. H. Corkin, and J. H. Growden, eds., *Alzheimer's Disease: Advances in Basic Re-*

search and Therapies. Zurich: Proceedings of the 3rd Meeting of the International Study Group on the Treatment of Memory Disorders Associated with Aging, 1984, p. 455l.

142. LAZARUS, L. H., BROWN, M. R., and PERRIN, M. H. "Distribution, Localization, and Characterization of Neurotensin Binding Sites in the Rat Brain," *Neuropharmacology,* 36 (1977):625–629.

143. LEHMANN, H., NAIR, N.P.V., and KLINE, N. S. "β-endorphin and Naloxone in Psychiatric Patients: Clinical and Biological Effects," *American Journal of Psychiatry,* 136 (1979):762–766.

144. LEVINE, J. D., et al. "The Narcotic Antagonist Naloxone Enhances Clinical Pain," *Nature,* 272 (1978):826–827.

145. LEVY, M. L., DENIGRIS, Y., and DAVIS, K. L. "Rapid Antidepressant Activity of Melanocyte Inhibiting Factor: A Clinical Trial," *Biological Psychiatry,* 17 (1982):259–263.

146. LEWIS, R. V., et al. "On β-Leu⁵-Endorphin and Schizophrenia," *Archives of General Psychiatry,* 36 (1979):237–239.

147. LINDSTRÖM, L. H., et al. "Endorphins in Human Cerebrospinal Fluid: Clinical Correlations to Some Psychotic States," *Acta Psychiatrica Scandinavica,* 57 (1978):153–169.

148. LINDSTRÖM, L. H., et al., "Cerebrospinal Content of Endorphins in Schizophrenia," in N. S. Shah and A. G. Donald, eds., *Endorphins and Opiate Antagonists in Psychiatry.* New York: Plenum Press, 1982, pp. 245–256.

149. LINDSTRÖM, L. H., et al. "Delta-sleep Inducing Peptide in Cerebrospinal Fluid from Schizophrenics, Depressives, and Healthy Volunteers," *Progress in Neuro-Psychopharmacology and Biological Psychiatry,* 8, in press.

150. LIPINSKI, J., et al. "Naloxone in Schizophrenia: Negative Result," *Lancet,* 2 (1979):1292–1293.

151. LO, C. W., WEN, H. L., and HO, W.K.K. "Cerebrospinal Fluid [Met⁵]-enkephalin Level in Schizophrenics During Treatment with Naloxone," *European Journal of Pharmacology,* 92 (1983):77–81.

152. LOH, Y. P., and GAINER, H. "Biosynthesis and Processing of Neuropeptides," in D. T. Krieger, M. J. Brownstein, and J. B. Martin, eds., *Brain Peptides.* New York: Wiley-Interscience, 1983, pp. 79–116.

153. LOOSEN, P. T., and PRANGE A. J., Jr. "Hormones of the Thyroid Axis and Behavior," in C. B. Nemeroff and A. J. Dunn, eds., *Peptides, Hormones and Behavior.* New York: Spectrum Publications, 1984, pp. 533–577.

154. LUTTINGER, D., et al. "Peptides and Nociception," in J. R. Smythies and R. J. Bradley, eds., *International Review of Neurobiology.* New York: Academic Press, 1984, pp. 185–241.

155. MACKAY, A. "Endorphins and the Psychiatrist," *Trends in Neuroscience,* 4 (1981):9–11.

156. MCKELVY, J. F. "Enzymatic Degradation of Brain Peptides," in D. T. Krieger, M. J. Brownstein, and J. B. Martin, eds., *Brain Peptides.* New York: Wiley-Interscience, 1983, pp. 117–133.

157. MCNICHOLS, L. F., and MARTIN, W. R. "New and Experimental Therapeutic Roles for Naloxone and Related Opioid Antagonists," *Drugs,* 27 (1984):81–93.

158. MANBERG, P. J., et al. "Regional Distribution of Neurotensin in Human Brain," *Journal of Neurochemistry,* 38 (1982): 1777–1780.

159. MANBERG, P. J., et al. "Cerebrospinal Fluid Levels of Neurotensin-like Immunoreactivity in Normal Controls and in Patients with Affective Disorder, Anorexia Nervosa and Premenstrual Syndrome (Abstract)," *Society of Neuroscience,* 9 (1983):1034.

160. MANCHANDRA, R., and HIRSCH, S. R. "(Des-tyr¹)-γ-endorphin in the Treatment of Schizophrenics," *Psychological Medicine,* 11 (1981):401–403.

161. MARSAN, C. A., and TRACZYK, W. Z. *Neuropeptides and Neural Transmission.* New York: Raven Press, 1980.

162. MARTIN, J. B. "Neuroendocrinology and Brain Peptides: An Emerging New Frontier in Neurobiology," in N. S. Shah and A. G. Donald, eds., *Psychoneuroendocrine Dysfunction.* New York: Plenum Press, 1984, pp. 15–40.

163. MATTES, J. A., et al. "Ceruletide for Schizophrenia: A Double-blind Study," *Biological Psychiatry,* 20 (1985):533–538.

164. MELTZER, H. Y., et al. "Effect of (des-tyr)-gamma-endorphin in Schizophrenia," *Psychiatry Research*, 6 (1982):313–326.

165. MENDELSON, J. H., et al. "Effects of Naltrexone on Mood and Neuroendocrine Function in Normal Adult Males," *Psychoneuroendocrinology*, 3 (1979):231–236.

166. METZ, J., BUSCH, D. A., and MELTZER, H. Y. "Des-tyrosine-γ-endorphin: H-reflex Response Similar to Neuroleptics," *Life Science*, 28 (1981):2003–2008.

167. MEYERSON, B. J. "Hypothalamic Hormones and Behavior," *Medical Biology*, 57 (1979):69–83.

168. MIELKE, D. H., and GALLANT, D. M. "An Oral Opiate Antagonist in Chronic Schizophrenia: A Pilot Study," *American Journal of Psychiatry*, 134 (1977): 1430–1431.

169. MILLAR, R. P. *Neuropeptides: Biochemical and Physiological Studies.* London: Churchill-Livingstone, 1981.

170. MILLER, L. H., SANDMAN, C. A., and KASTIN, A. J. *Neuropeptide Influences on the Brain and Behavior.* New York: Raven Press, 1977.

171. MOROJI, T., WATANABE, N., and ITOH, S. "Antipsychotic Effects of Caerulein on Chronic Schizophrenics," *Proceedings of the World Psychiatric Association,* (1982):165–169.

172. MOROJI, T., et al. "Antipsychotic Effects of Caerulein, a Decapeptide Chemically Related to Cholecystokinin Octapeptide, on Schizophrenia," *International Pharmacopsychiatry*, 17 (1982): 255–273.

173. MOROJI, T., et al. "Antipsychotic Effects of Ceruletide (Caerulein) on Chronic Schizophrenia," *Archives of General Psychiatry*, 39 (1982):485–486.

174. MUESER, K. T., and DYSKEN, M. W. "Narcotic Antagonists in Schizophrenia: A Methodological Review," *Schizophrenia Bulletin*, 9 (1983):213–225.

175. MUTT, V. "VIP, Motilin and Secretin," in D. T. Krieger, M. J. Brownstein, and J. B. Martin, eds., *Brain Peptides.* New York: Wiley-Interscience, 1983, pp. 871–902.

176. NABER, D., and LEIBL, K. "Repeated High Dosage Naloxone Treatment Without Therapeutic Efficacy in Schizophrenic Patients," *Pharmacopsychiatria*, 16 (1983):43–45.

177. NABER, D., and PICKAR, D. "The Measurement of Endorphins in Body Fluids," *Psychiatric Clinics of North America*, 6 (1983):443–456.

178. NABER, D., NEDOPIL, N., and EBEN, E. "No Correlation Between Neuroleptic-Induced Increase of β-endorphin Serum Level and Therapeutic Efficacy in Schizophrenia," *British Journal of Psychiatry*, 144 (1984):651–653.

179. NABER, D., et al. "CSF Opioid Activity in Psychiatric Patients," in C. Perris, G. Strüwe, and B. Jansson, eds., *Biological Psychiatry.* Amsterdam: Elsevier/North Holland Biomedical Press, 1981, pp. 372–375.

180. NABER, D., et al. "Endogenous Opioid Activity and β-endorphin Immunoreactivity in CSF of Psychiatric Patients and Normal Controls," *American Journal of Psychiatry*, 138 (1981):1457–1462.

181. NAIR, N.P.V., BLOOM, D. M., and NESTOROS, J. D. "Cholecystokinin Appears to Have Antipsychotic Properties," *Progress in Neuropsychopharmacology and Biological Psychiatry*, 6 (1982):509–512.

182. NEBES, R. D., REYNOLDS, C. F. III, and HORN, L. C. "The Effect of Vasopressin on Memory in the Healthy Elderly," *Psychiatry Research*, 11 (1984):49–59.

183. NEMEROFF, C. B. "The Interaction of Neurotensin with Dopaminergic Pathways in the Central Nervous System: Basic Neurobiology and Implications for the Pathogenesis and Treatment of Schizophrenia," *Psychoneuroendocrinology*, in press.

184. NEMEROFF, C. B., and CAIN, S. T. "Neurotensin-dopamine Interactions in the Central Nervous System," *Trends in Pharmacological Science*, 6 (1985):201–205.

185. NEMEROFF, C. B., and PRANGE, A. J., Jr. "Peptides in Psychoneuroendocrinology: A Perspective," *Archives of General Psychiatry*, 35 (1978):999–1010.

186. NEMEROFF, C. B., et al. "Cytoprotective Effect of Centrally Administered Neurotensin on Stress-induced Gastric Ulcers," *American Journal of Physiology*, 242 (1982):342–346.

187. NEMEROFF, C. B., et al. "Interactions of Neurotensin with Brain Dopamine Systems: Biochemical and Behavioral Studies," *Journal of Pharmacology and Experimental Therapeutics,* 225 (1983): 337–345.

188. NEMEROFF, C. B., et al. "Regional Brain Concentrations of Neuropeptides in Huntington's Chorea and Schizophrenia," *Science,* 221 (1983):972–975.

189. NEMEROFF, C. B., et al. "Regional Brain Concentrations of Neurotensin, Thyrotropin-releasing Hormone and Somatostatin in Alzheimer's Disease (Abstract)" *Society of Neuroscience,* 9 (1983):1052.

190. NEMEROFF, C. B., et al. "Behavioral Effects of Hypothalamic Hypophysiotropic Hormones, Neurotensin, Substance P and Other Neuropeptides," *Pharmacology and Therapeutics,* 24 (1984):1–56.

191. NEMEROFF, C. B., et al. "Effects of Hypothalamic Peptides on the Central Nervous System," in C. B. Nemeroff and A. J. Dunn, eds., *Peptides, Hormones and Behavior.* New York: Spectrum Publications, 1984, pp. 217–272.

192. NEMEROFF, C. B., et al. "Elevated Concentrations of CSF Corticotropin-releasing Factor-like Immunoreactivity in Depressed Patients," *Science,* 226 (1984):1342–1344.

193. ORAM, J. J., EDWARDSON, J., and MILLARD, P. H. "Investigation of Cerebrospinal Fluid Neuropeptides in Idiopathic Senile Dementia," *Gerontology,* 27 (1981):216–223.

194. ORR, M., and OPPENHEIMER, C. "Effects of Naloxone on Auditory Hallucinations," *British Medical Journal,* 1 (1978):481.

195. PERRY, R. H., et al. "Neuropeptides in Alzheimer's Disease, Depression and Schizophrenia," *Journal of Neurological Sciences,* 51 (1981):465–472.

196. PERT, A., et al. "Opiate Peptides and Brain Function," in H. M. van Praag et al., eds., *Handbook of Biological Psychiatry,* vol. 4: *Brain Mechanisms and Abnormal Behavior-Chemistry.* New York: Marcel Dekker, 1981, pp. 547–582.

197. PETHO, B., et al. "β-Endorphin and Schizophrenia," *Lancet,* 1 (1981):212–213.

198. PICKAR, D., and BUNNEY, W. E. "The Endogenous Opioid System and Psychiatric Illness: Effects of Naloxone Administration in Schizophrenic and Manic Patients," in C. Perris, G. Strüwe, and B. Jansson, eds., *Biological Psychiatry.* Amsterdam: Elsevier/North Holland Biomedical Press, 1981, pp. 394–397.

199. PICKAR, D., DUBOIS, M., and COHEN, M. R. "Behavioral Change in a Cancer Patient Following Intrathecal β-endorphin Administration," *American Journal of Psychiatry,* 141 (1984):103–104.

200. PICKAR, D., et al. "Behavioral and Biological Effects of Acute β-Endorphin Injection in Schizophrenic and Depressed Patients," *American Journal of Psychiatry,* 138 (1981):160–166.

201. PICKAR, D., et al. "Endorphins in the Cerebrospinal Fluid of Psychiatric Patients," *Annals of the New York Academy of Science,* 398 (1982):399–412.

202. PICKAR, D., et al. "Short-term Naloxone Administration in Schizophrenic and Manic Patients," *Archives of General Psychiatry,* 39 (1982):313–319.

203. POST, R. M., et al. "Effect of Carbamazepine on CSF Opioid Activity: Relationship to Antidepressant Response," *Psychiatry Research,* 5 (1981):59–66.

204. POST, R. M., et al. "Cerebrospinal Fluid as Neuroregulatory Pathway: Peptides in Neuropsychiatric Illness," in J. H. Wood, ed., *Neurobiology of Cerebrospinal Fluid.* New York: Plenum Press, 1983, pp. 107–141.

205. PRANGE, A. J., Jr., and LOOSEN, P. T. "Aspects of Thyroid Axis Function in Depression," in N. S. Shah and A. G. Donald, eds., *Psychoneuroendocrine Dysfunction.* New York: Plenum Press, 1984, pp. 431–442.

206. PRANGE, A. J., Jr., and WILSON, I. C. "Thyrotropin-releasing Hormone (TRH) for the Immediate Relief of Depression: A Preliminary Report," *Psychopharmacologia,* 26 (1972):82.

207. PRANGE, A. J., Jr., LOOSEN, P. T., and NEMEROFF, C. B. "Peptides: Application to Research in Nervous and Mental Disorders," in S. Fielding, ed., *Frontiers in Psychotropic Drug Research.* New York: Futura Publishing Company, 1979, pp. 117–189.

208. PRANGE, A. J., Jr., NEMEROFF, C. B., and LIPTON, M. A. "Behavioral Effects of Peptides: Basic and Clinical Studies," in M. A. Lipton, K. F. Killam, and A. DiMascio, eds., *Psychopharmacology: A Generation of Progress*. New York: Raven Press, 1977, pp. 441–458.

209. QUIRION, R., et al. "Autoradiographic Distribution of [^{3}H]Neurotensin Receptors in Rat Brain: Visualization by Tritium-sensitive Film," *Peptides*, 3 (1982):757–763.

210. REICHLIN, S. "Neuroendocrinology," in R. H. Williams, ed., *Textbook of Endocrinology*. Philadelphia: W. B. Saunders, 1981, pp. 589–671.

211. RIMON, R., TERENIUS, L., and KAMPMAN, R. "Cerebrospinal Fluid Endorphins in Schizophrenia," *Acta Psychiatrica Scandinavica*, 61 (1980):395–403.

212. RIMON, R., et al. "Elevation of Substance P-like Peptides in the CSF of Psychiatric Patients," *Biological Psychiatry*, 19 (1984):509–516.

213. ROBERTS, G. W., et al. "Peptides, the Limbic Lobe and Schizophrenia," *Brain Research*, 288 (1983):199–211.

214. ROSS, M., BERGER, P. A., and GOLDSTEIN, A. "Plasma β-endorphin Immunoreactivity in Schizophrenia," *Science*, 205 (1979):1163–1164.

215. ROSSOR, M. "Biological Markers in Mental Disorders: Post-mortem Studies," *Journal of Psychiatric Research*, 18 (1984):457–465.

216. ROSSOR, M. N., et al. "Reduced Amounts of Immunoreactive Somatostatin in the Temporal Cortex in Senile Dementia of Alzheimer Type," *Neuroscience Letter*, 20 (1980):373–377.

217. ROSSOR, M. N., et al. "Reduced Cortical Choline Acetyltransferase Activity in Senile Dementia of Alzheimer-type Is Not Accompanied by Changes in Vasoactive Intestinal Polypeptide," *Brain Research*, 201 (1980):249–253.

218. ROSSOR, M. N., et al. "Normal Cortical Concentration of Cholecystokinin-like Immunoreactivity with Reduced Choline Acetyltransferase Activity in Senile Dementia of Alzheimer Type," *Life Sciences*, 29 (1981):405–410.

219. ROSSOR, M. N., et al. "Patterns of Neuropeptide Deficits in Alzheimer's Disease," in R. J. Wurtman, S. H. Corkin, and J. H. Growden, eds., *Alzheimer's Disease: Advances in Basic Research and Therapies*. Zurich: Brain Sciences and Metabolites in Charitable Trust, 1984, pp. 29–37.

220. RUBINOW, D. R., et al. "CSF Somatostatin in Affective Illness," *Archives of General Psychiatry*, 40 (1983):409–412.

221. RUBINOW, D. R., et al. "Effects of Carbamazepine on Cerebrospinal Fluid Somatostatin," *Psychopharmacology*, 85 (1985):210–213.

222. SANDERS, D. J., ZAHEDI-ASI, S., and MARR, A. P. "Glucagon and CCK in Human Brain: Controls and Patients with Senile Dementia of Alzheimer Type," *Brain Research*, 55 (1982):465–471.

223. SAVOLDI, F. "Opioid Peptides in Alcoholics," in E. E. Muller and A. R. Gerazzani, eds., *Central and Peripheral Endorphins: Basic and Clinical Aspects*. New York: Raven Press, 1984, pp. 333–338.

224. SAWYNOK, J., PINSKEY, C., and LaBELLA, F. S. "On the Specificity of Naloxone as an Opiate Antagonist," *Life Sciences*, 9 (1979):213–225.

225. SCHNEIDER-HELMERT, D., and SCHOENENBERGER, G. A. "The Influence of Synthetic DSIP (delta-sleep-inducing peptide) on Disturbed Human Sleep," *Experentia*, 37 (1981):913–917.

226. ———. "Effects of DSIP in Man," *Neuropsychobiology*, 9 (1983):197–206.

227. SCHOENENBERGER, G. A., and SCHNEIDER-HELMERT, D. "Psychophysiological Functions of DSIP," *Trends in Pharmacological Science*, 4 (1983):307–310.

228. SERBY, M., et al. "CSF Somatostatin in Alzheimer's Disease," *Neurobiology of Aging*, 5 (1984):187–189.

229. SIMPSON, G. M., BRANCHEY, M. H., and LEE, J. H. "A Trial of Naltrexone in Chronic Schizophrenia," *Current Therapeutic Research*, 22 (1977):909–913.

230. SMITH, G. P. "Gut Hormones and Feeding Behavior: Intuitions and Experiments," in C. B. Nemeroff and A. J. Dunn, eds., *Peptides, Hormones, and Behavior*. New York: Spectrum Publications, 1984, pp. 497–532.

231. SNYDER, S. H. "The Opiate Receptor and Morphine-like Peptides in the Brain," *American Journal of Psychiatry*, 135 (1978):645–652.

232. ———. "Brain Peptides as Neurotransmitters," *Science*, 219 (1980):976–983.

233. SOININEN, H. S., et al. "Reduced Cholinesterase Activity and Somatostatin-like Immunoreactivity in the Cerebrospinal Fluid of Patients with Dementia of the Alzheimer Type," *Journal of Neurological Sciences*, 63 (1984):167–172.

234. SOININEN, H., et al. "Synthetic $ACTH_{4-9}$ (ORG 2766) in Treatment of Alzheimer's Disease," *Acta Neurologica Scandinavica*, 98 (Supplement) (1984): 236–237.

235. SORENSEN, P. S., et al. "CSF and Plasma Vasopressin Concentrations in Dementia," *Journal of Neurology, Neurosurgery, and Psychiatry*, 46 (1983):911–916.

236. STEARDO, L., et al. "CSF Somatostatin Immunoreactivity and GH Plasma Levels in Alzheimer's Disease," *Neuroendocrinology Letters*, 6 (1984):291–294.

237. STEIN, G., et al. "Vasopressin and Mood During the Puerperium," *Biological Psychiatry*, 19 (1984):1711–1717.

238. TAMMINGA, C. A., et al. "Des-tyrosine-γ-endorphin Administration in Chronic Schizophrenics," *Archives of General Psychiatry*, 38 (1981):167.

239. TERENIUS, L. "The Implications of Endorphins in Pathological States," in J. M. van Ree and L. Terenius, eds., *Characteristics and Function of Opioids*. Amsterdam: Elsevier/North Holland Biomedical Press, 1978, pp. 143–158.

240. TERENIUS, L., and NYBERG, F. "Multiple Forms of Neuropeptides in Human CSF and Their Significance," in G. Kock and D. Richter, eds., *Biochemical and Clinical Aspects of Neuropeptides: Synthesis, Processing and Gene Function*. New York: Academic Press, 1983, pp. 99–112.

241. TERENIUS, L., WAHLSTRÖM, A., and AGREN, H. "Naloxone Treatment in Depression. Clinical Observations and Effects on CSF Endorphins and Monoamine Metabolites," *Psychopharmacology*, 54 (1977):31–33.

242. TERENIUS, L., et al. "Increased CSF Levels of Endorphins in Chronic Psychosis," *Neuroscience Letters*, 3 (1976):157–162.

243. TERRY, R. D., and KATZMAN, R. "Senile Dementia of the Alzheimer Type," *Neurology*, 14 (1983):497–506.

244. TINKLENBERG, J. R., et al. "Vasopressin Peptides and Dementia," in S. C. Corkin et al., eds., *Alzheimer's Disease: A Report of Progress*. New York: Raven Press, 1982, pp. 463–468.

245. TSUJI, M., TAKAHASHI, S., and AKAZAWA, S. "CSF Vasopressin and Cyclic Nucleotide Concentrations in Senile Dementia," *Psychoneuroendocrinology*, 6 (1981):171–176.

246. UHL, G. R., and SNYDER, S. H. "Regional and Subcellular Distribution of Brain Neurotensin," *Life Sciences*, 19 (1977): 1827–1832.

247. UHL, G. R., BENNETT, J. P., Jr., and SNYDER, S. H. "Neurotensin, a Central Nervous System Peptide: Apparent Receptor Binding," *Brain Research*, 130 (1977):299–313.

248. UHL, G. R., GOODMAN, R. R., and SNYDER, S. H. "Neurotensin-containing Cell Bodies, Fibers, and Nerve Terminals in the Brainstem of the Rat: Immunohistochemical Mapping," *Brain Research*, 167 (1979):77–91.

249. UNGAR, G. "Peptides and Behavior," *International Review of Neurobiology*, 17 (1975):37–60.

250. VALE, W., and RIVIER, C. "Hypothalamic Hypophysiotropic Hormones," in L. L. Iversen, S. D. Iversen, and S. H. Snyder, eds., *Handbook of Psychopharmacology*, vol. 5. New York: Plenum Press, 1975, pp. 195–237.

251. VAN DER VELDE, C. D. "Rapid Clinical Effectiveness of MIF-I in the Treatment of Major Depressive Illness," *Peptides*, 4 (1983):297–300.

252. VAN KAMMEN, D. P., et al. "Spinal Fluid Vasopressin, Angiotensin I and II, β-endorphin and Opioid Activity in Schizophrenia: A Preliminary Evaluation," in C. Perris, G. Strüwe, and B. Jansson, eds., *Biological Psychiatry*. Amsterdam: Elsevier/North Holland Biomedical Press, 1981, pp. 339–344.

253. VAN PRAAG, H. M., and VERHOEVEN, W. M. A. "Endorphins and Schizophrenia," in D. DeWied and P.A. van Praag,

eds., *Hormones and the Brain*. Baltimore: University Park Press, 1980, pp. 141–153.

254. ———. "Neuropeptides: A New Dimension in Biological Psychiatry," in H. M. van Praag et al., eds. *Handbook of Biological Psychiatry*, vol. 4, *Brain Mechanisms and Abnormal Behavior-Chemistry*. New York: Marcel Dekker, 1981, pp. 511–545.

255. VAN REE, J. M., and DEWIED, D. "Endorphins in Schizophrenia," *Neuropharmacology*, 20 (1981):1271–1277.

256. ———. "Endorphins and Related Peptides in Schizophrenia," in E. E. Muiler and R. Genazzani, eds., *Central and Peripheral Endorphins: Basic and Clinical Aspects*. New York: Raven Press, 1984, pp. 325–332.

257. VAN REE, J. M., et al. "Antipsychotic Action of [Des-Tyr^1]-γ-endorphin (β-LPH$_{62\text{-}77}$)," in J. M. van Ree and L. Terenius, eds., *Characteristics and Functions of Opioids*. Amsterdam: Elsevier/North Holland Biomedical Press, 1978, pp. 181–184.

258. VEITH, J. L., et al. "Plasma β-endorphin, Pain Thresholds and Anxiety Levels Across the Human Menstrual Cycle," *Physiology and Behavior*, 32 (1984):31–34.

259. VERBANCK, P.M.P., et al. "Reduced Cholecystokinin Immunoreactivity in the Cerebrospinal Fluid of Patients with Psychiatric Disorders," *Life Sciences*, 34 (1983):67–72.

260. VEREBY, K., VOLAVKA, J., and CLOUET, D. "Endorphins in Psychiatry," *Archives of General Psychiatry*, 35 (1978):877–888.

261. VERHOEVEN, W.M.A., VAN PRAAG, H. M., and DE JONG, J.T.V.M. "Use of Naloxone in Schizophrenic Psychoses and Manic Syndromes," *Neuropsychobiology*, 7 (1981):159–168.

262. VERHOEVEN, W.M.A., VAN PRAAG, H. M., and VAN REE, J. M. "Repeated Naloxone Administration in Schizophrenia," *Psychiatry Research*, 12 (1984):297–312.

263. VERHOEVEN, W.M.A., et al. "[Des-Tyr^1]-γ-endorphin in Schizophrenia," *Lancet*, 1 (1978):1046–1047.

264. VERHOEVEN, W.M.A., et al. "Improvement of Schizophrenic Patients Treated with Des-Tyr^1-γ-endorphin (DTγE)," *Archives of General Psychiatry*, 36 (1979):294–298.

265. VERHOEVEN, W.M.A., et al. "Antipsychotic Properties of Des-enkephalin-γ-endorphinin Treatment of Schizophrenic Patients," *Archives of General Psychiatry*, 39 (1982):648–654.

266. VERHOEVEN, W.M.A., et al. "Clinical, Biochemical, and Hormonal Aspects of Treatment with Des-Tyr^1-Gamma Endorphin in Schizophrenia," *Psychiatry Research*, 11 (1984):329–346.

267. VOLAVKA, J., ANDERSON, B., and GOZ, G. "Naloxone and Naltrexone in Mental Illness and Tardive Dyskinesia," *Annals of the New York Academy of Science*, 398 (1982):97–102.

268. VOLAVKA, J., et al. "Naloxone in Chronic Schizophrenia," *Science*, 196 (1977): 1227–1228.

269. VOLAVKA, J., et al. "Naloxone Fails to Affect Short-term Memory in Man," *Psychiatry Research*, 1 (1979):89–92.

270. VOLAVKA, J., et al. "Short-lived Effect of (Des-Tyr)-Gamma-Endorphin in Schizophrenia," *Psychiatry Research*, 10 (1983):243–252.

271. VON GRAFFENRIED, B., et al. "Effects of the Synthetic Enkephalin Analogue FK-33-824 in Man," *Nature*, 272 (1978): 729–730.

272. VON KNORRING, L., et al. "Circannual Variation in Concentrations of Endorphins in Cerebrospinal Fluid," *Pain*, 12 (1982): 265–272.

273. WATSON, S. J., et al. "Effects of Naloxone on Schizophrenia: Reduction in Hallucinations in a Subpopulation of Subjects," *Science*, 201 (1978):73–76.

274. WEINGARTNER, H., et al. "Effect of Vasopressin on Human Memory Functions," *Science*, 211 (1981):601–603.

275. WEN, H. L., and HO, W.K.K. "Suppression of Withdrawal Symptoms by Dynorphin in Heroin Addicts," *European Journal of Pharmacology*, 82 (1982):183–186.

276. WEN, H. L., LO, C. W., and HO, W. K. "Met-enkephalin Levels in the Cerebrospinal Fluid of Schizophrenic Patients," *Clinical Chimica Acta*, 128 (1983):367–371.

277. WIDERLÖV, E., et al. "Subnormal CSF Levels of Neurotensin in a Subgroup of Schizophrenic Patients: Normalization After Neuroleptic Treatment," *American Journal of Psychiatry*, 139 (1982): 1122–1126.

278. WILSON, I. C., PRANGE, A. J., Jr., and LOOSEN, P. T. "Psychological and Thyroid Stimulating Hormone Changes After Thyrotropin-releasing Hormone in Normal Women: Antagonism by Pretreatment with Thyroid Hormones," *Psychiatry Research*, 2 (1980):211–222.

279. WILSON, I. C., et al. "TRH (Lopremone): Psychobiological Responses of Normal Women. I. Subjective Experiences," *Archives of General Psychiatry*, 29 (1973): 15–21.

280. WINOKUR, A., et al. "Improvement in Ratings of Tension after TRH Administration in Healthy Women," *Psychoneuroendocrinology*, 7 (1982):239–244.

281. WOOD, P. L., et al. "Reduced Lumbar CSF Somatostatin Levels in Alzheimer's Disease," *Life Sciences*, 31 (1982):2073–2079.

282. YATES, C. M., et al. "Thyrotropin-releasing Hormone and Substance P Immunoreactivity in Post-mortem Brain from Cases of Alzheimer-type Dementia and Down's Syndrome," *Brain Research*, 258 (1983):45–52.

283. ZUBENKO, G. S., and NIXON, R. A. "Mood-elevating Effect of Captopril in Depressed Patients," *American Journal of Psychiatry*, 141 (1984):110–111.

NEUROENDOCRINE FUNCTION IN PSYCHIATRIC DISORDERS AND BEHAVIOR

Herbert Y. Meltzer and Martin T. Lowy

¶ Introduction

The endocrine and nervous systems are the major mechanisms for the functional integration of the organ systems of the body and the maintenance of the stability of the internal milieu. Neuroendocrinology encompasses the study of the integrated activity of these two systems, both of which depend on the synthesis, release, action, and inactivation of neurotransmitters and hormones.

The central importance of neurotransmitter function and dysfunction for current theories of the pathophysiology of the major psychiatric disorders, the response to stress, and the mechanism of action of psychotropic drugs has been a principle reason for the investigation of neuroendocrine function in psychiatric disorders. As will be discussed, determination of the basal levels of hormones in blood and the hormonal response to psychotropic drugs permits the testing of specific hypotheses concerning neuronal function and receptor sensitivity in man and provides information that cannot be readily obtained by other means, if at all, at the current time. A second impetus for study of the neuroendocrine system in psychiatry comes from the numerous disturbances of endocrine function per se that have been reported to be present in various psychiatric disorders (e.g., decreased gonadal function in schizophrenia), some of which may be due to neuronal dysfunction. A third factor is the presence of various types of psychopathology in many endocrine disorders (e.g., depression in hypothyroidism and Cushing's syndrome), which may reflect endocrine influences on neuronal function.

This chapter will review the anatomy and physiology of the endocrine system; endocrine dysfunction in psychiatric disorders; studies that utilize the analysis of hormonal response to challenge agents for diagnostic purposes or to investigate the etiology of the psychiatric disorders; and studies that relate to the mechanism of action of psychotropic drugs or electroconvulsive therapy (ECT).

¶ Physiology of the Neuroendocrine System

The hypothalamus and the pituitary contain the major control mechanisms of the neuroendocrine system. In man the pituitary gland is divided into two lobes, the anterior pituitary, or adenohypophysis, and the posterior pituitary, or neurohypophysis. The median eminence of the hypothalamus is connected to the pituitary gland by a stalk that has three components: (1) a dense plexus of blood vessels called the hypophyseal portal system; (2) a glandular component called the pars tuberalis; and (3) a neural component containing the axons of several hypothalamic nuclei, which will be described subsequently.

Hypothalamic neurosecretory neurons secrete peptidergic substances from their nerve endings in the median eminence into the capillary plexus of the hypophyseal portal system. These substances are transported to the pituitary gland through these vessels, where they stimulate or inhibit the release of various trophic hormones. The major hypothalamic hormones that have been described include: corticotrophin- (ACTH) releasing factor (CRF), thyrotropin- (TSH) releasing hormone (TRH), gonadotropin-releasing hormone (GnRH), growth hormone (GH) release-inhibiting hormone (somatostatin), growth hormone–releasing factor (GHRF), melanocyte-stimulating hormone release–inhibiting factor (MIF), and melanocyte-stimulating hormone-releasing factor (MRF).[281] The amino acid composition of most of these hypothalamic hormones is known, which has

permitted their synthesis and intensive investigation, including administration to man. Prolactin secretion is directly inhibited by dopamine (DA),[167] which is released directly into the portal circulation from the terminals of the tuberoinfundibular dopaminergic neurons.[112] There is some evidence for a prolactin-releasing factor, which could be TRH, vasoactive intestinal peptide, or some other peptide.[199]

Neurotransmitters such as DA, serotonin (5HT), and norepinephrine (NE) regulate the release of the hypothalamic releasing hormones, thus permitting higher brain regions to influence the secretion of pituitary hormones. Table 4–1 is a list of most of the known neurotransmitter influences on the release of hypothalamic factors or direct effects on the release of pituitary hormones in the rat. Most of these relationships may be expected to carry over to man with the exception of the opiates, which inhibit cortisol secretion.[81] D-Ala^2-MePhe^4-met-enkephalin-(O)-ol (DAMME), a long-acting analogue of met-enkephalin, also increases GH, prolactin, and TSH secretion and decreases LH secretion.[81] Various opiate alkaloids have slightly different patterns of effects on hormone secretion in man.[81]

The pituitary hormones participate in their own regulation through direct influence on the secretion of hypothalamic releasing hormones and negative feedback at the pituitary itself. Further, some of the target gland hormones—for example, cortisol, estrogens, testosterone—can influence the activity of brain neurons and the release of hypothalamic and pituitary trophic hormones. Through these mechanisms, neural and endocrine activity can be fine-tuned to permit the organism to respond to internal and external stimuli.

The relationship between the hypothalamus and the secretion of posterior pituitary gland hormones, oxytocin and vasopressin (antidiuretic hormone, ADH), is quite different from what has just been described. The posterior pituitary contains the terminal regions of neurosecretory cells that originate in the supraoptic and paraventricular nuclei

TABLE 4–1
Effect of Neurotransmitters on Hypothalamic Releasing Factors and Pituitary Hormones

	Neurotransmitters							
	DA	NE	Epi	5HT	Ach	Hist	GABA	Opiate
Hypothalamic Factor								
CRF		↓		↑	↑		↓	
GHRF		↑						
Somatostatin	↑	↑		↓	↑		↓	↓
GnRH	↑	↑	→	→	→			↓
TRH	↑↓	→	→	↑↓	→	↑	→	
DA				↓				↓
AVP		↓		↑	↑			↓
Pituitary Hormone								
PRL	↓						↓	
α-MSH	↓		↑					
TSH	↓		↑					
ACTH/β-EP	↓	↑		↑	↑			↑

↑ = increase. ↓ = decrease. → = no effect. Abbreviations: α-MSH = alpha-melanocyte stimulating hormone. AVP = arginine vasopressin. β-EP = β-endorphin. Epi = epinephrine. GABA = gamma aminobutyric acid. Hist = histamine. PRL = prolactin.

and whose tracts descend through the neural part of the pituitary stalk. The posterior pituitary hormones are synthesized in the cell bodies of these neurons, reach the nerve terminals by axonal transport, and are secreted at the pituitary level after depolarization of these neurons. The regulation of the release of these hormones involves integrated effects of neurotransmitters, osmolality, suckling, and various reflexes. Because these cells convert neural information into hormonal output, they have been termed neuroendocrine transducers. Vasopressin and oxytocin appear to be secreted both into the bloodstream for direct peripheral action and centrally, where they may act as neurotransmitters or neuromodulators. The role of posterior pituitary peptides in psychiatric disorders and behavior is discussed elsewhere in this volume. (see chapter 3).

Other nuclei of the hypothalamus that are critical for endocrine function include the preoptic area and the suprachiasmatic, arcuate, and ventromedial nuclei. The preoptic region is associated with regulation of eating, body temperature, pituitary-thyroid responses to neural influences on body temperature, inhibition of gonadal function prior to puberty, and regulation of GnRH and somatostatin release. The suprachiasmatic nucleus has a major influence on circadian rhythms of various hormones, including melatonin from the pineal. The arcuate nucleus contains the cell bodies of the tuberoinfundibular dopaminergic neurons and the tuberohypophysial neurons, which synthesize many of the hypothalamic hormones. The ventromedial nucleus is important as a visceral regulator and as the source of GHRF. Abnormalities of the ventromedial nucleus cause animals to become hyperphagic, intensely irritable, prone to rage, and prone to decreased spontaneous activity. The function of these nuclei is, in part, integrated through neurons in the medial basal hypothalamus.

The other components of the limbic system—the amygdala, the hippocampus, the olfactory lobes, the cingulate gyrus, and ascending pathways from midbrain nuclei—also influence the hypothalamic neurons that serve the neuroendocrine transducer function. It is through the limbic nuclei that the hypothalamic nuclei can receive cortical and subcortical inputs and achieve the neuroendocrine integration necessary for appropriate responses to internal and external stimuli.

Endocrine Rhythms

It is well established that there are circadian rhythms in the secretion of cortisol,[147] prolactin,[94] and GH[209] and that nocturnal secretion of these hormones may be linked to sleep stages.[277] ACTH and cortisol levels are lowest in the first few hours of sleep, peak in the early-morning hours, and decline during the remainder of the twenty-four hour day.[147] In addition, there are six to eleven episodes of ACTH and cortisol secretion throughout the day superimposed on the circadian rhythm.[95] Peak GH levels occur during the early phase of sleep.[209] Episodic secretion of GH during the day as well as postprandially has been documented. The episodic secretion of serum prolactin during the day and the maximal secretory rate during the last half of the night have been described.[237] The gonadotrophins, luteinizing hormone (LH) and follicle-stimulating hormone (FSH) do not have a significant circadian rhythm in adults but do peak at night during puberty. Both are secreted episodically during the day. Testosterone has been reported to have a circadian rhythm with peak levels in the last hour of sleep and episodic secretion during the day.[132] The circadian rhythm of testosterone secretion is age-related, independent of the prolactin rhythm, and not DA-dependent.[253]

¶ Endocrine Disturbances in Affective Disorders

Introduction

The variety of vegetative symptoms in major depression—for example, loss of appetite, weight loss, sleep disturbances, and loss of interest in sex—as well as the high incidence of depressive symptomatology in endocrine disorders such as Cushing's syndrome, Addison's disease, and hypothyroidism,[171] strongly suggests that endocrine disturbances could play a key role in the etiology and pathophysiology of depression. Several decades of research involving the determination of serum levels of pituitary and target organ hormones have, in fact, unequivocally demonstrated a variety of endocrine abnormalities in major depression. These studies will be reviewed here. The interested reader is referred to excellent reviews of the earlier literature by Carroll and Mendels,[51] Sachar and associates,[235] and Rubin and Poland.[226]

The Hypothalamic-Pituitary-Adrenal Axis in Affective Disorders

Hypersecretion of cortisol is present in some, but not all, patients with primary major depression and has been demonstrated by various means, including: (1) increased twenty-four-hour urinary free cortisol, (2) increased plasma cortisol concentrations, (3) disturbance in the diurnal rhythm of cortisol secretion, (4) increased cerebrospinal fluid (CSF) cortisol concentrations, and (5) failure to suppress cortisol levels adequately after a low dose of the high-potency corticosteroid dexamethasone.[51]

The cortisol production rate as assessed by twenty-four-hour urinary 17-hydroxycorticosteroids, urinary free cortisol, or mean twenty-four-hour plasma cortisol is elevated in the acute stages of depression in about 50 percent of depressed patients.* Serum cortisol levels are elevated in major depressed patients as a group at most times of the day, but especially during the late evening, when cortisol secretion is normally lowest. Measurement of cortisol secretion at 1 to 4 P.M. or 3 to 6 P.M. has also been advocated as a means of demonstrating excessive hypothalamic-pituitary-adrenal (HPA) axis activity in major depression compared to normal controls.[63,117] These measures have been reported to correlate with severity of depression or twenty-four-hour serum cortisol levels.[19,63] Determination of the serum cortisol in plasma samples obtained via an indwelling catheter during the afternoon may have some value for following response to treatment, as these values return to normal

*See references 18, 47, 49, 104, 231, and 232.

following recovery from depression.[19,63] Increased plasma cortisol output during the 1 to 4 P.M. period also was associated with shortened rapid eye movement (REM) latency.[20]

Elevated glucocorticoids have usually been found in CSF in unipolar and bipolar patients and to a lesser extent in manic patients.[52,102,264] Levels have been reported to be highest in psychotic depressed patients and to normalize after treatment and recovery. CSF cortisol levels correlate with total plasma cortisol levels and urinary free cortisol excretion. However, no mean increase in CSF cortisol concentration in major depression was reported by Coppen and associates[66] or Jimerson and coworkers.[129] This may relate to the subtype of depression studied, severity of illness, duration of illness, the effects of stress, and sensitivity of the cortisol assays employed.

Carr and others[48] found that two of ten depressed patients had a paradoxical increase in plasma ACTH levels during a cortisol infusion, comparable to that frequently observed in Cushing's disease. This abnormality in the rate-sensitive component of the regulation of cortisol secretion was independent of the cortisol response to dexamethasone, which suggests an abnormality at the hypothalamic or pituitary level.

THE DEXAMETHASONE SUPPRESSION TEST

In recent years the greatest interest in the assessment of the HPA axis in depression has centered on the dexamethasone suppression test (DST). Following a test dose of dexamethasone of 1 mg orally at 11 P.M., normal controls will usually suppress serum cortisol levels at 8 A.M., 4 P.M., or 11 P.M. on the next day to less than 5 ug per dl, because dexamethasone activates feedback mechanisms at the hypothalamus and pituitary to decrease the release of CRF and ACTH, respectively. Carroll and associates.[54] studied a large number of depressed patients, other psychiatric patients, and normal controls and determined, with the competitive protein binding assay method of assaying cortisol, that 96 percent

of controls and nonmelancholic psychiatric patients suppressed serum cortisol to less than 5 ug per dl at 8 A.M., 4 P.M., or 11 P.M. the day following administration of 1 or 2 mg dexamethasone. However, 53 percent of the melancholic patients failed to suppress, giving a sensitivity (proportion of true positives among the melancholics) of 53 percent, a specificity (proportion of true negatives correctly identified) of 96 percent, and a diagnostic confidence (proportion of positive tests that are true positive) of 94 percent. The 1 mg DST procedure of Carroll and others[54] has become more or less standard, except that only the 8 A.M. and 4 P.M. sample have been utilized in more recent studies. If the cortisol concentration in either sample is equal to or greater than 5 ug per dl, the DST is considered abnormal. Elimination of the 11 P.M. sample has a minimal effect on sensitivity.

The DST is abnormal in a higher percentage of patients with major depression than any other psychiatric diagnosis, including mania. The sensitivity has ranged from 20 to 75 percent in various research studies.[50,113] There is now extensive evidence that the DST is not as specific for the melancholic subtype of depression as originally proposed by Carroll and associates.[54] For example, in a very careful study, Berger and coworkers[29] found the incidence of nonsuppression in endogenous depression was five of twenty (25 percent) and four of nineteen (21.1 percent) in nonendogenous depression. An average sensitivity for the DST over the better studies may be 40 percent with a specificity of 82 percent.[127] Using these figures, the predictive value of a positive DST for major depression in a consecutive cohort of newly admitted psychiatric patients, of whom as high as 50 percent are major depressives, would be only 69 percent, which in clinical practice means the DST should not be used as a laboratory test for melancholia or major depression.[127]

The DST has been reported to be abnormal in patients with borderline personality disorder or obsessive-compulsive disorder with secondary depression as frequently as in major depression.[128,254] The incidence of nonsuppression in schizophrenia, particularly in those patients with depressive symptoms, may be as high as 30 percent.[196] The rate of nonsuppression in schizo-affective disorder by Research Diagnostic Criteria has been reported to be less than that of major depression.[180]

There is mixed evidence concerning the relationship between the DST and symptom severity,[219] family history,[6,241] and bipolarity[6,261] and its utility as a predictor of treatment response. However, there is increasing evidence that abnormal DST tests are more common in primary depressed patients who have delusions or hallucinations,[225] have made a recent suicide attempt,[24,69] have sleep disturbances,[229] and have had a recent weight loss of approximately 10 percent or more.[83] However, some primary depressed patients without any of these four "risk factors" have abnormal DST tests.

In addition to weight loss, some of the other factors that produce false positive DST results are carbamazepine, diphenylhydantoin sodium, barbiturates, fever, pregnancy, diabetes, infection, and Cushing's syndrome.[50] Age per se is not associated with a false positive DST, but there is a high proportion of abnormal DST tests in both elderly depressed patients[77] and in patients with dementia, so the DST is of little use in the differential diagnosis of these two conditions.[218] The DST has been reported to be frequently abnormal in depressed prepubertal children.[213]

The DST in depression generally normalizes several weeks before clinical symptoms respond markedly to treatment.[124] Failure of the DST to normalize has been demonstrated by some investigators to be a harbinger of impending relapse in patients with symptomatic improvement.[110,124,259,261]

Despite the extensive investigation of the DST, it is not yet clear to what extent and how it should be used in general clinical practice. First, there is a significant problem in obtaining reliable determinations of serum cortisol in clinical laboratories around

the criterion value of 5 ug per dl.[178] Clinicians ordering the test need to be confident of the reliability of this determination in the laboratory they use. The DST should not be used to establish or confirm the diagnosis of major depression, because its low sensitivity and specificity lead to an unacceptable predictive value. However, it may be valuable as a marker of inadequate or unstable recovery when it remains abnormal in a depressed patient who has symptomatically recovered.[121] An abnormal DST does not define a subtype of depression such as melancholia, endogenous depression, or "vital" depression.

The biological basis for an abnormal DST has been sought by many investigators. The hypersecretion of cortisol during a twenty-four-hour period as indicated by elevated plasma cortisol levels in depressed patients is not necessarily associated with an abnormal DST.[18] Serum levels of ACTH have been found to be normal in both suppressors and nonsuppressors prior to the DST, but nonsuppressors fail to suppress ACTH adequately at 4 P.M.[87,125] Further, Yerevanian, Woolf, and Iker[291] reported that plasma ACTH levels, while not significantly elevated in depressed patients who were nonsuppressors, decreased after conversion to suppression but remained relatively high in those who did not convert. They interpreted this as evidence that ACTH was a major factor in nonsuppression. However, these results were confounded by possible medication effects. These findings also suggest that depressed patients could be secreting cortisol, in part via an enhanced response to ACTH or some non-ACTH dependent mechanism (e.g., vasopressin), and provide more direct evidence that the CRF-ACTH system fails to respond to the inhibitory signal provided by glucocorticoids.

The cortisol response to ACTH (cosyntropin, 250 ug) administration in sixteen women with major depression, endogenous subtype, has been found to be significantly greater and more rapid than normal,[8] suggesting adrenal hyperresponsiveness to ACTH could be a cause of increased cortisol secretion. Gold and coworkers[108] administered CRF, 1 ug per kg, to nine bipolar depressed patients, eight recovered bipolar patients, six manic patients, and fifteen controls. The basal ACTH levels were normal in all patients, but the ACTH response to CRF was blunted only in the depressed patients. Gold and associates[108] noted that the cortisol response to CRF was normal in depressed patients despite the low ACTH levels, consistent with the findings of Amsterdam and associates.[8]

A recent study has found that glucocorticoid receptors in the lymphocytes of nonsuppressors fail to respond to *in vivo* administration of dexamethasone in the expected fashion.[163] If this also occurred in other tissues, it would indicate that depressed patients who are nonsuppressors have a generalized insensitivity to glucocorticoids at the molecular level. This would help to explain why those depressed patients with greatly increased cortisol secretion do not develop the somatic symptoms of Cushing's disorder and might indicate that the many brain processes that are glucocorticoid-dependent might be inadequately stimulated in such patients. Since dexamethasone insensitivity is dose-dependent in depressed patients—that is, can be overcome by higher doses of dexamethasone—these findings suggest glucocorticoid treatment might be of value in such patients.

AMPHETAMINE AND CLONIDINE CHALLENGES OF THE HYPOTHALAMIC-PITUITARY-ADRENAL AXIS

Intravenous amphetamine or methamphetamine has been reported to suppress serum cortisol levels in depressed patients but to increase serum cortisol in normal controls.[60,236] The qualitative difference in response to methamphetamine or d-amphetamine was thought to be due to subsensitivity of postsynaptic alpha-2-adrenergic receptors and hence relevant to the putative decrease in noradrenergic activity in depression.[236] However, the difference in the cortisol response to amphetamine between depressed subjects and normal controls could not be replicated.[88]

Clonidine hydrochloride, an alpha-2-adrenergic agonist, has been used to further assess noradrenergic receptor sensitivity in depression. One study found no difference in the decrease in serum cortisol among groups of endogenous depressives, schizo-affective patients, schizophrenic patients, and normal control subjects following 150 ug clonidine.[174] However, Siever and associates[245] reported that the decrease in serum cortisol after an intravenous 2 ug per kg dose of clonidine was significantly greater in eighteen patients with major depressive disorder (ten bipolar, eight unipolar) than in normal controls. These results were attributed to either an enhanced effect of clonidine on postsynaptic noradrenergic receptors, which inhibit cortisol secretion in depressed patients, or an enhanced effect of clonidine on presynaptic alpha-2-adrenergic receptors, which inhibit the release of NE. Thus opposite conclusions about the status of postsynaptic alpha-2 receptors have been drawn from the studies with methamphetamine and clonidine, and further investigations are in order. The GH response to amphetamine and clonidine in depression is discussed later.

SEROTONERGIC CHALLENGES TO THE HYPOTHALAMIC-PITUITARY-ADRENAL AXIS

Administration of 5-hydroxytryptophan (5-HTP), the precursor of 5HT, has been reported to produce a greater stimulation of serum cortisol levels in patients with major depression and mania than in normal control subjects.[184] After an oral dose of 200 mg D,L-5-HTP, serum cortisol levels increased over the next three hours more than after placebo in unmedicated manic and depressed patients. No such difference in the cortisol response to placebo or 5-HTP has been noted in schizophrenic patients and controls. These findings suggest that in both of the major affective disorders, there could be an enhanced responsiveness to 5HT, possibly due to supersensitive 5HT receptors. The magnitude of the cortisol response to 5-HTP correlated with the severity of depression.[185]

The excessive cortisol response to 5-HTP may be an indication that the hypersecretion of cortisol in depression is related to increased serotonergic stimulation, since there is extensive evidence from animal studies that the secretion of corticosteroids is modulated by 5HT.

Following treatment with tricyclic; antidepressants for three weeks or longer, the cortisol response to 5-HTP usually decreased whereas following lithium carbonate treatment for four to eight weeks, the 5-HTP-induced cortisol response increased.[186] Chronic lithium may further augment 5HT release or increase 5HT receptor supersensitivity, while chronic antidepressant treatment may normalize the synthesis and release of 5HT, leading to down-regulation of the 5HT receptor that regulates cortisol secretion.

Charney, Heninger, and Reinhard[57] demonstrated that an intravenous infusion of tryptophan, 100 mg per kg, can stimulate serum prolactin and GH secretion in normal controls. Presumably tryptophan is converted to 5-HTP, which is then decarboxylated to 5HT. Heninger, Charney, and Sternberg[119] subsequently reported that the prolactin response to tryptophan was blunted in both male and female depressed patients. There was no relationship between the magnitude of the response and severity of depression. They also reported that the prolactin response to tryptophan normalized following treatment with desipramine hydrochloride or imipramine hydrochloride. It was suggested that the diminished prolactin response could be due to decreased 5HT receptor sensitivity, which was subsequently reversed by antidepressant treatment. We were initially unable to replicate these results,[188] but in a larger, unpublished series of subjects Koyama, of our group, found a diminished GH and cortisol response to tryptophan.

Siever and associates[246] recently reported that fenfluramine hydrochloride, a 5HT-releasing drug, produced a significantly smaller increase in serum prolactin levels in eighteen depressed patients compared to ten controls. We have not replicated these results.[188]

The challenge studies with serotonergic agents are in their earliest phases of development. The complete mechanism of action of 5-HTP, tryptophan, and fenfluramine with regard to stimulation of prolactin, GH, or cortisol is unknown. All three agents might directly or indirectly affect other neurotransmitters, such as NE or DA, which might affect hormonal responses. The status of the pre- and postsynaptic mechanisms that these agents affect need not be the same for the pathways that stimulate the three hormones studied to date. Finally, pharmacokinetic factors such as the rate of absorption of 5-HTP or fenfluramine, which are given orally, or the rate of clearance of tryptophan must be taken into account in subsequent studies. Direct-acting 5HT agonists are superior to these three agents for determining the status of 5HT receptor sensitivity in the neuroendocrine system.

The Thyroid Axis in Affective Disorders

The importance of the thyroid axis for depression has been appreciated for some time because depressive symptoms are so common in hypothyroidism[283] and because triiodothyronine (T_3) can potentiate the action of tricyclic antidepressant drugs in some female depressives.[217] These observations have stimulated extensive inquiry into the status of the hypothalamic-pituitary-thyroid axis in depression.[160,214]

The secretion of thyroxine (T_4) and T_3 is controlled by the anterior pituitary hormone TSH, which is in turn regulated by the hypothalamic tripeptide, TRH. The release of TSH is under feedback inhibition by T_3 and T_4. The TSH response to TRH is also inhibited by glucocorticoids and stimulated by estrogens. TRH can also stimulate prolactin release, which has led to speculation that it may be the prolactin-releasing factor.

Thyroid function, as indicated by serum T_3, T_4, and free T_4 index, has variously been reported to be normal, increased, or decreased in depression or mania.[160] These discrepancies are due to phase of illness, nutritional status of patients, stress, lack of adequate determination of normal limits, and heterogeneity in clinical populations. Serum concentrations of 3,3′,5′-triiodothyronine, reverse T_3, have been reported to be elevated in major depression and mania in some studies[159] but not in others.[142] However, even in the latter study, its concentration was correlated with the severity of psychopathology. Reverse T_3 may be an antagonist of T_3 and could account for the subtle hypothyroidism noted in some unipolar and bipolar patients. The majority of depressed patients are euthyroid in all studies. Those depressed patients who are hypothyroid need to be identified by appropriate laboratory measures and given replacement therapy.[106] Whybrow and Prange[284] have considered the possible effect of impaired thyroid function on noradrenergic function in major depression. Rapid-cycling bipolar patients appear to have a high incidence of hypothyroidism, possibly due to previous lithium treatment.[70] Despite these findings, there may be subtle marginal impairment of thyroid function, which, in interaction with other endocrine influences, could influence neuronal function in major depression. Antidepressant treatment does not systematically alter thyroid function.[158]

Administration of TRH to depressed patients has been reported to have an antidepressant effect in unipolar female depressed patients,[135,216] but other investigators have not been able to confirm this.[28,123]

There have been nearly fifty studies of the TSH response to TRH in depression.[160] Most but not all studies showed a significantly greater incidence of blunted responses in depressed patients compared to normal controls. With intravenous administration of 500 ug TRH, a blunted response is usually considered to be an increase equal to or less than 5 or 7 uU per ml. Blunted responses have been noted in about 25 percent of hospitalized unipolar depressed, bipolar depressed, and alcoholic patients.[160] The incidence of blunted TSH responses to TRH may not be greater than normal in outpatients with major depression.[165] A high incidence of blunted responses have also been reported in borderline patients.[97] The TSH response to TRH is usually normal in anorexia nervosa.[273] The TRH test has been reported to be blunted in manic patients as a group[141] and to have sufficient specificity and sensitivity to distinguish mania from schizophrenia.[86] However, there are reports of blunted TSH responses in schizophrenia also.[288] There is no correlation between severity of depression, serum cortisol levels, or basal thyroid levels and the magnitude of the TSH response.[160] The blunted TSH response usually normalizes during recovery, but it may persist, in which case it may predict a high degree of vulnerability to relapse unless treatment is continued.[149]

Loosen and Prange[160] have postulated that a blunted TSH response may be due to hypersecretion of TRH, leading to a decreased sensitivity to TRH. There is evidence that desensitization to TRH may occur in depressed patients during chronic TRH administration.[286] Decreased serotonergic activity or increased noradrenergic and dopaminergic activity have been postulated to be causally related to increased TRH secretion. Excessive release of somatostatin or neurotensin might also account for a blunted TSH response.[214]

Gonadotropin and Gonadal Steroid Hormones in Affective Disorders

Decreased libido is a prominent feature of major depression. Hence the levels of gonadotropins and gonadal steroids in the plasma of depressed patients have been of considerable interest. Basal plasma LH levels and the LH or FSH response to GnRH in depressed males have been reported to be within normal limits[5,25,84] or low in 20 to 30 percent of depressed subjects.[37,157,227] Altman and associates[4] reported decreased plasma LH levels in postmenopausal depressed women.

Plasma testosterone levels have been reported to be normal in depressed males and not to vary upon recovery.[5,233] However, Vogel, Klarber, and Broverman[275] found decreased total and free mean plasma testosterone levels and increased plasma estradiol in primary unipolar depressed males. Low plasma testosterone levels were also reported in the study of Rubin and associates.[227] Vogel, Klarber, and Broverman[275] also found increased plasma estradiol and testosterone concentrations in primary, unipolar premenopausal depressed women, but Amsterdam and coworkers[5] did not. These results suggest there may be modest abnormalities of the hypothalamo-pituitary-gonadal axis in some individuals with primary, unipolar depression, but their significance is obscure. Solid evidence relating decreased or increased levels of plasma gonadal steroids to decreased libido or severity of symptoms in major depression is lacking. Interpretation of borderline changes in plasma steroid levels is difficult without taking into account possible changes in receptor sensitivity.

Abnormal Response to Hypothalamic Hormones in Affective Disorder

Various investigators have reported that some depressed patients respond to TRH by releasing GH,[37,168] a response not found in normal subjects. Brambilla and associates,[37] proposed that in depression, hypothalamic releasing factor hormones may influence pituitary cells other than their normal targets because of a decrease in the inhibitory effect of neurohormonal mechanisms that normally convey specificity for a particular releasing factor. In a subsequent study, this pattern was noted to normalize during successful treatment with desipramine.[38] However, a GH increase after TRH may be a nonspecific finding or could be due to its spontaneous release. No differences in the incidence of GH or prolactin responses to GnRH were noted in bipolar or unipolar depressed patients when compared to normal controls.[7]

Interrelationships Between Neuroendocrine Abnormalities in Affective Disorders

With the diversity of neuroendocrine abnormalities in depressed patients, the issue of their interrelationships is of keen interest. Abnormal DST responses and blunted TSH responses to TRH are generally independent of each other; that is, they do not occur in the same patients more commonly than by chance alone.[76,259] Winokur and coworkers[285] and Amsterdam and others[8] carried out four neuroendocrine challenges (measuring two hormones after each challenge) in unipolar and bipolar depressed patients, respectively. These were the TRH test, the GnRH test, the insulin tolerance test, and the DST. No consistent patterns of abnormality of hormonal responses were observed. Twenty-five of twenty-six (96.2 percent) unipolar depressed patients had at least one abnormality compared to seven of twenty-four (29.2 percent) controls. Fifteen unipolar depressed patients had two or more abnormalities, but none of the control subjects did. A similar pattern was noted in the bipolar patients. These authors proposed that limbic system, pituitary, or hypothalamic receptor abnormalities might underlie these changes.

In a sample of twelve inpatients with major depression (eight primary, four secondary), Ansseau and associates[12] studied the DST, the GH responses to apomorphine and clonidine, and REM latency. Only blunted clonidine and apomorphine responses were associated with each other. The sensitivity of the clonidine test was much greater, however (75 percent versus 42 percent). Beck-Friis and coworkers[25] reported that the TSH and prolactin responses to TRH and the LH and FSH responses to GnRH were mainly normal in twenty-three patients with major depression. Several patients had phase advances of cortisol or prolactin secretion. Of most interest was a reciprocal relationship between plasma melatonin levels and DST nonsuppression. This was attributed to the inhibitory effect of melatonin on CRF release.

If one assumes that primary disturbances of neuronal mechanisms underlie neuroendocrine abnormalities in depression, the diversity of neuroendocrine disturbances among depressed subjects may be further evidence for the heterogeneity of neurotransmitter abnormalities within depression and the shift over time, within subjects, of neurotransmitter dysfunction. Studies relating biochemical abnormalities that may reflect specific neurotransmitters (e.g., CSF 5-hydroxyindoleacetic acid [5-HIAA], homovanillac acid [HVA], or urinary 3-methoxy-4-hydroxyphenylglycol [MHPG]) to the neuroendocrine abnormalities are of keen interest.

Growth Hormone Studies in Depression and Mania

GH secretion in man is stimulated by alpha-2- and inhibited by beta-adrenergic agonists, the former by a direct effect on GHRF and somatostatin, the latter via an effect on blood glucose and fatty acids. DA also stimulates GH secretion by inhibiting somatostatin release. GABA, 5HT, and acetylcholine (ACh) also stimulate GH secretion, but opiates and histamine appear not to have a direct effect.[61] GH secretion is enhanced by estrogens and inhibited by cortisol, both of which may be relevant factors in clinical studies.

The GH response to insulin-induced hypoglycemia in depression appears to be blunted,[111] whereas the response to levodopa[234] or the DA agonist apomorphine appears to be within normal limits.[55,187] The GH response to amphetamine or methamphetamine, which is probably mediated by release of NE, does not differ in depression when age and sex are accounted for.[60,116]

There has been extensive investigation of the GH response to clonidine in major depression, with all investigators reporting a decreased response.[58,62,174,244] This has been interpreted as evidence of subsensitive postsynaptic alpha-2-adrenergic receptors. The GH response to clonidine was significantly less than the response to apomorphine in eight drug-free patients with endogenous depression.[68] Treatment with tricyclic antidepressants or monoamine oxidase inhibitors (MAOIs) for four to six weeks had no effect on this response in responders or nonresponders, suggesting it is a trait marker for depression.[58,244]

Prolactin Studies in Affective Disorders

Normal, decreased, or increased basal serum prolactin levels have been reported in depressed patients.[67,156,168] In addition, Asnis and associates[17] reported that serum prolactin levels were slightly higher in depressed patients after clinical recovery than during illness, but were still within normal limits at both times. There is little evidence for prolactin differences between unipolar and bipolar patients. Halbreich, Grunhaus, and Ben-David[115] reported significantly increased serum prolactin levels during the evening, several hours before sleep, in a mixed group of depressed patients compared to control subjects. Morning serum prolactin levels were slightly higher among the depressive patients. Mendlewicz, Van Cauter, and Linkowski[190] found basal serum prolactin levels were increased in unipolar patients, mainly because of increased secretion during wakefulness, and lowered in bipolar patients because of a lack or reduction of the sleep-associated elevation. There was less variability in the twenty-four-hour profile of serum prolactin levels in both types of affective illness.

The TRH-induced prolactin response was reported to be blunted in seven of eight unipolar patients.[157] Linkowski, Brauman, and Mendlewicz[156] found that the TRH-induced prolactin response was blunted in postmenopausal unipolar and bipolar depressed patients, but not significantly different in premenopausal patients compared to control subjects. Coppen and coworkers[67] found normal responses in primary depression. The sporadic depressive disease subgroup had an enhanced response. Maeda and others[168] also found an enhanced prolactin response to TRH.

Oral levodopa has been demonstrated to reduce serum prolactin levels more in bipolar and less in unipolar depressed patients than in healthy volunteers.[107] These results were not confirmed by Mendlewicz, Linkowski, and Brauman.[189]

Two groups have reported a blunted prolactin response to morphine[85] or methadone[133] in depression. It is possible that this reflects an abnormality in the endogenous opiate regulation of prolactin secretion or a serotonergic abnormality, since there is strong evidence that morphine stimulates prolactin by promoting the release of 5HT.

Neuroendocrine Studies of Suicidal Behavior

There is some evidence that neuroendocrine disturbances may be particularly prominent in suicidal patients. Bunney and Fawcett[44] reported increased twenty-four-hour urinary 17-hydroxycorticosteroids in suicidal depressed patients compared to nonsuicidal patients. They attributed this association to unbearable psychic pain. In a subsequent report, Bunney and associates[45] reported longitudinal urinary 17-hydroxycorticosteroid data on nine patients who subsequently committed suicide or made a serious suicide attempt. Mean levels were elevated compared to 134 comparison subjects. Elevations were present for as long as one to two months prior to the suicidal act. Two small-scale studies failed to replicate these results,[92,155] but Ostroff and coworkers[207] recently confirmed the findings of Bunney and colleagues.

Krieger[148] reported elevated plasma cortisol levels in thirteen patients who subse-

quently committed suicide compared to thirty-nine patients who did not. Traskman and others[264] found no association between CSF cortisol and prior suicide attempts in a heterogeneous group of patients. However, Carroll, Greden, and Feinberg[53] reported an association between an abnormal DST and violent suicidal behavior in melancholic patients. Similar results were obtained by other investigators.[24,69] Increased CSF cortisol may also be associated with suicide.[53] There have been two reports of a small number of subjects who made serious suicidal attempts shortly after receiving dexamethasone.[15,26]

An association between violent suicidal behavior in depressed and manic patients and the magnitude of the 5-HTP increase in serum cortisol has been previously mentioned.[185] This may be related to reports of decreased 5-HIAA, the major metabolite of 5HT, in the CSF of depressed patients who made violent suicide attempts.[14]

Banki and associates[24] studied CSF levels of 5-HIAA, HVA, the major metabolite of DA, and cortisol, as well as the DST and the TSH response to TRH in 141 female psychiatric patients with diagnoses of major depression ($N = 36$), schizophrenia ($N = 46$), alcohol dependence ($N = 35$), and adjustment disorder ($N = 24$). Of these, thirty-three had recently made a nonviolent suicide attempt and eighteen, a violent one. CSF 5-HIAA was lower in the patients who made violent attempts in all four diagnostic groups. No relation between suicide and CSF cortisol was noted. CSF HVA was increased in those patients who made a nonviolent attempt. A positive DST was present in twelve of fifteen (80 percent) of the violent attempters and in seventeen of twenty-four (71 percent) of the nonviolent attempters, but in only thirty-eight of seventy-two (53 percent) of the nonsuicidal patients (chi-square = 6.12, $df = 2$, $p < 0.05$). The TSH response to TRH was greater in both types of suicidal patients. A significant negative correlation between CSF 5-HIAA and the TSH response was noted here and in the study by Gold, Pottash, and Extein.[106] Banki and Arato[23] have also reported significant correlations between

CSF 5-HIAA and various personality dimensions.

The direction of cause and effect in the apparently increased rate of endocrine disturbances in suicidal behavior is difficult to assess. It is possible that elevated cortisol secretion is a concomitant of decreased serotonergic activity, since there is evidence that 5HT may inhibit as well as stimulate cortisol secretion, probably via different 5HT pathways or excitatory and inhibitory postsynaptic effects.[184] In some patients glucocorticoid receptors may become partially insensitive to cortisol stimulation, which would convey protection from the deleterious consequences of excessive glucocorticoid stimulation. In those individuals who do not develop this mechanism, glucocorticoids may indeed be a risk factor contributing to suicide.

Summary of Endocrine Disturbance in Affective Disorders

There is unequivocal evidence of neuroendocrine disturbances in some patients with major depression. This is most clear-cut in studies of the HPA axis that reveal hypersecretion in many patients, perhaps associated with subsensitivity of glucocorticoid receptors. There is considerable evidence that these findings are not due to stress per se. While they do not identify a specific subtype of depression or provide guidance for treatment, these findings may be relevant as an indicator of potential for relapse and suicide.

Provocative tests, such as the 5-HTP- or ACTH-induced increase in cortisol, tryptophan-induced increase in prolactin, fenfluramine-induced increase in prolactin, clonidine-induced increase in GH, amphetamine-induced increase in cortisol, TRH-induced increase in TSH, and CRF-induced increase in ACTH, represent a new thrust in the endocrinology of depression. It is not yet clear whether these procedures will be clinically useful or help to clarify the pathophysiology of depression. Many more patients and control subjects, including patients with other psychiatric diseases, need to be studied before the findings we have reviewed can be accepted as established. The influence of prior treatment, stress, menstrual status, age, and circadian disturbances and other sources of variance need to be ascertained.

At the current time, the unstable, variegated pattern of neuroendocrine abnormalities in depressed patients suggests that more than one neurotransmitter is involved in both the neuroendocrine disturbances and the etiology of the depressive syndrome. Clearly, neuroendocrine assessment of depressed patients is a worthwhile procedure, both clinically and for the purpose of investigating neuronal mechanisms safely and conveniently using hormonal assays. If methods sensitive enough to determine the concentrations of hypothalamic releasing factors such as CRF or TRH in peripheral plasma are developed and prove to have some relationship to the production and release of these substances, the neuroendocrine strategy will move significantly closer to the stage of providing a window into the brain.

¶ Neuroendocrine–Immune System Relationships

Within the last decade, it has become increasingly clear that there are extensive relationships between the central nervous system and immune system. The neuroendocrine axis appears to play a major role in mediating communication between these two complex systems.[2,30,251] It is beyond the scope of this discussion to review this evidence, but several recent studies indicate various neuroendocrine-immune relationships that have important implications for psychiatry.

The role of glucocorticoids in modulating stress responses, as well as their role in the suppression of immune function, has been emphasized since the classic work of Selye. In view of the well-known dysfunction of the HPA axis in psychiatric disorders, particularly depression, elevations in cortisol levels may modify immune status in these individuals. Depressed patients with high serum cortisol levels have impaired responses to mitogen-induced lymphocyte proliferation (an *in vitro* assay that reflects immunocompetency) compared to healthy controls.[241] Psychiatric patients who have high loneliness scores have increased urinary cortisol levels compared to psychiatric patients with low scores on a standardized loneliness scale. The high-loneliness, elevated-cortisol group also had lower levels of natural killer cell activity and an impaired mitogen-induced lymphoproliferative response.[140] In addition, normal control subjects who have high scores on a stressful life events and loneliness scale also have lower natural killer cell activity.[139] These studies indicate that elevations in HPA activity can have significant adverse effects on immunocompetency in psychiatric patients. However, it should be noted that hormones other than glucocorticoids may be involved, since adrenalectomy does not block stress-induced immunosuppression in laboratory animals.[138]

Since lymphocytes possess receptors for a variety of neuromodulators, they may be useful peripheral markers to assess the receptor sensitivity and function of hormones and neuropeptides. Lowy and associates[163] have utilized circulating lymphocytes to assess glucocorticoid resistance in depressed patients during a standard DST. DST suppressors showed the expected dexamethasone-induced suppression of mitogenesis, while nonsuppressors were resistant to these immunosuppressive effects. This resistance may explain the lack of Cushingoid features in depressed patients with high cortisol levels. The dexamethasone-induced mitogen changes were significantly correlated with the highest post-dexamethasone cortisol values. Thus the neuroendocrine and immune systems show parallel sensitivity in their response to a glucocorticoid challenge.

It is becoming clear that not only can the neuroendocrine axis modify the immune system, but that products derived from immune tissue can have profound effects on neuroendocrine function. Blalock[32] has recently commented on the similarity between lympho-kines (hormonelike substances that provide communication between branches of the immune system) and endocrine hormones, as well as their interrelationships. Of particular note is the ability of lymphocytes to produce substances with ACTH- and endorphinlike activity.[249] It has been demonstrated that a lymphoid-adrenal axis that is sensitive to glucocorticoid modulation functions *in vivo*.[250] An apparent case of Cushing's syndrome due to lymphocyte-derived ACTH has also been reported.[210] These studies raise the possibility that an abnormality in lymphocyte function could activate the HPA axis, resulting in neuroendocrine abnormalities that are similar to those observed in depression.

The field of neuroendocrinology has provided enormous insights into the abnormalities and pathogenesis of psychiatric diseases. In future years the emerging field of psychoneuroimmunology may yield similar benefits.

¶ Neuroendocrine Effects of Electroconvulsive Therapy

The effects of ECT on the neuroendocrine system have been investigated mainly as a means of clarifying the mechanism of action of this treatment for severe depression. Numerous studies have documented increases in serum prolactin immediately following ECT,[13,206] but the effect on GH, TSH, and cortisol secretion is inconsistent.[13,230] The ECT-induced increase in serum cortisol in psychotic depressive patients was significantly smaller than in nonpsychotic depression,[79] further evidence that psychotic depression differs significantly from nonpsychotic depression. The acute effects of ECT on prolactin secretion show tolerance over a course of seven ECT treatments, but the cortisol response does not.[79] These effects of ECT on hormone release are short-lasting; however, since a variety of peptides may be released during ECT, mainly from the pituitary, and since the blood-brain barrier and the pattern of peptide transport and metabolism may be altered during ECT, it has been proposed that the clinical effects of ECT could be due to facilitation of the effects of behaviorally active peptides in the brain.[93] In this regard, plasma beta-endorphin levels increase following ECT.[3]

There have been a number of neuroendocrine studies designed to determine whether a course of ECT alters receptor sensitivity as indicated by the change in hormone response to challenge agents. Such studies should actually include a range of doses to determine whether there has been a shift in the dose-response curve, since changes in the magnitude of the endocrine response could reflect variations in pituitary stores or hormone clearance rates. Coppen and associates[67] found that the TRH-induced increase in serum prolactin was enhanced after ECT, which was related to increased sensitivity of 5HT receptors, since 5HT may mediate the TRH-induced increase in prolactin. Balldin and coworkers[21] found that the decrease in serum prolactin levels produced by the DA agonist apomorphine was enhanced after a course of ECT, but the increase in GH was not affected. Christie and others[64] found no difference in the prolactin or GH response following apomorphine after ECT. Slade and Checkley[248] reported the GH response to clonidine, an alpha-2 agonist, was not affected by a course of ECT. Since, as previously mentioned, four to six weeks of treatment with tricyclic antidepressant or MAOIs also did not alter the GH response to clonidine,[58,244] it appears that diminished GH response to clonidine may be a trait of some depressed patients.

¶ Endocrine Responses to Stress

Intense, frightening, novel, or unexpected stimuli that are experienced by an individual as stressful may be accompanied by a variety of effects on the secretion of hormones such as cortisol, prolactin, GH, beta-endorphin, vasopressin, and sex steroids. This has been reviewed in detail by Mason[172] and Rose.[221] Attempts to define stress or stressful stimuli

often lead to circular arguments. Ursin and Murison[265] have proposed that "all the physiological changes accompanying stress may be summarized as 'activation,' a normal response in normal individuals which prepares the body and the brain to meet the challenges of everyday life" (p. 124).

Anticipation of challenging or dangerous events such as a school examination,[172,257] hospital admission,[172] surgery,[74,202] or severe exercise[201,238,252] may produce large increases in cortisol and other stress-sensitive hormones, such as prolactin and GH. Not all serum hormones are modified by every stressful event. GH increases are less likely to occur during stress than cortisol increases.[221] Although prolactin may be secreted in response to stresses such as medical examination or surgery,[203,252] serum prolactin levels are even less likely to increase during stress than GH levels. Thus Curtis and associates[73] exposed phobic patients to their phobic objects (so-called flooding *in vivo*). Moderate, but not marked, elevations of serum cortisol were noted in only three of six subjects. No correlation with the degree of anxiety was noted. In a subsequent study, flooding produced no increase in serum prolactin levels in eight normal control subjects.[200] The cold-pressor test produces increases in serum cortisol without any effect on serum prolactin, GH, beta-endorphin, or opioid activity.[22] Miyabo, Asato, and Mizushima[192] noted that serum prolactin levels increased in females with anxiety and minor depression during a drawing test in which they drew a figure viewed in a mirror. No change in prolactin occurred in similar male patients or in male and female normal controls. GH increased in patients of both sexes, but not in normal controls. No increases in serum prolactin levels were found in severely disturbed schizophrenic patients with an acute exacerbation of their psychosis.[177] Testosterone levels decreased following some acute stresses, such as surgery, and other stressful events in man,[59,146] but also fell during the coping phases of chronic exposure to stressful stimuli, such as parachute jumping.[266] Sowers and coworkers[252] noted that treadmill exercise, diagnostic gastroscopy, and elective surgery under general anesthesia decreased serum TSH. Serum T_3 was also decreased after surgery. Adequate psychological defense, from denial to appropriate coping behavior, has been demonstrated to be associated with smaller endocrine responses to stress.[136,145]

Animal studies have demonstrated rapid development of adaptation to stress as indicated by neuroendocrine responses. For example, both rhesus monkeys[173] and rats[212] have no increase in adrenal corticoid output after multiple days of shock-avoidance trials. There are relatively few studies of this process in man, but the results are comparable to those observed in experimental animals.[221] The developmental adaptation of the endocrine response to challenging tasks after repetition and development of adequate skills for coping has been reported for pilots,[211] truck drivers,[72] and air traffic controllers.[222,223,224]

Given the complexity of the neurotransmitter regulation of the secretion of the hypothalamic peptides that regulate the pituitary or affect the secretion of pituitary hormones directly, it is clear that no single neurotransmitter can be implicated as the sole cause of the hormone response to stress. The influences of decreased noradrenergic inhibition of CRF or stimulation of CRF release by 5HT, histamine, ACh, or angiotensin II on the release of ACTH during stress has been discussed by Ganong.[96]

¶ Endocrine Studies in Schizophrenia

Introduction

The possibility that endocrine disturbances predispose to or actually cause schizophrenia has been considered because peaks in the age of onset and changes in the intensity of symptoms in schizophrenia parallel major shifts in neuroendocrine function and because diverse endocrine abnormalities

have been observed in schizophrenic patients.[34] Considering the modern view of schizophrenia as a syndrome with numerous underlying biological causes producing nonspecific changes in cognitive function, volition, and affect, perhaps through a few common pathways, it is not unreasonable to consider that some instances of the disorder might be related to primary disturbances of the endocrine system. If so, one would predict that when and if the endocrine disturbances were corrected, the syndrome would resolve, providing that no irreversible changes in the nervous system had occurred.

Numerous reports of patients with endocrine disturbances, such as Addison's disease (hypoadrenalism), Cushing's syndrome (hyperadrenalism), myxedema (hypothyroidism) or hyperthyroidism, and concomitant schizophreniform psychopathology, have, in fact, been published.[34] However, in all four conditions, depressive symptomatology is far more common.[191] The dependence of the psychopathology on the endocrinopathy is apparent in the temporal development of the psychopathology after the endocrine disturbances and in the resolution of the psychopathology with appropriate replacement therapy or surgery.[130] Abnormalities of the parathyroid gland, or pituitary, insulinomas, or diabetes mellitus are rarely associated with schizophrenialike symptoms.[204] Thus it is fair to conclude that major disturbances of the endocrine glands are possible without subsequent development of schizophrenia.[34,204] The incidence of endocrine disturbances such as Addison's disease, Cushing's syndrome, myxedema, thyrotoxicosis, hypo- and hyperparathyroidism, acromegaly, or hypopituitarism in schizophrenia does not differ from that of the general population,[34] indicating that the spectrum of those organic disturbances that comprise schizophrenia does not increase the risk of developing a gross abnormality of the endocrine organs.

Investigation of the serum or plasma concentrations of various pituitary and target organ hormones in schizophrenia have been carried out in order to assess endocrine function. More recently, the major aims of neuroendocrine research have been to obtain indirect evidence of the function of the neurotransmitters that regulate the secretion of these hormones, to assess drug action on neurotransmitter dynamics or receptors via effect on hormone release, and to assess whether hormone levels correlate with psychopathology or predict treatment response.

Secretion of prolactin and GH has received emphasis in schizophrenia research because the secretion of these hormones is influenced by DA. DA inhibits prolactin secretion and stimulates GH secretion. Increased dopaminergic activity has been postulated to be an element in the positive symptoms of schizophrenia and other psychoses, while decreased dopaminergic activity has been related to negative symptoms.[46,166,175,179] The major classes of psychotropic drugs also have important effects on DA; neuroleptic drugs block DA receptors, reserpine releases DA, alpha-methylparatyrosine inhibits DA synthesis, amantadine hydrochloride promotes DA release, antidepressants such as imipramine are weak inhibitors of DA uptake, chronic antidepressant treatment can decrease the sensitivity of DA receptors on cell bodies or terminals (DA autoreceptors), and lithium may affect DA receptor sensitivity.[179] Through these actions, the psychotropic drugs can affect basal prolactin or GH secretion or influence the prolactin or GH response to agents that stimulate or inhibit prolactin or GH secretion (e.g., the DA agonist, apomorphine). This review will concentrate on prolactin and GH but will also briefly discuss TRH, beta-endorphin, and cortisol.

Basal Hormone Levels in Schizophrenia

Prolactin concentrations in single blood samples obtained within one hour of awakening in schizophrenic patients were not significantly different from the levels found in normal controls.[182] Subsequent studies of the levels of prolactin in three catheter samples obtained between 9:30 and 10:00 A.M.

also revealed no significant differences between schizophrenic patients and control subjects.[175] Patients with tardive dyskinesia do not differ in basal serum prolactin levels from normal subjects or schizophrenic patients, nor do prolactin levels differ during chronic haloperidol treatment, serially after abrupt haloperidol withdrawal, or in response to an acute dose of 0.5 mg haloperidol intramusculary.[16]

A small proportion of schizophrenic patients have elevated serum prolactin levels,[131] but this may be due to the persistent effects of prior neuroleptic treatment, stress, or sleep-related elevations of serum prolactin levels. Normal serum prolactin levels suggest normal DA synthesis and/or release in the tuberoinfundibular DA neurons of the hypothalamus and no abnormalities of the DA receptors in the pituitary lactotrophes. This, of course, does not rule out the possibility that other factors that modulate prolactin secretion might account for the failure to find a difference in serum prolactin levels between schizophrenic patients and control subjects. Serum prolactin levels during sleep have been only minimally studied in schizophrenic patients but appear to show the normal pattern of an increase after sleep onset.[175]

There have been numerous attempts to relate basal serum prolactin levels in schizophrenic patients to demographic and biological variables. No significant correlations between serum prolactin levels and age, age of onset, duration of illness, presence of delusions, hallucinations, total psychotic symptoms, first-rank symptoms, anxiety ratings, total Brief Psychiatric Rating Scale (BPRS) scores, or total Global Assessment Scale scores were noted in twenty-three male and twenty-two female schizophrenic patients.[175] Lower serum prolactin levels were reported to predict relapse after withdrawal from neuroleptic drugs and subsequent good response to neuroleptic treatment.[42,152] Johnstone, Crow, and Mashiter[131] reported significant negative correlations between serum prolactin levels and incoherence of speech and total positive symptoms in sixteen very chronic male schizophrenic patients who had never received neuroleptic drugs. Of interest with regard to Crow's model of type I and II schizophrenia,[71] fourteen of the sixteen had both positive and negative symptoms. These investigators could not replicate the prolactin-psychopathology correlation in an independent group of schizophrenic patients.[90] Kleinman and associates[144] also reported a significant negative correlation between median plasma prolactin levels (three to seven determinations per subject over a one- to eleven-week drug-free period) and total BPRS score for seventeen chronic schizophrenic patients, especially the eight with normal ventricular size. We were unable to replicate these results.[164] CSF prolactin levels are also within normal limits.[175]

Basal serum GH levels have been found to be within normal limits in unmedicated chronic schizophrenic patients.[175] Some chronic schizophrenic patients do not show the expected increase in GH secretion during sleep.[34, 175, 274] This may be relevant to other instances of blunted GH secretion in schizophrenia.[186] Somatostatin levels have been reported to be normal in the CSF of schizophrenic patients[103] but decreased in the CSF of depressed patients.[228]

Extensive reviews of gonadal steroids in schizophrenia are available.[34, 175] Most studies have found serum testosterone, estrogen, and progesterone levels within normal limits, but there are significant exceptions.[35] Decreased serum FSH and LH levels in unmedicated schizophrenic patients have been noted by Brambilla and coworkers[35] and Ferrier and others,[90] but were not reported in a previous study from the latter group.[131] In Ferrier and associates'[90] study, the patients were elderly (mean age fifty-seven years) and the FSH and LH levels were low only in comparison with an age-matched control group. Despite this, testosterone levels were similar in both groups, suggesting normal feedback control in the schizophrenic patients. Ferrier and coworkers[90] noted a significant negative relationship between FSH levels and positive symptoms in these chronic schizophrenic patients.

There have been extensive studies of the levels of endogenous opioid substances,—for example, beta-endorphin—in unmedicated schizophrenia and following neuroleptic treatment. Some studies have found elevated levels in CSF or plasma or both, while others have not.[39,197] Differences in the assay, type and clinical state of patient studied, duration of neuroleptic withdrawal, and failure to separately assay beta-lipotropin (β-LPH) and beta-endorphin may account for these differences. Brambilla and associates[39] measured the concentrations of both peptides in thirty-seven chronic schizophrenic patients who had been withdrawn from medication for at least ten days. Basal β-LPH levels were increased in twenty patients, low in three, and normal in the others. Basal beta-endorphin levels were high in twenty-two patients and low in three others. Levels of either hormone were not related to age, psychopathology, duration of illness, or duration of treatment. There was a weak correlation between the levels of the two opioids. Haloperidol treatment did not significantly alter β-LPH or beta-endorphin levels. Brambilla and coworkers[39] suggested their data supported the theory of Volovka, Davis, and Ehrlich,[276] which related increased endogenous opioid activity to increased dopaminergic activity in schizophrenia through effects on DA_1 and DA_2 receptors. However, Naber, Nedopil, and Eben[197] reported that serum beta-endorphin levels were increased during neuroleptic treatment. In another study Naber and others[198] reported that plasma beta-endorphin levels increased after withdrawal of neuroleptics and that patients with low beta-endorphin levels during neuroleptic treatment were more likely to develop psychotic symptoms after neuroleptic withdrawal than were patients with high levels of beta-endorphin.

Naloxone hydrochloride has been reported to increase plasma prolactin and GH concentrations in chronic schizophrenic patients but not in normal controls.[144] The absence of major effects of administration of endogenous opioids or naloxone, the opioid antagonist, on the mental status of schizophrenic patients suggests these findings indicate the absence of important relationships between endogenous opioids and psychopathology in schizophrenia; however, further research with more potent and specific agents is clearly indicated.

Adrenal function in schizophrenia has been extensively reviewed by Brambilla and Penati. [34] Basal levels of serum or urinary glucocorticoids and ketosteroids have been found to be either above or below normal limits in some schizophrenic patients. The levels tend to be related to age or clinical state and to be highly variable within a given subject. More dynamic tests of adrenal function also reveal no consistent abnormalities in schizophrenia. Nonsuppression in the DST test has been observed in 10 to 20 percent of schizophrenic patients. [180, 255]

Thyroid function in schizophrenia may be somewhat decreased in some schizophrenic patients, but only occasional patients improve with thyroid treatment or TRH administration. [34, 217]

Plasma melatonin levels have been determined in aged chronic schizophrenic patients and control subjects. [91] The midnight melatonin level and midnight-to-8 A.M. melatonin ratio were significantly decreased in the schizophrenic patients, but this difference is partially accounted for by differences in body weight.

Effects of Apomorphine or Clonidine Administration on Growth Hormone and Prolactin in Schizophrenia

The GH responses of unmedicated patients with chronic schizophrenia following a single subemetic dose of apomorphine (0.5–1.0 mg) have been reported to be not significantly different from those of normal controls [183, 187] or to be significantly lower. [1, 89] These differences relate to age, duration of illness, sex, weight, and clinical state differ-

ences between the subjects in these studies. Meltzer and associates [187] reported that the GH response to apomorphine was inversely correlated with duration of illness and positively correlated with positive and negative symptoms. Ferrier and coworkers [89] also reported that the GH response was positively correlated with positive symptoms but inversely correlated with negative symptoms. The fifteen chronic schizophrenic patients in the study of Ferrier and associates [89] had been drug-free for more than a year and five had never been treated with neuroleptic drugs. Those in the study of Meltzer and others [187] were on average thirty-eight years younger than those in Ferrier and associates' study [89] and were drug-free for 23.2 ± 19.1 days. The possibility that abnormalities in the hypothalamus account for the decreased response to apomorphine over time was suggested in both these studies.

Hirschowitz, Zemlan, and Garver [122] reported that schizophreniform patients who had a robust GH response (≥ 20 ng/ml) to apomorphine had a positive response to treatment with lithium. Only one of twenty-five schizophrenics had a positive response to lithium, and only seven of the twenty-five (28 percent) had a GH response greater than or equal to 20 ng per ml. They proposed that this response might have utility for predicting clinical response.

There have been two studies of the GH response to clonidine in schizophrenia, one that reported a greater response than controls [174] and one that reported no difference. [151] Lal and associates [151] concluded that postsynaptic alpha-2-adrenergic receptor sensitivity was not altered in schizophrenia or by the effect of neuroleptic treatment.

Insulin-induced Hypoglycemia and Growth Hormone in Schizophrenia

Insulin-induced hypoglycemia stimulates GH secretion, possibly via a noradrenergic mechanism. [195] The GH response depends on the degree of hypoglycemia. There is considerable evidence of noradrenergic dysfunction in schizophrenia.[267] Schizophrenic patients have been reported to be resistant to hypoglycemia in some studies[194] but not in others.[41, 239] Normal GH response to insulin in chronic schizophrenia has been reported in three studies,[27,41,258] but a high proportion of blunted responses was observed in another study.[239] Brambilla and others[36] also noted a very variable GH response on test-retest in hebephrenic schizophrenic patients and a blunted response in patients with predominantly negative symptoms.

Effect of Gonadotrophin-releasing Hormone on LH and FSH in Schizophrenia

Brambilla and Penati[34] administered three doses of GnRH to fifteen adult male chronic hebephrenic patients and fifteen oligophrenic control subjects. The schizophrenic patients had greater FSH and LH responses. Ferrier and associates[90] administered 100 ug GnRH to eighteen chronic schizophrenic patients who had not received medication for at least a year, and observed a decreased FSH and LH response compared to nine normal controls. Nine of the eighteen schizophrenic patients also had a GH response to GnRH, whereas none of the control subjects did. This group of schizophrenic patients had normal basal levels of testosterone and estradiol but low levels of FSH and LH. GH responses following GnRH have also been noted in depression[37] and anorexia nervosa.[169] It is of interest that DA may inhibit gonadotrophin release[153] and block the effect of naloxone in man, suggesting a possible interaction between DA, opioid receptors, and gonadotrophin secretion in man.[80]

The Thyrotropin Stimulating Test in Schizophrenia

As previously discussed, the TSH response to TRH may be blunted in about 25 percent of depressed patients. The TSH response to TRH in schizophrenic patients is within normal limits.[86, 217] An abnormal GH increase after TRH has been found in adolescent schizophrenic boys,[105, 282] but not in adult schizophrenic subjects.[217] A GH response to TRH is not specific to schizophrenia, but is present in a variety of psychiatric and medical disorders. Its significance is unknown.

Effect of Neuroleptic Drugs on the Neuroendocrine System

The acute and chronic effects of neuroleptic drugs on the neuroendocrine system have been extensively reviewed elsewhere[175] and will only be briefly mentioned. The most important neuroendocrine effect of neuroleptic drugs is their ability to stimulate prolactin secretion by blockade of pituitary DA receptors. Tolerance does not develop during the first several years of neuroleptic administration but may appear after chronic administration. The prolactin response to neuroleptic drugs correlates significantly with plasma levels of neuroleptic drugs in most studies.[181] The increase in serum prolactin levels with neuroleptic treatment may correlate with clinical response and extrapyramidal side effects.[181] Determination of serum prolactin levels may be helpful in determining whether patients are ingesting and absorbing oral medication. The prolactin response is linear with doses of up to 800 mg per day chlorpromazine or its equivalent.[181] Females have higher serum prolactin levels during neuroleptic treatment than males. This is partially due to higher blood levels of neuroleptics, but is still present after this difference is accounted for.

Neuroleptic drugs do not affect basal serum GH levels. Levels of gonadotropins or testosterone may decrease slightly during treatment with neuroleptic drugs, especially thioridazine hydrochloride[43] or pimozide,[247] but these effects are minimal and probably not of clinical significance.

Short-term or chronic neuroleptic treatment does not adversely affect the HPA axis.[243] The excretion of 17-hydroxycorticosteroids and 17-ketosteroids was not affected by chronic haloperidol treatment.[36]

Thyroid function is also not affected in a clinically significant way by chronic neuroleptic treatment.[243] Chronic haloperidol treatment does not alter basal thyroid function.[36] Brief (four-week) treatment with chlorpromazine did not affect plasma or CSF concentrations of TSH,[287] suggesting that a subsequent report that chlorpromazine and clozapine treatment decreased serum thyroxine and free thyroxine index in twenty-four of forty-one schizophrenics did not signify an important antithyroid effect of these drugs.[220]

Summary of Neuroendocrine Studies in Schizophrenia

There appears to be minimal evidence of major neuroendocrine disturbances in schizophrenia. Unlike major depression, where one finds disturbances of the HPA axis in a large proportion of patients at the initial phase of the illness, endocrine function is largely spared in schizophrenia. Abnormal levels of hypothalamic, pituitary, and target gland hormones are infrequent either in unmedicated patients or after neuroleptic treatment, with the exception that serum prolactin levels are markedly elevated in the first few years of neuroleptic treatment, and they may return to normal limits after very prolonged neuroleptic treatment. Neuroendocrine challenge studies with drugs such as apomorphine or other neurotransmitter agonists and antagonists are useful research tools to study receptor abnormalities in schizophrenia.

¶ Neuroendocrine Function in Anorexia Nervosa

Introduction

Anorexia nervosa is a feeding disorder characterized by self-induced weight loss through starvation and/or increased physical activity. Anorexic patients also have greatly distorted perceptions of their own body image and eating habits, as well as obsessive thoughts about food and self-image. The weight loss can be severe enough to result in morbidity or mortality due to electrolyte changes and cardiovascular irregularities. Young females make up the majority of anorexia nervosa patients, but a small percentage of males are also afflicted.

While anorexia nervosa has long been considered to be a psychiatric disorder, recent evidence suggests a strong relationship between this eating disorder and affective disease. Similarities between these two disorders include depressed mood, positive family history, sleep abnormalities, response to pharmacological treatment, and endocrine abnormalities.[137] This section will discuss the multiple neuroendocrine abnormalities present in patients with anorexia nervosa. Several recent papers and chapter 27 in this volume have extensively reviewed the early neuroendocrine studies[31,40,79,98,279] of anorexia. It should be emphasized from the start that the dramatic loss of body weight in anorexia nervosa patients may contribute to many of the reported neuroendocrine changes, since body weight loss due to malnutrition is known to alter endocrine function.

Gonadal Function in Anorexia Nervosa

Menstrual disturbance, usually amenorrhea, is an invariant feature of anorexia nervosa in postpubertal females. It may precede the weight loss itself. The amenorrhea is due to the absence of the normal cyclic circulating levels of the sex steroids, estradiol and progesterone. The mechanism for this deficiency has been extensively investigated and appears to be due to hypogonadotropic hypogonadism.[272] It has been repeatedly demonstrated that serum LH and FSH levels are depressed in anorexia nervosa and, furthermore, that levels of these hormones are correlated with body weight loss. When body weight recovers, circulating levels of LH and FSH also normalize, but amenorrhea may persist.

While both hypothalamic and pituitary sites have been implicated in this abnormality, recent work suggests a hypothalamic locus as the primary site of dysfunction. The response of LH and FSH to GnRH has been intensively studied and generally, normal responses have been obtained, although not infrequently the response is blunted or of a prepubertal nature (e.g., the FSH response is greater than that of LH). Chronic GnRH infusions may induce ovulation in some anorexic patients, indicating a functional pituitary and ovary. Thus a hypothalamic basis for the amenorrhea in anorexia nervosa is suggested. However, it should be pointed out that stress and increased physical activity, both of which are present in anorexic patients, also produce amenorrhea. Further research is necessary to clarify the relative contribution of these parameters and whether these changes are related to dysfunctional hypothalamic neurotransmitter systems.

Hypothalamic-Pituitary-Adrenal Axis in Anorexia Nervosa

A large body of evidence suggests increased activity of the HPA axis in anorexia nervosa.[280] Daily excretion of urinary free cortisol is elevated, as is the circadian rhythm of serum cortisol levels. The elevated serum cortisol levels are due to both an increase in cortisol secretion and a decrease in cortisol metabolism. The increased cortisol production declines as body weight gain occurs. These elevations in HPA axis activity are quite similar to those observed in major depression.[51]

The DST provides a more dynamic means of assessing the activity of the HPA axis. As discussed, the DST has been proposed to be a putative biological marker for major depression. Patients with anorexia nervosa fail to show adequate suppression of serum cortisol following low oral doses of dexamethasone.[101] Since patients with major depression also show a high rate of DST nonsuppression, these results may provide additional evidence for an association between anorexia

nervosa and affective disorder. However, not all of the nonsuppressor anorexic patients are depressed,[101] and, as previously mentioned, weight loss per se has been reported to result in DST nonsuppression.[83]

Donohue[82] has discussed the possibility that CRF, the hypothalamic hypophyseal hormone that regulates ACTH release, may itself be a cause of anorexia. The interactions among the HPA axis, 5HT, and stress were suggested as a possible cause of appetite suppression.

Thyroid Function in Anorexia Nervosa

Patients with anorexia nervosa often show features suggestive of hypothyroidism, but their thyroid status is generally different from true cases of hypothyroidism.[31] T_4 levels are normal or slightly below normal in anorexic patients.[98] However, T_3 levels are consistently reported to be depressed in anorexic patients, which is associated with an increase in the inactive reverse form of T_3.[154] The levels of T_3 are correlated with the percentage of ideal body weight. When body weight is increased, the T_3 and reverse T_3 levels normalize. Similar changes in T_3 levels also occur in other states of starvation. Basal levels of TSH are normal in anorexia nervosa and show no correlation with body weight.[154] The TRH-induced release of TSH is normal in anorexia, but may be temporarily delayed.[273] The available data suggest that the changes in pituitary-thyroid function are adaptive responses to the state of chronic starvation.[98]

Growth Hormone and Prolactin in Anorexia Nervosa

Resting basal daytime levels of GH are generally elevated in anorexia nervosa and return to normal following recovery.[99] The elevated GH levels are not related to body weight, but rather are influenced by the caloric intake of the patient. Since other states of decreased food intake are also associated with increased serum GH levels, starvation appears to be responsible for the elevated GH levels.

A variety of studies have examined the effect of provocative challenges on GH levels in anorexia nervosa.[31,40,98,279] Blunted responses to bromocriptine, levodopa, insulin-induced hypoglycemia, and slow-wave sleep have been reported, although not all studies agree. The GH response to arginine administration is intact, and a paradoxical increase in GH levels following TRH has also been reported.

Basal daytime levels of prolactin are normal in anorexic patients, and there is no correlation between these prolactin levels and weight, gonadotropin levels, or estradiol levels.[278] Prolactin responses to dopaminergic compounds are normal, as are responses to TRH, although the TRH responses may be somewhat delayed.[98] However, there may be subtle alterations in the circadian regulation of prolactin, as anorexic patients display a blunting of the nocturnal rise in serum prolactin levels compared to controls.[134]

Bulimia and Neuroendocrine Function

Bulimia is a feeding disorder characterized by uncontrolled eating binges followed by self-induced vomiting or laxative abuse. The behaviors are frequently followed by depression and self-deprecatory thoughts. The exact diagnostic relationship between bulimia and anorexia nervosa has not been established, but bulimic patients do appear to form a subgroup distinct from typical anorexic patients.

Accumulating evidence suggests a strong association between bulimia and affective disorders, as indicated by phenomenology, positive family history, response to antidepressants, and neuroendocrine abnormalities. Two recent reports have studied DST results in bulimic patients; nonsuppression rates of 47 and 67 percent have been demonstrated.[114,126] In addition, a large majority of bulimic patients display a blunted TSH response to TRH infusions.[114] In contrast to the studies of anorexia nervosa, bu-

limic patients are not severely underweight. Thus it would appear that weight loss per se is not a major factor contributing to the abnormal DST results. Further neuroendocrine testing in bulimia should provide a powerful tool to examine the relationship between this disorder and affective disease.

¶ Neuroendocrinology of Alcoholism

Introduction

Alcohol is one of the oldest and most widely used psychoactive substances. However, the molecular basis for its physiological actions and, especially, its effect on endocrine function are not well understood. Several factors account for the large amount of contradictory evidence on the effect of ethanol on neuroendocrine parameters in man. First, it is necessary to differentiate between the effects of acute ethanol administration to normal volunteers versus the chronic alcohol ingestion observed in alcoholic subjects. However, studies utilizing an alcoholic population are often difficult to interpret. It is well known that chronic ethanol intoxication is associated with organic tissue damage, particularly of the liver. Since a variety of hormones and agents used to challenge endocrine systems are metabolized by the liver, any observed hormonal abnormalities may be secondary to liver damage rather than specific neuroendocrine effects.

Alcoholism is often associated with depression, and a variety of neuroendocrine abnormalities are present in depression (see section entitled "Endocrine Disturbances in Affective Disorders"). Thus altered hormonal responses in alcoholic patients may reflect the depressed rather than the alcoholic condition. In addition, many studies are done on alcoholic patients during the withdrawal period, the stressful nature of which may itself affect endocrine function. Finally, many alcoholic patients are polydrug users and suffer from various nutritional deficits, which can further confound the interpretation of endocrine findings.

This section will focus on neuroendocrine function in alcoholic patients, primarily during the drinking phase or during withdrawal. More extensive reviews of neuroendocrine studies in alcoholism are available elsewhere.*

Gonadal Function in Alcoholism

One of the most common endocrine consequences of chronic ethanol intake is alteration in gonadal function.[10, 268] Chronic alcoholic men show decreased libido, impotence, and testicular atrophy, along with various altered endocrine parameters. While these abnormalities have multiple causes, including hepatic, testicular, hypothalamic, and pituitary dysfunction,[65] some general statements can be made concerning their pathogenesis. Alcohol and its metabolite, acetaldehyde, are clearly testicular toxins. This probably accounts for the well-documented decrease in serum levels of testosterone in alcoholic patients,[269] although increased liver metabolism of testosterone is also a contributing factor.[10,65] Serum LH and FSH levels in alcoholic patients are generally normal to slightly elevated.[269] The results of GnRH stimulation tests have been conflicting, with both normal, blunted, and exaggerated responses being reported.[268,289,291] These varied results make it difficult to interpret whether the impaired gonadal function in alcoholic patients involves a hypothalamic-pituitary mechanism. However, as Cicero[65] points out, the fact that basal or stimulated gonadotropin levels can be relatively normal despite marked reductions in serum testosterone levels strongly suggests that alcohol can cause a disturbance of the hypothalamic-pituitary feedback mechanisms. In addition, a large body of evidence from animal studies suggests a hypothalamic-pituitary effect of ethanol, as well as a direct effect on gonadal function.[65] While the studies mentioned emphasize the effect of ethanol on male gonadal function, there is evidence that alcohol also disrupts female sexual function.[268]

The Hypothalamic-Pituitary-Adrenal Axis in Alcoholism

There is an abundance of evidence indicating that ethanol intake can modulate the activity of the HPA axis,[193,205] but, as with the gonadal axis, the sites and mechanism of action are not well defined. The stress of chronic alcoholic intoxication or of abrupt withdrawal from alcohol may indirectly activate the HPA axis. Moreover, a large percentage of alcoholic subjects are depressed, and as we have reviewed, depression is frequently associated with increased HPA activity.

Although very early reports suggested that alcoholic patients had adrenocortical insufficiency,[170] more recent studies indicate a hyperactivity of the HPA axis in a subpopulation of alcoholic patients. Several studies indicate that some chronic alcoholic patients develop a Cushingoid syndrome that is reversed when alcohol intake is stopped.[205] Features include moon face, buffalo hump, central obesity, and skin changes. These subjects often have biochemical indices of Cushing's syndrome, such as elevated serum cortisol and resistance to dexamethasone-induced cortisol suppression.[193] However, Hasselbalch and associates[118] reported several chronic alcoholic patients who had Cushingoid features with normal serum cortisol levels and dexamethasone suppression.

Alcoholic patients free of liver disease have normal to elevated serum cortisol levels, while those with significant liver disease have normal to low serum cortisol levels. The circadian rhythm in serum cortisol is intact in both conditions.[193] The effect of ethanol on the HPA axis of normal subjects is variable, and it has been suggested that any acute alcohol-induced increase in serum cortisol may be stress-related.[78]

With the increased use of the DST in psy-

---

*See references 65, 170, 193, 205, 289, and 291.

chiatry, it has become important to evaluate the clinical utility of the DST as a biological marker for depression in alcoholic populations. Depressed alcoholic patients, when tested during withdrawal, have a rate of nonsuppression (64 percent) comparable to that observed in nonalcoholic depressed populations.[262] In nondepressed alcoholic patients tested during the early phase of withdrawal (less than one week), rates of nonsuppression between 19 and 33 percent have been reported.[75,256,263] Thus acute alcoholic withdrawal can produce false positive DST results. When DST testing is done later (three to four weeks) in the withdrawal period, lower rates of nonsuppression, approaching those in the general population, are noted.[75,150] In summary, if the proper clinical considerations are used, the DST can be a useful laboratory tool to assess depression in alcoholic populations.[150]

Thyroid Function in Alcoholism

Alcoholic patients generally show no clinical signs of thyroid dysfunction, although laboratory tests often indicate thyroid irregularities. In particular, alcoholic patients with liver disease have normal serum T_4 levels, decreased serum T_3 levels, increased serum levels of reverse T_3, normal to high serum TSH levels, and variable TSH responses to TRH.[193,208] Many of the serum thyroid abnormalities are due to altered peripheral metabolism as a result of liver damage.

The TRH stimulation test has been studied in alcoholic patients undergoing withdrawal and in abstinent alcoholic patients. Approximately 50 percent of alcoholic patients without major depression undergoing acute withdrawal have blunted TSH responses to TRH. A smaller number[75,161] of alcoholic patients maintain a blunted response after withdrawal. Loosen and associates[162] studied a group of abstinent (six years) alcoholic subjects for thyroid status and TRH responses. A "euthyroid sick syndrome" was described,

which consisted of low T_3 levels, high levels of reverse T_3, and normal T_4 levels. In this nondepressed population, 31 percent of the abstinent alcoholic individuals had a blunted TRH response. This suggests that an abnormal TRH test may be a trait as well as a state marker for alcoholism.

Growth Hormone and Prolactin in Alcoholism

There is no evidence that GH abnormalities in alcoholic patients have any clinical significance. As with the other endocrine systems, there are a number of conflicting studies describing the effect of ethanol on GH levels. In general, the most profound disruptions of the GH system occur in alcoholic patients with significant liver disease. Such individuals generally have increased basal levels of serum GH and show more pronounced deficits to various provocative challenges, including arginine, levodopa, and insulin-induced hypoglycemia.[193,289] A paradoxical increase in GH following TRH has also been reported.[271]

Normal to slightly increased basal levels of GH in alcoholic patients free of liver disease have been reported. The GH response to hypoglycemia is intact, but the responses to other provocative tests may be impaired in some alcoholic patients.[193] Of particular note is the recent report that DA infusions in healthy alcoholic patients undergoing withdrawal elicits a dramatic increase in serum GH levels compared to controls. This indicates that an increased sensitivity of DA receptors develops during acute alcohol withdrawal.[11] Loosen, Prange, and Wilson[161] have also suggested a hyperfunctioning of central DA systems during acute withdrawal.

As previously mentioned, the gonadal system in chronic alcoholic patients is severely impaired. Some alcoholic patients also show signs of feminization, including gynecomastia. Alcoholic patients with liver disease have a two-fold elevation in serum levels of prolactin and estrone. In addition, those alcoholic patients with gynecomastia had markedly increased prolactin levels compared to alcoholic subjects without gynecomastia, which suggests a possible role for prolactin in alcohol-induced feminization.[270]

During acute withdrawal, serum prolactin levels are decreased,[161] and blunted prolactin responses to TRH during and after withdrawal have been reported.[291] A decreased prolactin response to insulin-induced hypoglycemia also occurs.[56]

Ethanol administration usually increases serum prolactin levels in normal subjects.[65] A recent study considered possible genetic influences on alcohol-induced changes in serum prolactin levels.[242] Normal subjects with either positive or negative family history of alcoholism increased serum prolactin levels at thirty minutes following a test dose of alcohol. However, at later times, subjects with a positive family history had significantly lower levels of prolactin.

Opiates and Alcohol

Since the discovery of endogenous opiate peptides and opiate receptors, there has been a great deal of speculation about their role in both normal physiology as well as pathological conditions. Recent work indicates a possible link between the effects of alcohol and endogenous opiate systems. Ethanol itself appears to compete for opiate receptor binding sites,[120] and the opiate antagonist naloxone has been shown to attenuate several effects of ethanol.[33] Recent studies indicate that alcoholic subjects have altered levels of endogenous opiate peptides. Circulating levels of pro-opiomelanocortin-derived peptides, including beta-endorphin, ACTH, and β-LPH are normal in alcoholic patients. However, CSF levels of beta-endorphin are markedly suppressed, despite increased levels of CSF ACTH.[100] In addition, plasma levels of met-enkephalin are lower in alcoholic patients compared to normal control subjects.[109] The significance of these findings awaits further clarification, but could be due to ethanol-induced opiate receptor alterations or changes in feedback regulation of endorphin synthesis.

Summary of the Neuroendocrinology of Alcoholism

In conclusion, there is definitive clinical and laboratory evidence that chronic alcohol intake adversely influences the gonadal and HPA axis. The effect of alcohol on other endocrine systems is less clear. It is important to consider the effects of liver damage and the concomitant presence of depression when evaluating neuroendocrine studies of alcoholism.

¶ Conclusions

This review, despite its length, is necessarily circumscribed and can give only an introductory and summary approach to the dynamic field of neuroendocrine investigation of psychiatric disorders and behavior. We have particularly underemphasized studies of the effect of hormones on behavior because this is included in the chapter on the effect of peptides on behavior (see Chapter 3). The neuroendocrine contribution to the study of the effect of psychotropic drugs in man has also been underemphasized because of space limitations, but it is one of the most important types of research in psychopharmacology.

It is our hope that this review will have provided the reader with an introduction to the literature of neuroendocrinology and the concepts that will stimulate and permit an intensive exploration of this area. In the years to come, neuroendocrine assessment will be of certain importance for diagnosis of many psychiatric disorders, especially the affective disorders. It is also probable that neuroendocrine assessment will be valuable for monitoring the effects of treatment and for prognosis. Whether neuroendocrinology will play an equally important role in deciphering basic disease mechanisms in the major forms of mental illness is not as certain. Many promising beginnings along these lines have been cited in this chapter, but it remains to be determined if they will stand the test of time.

¶ Acknowledgements

Research for this chapter was supported, in part, by U.S. Public Health Service Mental Health grants 30059, 40206, and 14651. The assistance of Dr. James Koenig in preparing table 4–1 and the excellent secretarial support of Ms. Georgia Gilbert is gratefully acknowledged.

¶ Bibliography

1. ACKENHEIL, M. "Biochemical Effects of Apomorphine: Contribution to Schizophrenia Research in Apomorphine and Other Dopaminomimetics," in G. U. Corsini et al., eds., *Clinical Pharmacology*, vol. 1. New York: Raven Press, 1981, pp. 215–229.

2. ADER, R. *Psychoneuroimmunology.* New York: Academic Press, 1981.

3. ALEXOPOULOS, G.S., et al. "Plasma Immunoreactive β-Endorphin Levels in Depression. Effect of Electroconvulsive Therapy," *Archives of General Psychiatry*, 40 (1983):181–183.

4. ALTMAN, N., et al. "Reduced Plasma LH Concentration in Post-Menopausal Depressed Women," *Psychosomatic Medicine*, 37 (1975):274–276.

5. AMSTERDAM, J. D., et al. "Gonadotropin Release After Administration of GnRH in Depressed Patients and Healthy Volunteers," *Journal of Affective Disorders*, 3 (1981):367–380.

6. AMSTERDAM, J. D., et al. "The Dexamethasone Suppression Test in Outpatients with Primary Affective Disorder and Healthy Control Subjects," *American Journal of Psychiatry*, 139 (1982):287–291.

7. AMSTERDAM, J. D., et al. "Growth Hormone, Prolactin and Thyrotropin Responses to Gonadotropin-Releasing Hormone in Depressed Patients and Healthy Volunteers," *Psychoneuroendocrinology*, 7 (1982):177–184.

8. AMSTERDAM, J. D., et al. "Cosyntropin ($ACTH_{1-24}$) Stimulation Test in Depressed Patients and Healthy Subjects," *American Journal of Psychiatry*, 140 (1983):907–909.

9. AMSTERDAM, J. D., et al. "A Neuroendocrine Test Battery in Bipolar Patients and Healthy Subjects," *Archives of General Psychiatry*, 40 (1983):515–521.

10. ANDERSON, R. A., et al. "Male Reproductive Tract Sensitivity to Ethanol: A Critical Overview," *Pharmacology, Biochemistry, Behavior*, 18 (1983):305–310.

11. ANNUNZIATO, L., et al. "Increased GH Responsiveness to Dopamine Receptor Stimulation in Alcohol Addicts During the Late Withdrawal Syndrome," *Life Sciences*, 33 (1983):2651–2655.

12. ANSSEAU, M., et al. "Concurrent Use of REM Latency, Dexamethasone Suppression, Clonidine and Apomorphine Tests as Biological Markers of Endogenous Depression: A Pilot Study," *Psychiatry Research*, 12 (1984): 261–272.

13. ARATO, M., et al. "Studies on the Prolactin Response Induced by Electroconvulsive Therapy in Schizophrenics," *Acta Psychiatrica Scandinavica*, 61 (1980):239–244.

14. ASBERG, M., et al., "Serotonin Depression —A Biochemical Subgroup Within the Affective Disorders?" *Science*, 191 (1976):478–480.

15. ASBERG, M., et al. "Suicidal Behavior and the Dexamethasone Suppression Test," *American Journal of Psychiatry*, 138 (1981):994–995.

16. ASNIS, G. M., et al. "Normal Prolactin Responses in Tardive Dyskinesia," *Psychopharmacology*, 66 (1979):247–250.

17. ASNIS, G. M., et al. "Prolactin Changes in Major Depressive Disorders," *American Journal of Psychiatry*, 137 (1980):1117–1118.

18. ASNIS, G. M., et al. "Cortisol Secretion and Dexamethasone Response in Depression," *American Journal of Psychiatry*, 138 (1981):1218–1221.

19. ASNIS, G.M., et al. "Relationship of Dex-

amethasone (2 mg) and Plasma Cortisol Secretion in Depressive Illness: Clinical and Neuroendocrine Parameters," *Psychopharmacology Bulletin*, 18 (1982):-122–126.

20. ASNIS, G. M., et al., "Plasma Cortisol Secretion and REM Period Latency in Adult Endogenous Depression," *American Journal of Psychiatry*, 140 (1983):-750–753.

21. BALLDIN, S., et al. "Neuroendocrine Evidence for Increased Responsiveness of Dopamine Receptors in Humans Following Electroconvulsive Therapy," *Psychopharmacology*, 76 (1982):371–376.

22. BALLENGER, M., et al. "Endocrine Effects of the Cold Pressor Test: Relationships to Subjective Pain Appraisal and Coping," *Psychiatry Research*, 12 (1984):-227–233.

23. BANKI, C. M., and ARATO, M. "Relationship Between Cerebrospinal Fluid Amine Metabolites, Neuroendocrine Findings and Personality Dimensions (Marke-Nyman Scale Factors) in Psychiatric Patients," *Acta Psychiatrica Scandinavica*, 67 (1983):272–280.

24. BANKI, C. M., et al. "Biochemical Markers in Suicidal Patients: Investigations with Cerebrospinal Fluid Amine Metabolites and Neuroendocrine Tests," *Journal of Affective Disorders*, 6 (1984):341–350.

25. BECK-FRIIS, J., et al. "Hormonal Changes in Acute Depression," in C. Perris et al., eds., *Biological Psychiatry*. Amsterdam: Elsevier North Holland Biomedical Press, 1981, pp. 1244–1248.

26. BECK-FRIIS, J., et al. "Suicidal Behavior and the Dexamethasone Suppression Test," *American Journal of Psychiatry*, 138 (1981):993–994.

27. BEG, A. A., et al. "Effect of Chlorpromazine on Human Growth Hormone," *American Journal of Psychiatry*, 136 (1979):914–917.

28. BENKERT, O., GORDON, A., and MARTSCHKE, D. "The Comparison of Thyrotropin Releasing Hormone, Luteinizing Hormone-Releasing Hormone and Placebo in Depressive Patients Using a Double-Blind Cross-Over Technique," *Psychopharmacologia*, 90 (1974):191–198.

29. BERGER, M., et al. "Neuroendocrinological and Neurophysiological Studies in Major Depressive Disorders: Are There Biological Markers for the Endogenous Subtype?" *Biological Psychiatry*, 17 (1982):1217–1242.

30. BESEDOVSKY, H., and SORKIN, E. "Network of Immune Neuroendocrine Interactions," *Clinical and Experimental Immunology*, 27 (1977):1–12.

31. BEUMONT, P.J.V., and RUSSELL, J. "Anorexia Nervosa," in P.J.V. Beumont et al., eds., *Handbook of Psychiatry*. New York: Elsevier Biomedical Press, 1982, pp. 63–96.

32. BLALOCK, J. E. "Relationship Between Neuroendocrine Hormones and Lymphokines," *Lymphokines*, 9 (1984):1–13.

33. BLUM, K., et al. "Naloxone-Induced Inhibition of Ethanol Dependence in Mice," *Nature*, 165 (1977):49–51.

34. BRAMBILLA, F., and PENATI, G. "Schizophrenia: Endocrinological Review," in F. Brambilla et al., eds., *Perspectives in Endocrine Psychobiology*. London: John Wiley & Sons, 1978, pp. 309–422.

35. BRAMBILLA, F., et al. "Psychoendocrine Investigation in Schizophrenia: Relationship Between Pituitary-Gonadal Function and Behavior," *Diseases of the Nervous System*, 35 (1974):362–367.

36. BRAMBILLA, F., et al. "Growth Hormone Secretion in Chronic Schizophrenia," *Neuropsychobiology*, 1 (1975):267–276.

37. BRAMBILLA, F., et al. "Deranged Anterior Pituitary Responsiveness to Hypothalamic Hormones in Depressed Patients," *Archives of General Psychiatry*, 35 (1978):1231–1238.

38. BRAMBILLA, F., et al. "Abnormal Anterior Pituitary Responsiveness to Hypothalamic Hormones in Primary Affective Disorders," *Neuropsychobiology*, 8 (1982):269–275.

39. BRAMBILLA, F., et al. "Endogenous Opioid Levels in Chronic Schizophrenia," in E. Endroczi et al., eds., *Integrative Neurohumoral Mechanisms*. Amsterdam: Elsevier Science Publishers, 1983, pp. 515–524.

40. BROWN, G. M. "Endocrine Alterations in Anorexia Nervosa," in P. L. Darby et al., eds., *Anorexia Nervosa: Recent Devel-

opments in Research. New York: Alan R. Liss, 1983, pp. 231–247.

41. BROWN, G. M., et al. "Growth Hormone Responses in Schizophrenia," in E. Endroczi et al., eds., *Integrative Neurohumoral Mechanisms.* Amsterdam: Elsevier Science Publishers, 1983, pp. 539–550.

42. BROWN, W. K., and LAUGHREN, T. "Low Serum Prolactin and Early Relapse Following Neuroleptic Withdrawal," *American Journal of Psychiatry,* 138 (1981):237–239.

43. BROWN, W. K., LAUGHREN, T. P., and WILLIAMS, B. "Differential Effects of Neuroleptic Agents on the Pituitary-Gonadal Axis in Men," *Archives of General Psychiatry,* 38 (1981):1270–1272.

44. BUNNEY, W. E., JR., and FAWCETT, J. A. "Possibility of a Biochemical Test for Suicidal Potential," *Archives of General Psychiatry,* 13 (1965):232–239.

45. BUNNEY, W. E., JR., et al. "Further Evaluation of Urinary 17-Hydroxycorticosteroids in Suicidal Patients," *Archives of General Psychiatry,* 21 (1969):138–150.

46. CARLSON, A. "Antipsychotic Drugs, Neurotransmitters and Schizophrenia," *American Journal of Psychiatry,* 135 (1978):164–173.

47. CARPENTER, W. T., and BUNNEY, W. E. "Adrenal Cortical Activity in Depressive Illness," *American Journal of Psychiatry,* 128 (1971):65–71.

48. CARR, D. B., et al. "Rate-Sensitive Inhibition of ACTH Release in Depression," *American Journal of Psychiatry,* 141 (1984):590–592.

49. CARROLL, B. J. "Limbic System-Adrenal Cortex Regulation in Depression and Schizophrenia," *Psychosomatic Medicine,* 38 (1976):106–121.

50. ———. "Neuroendocrine Diagnosis of Depression: The Dexamethasone Suppression Test," in P. J. Clayton et al., eds., *Treatment of Depression: Old Controversies and New Approaches.* New York: Raven Press, 1983, pp. 1–27.

51. CARROLL, B. J., and MENDELS, J. "Neuroendocrine Regulation in Affective Disorders," in E. J. Sachar, ed., *Hormones, Behavior* and *Psychopathology.* New York: Raven Press, 1976, pp. 193–224.

52. CARROLL, B. J., CURTIS, G. C., and MEN-DELS, J. "Cerebrospinal Fluid and Plasma Free Cortisol Concentrations in Depression," *Psychological Medicine,* 6 (1976):235–244.

53. CARROLL, B. J., GREDEN, J. F., and FEINBERG, M. "Suicide, Neuroendocrine Dysfunction and CSF 5-HIAA Concentrations in Depression," in B. Angrist et al., eds., *Recent Advances in Neuropsychopharmacology,* vol. 31. Oxford: Pergamon Press, 1981, pp. 307–313.

54. CARROLL, B. J., et al. "A Specific Laboratory Test for the Diagnosis of Melancholia," *Archives of General Psychiatry,* 38 (1981):15–22.

55. CASPAR, R. C., et al. "Neuroendocrine and Amine Studies in Affective Illness," *Psychoneuroendocrinology,* 2 (1977):-105–114.

56. CHALMERS, R. J., et al. "Growth Hormone, Prolactin and Corticosteroid Responses to Insulin Hypoglycemia in Alcoholics," *British Medical Journal,* 1 (1978):745–748.

57. CHARNEY, D. S., HENINGER, G. R., and REINHARD, J. F. "The Effect of Intravenous L-Tryptophan on Prolactin and Growth Hormone and Mood in Healthy Subjects," *Psychopharmacology,* 77 (1982):217–222.

58. CHARNEY, D. S., HENINGER, G. R., and STERNBERG, D. E. "Alpha-2 Adrenergic Receptor Sensitivity and the Mechanism of Action of Antidepressant Therapy: The Effect of Long-Term Amitriptyline Treatment," *British Journal of Psychiatry,* 142 (1983):265–275.

59. CHARTERS, A. C., ODELL, W. D., and THOMPSON, J. C. "Anterior Pituitary Function During Surgical Stress and Convalescence. Radioimmunoassay Measurements of Blood TSH, LH, FSH and Growth Hormone," *Journal of Clinical Endocrinology and Metabolism,* 29 (1969):63–71.

60. CHECKLEY, S. A. "Corticosteroid and Growth Hormone Responses to Methylamphetamine in Depressive Illness," *Psychological Medicine,* 9 (1979):107–116.

61. CHECKLEY, S. A., and ARENDT, J. "Pharmacoendocrine Studies of G.H., PRL, and Melatonin in Patients with Affective Illness," in G. M. Brown et al., eds.,

Neuroendocrinology and Psychiatric Disorders. New York: Raven Press, 1984, pp. 165–190.

62. CHECKLEY, S. A., SLADE, A. P., and SHUR, E. "Growth Hormone and Other Responses to Clonidine in Patients with Endogenous Depression," *British Journal of Psychiatry,* 138 (1981):51–55.

63. CHRISTENSEN, L., et al. "Afternoon Plasma Cortisol in Depressed Patients: A Measure of Diagnosis or Severity," *Life Sciences,* 32 (1983):617–623.

64. CHRISTIE, J. E., et al. "Effect of ECT on the Neuroendocrine Response to Apomorphine in Severely Depressed Patients," *British Journal of Psychiatry,* 140 (1982):268–273.

65. CICERO, T. J. "Neuroendocrinological Effects of Alcohol," *Annual Review of Medicine,* 32 (1981):123–142.

66. COPPEN, A., et al. "Cortisol in the Cerebrospinal Fluid of Patients Suffering from Affective Disorders," *Journal of Neurology, Neurosurgery, and Psychiatry,* 34 (1971):432–435.

67. COPPEN, A., et al. "Neuroendocrine Studies in Affective Disorders. Part 1. Plasma Prolactin Response to Thyrotropin-Releasing Hormone in Affective Disorders: Effect of ECT," *Journal of Affective Disorders,* 2 (1980):311–315.

68. CORN, T. H., et al. "A Comparison of the Growth Hormone Responses to Clonidine and Apormorphine in the Same Patients with Endogenous Depression," *British Journal of Psychiatry,* 144 (1984):636–639.

69. CORYELL, W., and SCHLESSER, M. A. "Suicide and the Dexamethasone Suppression Test in Unipolar Depression," *American Journal of Psychiatry,* 138 (1981):1120–1121.

70. COWDRY, R. W., et al. "Thyroid Abnormalities Associated with Rapid-Cycling Bipolar Illness," *Archives of General Psychiatry,* 40 (1983):414–420.

71. CROW, T. J. "Molecular Pathology of Schizophrenia: More Than One Disease Process," *British Medical Journal,* 280 (1980):66–68.

72. CULLEN, J., FULLER, R., and DOLPHIN, C. "Endocrine Stress Responses of Drivers in a 'Real-Life' Heavy-Goods Vehicle Driving Task," *Psychoneuroendocrinology,* 4 (1979):107–115.

73. CURTIS, G. C., et al. "Anxiety and Plasma Cortisol at the Crest of the Circadian Cycle: Reappraisal of a Classical Hypothesis," *Psychosomatic Medicine,* 40 (1978):368–378.

74. CZEISLER, C. A., et al. "Episodic 24-Hour Cortisol Secretory Patterns in Patients Awaiting Elective Cardiac Surgery," *Journal of Clinical Endocrinology and Metabolism,* 42 (1976):273–283.

75. DACKIS, C. A., et al. "Specificity of the DST and the TRH Test for Major Depression in Alcoholics," *American Journal of Psychiatry,* 141 (1984):680–683.

76. DAVIS, K. L., et al. "Neuroendocrine and Neurochemical Measurements in Depression," *American Journal of Psychiatry,* 138 (1981):1555–1562.

77. DAVIS, K. L., et al. "Age and the Dexamethasone Suppression Test in Depression," *American Journal of Psychiatry,* 141 (1984):872–874.

78. DAVIS, J. R. E., and JEFFCOATE, W. J. "Lack of Effect of Ethanol on Plasma Cortisol in Man," *Clinical Endocrinology,* 19 (1983):461–466.

79. DEAKIN, J. F. W., et al. "Effects of ECT on Pituitary Hormone Release: Relationships to Seizure, Clinical Variables and Outcome," *British Journal of Psychiatry,* 143 (1983):618–624.

80. DELITALA, G., DEVILLA, L., and DIBIASO, D. "Dopamine Inhibits the Naloxone-Induced Gonadotrophin Rise in Man," *Clinical Endocrinology,* 13 (1980):515–518.

81. DELITALA, G., GROSSMAN, A., and BESSER, M. "Differential Effects of Opiate Peptides and Alkaloids on Anterior Pituitary Hormone Secretion," *Neuroendocrinology,* 37 (1983):275–279.

82. DONOHOE, T. P. "Stress-Induced Anorexia: Implications for Anorexia Nervosa," *Life Sciences,* 34 (1984):203–218.

83. EDELSTEIN, C. K., et al. "Effect of Weight Loss on the Dexamethasone Suppression Test," *American Journal of Psychiatry,* 140 (1983):338–341.

84. ETTIGI, P. G., BROWN, G. M., and SEGGIE, J. A. "TSH and LH Responses in Sub-

types of Depression," *Psychosomatic Medicine,* 41 (1979):203–208.

85. EXTEIN, I., et al. "Deficient Prolactin Response to Morphine in Depressed Patients," *American Journal of Psychiatry,* 137 (1980):845–846.

86. EXTEIN, I., et al. "Using the Protirelin Test to Distinguish Mania from Schizophrenia," *Archives of General Psychiatry,* 39 (1982):77–81.

87. FANG, V. S., et al. "Plasma ACTH and Cortisol Levels in Depressed Patients: Relation to Dexamethasone Suppression Test," *Life Sciences,* 29 (1981):931–938.

88. FEINBERG, M., GREDEN, J. F., and CARROLL, B. J. "The Effect of Amphetamine on Plasma Cortisol in Patients with Endogenous and Non-Endogenous Depression," *Psychoneuroendocrinology,* 6 (1981):355–357.

89. FERRIER, I. N., JOHNSTONE, E. C., and CROW, T. J. "Hormonal Effects of Apomorphine in Schizophrenia," *British Journal of Psychiatry,* 144 (1984):349–357.

90. FERRIER, I. N., et al. "Gonadotrophin Secretion Abnormalities in Chronic Schizophrenia," *Psychological Medicine,* 12 (1982):263–273.

91. FERRIER, I. N., et al. "Reduced Nocturnal Melatonin Secretion in Chronic Schizophrenia: Relationship to Body Weight," *Clinical Endocrinology,* 17 (1982):181–187.

92. FINK, E. B., and CARPENTER, W. T. "Further Examination of a Biochemical Test for Suicide Potential," *Diseases of the Nervous System,* 37 (1976):341–343.

93. FINK, M. "Neuroendocrinology and ECT. A Review of Recent Developments," *Comprehensive Psychiatry,* 21 (1980):450–459.

94. FRANTZ, A. G. "Rhythm in Prolactin Section," in D. T. Krieger, ed., *Endocrine Rhythms.* New York: Raven Press, 1979, pp. 175–186.

95. GALLAGHER, T. F., et al. "ACTH and Cortisol Secretory Patterns in Man," *Journal of Clinical Endocrinology and Metabolism,* 36 (1973):1058–1073.

96. GANONG, W. F. "Neurotransmitter Mechanisms Underlying Stress Responses," in G. M. Brown et al., eds., *Neuroendo-crinology and Psychiatric Disorders.* New York: Raven Press, 1984, pp. 133–143.

97. GARBUTT, J. C., et al. "The TRH Test in Patients with Borderline Personality Disorder," *Psychiatry Research,* 9 (1983):107–114.

98. GARFINKEL, P. E. "Anorexia Nervosa: An Overview of Hypothalamic-Pituitary Function," in G. M. Brown et al., eds., *Neuroendocrinology and Psychiatric Disorder.* New York: Raven Press, 1984, pp. 301–314.

99. GARFINKEL, P. E., et al. "Hypothalamic-Pituitary Function in Anorexia Nervosa," *Archives of General Psychiatry,* 32 (1975):739–744.

100. GENAZZANI, A. R., et al. "Central Deficiency of β-Endorphin in Alcohol Addicts," *Journal of Clinical Endocrinology and Metabolism,* 55 (1982):583–586.

101. GERNER, R. H., and GWIRTSMAN, H. E. "Abnormalities of Dexamethasone Suppression Test and Urinary MHPG in Anorexia Nervosa," *American Journal of Psychiatry,* 138 (1981):650–653.

102. GERNER, R. H., and WILKINS, J. N. "CSF Cortisol in Patients with Depression, Mania, or Anorexia Nervosa and in Normal Subjects," *American Journal of Psychiatry,* 140 (1983):92–94.

103. GERNER, R. H., and YAMADA, T. "Altered Neuropeptide Concentrations in Cerebrospinal Fluid of Psychiatric Patients," *Brain Research,* 238 (1982):298–302.

104. GIBBONS, J. L. "Cortisol Secretion Rate in Depressive Illness," *Archives of General Psychiatry,* 10 (1964):572–575.

105. GIL-AD, I., et al. "Abnormal Growth Hormone Response to LRH and TRH in Adolescent Schizophrenic Boys," *American Journal of Psychiatry,* 138 (1981):357–360.

106. GOLD, M. S., POTTASH, L. C., and EXTEIN, I. "Hypothyroidism and Depression: Evidence from Complex Thyroid Function Evaluation," *Journal of American Medical Association,* 245 (1981):1919–1922.

107. GOLD, P. W., et al. "Growth Hormone and Prolactin Response to Levodopa in

Affective Illness," *Lancet,* 2 (1976):1308–1309.

108. GOLD, P. W., et al. "Psychiatric Implications of Basic and Clinical Studies with Corticotropin-Releasing Factor," *American Journal of Psychiatry,* 141 (1984):619–627.

109. GOVANI, S., et al. "Immunoreactive Met-Enkephalin Plasma Concentrations in Chronic Alcoholics and in Children Born from Alcoholic Mothers," *Life Sciences,* 33 (1983):1581–1586.

110. GREDEN, J. F., et al. "Normalization of Dexamethasone Suppression Test: A Laboratory Index of Recovery from Endogenous Depression," *Biological Psychiatry,* 15 (1980):449–458.

111. GRUEN, P. H., et al. "Growth Hormone Response to Hypoglycemia in Post-Menopausal Depressed Women," *Archives of General Psychiatry,* 32 (1975):31–33.

112. GUDELSKY, G. A., and PORTER, J. C. "Release of Newly Synthesized Dopamine into the Hypophysial Portal Vasculature of the Rat," *Endocrinology,* 104 (1979):583–587.

113. GWIRTSMAN, H., GERNER, R. H., and STERNBACH, H. "The Overnight Dexamethasone Suppression Test. Clinical and Theoretical Review," *Journal of Clinical Psychiatry,* 43 (1982):321–327.

114. GWIRTSMAN, H. et al. "Neuroendocrine Abnormalities in Bulimia," *American Journal of Psychiatry,* 140 (1983):559–563.

115. HALBREICH, U., GRUNHAUS, L., and BEN-DAVID, M. "Twenty-Four-Hour Rhythm of Prolactin in Depressive Patients," *Archives of General Psychiatry,* 36 (1979):1183–1186.

116. HALBREICH, U., et al. "Growth Hormone Response to Dextroamphetamine in Depressed Patients and Normal Subjects,"*Archives of General Psychiatry,* 39 (1982):189–192.

117. HALBREICH, U., et al. "The Mean 1300–1600 h Plasma Cortisol Concentrations as a Diagnostic Test for Hypercortisolism," *Journal of Clinical Endocrinology and Metabolism,* 54 (1982):1262–1264.

118. HASSELBALCH, H., et al. "Hypothalamic-Pituitary-Adrenocortical Function in Chronic Alcoholism," *Clinical Endocrinology,* 16 (1982):73–76.

119. HENINGER, G. R., CHARNEY, D. S., and STERNBERG, D. E. "Serotonergic Function in Depression. Prolactin Response to Intravenous Tryptophan in Depressed Patients and Healthy Subjects," *Archives of General Psychiatry,* 41 (1984):398–402.

120. HILLER, J. M., ANGEL, L. M., and SIMON, E. J. "Multiple Opiate Receptors: Alcohol Selectively Inhibits Binding to Delta Receptors," *Science,* 214 (1981):468–469.

121. HIRSCHFELD, R.M.A., KOSLOW, S. H., and KUPFER, D. J. "The Clinical Utility of the Dexamethasone Suppression Test in Psychiatry," *Journal of the American Medical Association,* 250 (1983):2172–2174.

122. HIRSCHOWITZ, J., ZEMLAN F. P., and GARVER, D. L. "Growth Hormone Levels and Lithium Ratios as Predictors of Success of Lithium Therapy in Schizophrenia," *American Journal of Psychiatry,* 139 (1982):646–649.

123. HOLLISTER, L., DAVIS, K., and BERGER, P. "Pituitary Response to Thyrotropin-Releasing Hormone in Depression," *Archives of General Psychiatry,* 33 (1976):1393–1396.

124. HOLSBOER, F., LIEBL, R., and HOFSCHUSTER, E. "Repeated Dexamethasone Suppression Test During Depressive Illness," *Journal of Affective Disorders,* 4 (1982):93–101.

125. HOLSBOER, F., et al. "Cortisol, 11-Deoxycortisol and ACTH Concentrations After Dexamethasone in Depressed Patients and Healthy Volunteers," *Psychiatry Research,* 11 (1984):15–23.

126. HUDSON, J. I., et al. "Hypothalamic-Pituitary-Adrenal-Axis Hyperactivity in Bulimia," *Psychiatry Research,* 8 (1983):111–117.

127. INSEL, T. R., and GOODWIN, F. K. "The Dexamethasone Suppression Test: Promises and Problems of Diagnostic Laboratory Tests in Psychiatry," *Hospital and Community Psychiatry,* 34 (1983):1131–1138.

128. INSEL, T. R., et al. "The Dexamethasone Suppression Test in Patients with Primary Obsessive-Compulsive Disorder," *Psychiatry Research,* 6 (1982):153–160.

129. JIMERSON, D. C., et al. "Cerebrospinal Fluid Cortisol Levels in Depression and Schizophrenia," *American Journal of Psychiatry*, 137 (1980):979–980.

130. JOHNSON, J. "Schizophrenia and Cushing's Syndrome Cured by Adrenalectomy," *Psychological Medicine*, 5 (1975):165–168.

131. JOHNSTONE, E. C., CROW, T. J., and MASHITER, K. "Anterior Pituitary Hormone Secretion in Chronic Schizophrenia—An Approach to Neurohumoral Mechanisms," *Psychological Medicine*, 7 (1977):223–228.

132. JUDD, H. L. "Biorhythms of Gonadotropins and Testicular Hormone Secretion," in D. T. Krieger, ed., *Endocrine Rhythms.* New York: Raven Press, 1979, pp. 299–324.

133. JUDD, L. L., et al. "Blunted Prolactin Response. A Neuroendocrine Abnormality Manifested by Depressed Patients," *Archives of General Psychiatry*, 39 (1982):1413–1416.

134. KALUCY, R. S., et al. "Nocturnal Hormonal Profiles in Massive Obesity, Anorexia Nervosa and Normal Females," *Journal of Psychosomatic Research*, 20 (1976):595–604.

135. KASTIN, A. J., et al. "Improvement in Mental Depression with Decreased Thyrotropin Response After Administration of Thyrotropin-Releasing Hormone," *Lancet*, 2 (1972):740–742.

136. KATZ, J. L., et al. "Stress, Distress, and Ego Defenses," *Archives of General Psychiatry*, 23 (1970):131–142.

137. KATZ, J. L., et al. "Is There a Relationship Between Eating Disorder and Affective Disorder? New Evidence from Sleep Recordings," *American Journal of Psychiatry*, 141 (1984):753–759.

138. KELLER, S. E., et al. "Stress-Induced Suppression of Immunity in Adrenalectomized Rats," *Science*, 221 (1983):1301–1304.

139. KIECOLT GLASER, J. K., et al. "Psychosocial Modifiers of Immunocompetence in Medical Students," *Psychosomatic Medicine*, 46 (1984):7–14.

140. KIECOLT-GLASER, J. K., et al. "Urinary Cortisol Levels, Cellular Immunocompetency and Loneliness in Psychiatric Inpatients," *Psychosomatic Medicine*, 46 (1984):15–23.

141. KIRKEGAARD, C., et al. "Thyrotropin-Releasing-Hormone (TRH) Stimulation Test in Manic-Depressive Illness," *Archives of General Psychiatry*, 35 (1978):1017–1021.

142. KJELLMAN, B. F., et al. "Reverse T_3 Levels in Affective Disorders," *Psychiatry Research*, 10 (1983):1–9.

143. KLEINMAN, J. E., et al. "Naloxone in Chronic Schizophrenic Patients: Neuroendocrine and Behavioral Effects," *Psychiatry Research*, 7 (1982):1–7.

144. KLEINMAN, J. E., et al. "Plasma Prolactin Concentration and Psychopathology in Chronic Schizophrenia," *Archives of General Psychiatry*, 39 (1982):655–657.

145. KNIGHT, R. B., et al. "Psychological Stress, Ego Defenses, and Cortisol Production in Children Hospitalized for Elective Surgery," *Psychosomatic Medicine*, 4 (1979):40–49.

146. KREUZ, L. E., ROSE, R. M., and JENNINGS, J. R. "Suppression of Plasma Testosterone Levels and Psychological Stress," *Archives of General Psychiatry*, 26 (1972):479–482.

147. KRIEGER, D. T. "Rhythms in CRF, ACTH, and Corticosteroids," in D. T. Krieger, ed., *Endocrine Rhythms.* New York: Raven Press, 1979, pp. 123–142.

148. KRIEGER, J. "The Plasma Level of Cortisol as a Predictor of Suicide," *Journal of Diseases of the Nervous System*, 35 (1974):237–240.

149. KROG-MEYER, I., et al. "Prediction of Relapse with the TRH Test and Prophylactic Amitriptyline in 39 Patients with Endogenous Depression," *American Journal of Psychiatry*, 141 (1984):945–948.

150. KROLL, P., PALMER, C., and GREDEN, J. F. "The Dexamethasone Suppression Test in Patients with Alcoholism," *Biological Psychiatry*, 18 (1983):441–450.

151. LAL, S., et al. "Clonidine-Induced Growth Hormone Secretion in Chronic Schizophrenia," *Acta Psychiatrica Scandinavica*, 68 (1983):82–88.

152. LAUGHREN, T. P., BROWN, W. A., and WILLIAMS, B. W. "Serum Prolactin and Clinical State During Neuroleptic Treatment and Withdrawal," *American*

Journal of Psychiatry, 136 (1979):108–110.

153. LEBLANC, H., et al. "Effect of Dopamine Infusion on Pituitary Secretion in Humans," _Journal of Clinical Endocrinology and Metabolism,_ 43 (1976):668–672.

154. LESLIE, R.D.G., et al. "Hypothalamo-Pituitary-Thyroid Function in Anorexia Nervosa: Influence of Weight Gain. _British Medical Journal,_ 2 (1978):526–528.

155. LEVY, B., and HANSEN, E. "Failure of the Urinary Test for Suicide Potential: Analysis of Urinary 17-OH-CS Steroid Findings Prior to Suicide in Two Patients," _Archives of General Psychiatry,_ 20 (1969): 415–418.

156. LINKOWSKI, P., BRAUMAN, H., and MENDLEWICZ, J. "Prolactin Secretion in Women with Unipolar and Bipolar Depression," _Psychiatry Research,_ 3 (1980):265–271.

157. LINNOILA, M., et al. "Thyroid Hormones and TSH, Prolactin and LH Responses to Repeated TRH and LRH Injections in Depressed Patients," _Acta Psychiatrica Scandinavica,_ 59 (1979):536–544.

158. LINNOILA, M., et al. "Tricyclic Antidepressants Do Not Alter Thyroid Hormone Levels in Patients Suffering From a Major Affective Disorder," _Psychiatry Research,_ 4 (1981):357–360.

159. LINNOILA, M., et al. "High Reverse T_3 Levels in Manic and Unipolar Depressed Women," _Psychiatry Research,_ 6 (1982):271–276.

160. LOOSEN, P. T., and PRANGE, A. J., JR. "Serum Thyrotropin Response to Thyrotropin-Releasing Hormone in Psychiatric Patients: A Review," _American Journal of Psychiatry,_ 139 (1982):405–416.

161. LOOSEN, P. T., PRANGE, A. J., JR., and WILSON, I. C. "TRH (Protirelin) in Depressed Alcoholic Men," _Archives of General Psychiatry,_ 36 (1979):540–547.

162. LOOSEN, P. T., et al. "Thyrotropin-Releasing Hormone (TRH) in Abstinent Alcoholic Men," _American Journal of Psychiatry,_ 140 (1983):1145–1149.

163. LOWY, M. T., et al. "Glucocorticoid Resistance in Depression: Relation Between the DST and Lymphocyte Sensitivity to Dexamethasone," _American Journal of Psychiatry,_ 141 (1984):1365–1370.

164. LUCHINS, D. J., ROBERTSON, A. G., and MELTZER, H. Y. "Serum Prolactin, Psychopathology and Ventricular Size in Chronic Schizophrenia," _Psychiatry Research,_ 12 (1984):149–154.

165. MCGRATH, P. J., et al. "A Comparative Study of the Pituitary TSH Response to Thyrotropin in Outpatient Depressives," _Psychiatry Research,_ 12 (1984):185–194.

166. MACKAY, A.V.P. "Positive and Negative Schizophrenic Symptoms and the Role of Dopamine," _British Journal of Psychiatry,_ 137 (1980):374–383.

167. MACLEOD, R. M. "Regulation of Prolactin Secretion," in L. Martini et al., eds., _Frontiers in Neuroendocrinology._ New York: Raven Press, 1976, pp. 169–194.

168. MAEDA, K., et al. "Growth Hormone and Prolactin Release After Injection of TRH in Patients with Depression," _Journal of Clinical Endocrinology and Metabolism,_ 40 (1975):501–503.

169. MAEDA, K., et al. "Growth Hormone Release Following Thyrotropin Releasing Hormone Injection Into Patients with Anorexia Nervosa," _Acta Endocrinologica,_ 81 (1976):1–8.

170. MARKS, V., and WRIGHT, J. W. "Endocrinological and Metabolic Effects of Alcohol," _Proceedings of the Royal Society of Medicine,_ 70 (1977):337–344.

171. MARTIN, J. B., REICHLIN, S., and BROWN, G. M. "Effects of Hormones on Brain," in _Clinical Neuroendocrinology._ Philadelphia: F.A. Davis Co., 1977, pp. 275–304.

172. MASON, J. W. "A Review of Psychoendocrine Research on the Sympathetic-Adrenal Medullary System," _Psychosomatic Medicine,_ 30 (1968):631–653.

173. MASON, J. W., BRADY, J. V., and TOLLIVER, G. A. "Plasma and Urinary 17-Hydroxycorticosteroid Responses to 72-Hour Avoidance Sessions in the Monkey," _Psychosomatic Medicine,_ 30 (1968):608–630.

174. MATUSSEK, N., et al. "Effect of Clonidine on Growth Hormone Release in Psychiatric Patients and Controls," _Psychiatry Research,_ 2 (1980):25–36.

175. MELTZER, H. Y. "Neuroendocrine Abnor-

malities in Schizophrenia: Prolactin, Growth Hormone and Gonadotrophins," in G. M. Brown et al., eds., *Neuroendocrinology and Psychiatric Disorder.* New York: Raven Press, 1984, pp. 1–28.

176. ———. "Dopamine and Negative Symptoms in Schizophrenia. I. Critique of the Type I–II Hypothesis," in M. Alpert, ed., *Controversies in Schizophrenia: Changes and Constancy.* New York: Guilford Press, forthcoming.

177. MELTZER, H. Y., and FANG, V. S. "The Effect of Neuroleptics on Serum Prolactin in Schizophrenic Patients," *Archives of General Psychiatry,* 33 (1976):279–286.

178. ———. "Cortisol Determination and the Dexamethasone Suppression Test: A Review," *Archives of General Psychiatry,* 40 (1983):501–505.

179. MELTZER, H. Y., and STAHL, S. M. "The Dopamine Hypothesis of Schizophrenia: A Review," *Schizophrenia Bulletin,* 2 (1976):19–76.

180. MELTZER, H. Y., ARORA, R. C., and METZ, J. "Biological Studies of Schizoaffective Disorders," *Schizophrenia Bulletin,* 10 (1984):49–70.

181. MELTZER, H. Y., KANE, J. M., and KOLAKOWSKA, T. "Plasma Levels of Neuroleptics, Prolactin Levels and Clinical Response," in J. T. Coyle et al., eds. *Neuroleptics: Neurochemical, Behavioral and Clinical Perspectives.* New York: Raven Press, 1983, pp. 255–279.

182. MELTZER, H. Y., SACHAR, E. J., and FRANTZ, A. G. "Serum Prolactin Levels in Unmedicated Schizophrenic Patients," *Archives of General Psychiatry,* 31 (1974):564–569.

183. MELTZER, H. Y., et al. "Dopamine and Schizophrenia," *Lancet,* 2 (1976):1142.

184. MELTZER, H. Y., et al. "Effect of 5-Hydroxytryptophan on Serum Cortisol Levels in the Major Affective Disorders and Normal Controls. I. Enhanced Response in Depression and Mania," *Archives of General Psychiatry,* 41 (1984):366–374.

185. MELTZER, H. Y., et al. "Effect of 5-Hydroxytryptophan on Serum Cortisol Levels in the Major Affective Disorders.

II. Relation to Suicide, Psychosis and Depressive Syndrome," *Archives of General Psychiatry,* 41 (1984):379–387.

186. MELTZER, H. Y., et al. "Effect of 5-Hydroxytryptophan on Serum Cortisol Levels in the Major Affective Disorders. III. Effect of Antidepressants and Lithium," *Archives of General Psychiatry,* 41 (1984):391–402.

187. MELTZER, H. Y., et al. "Growth Hormone and Prolactin Response to Apomorphine in Schizophrenia and the Major Affective Disorders: Relation to Duration of Illness and Depressive Symptoms," *Archives of General Psychiatry,* 41 (1984):512–519.

188. MELTZER, H. Y., et al. "Stimulation of Adrenal and Pituitary Hormone Secretion by Serotonergic Agents in the Affective Disorders," *Clinical Neuropharmacology,* 7 (Supplement) (1984):154–155.

189. MENDLEWICZ, J., LINKOWSKI, P., and BRAUMAN, H. "Growth Hormone and Prolactin Response to Levodopa in Affective Illness," *Lancet,* 1 (1977):652–653.

190. MENDLEWICZ, J., VAN CAUTER, E., and LINKOWSKI, P. "Current Concepts: I. The 24-Hour Profile of Prolactin in Depression," *Life Sciences,* 27 (1980):2014–2024.

191. MICHAEL, R. P., and GIBBONS, J. L. "Interrelationships Between the Endocrine System and Neuropsychiatry," *International Review of Neurobiology,* 5 (1963):243–302.

192. MIYABO, S., ASATO, T., and MIZUSHIMA, N. "Prolactin and Growth Hormone Responses to Psychological Stress in Normal and Neurotic Subjects," *Journal of Clinical Endocrinology and Metabolism,* 44 (1977):947–957.

193. MORGAN, M. Y. "Alcohol and the Endocrine System," *British Medical Bulletin,* 38 (1982):35–42.

194. MUELLER, P. S. "Plasma Free Fatty Acid Response to Insulin in Schizophrenia," *Archives of General Psychiatry,* 7 (1962):140–146.

195. MULLER, E. E., et al. "Hypoglycemia, Stress and Growth Hormone Release: Blockage of Growth Hormone Release by Drugs Acting on the Central Ner-

vous System," *Endocrinology,* 80 (1967):109–117.

196. MUNRO, J. G., HARDIKER, T. M., and LEONARD, D. P. "The Dexamethasone Suppression Test in Residual Schizophrenia with Depression," *American Journal of Psychiatry,* 141 (1984):250–252.

197. NABER, D., NEDOPIL, N., and EBEN, E. "No Correlation Between Neuroleptic-Induced Increase of β-Endorphin Serum Level and Therapeutic Efficacy in Schizophrenia," *British Journal of Psychiatry,* 144 (1984):651–653.

198. NABER, D., et al. "β-Endorphin, Cortisol and Prolactin in Serum of Schizophrenic Patients During Long-Term Neuroleptic Treatment and After Withdrawal: Relation to Psychopathology," *Psychopharmacology Bulletin,* 18 (1982):224–226.

199. NEILL, J. D. "Neuroendocrine Regulation of Prolactin Secretion," in L. Martin et al., eds., *Frontiers in Neuroendocrinology.* New York: Raven Press, 1980, pp. 129–155.

200. NESSE, R. N., et al. "Anxiety Induced by Flooding Therapy for Phobias Does Not Elicit Prolactin Secretory Response," *Psychosomatic Medicine,* 42 (1980):25–31.

201. NEWMARK, S. R., et al. "Adrenocortical Response to Marathon Running," *Journal of Clinical Endocrinology and Metabolism,* 42 (1976):393–394.

202. NEWSOME, H. H., and ROSE, J. C. "The Response of Human Adrenocorticotrophic Hormone and Growth Hormone to Surgical Stress," *Journal of Clinical Endocrinology and Metabolism,* 33 (1971):481–487.

203. NOEL, G. L., et al. "Human Prolactin and Growth Hormone Release During Surgery and Other Conditions of Stress," *Journal of Clinical Endocrinology and Metabolism,* 35 (1972):840–851.

204. NORMAN, T. R., and BURROWS, G. D. "Clinical Endocrinology of Schizophrenia," in P.J.V. Beumont et al., eds., *Handbook of Psychiatry and Endocrinology.* Amsterdam: Elsevier Biomedical Press, 1982, pp. 97–122.

205. NOTH, R. H., and WALTER, R. M. "The Effects of Alcohol on the Endocrine System," *Medical Clinics of North America,* 68 (1984):133–146.

206. OHMAN, R., et al. "Prolactin Response to Electroconvulsive Therapy," *Lancet,* 2 (1976):936–937.

207. OSTROFF, R., et al. "Neuroendocrine Risk Factors of Suicidal Behavior," *American Journal of Psychiatry,* 139 (1982):1323–1325.

208. PAMENTER, R. W., and BOYDEN, T. W. "Interactions of Ethanol with the Hypothalamic-Pituitary-Thyroid Axis," *Life Sciences,* 34 (1984):707–712.

209. PARKER, D. C., et al. "Rhythmicities in Human Growth Hormone Concentrations in Plasma," in D. T. Krieger, ed., *Endocrine Rhythms.* New York: Raven Press, 1979, pp. 143–174.

210. PFLUGER, K. H., et al. "Ectopic ACTH Production with Autoantibody Formation in a Patient with Acute Myeloblastic Leukemia," *New England Journal of Medicine,* 305 (1981):1632–1636.

211. PINTER, E. J., et al. "Hormonal and Free Fatty Acid Changes During Strenuous Flight in Novices and Trained Personnel," *Psychoneuroendocrinology,* 4 (1979):79–82.

212. POLLARD, I., BASSETT, J.R., and CAIRNS-CROSS, K. D. "Plasma Glucocorticoid Elevation and Ultrastructural Changes in the Adenohypophysis of the Male Rat Following Prolonged Exposure to Stress," *Neuroendocrinology,* 21 (1976):-312–330.

213. POZNANSKI, E. O., et al. "The Dexamethasone Suppression Test in Prepubertal Depressed Children," *American Journal of Psychiatry,* 139 (1982):321–324.

214. PRANGE, A. J., JR., and LOOSEN, P. T. "Findings in Affective Disorders Relevant to the Thyroid Axis, Melanotropin, Oxytocin and Vasopressin," in G. M. Brown et al., eds., *Neuroendocrinology and Psychiatric Disorder.* New York: Raven Press, 1984, pp. 191–200.

215. PRANGE, A. J., JR., et al. "Enhancement of Imipramine Antidepressant Activity by Thyroid Hormone," *American Journal of Psychiatry,* 126 (1969):452–469.

216. PRANGE, A. J., JR., et al. "Effects of Thyrotropin-Releasing Hormone in Depression," *Lancet,* 2 (1972):999–1002.

217. PRANGE, A. J., JR., et al. "Behavioral and

Endocrine Responses of Schizophrenic Patients to TRH (Protirelin)," *Archives of General Psychiatry,* 36 (1979):1086–1093.

218. RASKIND, M., et al. "Dexamethasone Suppression Test and Cortisol Circadian Rhythm in Primary Degenerative Dementia," *American Journal of Psychiatry,* 139 (1982):1469–1470.

219. REUS, V.I., JOSEPH, M., and DALLMAN, M. "Regulation of ACTH and Cortisol in Depression," *Peptides,* 4 (1983):785–788.

220. RINIERIS, P., et al. "Free-Thyroxine-Index in Schizophrenic Patients Before and After Neuroleptic Treatment," *Neuropsychobiology,* 6 (1980):29–33.

221. ROSE, R. M. "Overview of Endocrinology of Stress," in G. M. Brown et al., eds., *Neuroendocrinology and Psychiatric Disorder.* New York: Raven Press, 1984, pp. 95–128.

222. ROSE, R. M., et al. "Endocrine Activity in Air Traffic Controllers at Work. I. Characterization of Cortisol and Growth Hormone Levels During the Day," *Psychoneuroendocrinology,* 7 (1982):101–111.

223. ROSE, R. M., et al. "Endocrine Activity in Air Traffic Controllers at Work. II. Biological, Psychological and Work Correlates," *Psychoneuroendocrinology,* 7 (1982):113–123.

224. ROSE, R. M., et al. "Endocrine Activity in Air Traffic Controllers at Work. III. Relationship to Physical and Psychiatric Morbidity," *Psychoneuroendocrinology,* 7 (1982):123–134.

225. ROTHSCHILD, A. J., et al. "The Dexamethasone Suppression Test as a Discriminator Among Subtypes of Psychotic Patients," *British Journal of Psychiatry,* 141 (1982):471–474.

226. RUBIN, R. T., and POLAND, R. E. "Pituitary-Adrenocortical and Pituitary-Gonadal Function in Affective Disorder," in G. M. Brown, et al., *Neuroendocrinology and Psychiatric Disorder.* New York: Raven Press, 1984, pp. 151–164.

227. RUBIN, R. T., et al. "Hypothalamo-Pituitary-Gonadal Function in Primary Endogenously Depressed Men: Preliminary Findings," in K. Fuxe et al., eds., *Steroid Hormone Regulation of the Brain.* Oxford: Pergamon Press, 1981, pp. 387–396.

228. RUBINOW, D. R., et al. "CSF Somatostatin in Affective Illness," *Archives of General Psychiatry,* 40 (1983):409–412.

229. RUSH, A. J., et al. "Sleep EEG and Dexamethasone Suppression Test Findings in Outpatients with Unipolar Major Depressive Disorders," *Biological Psychiatry,* 17 (1982):327–341.

230. RYAN, R. J., et al. "Effect of Convulsive Electroshock on Serum Concentrations of Follicle Stimulating Hormone, Luteinizing Hormone, Thyroid Stimulating Hormone and Growth Hormone," *Journal of Clinical Endocrinology and Metabolism,* 30 (1970):51–58.

231. SACHAR, E. J., et al. "Cortisol Production in Depressive Illness: A Clinical and Biochemical Classification," *Archives of General Psychiatry,* 23 (1971):289–298.

232. SACHAR, E. J., et al. "Disrupted 24-Hour Patterns of Cortisol Secretion in Psychotic Depression," *Archives of General Psychiatry,* 28 (1973):19–24.

233. SACHAR, E. J., et al. "Plasma and Urinary Testosterone Levels in Depressed Men," *Archives of General Psychiatry,* 28 (1973):15–18.

234. SACHAR, E. J., et al. "Human Growth Hormone Responses to Levodopa: Relation to Menopause, Depression and Plasma Dopa Concentration," *Archives of General Psychiatry,* 32 (1975):502–503.

235. SACHAR, E. J., et al. "Recent Studies in the Neuroendocrinology of Major Depressive Disorders," *Psychiatric Clinics of North America,* 3 (1980):313–326.

236. SACHAR, E. J., et al. "Paradoxical Cortisol Responses to Dextroamphetamine in Endogenous Depression," *Archives of General Psychiatry,* 38 (1981):1113–1117.

237. SASSIN, J. F., et al. "The Nocturnal Rise of Human Prolactin Is Dependent on Sleep," *Journal of Clinical Endocrinology and Metabolism,* 37 (1973):436–440.

238. SCHALCH, D. S. "The Influence of Physical Stress and Exercise on Growth Hormone and Insulin Secretion in Man," *Journal of Laboratory and Clinical Medicine,* 69 (1967):256–269.

239. SCHIMMELBUSCH, W. H., MUELLER, P. S., and SHEPS, J. "The Positive Correlation

Between Insulin Resistance and Duration of Hospitalization in Untreated Schizophrenia," *British Journal of Psychiatry*, 118 (1971):429–436.

240. SCHLEIFER, S. J., et al. "Lymphocyte Function in Major Depressive Disorder," *Archives of General Psychiatry*, 41 (1984):484–486.

241. SCHLESSER, M. A., WINOKUR, G., and SHERMAN, B. M. "Genetic Subtypes of Unipolar Primary Depressive Illness Distinguished by Hypothalamic-Pituitary-Adrenal Axis Activity," *Lancet*, 1 (1979):739–741.

242. SCHUCKIT, M. A., PARKER, D. C., and ROSSMAN, L. R. "Ethanol-Related Prolactin Responses and Risk for Alcoholism," *Biological Psychiatry*, 18 (1983):1153–1159.

243. SHADER, R. I., and DE MASCIO, A. *"Psychotropic Drug Side Effects.* Baltimore: Williams & Wilkins, 1970.

244. SIEVER, L. J., et al. "Growth Hormone Response to Clonidine Unchanged by Chronic Clorgyline Treatment," *Psychiatry Research*, 7 (1982):139–144.

245. SIEVER, L. J., et al. "Plasma Cortisol Responses to Clonidine in Depressed Patients and Controls," *Archives of General Psychiatry*, 41 (1984):63–68.

246. SIEVER, L. J., et al. "Plasma Prolactin Changes Following Fenfluramine in Depressed Patients Compared to Controls: An Evaluation of Central Serotonergic Responsivity in Depression," *Life Sciences*, 34 (1984):1029–1039.

247. SIRIS, S. G., et al. "Effect of Dopamine Blockade on Gonadotropins and Testosterone in Men," *American Journal of Psychiatry*, 137 (1980):211–215.

248. SLADE, A. P., and CHECKLEY, S. A. "A Neuroendocrine Study of the Mechanism of Action of ECT," *British Journal of Psychiatry*, 137 (1980):217–221.

249. SMITH, E. M., and BLALOCK, J. E. "Human Lymphocyte Production of Corticotropin and Endorphin-like Substances: Association with Leukocyte Interferon," *Proceedings of the National Academy of Science*, 78 (1981):7530–7534.

250. SMITH, E. M., MEYER, W. M., III, and BLALOCK, J. E. "Virus-Induced Corticosterone in Hypophysectomized Mice: A Possible Lymphoid Adrenal Axis," *Science*, 218 (1982):1311–1312.

251. SOLOMON, G. F., and AMKRAUT, A. A. "Psychoneuroendocrinological Effects on the Immune Response," *Annual Review of Microbiology*, 35 (1981):155–184.

252. SOWERS, J. R., et al. "The Effect of Stressful Diagnostic Studies and Surgery on Anterior Pituitary Hormone Release in Man," *Acta Endocrinologica*, 86 (1977):25–32.

253. SOWERS, J. R., et al. "Influence of Dopaminergic Mechanisms on 24-Hour Secretory Patterns of Prolactin, Luteinizing Hormone and Testosterone in Recumbent Men," *Journal of Endocrine Investigation*, 6 (1983):9–15.

254. STERNBACH, H. A., et al. "The Dexamethasone Suppression and Thyrotropin-Releasing Hormone Tests in Depressed Borderline Patients," *Psychoneuroendocrinology*, 8 (1983):459–462.

255. STOKES, P. E., et al. "Pretreatment DST and Hypothalamic-Pituitary-Adrenocortical Function in Depressed Patients and Comparison Groups," *Archives of General Psychiatry*, 41 (1984):257–267.

256. SWARTZ, C. M., and DUNNER, F. J. "Dexamethasone Suppression Testing of Alcoholics," *Archives of General Psychiatry*, 39 (1982):1309–1312.

257. SYVLAHTI, E., LAMMINTAUSTA, R., and PEKKARINEN, D. "Effect of Psychic Stress of Examination on Serum Growth Hormone, Serum Insulin and Plasma Renin Activity," *Acta Pharmacologica et Toxicologica*, 38 (1976):344–352.

258. TAKAHASHI, Y., KIPNIS, D. M., and DAUGHADAY, W. J. "Growth Hormone Secretion During Sleep," *Journal of Clinical Investigation*, 47 (1968):2079–2080.

259. TARGUM, S. D. "The Application of Serial Neuroendocrine Challenge Studies in the Management of Depressive Disorder," *Biological Psychiatry*, 18 (1982):3–19.

260. TARGUM, S. D. "Persistent Neuroendocrine Dysregulation in Major Depressive Disorder: A Marker for Early Relapse," *Biological Psychiatry*, 19 (1984):305–318.

261. TARGUM, S. D., BYRNES, S. M., and SULLIVAN, A. C. "Subtypes of Unipolar De-

pression Distinguished by the Dexamethasone Suppression Test," *Journal of Affective Disorders*, 4 (1982):21–27.

262. TARGUM, S. D., et al. "Dysregulation of Hypothalamic-Pituitary-Adrenal Axis Function in Depressed Alcoholic Patients," *Journal of Affective Disorders*, 4 (1982):347–353.

263. TARGUM, S. D., et al. "Abnormal Dexamethasone Tests in Withdrawing Alcoholic Patients," *Biological Psychiatry*, 19 (1984):401–405.

264. TRASKMAN, L., et al. "Cortisol in the CSF of Depressed and Suicidal Patients," *Archives of General Psychiatry*, 37 (1980):761–767.

265. URSIN, H., and MURISON, R.C.C. "Classification and Description of Stress," in G. M. Brown et al., eds., *Neuroendocrinology and Psychiatric Disorder*. New York: Raven Press, 1984, pp. 123–131.

266. URSIN, H., BAADE, E., and LEVINE, S., eds. *Psychobiology of Stress. A Study of Coping Men*. New York: Academic Press, 1978.

267. VAN KAMMEN, D. P., and ANTELMAN, S. "Impaired Noradrenergic Transmission in Schizophrenia," *Life Sciences*, 34 (1984):1403–1413.

268. VAN THIEL, D. H., and LESTER, R. "The Effect of Chronic Alcohol Abuse on Sexual Function," *Clinical Endocrinology and Metabolism*, 8 (1979):499–510.

269. VAN THIEL, D. H., LESTER, R., and VAITUKAITUS, J. "Evidence for a Defect in Pituitary Secretion of Luteinizing Hormone in Chronic Alcoholic Men," *Journal of Clinical Endocrinology and Metabolism*, 47 (1978):499–507.

270. VAN THIEL, D. H., et al. "Plasma Estrone, Prolactin, Neurophysin, and Sex Steroid-Binding Globulin in Chronic Alcoholic Men," *Metabolism*, 24 (1975):1015–1019.

271. VAN THIEL, D. H., et al. "Abnormal Prolactin and Growth Hormone Responses to Thyrotropin Releasing Hormone in Chronic Alcoholic Men," in M. Galanter, ed., *Currents in Alcoholism*. New York: Grune & Stratton, 1979, pp. 71–79.

272. VIGERSKY, R. A. "Hypothalamic Hypogonadotropism in Weight-Loss-Associated Amenorrhea," in G. M. Brown et al., *Neuroendocrinology and Psychiatric Disorder*. New York: Raven Press, 1984, pp. 291–300.

273. VIGERSKY, R. A., et al. "Delayed Pituitary Hormone Response to LRF and TRF in Patients with Anorexia Nervosa and with Secondary Amenorrhea Associated with Simple Weight Loss," *Journal of Clinical Endocrinology and Metabolism*, 43 (1976):893–906.

274. VIGNERI, R., et al. "Sleep-Associated Growth Hormone (GH) Release in Schizophrenia," *Neuroendocrinology*, 14 (1974):356–361.

275. VOGEL, W., KLARBER, E. L., and BROVERMAN, O. H. "Gonadal Function in Depression," *Progress in Neuropsychopharmacology*, 2 (1978):487–503.

276. VOLOVKA, J., DAVIS, L. G., and EHRLICH, Y. H. "Endorphins, Dopamine, and Schizophrenia," *Schizophrenia Bulletin*, 5 (1979):227–250.

277. WAGNER, D. R., and WEITZMAN, E. D. "Neuroendocrine Secretion and Biological Rhythms in Man," *Psychiatric Clinics of North America*, 3 (1980):223–250.

278. WAKELING, A., et al. "Amenorrhea, Body Weight, and Serum Hormone Concentrations, with Particular Reference to Prolactin and Thyroid Hormones in Anorexia Nervosa," *Psychological Medicine*, 9 (1979):265–272.

279. WALSH, B. T. "The Endocrinology of Anorexia Nervosa," *Psychiatric Clinics of North America*, 3 (1980):299–312.

280. WEINER, H., and KATZ, J. L. "The Hypothalamic-Pituitary-Adrenal Axis in Anorexia Nervosa: A Reassessment," in P. L. Darby et al., eds., *Anorexia Nervosa: Recent Developments in Research*. New York: Alan R. Liss, 1983, pp. 249–270.

281. WEINER, R., and GANONG, W. F. "Role of Brain Monoamines and Histamine in Regulation of Anterior Pituitary Hormone Secretion," *Physiological Review*, 58 (1978):905–976.

282. WEIZMAN, R., et al. "Abnormal Growth Hormone Response to TRH in Chronic Adolescent Schizophrenic Patients," *British Journal of Psychiatry*, 141 (1982):583–585.

283. WHYBROW, P. C., and HURWITZ, T. "Psychological Disturbances Associated

with Endocrine Disease and Hormone Therapy," in E. J. Sachar, ed., *Hormones, Behavior and Psychopathology.* New York: Raven Press, 1976, pp. 125–143.

284. WHYBROW, P. C., and PRANGE, A. J., JR. "A Hypothesis of Thyroid-Catecholamine-Receptor Interaction," *Archives of General Psychiatry,* 38 (1981):106–113.

285. WINOKUR, A., et al. "Variability of Hormonal Responses to a Series Neuroendocrine Challenge in Depressed Patients," *American Journal Psychiatry,* 139 (1982):39–44.

286. WINOKUR, A., et al. "Administration of Thyrotropin-Releasing Hormone at Weekly Intervals Results in a Diminished Thyrotropin Response," *Biological Psychiatry,* 19 (1984):695–702.

287. WODE-HELGODT, B., et al. "Effect of Chlorpromazine Treatment on Prolac-tin Levels in Cerebrospinal Fluid and Plasma of Psychotic Patients," *Acta Psychiatrica Scandinavica,* 56 (1977):280–293.

288. WOLKIN, A., et al. "TRH Test Abnormalities in Psychiatric Disorders," *Journal of Affective Disorders,* 6 (1984):273–281.

289. WRIGHT, J. "Endocrine Effects of Alcohol," *Clinical Endocrinology and Metabolism,* 7 (1978):351–367.

290. YEREVANIAN, B. I., WOOLF, P. D., and IKER, H. P. "Plasma ACTH Levels in Depression Before and After Recovery: Relationship to the Dexamethasone Suppression Test," *Psychiatry Research,* 10 (1983):175–181.

291. YLIKAHRI, R. H., HUTTUNEN, M. O., and HARKANEN, M. "Hormonal Changes During Alcohol Intoxication and Withdrawal," *Pharmacology, Biochemistry, Behavior,* 13 (1980):131–137.

CHAPTER 5

THE NEUROPATHOLOGY OF PSYCHIATRIC DISORDERS

Steven Matthysse and Alfred Pope

Despite the failure of classical neuropathology to demonstrate specific lesions in the major neuropsychiatric diseases,[10,34] in a review published ten years ago[19] we concluded that

in the light of impressive recent advances in the neurosciences it may well be that comparative studies of morphology and biochemistry of the human brain, interpreted in terms of physiological circuitry determined in animal models, will provide some genuine insights concerning the pathologic physiology of schizophrenia. (P. 759)

Recent years have, indeed, witnessed a remarkable expansion of research on the neuropathology (broadly defined as comparative neurobiology) of the human brain in mental disease. Four factors have contributed to this renewal of interest: (1) the intellectual appeal of the current hypotheses in biological psychiatry (e.g., the catecholamine theories of schizophrenia and affective disorders), which, although far from established, have motivated studies of human brain chemistry and have narrowed the potentially bewildering array of substances that could be investigated; (2) the recognition that although studies of the biochemistry of the human brain are fraught with potential artifacts, not all constituents are equally susceptible; (3) the steady refinement of biochemical techniques, which now have far greater versatility, specificity, and sensitivity than has been possible in the past; and (4) the development of facilities, such as the Brain Tissue Banks at McLean Hospital in Massachusetts and the Wadsworth Veterans' Hospital in California, which have been mandated to acquire, dissect, and distribute human brain tissue, with clinical and pathological documentation, to interested investigators on a worldwide basis.

The results of this effort have been comprehensively reviewed.[13,32] Despite many provocative findings, an impartial reading of the recent literature does not provide the hoped-for clarification of the catecholamine hypotheses, nor does compelling evidence emerge for other biological differences that may characterize the brains of patients with mental disease.

To be sure, uncontroverted findings and unambiguous interpretations are not to be expected quickly in a field as complex as human neurobiology related to mental disease; but there are also systematic reasons for the inconclusiveness of the recent literature, which might be corrected by improved experimental designs. This chapter will focus on design issues. We hope to offer the nonspecialist reader a guide to those aspects of experimental design that are required for studies of the postmortem human brain to be interpretable and replicable; in a word, to be taken seriously. We will illustrate these principles with examples from the literature in which that aspect of experimental design has been used effectively. Our references are not intended to be exhaustive.

¶ Ambiguities of Diagnosis

The problem of nosology in psychiatric disease is a very difficult one, which has been discussed in other chapters. In addition to the vagueness of diagnostic boundaries, the possibility exists that syndromes, as currently defined, are actually heterogeneous groups of illnesses. If a particular brain abnormality is present in only one diagnostic subtype, mixing that subtype together with other cases will decrease the probability of uncovering a significant difference. Elevations in norepinephrine, for example, have been observed in the ventral septum, bed nucleus of the stria terminalis, nucleus accumbens, and mammillary body in the chronic paranoid subtype of schizophrenia, as opposed to other types[12] (see also Kleinman et al.[16]). The more minutely a syndrome is divided into subtypes, however, the more vital becomes replication of findings in an independent sample, since chance fluctuations can the more easily mimic heterogeneity among subtypes.

The provisional nature of psychiatric diagnosis underscores the importance of obtaining as much descriptive data as possible about the patient. Not only do diagnostic terms not have universal meanings, but in the future it may become useful to group patients according to symptoms and signs not considered crucial at present. Data concerning the patient's family is also valuable, because heritable and nonheritable forms of an illness may be etiologically distinct. Even data on illnesses in the family other than that presented by the patient may be relevant, since shared genes may express themselves in varied ways in different family members. Neuropathology must make use of the most rigorous and consensually validated criteria available, but at the same time must regard its own data as contributing ultimately to the refinement of diagnostic criteria. Attentiveness to outliers and nonunimodal distributions of neurochemical and morphological variables may be very rewarding.

A common defect in the design of studies of the postmortem human brain is the absence of an adequate range of diagnostic groups for comparison. It is tempting to focus exclusively on the neuropsychiatric disease of interest and on "controls," which are usually brains of "normal" individuals of approximately the same age. Reports of positive findings, without a range of comparison groups, are not only difficult to interpret but also tend to distort subsequent work in the field. Once one or two reports are published claiming an abnormality based on studies of a single diagnostic group, these reports attract other investigators, and soon the literature grows; the phenomenon becomes the "property" of the disease that was the subject of the first publications. Since psychiatric diagnoses overlap, the relationship might have been stronger all along in other conditions, but the absence of a range of comparison groups militates against making that discovery.

Psychiatric research is familiar with this problem in studies of peripheral metabolism. The early reports of decreased platelet monoamine oxidase (MAO) in schizophrenia led to a copious flow of publications on the subject, most of which ignored the possibility that platelet MAO might be equally abnormal in other psychiatric conditions. When a study finally appeared that avoided any bias toward schizophrenia (subjects were selected by MAO values and interviewed later), antisocial behavior and suicide were at least as strong correlates of low MAO as schizophrenia.[6] Similarly, absence of suppression of serum cortisol by oral dexamethasone (the "dexamethasone suppression test") became the "property" of affective illness, and nearly all subsequent studies confined themselves to comparing depressed patients with normal "controls." A more thorough analysis, which included a wide variety of diagnostic groups, clearly demonstrates that nonsuppression occurs in many physical illnesses and is by no means a specific correlate of affective disorder.[8]

A few reports on the postmortem human brain in neuropsychiatric conditions do make use of an adequate range of comparison groups. Stevens[30] studied fibrillary gliosis in schizophrenia (as defined by *International Classification of Diseases* criteria). Using Holzer's stain for glial fibrils, she observed patchy gliosis, especially in periventricular regions (seventeen out of twenty-eight cases). Among her comparison groups were twenty-eight patients with neurologic and psychiatric disorders other than schizophrenia, similar in the range of ages at death. The diagnoses of these patients included a broad spectrum of infectious, degenerative, deficiency, vascular, neoplastic, and "functional" neuropsychiatric disorders. Gliosis was also common in this material. Alcoholic encephalopathy, like schizophrenia, was associated with periaqueductal and hypothalamic gliosis. Huntington's chorea patients also had fibrillary gliosis around the lateral and third ventricles. The nonspecificity of the findings in this study is not surprising, since gliosis is a sign of tissue reaction to injury rather than a specific lesion. A lesion uniquely found in a particular neuropsychiatric disease would, of course, be of great importance in tracing the etiology of that disease; but such a claim carries with it the burden of proof of specificity through comparison with other disorders. The importance of establishing diagnostic specificity was already stressed by Adolf Meyer[20] at the turn of the century: "It seems quite obvious that for a pathological anatomy of the nervous system all possible disorders, whether or not accompanied by mental diseases, must first be subjected to a sufficient study before the special cases which show mental disorders can be expected to furnish sufficient material for comparison" (P. 304).

¶ Drug and Age Effects

The wide spectrum of actions of the commonly used antipsychotic drugs—affecting many enzymes and neurotransmitter systems, as well as having pronounced physicochemical actions on biological membranes—makes their possible confounding effects in postmortem studies of psychotic patients a major concern.

Nearly all schizophrenic patients have been treated with neuroleptics at some time in the course of their illness. Working with patients certified to be "drug-free" for several months before death, or even a year, is likely to be a disappointing strategy, since the biochemical sequelae of neuroleptic treatment may well outlast the persistence of detectable concentrations of the neuroleptic drug itself in the brain.[1] The most promising strategy for assessing this problem is long-term experimentation in animals. Comparison of neurochemical changes in several brain regions as a way of compensating for neuroleptic effects is hazardous, since regional specificity may be an integral part of the therapeutic action of these drugs. Treatment of rats with haloperidol for six months, for example, causes increases of dopamine and norepinephrine in the nucleus accumbens and septum, but not in the basal ganglia.[18]

Adequate studies of neuroleptic drug effects require patience. An example is Bird and Anton's[3] twenty-month, daily administration of prochlorperazine to monkeys by naso-gastric tube, which showed a decrease of dopamine concentration in the basal ganglia after this period of time. Some schizophrenic patients may be withdrawn from neuroleptic medication while in a late residual phase, or during their terminal illness, and strict control for drug effects in these cases requires that the animals also undergo withdrawal. Such an experiment was carried out by Clow,[7] who treated rats with neuroleptics for a year and allowed a three-month withdrawal period. This procedure resulted in an increase in striatal dopamine receptor concentration that remained unaltered after the drug-free period.

Age is a confounding factor that is difficult to eliminate, since most patients with mental illness have a normal life span. Age-matching can, of course, be used to eliminate bias, but the problem remains that age changes may be so pronounced that they obscure effects due to the disease process itself. On the other hand, suicide is not rare among young patients with major psychiatric illnesses, and a greater effort should be made to study brain specimens from suicide victims. A very interesting recent study compared imipramine binding in the frontal cortex of suicide victims and patients dying from other causes (homicide and myocardial infarction) in the same age range. The mean number of imipramine binding sites appeared to be lower in the suicide victims.[29] Since suicide occurs in both schizophrenia and affective disorder, comparison between diagnostic groups can be made.

¶ Artifacts Related to Specimen Acquisition

Changes caused by aging, the terminal illness, drug treatment, or the state of chemical preservation of the brain can all masquerade as abnormalities related to the disease under study. While it is obviously dangerous to ignore these artifacts, it is also unfortunate if concern about them leads to neglect of postmortem neurochemistry and neuroanatomy. The responsible course is to estimate the magnitude of confounding effects as directly as possible; to determine which substances and structures are most, and which are least, sensitive; and to establish criteria for assessing the suitability of tissue from any given human brain for investigation. The confounding effects have to be studied separately for each biochemical or morphological

variable to be investigated. Fortunately, knowledge is accumulating slowly but steadily about potential artifacts (see Bird and Iversen[4] for a review).

The nature and duration of the terminal illness has a pronounced effect on the level of brain glutamic acid decarboxylase (prolonged illness is associated with lower values than sudden death), but norepinephrine, dopamine, and choline acetyltransferase seem to be relatively insensitive to this factor.[27] Phosphofructokinase and pH are also sensitive to the duration of the terminal illness.[21]

Time from death to refrigeration and from refrigeration to freezing or fixation of the brain is a major factor influencing postmortem morphology and biochemistry. In morphology, there are few systematic studies of the effects of time from death to fixation. Williams and colleagues[33] found that mouse brains fixed after six hours still permitted neuronal Golgi impregnations of good quality, although the number of stained cells diminished; but specimens fixed after twenty-four hours were not useful for the Golgi method. In the case of neurochemical variables, there is evidence that gamma-aminobutyric acid rises rapidly following death, then stabilizes for forty-eight hours or more.[22] Dopamine falls by 30 to 40 percent during the first four hours, then becomes relatively constant, with a further 10 percent decline occurring over the next sixty-eight hours.[28] Glutamic acid decarboxylase falls slowly for the first twelve hours to about 80 percent of its initial value, then stabilizes. Choline acetyltransferase, on the other hand, is reported to be essentially unchanged for seventy-two hours postmortem.[28] Since most human brain specimens are obtained on the plateaus of these curves, one might conclude that deterioration artifacts are not likely to be major confounding factors in disease, at least for the substances that have been examined thus far. It might even be argued that a short period of autolysis is preferable to rapid freezing, since it permits substances to be measured during a less rapidly changing phase. This procedure would not be well advised, however; precisely because a plateau has been reached, neurochemical measurements after a period of autolysis may no longer reflect the conditions prevailing in the brain at the time of death, so the possibility of detecting real differences between diagnostic groups would be compromised. On the contrary, the effort to obtain specimens frozen as rapidly as possible after death is well worthwhile, although the exact estimation of postmortem change then becomes more critical. In some instances direct comparison of biopsy and autopsy specimens from the human brain is possible, and this technique can provide useful information about stability, as long as the indications for intracranial surgery and the effects of anesthesia, use of electrocautery, and other confounding factors are taken into account.[23]

Experiments using animals to determine the characteristics of the rapidly changing phase of postmortem autolysis run into difficulty because the human brain, being so much larger, will have different heat exchange and diffusion characteristics. In the study by Spokes referred to earlier,[28] even though mice were used as experimental models, the investigators cleverly designed environmental conditions that made the cooling curves similar to those of human brain. They first measured the depth and surface temperatures of the human brain for thirty-two hours after death while the cadaver remained refrigerated; they then placed the mouse brain in an incubator programmed so that its temperature, as a function of time, approximated the cooling curve of human brain.

E. Perry[21] has suggested that particularly sensitive neurochemical parameters be used as internal indices of the general state of biochemical integrity of the brain. Internal indices may be useful in practice, because postmortem conditions, such as the number of hours from death to freezing, may be uncertain unless patients are under continuous nursing surveillance. Of course, these measures can only be used as indices of chemical integrity if there are no specific hypotheses implicating them in the disease process under study. Another relatively simple and effective approach is to use the brain as its own control: to compare substances of interest in brain regions postulated to be, and those regions postulated not to be, involved in the disease process. For example, in the study of norepinephrine in chronic paranoid schizophrenia referred to earlier,[12] the increase in norepinephrine in regions of the limbic forebrain was not accompanied by corresponding changes in other parts of the limbic system. While it is conceivable that postmortem degenerative processes might differentially affect the components of a specific anatomical system, it seems more likely that such processes would act across regions. Similarly, the increases in dopamine in the nucleus accumbens and anterior perforated substance observed by Bird, Spokes, and Iversen[5] were not reflected by changes in other limbic brain areas.

¶ Problems of Observation

Even when specimens from well-documented cases are acquired under optimal conditions, the difficulties are not over. Subjective bias is a constant danger in the microscopic examination of brain tissue. It is curious that an investigation of neuropathology in mental disease carried out sixty years ago[10] used unbiased quantitative methods (e.g., cell counts tabulated by four different observers), whereas many subsequent studies have been more subjective. Even work by influential neuropathologists like C. and O. Vogt came under criticism for subjective and selective reporting. Wolf and Cowen[35] showed decisively that loss of neurons and cytological changes like "shrinkage and sclerosis" could be demonstrated in selected samples of normal, as well as schizophrenic, brain.

Recent years have brought a much more objective and quantitative approach to the neuropathology of mental disease. Measurements have been made of neuron number, volume of neuropil, thickness of the cortical layers, volume of cortex and subcortical nuclei, and other potentially important morphological parameters. There are now very well developed principles of random sampling and statistical analysis (stereology) that can be used to estimate three-dimensional quantities such as volume, size distribution, and cell density from measurements on two-dimensional sections.[31] Benes, Davidson, and Bird[2] have recently applied these principles in a study of schizophrenia. Processing of large numbers of tissue sections in an objective manner would be greatly facilitated if computer-coupled microscopes could be used to classify and count neurons and glia. This task is very difficult to carry out accurately, partly because the subtleties of human feature recognition are not easily imitated by computer and partly because thin sections may cut neurons in profiles small enough to be mistaken for glia, whereas thick sections create a focusing and overlap problem. The development of specific markers for cell types (e.g., antibodies to tyrosine hydroxylase) may make the automated cell recognition problem more tractable.

Kovelman and Scheibel[17] have applied quantitative methods in an interesting way to study cell orientation in hippocampal specimens from schizophrenic patients. Diagonal lines were drawn between the corners of photographs of sections of the hippocampus, and the three pyramidal cells in each quadrant closest to the intersection point were chosen. The absolute value of the angular deviation of the long axis of each pyramidal cell, relative to a perpendicular drawn from the border of the ventricle, was measured. These deviations were small, but significantly greater in ten schizophrenic patients than in eight control subjects. None of the control subjects had neurological or psychiatric illness, so the specificity of these changes for schizophrenia remains uncertain. In a previous, nonquantitative study more dramatic differences were found, and there was evidence of specificity, in that patients with other neuropsychiatric diagnoses were included among the control group.[26] The findings are intriguing and warrant further exploration.

Just as subjective bias complicates microscopic observation of human brain tissue, regional heterogeneity poses a problem for biochemical analysis. When human brain dissection technique varies from laboratory to laboratory, comparability of results is impossible to achieve. A striking example is the finding of tenfold higher norepinephrine concentration in the nucleus accumbens by the Hornykiewicz group than the concentration found by other competent laboratories because of differences in definition of the boundaries of the nucleus.[11] There has been an international effort, extending over several years, to define nuclear boundaries in the human brain in universally accepted operational terms (e.g., Pope[24]).

Despite the obvious utility of this approach, it masks a deeper problem. In the animal brain, nuclei can be defined by input-output relations, as established by anterograde and retrograde tracing techniques. In the human brain, no such absolute definitions are possible. Demarcation of regions in terms of landmarks such as fiber tracts or the ventricular surface is convenient, but there is no guarantee that regions so defined will contain the same classes of synaptic terminals in two different individuals. Consequently, there may be variation from brain to brain, not because of true biochemical differences but because the homologous pathways are not precisely correlated with the landmarks. One approach to overcoming this problem is the use of biochemical coordinates to locate regions of interest. For example, to sample the zone of terminations of the mesocortical dopamine system, one would not proceed by dissecting the appropriate gyrus and measuring a certain number of microns below the pial surface, but rather by selecting that region of prefrontal cortex that had the highest density of spiroperidol binding sites. In such an experiment dopamine receptor binding would not be the object of comparison between patients and controls, but would instead be the parameter used to locate homologous regions to be compared in other ways. Appropriate techniques combining microdissection and ultramicrochemical analysis are available for study of the human brain (for a summary review see Matthysse and Pope[19]).

¶ Requirements for Interpretation

When pathological phenomena have been reported from several laboratories, it is encouraging if, taken together, they can be interpreted as presenting a consistent picture. To be sure, the history of science is full of instances of apparently inconsistent observations that became resolved by a brilliant theoretical stroke; and the same could happen in the neuropathology of mental diseases. An apparently inconsistent picture should, however, motivate efforts toward replication of each of the empirical findings and explication of divergent results.

There have been, for example, at least six reports of positive findings concerning catecholamine concentrations in specific regions of schizophrenic brain:

1. Farley and associates[12] found norepinephrine elevated in the ventral septum, bed nucleus of the stria terminalis, nucleus accumbens, and mammillary body.
2. Bird, Spokes, and Iversen[5] found dopamine elevated in the nucleus accumbens and anterior perforated substance.
3. Crow and others[9] found elevations of dopamine in the caudate and putamen and of norepinephrine in the putamen. Comparable measurements by Winblad and coworkers,[34] however, did not show differences.
4. Kleinman and associates[16] found elevated free 3-methoxy-4-hydroxy-phenylglycol in the hypothalamus.
5. Farley, Shannak, and Hornykiewicz[11] found elevated dopamine only in the ventral septum.
6. Reynolds[25] found increased dopamine in the left amygdala.

These diverse findings, each implicating a different region or substance, do not lend themselves to a consistent interpretation. The interested reader may find the debate between Hornykiewicz[14] and Iversen, Reynolds, and Snyder[15] illuminating. Certainly,

however, these apparent inconsistencies are not grounds for discouragement at this stage of development of human neurochemistry. Replication, with attention to the methodological problems that have been discussed, seems called for.

¶ Conclusion

The field of neuropathology of mental disease has provocative hypotheses to test and reasonably effective ways of testing them. Artifacts abound, but there are relatively simple principles that can make studies more convincing. Each of these principles has been applied by a few investigators with good results, but it is still difficult to find studies that have applied them all. As methodology improves, it is likely that the uncertainties and controversies surrounding the neuropathology of the human brain in neuropsychiatric disease will gradually become resolved.

¶ Acknowledgments

The authors wish to acknowledge the support of Collaborative Biological Research in Schizophrenia, grant 5 P01 MH 31154.

¶ Bibliography

1. ANTELMAN, S. M., et al. "Haloperidol Catalepsy Shows Sensitization Which Depends on the Passage of Time Rather Than Repeated Treatment," *Neuroscience Abstracts*, 9 (1983):556.
2. BENES, F. M., DAVIDSON, J., and BIRD, E. D. "Quantitative Cytoarchitectural Studies of the Cerebral Cortex of Schizophrenics," *Archives of General Psychiatry*, in press.
3. BIRD, E. D., and ANTON, A. H. "Phenothiazine Biphasic Effect on Dopamine Concentrations in the Basal Ganglia of Subhuman Primates," *Psychiatry Research*, 6 (1982):1–6.
4. BIRD, E. D., and IVERSEN, L. L. "Human

Brain Postmortem Studies of Neurotransmitters and Related Markers," in A. Lajtha, ed., *Handbook of Neurochemistry*, vol. 2, 2nd ed. New York: Plenum Press, 1982, pp. 225–251.

5. BIRD, E. D., SPOKES, E. G. S., and IVERSEN, L. L. "Increased Dopamine Concentration in Limbic Areas of Brain from Patients Dying with Schizophrenia," *Brain*, 102 (1979):347–360.

6. BUCHSBAUM, M. S., COURSEY, R. D., and MURPHY, D. L. "The Biochemical High-risk Paradigm: Behavioral and Familial Correlates of Low Platelet Monoamine Oxidase Activity," *Science*, 194 (1976): 339–341.

7. CLOW, A., et al. "Neuroleptic Drugs and the Dopamine Hypothesis," *Lancet*, 1 (1979):934.

8. CRAPO, L. "Cushing's Syndrome: A Review of Diagnostic Tests," *Metabolism*, 28 (1979):955–977.

9. CROW, T. J., et al. "Monoamine Mechanisms in Chronic Schizophrenia: Postmortem Neurochemical Findings," *British Journal of Psychiatry*, 134 (1979):249–256.

10. DUNLAP, C. B. "Dementia Praecox: Some Preliminary Observations on Brains from Carefully Selected Cases, and a Consideration of Certain Sources of Error," *American Journal of Psychiatry*, 3 (1924):403–421.

11. FARLEY, I. J., SHANNAK, K. S., and HORNYKIEWICZ, O. "Brain Monoamine Changes in Chronic Paranoid Schizophrenia and Their Possible Relation to Increased Dopamine Receptor Sensitivity," in G. Pepeu, M. J. Kuhar, and S. J. Enna, eds., *Receptors for Neurotransmitters and Peptide Hormones*. New York: Raven Press, 1980, pp. 427–433.

12. FARLEY, I. J., et al. "Norepinephrine in Chronic Paranoid Schizophrenia: Above-Normal Levels in Limbic Forebrain," *Science*, 200 (1978):456–458.

13. HORACZ, J. L. "The Dopamine Hypothesis: An Overview of Studies with Schizophrenic Patients," *Schizophrenic Bulletin*, 8 (1982):438–469.

14. HORNYKIEWICZ, O. "Brain Catecholamines in Schizophrenia—A Good Case for Noradrenaline," *Nature*, 299 (1982): 484–486.

15. IVERSEN, L. L., REYNOLDS, G. P., and SNYDER, S. H. "Pathophysiology of Schizophrenia—Causal Role for Dopamine or Noradrenaline?" *Nature*, 305 (1983):577 (with reply by Hornykiewicz, ibid., 577–578).

16. KLEINMAN, J. E., et al. "Chronic Schizophrenia: Postmortem Studies," in C. Baxter and T. Melnechuk, eds., *Perspectives in Schizophrenia Research*. New York: Raven Press, 1980, pp. 227–236.

17. KOVELMAN, J. A., and SCHEIBEL, A. B. "A Neurohistological Correlate of Schizophrenia," *Biological Psychiatry*, 19 (1984):1601–1621.

18. LLOYD, K. G., et al. "Chronic Neuroleptic Therapy: Tolerance and GABA Systems," in E. Costa and G. L. Gessa, eds., *Advances in Biochemical Psychopharmacology*, vol. 16. New York: Raven Press, 1977, pp. 409–415.

19. MATTHYSSE, S., and POPE, A. "The Approach to Schizophrenia Through Molecular Pathology," in R. A. Good, S. B. Day, and J. J. Yunis, eds., *Molecular Pathology*, Springfield, Ill.: Charles C Thomas, 1975, pp. 744–768.

20. MEYER, A. *Collected Papers*, vol. 2. Baltimore: Johns Hopkins Press, 1951.

21. PERRY, E. "Brain Markers," in A. Pope, ed., *Human Brain Dissection*. Washington, D.C.: U. S. Government Printing Office, 1983, pp. 43–44.

22. PERRY, T. L., et al. "γ-Aminobutyric-Acid Deficiency in Brain of Schizophrenic Patients," *Lancet*, (1979):237–239.

23. POPE, A. "Problems of Interpretation in the Chemical Pathology of Schizophrenia," *Journal for Psychiatric Research*, 11 (1974):265–272.

24. POPE, A., ed. *Human Brain Dissection*. Washington, D.C.: U. S. Government Printing Office, 1983.

25. REYNOLDS, G. P. "Increased Concentrations and Lateral Asymmetry of Amygdala Dopamine in Schizophrenia," *Nature*, 305 (1983):527–529.

26. SCHEIBEL, A. B., and KOVELMAN, J. A. "Disorientation of the Hippocampal Pyramidal Cell and Its Processes in the Schizophrenic Patient," *Biological Psychiatry*, 16 (1981):101–102.

27. SPOKES, E. G. S. "An Analysis of Factors Influencing Measurements of Dopa-

mine, Noradrenaline, Glutamate Decarboxylase and Choline Acetylase in Human Post-mortem Brain Tissue," *Brain*, 102 (1979):333–346.

28. SPOKES, E. G. S., and KOCH, D. J. "Post-mortem Stability of Dopamine, Glutamate Decarboxylase and Choline Acetyltransferase in the Mouse Brain under Conditions Simulating the Handling of Human Autopsy Material," *Journal of Neurochemistry*, 31 (1978):381–383.

29. STANLEY, M., VIRGILIO, J., and GERSHON, S. "Tritiated Imipramine Binding Sites are Decreased in the Frontal Cortex of Suicides," *Science*, 216 (1982):1337–1339.

30. STEVENS, J. R. "Neuropathology of Schizophrenia," *Archives of General Psychiatry*, 39 (1982):1131–1139.

31. WEIBEL, E. R. *Stereological Methods*. London: Academic Press, 1979.

32. WEINBERGER, D. R., WAGNER, R. L., and WYATT, R. J. "Neuropathological Studies of Schizophrenia: A Selective Review," *Schizophrenic Bulletin*, 9 (1983):193–212.

33. WILLIAMS, R. S., FERRANTE, R. J., and CAVINESS, V. S., JR. "The Golgi-Rapid Methods in Clinical Neuropathology: I. Morphologic Consequences of Suboptimum Fixation," *Neurology*, 37 (1978): 1333.

34. WINBLAD, B., et al. "Monoamines and Monoamine Metabolites in Brains from Demented Schizophrenics," *Acta Psychiatrica Scandinavica*, 60 (1979):17–28.

35. WOLF, A., and COWEN, D. "Histopathology of Schizophrenia and Other Psychoses of Unknown Origin," in S. Cobb, ed., *The Biology of Mental Health and Disease*. New York: P. B. Hoeber, 1952, pp. 469–497.

CHAPTER 6

THE GENETICS OF PSYCHIATRIC DISORDERS

Steven Matthysse and Seymour S. Kety

¶ Introduction

Elucidation of the significance and mode of genetic transmission in the etiology of the major psychoses is hampered by the absence of objective diagnostic criteria and the lack of agreement regarding the boundaries of each disorder. Early in this century, schizophrenia and manic-depressive illness were described and differentiated by Kraepelin and Bleuler in terms of course and symptoms; in the absence of definitive evidence regarding etiology and pathogenesis, they have remained phenomenological syndromes. There is little to support a presumption that they are homogeneous disease entities.

¶ Genetic Correlates of Psychopathology

Another methodological difficulty in evaluating the magnitude of the genetic contribution to mental disorders generally is the ne-

cessity of removing, controlling, or randomizing environmental influences. Study of the prevalence of a disorder in families is the least successful strategy in this regard; the short-lived genetic hypotheses of pellagra and kuru, based upon the familial tendency of these disorders, failed to recognize environmental influences (peculiarities of diet in both disorders) that a family shares. Several classical studies of the risk for schizophrenia in the relatives of schizophrenic patients have found the risk to lie between 10 and 15 percent in the siblings and offspring of a schizophrenic patient. Parents, the other first-degree relatives, have a lower risk, probably because of the reduced fertility of schizophrenics and the diminished likelihood that they will become parents. The offspring of two schizophrenic parents have a 30 to 40 percent risk of developing the disorder.[35]

Recent studies have found a lower risk in first-degree relatives; for example, Tsuang's careful epidemiological study concluded that the risk was 3.2 percent.[38] These studies used narrower criteria than those in the past

(Tsuang relied upon Feighner's criteria), which also entailed a lower incidence in the general population (0.6 percent in Tsuang's survey, compared to about 1 percent in the classical studies). "Heritability," as estimated from the relation between risk to first-degree relatives and incidence in the general population, seems not to be changed by the narrowing of diagnostic criteria.

Because of the difference in genetic congruence between monozygotic and dizygotic twins, comparison of their respective rates of concordance for schizophrenia offers a better means of dissociating genetic from environmental variables than family prevalence. The larger number of environmental influences that monozygotic twins share makes the dissociation imperfect, although recent studies challenge this objection.[17] In more than fourteen studies of schizophrenia in twins, monozygotic pairs have a high concordance rate for the disorder (40 to 50 percent in the more rigorous studies), while the concordance in dizygotic twins is not different from that found in siblings.[6] These findings are compatible with the operation of genetic factors in a major segment of schizophrenic illness, while the considerably less than 100 percent concordance in monozygotic twins indicates the importance of environmental influences.

Adopted individuals, who share their genes with their biological family and their environment with the adoptive family, offer what may be the best means of disentangling genetic and environmental influences. When selective placement occurs, it can reduce the randomization of environmental factors; assortative mating may enhance the expression of genetic factors when they are present[31]; and knowledge of mental illness in the biological family may affect the development, ascertainment, or diagnosis of mental illness in the adoptee. These confounding influences operate to a greater or lesser extent in different studies and should be taken into account. In each of the relatively small number of studies that have been completed, the prevalence of schizophrenic illness in the offspring, parents, and siblings of schizophrenic patients who have been reared apart from them remains significantly higher than that in the general population, whereas the adoptive relatives of schizophrenics show no enhanced prevalence.* Although this indicates that genetic factors operate significantly in the transmission of schizophrenia, they do not appear to do so uniformly but are clustered in some biological families and apparently absent in others. The genetic heterogeneity that is thus suggested may explain the absence of a consistent and generally accepted mode of genetic transmission in schizophrenia. The family, twin, and adoption studies all find evidence for the existence of a milder, schizophrenialike syndrome (Kraepelin and Bleuler called it "latent schizophrenia") that is genetically related to classical schizophrenia.

Among the environmental influences that have been suggested as etiological factors in schizophrenic illness are the psychosocial interactions associated with rearing, although two well-controlled studies were unable to find an effect of widely differing rearing environments on the development of schizophrenia in the offspring of schizophrenic mothers.[10,11] Viral infection and dietary factors have been suggested by provocative observations but remain to be further established. Two well-designed studies have found a significant association between birth complications and the later development of schizophrenia.[15,23]

Regarding the affective disorders, there have been a substantial number of family studies but comparatively few that have used the twin or adoptive strategies.† When affective disorder is defined narrowly and restricted to severe depression or clear manic-depressive illness, the strong concentration in biological families of affected individuals is compatible with a significant genetic influence on transmission. On the other hand, when affective disorder is defined more broadly, it is found at a relatively high prevalence in the population, the evidence for ge-

*See references 9, 19, 20, 32, and 40.
†See references 2, 4, 27, 39, and 41.

netic transmission is diminished, and cultural factors appear to have considerable weight. An overlap between major affective disorder and schizophrenia in family, twin, or adoption studies has usually been found, but it is reduced when syndromes are defined carefully.[18] There is a consistent overlap between manic-depressive and severe depressive symptomatology (bipolar and unipolar disorder). The high rate of unipolar illness in the relatives of bipolar probands is compatible with genetic models in which bipolar illness is a genetically more severe form of the same disorder. Absence of father-to-son transmission, which has been reported, is not found generally, and if X-linkage occurs, it is probably restricted to a relatively small subgroup.

An increased prevalence of alcoholism, cyclothymic personality disorder, and suicide is found in the families of patients with affective disorder. Because of the obvious cultural and environmental determinants of suicide, its high familial incidence is usually assumed to be an expression of those factors. However, suicide rates that are ten to fifteen times higher than control levels have been found in the biological relatives of adoptees with clear-cut affective disorders or suicide per se, indicating a strong genetic predisposition in addition to environmental precipitants.[34,41]

¶ Major Gene Versus Polygenic Inheritance

From the perspective of biological research, diseases transmitted by major genes, or in which major genes control important risk factors, are the most tractable; for then the full power of modern biological techniques can be brought to bear to understand the role of each major gene. Our hopes of using the new possibilities created by contemporary molecular biology to elucidate the basic mechanisms of psychiatric disorders would come to a premature end, however, if it turned out that there were no major loci for schizophrenia or affective illness. If a trait like schizophrenia resulted

from the additive effects of many loci, each of small effect, there would be no major loci, yet the trait would still be heritable. Indeed, in a mathematically sophisticated paper, O'Rourke and associates[29] show that the well-known data sets on incidence rates in relatives of various degrees cannot be fit by any parameter choices (gene frequency, phenocopy rate, dominance, penetrance) available to the single-major-locus model. The frequencies that spoil the fit are the incidences in monozygotic twins and offspring of dual matings, which are too high to conform to the model (see also Matthysse and Kidd[25]).

The goodness-of-fit difficulties encountered by the single-major-locus model do not really amount to a refutation. O'Rourke and coworkers consider all schizophrenia to be the result of a single etiology, an assumption that is now widely doubted. They also found that rejection of the single-major-locus model was not possible when broader criteria were used.[29] Although DSM-III is a great step forward from the point of view of uniformity and reliability, the lack of external validation of its diagnostic rules prevents it from being used for a decisive test of the single-major-locus model of schizophrenia. Such a test would inevitably be confounded with the validity of the diagnostic scheme.

Even if the single-major-locus model were rejected, it would not follow that the polygenic hypothesis is true. A number of models that do allow major loci make predictions that are extremely difficult to distinguish from the predictions of the polygenic theory. For example, a model with a large number of loci, decreasing geometrically in effect as powers of two (one, one half, one fourth, one eighth, etc.), predicts a triangular instead of a normal distribution of trait values (as in the polygenic model) but for the most part behaves in a very similar way.[26] In the decreasing-effect model, the first locus is as important as all the other loci put together, so it would give rise to a genetic effect suitable for molecular study. Gottesman and Shields[6] reach a very similar conclusion: "It is heuristically important for us to learn that whenever polygenic variation has been studied under *laboratory conditions* . . . a few handleable genes have proved to mediate a large part of the genetic variance . . ." (pp. 225–226). It is clear, however, that schizophrenia and most other mental disorders are not transmitted as classical Mendelian traits.

¶ The Power of Linkage Analysis for Non-Mendelian Traits

The discovery of genetic linkage—cosegregation with a Mendelian marker trait within families—provides unequivocal evidence for genetic transmission. It also demonstrates that a major locus is involved; it potentially offers the opportunity for prenatal detection; it can ultimately lead to identification of the gene, by mapping to a well-understood region of a chromosome.

The obstacles for discovering linkage for non-Mendelian traits are much greater than for traits that obey the classical laws of genetic segregation. Both "reduced penetrance" (or multigenic effects, which have the same consequences for linkage analysis) and heterogeneity militate against success. Lange, Spence, and Frank[22] have simulated the effect of uncontrolled phenotypic variance on the power of linkage analysis. Adding random noise to one of the phenotypes substantially decreases the power to detect linkage in cases that would otherwise be unambiguous, but as long as a major locus is strongly involved and an adequate sample of informative families is available, linkage analysis is still possible.

Like reduced penetrance, heterogeneity is also an obstacle to linkage analysis, as an example will illustrate. In 1978 strong linkage between cerebellar ataxia and HLA was reported.[14] In the next few years families were found in which the gene did not appear to be linked to the histocompatibility locus HLA, although other families with HLA linkage continued to be observed. A review of all available data by Morton and associates[28] suggested that these apparently contradictory results could be consistently interpreted if the HLA–linked gene determined not ataxia in general but the so-called Menzel type, in which degeneration occurs primarily in the tracts ascending to the cerebellum, with concomitant loss of aspartate in the cerebellar cortex. Had a neuropathological scheme that permitted ataxia to be subdivided into more homogeneous entities not been available, the search for linkage might have foundered.

¶ The Search for Underlying Mendelian Traits

Whenever a disease has non-Mendelian transmission characteristics, the possibility has to be considered that the disease itself is not the most appropriate trait for genetic investigation. "Partial penetrance" is not an explanation at all, but a confession of ignorance; it is a sure sign that the list of causal factors is incomplete. The challenge to psychiatric genetics is to elucidate the traits that are directly inherited and to find out how they create a predisposition for disease. Gottesman and Shields[7] also recommend "focusing on partitionable facets of the syndrome such as neurotransmitter receptor morphology, number, and subtype, paranoid features, genetic polymorphisms of proteins in brain and blood, variation in brain scans, and neurophysiology, on the chance that ordinary twin, adoption, and family studies will reveal one or more of the high-value genes segregating in a clear Mendelian pattern" (p. 226).

Two recent studies of schizophrenia have adopted this point of view. DeAmicis and Cromwell[3] examined schizophrenic patients who showed reaction time "crossover" (a paradoxical worsening of reaction time when warning cues are given at a constant interval before the test stimulus, frequently found in schizophrenic subjects but rarely in normal subjects). Their first-degree relatives had a tendency to show crossover, even though they had no psychotic symptoms. Holzman and coworkers[12] examined smooth-pursuit visual tracking, which is disturbed in about 50 percent of schizophrenic patients but only infrequently in normal subjects. Schizophrenic patients who had no disturbance in visual tracking were also included in the sample, and their relatives tended to have bad tracking even if they were nonpsychotic.

Numerous examples could be cited of the value of uncovering major genes to progress in medical genetics. One of the best is the discovery of the role of the low-density lipoprotein (LDL) receptor in atherosclerotic heart disease. Heart disease is a complex trait that shows no Mendelian pattern of inheritance. Yet the conclusion that it is polygenic, caused by many loci with effects too small to be separately isolated, would have been unduly pessimistic. Most plasma cholesterol is contained in LDL. LDL binds to the "LDL-receptor" on cell surfaces and is internalized, whereupon it suppresses cholesterol synthesis. Several types of hypercholesterolemia have been delineated, each traced to a different mutation in this system. In one type the LDL receptors are missing, so the cells continue to synthesize cholesterol even when it is at high levels in the serum. In another the receptor is present but the cell is unable to internalize the bound LDL. In a third (abetalipoproteinemia), LDL is not synthesized, so the feedback regulation pathway is ineffective.[5] Similar regulatory genetic defects in neurotransmitter receptors would be of obvious interest in psychiatry.

A dramatic example of major loci underlying an apparently polygenic trait—not, perhaps, a typical case, but one that illustrates the potential power of the technique—concerns overall size in mice. Palmiter and co-workers[30] have coupled the structural gene for human growth hormone with the transcription initiation site, or promoter, for metallothionein in the mouse and obtained expression of the fusion gene in fertilized eggs. The mice expressing the gene for human growth hormone grew larger than their littermates, as much as twice normal (retaining normal proportions), and passed the trait on to their progeny. Moreover, since the synthesis of metallothionein is stimulated by heavy metals, the investigators added zinc sulfate to the drinking water and found that the level of human growth hormone in the mice increased. Size is a classical example of a trait believed to be polygenic, but this experiment shows that it has major gene components and that these components lend themselves to experimental manipulation.

It may turn out that no single manifest trait detectable at the present state of technology is the sought-for Mendelian risk factor, but that an unobservable or latent trait with Mendelian characteristics underlies both the disease in question and the other manifest traits that seem related to it. A neurological disease process might produce unpredictable combinations of symptoms—some mental, some physical—depending on where it happened to strike in the nervous system; the vulnerability of different target areas might be influenced by multigenic factors distinct from the disease process itself. For example, smooth-pursuit visual tracking disturbance and schizophrenia might both be manifestations of a yet unknown latent trait, and this trait might be determined by a major gene with higher penetrance than either smooth pursuit or schizophrenia. Eventually such a latent trait might be made concrete (e.g., as an abnormality in some neurotransmitter system), but it is not necessary to wait for that to occur to use it in genetic analysis. Once a latent Mendelian structure model has been worked out for a set of associated traits, the Bayesian probability that each member of a pedigree has the latent trait can be calculated from the pattern of the person's manifest traits, position in the pedigree, and the manifest traits of the other family members.[24] This computed probability can then be used in linkage analysis, just as if the underlying trait could be directly measured.

¶ Steps in the Isolation of Major Genes

The first step in isolating a major gene is mapping to a chromosomal region by demonstrating linkage. Ideally, segregation analysis will already have provided strong evidence for a major locus. Even if the evidence is not strong, linkage studies can be pursued profitably providing that the illness, some subtype of it, or some associated manifest or latent trait has familial patterns consistent with major gene transmission with reasonably high penetrance.

Genetic linkage analysis has been revolutionized by the discovery of restriction fragment length polymorphisms (RFLPs). For an excellent discussion of RFLP theory, see Botstein.[1] The technique rests upon the existence of certain enzymes in bacteria, which cut foreign deoxyribonucleic acid (DNA) at points where they encounter precisely specified sequences. Variations in the DNA sequence from individual to individual will cause the cuts to occur at different places, resulting in fragments of different length. These variations can be used for linkage analysis in just the same way that traditional blood group markers or HLA polymorphisms are used. They have the advantage that variation in the sequences of DNA that do not code for protein ("introns" and "flanking sequences") can also provide linkage markers. The noncoding regions may have more variability from person to person than the coding regions because of diminished pressure from natural selection.

The potential power of the RFLP technique is illustrated by a calculation carried out by Lange and Boehnke.[21] They show that from approximately 1,500 randomly derived RFLPs, a subset can be selected that will divide the human chromosomes (excluding X and Y) into regions not exceeding 10 centimorgans (cM) in length. (One cM is the distance along a chromosome that corresponds to 1 percent probability of recombination at meiosis.) Were such a library available, any major gene could be mapped to within 5 cM. If RFLPs are to become a complete method for genetic analysis, the actual number of RFLP markers must exceed the minimum necessary to span the genome, since not all markers will be informative in a given family. A comprehensive library of RFLP markers will become available in the forseeable future.

The recent success of RFLP methods in mapping the gene for Huntington's disease to the short arm of chromosome 4 has drawn the attention of investigators in psychiatric research.[8] Gusella and associates initially worked with an American pedigree and a very large Venezuelan pedigree. To detect polymorphisms, they used a recombinant phage probe, G8 (among others), derived from a human gene library. The mapping of G8 to chromosome 4 was accomplished using human-mouse somatic cell hybrids; only those hybrids retaining human chromosome 4 had the ability to bind G8. When human DNA is cut with a restriction enzyme such as Hind III, the fragments within the G8-binding region differ from person to person. The restriction fragment data revealed the existence of two "sites"—small regions of DNA whose exact sequence determines susceptibility to cutting by Hind III—that are variable ("polymorphic") in the population. Cutting or noncutting sequences can occur independently at the two sites, so there are four possible combinations, or haplotypes. In both the American and Venezuelan pedigrees, Huntington's disease co-segregated with the G8-detectable restriction sites (the haplotype associated with Huntington's disease was not the same in the two families; linkage requires association between a trait and a marker locus within families, except for recombinants, but not across families). It was possible to determine an upper limit for the distance between the Huntington's disease gene and the restriction polymorphism sites detected by G8; the limit was 10 cM.

Once an approximate mapping has been achieved, there are a number of techniques for obtaining markers still closer to the gene. These methods of "chromosome walking" in the vicinity of a gene are discussed in reviews by Botstein[1] and Ruddle.[33] There are, however, potential limitations in pursuing a human gene to its exact location by this method. As mentioned, one cM corresponds to 1 percent probability of recombination at each meiosis and to approximately 10^6 base pairs. A single coding sequence is about 1,000 base pairs in length, which would correspond, approximately, to a recombination rate of 0.001 percent. In most human diseases there will not be enough informative matings to measure a recombination rate this small. In other words, given two markers both sufficiently close to the gene, it will not be possible by linkage techniques to determine which is closer.

In order to obtain finer resolution, methods other than linkage analysis have to be called upon. In principle, sequences can be directly compared between groups of trait-positive and trait-negative individuals, although sequencing all 10^6 bases in a 1-cM region would be a costly procedure. The locus for the trait would be expected to be altered from its most common form more frequently in the trait-positive than in the trait-negative group. The large number of loci to be compared creates a risk of false positives, and the existence of genes with a high degree of natural polymorphism creates a risk of false negatives. To complete the localization process, there must be a decision procedure for choosing among the candidates for the gene. Pathoanatomy and pathophysiology may be crucial for deciding among candidates for a trait-related gene after linkage and sequence analysis have accomplished all that they can.

¶ The Significance of Pathoanatomy and Pathophysiology for Gene Isolation

If there is some knowledge of the anatomical pathways and physiological mechanisms underlying the trait for which a genetic locus is sought, functional considerations can be used to make a selection among candidate genes. Either complementary (cDNA) DNA or peptides coded by each gene can be used to construct histochemical stains, and if these stains show that the gene product is normally present in brain regions known to be relevant to the trait in question, the likelihood that the right gene has been found will be enhanced.

Two examples of *in situ* hybridization and peptide immunohistochemistry techniques will illustrate their potential power. In one study an 800-base pair DNA fragment corresponding to the structural gene for rat growth hormone was cloned and used as a template for synthesis of cDNA labeled with radioactive phosphorus (^{32}P). Hybridization to the cDNA *in situ* revealed specific labeling in the anterior pituitary.[13] In another study Sutcliffe and others[36] selected cDNA clones hybridizing only to brain messenger ribonucleic acid (mRNA). After sequencing, they translated them into amino acid sequences (according to the genetic code) and chemically synthesized short peptides included within those sequences. Antibodies were raised against the synthetic peptides, and these were made into histochemical stains by the indirect immunoperoxidase method. One such stain derived from a cDNA clone reacted with a previously unknown fiber system that is widely distributed in the brain. Viral and plasmid vectors can also be used to synthesize peptides in bacteria from DNA clones. Complete proteins will not be made in the bacterial host because of intervening nontranslated sequences (introns), but in some cases the antibodies needed for the histochemical technique can be made using a single exon as antigen.[16]

An intriguing method for selecting genes that are expressed in the brain is suggested by the discovery of an eighty-two-nucleotide ("ID") sequence in several cDNA clones derived from brain mRNA. The sequence is less abundant in the mRNA of other organs.[37] Conceivably genes relevant to brain function could be identified by the presence of such sequences and singled out from the other candidates for more thorough consideration.

It is possible that analysis of clones derived from a 1-cM linkage-defined region of DNA by *in situ* hybridization, peptide histochemistry, and hybridization to ID probes could be used *before* direct sequence comparison in trait-positive and trait-negative groups to limit the amount of sequencing required. The success of a prescreening procedure depends on the relative concentration of the trait-related mRNA or protein in the brain. A great decrease in the labor required to isolate the gene would result if prescreening was successful; but the signal-to-noise ratio would be very unfavorable for low-concentration mRNAs and peptides. Whatever the order, it appears that both functional analysis and sequence comparison are necessary steps in the isolation of genes.

¶ Conclusion

The isolation of major genes contributing to the risk for mental illness is the crucial long-term task of psychiatric genetics. Completion of that task requires a partnership between classical genetics and pathobiology on one hand and molecular biology on the other. Classical genetics is indispensible for refining the concepts of mental diseases, resolving heterogeneity, and uncovering disease-related processes with more nearly Mendelian transmission than the symptoms themselves. Without these achievements, linkage analysis is not likely to succeed, and the subsequent steps in the process cannot be carried out. The more thoroughly understood the pathoanatomy and pathophysiology of the disease, the more successfully can *in situ* hybridization and peptide histochemistry techniques be used to prescreen clones prior to sequencing or to rule out false positives in sequence-comparison tests. The task is a daunting one, but it must eventually be carried out if molecular understanding of mental illness is to be achieved.

¶ Bibliography

1. BOTSTEIN, D., et al. "Construction of a Genetic Linkage Map in Man Using Restriction Fragment Length Polymorphisms," *American Journal of Human Genetics*, 32 (1980):314–331.

2. CADORET, R. J. "Evidence for Genetic Inheritance of Primary Affective Disorder in Adoptees," *American Journal of Psychiatry*, 135 (1978):463–466.

3. DEAMICIS, L. A., and CROMWELL, R. L. "Reaction Time Crossover in Schizophrenic Patients, Their Relatives, and Control Subjects," *Journal of Nervous and Mental Disease*, 167 (1979):593–600.

4. GERSHON, E. S. *Genetics of the Major Psychoses*, Proceedings of the 60th Annual Meeting of the Association for Research in Nervous and Mental Disorders. New York: Raven Press, 1983.

5. GOLDSTEIN, J. L., and BROWN, M. S. "The Low-density Lipoprotein Pathway and Its Relation to Atherosclerosis," *Annual Review of Biochemistry*, 46 (1977):897–930.

6. GOTTESMAN, I. I., and SHIELDS, J. *Schizophrenia and Genetics: A Twin Study Vantage Point*. New York: Academic Press, 1972.

7. ———. *Schizophrenia: The Epigenetic Puzzle*. Cambridge: Cambridge University Press, 1982.

8. GUSELLA, J. F., et al. "A Polymorphic DNA Marker Genetically Linked to Huntington's Disease," *Nature*, 306 (1983):234–238.

9. HESTON, L. L. "Psychiatric Disorders in Foster Home Reared Children of Schizophrenic Mothers," *British Journal of Psychiatry*, 112 (1966):819–825.

10. HESTON, L. L., and DENNEY, D. "Interactions Between Early Life Experience and Biological Factors in Schizophrenia," in D. Rosenthal and S. S. Kety, eds., *The Transmission of Schizophrenia*. Oxford: Pergamon Press, 1968, pp. 363–376.

11. HIGGINS, J. "Effect of Child Rearing by Schizophrenic Mothers," *Journal of Psychiatric Research*, 4 (1966):153–167.

12. HOLZMAN, P. S., et al. "Pursuit Eye Movement Dysfunctions in Schizophrenia: Family Evidence for Specificity," *Archives of General Psychiatry*, 41 (1984): 136–139.

13. HUDSON, P., et al. "Hybridization Histochemistry: Use of Recombinant DNA as a 'Homing Probe' for Tissue Localization of Specific mRNA Populations," *Endocrinology*, 108 (1981):353–356.

14. JACKSON, J. F., et al. "Genetic Linkage and Spinocerebellar Ataxia," In: R.A.P. Kark, R. N. Rosenberg, and L. J. Schut, eds., *Advances in Neurology*, vol. 21. New York: Raven Press, 1978, pp. 315–318.

15. JACOBSEN, B., and KINNEY, D. K. "Perina-

tal Complications in Adopted and Nonadopted Schizophrenics and Their Controls: Preliminary Results," *Acta Psychiatrica Scandinavica*, 62 (Supplement 285) (1980):337–346.

16. KAUFMAN, D. L., and TOBIN, A. J. "Prospects for the Isolation of Genes for Receptors and Other Proteins of Pharmacological and Neurobiological Interest," in J. C. Venter and L. C. Harrison, eds., *Membrane Receptor Purification and Characterization Techniques*. New York: Alan Liss, 1984, pp. 241–259.

17. KENDLER, K. S. "Overview: A Current Perspective on Twin Studies of Schizophrenia," *American Journal of Psychiatry*, 140 (1983):1413–1425.

18. KENDLER, K. S., GRUENBERG, A. M., and TSUANG, M. T. "Psychiatric Illness in First-degree Relatives of Schizophrenic and Surgical Control Patients," *Archives of General Psychiatry*, 42 (1985): 770–779.

19. KETY, S. S., et al. "The Types and Prevalence of Mental Illness in the Biological and Adoptive Families of Adopted Schizophrenics," in D. Rosenthal and S. S. Kety, eds., *The Transmission of Schizophrenia*. Oxford: Pergamon Press, 1968, pp. 345–362.

20. KETY, S. S., et al. "Mental Illness in the Biological and Adoptive Families of Adopted Individuals Who Have Become Schizophrenic: A Preliminary Report Based on Psychiatric Interviews," in R. R. Fieve, D. Rosenthal, and H. Brill, eds., *Genetic Research in Psychiatry*. Baltimore: Johns Hopkins University Press, 1975, pp. 147–165.

21. LANGE, K., and BOEHNKE, M. "How Many Polymorphic Marker Genes Will It Take to Span the Human Genome?" *American Journal of Human Genetics*, 34 (1982):842–845.

22. LANGE, K., SPENCE, M. A., and FRANK, M. B. "Application of the Lod Method to the Detection of Linkage Between a Quantitative Trait and a Qualitative Marker: A Stimulation Experiment," *American Journal of Human Genetics*, 28 (1976):167–173.

23. McNEIL, T. F., and KAIJ, L. "Obstetric Factors in the Development of Schizophrenia: Complications in the Births of Preschizophrenics and in Reproduction by Schizophrenic Parents," in L. D. Wynne, R. L. Cromwell, and S. Matthysse, eds., *The Nature of Schizophrenia*. New York: John Wiley and Sons, 1978, pp. 401–429.

24. MATTHYSSE, S. "Genetic Latent Structure Analysis," in T. Sakai and T. Tsuboi, eds., *Genetic Aspects of Human Behavior*. Tokyo: Igaku-Shoin Ltd., 1985, pp. 103–111.

25. MATTHYSSE, S. W., and KIDD, K. K. "Estimating the Genetic Contribution to Schizophrenia," *American Journal of Psychiatry*, 133 (1976):185–191.

26. MATTHYSSE, S. W., LANGE, K., and WAGENER, D. K. "Continuous Variation Caused by Genes with Graduated Effects," *Proceedings of the National Academy of Sciences* (U.S.), 76 (1979): 2862–2865.

27. MENDLEWICZ, J., and RAINER, J. D. "Adoption Study Supporting Genetic Transmission in Manic-Depressive Illness," *Nature*, 268 (1977):327–329.

28. MORTON, N. E., et al. "Linkage Studies in Spinocerebellar Ataxia," *American Journal of Medical Genetics*, 6 (1980): 251–257.

29. O'ROURKE, D. H., et al. "Refutation of the General Single-locus Model for the Etiology of Schizophrenia," *American Journal of Human Genetics*, 34 (1982):-630–649.

30. PALMITER, R. D., et al. "Metallothionein-human GH Fusion Genes Stimulate Growth of Mice," *Science*, 222 (1983): 809–814.

31. PLOMIN, R., DeFRIES, J. C., and ROBERTS, M. K. "Assortative Mating by Unwed Biological Parents of Adopted Children," *Science*, 196 (1977):449–450.

32. ROSENTHAL, D., et al. "Schizophrenics' Offspring Reared in Adoptive Homes," in D. Rosenthal and S. S. Kety, eds., *The Transmission of Schizophrenia*. Oxford: Pergamon Press, 1968, pp. 377–391.

33. RUDDLE, F. H. "Reverse Genetics as a Means of Understanding and Treating Genetic Disease," in A. J. Friedhoff and T. N. Chase, eds., *Gilles de la Tourette Syndrome*. New York: Raven Press, 1982, pp. 239–242.

34. SCHULSINGER, F., et al. "A Family Study of Suicide," in M. Schou and E. Stromgren, eds., *Origin, Prevention and Treatment of Affective Disorders*. New York: Academic Press, 1979, pp. 277–287.

35. SLATER, E. "A Review of Earlier Evidence on Genetic Factors in Schizophrenia," in D. Rosenthal and S. S. Kety, eds., *The Transmission of Schizophrenia*. Oxford: Pergamon Press, 1968, pp. 15–26.

36. SUTCLIFFE, J. G., et al. "Identifying the Protein Products of Brain-Specific Genes with Antibodies to Chemically Synthesized Peptides," *Cell*, 33 (1983): 671–682.

37. SUTCLIFFE, J. G., et al. "Identifier Sequences Are Transcribed Specifically in Brain," *Nature*, 308 (1984):237–241.

38. TSUANG, M. T., WINOKUR, G., and CROWE, R. R. "Morbidity Risks of Schizophrenia and Affective Disorders Among First Degree Relatives of Patients with Schizophrenia, Mania, Depression and Surgical Conditions," *British Journal of Psychiatry*, 137 (1980):497–504.

39. VON KNORRING, A. L., et al. "An Adoption Study of Depressive Disorders and Substance Abuse," *Archives of General Psychiatry*, 40 (1983):943–950.

40. WENDER, P. H., et al. "Cross-fostering: A Research Strategy for Clarifying the Role of Genetic and Experiential Factors in the Etiology of Schizophrenia," *Archives of General Psychiatry*, 30 (1974):121–128.

41. WENDER, P. H., et al. "Psychiatric Disorders in the Biological and Adoptive Families of Adopted Individuals with Affective Disorders," unpublished.

PART TWO

Scientific Approaches to
Biological Investigation
in Psychiatry

CHAPTER 7

ANIMAL MODELS IN
PSYCHIATRIC RESEARCH

Steven Matthysse

¶ Introduction

To make rational use of animal models in psychiatric research, the experimenter must have a clear concept of the purpose for which the model is intended. Much confusion arises in the literature because behavioral models are used that resemble psychoses only in that they are maladaptive for the species concerned or involve one of the hundreds of mental processes that are disturbed in psychiatric disease; or they are admitted as models just because they are known to be affected by dopamine-blockers or to require intactness of the dopamine tracts for their expression. In this chapter I will attempt to outline a more logical rationale, to classify models into types, and to give a few examples of each type.

As of this writing, animal models in psychiatric research can be conveniently classified into four types, based on principles of: (1) pharmacological isomorphism, (2) symptom similarity, (3) gene transfer, and (4) cross-species psychological processes. I will discuss each in turn.

¶ Pharmacological Isomorphism

Models of pharmacological isomorphism depend on the existence of a class of drugs that ameliorate (exacerbate, or mimic) psychoses in humans. To the extent that the pharmacological responses of an animal model parallel those of psychotic patients to this class of drugs, the model may be useful for screening new members of the class and even for identifying brain regions or circuits that these drugs act upon. At the outset, it must be emphasized that the model will not be more useful than the drug class on which it is based. This limitation is especially important in evaluating models that are derived from the antipsychotic drugs in current use, since these drugs make patients "better but not well"[19] and, moreover, affect the various

This chapter appears in a different form in *Progress in Brain Research*, vol. 65, *Psychiatric Disorders: Neurotransmitters and Neuropeptides*, S. Matthysee and J. M. Van Ree, eds. (Amsterdam, The Netherlands: Elsevier, 1986), pp. 259–270.

psychotic symptoms unequally. The class of drugs with effects like chlorpromazine and haloperidol is already rather large, and it is not evident that further additions to it will make any fundamental difference in the treatment of psychotic patients. Pharmacological isomorphism, in principle, cannot step outside the circle to guide the development of a genuinely new class of drugs. It can, however, be very useful in understanding the mechanism of action of the drugs in current use.

Now let us define pharmacological isomorphism more exactly. Isomorphism, in mathematics, refers to a correspondence between two different systems of objects that preserves the natural relationships within each system. For example, the complex numbers $(a + b\sqrt{-1})$ have a one-to-one correspondence with vectors drawn radially outward from the origin of coordinates in two dimensions. Each complex number corresponds to a vector, and vector addition (for example) is fully consistent with the laws of addition of complex numbers. The concept of "isomorphism" is extended somewhat when applied to the pharmacological context, but the basic idea is very similar to the mathematical use of the term. All the relationships among drugs in the relevant class should faithfully correspond to parallel relationships in the animal model (for a general reference, see Matthysse and Haber[22]).

Specifically:

1. Potency in the animal model should parallel potency in the treatment of psychoses.
2. Drugs closely related in chemical structure to antipsychotics, but without efficacy in the treatment of psychosis, should also be without efficacy in the animal model.
3. Tolerance should not develop in the animal model.
4. Anticholinergics should not block the effects of antipsychotic drugs in the animal model.

The last two principles arise because tolerance does not develop to the antipsychotic effects of antipsychotic drugs, and those effects are not blocked by anticholinergics

(although some of their side effects do show tolerance and are antagonized by anticholinergics).

A case could be made for strengthening the third principle: Not only should tolerance not develop, but the pharmacological effect should grow stronger with time. It is often said that antipsychotic effects take weeks to develop, whereas many dopaminergic effects in animals, for example, occur almost instantaneously. Thus Cotes and associates[8] found that delusions, hallucinations, and incoherence of speech improved gradually over a four-week period of treatment with flupenthixol, whereas a dopaminergic sign (serum prolactin) responded more rapidly. It is possible, however, that one's judgment about delayed onset of improvement will depend on the processes being followed. It may be that the more "molecular" the process (attention, formal thought disorder), the less the lag period, and the more "molar" (delusions, withdrawn behavior), the greater. Certainly, to observe rapid actions one must make early ratings. The earliest reported rating in the Cotes and coworkers study was at one week. Hurt, Holzman, and Davis[16] arranged their first testing session after haloperidol at three days, and at that point, they observed measurable improvement in

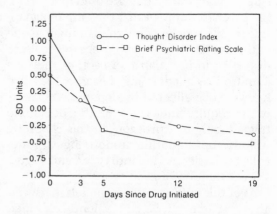

Figure 7–1. Early effects of haloperidol on thought disorder and psychiatric symptoms.

NOTE: Reprinted, by permission of the publisher, from S. W. Hurt, P. S. Holzman, and J. M. Davis, "Thought Disorder: The Measurement of Its Changes," *Archives of General Psychiatry*, 40 (1983):1281–1285.

the thought disorder index as well as in several scales on the Brief Psychiatric Rating Scale (see figure 7–1).

The second principle is particularly important, because many of the non-antipsychotic analogues of common antipsychotic drugs are potent pharmacological agents in their own right. For example, the non-antipsychotic phenothiazines (see figure 7–2) include cholinergic, histaminergic, and noradrenergic blockers. Thus the absence of efficacy of these drugs in an animal model restricts the range of neurochemical processes that may be involved. In the same way, absence of tolerance tends to rule out sedative effects (animal behavior is particularly sensitive to disruption by sedation).

Example of an Isomorphism Model: Depolarization Block in Mesolimbic Dopamine Neurons

White and Wang[39] and Chiodo and Bunney[6] have discovered and characterized a model system that admirably illustrates the principles of pharmacological isomorphism.

Rather than broadly survey models of this type, I will review the depolarization block model in some depth, in order to clarify how the isomorphism principles may be used. Data from both laboratories will be combined in this summary.

Acutely, systemic chlorpromazine and haloperidol increase the rate and number of active dopamine neurons in the substantia nigra and the mesolimbic dopamine area ("A10"). These neurons can be detected by their slow (regular or bursting) firing patterns and long-duration action potentials.[37] The procedure in these experiments is different. In both areas, chronic administration (three to four weeks) silences the dopamine neurons. The cause seems to be depolarization block, since they can be reactivated by iontophoretic application of hyperpolarizing substances (gamma-aminobutyric acid, apomorphine, dopamine) but not by the depolarizing agent glutamate. Membrane potential was not, however, directly measured.

It is the mesolimbic area that shows the most convincing pharmacological isomorphism, not the substantia nigra; this

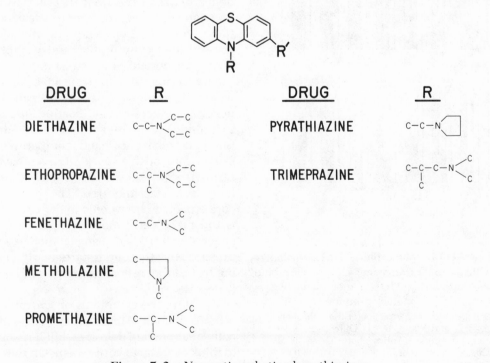

Figure 7–2. Non-antipsychotic phenothiazines.

summary will be confined to that area. Chlorpromazine, haloperidol, thioridazine hydrochloride, clozapine, sulpiride, and molindone—active antipsychotics of several chemical types—all caused depolarization block. Promethazine, d-sulpiride, metaclopramide, and desipramine—chemically similar to antipsychotic drugs but without efficacy—all failed to cause depolarization block (see figure 7–3).

A number of the isomorphism criteria are satisfied. The active antipsychotics tested produce the effect in rough proportion to their antipsychotic efficacy (not in proportion to their tendency to cause parkinsonian side effects). The non-antipsychotics tested do not produce the effect—although there are a number of others that could also be

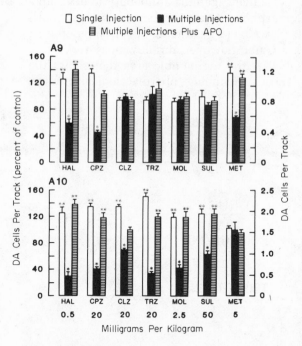

Figure 7–3. Depolarization block in dopamine neurons. APO = apomorphine: HAL = haloperidol; CPZ = chlorpromazine; CLZ = clozapine; TRZ = thioridazine; MOL = molindone; SUL = sulpiride; MET = metaclopromide.

NOTE: Reprinted, by permission of the publisher, from White, F. J., and Wang, R. Y. "Differential Effects of Classical and Atypical Antipsychotic Drugs in A9 and A10 Dopamine Neurons," *Science,* 221 (1983).

tested for completeness. Tolerance does not develop; indeed, it seems that just the opposite happens (in accord with the extension of the tolerance criterion discussed earlier). Longer time periods would be worth examining. The fourth criterion, absence of blockade of the antipsychotic effect by anticholinergics, was not tested. This set of studies illustrates nicely what can be done with the isomorphism criteria.

¶ Symptom Similarity

As a principle in the construction of models, symptom similarity is treacherous, because nearly all aspects of behavior are disturbed in the major psychoses, so practically any abnormal behavior in an animal can be said to be a model. One of the most conscientious applications of this principle is the uncontrollable-shock model of depression, especially as developed by Weiss and associates.[38] Rats are yoked to controls and receive inescapable shock. As shown in figure 7–4, there is an intriguing correspondence between the DSM-III criteria for depression and the behavior disturbance of these animals. Their symptoms include decreased food consumption and weight loss, poor performance in stress-coping tasks (such as trying to escape from a tank of water, where they adopt a passive instead of the normal, active strategy, floating instead of swimming), decreased grooming, and diminished aggressiveness and competitiveness. The uncontrollable-shock rats even have the DSM-III symptoms of sleep loss as long as four weeks after the stress. The insomnia occurs especially between 7 and 9 P.M., which is the rat's "early morning"! There are, of course, well-studied primate models of depression, but this one is particularly intriguing from a theoretical point of view, because it uses the rat.

Modeling the symptoms of schizophrenia is more difficult. Animals may be capable of hallucinations and delusions, but it is not easy to think of a way to verify them. On the other

Uncontrollable Shock Produces the Following Symptomatology:	DSM-III Criteria for Depression (four of the following):
1. Decreased Food and/or Water Consumption	1. Poor Appetite and Significant Weight Loss
2. Weight Loss	2. Psychomotor Alterations
3. Poor Performance in Tasks Requiring Active Motor Behavior (shuttle avoidance-escape, lever-press escape, water-escape, open-field activity, etc.)	3. Loss of Energy or Fatigue
	4. Loss of Interest in Usual Activities
	5. Sleep Changes
4. Loss of normal aggressiveness or Competitiveness	6. Indecisiveness, Evidence of Decreased Ability to Think
	7. Feelings of Worthlessness
5. Loss of Normal Grooming or Play Activity	8. Recurrent Thoughts of Death and Suicide
6. Decreased Sleep	

Figure 7–4.   Correspondence between symptoms of uncontrollable shock and clinical depression.
SOURCE: J. M. Weiss et al., "A Model for Neurochemical Study of Depression," in M. Y. Speigelstein and A. Levy, eds., *Behavioral Models and the Analysis of Drug Action* (Amsterdam: Elsevier, 1982), pp. 195–223.

hand, some very bizarre behavior has been observed in monkeys subjected to prolonged isolation, as this excerpt[24] illustrates:

One 6-month enclosed isolate male slowly moved his right arm toward his head while in a rigid seated pose and, upon seeing his own approaching hand, suddenly appeared startled by it. His eyes slowly widened and he would at times fear, grimace toward, threaten, or even bite the hand "sneaking up on him." If he did not look directly at the hand or did not bite it, "it" would continue to move toward him as he looked at "it" out of the corner of his eyes. As "it" approached him, his eyes became wider and wider until the hand was entirely clasping his face. There he would sit for a second or two, with saucer-sized eyes staring in terror between clutching fingers. (p. 228)

This vivid description certainly reminds us of some of the bizarre behavior seen in schizophrenic patients, but it is difficult to know whether the mental state (delusion that the hand was "sneaking up on him"), which suggested itself to the observer, was really present in the animal. (I will defend later the view that some mental states in animals can be inferred and suggest paradigms for making such inferences.)

Despite the ambiguities of models based on symptom similarity, workers in the psychiatric field are reluctant to give them up because of frustration with the limitations of the isomorphism principles. The problem of "negative symptoms" is a case in point. Since the current generation of antipsychotic drugs is relatively ineffective on symptoms such as lack of motivation and flat affect, isomorphism models will not capture these aspects of the syndrome, hence will not be useful in pointing toward brain regions that may be involved in the genesis of negative symptoms or in discovering new drugs effective against them. If negative symptoms could be modeled in an animal, the prospects for research in this area would be brighter.

Animal models of negative symptoms do exist. In the 1950s and 1960s, because of concern about the dangers of nuclear radiation, there were numerous experiments on the long-term effects of radiation damage in monkeys. In general, effects on problem-solving ability were small, but there were profound consequences for social interest, curiosity, and motivation.[15] The radiation-damaged monkeys were less responsive to monkey or human sounds. They would not work as hard to open a window that would give them a view of other monkeys or interesting objects. They became self-preoccupied and less social; they initiated sexual and aggressive activity less often.[10] High-motivation activities (manipulating puzzles, working for food reward) are least impaired, but activities that are less motivating are very much reduced after radiation damage.[21] It would be interesting to compare alternative ways of producing these motivational defects, to see what brain pathways they affect in common.

¶ Gene Transfer

The possibility, just alluded to, that similar symptoms could be produced by a variety of causes is an inevitable limitation of symptom similarity models. Ultimately, one would like to hold the etiology constant and let the form of symptom expression vary, rather than holding the symptoms constant and accepting the possibility of divergent etiologies. In other words, one would like to instigate in an animal the very same pathological process that occurs in the human disease. While this possibility definitely looks toward the future, it is not too far-fetched to be considered. Suppose that one could isolate a gene for a mental disease (without necessarily knowing its mode of action); there are several precedents for transferring genes into foreign species and obtaining expression.

A bacterial gene for resistance to the antibiotic kanamycin sulfate has been transferred effectively to tobacco, using a plasmid vector. The structural gene coding for human growth hormone has been successfully transferred to mice. The mice grow to as much as twice the size of their littermates, while remaining normally proportioned; moreover, their enhanced growth rate is passed on to their own progeny.[26] In both these cases of successful transfer, transcription promoters from the host were included to initiate effective expression. For example, the human growth hormone sequence was transferred as a fusion gene with mouse metallothionein promoter. Metallothionein is a metal-binding protein that is stimulated by heavy metals. The activity of the promoter was increased by adding zinc sulfate to the drinking water, leading to higher levels of human growth hormone in the mice.

Although in these cases a similar phenotype was obtained in the donor and host by gene transfer, similarity of expression is not guaranteed. Gene transfer, to be sure, is a rare experiment; but differences in the phenotypic expression of single genes, depending on genetic background, can be readily studied. The influence of genetic background can be quite strong. The "Reeler" gene in the mouse is an autosomal recessive causing defective neuronal migration. On the C57BL/6J background, these mice are frail and rarely survive weaning. Ataxia is severe; the animal may not be able to right itself if turned on its side. The same gene, on a C3H/HeJ background, results in only moderate ataxia, and the animal is vigorous enough to be used for breeding.[5]

Fascinating as gene transfer models are, they remain impractical for psychiatric research, because isolation of single genes is very difficult. Even the recent discovery of close linkage between the G8 restriction fragment length polymorphism marker and Huntington's disease[14] localizes the gene only within 10 centimorgans (i.e., 10 percent probability of recombination) at a 99 percent confidence level, a length of deoxyribonucleic acid containing about 10,000,000 base pairs (approximately 10,000 coding sequences).[3] Nevertheless, it is worth keeping the possibility of gene transfer models in mind.

¶ Cross-Species Psychological Processes

Instead of attempting to mimic individual symptoms, more convincing animal models of a psychiatric illness can be constructed by formulating a psychological theory of the disorder, in which symptoms are accounted for in terms of a more fundamental psychological process. If the psychological process is one common to both animals and humans, it may lend itself to cross-species comparison. In fact, the experimental paradigms that translate the psychological theory into operational terms, for work with humans, may have direct analogs in paradigms appropriate for animals. Models constructed in this way will be more rational and less arbitrary than symptom-similarity models, while escaping the dependence of isomorphism models on the current generation of antipsychotic drugs. Two examples, the "attentional perseveration" model of schizophrenia and a new psychological process model of affective disorder, will clarify the "psychological process" category of models.

"Attentional Perseveration" Models of Schizophrenia

Cromwell and Dokecki[9] suggested the simple but useful generalization that, in schizophrenia, there is an inability to withdraw attention from the stimulus or idea on which it is focused. There is abundant evidence that this is an important basic disturbance in schizophrenia, although it would be claiming too much to suggest that it accounts for the whole syndrome. Kraepelin noted that patients stare at the same point or object and continue the same line of thought. The inability to withdraw attention can affect various levels of integration of behavior—from obsessional pursuit of inappropriate goals, to perseveration in speech, and even to stereotypic motor behavior, as illustrated in this excerpt from Bleuler[2]: "Many years before his illness became manifest, a physician had made deep holes in the hardwood floor of his room because he always turned on his heels at exactly the same place on the floor" (p. 186). Corresponding to this hierarchy of levels at which "inability to withdraw attention" can be manifested, there is a continuum of animal models of attentional perseveration, from "motor" to "mental." I will review this continuum, because it illustrates the "psychological process" category of models and also has profound implications for drug-screening paradigms.

The classical study of motor perseveration induced by dopamine agonists was by Randrup and Munkvad.[29] In this paradigm, the path traced by a freely moving rat, placed in a box with no exit, was recorded. As can be seen in figure 7–5, the untreated animal (bottom) efficiently explores all the walls and corners of the box, whereas the drug-treated animal (top)—like Bleuler's patient—paces back and forth in a constricted area, never succeeding in exploring the whole boundary. This form of stereotypy can be said to be closer to the "motor" than the "mental" end of the hierarchy, since the drugged animal seems not to be pursuing a goal at all, but is deflected by its motor automatism from the normal goal of looking for a way out. Many other motor stereotypies have been studied: for example, gnawing, sniffing, and licking in rodents, and head bobbing, gaze shifting, and circling in dogs. None of these motor stereotypies fares well by the isomorphism criteria.[18,22]

Slightly higher up the hierarchy from "motor" to "mental" is stereotyped posturing in squirrel monkeys. These animals assume a submissive (or juvenile) posture when dopamine, potentiated by a monoamine oxidase inhibitor, is injected into the mesolimbic forebrain.[13] Here a goal is more in evidence, since posturing is a social gesture. Dr. Suzanne Haber has observed a pair of monkeys in a cage, one of whom received amphetamine and the other who did not. The drugged male pursued the undrugged female all around the cage in order to stare at

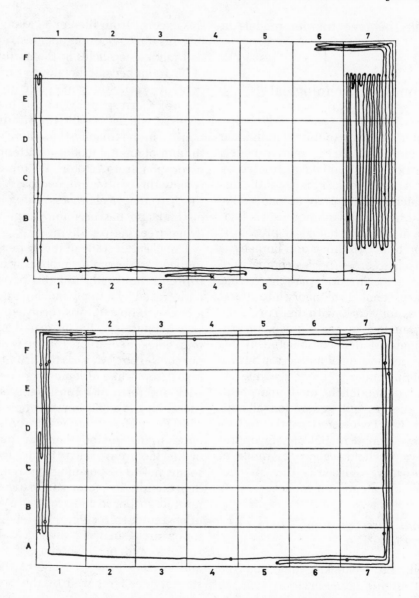

Figure 7–5. Motor stereotypy induced by amphetamine.

NOTE: Reprinted, by permission of the publisher, from A. Randrup and I. Munkvad, "Pharmacology and Physiology of Stereotyped Behavior," *Journal of Psychiatric Research*, 11 (1974):110.

her; as she moved to escape his gaze, he continuously repositioned himself in order to renew eye contact. Here there is no motor perseveration, but rather motor flexibility in pursuit of a fixed goal.

Advancing upward in the hierarchy, we come to paradigms that test more directly the concept of switching attention from one object to another. In humans, there is an ele-

gant paradigm developed by Kristofferson and Allan.[20] Two stimuli are presented in different channels (visual and auditory). There are two such pairs, one in which the stimuli terminate successively and one in which they terminate simultaneously. The subject's task is to guess which pair is which. This forced-choice design circumvents response biases. Kristofferson and Allan's theory is that a minimum switching time, or "quantum," must elapse between the termination times for discrimination to be better than chance. This is the interval required to switch attention between the two channels. Schizophrenic patients may have a longer "quantum" than normal subjects.[1] This paradigm has not been carried over into animal work, but it probably could be adapted.

Two simple behavioral switching paradigms have been developed for the rat that show that much can be done to study relevant attentional processes without requiring primate species. When placed in a chamber with several water-filled burettes, normal rats will sample each of them. Rats with a lesion in the nucleus accumbens spend a greater proportion of time drinking from their most-preferred burette, although total water consumption is not changed and general locomotor activity seems not to be impaired.[30] A related paradigm required rats to search for four food pellets under holes in a sixteen-hole board. The behavioral switching rate was estimated by the frequency with which the animals changed their hole-visit sequences.[24]

An ingenious and lifelike behavioral switching paradigm for animal experimentation has been recently developed by Cools.[7] Rats are placed in a tank of water, from which there is no escape. Immediately the animals swim to the side and explore the tank, then tread water and investigate the area above it. Then they typically plunge to the bottom several times and swim back up. After that, they may engage in a variety of behaviors: swimming in circles, kicking with hindlimbs, and floating (filling their lungs with air). Switching behavior was evaluated by estimating the number of different strategies and the duration of each. Floating, while not affording a means of escape, is at least a means of surviving indefinitely. When that strategy was achieved, the experimenter threw the animals a rope. With this design the question could be asked: Would the animals switch from a partially satisfactory strategy to a still more adequate one? To be sure,

multiple interpretations of behavior in such a complex design must be considered, but the paradigm has the virtue of approximating real-life behavior.

Before continuing this survey of attentional perseveration paradigms, let us reflect on the psychiatric conditions that motivated this discussion. Schizophrenic patients have attentional perseveration, but how much of the symptomatology can this process explain? "Inability to withdraw attention from the stimulus or idea on which it is focused" could explain how delusions grow to become morbid preoccupations or how a thought—experienced as subvocal—could grow in intensity until it became a voice. There seems to be a missing element in this formulation: the role of reality-testing. A misinterpretation, a sensory aberration, a peculiar fantasy, can occur to anyone. In normal people, these are rejected as unreal or untrue. In psychosis, they are not only accepted but held tenaciously in the face of contradictory evidence. The perseveration is not only of attending, but of hypothesis-maintaining.

None of the paradigms reviewed so far is concerned with hypothesis formation and maintenance. This behavior, however, can also be operationalized. Isaacson and Kimble[17] define the behavior of rats in a Y-maze as manifesting a "spatial hypothesis" if they make three or more consecutive responses to one of the goal arms (despite varying illumination levels) and a "brightness hypothesis" if they make three or more consecutive responses to one of the brightness levels (the maze arms are either illuminated or dark), independent of position. Figure 7–6 summarizes the hypothesis behavior of normal, cortical-lesioned, and hippocampal-lesioned rats on acquisition trials. Black bars indicate brightness hypotheses; white bars indicate spatial hypotheses. The hippocampal animals shifted hypotheses less often than the others. Figure 7–7 is a similar representation of data obtained under extinction conditions. "X" stands for nonentry into the maze. Again, the hippocampal rats switched hypotheses less often than the other groups. The main differ-

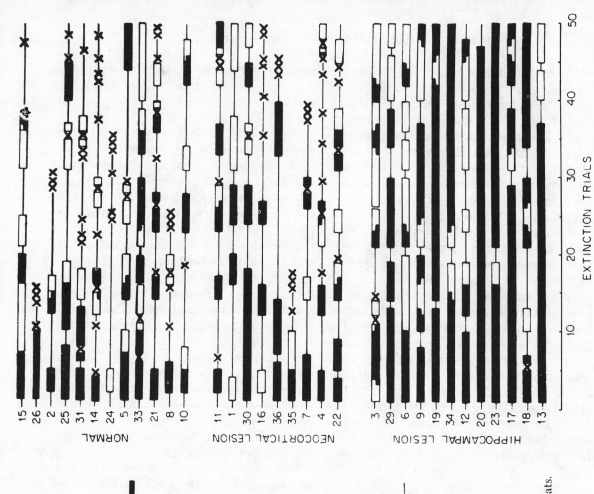

Figure 7-6. "Hypothesis acquisition" by hippocampal-lesioned rats.

NOTE: Reprinted, by permission of the publisher, from R. L. Isaacson and D. P. Kimble, "Lesions of the Limbic System. Their Effects upon Hypotheses and Frustration," *Behavioral Biology* 7 (1972).

Figure 7-7. "Hypothesis extinction" by hippocampal-lesioned rats.

NOTE: Reprinted, by permission of the publisher, from R. L. Isaacson and D. P. Kimble (1972).

ence from acquisition is that, whereas during acquisition they are slow to abandon their instinctive spatial hypothesis, under extinction they perseveratively maintained the brightness hypothesis they had learned.

By broadening the concept of perseveration to include hypothesis maintenance in the face of contradictory evidence, we ascend still higher along the "motor-mental" continuum and still closer to psychological processes underlying psychosis. Yet there remains an inadequacy. Patients with frontal lobe damage have marked difficulty in switching hypotheses, as judged by the Wisconsin Card Sorting Test. There are three possible sorting criteria (color, shape, or number of the figures shown on the cards). In the middle of the test, the examiner changes the sorts that will be rewarded but does not inform the subject that a change has taken place. Frontal lobe patients are slow to change their sorting criteria to match the examiner's. Their hypothesis perseveration does not seem at all like that of psychotic patients, however. These patients often seem to be aware of what their responses should be. According to Milner,[23] some "were able themselves to say 'right' or 'wrong' as they placed the cards, and yet did not modify their responses accordingly" (p. 99). The defect seems to be "failure to suppress an ongoing reaction tendency, despite growing proof of its inadequacy" (p. 99) rather than the vigorous defense of an incorrect hypothesis, as in psychosis.

The contrast with frontal lobe hypothesis perseveration helps clarify the psychological process we are trying to model in psychosis. It is an active tendency to form hypotheses, with resistance to giving them up, however contradictory the evidence may be. The animal behavior that comes closest to this trait is "superstition," first described by Skinner.[32] Pellets were made available to a pigeon, completely independent of its behavior. Each bird developed a characteristic pattern of behavior.

One bird was conditioned to turn counter-clockwise about the cage, making two or three turns between reinforcements. Another repeatedly thrust its head into one of the upper corners of the cage. A third developed a "tossing" response, as if placing its head beneath an invisible bar and lifting it repeatedly. Two birds developed a pendulum motion of the head and body . . . Another bird was conditioned to make incomplete pecking or brushing movements directed to but not touching the floor (p. 168).

Skinner used the term superstition because "the bird behaves as if there were a causal relation between its behavior and the presentation of food, although such a relation is lacking" (p. 171). Similar behavior occurs in rats, but, unlike in pigeons, in rats it rapidly becomes extinguished. Rats with hippocampal lesions, however, fail to extinguish "superstitious" behavior.[11] In Devenport's experiment, food pellets were offered to rats every 100 seconds, independent of their behavior. The "superstitious" response was bar-pressing. There is a tendency among contemporary behaviorists to substitute the term schedule-induced behavior for superstition[33] because it is more noncommittal about the animal's cognitive state; however, a cognitive interpretation seems at least plausible in this case because (1) the cumulative response record shows an increase just prior to reinforcement ("scalloping") that is observed in normal operant responding on a fixed interval schedule (see figure 7–8) and (2) extinction trials before beginning noncontingent reinforcement, which reduce the rate of spontaneous lever-pressing, delay the acquisition of the "superstitious" response, as if coincidental reinforcement were the cause.[12]

While the interpretation is not completely unambiguous, it is possible that the "superstition" model is a reasonably faithful analogue of active hypothesis formation without adequate rejection when the evidence is contradictory. It is not simply a matter of inability to inhibit responding, because the "superstitious" responses cease when reinforcement is withdrawn. Devenport suggests that the animal never relaxes its commitment to the "superstitious" hypothesis long enough to compare reinforcement rates with and with-

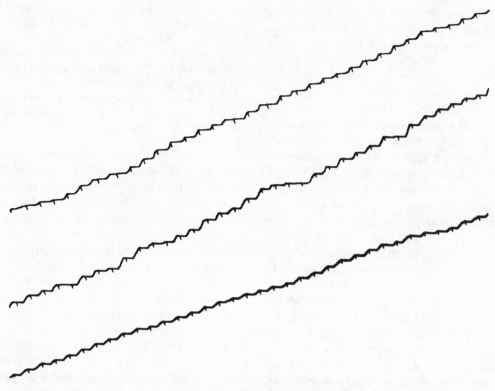

Figure 7–8. "Superstitious behavior" in hippocampal-lesioned rats.

NOTE: Reprinted, by permission of the publisher, from L. D. Devenport, "Superstitious Bar-pressing in Hippocampal and Septal Rats," *Science,* 205 (1979).

out lever-pressing. In psychiatric terms, one might say that delusional patients fail to disconfirm incorrect hypotheses because they never withdraw attention from them long enough to evaluate alternatives. From this point of view, the "superstition" model is continuous with, although an extension of, the attentional models already reviewed.

In summary, there seems to be a hierarchy of attentional models, from the most "motor" to the most "mental": (1) locomotor perseveration, repetitive performance of simple motor acts; (2) stereotyped social gesturing; (3) behavioral switching; (4) perseverative maintenance of hypotheses; and (5) active acquisition and perseverative maintenance of false hypotheses. One immediate consequence of the hierarchy is that it offers hope of distinguishing between antipsychotic and extrapyramidal effects of drugs being screened for antipsychotic activity. The higher up in the hierarchy, the better the

distinction is likely to be. This somewhat bewildering proliferation of models also shows how fruitful the "cross-species psychological process" type of model can be.

Problems of Interpretation of Animal Behavior

This review of attentional models underscores the difficulty of interpreting animal behavior. The functional significance for the animal of any one behavior, considered in isolation, may be impossible to determine with certainty. When it is taken together with other responses or when evoking conditions are varied, more convincing interpretations become possible.

As an example, consider the stimulation of locomotor activity evoked by injecting dopamine or dopamine agonists into the nucleus accumbens. This effect has been known for over a decade,[27,28] and a rich literature has grown out of it, particularly with respect to pharmacological variation. On the whole, the behavioral analysis is quite weak. What is the significance of increased locomotor activity? Is it a primary motor effect, like akathisia? Is it caused by a state of increased arousal? Is it related to distractibility or failure to habituate? It is interesting that the first authors to explore the locomotor stimulation phenomenon were more sensitive to the problem of interpretation than those who followed. Pijnenburg and van Rossum[27] noted, for example, that the stimulated animals "showed no sign of aggressiveness but, on the contrary, could be handled very easily without resistance. When they were handled, they stopped their activity and after they had been replaced in the observation cage they resumed their running" (p. 298).

There is some evidence to support the hypothesis that locomotor hyperactivity after intra-accumbens injections represents interference with habituation. Wachtel, Ahlenius, and Anden[36] took the simple step of dividing the observation period into three three-minute intervals. Dopamine was injected into the nucleus accumbens ten minutes before the first observation period. During the first three-minute interval, dopamine-treated animals actually moved less than controls, whereas during the last interval they moved more. The authors concluded that normal animals decline in activity over the nine-minute period of observation because they habituate to the test environment, whereas the dopamine-treated animals maintain their initial high level of activity because they fail to habituate. Van Ree and associates[35] found decreased habituation after chronic injection of gamma-endorphin antiserum into the nucleus accumbens. As they point out, the decreased habituation could itself be understood in several different ways (e.g., increased exploratory drive, increased awareness of sensory stimuli, impaired memory), but interpreting locomotor hyperactivity as decreased habituation is a step toward specificity.

A sophisticated behavioral analysis by Solomon and Staton[33] strengthens the habituation interpretation. They studied latent inhibition, which is the retarding effect of preexposure to a stimulus, without reinforcement, on subsequent conditioning to that stimulus. A tone served as a cue for the animal to run from one side of a shuttlebox to the other to avoid an electric shock. The preexposure experience was thirty five-second presentations of the tone, without reinforcement. After five days of bilateral amphetamine injections into the nucleus accumbens, the latent inhibition effect was decreased relative to controls. There did not appear to be changes in either auditory or shock sensitivity. These relatively simple manipulations show that behavioral analysis can substantially clarify the interpretation of experimental modification of behavior and therefore increase its usefulness in developing animal models for neuropsychiatric disease.

A Psychological Process Model of Affective Disorder

Despite their clinical and experimental utility, the biogenic amine theories of affective disorders—in their present formulation —fall short of a psychological process model. This gap in explanation was evident to some of the originators of the amine hypothesis,[31] who wrote: "The interactions between . . . environmental determinants of affect, various physiological factors, and the complexity of psychological determinants, including cognitive factors derived from the individual's remote and immediate past experiences, have received only limited study . . . only within such a multifactorial framework may one expect to understand fully the relationship of the biogenic amines to emotional state" (p. 28).

It is plausible to postulate that a person vulnerable to affective disorder differs from normal, primarily in the organization of his or her memory storage. Associations between memories, in normal persons, are based partly on affect, partly on content, and partly on temporal contiguity. Thus an unpleasant experience involving a certain person may be linked to other unpleasant experiences, to other memories of that person, or to other experiences occurring at the same time. Suppose that an external event, even a minor one, rekindles a certain unpleasant memory. If the associative links between this memory and others are almost exclusively affective, other unpleasant memories will be rekindled, and mood can spiral downward. If there is a balance of affect- and content-associations, mood will be stabilized because some of the content-associations may have positive affective tone and prevent retrieval of more and more negative memories. Affective disorder, in this hypothesis, is not a periodicity in mood paced by an internal clock but an instability that causes escalation of minor perturbations of the system from external causes.

The clinical evidence for this theory and the relation between these psychological processes and biogenic amines will be omitted here, since the primary question concerns how a theory of this kind can be used to devise an animal model. Paradigms based on psychological processes ought to be roughly translatable across species, so let us first imagine an experimental design suitable for humans. Suppose it is wished to subdivide a sample of subjects into two groups, one vulnerable to affective disorder (according to this theory) and one not. Present each subject with two levers, A and B, and reward the "correct" lever as cued by a visual stimulus. The rules will be: Reward A when a smiling female face is shown; reward B when a frowning male face is shown. No verbal description of these contingencies is given. After the task has been learned, present mixed stimuli—that is, frowning females or smiling males. If the subject's proclivity is to associate by affect, he or she will press lever B for frowning females and A for smiling males, but if the subject tends to associate by content, his or her behavior in response to the ambiguous cues will be the opposite.

This is only a schematic sketch of an experiment, but it provides a rationale for a more serious attempt to design an animal model. A rat is placed in a Y-maze and rewarded if it makes the "correct" choice as cued by an auditory stimulus. Three auditory stimuli are used: A, a high-frequency tone that has, in a preparatory conditioning step, been a cue for the availability of food; B, a low-frequency tone that has been presented an equal number of times in the preparatory step, but randomly with respect to the availability of food; and X, a tone of intermediate frequency (between A and B) that has also been used in the preparatory step, but with partial cue value (presented more often than chance in association with food but not as predictably as A).

In the Y-maze step, A is used as a cue for reward on the left, B for reward on the right. After training is complete and the animal makes the correct choices to A and B, X is presented under extinction conditions. Will the animal go to the left or the right? Suppose the frequency and cue value of X are adjusted so the animal makes exactly 50 percent responses to the left and to the right. Then we know how much affective similarity (cue value for rewarding contingencies) is equivalent to a given amount of content-similarity (intrinsic stimulus properties) in the animal's associative scheme. The next step is to subdivide animals, either by strain or by individual differences, into affect- and content-associators according to this paradigm and then subject them all to a depression-inducing stress (e.g., separation). The theory predicts that the affect-associators will be especially vulnerable to depression, even though they were not any more depressed before the separation experience.

¶ Conclusion

Each type of animal model has its own functions and limitations. Isomorphism models are useful for elucidating mechanisms of drug action, but are not able to step outside the existing class of therapeutic agents. Symptom similarity models escape this circularity, but suffer from an inherent arbitrariness because of the multiplicity of behaviors that are disturbed in the major psychoses. Gene transfer models focus more directly on etiology, but require isolation of single genes, a very difficult task. Psychological process models—cross-species paradigms developed by analyzing the underlying psychological disturbance in the human illness —seem to offer the best hope for modeling psychiatric illness at the present time.

¶ Bibliography

1. ALLAN, L. G. "The Attention Switching Model: Implications for Research in Schizophrenia," *Journal of Psychiatric Research*, 14 (1978):195–202.

2. BLEULER, E. *Dementia Praecox or the Group of Schizophrenias.* New York: International Universities Press, 1950.

3. BOTSTEIN, D., et al. "Construction of a Genetic Linkage Map in Man Using Restriction Fragment Length Polymorphisms," *American Journal of Human Genetics*, 32 (1980):314–331.

4. CAPLAN, A., et al. "Introduction of Genetic Material into Plant Cells," *Science*, 222 (1983):815–821.

5. CAVINESS, V. S., SO, D. K., and SIDMAN, R. L. "The Hybrid Reeler Mouse," *Journal of Heredity*, 63 (1972):241–246.

6. CHIODO, L. A., and BUNNEY, B. S. "Typical and Atypical Neuroleptics: Differential Effects of Chronic Administration on the Activity of A9 and A10 Midbrain Dopamine Neurons," *Journal of Neuroscience*, 3 (1983):1607–1619.

7. COOLS, A. R. "Role of the Neostriatal Dopaminergic Activity in Sequencing and Selecting Behavioral Strategies: Facilitation of Process Involved in Selecting the Best Strategy in a Stressful Situation," *Behavioural Brain Research*, 1 (1980):361–378.

8. COTES, P. M., et al. "Neuroendocrine Changes in Acute Schizophrenia as a Function of Clinical State and Neuroleptic Medication," *Psychological Medicine*, 8 (1978):657–665.

9. CROMWELL, R. L., and DOKECKI, P. "Schizophrenic Language: A Disattention Interpretation," in S. Rosenberg and J. H. Koplin, eds., *Developments in Applied Psycholinguistics Research*. New York: Macmillan, 1968, pp. 209–260.

10. DAVIS, R. T. "The Radiation Syndrome," in A. M. Schrier, H. F. Harlow, and F. Stollnitz, eds., *Behavior of Nonhuman Primates: Modern Research Trends*, vol. 2. New York: Academic Press, 1965, pp. 503–508.

11. DEVENPORT, L. D. "Superstitious Barpressing in Hippocampal and Septal Rats," *Science*, 205 (1979):721–723.

12. DEVENPORT, L. D., and HOLLOWAY, F. A. "The Rat's Resistance to Superstition: Role of the Hippocampus," *Journal of Comparative and Physiological Psychology*, 94 (1980):691–705.

13. DILL, R. E., et al. "Comparison of Behavioral Effects of Systemic L-DOPA and Intracranial Dopamine in Mesolimbic Forebrain of Nonhuman Primates," *Pharmacology, Biochemistry and Behavior*, 10 (1979):711–716.

14. GUSELLA, J. F., et al. "A Polymorphic DNA Marker Genetically Linked to Huntington's Disease," *Nature*, 306 (1983):234–238.

15. HARLOW, H. F. "Effects of Radiation on the Central Nervous System and on Behavior—General Survey," in T. J. Haley and R. S. Snider, eds., *Response of the Nervous System to Ionizing Radiation*. New York: Academic Press, 1962, pp. 627–644.

16. HURT, S. W., HOLZMAN, P. S., and DAVIS, J. M. "Thought Disorder: The Measurement of Its Changes," *Archives of General Psychiatry*, 40 (1983):1281–1285.

17. ISAACSON, R. L., and KIMBLE, D. P. "Lesions of the Limbic System. Their Effects upon Hypotheses and Frustration," *Behavioral Biology*, 7 (1972):767–793.

18. IVERSEN, S. D., and KOOB, G. F. "Behavioral Implications of Dopaminergic Neurons in the Mesolimbic System," *Advances in Biochemical Psychopharmacology*, 16 (1977):209–214.

19. KLERMAN, G. "Better But Not Well: Sociological and Ethical Issues in the Deinstitutionalization of the Mentally Ill," *Schizophrenia Bulletin*, 3 (1977):617–631.

20. KRISTOFFERSON, A. B., and ALLAN, L. G. "Successiveness and Duration Discrimination," in S. Kornblum, ed., *Attention and Performance*, vol. 4. New York: Academic Press, 1973, pp. 737–749.

21. LEARY, R. W., and RUCH, T. C. "Activity, Manipulation Drive, and Strength in Monkeys Subjected to Low-level Irradiation," *Journal of Comparative and Physiological Psychology*, 48 (1955): 336–342.

22. MATTHYSSE, S., and HABER, S. "Animal Models of Schizophrenia," in D. Ingle and H. Shein, eds., *The Use of Model Systems in Biological Psychiatry*. Cambridge, Mass.: MIT Press, 1975, pp. 4–25.

23. MILNER, B. "The Effects of Different Brain Lesions on Card Sorting: The Role of the Frontal Lobes," *Archives of Neurology*, 9 (1963):90–100.

24. MITCHELL, G. "Abnormal Behavior in Primates," in L. A. Rosenblum, ed., *Primate Behavior: Developments in Field and Laboratory Research*, vol. 1. New York: Academic Press, 1970, pp. 195–249.

25. OADES, R. D. "Dopaminergic Agonistic and Antagonistic Drugs in the Ventral Tegmentum of Rats Inhibit and Facilitate Changes of Food Search Behavior," *Neuroscience Letters* 27 (1981):75–80.

26. PALMITER, R. D., et al. "Metallothionein—Human GH Fusion Genes Stimulate Growth of Mice," *Science*, 222 (1983): 809–814.

27. PIJNENBURG, A.J.J., and VAN ROSSUM, J. M. "Ergometrine-induced Locomotor Activity Following Intra-cerebral Injection into the Nucleus Accumbens," *Brain Research*, 59 (1973):289–302.

28. ———. "Stimulation of Locomotor Activity Following Injection of Dopamine into the Nucleus Accumbens," *Journal of Pharmacy and Pharmacology*, 25 (1973):1003–1005.

29. RANDRUP, A., and MUNKVAD, I. "Pharmacology and Physiology of Stereotyped Behavior," *Journal of Psychiatric Research*, 11 (1974):110.

30. ROBBINS, T. W., and KOOB, G. F. "Selective Disruption of Displacement Behavior by Lesions of the Mesolimbic Dopamine System," *Nature*, 285 (1980):409–412.

31. SCHILDKRAUT, J. J., and KETY, S. S. "Biogenic Amines and Emotion," *Science*, 156 (1967):21–30.

32. SKINNER, B. F. " 'Superstition' in the Pigeon," *Journal of Experimental Psychology*, 38 (1948):168–172.

33. SOLOMON, P. R., and STATON, D. M. "Differential Effects of Microinjections of d-amphetamine into the Nucleus Accumbens or the Caudate Putamen on the Rat's Ability to Ignore an Irrelevant Stimulus," *Biological Psychiatry*, 17 (1982):743–756.

34. STADDON, J.E.R. "Schedule-induced Behavior," in W. K. Honig, and J.E.R. Staddon, eds., *Handbook of Operant Behavior*. Englewood Cliffs, N.J.: Prentice-Hall, 1977, pp. 125–152.

35. VAN REE, J. M., et al. "Non-opiate Beta-endorphin Fragments and Dopamine IV. Gamma-type Endorphins May Control Dopaminergic Systems in the Nucleus Accumbens," *Neuropharmacology* 21 (1982):1119–1127.

36. WACHTEL, H., AHLENIUS, S., and ANDEN, N. E. "Effects of Locally Applied Dopamine to the Nucleus Accumbens on the Motor Activity of Normal Rats and Following Alpha-methyltyrosine or Reserpine," *Psychopharmacology*, 63 (1979): 203–206.

37. WANG, R. Y. "Dopaminergic Neurons in the Rat Ventral Tegmental Area: I. Identification and Characterization," *Brain Research Reviews* 3 (1981):123–140.

38. WEISS, J. M., et al. "A Model for Neurochemical Study of Depression," in M. Y. Speigelstein and A. Levy, eds., *Behavioral Models and the Analysis of Drug Action*. Amsterdam: Elsevier, 1982, pp. 195–223.

39. WHITE, F. J., and WANG, R. Y. "Differential Effects of Classical and Atypical Antipsychotic Drugs in A9 and A10 Dopamine Neurons," *Science*, 221 (1983):1054–1057.

CHAPTER 8

HUMAN BRAIN ELECTRICAL POTENTIALS IN PSYCHIATRIC DISORDERS

Walton T. Roth and Adolf Pfefferbaum

¶ Introduction

The ability to record the constantly changing electrical potentials of the human brain from the scalp has captured the interest of researchers in neurology and psychiatry since the late 1930s. In the last ten years the increasing availability of computers in the laboratory has made complex analyses such as digital spectral analysis and signal averaging commonplace. It has become easier and easier to analyze data from multiple leads, to display it in elegant formats, and to submit it to sophisticated multivariate statistical analysis. Event-related potentials (ERPs) now play a clinical role in neurology—for example, in the diagnosis of multiple sclerosis and the measurement of nerve conduction. Click ERPs are now being used to diagnose hearing deficits in neonates. In psychiatry, however, no generally accepted clinical role for electrophysiology has yet been established.

This chapter will outline some current hypotheses and research strategies used in psychiatric electrophysiological research, summarize relevant experimental findings, and provide a critique of this field. Finally, we will discuss some general reasons for the gap between the laboratory and clinic. This review is not exhaustive, but is instead an introduction to ideas that are of current interest. The interested reader may want to consult other more comprehensive and specialized reviews and books.*

*See references 8, 12, 19, 20, 25, 37, 40, 44, 45, 76, 79, 82, 89, 91, 98, and 103.

¶ Spontaneous Activity in the Electroencephalogram

Regardless of the presence or absence of outside stimulation and regardless of whether the subject is awake or asleep, electrical activity from the brain can be recorded from the scalp. This activity is usually recorded as potential differences between various points on the head, although recently the recording of the magnetic fields produced by ionic current flow has become feasible.[51,69] In most people the electroencephalogram (EEG) consists of gradually waxing and waning rhythmic activity, often with a peak frequency around 10 Hertz (Hz; alpha rhythm). Dominant frequencies vary depending on the subject's alertness and whether his or her eyes are open. In a few people sporadic bursts of rhythmic activity at subalpha frequencies, or spikes, can be observed; these paroxysms of activity are especially prevalent in those suffering from seizure disorders. The absence of any brain electrical activity is, under most circumstances, evidence of brain death.

Features of the spontaneous EEG can be evaluated qualitatively by trained observers or quantitatively by mathematical methods. Rhythmic activity is analyzed into power spectra by Fourier transformations; paroxysmal activity is detected by pattern recognition algorithms. Spectral analysis can give the spectrum of the EEG at a single pair of electrodes or of EEG activity shared between two pairs of electrodes. Figure 8–1 illustrates the application of spectral analysis to EEG activity recorded between an occipital electrode (o2) and the right earlobe (A2) in a normal subject before and after administration of chlorpromazine. The bars show the relative power of the EEG in six frequency bands from 1.5 to 30 Hz.

Calculating relative rather than absolute power has the theoretical advantage of minimizing irrelevant individual differences, such as those due to skull thickness,[53] but can be misleading if, for example, a relative increase in lower frequencies produced by a

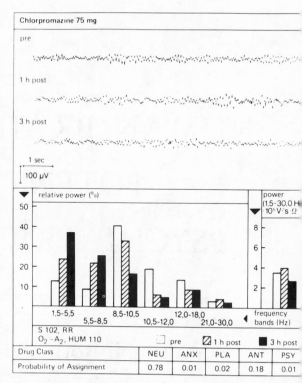

Figure 8–1. The upper part of the figure shows sample EEG tracings from a subject before and after receiving 75 mg chlorpromazine orally. Electrodes were attached to the scalp in the right occipital area (O2) and the right ear (A2). The power calculations are averages from multiple 10-second segments of EEG recorded during a 5-minute period. Probability of Assignment refers to the results of a multivariate classification procedure. In this case, chlorpromazine was correctly classified as a neuroleptic (NEU) with a probability of 0.78. The other classes of drugs evaluated were anxiolytic (ANX), placebo (PLA), and psychostimulant (PSY).

NOTE: Reprinted, by permission of the publisher, from W. M. Herrmann, ed., *Electroencephalography in Drug Research* (Stuttgart: Gustav Fischer, 1982), p. 328.

reduction in higher frequencies is not distinguished from an absolute increase in lower frequencies.

Figure 8–2 demonstrates that the spatial distribution of EEG activity is not uniform over the scalp. For normal subjects, power in

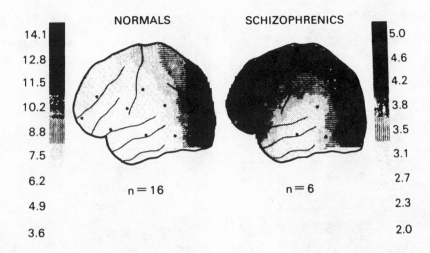

Figure 8–2.   Distribution of alpha activity in sixteen normal subjects and six medication-free schizophrenic patients meeting DSM-III criteria. After spectral analysis, averages were computed for each of sixteen leads, and these mean values were mapped. The gray scale shows alpha activity in microvolts. Note that this scale is set to be almost three times more sensitive for normal subjects than for schizophrenic patients. In normal subjects, alpha activity is confined to occipital and posterior parietal regions. Schizophrenic patients have lower-amplitude alpha activity with approximately equal intensity over a wide area.

NOTE: Reprinted, by permission of the publisher, from M. S. Buchsbaum, R. Coppola, and J. Cappelletti, "Positron Emission Tomography, EEG and Evoked Potential Topography: New Approaches to Local Function in Pharmaco-Electroencephalography," in W. M. Herrmann, ed., *Electroencephalography in Drug Research* (Stuttgart: Gustav Fischer, 1982), p. 199.

the alpha (8–12 Hz) band is concentrated in the occipital region. Different distributions apply to other frequency bands. Figure 8–3 reveals how much temporal variability there can be in EEG spectra over consecutive eight-second periods. For this subject, the spectra stabilized in the 10 Hz region after 10 mg dextroamphetamine. Because of this variability, it is common to average spectral values across successive analysis epochs.

Whatever the method of EEG analysis, artifacts can invalidate the results. Over the anterior scalp, eye blinks and shifts in gaze produce voltages generated by the eye that are much larger than those generated by the brain. Contractions of the scalp muscles give electromyographic signals and movement artifacts that can be confused with fast EEG activity. In psychiatric patients especially, these nonbrain electrical artifacts cannot be avoided completely, and analysis methods

have to estimate the amount of distortion they produce.

Statistical Deviance

A simple and general hypothesis for the study of psychiatric disorders is that since the EEG reflects functioning of the brain, the organ of the mind, mental abnormality will be reflected in differences between EEGs of patients with psychopathology and those of normal subjects. Furthermore, since different psychiatric disorders have different manifestations and are affected by different drugs, they may be assumed to have different biological or psychological natures. The specific nature of the psychiatric disorder must be expressed at some point in abnormalities of brain function reflected in the EEG. These abnormalities may be present even when the psychiatric disturbance is in remission, corre-

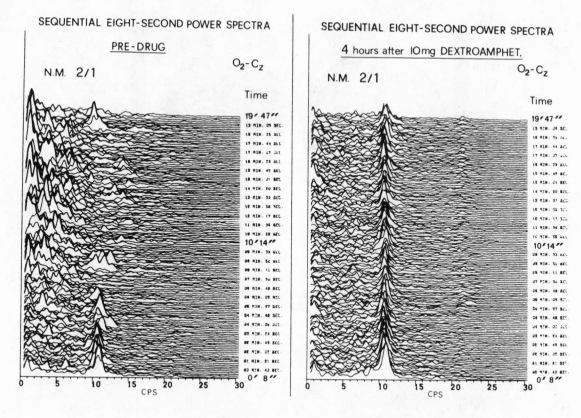

Figure 8–3. EEG power at different cycles per second (CPS) evaluated at 8-second intervals over a 19-minute period in a single subject before and after receiving dextroamphetamine. Recordings are made from scalp electrodes at the right occipital area (O2) and the top of the head at the midline of the saggital plane (Cz).

NOTE: Reprinted, by permission of the publisher, from M. Matejcek, "Vigilance and the EEG: Psychological, Physiological and Pharmacological Aspects," in W. M. Herrmann, ed., *Electroencephalography in Drug Research* (Stuttgart: Gustav Fischer, 1982), p. 442.

sponding to a "trait," or stable characteristic, or they may depend on symptoms being present, thus reflecting a "state," or temporary characteristic. EEG abnormalities might be specific to disease entities, such as schizophrenia or manic-depressive disease, or they might be specific to psychological states or to symptoms, such as auditory hallucinations, that cross-cut these diseases. Psychoactive drugs will produce changes in the EEG corresponding to their mental effects. If a drug counteracts a mental abnormality, it can be expected that it would normalize the EEG deviance reflecting that abnormality.

This line of reasoning is used to justify empirical, exploratory EEG investigations of psychiatric patients and psychoactive drugs. It does not require a commitment as to what specific EEG differences are expected or whether they reflect biological or psychological factors. Some researchers believe that enough remains unknown about psychiatric illness and the EEG to make more specific hypotheses speculative at best.

Statistical differences have often been found between chronic schizophenic patients and control subjects in the power spectrum of the EEG: With either absolute or relative power measures, schizophrenic patients usually have less power in the fast alpha range (11–13 Hz), more power in the fast beta range (20+ Hz), and slightly more power in the theta and delta bands (8 Hz and less).* Figure 8–2 shows that the distribution of alpha power may also be different.

Unfortunately, these features are not found in all schizophrenic patients. Acute schizophrenic patients may only have reduced alpha activity.[24] Familial cases of schizophrenia in which a first-degree relative is also schizophrenic are less likely to have increased or asymmetric theta activity than are sporadic cases.[52] Unfortunately, these features are also found in nonschizophrenic subjects. Chronic alcoholic patients show the alpha, beta, and theta and delta findings mentioned earlier,[16] and demented subjects show decreased alpha and increased theta and delta activity.[44] Certain demented subjects show decreased beta activity,[21] and others show increased beta activity.[44]

Variability of EEG power over time has often been found to be reduced in chronic schizophrenia.† Recordings were made from occipital electrodes in subjects whose eyes were closed. Acute schizophrenic patients who were hallucinating were also less variable than controls.[61] In one study lowered variability in the 18-to-32 Hz band was the most powerful discriminator between schizophrenic patients and control subjects.[56] A study with twelve EEG leads showed that the reduced variability was greatest in posterior leads.[93] This finding is not due to medication, since it was present in unmedicated schizophrenic patients. However, it is not limited to schizophrenic patients, as variability is also reduced in manic patients.[93] Reduced amplitude variability can be accompanied by increased frequency variability.[93]

A number of studies have shown that psychoactive drugs cause statistically significant changes in the EEG spectrum. Antipsychotic drugs such as haloperidol, thiothixene, and fluphenazine hydrochloride increase power in the theta range and decrease beta activity.[40] Schizophrenic patients resistant to treatment with antipsychotic drugs tend to

have more alpha and less beta activity before treatment,[43] which suggests that their pretreatment EEGs are more like those of normal subjects. Anxiolytics produce an increase in slow beta activity. Stimulants produce an increase in total power, particularly in the alpha range.[36] Antidepressants cause increases in delta power and decreases in alpha power.[36] Anticholinergic hallucinogens produce increases in delta and beta activity and a decrease in alpha activity.[40] Cholinergic drugs, such as physostigmine, in large doses also produce increased delta activity.[73]

One criticism of the studies just detailed is that, although statistically significant differences can be seen between diagnostic groups and between people on and off medication, these differences are not specific to a particular diagnostic group and are not universal within a group. There is much individual variation in EEGs that is unrelated to known psychological or physical differences. For example, a substantial minority of normal subjects fail to produce alpha activity.

A second criticism is that the strength of the statistical approach is also its weakness: It requires no knowledge of what the EEG parameters measured mean in biochemical, physiological, or psychological terms. However, without this knowledge it is impossible to integrate EEG findings with other scientific findings. Without clear hypotheses, a stepwise improvement in experiments cannot occur. This second criticism is blunted by the fact that, as will be discussed, at least some EEG parameters can be interpreted in terms of arousal or cerebral insufficiency.

Another problem with the studies just cited is that, although the recent literature reflects a general awareness of the possible role of artifacts in generating the spectral and variability differences between patients and control subjects, quantitative estimates are lacking of how much artifact remains after specific editing procedures. Frontal delta activity can be due to eye or head movements. Topographic analysis can help determine if potentials originate in the eye.[84] Beta activity can be due to muscle

*See references 10, 16, 24, 38, 42, 65, and 100.
†See references 31, 55, 56, 61, and 93.

artifact,[56] which has a higher peak frequency but can spill down into lower bands. The presence of more beta activity in schizophrenic patients during rapid-eye-movement sleep, when neck muscle tension is low, and the reduction of beta activity after administration of antipsychotic drugs that increase muscle tension have been used as general arguments for independence of beta activity from muscle artifact,[40] but quantification of the impact of this artifact on individual records would be more convincing.

Arousal Abnormality

A central concept in psychophysiology is arousal. The EEG has been considered an index of "cortical arousal," which is sometimes contrasted with "autonomic arousal." At first approximation, high arousal is characterized by an absence of rhythmic EEG activity and low arousal by an abundance. High arousal is also associated with higher-frequency activity than is low arousal. In the awake subject, decreasing arousal might first be reflected by an increase in alpha activity, which is then replaced by an increase in theta activity. Psychological theories of schizophrenia have often argued that at least some subgroups of schizophrenia show hyperarousal,[7] and investigators have looked for confirmation of that idea from the EEG.

The increased beta activity in the power spectrum of chronic schizophrenic patients is consistent with higher arousal, since increased beta activity is a consequence of reticular formation stimulation in animals[40]; however, the relation between beta activity and arousal in man may be less straightforward.[56] Lower variability of total EEG power over time is also associated with higher arousal. However, delta power increases as people fall asleep,[58] so the increased slow activity seen in chronic schizophrenic patients is more consistent with decreased arousal.[55] Thus the signs of abnormal arousal point in opposite directions. The reported decreases in alpha activity are ambiguous: They can be a sign of either increased or decreased arousal.

Even when indicators of arousal are consistent, deviant arousal levels are not confined to a single diagnostic group. In one study the change in EEG measures between eyes-closed and eyes-opened states was used as an index of arousal increase,[93] an only partially satisfactory index, because differences in visual input decisively influence the EEG. In any case, three groups—overt schizophrenic, latent schizophrenic, and manic patients—were found to be more aroused than control subjects, and two groups—major depressive and personality-disorder patients—were less aroused. Neurotic subjects did not differ from control subjects.

To some extent, the spectral changes caused by psychoactive drugs may be simply a reflection of changes in arousal. The increase in total spectral power with stimulants may be because they prevent drowsiness and the disappearance of alpha activity. The greater stability of the spectra after amphetamine in figure 8–3 could occur because amphetamine prevents the subject from periodically drifting into sleep. The increased theta activity and decreased beta activity produced by antipsychotics is consistent with lower arousal, but the increased beta activity produced by anxiolytics is not.

Although the concept of arousal abnormality has been fruitful in inspiring experiments and integrating diverse findings, it has major limitations. The validity of the concept of a single arousal continuum has been questioned generally, and the ability of the EEG to index it has been challenged specifically. There is neuropharmacological evidence for separate cholinergic and aminergic arousal systems.[104] The existence of different sleep stages is proof that there is no simple EEG continuum from excitement through relaxation to deep sleep and finally coma, as was first suggested. During the waking state, skin conductance level may correspond better to fluctuations of excitement and alertness than the EEG.

Another problem is that, from a clinical perspective, arousal abnormalities are secondary and nonspecific features of disorders such as schizophrenia, depression, mania, and dementia. In contrast, the subjective awareness of heightened arousal is a primary, defining characteristic of patients with anxiety disorders such as panic attacks with agoraphobia.

Although not central to their psychosis, differences in arousal between psychotic patients and control subjects may nonetheless be crucial in explaining EEG differences between them in a specific experiment. For example, unmedicated schizophrenic patients, especially those with positive symptoms, are less likely to relax and begin to fall asleep when they sit with their eyes closed in a laboratory setting than are control subjects. Anxiety is a common secondary reaction to perceptual distortions and disorganization in thinking during acute exacerbations of schizophrenia.

Cerebral Insufficiency

Engel and Romano coined the term cerebral insufficiency more than twenty-five years ago in analogy with renal or hepatic insufficiency.[23] They thought it expressive of the generalized and undifferentiated syndrome of decreased mental functioning and EEG slowing common to alcoholic intoxication, hypoglycemia, hypoxia, and other organic causes of what has been called delirium or acute brain syndrome. When this syndrome was induced experimentally, the dominant frequency of the EEG was observed to slow reversibly in proportion to cognitive impairment. Irreversible damage led to "dementia" or "chronic brain syndrome," in which the EEG might continue to be slow or might normalize.

Until recently, the concept of cerebral insufficiency seemed irrelevant to major psychoses. Central to the clinical definition of schizophrenia was the concept that cognitive functions were essentially intact, although deficits in motivation and attention might give the appearance of deficit. However, studies demonstrating radiological signs of enlarged cerebral ventricles and cerebral atrophy in certain groups of chronic schizophrenic patients[46,107] have revived notions of schizophrenia as a diffuse brain disease with characteristics in common with other dementias. This concept suggests an interpretation of the EEG characteristics of schizophrenia in terms of their similarities with dementia rather than in terms of arousal. Certainly the EEG findings in chronic schizophrenic patients deviate from those of control subjects in many of the same ways that the EEGs of patients with senile cognitive impairment do: increased delta activity and less alpha activity.[44] Unfortunately, demented and schizophrenic patients have not been directly compared in recent EEG studies. Of course, even if these two patient groups have the same structural and EEG abnormalities, the causes of the abnormalities may not be the same.

The partial vindication of the cerebral insufficiency hypothesis in schizophrenia by new radiological evidence is both exciting and disappointing. The excitement comes from the fact that statistically demonstrable abnormalities in brain structure that had eluded investigators for more than a century have been found. The disappointment lies in the fact that although the brain is a highly differentiated organ with regional specialization of functions, the radiological abnormalities that have been observed in schizophrenic patients suggest only nonspecific, diffuse loss of neurons. Such losses are usually associated with generalized deficits in memory and problem-solving ability, rather than with features more characteristic of schizophrenia, such as auditory hallucinations or bizarre thinking. Concepts less global than cerebral insufficiency are needed for understanding these more specific features.

Epileptiform Abnormality

The relationship between the major psychoses and epilepsy is an area of continuing interest. Evidence has been advanced that spiking in the limbic area is related to schizophrenia.[35] The symptoms of temporal lobe epilepsy can be similar to those of schizophrenia or affective disorder.[78] Carbamazepine is a drug commonly used for treating temporal lobe epilepsy, but it is also effective in manic-depressive disease. Therefore, EEG researchers have continued to search for paroxysmal electrical discharges in psychiatric patients.

Studies have been made correlating the free behavior on psychiatric wards of unmedicated schizophrenic patients with events in their telemetered EEG. In one study,[101] 40 percent of the schizophrenic patients and none of the control subjects had focal slow or spike activity in the temporal regions, but these EEG events did not correspond to episodes of abnormal behavior. In a subsequent study using similar methods, power spectra were compared between normal behavior and episodes of abnormal behavior such as psychomotor blocking, automatisms, or hallucinations.[100] A spectral pattern of a smooth decline in power from lower to high frequencies (0.5–35 Hz) was seen in half of the schizophrenic patients and none of the control subjects and was twice as common during abnormal behaviors as during normal ones. This spectral pattern has been associated with subcortical spiking in other studies comparing the effects of epileptic foci on surface and depth electrodes. Artifact control as was attempted in this study is crucial, since slow transients from the eye or from body movements can produce the same spectral pattern.

Aside from these studies, there is little evidence that schizophrenia is associated with paroxysmal electrical disturbances. Except in unusual cases, the symptoms of the type of epilepsy most similar to schizophrenia, temporal lobe epilepsy, are distinct from schizophrenic symptoms. The scalp EEG findings characteristic of epilepsy are rare in psychoses.

Regional Differences

The EEG is capable of localizing brain lesions to a certain extent, both in anterior-posterior planes and in transverse planes. For this reason the EEG has been used to test hypotheses of regional brain disturbance in psychiatric disorders. It is plausible to hypothesize that psychiatric entities can be differentiated by the brain region most disturbed. One hypothesis, derived from studies of regional blood flow, postulates that schizophrenic patients and possibly other patient groups are characterized by hypofrontality—that is, decreased frontal lobe activity. Increased frontal delta power in schizophrenic patients has been interpreted as supporting the idea of hypofrontality.[65]

A second hypothesis is that right-left brain functional asymmetries are responsible for the predominance of schizophrenic or affective symptoms. Schizophrenia is postulated to be a disturbance of language and analytical thinking involving the left side of the brain, while affective disorders are postulated to be a disturbance of emotion involving the right side. Evidence for this hypothesis is that in patients with temporal lobe epilepsy, foci on the left are more often associated with symptoms of schizophrenia and foci on the right with psychotic depression (for a review, see Flor-Henry[25]).

In the absence of foci, however, it is uncertain what the EEG evidence for disturbance should be. Studies of power ratios have given contradictory results. In one report the right-left ratio in the higher-frequency bands at temporal electrodes was greater than one in patients with depressive psychosis and less than one in schizophrenic patients.[26] However, two later studies[63,106] from other centers found exactly the opposite asymmetries. The reason for these discrepancies is unclear, but it is relevant to emphasize that right-left power ratios are not fixed individual traits. When power ratios between hemispheres are examined millisecond by millisecond, they are observed to be constantly in flux. Ratios can be influenced by the nature of the subject's mental activities.[25] Furthermore, it cannot be taken for granted that asymmetries originate in the brain. Masseter and temporalis muscle artifacts spill down into the frequency bands above alpha, and asymmetries in these artifacts were reported by Flor-Henry.[25]

In sum, hypotheses of regional differences have generated much enthusiasm and EEG experimentation, but meager results. Ingenious measures of regional coupling have been developed (e.g., see Gevins et al.[30]), but their applicability is uncertain. It is a mistake, of course, to assume that the activity measured by an electrode on the scalp indicates solely the activity of subadjacent cortex. The fact that electrical potential is volume-conducted means that it cannot be used to construct three-dimensional maps as x-rays can. The electrical source might be shallow or deep, diffuse or localized. For example, a small region could contribute activity at a certain frequency that would appear in many locations. In the future, additional information provided by the new methods of magnetic field recording may be used to locate dipole sources more accurately.[51]

¶ Event-related Potentials

Signal averaging methods have made it possible to study scalp EEG potentials time-locked to specific, repeated external events. Averaging effectively improves the signal-to-noise ratio, since the "signal," or ERP, is time-locked to the stimuli and the "noise," or spontaneous EEG, is not. One way to visualize the mathematics of signal averaging is to imagine that each stimulus (or "trial") generates a row of numbers representing the digital value of EEG voltage at consecutive time points following it. For example, following each stimulus, 100 voltage points at intervals of 1 millisecond might be digitized. The rows generated by successive stimuli are written down the page so that the values representing a given time point fall in columns. The numbers in each column are averaged separately, and the averages are written as a new row of numbers. This new row is the signal average. The number of trials needed for adequate enhancement of the signal-to-noise ratio varies widely, from just a few to thousands, depending on the relative size of the ERP and the background EEG. In some cases it is even possible to measure ERPs to single events without averaging.

The ERP is often complex, including both multiple components that represent activity in simple sensory pathways and multiple components that represent complicated cognitive activity. Cognitive components are very sensitive to task instructions and are usually measured in reaction time paradigms of the type used by cognitive psychologists to investigate what is sometimes called human information processing.

ERPs often look like a series of peaks and valleys and can be quantified by measuring maximum and minimum voltages in specified latency ranges. Alternatively, the ERP can be decomposed with a multivariate statistical method called Principal Components Analysis or by pattern recognition algorithms.

Figure 8–4 contains ERP curves from four different electrode pairs for two kinds of stimuli. The curves to the frequent type of stimuli have only one negative and one positive peak, while the curves to the infrequent type have two early negative peaks, a later positive peak (P3 or P300), and a final voltage shift that is slightly negative at the frontal region (Fz) and positive at the parietal region (Pz). As with spectral analysis of the spontaneous EEG, voltages from several sources other than the brain can mislead the ERP researcher. Eye blinks and gaze shifts are the most important of these, and there are several methods of reducing their influence.[84] The influence of eye movement and blinks was eliminated from the curves in the figure.

ERP peaks or components are either labeled by numbering them consecutively or by giving their polarity and average peak latency in milliseconds. Here we will use the latter system, labeling a negative peak at 100 milliseconds N100 and a positive peak at 300 milliseconds P300. Figure 8–4 used a version of a system of consecutive numbering. To translate it to the millisecond system, N1 is N100, N2 is N200, P2 is P180, and P3 is P300. A drawback of this nomenclature is that certain later peaks, like P300, can have widely differing latencies depending on the stimuli and experimental conditions, although they are from a single brain source. Slow potentials with no definite peak latency receive

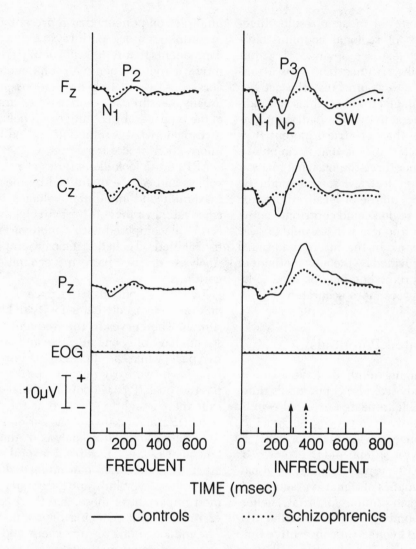

Figure 8–4. ERP averages made from scalp electrodes at the frontal region (Fz), the top of the head (Cz), and the parietal region (Pz), all in the saggital midline. The voltages from these electrodes were referenced to the voltage of the ears. The electro-oculogram (EOG) was recorded from electrodes above and below the right eye. The 10 μuV scale applies to the EEG leads and is equivalent to 50 μuV for the EOG. The EEG leads have been corrected for any eye artifact detected in the EOG lead. The stimuli were tone pips given at one-second intervals. The frequent stimuli were 800 cycles-per-second tone pips with a probability of occurrence of 0.85, and the infrequent stimuli were 1,200 cycles per second with a probability of 0.15. Subjects were instructed to press quickly to the higher-pitch stimuli. The vertical arrows on the time scale of the ERPs to infrequent stimuli indicates the mean reaction time of the controls and schizophrenics.

These ERP averages were calculated across subjects as well as trials. The averages to frequent stimuli are based on 430 trials per subject for fifteen subjects, and the averages to infrequent stimuli on 75 trials per subject for fifteen subjects. This kind of average is used as a pictorial summary of an experiment. The actual peak measurements and statistical analysis are based on the averages of individual subjects.

NOTE: Reprinted, by permission of the publisher, from W. T. Roth et al., "Event-related Potentials in Schizophrenics," *Electroencephalography and Clinical Neurophysiology,* 48 (1980): 132.

more arbitrary designations. Slow wave (SW) in figure 8–4 is a slow potential.

The hypotheses motivating experiments with the spontaneous EEG find some currency in ERP research. ERP research has focused on an empirical search for statistical deviations from normality, on temporal recovery properties as evidence of changes in excitability or arousal, on ERP components indicating general cerebral insufficiency, on increasing ERP amplitude with repeated stimulation in analogy to photic driving in epileptics, and on right-left hemisphere differences.

In addition to these common themes, ERP research is also motivated by specific hypotheses about how the mind processes information from stimuli. ERPs are different from the spontaneous EEG in that they are elicited by specific stimuli presented in a specific way. Paradigms for evoking ERPs and the resulting ERPs are very diverse. Some ERPs depend almost entirely on how the subject interprets the stimuli that evoke them, while others are almost completely automatic. Other components lie somewhere in between. Clinical ERP investigations tend to polarize into those exploiting the neurological or automatic aspects of ERP phenomena and those exploiting their psychological aspects. The motivating hypotheses of these two types are quite different.

Deficits in Automatic Processes

Neurologically oriented research efforts, or those seeking to uncover what has been called pathophysiology as opposed to psychophysiology,[92] aim to find pathognomonic characteristics of specific psychiatric diseases. Occasionally a specific anatomical or chemical hypothesis is proposed. For example, visual pattern reversal P100 latency may be dependent on dopaminergic activity[5] and thus could be used to test the hypothesis of dopamine excess in certain kinds of schizophrenia.

Investigations designed to find neural lesions tend to focus on early ERP components that are relatively impervious to the influence of attention and task. In some cases the neuroanatomic origin of these early components have been localized. From this point of view, variability due to psychological states is a source of error that compromises the accuracy of measurements of the specific, basic features of psychiatric disease.

An early series of ERP studies motivated by this approach concentrated on the temporal recovery of somatosensory ERPs.[91] When two stimuli are given within a hundred milliseconds, certain ERP peaks associated with the second stimulus are smaller than they would be if the interval between the stimuli were longer. The relationship between ERP amplitude and interstimulus interval (ISI) was felt to represent some basic property of the nervous system.

Psychiatric patient groups were found to have less temporal recovery of peaks in a 20- to 30-millisecond latency range when ISIs were less than 20 milliseconds, but there were few differences between diagnostic groups. To a certain extent, recovery function abnormalities reflected states rather than traits, since the functions of severely depressed patients normalized as they improved clinically.

More recently, abnormalities in the temporal recovery of a P50 component to auditory clicks have been reported for schizophrenic patients, both on and off medication.[1,28] The ratio of P50 amplitude after 0.5-second ISI to P50 amplitude after 10-second ISI is greater in schizophrenic patients than in control subjects. This finding is not limited to the schizophrenic state, because it is also seen more frequently in the clinically well first-degree relatives of schizophrenic patients,[97] and is present in patients with manic-depressive disease.[27]

Early components of the ERPs to unpaired somatosensory stimuli also differ between patient groups. Chronic schizophrenic patients have larger N60s at central leads.[94] However, in the auditory modality even earlier ERPs—the "brainstem potentials" occurring with latencies less than 10 milliseconds—are identical in schizophrenic patients and control subjects.[74]

Interpretation of altered recovery or amplitude changes in these early components at a neurophysiological level is uncertain, though to some extent somatosensory recovery is influenced by reticular system activation.[90] "Sensory gating" hypotheses have been advanced for explaining amplitude changes. Psychotic patients, especially chronic schizophrenic patients, have been postulated to have difficulty filtering out somatosensory stimuli, which produces an increase in the amplitude of early components and a reduction in the amplitude of later components.[92] Both increased and decreased recovery can be interpreted as evidence for pathological sensory gating. Less recovery suggests less ability to process a rapid stream of stimuli, while more recovery might indicate a vulnerability to flooding by an overabundance of sensory impressions.[97]

Although the aim of this kind of research was to study components that were independent of attention and task, many of the components investigated have turned out to be attention-sensitive. The filtering interpretations proposed earlier are attentional theories, as are the ones that motivate the experiments discussed in the next section. Often the false assumption is made that early-latency physiological events must reflect automatic processes alone and that late-latency events reflect the controlled focusing of attention. The facts are otherwise. Somatosensory peaks as early as P_{45}[49] or auditory peaks as early as P_{50}[83] can be sensitive to attention, while under some circumstances the later P_{300} can be triggered automatically in spite of distraction.[83,88]

On the one hand, it is efficient for humans to have neurophysiological mechanisms permitting task-sensitive attentional filtering early in the afferent sensory pathways. On the other hand, it would be maladaptive for attention filtering to have such power that loud, unexpected noises would fail to be analyzed because attention was directed elsewhere. The orienting response to novel stimuli of even low intensity is another example of the biologically adaptive automatic invocation of complex late processing that,

under other circumstances, is associated only with voluntary effort.[67] The attention-sensitivity of an ERP component in general or in a specific situation is always an empirical question.

The quest for an attention-independent ERP component that is diagnostic of a psychiatric disease is a worthy one. The alternative of studying attention-sensitive components has many drawbacks, as we shall discuss in later sections. However, this quest has the quixotic quality of flying in the face of the phenomenology of the diseases being studied: Preattentional components tend to be related to primary sensory pathways or elementary perception, which do not appear to be disturbed in psychiatric diseases.

Attentional Deficits

Psychologically oriented investigations are not interested in ERPs unaffected by attention and task, except perhaps as a way to prove the integrity of sensory pathways. They have hailed ERPs as a way to measure attention objectively without requiring overt behavioral responses and have often regarded abnormalities of attention as characteristic of disorders such as schizophrenia. Concentrating on components with latencies greater than 75 milliseconds, they have sought to confirm the idea that schizophrenic patients have a deficit in selective attention.[59,66] Attentional filtering may be less efficient in acute schizophrenic and manic patients because of increased distractibility by external stimuli[70,71] or by internal stimuli.[11]

Early studies demonstrated that the spontaneous variability of attention-sensitive ERPs to auditory stimuli was greater in schizophrenic patients than in control subjects.[47] This variability was greatest in thought-disordered schizophrenic patients and supported the theory that internal disruptions of attention were occurring in these patients. Several subsequent investigations have confirmed that schizophrenic ERPs are more variable than those of control subjects[9,11,95] (for reviews, see Buchsbaum[8] and Callaway[12]). However, this variability is not specific to schizophrenia; patients with Korsokoff's syndrome have the same amount of variability as schizophrenic patients.[60]

An important aspect of attention is selectivity, the ability to focus on certain features of the environment while filtering out other features. Listening to a train of stimuli coming into a certain ear makes the ERPs associated with them different from the ERPs associated with the unattended stimuli coming into the other ear (for a review, see Hillyard and Kutas[37]). A comparison of the ERPs of schizophrenic and control subjects in this paradigm shows that schizophrenic subjects are less able to attend selectively when ISIs were 500 to 1500 milliseconds.[2] The attention effect was present in a frontocentral negative wave peaking at 125 milliseconds.

Many investigators have noted decreased ERP peak amplitudes in the 75- to 250-millisecond range in psychotic patients (for a review, see Buchsbaum[8]). From experiments on normal subjects, it is known that direction of attention away from stimuli decreases ERP amplitude in this latency range. Thus it is plausible that amplitude decreases in these patients are due to inattention to their surroundings. It might be assumed that more intense stimuli would break through this barrier of inattention, but, paradoxically, some groups of schizophrenic patients seem to be able to pay even less attention to more intense stimuli.

Individual differences in the tendency to modulate reactions to the intensity of stimuli in the direction of "augmentation" (disproportionately strong reactions to intense stimuli) or "reduction" (disproportionately weak reactions to intense stimuli) have been investigated extensively using the functional relationship between stimulus intensity and ERP amplitude as a principal variable. For example, schizophrenic patients were given a train of shocks of four intensities in random order to their left forearm. They rated the higher-intensity shocks as less painful and had smaller N120 ERPs associated with them than did control subjects. There is some indication that naltrexone, an opiate antagonist,

increases schizophrenic sensitivity and ERPs to normal levels.[18]

Other studies have attempted to relate individual differences in stimulus-intensity modulation to personality dimensions, platelet monoamine oxidase enzyme activity, and clinical subtypes of affective disorder. This literature has been criticized severely in recent years because of its inconsistency as to which peaks are the best indicators of augmenting-reducing,[17] inadequate control for eye-blink artifact,[39] and the lack of generalizability of stimulus-intensity modulation functions across modalities.[77]

Another ERP phenomenon whose deviations in psychiatric patients have been interpreted in terms of attention is the Contingent Negative Variation (CNV). The subject is given a pair of stimuli, the first of which is a warning and the second a signal to press a button. The two stimuli are separated by fixed intervals, ranging from one to four seconds in different paradigms. At least two negative waves compose the broad CNV elicited by this procedure: one following and in response to the warning stimuli and another preceding and in preparation for the button press (for a review, see Rohrbaugh and Gaillard[78]). These two waves overlap, especially when intervals are shorter than two seconds. Both waves are reduced by distraction.

Patients with schizophrenia, depression, dementia, and head trauma have smaller negative waves in this paradigm (for reviews, see Dongier, Dubrovsky, and Englesmann[20]; Roth[79]; Spohn and Patterson[98]; and Timsit-Berthier[103]), probably because they do not concentrate their attention on the task. This is usually also reflected in slower reaction times. The same kinds of patients who have smaller negative waves, especially acute psychotic patients, also tend to have a slow return of the negativity to baseline after the second stimulus is given and the response is made.[103] This slow return suggests a delay in demobilizing the attentional resources mustered for pressing the button at the proper time.

Three general criticisms of attentional ERP studies can be made. First, attentional deficits are unlikely to be specific to any of the psychiatric entities that have been investigated. Attention is disturbed in schizophrenia, depression, mania, dementia, anxiety states, and other psychiatric disorders. Bleuler recognized that attentional disturbances were secondary in schizophrenia. Hyperactive children are in many ways the best candidates for a group whose salient characteristic is inability to maintain attention. Second, although ERPs can reveal features of attention that reaction time and other behavioral paradigms cannot, there have been no demonstrations that ERP measures of attention are more specific or sensitive to psychopathology than the best available behavioral measures. Thus a special practical role of ERPs in clinical attention tests has never been established. Third, neither ERPs nor behavioral paradigms measure attention independently from motivation when they require some kind of cooperation from the subject. These paradigms have difficulty making the elementary distinction between whether a subject cannot or will not do a task. ERP paradigms can have an advantage here: When the subject is given no task, ERPs can be used to assess spontaneous qualities of attention, such as whether attention fluctuates or can be attracted by novel stimuli.

Stage or Process Deficits

Cognitive psychologists construct models of information processing based on distinctions between various stages and processes. Examples are stimulus evaluation and response production stages in reaction time (RT) tasks, storage and retrieval in memory tasks, and the general characterization of processes as either automatic or controlled. The conceptual and experimental independence of certain stages leads to the hope that investigation can show that particular lesions or diseases affect specific stages. This hope has been realized in part for certain amnesias: Specific diencephalic and bitemporal lesions affect, respectively, the establishment of memories at the time of learning and the consolidation of memory for a time

afterward, while both lesions leave intact the retrieval of memories laid down before the lesions existed (for a review, see Squire[99]). It is reasonable to ask whether particular stages or processes are selectively vulnerable to anatomically undefined diseases like schizophrenia. Since ERPs efficiently index some of these processes, they should be suited for testing their vulnerabilities.

Some mental processes occur in serial stages—that is, each depends on the completion of the previous process in the chain. The last process in many of the chains is the execution of a button press, signaling that a unit of the task is completed. If any previous process is slowed, RT is slowed. The latency of a specific ERP associated with a specific processing stage indicates whether a delay in that stage is contributing to the longer RT. RT slowing is seen in many psychologically abnormal groups, and so it is logical to apply ERPs to the measurement and specification of the locus of this slowing. For example, there is considerable evidence that P300 latency is a measure of the time taken for stimulus evaluation and is independent of response preparation and execution; thus P300 latency gives more specific information than RT would in the same paradigms (for reviews, see Donchin[19] and Pritchard[76]).

A common paradigm for eliciting P300 is to present a train of stimuli of which 20 percent or fewer deviate from the others in some feature. Subjects are usually required either to count the "oddball" stimuli or to press a button whenever they occur. Figure 8–4 shows ERPs from this kind of paradigm. The frequent stimuli were 800 cycles-per-second tone pips given with a probability of occurrence of 0.85, and the infrequent stimuli were 1,200 cycles-per-second tone pips with a probability of 0.15. Subjects were told to press to the higher-pitch tone.

In such paradigms, P300 latencies in schizophrenic patients are often close to control values, although schizophrenic RTs are significantly later.[85] This implies that most of their slowness occurs after stimulus evaluation, probably at the motor preparation or execution stages. Demented patients show distinctly later P300s than control subjects, indicating delay in the stimulus evaluation stage. Unfortunately for diagnostic purposes, later P300s occur regardless of whether the dementia is due to Alzheimer's disease,[102] Huntington's disease,[33] or Parkinson's disease.[34] Furthermore, the differences between demented patients, schizophrenic patients, and age-matched controls are more statistical and quantitative than categorical and qualitative, in that some subjects who are demented have P300 latencies equal to those of controls, while some schizophrenic patients have significantly longer latencies.[75] Some of this variability can be attributed to differences in the degree of cognitive impairment.[34,75]

Hyperactive children have slower reaction times than control children. Reaction times become shorter as the child gets older or if the child is treated with methylphenidate hydrochloride. A comparison of P300 latency and RT in a paradigm of the type just described showed that RT speeding with maturation has a different mechanism from that of RT speeding after methylphenidate.[32] As children age, their P300 latency gets shorter, showing that they can process the stimuli more quickly. Methylphenidate, on the other hand, does not shorten P300. It reduces RT solely by affecting motor preparation or execution. The latency of other ERP components also changes with age. A comparison of these changes in hyperactive and normal children does not support a simple hypothesis of maturational lag in hyperactive children.[13]

P300 amplitude is often markedly reduced in psychiatric patients. One of the most reproducible findings of biological psychiatry is the reduction of P300 amplitude in schizophrenic patients.* Figure 8–4 is an example of schizophrenic and control P300s. What is the reason for this reduction? Some possible reasons have already been ruled out. First, it was possible to demonstrate with special averaging methods that P300 reduction was not a simple consequence of greater latency variability underlying trials that make up the ERP average.[86] Second, P300 reduction in schizophrenic patients cannot be explained by deficits in probability perception, a cognitive process important for determining P300 amplitude. This amplitude is inversely related to the subjective probability of the stimulus eliciting it.[76] Subjective probability is influenced by the sequence of events in a series, even when the series is completely random and has a constant global probability. For example, normal subjects react to a new stimulus type with a larger P300 when it has been preceded by a run of five of the old stimulus type than when it has been preceded by a run of only two. Schizophrenic patients react in exactly the same way, although their overall P300 amplitude is lower.[22] Incidentally, these sequential effects imply the existence of an intact short-term memory to keep track of the number of recent repetitions of each stimulus type. Third, P300 reduction is unlikely to be a direct or indirect effect of antipsychotic medication. Such medication tends to increase rather than to decrease P300 amplitude.[50]

Why then is P300 amplitude less in schizophrenic patients? One possibility is that smaller P300s result from an affective-motivational disinterest or uninvolvement in the experimental task. In experiments with normal subjects, P300s to stimuli of low or moderate intensity are greatly increased in amplitude when the stimuli are made task-relevant. Yet, whatever the motivating task, P300 amplitude in schizophrenic patients falls below control levels. For example, when monetary rewards were linked to certain stimuli, those stimuli evoked larger P300s in control subjects but not in schizophrenic patients.[6] This kind of effect may be mediated through the attentional differences we have discussed; less involved or motivated subjects may be less attentive. The inattention and uninvolvement may be manifested by smaller P300s even when no explicit task is given.[81]

A second possibility is that the P300 reduction in schizophrenic patients cannot be explained in terms of these psychological varia-

*See references 2, 22, 48, 54, 72, 81, 85, 87, 94, and 105.

bles but represents some new, not understood psychophysiological aberration. Some evidence for this possibility comes from an experiment in which only trials falling within a single, common latency range were selected from each schizophrenic and control subject series, counteracting the overall tendency for mean reaction times to be longer in schizophrenic patients than in control subjects.[86] Schizophrenic patients had smaller P300s than control subjects even on these selected trials, trials for which involvement and motivation were presumably more nearly equal between the groups. This finding has been replicated in another laboratory.[2]

P300 reduction has much in common with another psychophysiological characteristic of schizophrenia, skin conductance response (SCR) nonresponding.[82] Over 50 percent of schizophrenic patients give no SCR to moderate-intensity auditory stimuli, while only 15 percent of control subjects fail to do so.[3,68] Both SCR and P300 are affected by many of the same task and stimulus variables,[80] although P300 tends to habituate more slowly.[83] Task-relevant stimuli elicit larger P300s and SCRs than task-irrelevant stimuli in both schizophrenic patients and control subjects, but both responses to task-relevant stimuli remain smaller in schizophrenic subjects.[4,85] Both P300 and SCR are examples of responses associated with complex stimulus processing that can be evoked either by tasks or automatically by novel or salient stimuli. The failure of novel stimuli to evoke P300 and SCR in schizophrenic patients must mean a deficit somewhere in this orienting response mechanism.

Whatever the cause of P300 or SCR nonresponsivity, neither phenomenon is specific to schizophrenic patients. In a comparison of demented, schizophrenic, and depressed patients with age-matched controls, all of the patient groups had reduced P300 roughly in relation to the global severity of their mental disturbance.[75] P300 latency also increased in proportion to severity. Others have found P300 amplitude to be reduced in hyperactive children[64] and children at high risk for schiz-

ophrenia.[29] Similarly, SCR nonresponding occurs in children at risk for schizophrenia and in depressed patients.[68] Thus both responses represent some kind of general deficit, whose basis and extent in disabled populations is unknown.

The criticisms of attentional ERP paradigms apply to stage or process deficit paradigms as well: lack of diagnostic specificity for any known stage or process deficit, absence of practical examples of ERPs measuring what RT cannot, and the overriding influence of motivational factors on supposedly specific ERP and behavioral outcome measures. One of the reasons that the same criticisms apply is that attentional deficits may mediate many of the stage or process deficits observed. What appear to be deficits in a specific process may merely be consequences of the ordering of that process on a general difficulty dimension on which certain processes are vulnerable not because of their specific natures, but because they take more processing resources.

Certain of these criticisms have been met, at least in part, by ERP researchers and others. For example, even though RT or other behavioral paradigms are able to distinguish deficits in stimulus and response stages of processing, ERPs may be able to make this distinction more quickly with fewer experimental conditions. P300 amplitude is empirically superior to RT in distinguishing schizophrenic from control subjects in simple paradigms where both are measured. Finally, by administering a combination of ERP tests with the proper cognitive and psychometric properties, it should be possible to distinguish general from specific deficits.[15]

¶ Multivariate Classification

Although unstimulated EEG data from single-frequency bands and single derivations show much overlap between groups, a multivariate combination can be more successful. The same applies to the parameters of ERPs. A general rationale for a multivariate approach is that since the clinical phenomenology on which clinical groupings are made is complex and takes into account a constellation of features, no one EEG feature is likely to separate one group from all the others. Whatever the theoretical validity of such justifications, empirically it has been shown that multiple EEG features give better group separations, even after removing their statistical biases.

One of the most ambitious neurophysiological testing and analysis systems uses a battery of forty-seven different test scores taken from various spontaneous EEG, auditory, visual, and somatosensory ERP measures.[44,45] The battery does not require verbal interactions or behavioral response, and thus is suitable for subjects who are capable of only minimal cooperation. Recording is made from multiple scalp electrodes. Multivariate methods create statistics that can discriminate among neurological diseases such as brain tumors, cerebrovascular accidents, and epilepsy; between learning disabled and normal children; and between normal elderly and demented elderly. About 84 percent of the demented and normal elderly were classified correctly when each case was classified on the basis of a function developed from the rest of the subjects. Prominent individual discriminating variables were auditory ERP interhemispheric asymmetry and delta power, both of which were increased in demented subjects. A classification of a new group of demented patients by the old function was equally accurate. A multivariate method known as cluster analysis was used to subdivide broad diagnostic categories on the basis of EEG and ERP variables. This method showed that the demented elderly could be differentiated into at least four subgroups, one of which did not have excessive slow waves.

Another multivariate testing and analysis system was able to distinguish medicated and unmedicated schizophrenic patients from control subjects.[65] The test battery included eyes-open and eyes-closed recording of the spontaneous EEG and visual and auditory stimulus presentation while the subjects sat passively with their eyes closed. Twenty EEG leads with ear references and eye leads picked up electrical activity. The success rate of classification into controls and patients was 84 percent for medicated schizophrenic patients and 82 percent for unmedicated schizophrenic patients. Features important in the classification were that in certain leads, compared to control subjects, schizophrenic patients had decreased alpha power, decreased theta variability, increased beta variability, and decreased auditory ERP amplitudes in the 104- to 124-millisecond range.

In another study a combination of somatosensory ERP measures were able to distinguish between psychotic depressive and chronic schizophrenic patients.[96] A selection of 7 measurements taken from 135 (nine peaks times fifteen leads) could classify thirty-one of thirty-two patients correctly, half of whom were depressive and half, schizophrenic, and three measurements could classify thirty of thirty-two. The four earlier peaks (P_{12}, N_{20}, P_{45}, and N_{60}) were larger in the schizophrenic patients, and three later ones (P_{90}, N_{130}, and P_{185}) were larger in the depressed patients. Since the classifying measures were selected retrospectively from a large number of possibilities, the validity of their discriminatory power awaits confirmation in a new patient sample.

Multivariate methods have also been used to classify psychoactive drugs. One proprietary system classifies them on the basis of EEG and auditory ERP data recorded before and after drug administration to normal subjects.[41] Only healthy subjects with EEGs containing alpha activity are used in these studies. EEG parameters are derived by spectral analysis and analysis of the period of baseline crossings. Using two methods, stepwise discriminant analysis and correlation of profiles of variables, drugs are classified into five classes: anxiolytic, antidepressant, psychostimulant, neuroleptic, or placebo. A variety of known active drugs from each class were classified retrospectively with an accuracy of 100 percent using discriminant analysis. The accuracy of prospective classification of additional known active drugs is about 60 percent. Figure 8–1 is an illustration of the correct classification of chlorpromazine as a neuroleptic. Correlation of profiles has a similar accuracy. The properties of several new possibly psychoactive drugs were correctly predicted by this system.

Most criticisms of multivariate methods revolve around two issues: their lack of generalizability and the apparent randomness of the variables that are given weight. First, a generalizable discrimination function is one that is successful in classifying samples other than the ones from which the function was developed. Although authors are all aware of the weakness of solely retrospective classification, they are less sensitive to the fact that individuals in one sample of patients from a given diagnostic population have more in common with each other, not only on the variables relevant to their pathology but also on irrelevant variables, than individuals from different samples drawn at a different time and place from the same population. As a result, validation of discriminant functions by leaving out the subject being classified (the jackknife procedure) is usually more encouraging than cross-validation between separately recruited samples at the same place, which in turn is more encouraging than cross-validation between research centers. A false optimism can also result from the fact that in some statistical packages the jackknife procedure uses a formula that puts undue weight on variables already chosen.

The apparent randomness of some variables selected by multivariate methods may in fact represent random statistical artifact. On the other hand, they may represent independent unknown features of the classification. Constraining the numbers of variables entered into analysis on the basis of some prior anatomical or neurophysiological knowledge will increase the likelihood that the ones chosen by the statistical procedure will be valid and interpretable. Multivariate statistics alone, without hypotheses or knowledge from separate parametric experiments, provide no guarantee that the variables chosen will be meaningful and do not tell the experi-

menter what new measures to add to improve the classification.

¶ Clinical Implications

During the last decade there have been numerous studies of the human neurophysiology of psychiatric patients and drug states. The methodology of these studies has often been of a very high quality; patient groups have been well defined, electrophysiological recording has been extensive in time and space, artifacts have been controlled or taken into account, and the behavior of the subject during recording has been observed. Yet no practical clinical application of these techniques has yet emerged.

The reasons for the experimental rather than clinical status of human neurophysiology in psychiatry can be understood in terms of two concepts: sensitivity and specificity. By sensitivity is meant the ability of these techniques to separate patients from controls or medicated subjects from unmedicated subjects. Often neurophysiological methods are less sensitive than clinical observation in detecting minor amounts of mental deviance. Even with severely ill patients and well-screened controls, misclassification of subjects often reaches unacceptable levels. Specificity is the ability of these techniques to distinguish between subjects with different diagnoses or between subjects who received different drugs. Our studies of P300 and our reading of the clinical P300 literature, for example, lead us to believe that a general cognitive impairment present to some degree in patients with schizophrenia, affective disorder, and dementia affects P300 similarly in all of them. Therefore, P300 deviance in the paradigms used so far cannot help us in making diagnostic distinctions that are important clinically. Perhaps existing multivariate techniques can make these distinctions, but demonstration of their effectiveness in hands other than those of their originators is needed before they can be generally adopted.

The clinical success of neurophysiological techniques in neurology and in the evaluation of sleep is a demonstration that the fault does not lie in the techniques themselves, but in what they are being asked to do. Neurological diseases are characterized by distinct lesions that affect neural pathways whose functions are fairly well understood. A good example is multiple sclerosis, with its optic tract lesions. EEG and other physiological channels are useful in evaluating sleep disorders because they reflect the phenomenology of sleep so closely and objectively. Unlike neurological disorders, psychiatric disorders are usually without distinct lesions, and the neurological mechanisms underlying the complex mental behavior that is disturbed by these diseases are unknown.

The problems of specificity and sensitivity are not those of human electrophysiology alone. Behavioral tests of mental disorder have the same failings. What appeared to be the first practical physiological test for mental disease, the dexamethasone suppression test, has turned out to be limited in exactly the same ways—specificity and sensitivity, as described in chapter 35. Many postulated biochemical abnormalities in schizophrenia and affective disorders have fallen by the wayside for the same reasons. The chief advantage of biochemical theories lies not in their ability to develop tests for psychiatric diseases but in their stimulating influence on the development of new psychotherapeutic drugs.

These problems do not mean that there is any intrinsic reason that human neurophysiology will never have practical clinical applications, only that specific and sensitive tests are a matter for future development. ERPs in particular provide a window on the functioning human brain that is unparalleled in its temporal resolution. Millisecond-by-millisecond monitoring of electrical activity accompanying mental events is possible. A convergence of insights from new brain imaging techniques, some of which permit the observation of regional metabolism, and more extensive spatial mapping of the spontaneous EEG and ERPs in terms of both electrical potential and magnetic field should lead to a better understanding of psychiatric disorders and to new ways of diagnosing and quantifying them.

¶ Acknowledgments

Preparation of this manuscript was supported by the Veterans Administration. We thank Margaret Rosenbloom for her assistance. Drs. Callaway, Gevins, Itil, and Shagass made helpful comments on an earlier draft.

¶ Bibliography

1. ADLER, L. E., et al. "Neurophysiological Evidence for a Defect in Neuronal Mechanisms Involved in Sensory Gating in Schizophrenia," *Biological Psychiatry,* 17 (1982):639–654.
2. BARIBEAU-BRAUN, J., et al. "Schizophrenia: A Neurophysiological Evaluation of Abnormal Information Processing," *Science,* 219 (1983):874–876.
3. BERNSTEIN, A. S., et al. "An Analysis of the Skin Conductance Orienting Response in Samples of American, British, and German Schizophrenics," *Biological Psychology,* 14 (1982):155–211.
4. BERNSTEIN, A. S., et al. "A Limiting Factor in the Normalization of Schizophrenic Orienting Response Dysfunction," *Schizophrenia Bulletin,* 1985, in press.
5. BODIS-WOLLNER, I., et al. "Dopaminergic Deficiency and Delayed Visual Evoked Potentials in Humans," *Annals of Neurology,* 11 (1982):478–483.
6. BRECHER, M., and BEGLEITER, H. "Event-related Brain Potentials to High Incentive Stimuli in Unmedicated Schizophrenics," *Biological Psychiatry,* 18 (1982):661–674.
7. BROEN, W. E. *Schizophrenia Research and Theory.* New York: Academic Press, 1968.
8. BUCHSBAUM, M. S. "The Middle Evoked

Response Components and Schizophrenia," *Schizophrenia Bulletin,* 3 (1977): 93–104.

9. BUCHSBAUM, M. S., and COPPOLA, R. "Signal-to-Noise Ratio and Response Variability in Affective Disorders and Schizophrenia," in H. Begleiter, ed., *Evoked Brain Potentials and Behavior.* New York: Plenum Press, 1979, pp. 447–466.

10. BUCHSBAUM, M. S., COPPOLA, R., and CAPPELLETTI, J. "Positron Emission Tomography, EEG and Evoked Potential Topography: New Approaches to Local Function in Pharmaco-Electroencephalography," in W. M. Herrmann, ed., *Electroencephalography in Drug Research.* Stuttgart: Gustav Fischer, 1982, pp. 193–207.

11. CALLAWAY, E. "Schizophrenia and Interference," *Archives of General Psychiatry,* 22 (1970):193–208.

12. ———. *Brain Electric Potentials and Individual Psychological Differences,* New York: Grune & Stratton, 1975.

13. CALLAWAY, E., HALLIDAY, R., and NAYLOR, H. "Hyperactive Children's Event-Related Potentials Fail to Support Underarousal and Maturational-Lag Theories," *Archives of General Psychiatry,* 40 (1983):1243–1248.

14. CALLAWAY, E., JONES, R. T., and DONCHIN, E. "Auditory Evoked Potential Variability in Schizophrenia," *Electroencephalography and Clinical Neurophysiology,* 29 (1970):421–428.

15. CHAPMAN, L. J., and CHAPMAN, J. P. "The Measurement of Differential Deficit," *Journal of Psychiatric Research,* 14 (1978):303–311.

16. COGER, R. W., DYMOND, A. M., and SERAFETINIDES, E. A. "Electroencephalographic Similarities between Chronic Alcoholics and Chronic, Nonparanoid Schizophrenics," *Archives of General Psychiatry,* 36 (1979):91–94.

17. CONNOLLY, J. F., and GRUZELIER, J. H. "Amplitude and Latency Changes in the Visual Evoked Potential (VEP) to Different Stimulus Intensities," *Psychophysiology,* 19 (1982):599–608.

18. DAVIS, G. C., et al. "Analgesia to Pain Stimuli in Schizophrenics and Its Reversal by Naltrexone," *Psychiatry Research,* 1 (1979):61–69.

19. DONCHIN, E. "Surprise! . . . Surprise?" *Psychophysiology,* 18 (1981):493–513.

20. DONGIER, M., DUBROVSKY, B., and ENGELSMANN, F. "Event-Related Slow Potentials in Psychiatry," in C. Shagass, S. Gershon, and A. J. Friedhoff, eds., *Psychopathology and Brain Dysfunction.* New York: Raven Press, 1977, pp. 339–352.

21. DUFFY, F. H., ALBERT, M. S., and McANULTY, G. "Brain Electrical Activity in Patients with Presenile and Senile Dementia of the Alzheimer's Type," *Annals of Neurology,* 16 (1984):439–448.

22. DUNCAN-JOHNSON, C. C., ROTH, W. T., and KOPELL, B. S. "Effects of Stimulus Sequence on P300 and Reaction Time in Schizophrenics: A Preliminary Report," in R. Karrer, J. Cohen, and P. Tueting, eds., *Brain and Information: Event-Related Potentials. Annals of the New York Academy of Science,* 425 (1984):570–577.

23. ENGEL, G. L., and ROMANO, J. "Delirium, A Syndrome of Cerebral Insufficiency," *Journal of Chronic Disease,* 9 (1959): 260–277.

24. FENTON, G. W., et al. "EEG Spectral Analysis in Schizophrenia," *British Journal of Psychiatry,* 136 (1980):445–455.

25. FLOR-HENRY, P. *Cerebral Basis of Psychopathology.* Boston: John Wright, 1983.

26. FLOR-HENRY, P., et al. "Neurophysiological Studies on Schizophrenia, Mania, and Depression," in J. Gruzelier and P. Flor-Henry, eds., *Hemisphere Asymmetries of Function in Psychopathology.* Amsterdam: Elsevier/North Holland Biomedical Press, 1979, pp. 189–222.

27. FRANKS, R. D., et al. "Neurophysiological Studies of Sensory Gating in Mania: Comparison with Schizophrenia," *Biological Psychiatry,* 18 (1983):989–1005.

28. FREEDMAN, R., et al. "Neurophysiological Evidence for a Defect in Inhibitory Pathways in Schizophrenia: Comparison of Medicated and Drug-free Patients," *Biological Psychiatry,* 18 (1983): 537–551.

29. FRIEDMAN, D., VAUGHAN, H. G., and ERLENMEYER-KIMLING, L. "Cognitive Brain Potentials in Children at Risk for

Schizophrenia: Preliminary Findings and Methodological Considerations," *Schizophrenia Bulletin,* 8 (1982):514–531.

30. GEVINS, A. S., et al. "Shadows of Thought: Shifting Lateralization of Human Brain Electric Patterns During Brief Visuomotor Task," *Science,* 220 (1983):97–99.

31. GOLDSTEIN, L., et al. "Electro-cerebral Activity in Schizophrenics and Nonpsychotic Subjects: Quantitative EEG Amplitude Analysis," *Electroencephalography and Clinical Neurophysiology,* 19 (1965):350–361.

32. HALLIDAY, R., CALLAWAY, E., and NAYLOR, H. "Visual Evoked Potential Changes Induced by Methylphenidate in Hyperactive Children: Dose/Response Effects," *Electroencephalography and Clinical Neurophysiology,* 55 (1983):258–267.

33. HANSCH, E. C., et al. "Event-Related Potentials in Huntington's Disease: Preliminary Data (Abstract)," *Bulletin of the Los Angeles Neurological Society,* 45 (1980):61.

34. HANSCH, E. C., et al. "Cognition in Parkinson's Disease: An Event-Related Potential Perspective," *Annals of Neurology,* 11 (1982):599–607.

35. HEATH, R. G. *Studies in Schizophrenia.* Cambridge, Mass.: Harvard University Press, 1954.

36. HERRMANN, W. M. "Development and Critical Evaluation of an Objective Procedure for the Electroencephalographic Classification of Psychotropic Drugs," in W. M. Herrmann, ed., *Electroencephalography in Drug Research.* Stuttgart: Gustav Fischer, 1982, pp. 249–351.

37. HILLYARD, S. A., and KUTAS, M. "Electrophysiology of Cognitive Processing," *Annual Review of Psychology,* 34 (1983):33–61.

38. IACONO, W. G. "Bilateral Electrodermal Habituation-dishabituation and Resting EEG in Remitted Schizophrenics," *Journal of Nervous and Mental Disease,* 170 (1982):91–101.

39. IACONO, W. G., GABBAY, F. H., and LYKKEN, D. T. "Measuring the Average Evoked Response to Light Flashes: The Contribution of Eye-Blink Artifact to Augmenting-Reducing," *Biological Psychiatry,* 17 (1982):897–911.

40. ITIL, T. M. "Qualitative and Quantitative EEG Findings in Schizophrenia," *Schizophrenia Bulletin,* 3 (1977):61–79.

41. ———. "The Significance of Quantitative Pharmaco-EEG in the Discovery and Classification of Psychotropic Drugs," in W. M. Herrmann, ed., *Electroencephalography in Drug Research.* Stuttgart: Gustav Fischer, 1982, pp. 131–157.

42. ITIL, T. M., SALETU, B., and DAVIS, S. "EEG Findings in Chronic Schizophrenics Based on Digital Computer Period Analysis and Analog Power Spectra," *Biological Psychiatry,* 5 (1972):1–13.

43. ITIL, T. M., et al. "Computerized EEG as a Predictor of Drug Response in Treatment Resistant Schizophrenics," *Journal of Nervous and Mental Disease,* 169 (1981):629–637.

44. JOHN, E. R. *Functional Neuroscience,* vol. 2 of E. R. John and R. W. Thatcher, eds., *Neurometrics: Clinical Applications of Quantitative Electrophysiology.* Hillsdale, N.J.: Lawrence Erlbaum Associates, 1977, pp. 143–174.

45. JOHN, E. R., et al. "Neurometrics," *Science,* 196 (1977):1393–1410.

46. JOHNSTONE, E. C., et al. "Cerebral Ventricular Size and Cognitive Impairment in Chronic Schizophrenics," *Lancet,* 2 (1976):924–926.

47. JONES, R. T., BLACKER, K. H., and CALLAWAY, E. "Perceptual Dysfunction in Schizophrenia: Clinical and Auditory Evoked Response Findings," *American Journal of Psychiatry,* 123 (1966):639–645.

48. JOSIASSEN, R. C., et al. "The Attention-related Somatosensory Evoked Potential Late Positive Wave in Psychiatric Patients," *Psychiatry Research,* 5 (1981):147–156.

49. JOSIASSEN, R. C., et al. "Somatosensory Evoked Potential Changes with a Selective Attention Task," *Psychophysiology,* 19 (1982):146–159.

50. JOSIASSEN, R. C., et al. "Psychiatric Drugs and the Somatosensory P400 Wave," *Psychiatry Research,* 11 (1984):151–162.

51. KAUFMAN, L., and WILLIAMSON, S. F.

"Magnetic Location of Cortical Activity," in I. Bodis-Wollner, ed. *Evoked Potentials. Annals of the New York Academy of Sciences*, 388 (1982):197–213.

52. KENDLER, K. S., and HAYS, P. "Familial and Sporadic Schizophrenia: A Symptomatic, Prognostic, and EEG Comparison," *American Journal of Psychiatry*, 139 (1982):1557–1562.

53. LEISSNER, P., LINDHOLM, L. D., and PETERSEN, I. "Alpha Amplitude Dependence on Skull Thickness as Measured by Ultrasound Technique," *Electroencephalography and Clinical Neurophysiology*, 29 (1970):392–399.

54. LEVIT, R. A., SUTTON, S., and ZUBIN, J. "Evoked Potential Correlates of Information Processing in Psychiatric Patients," *Psychological Medicine*, 3 (1973):487–494.

55. LIFSHITZ, K., and GRADIJAN, J. "Relationship Between Measures of the Coefficient of Variation of the Mean Absolute EEG Voltage and Spectral Intensities in Schizophrenic and Control Subjects," *Biological Psychiatry*, 5 (1972):149–163.

56. ———. "Spectral Evaluation of the Electroencephalogram: Power and Variability in Chronic Schizophrenics and Control Subjects," *Psychophysiology*, 11 (1974):479–490.

57. LISHMAN, W. A. *Organic Psychiatry*, Oxford: Blackwell Scientific Publications, 1978.

58. LUBIN, A., JOHNSON, L. C., and AUSTIN, M. T. "Discrimination Among States of Consciousness Using EEG Spectra," *Psychophysiology*, 6 (1969):122–132.

59. McGHIE, A., and CHAPMAN, J. "Disorders of Attention and Perception in Early Schizophrenia," *British Journal of Medical Psychology*, 34 (1961):103–116.

60. MALERSTEIN, A. J., and CALLAWAY, E. "Two-tone Average Evoked Response in Korsakoff Patients," *Journal of Psychiatric Research*, 6 (1969):253–260.

61. MARJERRRISON, G., KRAUSE, A. E., and KEOGH, R. P. "Variability of the EEG in Schizophrenia: Quantitative Analysis with a Modulus Voltage Integrator," *Electroencephalography and Clinical Neurophysiology*, 24 (1968):35–41.

62. MATEJCEK, M. "Vigilance and the EEG: Psychological, Physiological and Pharmacological Aspects," in W. M. Herrmann, ed., *Electroencephalography in Drug Research*. Stuttgart: Gustav Fischer, 1982, pp. 405–508.

63. MATOUSEK, M., CAPONE, C., and OKAWA, M. "Measurement of the Inter-Hemispheral Differences as a Diagnostic Tool in Psychiatry," in C. Perris, D. Kemali, and L. Vacca, eds., *Advances in Biological Psychiatry*, vol. 6. Basel: S. Karger, 1981, pp. 76–80.

64. MICHAEL, R. L., et al. "Normalizing Effects of Methylphenidate on Hyperactive Children's Vigilance Performance and Evoked Potentials," *Psychophysiology*, 18 (1981):665–667.

65. MORIHISA, J. M., DUFFY, F. H., and WYATT, R. J. "Brain Electrical Activity Mapping (BEAM) in Schizophrenic Patients," *Archives of General Psychiatry*, 40 (1983):719–728.

66. NEALE, J. M., and OLTMANNS, T. F. *Schizophrenia*. New York: John Wiley & Sons, 1980.

67. ÖHMAN, A. "The Orienting Response, Attention, and Learning: An Information Processing Perspective," in H. D. Kimmel et al., eds., *The Orienting Reflex in Humans*. Hillsdale, N.J.: Lawrence Erlbaum Associates, 1979, pp. 443–471.

68. ———. "Electrodermal Activity and Vulnerability to Schizophrenia: A Review," *Biological Psychology*, 2 (1981):87–145.

69. OKADA, Y. C., KAUFMAN, L., and WILLIAMSON, S. L. "The Hippocampal Formation as a Source of the Slow Endogenous Potentials," *Electroencephalography and Clinical Neurophysiology*, 55 (1983):417–426.

70. OLTMANNS, T. F. "Selective Attention in Schizophrenic and Manic Psychoses: The Effect of Distraction on Information Processing," *Journal of Abnormal Psychology*, 87 (1978):212–225.

71. OLTMANNS, T. F., and NEALE, J. M. "Schizophrenic Performance When Distractors Are Present: Attentional Deficit or Differential Task Difficulty?" *Journal of Abnormal Psychology*, 84 (1975):205–209.

72. PASS, H. L., et al. "The Late Positive Component of the Evoked Response in Acute Schizophrenics During a Test of

Sustained Attention," *Biological Psychiatry,* 15 (1980):9–20.

73. PFEFFERBAUM, A., et al. "EEG Effects of Physostigmine and Choline Chloride in Humans," *Psychopharmacology,* 62 (1979):225–233.

74. PFEFFERBAUM, A., et al. "Auditory Brain Stem and Cortical Evoked Potentials in Schizophrenia," *Biological Psychiatry,* 15 (1980):209–223.

75. PFEFFERBAUM, A., et al. "Clinical Application of the P3 Component of Event-related Potentials. II. Dementia, Depression and Schizophrenia," *Electroencephalography and Clinical Neurophysiology,* 59 (1984):104–124.

76. PRITCHARD, W. S. "Psychophysiology of P300," *Psychological Bulletin,* 90 (1981):506–540.

77. RAINE, A., MITCHELL, D. A., and VENABLES, P. H. "Cortical Augmenting-Reducing—Modality Specific?" *Psychophysiology,* 18 (1981):700–708.

78. ROHRBAUGH, J. W., and GAILLARD, A.W.K. "Sensory and Motor Aspects of the Contingent Negative Variation," in A.W.K. Gaillard and W. Ritter, eds., *Tutorials in ERP Research: Endogenous Components.* Amsterdam: North Holland Publishing Company, 1983, pp. 269–310.

79. ROTH, W. T. "Late Event-related Potentials and Psychopathology," *Schizophrenia Bulletin,* 3 (1977):105–120.

80. ———. "A Comparison of P300 and Skin Conductance Response," in A.W.K. Gaillard and W. Ritter, eds., *Tutorials in ERP Research: Endogenous Components.* Amsterdam: North-Holland Publishing Company, 1983, pp. 177–199.

81. ROTH, W. T., and CANNON, E. H. "Some Features of the Auditory Evoked Response in Schizophrenics," *Archives of General Psychiatry,* 27 (1972):466–471.

82. ROTH, W. T., and TINKLENBERG, J. R. "A Convergence of Findings in the Psychophysiology of Schizophrenia," *Psychopharmacology Bulletin,* 18 (1982):78–83.

83. ROTH, W. T., DORATO, K. H., and KOPELL, B. S. "Intensity and Task Effects on Evoked Physiological Responses to Noise Bursts," *Psychophysiology,* 21 (1984):466–481.

84. ROTH, W. T., PFEFFERBAUM, A., and

WENEGRAT, B. "Eye Artifact in EEG Research," in preparation.

85. ROTH, W. T., et al. "Event-related Potentials in Schizophrenics," *Electroencephalography and Clinical Neurophysiology,* 48 (1980):127–139.

86. ROTH, W. T., et al. "P3 Reduction in Auditory Evoked Potentials of Schizophrenics," *Electroencephalography and Clinical Neurophysiology,* 49 (1980):497–505.

87. ROTH, W. T., et al. "Auditory Event-related Potentials in Schizophrenia and Depression," *Psychiatry Research,* 4 (1981):199–212.

88. ROTH, W. T., et al. "Auditory Stimulus Intensity Effects on Components of the Late Positive Complex," *Electroencephalography and Clinical Neurophysiology,* 54 (1982):132–146.

89. ROTH, W. T., et al. "ERPs and Psychopathology: Behavior Process Issues," in R. Karrer, J. Cohen, and P. Tueting, eds., *Brain and Information: Event-Related Potentials. Annals of the New York Academy of Science,* 425 (1984):496–522.

90. SCHWARTZ, M., and SHAGASS, C. "Reticular Modification of Somatosensory Cortical Recovery Function," *Electroencephalography and Clinical Neurophysiology,* 15 (1963):265–271.

91. SHAGASS, C. *Evoked Brain Potentials in Psychiatry.* New York: Plenum Press, 1972.

92. ———. "An Electrophysiological View of Schizophrenia," *Biological Psychiatry,* 11 (1976):3–30.

93. SHAGASS, C., ROEMER, R. A., and STRAUMANIS, J. J. "Relationships Between Psychiatric Diagnosis and Some Quantitative EEG Variables," *Archives of General Psychiatry,* 39 (1982):1423–1435.

94. SHAGASS, C., et al. "Evoked Potential Correlates of Psychosis," *Biological Psychiatry,* 13 (1978):163–184.

95. SHAGASS, C., et al. "Temporal Variability of Somatosensory, Visual, and Auditory Evoked Potentials in Schizophrenics," *Archives of General Psychiatry,* 35 (1979):1341–1351.

96. SHAGASS, C., et al. "Differentiation of Depressive and Schizophrenic Psychoses

by Evoked Potentials," in C. Perris, D. Kemali, and L. Vacca, *Advances in Biological Psychiatry,* vol. 6. Basel: S. Karger, 1981, pp. 173–179.

97. SIEGEL, C., et al. "Deficits in Sensory Gating in Schizophrenic Patients and Their Relatives," *Archives of General Psychiatry,* 41 (1984):607–612.

98. SPOHN, H. E., and PATTERSON, T. "Recent Studies of Psychophysiology in Schizophrenia," *Schizophrenia Bulletin,* 5 (1979):581–611.

99. SQUIRE, L. R. "The Neuropsychology of Human Memory," *Annual Review of Neuroscience,* 5 (1982):241–273.

100. STEVENS, J. R., and LIVERMORE, A. "Telemetered EEG in Schizophrenia: Spectral Analysis During Abnormal Behavior Episodes," *Journal of Neurology, Neurosurgery, and Psychiatry,* 45 (1982):385–395.

101. STEVENS, J. R., et al. "Telemetered EEG-EOG During Psychotic Behaviors of Schizophrenia," *Archives of General Psychiatry,* 36 (1979):251–262.

102. SYNDULKO, K., et al. "Long Latency Event-Related Potentials in Normal Aging and Dementia," in J. Courjon, F. Mauguiere, and M. Revol, eds., *Clinical Applications of Evoked Potentials in Neurology.* New York: Raven Press, 1982, pp. 279–285.

103. TIMSIT-BERTHIER, M. "Contingent Negative Variation (CNV) in Psychiatry," *Electroencephalography and Clinical Neurophysiology* (Supplement), in press.

104. VANDERWOLF, C. H., and ROBINSON, T. E. "Reticulo-Cortical Activity and Behavior: A Critique of the Arousal Theory and a New Synthesis," *Behavioral and Brain Sciences,* 43 (1981):459–476.

105. VERLEGER, R., and COHEN, R. "Effects of Certainty, Modality Shift, and Guess Outcome on Evoked Potentials and Reaction Times in Chronic Schizophrenics," *Psychological Medicine,* 8 (1978):81–93.

106. VOLAVKA, J., et al. "Hemispheric Lateralization of Fast EEG Activity in Schizophrenia and Endogenous Depression," in C. Perris, J. Kemali, and L. Vacca, eds., *Advances in Biological Psychiatry,* vol. 6. Basel: S. Karger, 1981, pp. 72–75.

107. WEINBERGER, D. R., et al. "Lateral Cerebral Ventricular Enlargement in Chronic Schizophrenia," *Archives of General Psychiatry,* 36 (1979):735–739.

CHAPTER 9

ANATOMICAL AND CT SCAN STUDIES OF PSYCHIATRIC DISORDERS

Terry L. Jernigan

¶ Introduction

For many years, investigators have searched for neuroanatomical features that distinguish the primary disorders of personality and cognition. Histopathological studies have produced many reported abnormalities in the brains of psychiatric patients,[30,151,165] but only in dementia of the Alzheimer's type (DAT) have these findings proven to be reliable and reasonably specific to the disorder.[12,139,156] The findings in other psychiatric disorders clearly do not yet point to specific, pathognomonic alterations in cerebral structure. When a promising finding has emerged, it has sometimes been challenged because of uncertainty about agonal or postmortem effects. Nevertheless, postmortem studies, with rapidly improving methodology, continue to lead to speculations about neuropathological factors in psychiatric disorders (see chapter 5). Stevens[151] recently reported fibrillary gliosis in periventricular, periaqueductal, and basal forebrain structures in schizophrenic patients and hypothesizes that this may be related to inflammation.

In vivo anatomical studies began when pneumoencephalography (PEG) became available. In psychiatric disorders, findings of enlarged cerebral fluid spaces began to emerge from PEG investigations.[64,69] Unfortunately, these were followed by inconsistent results.[4] Because of associated morbidity, PEG has rarely been applied to a representative sample of psychiatric patients and controls, so inferences based on such studies have questionable generality.

Computed tomography (CT) of the brain

provided the first benign *in vivo* technique for assessing brain structure. Since its development, a great many investigations of psychiatric disorders have been undertaken with CT. Nowhere has the use of the technique generated as much controversy as in studies of schizophrenia. The discussion to follow will concentrate on this literature especially, in an attempt to outline some of the potential sources of confusion. After results from schizophrenia studies, those from studies of other psychiatric disorders not considered "organic" will be discussed. Finally, a brief summary of CT studies of dementia will be provided.

¶ CT in the Functional Disorders

Schizophrenia

NATURE AND PREVALENCE OF ABNORMALITIES

The first report of CT abnormalities in schizophrenic patients came from Johnstone and associates.[88,89] Seventeen older, institutionalized patients were compared to volunteers on planimetric area measures of the ventricles. The patients had significantly larger ventricles, and ventricular size was strongly related to measures of cognitive impairment. Because of the subjects' advanced age, their need for virtually continuous hospitalization, and their significant intellectual deficits, the generalizability of this finding to the larger schizophrenic population was uncertain.

Weinberger and associates,[166] also using a planimetric area measurement of the ventricles (ventriculo-brain ratio [VBR]), reported a similar high prevalence of ventricular enlargement in a younger group of chronic schizophrenic patients. Again, the schizophrenic group showed significant intellectual impairment, and in subsequent reports,[86] this population of patients (at the National Institute of Mental Health [NIMH]) was described as largely consisting of treatment-recalcitrant patients. Again, such char-

acteristics suggest that the sample may be unrepresentative; however, the finding stimulated much interest in the basis for such abnormalities. In neither of these early studies was any evidence found for an association between neuroleptic treatment and ventricular enlargement, nor did the abnormalities appear to relate exclusively to electroconvulsive therapy or leucotomy.

Subsequent studies of ventricular size in schizophrenia yielded highly variable results. Gluck and associates[55] found no difference between a large group of chronic schizophrenic patients and their controls on linear measures of the ventricles; however, Okasha and Madkour,[125] also using linear measures, did observe ventricular enlargement in schizophrenic patients. The diagnostic criteria, however, were not given in either of these studies. Tanaka and coworkers[153] also found no difference in their young (twenty-one to forty years) patients, but found significant ventricular enlargement in older schizophrenic patients and a correlation of third ventricular width with duration of illness. Unfortunately, the possibility that age may have been confounded with duration of illness and that age mediated this effect was not examined in their study. Andreasen[2] studied a group of chronic schizophrenic patients of comparable age to those in the study by Weinberger and associates. The patients were not chronically institutionalized, however, and were probably a more representative sample. In this study, ventricular enlargement was observed in only a small percentage of patients (6 percent).

Jernigan and associates[84] studied chronic schizophrenic patients in a veterans' hospital with a variety of measures of ventricular volume and area. The patients were somewhat older than the NIMH patients, with slightly later onset of the disorder. Two-thirds of the patients were inpatients, but all spent some time in the community. No differences were observed between these patients and volunteer controls on any CT measure. The subjects' scans were measured blindly (with a planimeter) by the NIMH group and by C. J. Golden[60] in Nebraska. No group differences were detected with these measurements either. The VBR values obtained from the two groups were dramatically different, conclusively demonstrating that control values from other studies should not be used as criteria in new studies. Nevertheless, all measures of ventricular size were highly intercorrelated, suggesting that among area and volume measures, measurement variability probably accounts for little of the discrepancy in observed prevalence of ventricular enlargement. It was concluded that differences between the patient samples probably led to disparate findings, although the critical variables could not be identified.

A possible explanation of the differences was that the NIMH patients were from a severely disturbed population of patients requiring long-term institutionalization. Certainly the proportion of patients with abnormal scans found by Andreasen and associates was much closer to that found by Jernigan and coworkers, with both of the latter patient groups fitting the more typical "revolving door" description. A number of other studies have emerged in which the patient groups had mean ages of approximately thirty and hospitalization was intermittent rather than long-term. Dewan, Pandurangi, and their associates[37] studied twenty-three schizophrenic patients not requiring chronic hospitalization and found no lateral ventricular enlargement with the VBR. They did observe enlargement of the third ventricle, however. A similar result occurred in a study by Smith and others:[146] Schizophrenic patients did not show enlarged lateral ventricles but did show some enlargement of the third ventricle and bicaudate ratio. Unfortunately, in this report the subjects were poorly described. Luchins, Lewine, and Meltzer[105] found abnormal VBRs in 11 percent of a similar sample of chronic schizophrenic patients. In a sample from a university hospital, Weinberger and coworkers[172] found that 24 percent of chronic schizophrenic patients showed ventricular enlargement. Finally, Nasrallah and associates[119] studied a group of veterans quite similar to the patients studied by Jernigan and coworkers but found that 35

percent had abnormal VBRs. Although most of the later studies have yielded considerably lower prevalence estimates than the earliest reports, the range (3 to 35 percent) is still large considering that the reported clinical characteristics of these patient groups are quite similar.

Because Johnstone and associates' original dramatic findings were in a group of older patients, many have suggested that ventricular enlargement may develop over the course of the disease in some subset of patients.[27] Woods and Wolf[175] argue forcefully that ventricular enlargement results from an inherited and progressive degenerative form of schizophrenia. Their own finding of a very small difference between the bicaudate ratios in young (mean age twenty-three) schizophrenic patients and controls is offered in support of this hypothesis. Most of the argument, however, is based on studies of twins discordant for schizophrenia,[133] in which duration of illness strongly predicts both the VBR of the schizophrenic twin and that of the normal cotwin. Consistent with this hypothesis, Benes and associates[10] found no difference in ventricular size between a group of young schizophrenic patients (mean age twenty-one) and controls. However, in a group of young (mean age twenty-one) patients with schizophreniform disorder, 20 percent showed ventricular enlargement; and Schulz and others[142,143] reported a 53 percent rate of abnormality in a group of teen-age schizophrenic patients whose duration of illness was less than twenty-four months. The authors of the latter report point out, however, that their setting is a tertiary referral source, receiving patients who are more severely affected than typical patients.

In schizophrenic patients, ventricular enlargement is the most commonly reported abnormality on CT. However, cortical atrophy, as reflected in sulcal widening, has also been observed. Weinberger and coworkers[167] found increased width of the sylvian fissure, interhemispheric fissure, and convexity sulci. They noted that ventricular enlargement and cortical atrophy were not highly correlated. Reider and associates[134] rated cortical atrophy in a group of schizophrenic patients. Although no controls were rated, neuroradiological assessment suggested that four of seventeen patients had prominent sulci. These four were age-matched to patients without prominent sulci. The patients with cortical atrophy performed much worse on neuropsychological tests. In one study,[153] more cortical atrophy was present in schizophrenic patients than controls, but only in an older group of patients (aged forty to sixty). In another study,[121] however, this finding was obtained in a group of younger patients (mean age thirty). In this study, the independence of cortical atrophy and ventricular enlargement and the association of cortical atrophy with cognitive dysfunction were again noted. Enlargement of the sylvian fissures was observed in a group of twenty-three chronic schizophrenic patients compared to headache controls,[37] and cortical atrophy occurred more frequently in a group of poorly described schizophrenic patients.[171]

Several studies could not detect any increase in cortical atrophy in schizophrenic patients. Gluck and coworkers[55] found no difference between patients and controls, but the measure of cortical atrophy—the number of enlarged sulci—was fairly crude. Jernigan and coworkers, using a measure of sulcal fluid volume previously validated in studies of aging, also found no increase in schizophrenic patients.[84] Okasha and Madkour,[125] using the same cortical measures as those used in several positive studies, found no difference between forty-three chronic schizophrenic patients and their controls.

The presence of cerebellar atrophy in schizophrenic patients was originally suggested by two uncontrolled studies,[70,164] but in an initial controlled study of vermian atrophy,[23] no differences were detected in a group of fourteen patients and twenty-one controls. Nasrallah and associates[120] also found no difference between schizophrenic patients and controls in cerebellar atrophy. Lippmann and others[100] found more vermian atrophy in a group of fifty-four schizo-

phrenic patients than in controls, and Dewan and coworkers[36] found reduced vermian width in twenty-three schizophrenic patients. Snider[147] has reviewed this research and outlines some mechanisms by which cerebellar dysfunction may contribute to schizophrenic behavior.

Another CT abnormality reported in an early study of schizophrenic patients is reversed cranial asymmetry. Earlier studies of nonschizophrenic patients[98] had demonstrated that on CT scans, the left hemicranium is usually wider and longer in the posterior areas and the right hemicranium is often larger in the frontal areas. Luchins, Weinberger, and Wyatt[106] found that in schizophrenia, a reversal of this pattern is more prevalent than in controls, especially in those schizophrenic patients without cerebral atrophy. Andreasen and associates[1] and Jernigan and others[85] were unable to confirm this finding in subsequent studies. In one study, schizophrenic patients had more cranial reversals than did a group of manic patients,[159] but no controls were studied. A second study by Luchins,[105] in which forty-five patients were compared to headache controls, yielded no differences in the incidence of reversals. Various methods have been devised to attempt to measure cranial asymmetries, and most authors agree that different methods give quite variable estimates of the prevalence of reversals. Nevertheless, it is unlikely that such measurement variability accounts for the number of negative studies. It is more likely that reversal of cranial asymmetry is not substantially more common in schizophrenic patients than in normal subjects.

Golden and coworkers[56,59] reported decreased CT attenuation values, particularly in the left anterior region, in the cerebral hemispheres of a group of twenty-one chronic schizophrenic patients compared to twenty-two controls. The method of measuring the brain attenuation values, however, was to take every fourth pixel value throughout the entire hemisphere. With this method, areas of ventricular and sulcal fluid are sampled, as well as parenchymal areas, and group differences can occur because of increased cerebrospinal fluid (CSF) spaces in the patients. Also, the patients were included only if they performed abnormally on a neuropsychological test battery, while no such criterion was applied to the controls. The relation of this finding to schizophrenia per se is therefore suspect. A subsequent study by this group[110] showed significant correlations between CT values in posterior quadrants of CT sections and lifetime neuroleptic use in schizophrenic patients. Again, whether this should be interpreted as a correlation with enlarging fluid spaces or with parenchymal values is unclear. Jernigan and associates[84] found no difference between schizophrenic patients and controls on a measure of CT values from a carefully selected sample of the centrum semiovale. Largen, Calderon, and Smith[97] also found no differences between schizophrenic patients and controls in the density of gray or white matter samples. They did observe that in schizophrenic patients the density of left-hemisphere samples was sometimes significantly lower than that of right-hemisphere samples, while significant hemispheric differences did not occur in the control subjects. Unfortunately, the group difference on this density asymmetry was not directly significance tested.

PSYCHOPATHOLOGICAL CORRELATES OF CT ABNORMALITIES

In the early reports by Johnstone and coworkers[88,89] of ventricular enlargement in schizophrenic patients, it was noted that this finding was strongly related to cognitive impairment, and that the presence of negative symptoms (such as flat affect, impoverished speech, and psychomotor retardation) was also associated with cognitive impairment. This led the authors to speculate that the cerebral abnormality might be related to the negative symptoms of schizophrenia, although this could not be demonstrated directly with their data. Soon afterward Weinberger and associates[169] found that a measure of premorbid adjustment was correlated with CT results in a group of schizophrenic patients.

Poor premorbid adjustment, especially in childhood, was associated with abnormal CT scans in adult patients.

A number of subsequent studies have examined the relationship of certain psychopathological features to CT abnormalities. Gluck and others[55] did not observe differences on CT between patients described as having "loss of potential . . . lack of impulse" and patients without these features. Andreasen and coworkers[3] attempted a systematic investigation of positive and negative symptoms in their patients. They compared sixteen patients with large ventricles (VBR > control mean + 1 standard deviation) to the sixteen patients with smallest ventricles. The large-ventricle group was significantly older than the small-ventricle group. A measure of premorbid adjustment did not show a group difference. Only one of ten measured symptoms differentiated the groups: "bizarre behavior" was more prevalent in the small-ventricle group. Composite scores were constructed from combinations of the positive and negative scores (chosen based on the degree to which they separated the groups), and a difference score between the positive and negative composite scores was computed. The positive-symptom score and the difference score were higher in the small-ventricle group. The interpretation of this study is complicated, because the symptom patterns were constructed post hoc. A study by Luchins, Lewine, and Meltzer[105] only weakly supported this finding. A measure of positive symptoms was higher in small-ventricle than large-ventricle patients, but the group difference did not reach significance. A negative symptom score was not different between the groups. The measures used were not Andreasen's, however.

Several studies have examined subgroups of the schizophrenic population to address questions raised by the findings just reviewed. Kling and associates[94] found that among schizophrenic patients in a veterans' hospital population, chronic residual patients, with more negative symptoms, had significantly larger VBRs, widened sylvian fissures, and reversed frontal asymmetry.

The chronic paranoid group was not different from controls. In another study, however, paranoid and hebephrenic subgroups showed significantly larger VBRs than an undifferentiated subgroup.[119] No correlations were found in this study between VBR and premorbid adjustment, duration of illness, or any treatment variable. In a similar study, Frangos and Athanassenas[44] found larger VBRs in paranoid patients than in hebephrenic or undifferentiated patients. Although the paranoid patient group was also older than the other groups, regression analyses suggested that age did not account for the difference on VBR. Since paranoid patients have many positive symptoms, the latter findings would seem to challenge the hypothesis that schizophrenics with CT abnormalities have predominantly negative symptoms. Frangos and Athanassenas point out, however, that their chronically hospitalized paranoid patients are treatment-resistant and may have a particularly severe form of the disorder.

Recently two additional reports have appeared linking CT abnormalities to clinical course in schizophrenia. DeLisi and associates[35] report that among first-episode schizophreniform patients, poor premorbid adjustment predicts the presence of enlarged VBR. When the large-ventricle patients were compared to the smallest-ventricle group, outcome scores taken at follow-up were also poorer for the large-ventricle patients. In the second report,[99] a strong association was noted between abnormal VBRs and previous suicide attempts. Ten of twelve patients with large VBRs had attempted suicide, while only two of twenty small-VBR patients had. The authors felt that the result was not due to the suicide attempts themselves, as only one of the patients had lost consciousness in the attempt. They speculated that the suicidal ideation might be a result of the process by which the ventricular enlargement occurs.

Since the early report by Johnstone and others,[88] several studies have specifically examined the relationship between neuropsychological test scores and CT abnormalities. Donnelly and coworkers[39] studied fifteen patients with a series of intellectual and neuropsychological tests and found that those patients with abnormal CT scans had much poorer scores. The authors concluded that these test scores reliably predict which patients have CT abnormalities. However, the clinical utility of the test scores in predicting CT abnormality may not be inferred from this study unless the study sample is representative of the schizophrenic population. This is due to the dependence of such utility estimates on the base rate of abnormality (as defined by these authors) in the population of schizophrenic patients. If the rate is lower than the high rate of abnormality in this sample, the prediction will be weaker (see the section entitled "Interpretive Issues").

In a series of papers, Golden and associates[57,58,60] have attempted to discriminate schizophrenic patients with ventricular enlargement from those without on the basis of performance on the Luria-Nebraska Neuropsychological Battery (LNNB). In their first two papers, the correlation of VBR with the scores on the fourteen LNNB subtests was assessed. An attempt was made to design decision rules combining the scores to predict the presence of abnormal VBRs. The results were that high levels of discrimination were obtained. The interpretation of these findings, however, is complicated by two factors. First, no controls were studied, and the abnormality criterion for the VBR was based on published measurements by other investigators. A later study called into question the comparability of such VBRs.[84] Also, the discrimination rate given was inflated over what could be expected in an independent sample, because the design of the rules was done on a post-hoc basis. It is a statistical fact that optimizing group discrimination by linearly combining fourteen variables results in substantial spurious inflation of the hit rate in the original sample. In a cross-validation study,[60] however, discrimination of patients with large VBRs from others was achieved with suprisingly high accuracy. It appears that among studies in which CT abnormalities are noted in schizophrenic patients, cognitive deficits usually are associated with these abnormalities.

RELATIONSHIP OF CT ABNORMALITY TO TREATMENT RESPONSE

In an early study Weinberger and associates[168] found that schizophrenic patients with enlarged ventricles showed significantly less improvement after two months of oral neuroleptic medication than did patients with normal ventricles. This finding suggested that patients with enlarged ventricles may have a different illness than other patients. Unfortunately, these investigators later had difficulty confirming the finding in another group of schizophrenic patients.[171] In some studies, neuroleptic responsiveness has been estimated retrospectively, and no correlation with VBR[94,118] has been obtained. However, Schulz and others,[144] studying very young schizophrenic patients, and Luchins, Lewine, and Meltzer,[105] in older patients, found that those with abnormal VBRs responded less well to neuroleptic treatment than those with normal VBRs.

Jeste and coworkers[87] recently reported a difference between schizophrenic patients with ventricular enlargement and those without in their response to apomorphine. The patients with normal CT scans tended to worsen on the drug, whereas patients with ventricular enlargement tended to improve or remain unchanged. These findings, though in a small sample, are intriguing and merit further investigation.

GENETIC AND BIOCHEMICAL CORRELATES OF CT ABNORMALITY

Two studies have dealt directly with genetic factors as they relate to ventricular enlargement in schizophrenia. In the first, Weinberger and associates[170] studied schizophrenic patients and their nonschizophrenic siblings, as well as a group of normal sibships. They found no difference in the prevalence of schizophrenia in first-degree relatives between patients with large ventricles and those with normal ventricles. They did observe, however, that ventricular size seemed to be correlated in the normal siblings, suggesting a genetic influence on ventricular size. They also found that all of the schizophrenic patients had larger ventricles than their siblings, and the nonschizophrenic siblings had larger ventricles than the subjects from the normal sibships.

Reveley and others[133] studied normal monozygotic and dizygotic twin pairs and a group of monozygotic pairs discordant for schizophrenia. Their findings were supportive of those of Weinberger and coworkers.[170] Ventricular size was highly correlated in normal monozygotic twins, somewhat less so in the schizophrenic twins, and considerably less so in the dizygotic twins. Again, the schizophrenic subjects had significantly higher VBRs than their cotwins, and there was a trend toward higher VBRs in the cotwins of schizophrenic patients relative to the normal twins. The results of these studies suggest that although there are genetic influences on ventricular size and normal siblings in schizophrenic families may "inherit" mild ventricular enlargement, some environmental factor results in larger ventricles in the affected sibling. It is possible that the isolation of sibships discordant for schizophrenia selects for cases in which an environmental insult has influenced the emergence of the disorder; and these cases may represent a relatively small proportion of schizophrenic patients. Therefore, no inferences about the prevalence of atrophy in schizophrenia can be made from these studies.

In two studies by Luchins and associates,[108,109] a link was hypothesized between HLA antigens and cerebral abnormalities in schizophrenia. Significant correlations were found among black patients between increases in HLA-A2 and the absence of cerebral atrophy. Also in this group, the presence of reversed cranial asymmetry was associated with the increased HLA-A2. Within the white schizophrenic group, these effects did not reach significance. Frangos and others[45] did not observe an increase in HLA-A2 in their schizophrenic patients without cerebral atrophy; however, their CT abnormality criterion, based on data from another investigator, renders a comparison of the two studies very difficult.

DeLisi and coworkers[34] reported that whole-blood serotonin concentrations were significantly higher in schizophrenic patients with enlarged ventricles than in either schizophrenic patients without ventricular enlargement or normal controls. Potkin and associates,[131] from the same group, found an association within schizophrenic patients of enlarged VBRs and decreased CSF 5-hydroxyindoleacetic acid (5-HIAA) concentrations. They explained the apparent discrepancy between the results of these two studies by postulating an inverse relationship between blood serotonin and CSF 5-HIAA.

Decreased CSF concentrations of homovanillic acid and dopamine-beta-hydroxylase activity have been reported in schizophrenic patients with brain atrophy relative to those without atrophy.[161] These findings were interpreted to support the hypothesis that a subgroup of schizophrenic patients have disturbed dopamine neurotransmission and to refute the hypothesis that schizophrenic patients with atrophy have a "nondopamine-related" disorder.

In one last study linking CT abnormalities to biochemical factors in schizophrenia, Kleinman and others[93] reported that relationships between plasma prolactin levels and psychopathological dimensions measured on the Brief Psychiatric Rating Scale were weaker in patients with large ventricles. Such relationships, however, appeared to be present in both groups.

Affective Disorders

Three years after the first report of CT abnormalities in schizophrenic patients, a group from Johns Hopkins presented data suggesting that patients with manic-depressive illness also had enlarged VBRs.[127,128] A similar result was obtained by Nasrallah, McCalley-Whitters, and Jacoby in a group of twenty-four patients with bipolar affective disorder.[117] These authors also reported that VBR was larger in their manic-depressive patients with cerebellar atrophy than in those without[121]; however, many tests were performed in this study and the effect size was not large. Fifty patients with affective disorder were studied with PEG and CT, and the authors felt that the results showed increased ventricular size in their sample.[150] The conclusion was drawn, however, on the basis of comparisons with control data from other reports. Reider and associates[135] compared patients with bipolar affective disorder to groups of schizophrenic and schizo-affective patients and found comparable distributions of VBRs in all groups. Unfortunately, no controls were measured in this study. Lippmann and others reported an increased prevalence of cerebellar abnormalities on CT in bipolar patients, but this occurred only in the subgroup of patients with alcoholism.[100] The Johns Hopkins group recently replicated their finding of increased VBRs in bipolar patients and found in post-hoc analyses that large-VBR patients had a history of more hospitalizations and more persistent unemployment than small-VBR patients.[129]

Ventricular enlargement has also been reported in patients with major unipolar depression.[145] The patients in this study all had delusions or hallucinations. Targum and coworkers[154] found that delusional patients with major depressive disorders had significantly higher VBRs than controls and that the prevalence of VBRs greater than two standard deviations from the control mean was higher in delusional than in nondelusional patients. Kellner and others[92] found that urinary-free cortisol levels were highly correlated with VBR in a small group of mixed patients with major affective disorders. The authors hypothesized that cortisol hypersecretion might produce ventricular enlargement.

Although no studies of patients with primary affective disorders have suggested localized CT abnormalities, it is of some interest that in two studies of patients with stroke or brain trauma, depression was associated with location of lesion.[101,137] The proximity of the lesion to the left frontal pole seemed to predict the presence of significant dysthymia. Attempts were made to control for the degree of functional impairment suffered by the patients secondary to the brain insults when evaluating the relationship of lesion site to depression.

Obsessive-Compulsive Disorder

There have been two CT studies of patients with obsessive-compulsive disorders and controls. In the first, by Insel and associates,[75] no differences were observed between the patients and controls despite the fact that patients were explicitly selected for the presence of electroencephalogram, neurological, or neuropsychological abnormality. VBR and cranial asymmetry measures were examined.

In a second report, Behar and others[9] described a group of sixteen adolescent obsessive-compulsive patients. The patients were found to have significant neuropsychological impairment and higher VBRs than controls. This finding is difficult to interpret, however, because the control scans were clearly screened differently for inclusion in the study than were patient scans.

Childhood Disorders

In an early report by Hier, LeMay, and Rosenberger,[71] an increased incidence of reversed cranial asymmetry in the parieto-occipital region was found in a group of sixteen autistic patients relative to mentally retarded patients and a mixed neurological population. The authors hypothesized that this morphological difference near the language areas might be related to the disordered language acquisition in autistic children.

Damasio and associates[29] studied seventeen autistic patients with CT. A variety of CT abnormalities were noted, including intraparenchymal lesions, hydrocephalus, and frontal horn enlargement. No differences were observed, however, in any measure of cranial asymmetry between these patients and controls.

In two studies from Tsai and others,[158,160] no differences in cranial asymmetry were observed between autistic patients and controls. These authors discuss problems in the measurement of cranial asymmetry and point out that the discrepancy between studies appears to be in the values for controls rather than patients.

Campbell and coworkers[19] conducted a CT study of forty-five young autistic children. Controls were selected from radiology files considered normal. The difference between the two groups on CT measures is not given and is assumed to be nonsignificant. The authors subjectively separated patients into groups on the basis of ventricular size, but the groups did not appear to differ clinically.

Hier and associates[72] have also examined patients with developmental dyslexia for evidence of cranial reversals. They reported increased prevalence of such reversals in the parieto-occipital region relative to controls. In another report by this group, delayed speech was associated with reversal in patients with learning disabilities.[138] Posterior cranial reversals were not associated with reading disability, however, in developmental dyslexic patients studied by Haslam and others.[68]

A largely descriptive study of eighty-five patients with childhood-onset neuropsychiatric disorders showed that many of these patients had clinically detected CT abnormalities.[21] The nature of the abnormalities varied, and both focal and diffuse findings occurred. Patients with primary cognitive disorders had particularly high rates of CT abnormalities.

A similar study was conducted by Reiss and associates.[132] Twenty children with mixed psychiatric diagnoses, referred for scanning because of suspicion of neurologic involvement, were studied and compared to controls with scans read as normal. VBR was higher in the patients than in the controls.

¶ Interpretive Issues: Experimental Design and Methods

Discrepancies in Prevalence Estimates

MEASUREMENT DIFFERENCES

There are at least two ways in which measurement differences may result in discrepant estimates of the prevalence of an abnormality. First, different measurements may actually quantify different aspects or subcomponents of the measured object. For example, suppose one intends to measure lateral ventricular size. Since the lateral ventricles are three-dimensional structures, one is attempting to estimate a volume. A measure of the width of the frontal horns at their widest point may be considered an estimate of this volume, as might a measure of the area of the lateral ventricles on a section through the bodies. However, if the frontal horns are focally enlarged in schizophrenia, then the prevalence of ventricular enlargement estimated from the former measure might be considerably higher than that estimated with the latter.

A second way that measurement differences give rise to discrepant prevalence estimates involves the sensitivity of the measures. If, following the example just given, the linear measure is substantially less sensitive to ventricular size (i.e., a greater proportion of its variability is irrelevant to ventricular size), then a lower prevalence estimate will result from its use, because the variability about the mean of this measure in controls will be greater than with the area measure. This will lead to a larger confidence interval around the control mean and a more conservative labeling of patient scans as abnormal. In other words, a patient scan will have to be more abnormal to be labeled as abnormal. Evidence [84] suggests that among area and volumetric measures, differences of this sort are unlikely to account for discrepancies in this literature. Linear measurements, however, have lower sensitivity.

These considerations may be particularly relevant in explaining apparent discrepancies in the prevalence of cortical atrophy. In most studies, what is meant by "cortical atrophy" is not clearly defined; and the measurements used are often very crude. Also, the areas of the CT scan in which cortical sulci appear are among those in which artifacts are most often present.

SAMPLING ERROR

Sampling error arises because in successive sampling of a population, a statistic computed from the samples will not be the same each time but will vary around the population parameter. By making certain assumptions, it is possible to evaluate whether given sets of sample values, such as mean group differences on VBR, are likely to be generated by sampling error. Power analyses like those described in Rothpearl, Mohs, and Davis [140] are very helpful in this regard. Using these calculations, it is clear that differences as large as those between the Weinberger and others study [166] and the Jernigan and associates study [84] are very unlikely to occur due to sampling error alone. Nevertheless, a certain amount of variation from study to study is a result of sampling fluctuation.

CONTROL GROUP DEFINITION

Ideally, the control group for any clinical study of a disease should be one that is randomly sampled from a population of people who are as much like the patients as possible in all respects except for the presence of the disease. Additionally, power is added to the analysis when potential subjects are omitted who have other diseases known to affect the criterion variable. In all cases, however, it is critical that the selection of subjects for the experimental and control groups be identical after the diagnostic distinction is made.

Many studies just reviewed used as controls patients who had been scanned for clinical reasons but who did not have the psychiatric diagnosis of interest. Patients were omitted from this group if they were diagnosed as having some other central nervous system (CNS) or psychiatric disease or if their CT scans were read as abnormal. There are two dangers inherent in this practice. First, if subjects with occult CNS diseases are included in these control groups, the group comparison will have less power; the null hypothesis of "no difference" may be inaccurately retained.

A second possibility is that this practice will actually produce spurious group "differences," leading the investigator to infer that abnormalities are more common in psychiatric patients than they actually are. This happens because the scans of the psychiatric patients are not screened for abnormalities on CT while those of the control subjects are. "Abnormalities" on CT occur in the otherwise normal population with a certain frequency. Suppose that people with these abnormalities were omitted from one group of normals and not from another. Given a large enough sample size, even these two normal groups would be significantly different. If the dependent variable—in this case the presence of CT abnormalities—is made a screening variable for the control group and not for the experimental group, any differences between the groups on this variable may not be interpreted to be due to the diagnostic distinction.

POPULATION DIFFERENCES

The most likely explanation for the large discrepancies in this literature is that the samples are actually being drawn from different patient populations and are not random samples of the universal population of patients with a given diagnosis. Certain restrictions of the target population are made by consensus. If, for example, it is known that there is an increased incidence of alcoholism among schizophrenic patients and that alcoholism is associated with cerebral atrophy, then it is reasonable to sample only nonalcoholic schizophrenic subjects in an attempt to establish the association of cerebral atrophy with schizophrenia per se. Beyond such

explicit restrictions, however, one would like to assume that a sample is representative of the otherwise unrestricted population of cases. It is this assumption that would appear frequently to be in error. Presumably, since investigators rarely stipulate that the target population is further restricted, they are often unaware that their patients are not typical. Even if the bias in the sample is not explicit, it is sometimes possible to detect from the summary clinical variables published with the results. For example, the sample of Johnstone and associates[88] was older than most. Unfortunately, inspection of clinical or demographic characteristics of the samples does little to clarify why the populations sampled by some investigators have a high prevalence of cerebral abnormalities, while those sampled by others do not. Both old and young patient groups have shown high proportions of abnormal scans. This is also true for groups with long- and short-term illnesses, long- and short-term neuroleptic use, prominent negative and prominent positive symptoms, and early and late onset of illness. Although it has not been established, many investigators suspect that tertiary treatment settings, serving many anomalous, severely ill, or treatment-recalcitrant patients, have more patients with cerebral abnormalities. Even if this is the case, it is not clear how it should be interpreted.

Unreliability of Clinical Correlates

INFERENCES BASED ON POST-HOC ANALYSES

Often when clinical correlates of brain abnormalities have been reported, they have emerged from studies that were not designed specifically to test the hypothesis that the reported relationship was present. More commonly, a group of patients has been studied in a clinical research setting where many protocols are underway and many, sometimes hundreds, of measurements are taken. In this context, there is great temptation to look at the relationship of each variable to every other, and indeed it is sound practice to do so in the service of generating new hypotheses. When evaluating the results, it is essential, however, to keep the statistical implications in mind. Statistical "significance" has little meaning here; certainly it is no longer grounds for publishing the result as a finding. Inferences may be drawn only from results that are tested for significance in prospective studies. Cohen and Cohen[24] present an excellent summary of this problem in multivariate research and suggest some things to do about it.

The practical problems generated by the publication of post-hoc results are that a few apparent relationships will emerge from each large study, the spurious ones will be indistinguishable from the others, and generally very few effects will be replicable.

LOW CONVERGENT VALIDITY OF CLINICAL MEASURES

Another source of unreliability in clinical correlations has to do with convergent validity. If a clinical construct is a useful, clearly defined, and valid one, then measures used by the psychiatric community to measure it should be in agreement. Unfortunately, many constructs in clinical psychiatry do not enjoy this status. Treatment response, for example, is measured by some using current behavioral rating scales, whereas others may extract historical information from charts. These methods may lead to discrepant evaluations that would be likely to correlate differently with cerebral abnormalities. The definition of "positive" and "negative" symptoms is another example that is particularly relevant in this literature. While some investigators have attempted to define these different symptom types more concretely, the arguments about the cerebral correlates of positive versus negative symptom disorders continue to be conducted without good agreement about what the constructs mean. To the extent that they mean different things to different investigators, different phenomena will be correlated with CT abnormalities, and apparent discrepancies will

inevitably occur. Another way of describing this problem is to say that investigators are measuring different things, but giving them the same name.

¶ Interpretive Issues: Theoretical and Clinical

Etiological Hypotheses

A number of investigators have speculated about the significance of cerebral abnormalities in "functional" psychiatric disorders. Only in schizophrenia has enough relevant evidence accumulated to support elaboration of such speculations. From the schizophrenia literature, two points of view have been extracted for discussion here. These are primarily distinct from each other in that (1) they predict different things about the onset of structural abnormalities relative to the onset of the illness, and (2) while one suggests that CT abnormalities reflect a primary degenerative process, the other views the structural changes as sequelae to a nonspecific cerebral insult.

Crow[26,27] and others[133,175] have suggested that untimely cerebral atrophy in schizophrenia may be, as in primary degenerative dementia, the result of a progressive degenerative cerebral pathology. Labeled the type II syndrome, this process results in negative symptoms, intellectual impairment, and deterioration to the "defect state." Crow suggests that while the type I syndrome, characterized primarily by positive symptoms, is neurochemically based and reversible, type II schizophrenia is anatomically based and irreversible. Correlations of structural abnormalities with negative symptoms, high prevalence estimates in older samples of schizophrenic patients, correlations of ventricular size with duration of illness, and lack of neuroleptic response in patients with abnormalities are supportive of this hypothesis. Findings of high prevalence of CT abnormalities in samples of very young patients with recent onset, however, suggest that many structural abnormalities in schizophrenia are not of this type.

Weinberger, Wagner, and Wyatt,[165] have suggested a different explanation. They review the neuropathological literature and make the argument that diffuse, nonspecific limbic and diencephalic pathology is present in a subgroup of the schizophrenic population. Based on the observation of structural abnormalities in recent-onset cases, they speculate that early CNS insults are responsible. In some as yet undefined way, this deep cerebral pathology affects the pathogenesis of the disorder.

Both groups of investigators consider the possibility that viral processes may be involved in the pathology, and neither attempts to predict the pathophysiology more specifically. The distinctions between them, again, are found in the proposed time of onset of the cerebral pathology and the extent to which the process is seen as progressive and degenerative.

Base Rates and Prevalence Estimates

An important question that arises in the interpretation of the findings just reviewed regards the extent to which they can or should influence the diagnostic and therapeutic process in the clinic. Many complex factors bear on this question. One that is particularly pertinent is prevalence, or the base rate of an abnormality in the clinical population. The following example illustrates the impact on clinical utility of uncertainty about this factor.

The report by Donnelly and associates[39] is used here as an example, but similar reasoning may be applied in the interpretation of most clinical reports in this literature. To review, the study involved the administration of the Halstead-Reitan Neuropsychological Test Battery (HRB) to a group of fifteen schizophrenic patients. On the basis of previous CT scans, the patients had been classified as showing either normal or abnormal cerebral morphology. The scores on an index

from the HRB were compared to this classification. Using a published cutoff for the HRB index to predict abnormality, the authors found that for twelve of fifteen patients the HRB and the CT results agreed. They stated in the abstract, "These results supported our hypothesis that impairment on the HRB in chronic schizophrenic patients was associated with morphological abnormalities on the CT scan, and that the positive and negative CT scans of these patients could be predicted accurately" (p. 305). On first impressions it may appear that, with an 80 percent chance of succeeding, one could use the HRB index in the clinic to identify patients with cerebral abnormality and then alter their treatment or diagnosis accordingly. Closer inspection, however, suggests otherwise. In the Donnelly sample, eight of the fifteen patients (53 percent) had abnormal CT scans. Among the reported prevalence estimates in the literature, this is a very high one, suggesting that in many settings the proportion of patients with cerebral abnormalities is considerably lower. Also, in this study the error rate for the abnormal patients (one of eight, or 12.5 percent) was considerably lower than for the normal patients (two of seven, or 28.5 percent). Suppose that a clinician is working in a setting in which 20 percent of the chronic schizophrenic patients have cerebral abnormalities (a considerably more representative figure), and he or she applies the HRB to the prediction of these abnormalities in one hundred patients. Only three of the twenty abnormal patients will be incorrectly classified as normal, but twenty-three of the eighty normal patients will be misclassified as abnormal. The total misclassification rate will be 26 percent. If all of the patients had simply been considered normal and no assessments had been done, only 20 percent would have been misclassified. The use of the index has reduced the accuracy of prediction below that obtained by doing nothing! If, as in the samples by Andreasen and coworkers or Jernigan and others, the prevalence in the clinician's setting was closer to 10 percent, the misclassification rate would be 27 percent, while doing nothing would yield a 10 percent misclassification rate. From these examples, it should be clear that the clinical utility of findings of group differences depends strongly on the composition of the target patient population.

¶ CT Abnormality in Primary Degenerative Dementias

CT studies of cerebral atrophy in normal aging have shown that average ventricular and sulcal sizes remain relatively constant until about age sixty and increase rapidly thereafter.* Studies in our laboratory were the first to suggest a decrease in parenchymal CT values in normal aging,[178] although such changes had been reported in the demented elderly.[114] Such studies demonstrate that abnormalities observed on CT that are putatively related to dementia must be carefully differentiated from normal age changes.

Cognitive declines in the elderly have also been well documented.[15,25,53,92] In elderly subjects, a clinical evaluation of "memory and information" was correlated with maximum ventricular area but not with an undescribed measure of cortical atrophy.[136] In another study, however, a clinical "memory and orientation" assessment correlated with ratings of cortical atrophy but not measures of ventricular enlargement.[79] The visual reproduction score from the Wechsler Memory Scale correlated weakly with sulcal and ventricular width in another study of people sixty to one hundred years old.[40] When an otherwise unselected group of elderly people with diffuse cerebral atrophy was studied, correlations were obtained between a measure of delayed recall of words and frontal ventricular width. In the same study, the score on the Squire Television Test of remote memory correlated with sylvian fissure width, which is thought to reflect anterior temporal atrophy.[176]

The interpretation of studies such as these is problematic. Perhaps to some extent the findings are due to inclusion of subjects with occult dementing processes. It is likely, however, that the processes responsible for these clinico-anatomical correlations in normal elderly are distinct from the malignant degenerative processes occurring in primary dementias. Any CT study of dementia, then, must attempt to unravel the clinico-anatomic correlations of the disease from those of aging.

Increased cerebral atrophy has now been observed repeatedly in groups of demented patients relative to age controls,* although in some early studies no increases were observed.[46,113] Correlations of degree of dementia or psychometric cognitive assessments with degree of atrophy have usually been obtained,† although, again, such relationships are not invariably found.[11,22,46,174]

Attempts to use local density measures to predict presence of dementia or degree of cognitive impairment have also yielded mixed results. In some studies, no relationship between local density measures and cognitive status was found[174]; in other studies, increased density was associated with cognitive changes[49,51]; and in others, decreased density was associated with cognitive deterioration.[14,81,114] The discrepancies may be related to the spectral shift artifact in CT. CT values nearer to the skull are artifactually elevated. If demented patients have ventricular enlargement, samples of tissue density may be taken more peripherally to avoid sampling in ventricular fluid. A concomitant artifactual increase in the sampled values may cause what appears to be no difference, or even increased values in dementia, when actual tissue values may be decreased.

In Huntington's disease, ventricular and sulcal enlargement and specific striatal atrophy have been demonstrated with PEG[13] and with CT.‡ Sax and associates[141] have also demonstrated that within Huntington's disease patients, increasing atrophy predicts de-

---

*See references 8, 18, 40, 61, 66, 76, 79, 112, and 177.

*See references 17, 43, 49, 65, 77, and 174.
†See references 17, 32, 42, 65, 79, 90, 91, and 136.
‡See references 7, 96, 124, 141, and 155.

gree of dementia as well as degree of chorea. The CT correlates of the dementia of Parkinson's disease were studied by Sroka and coworkers. [149] They found an association between the presence of an "organic mental syndrome" and an abnormal degree of cerebral atrophy. In his review, Wells describes an argument that dementia, when it occurs in Parkinson's disease, may be a form of Alzheimer's disease. [173]

A few cases of Pick's disease have been reported for which CT was available. [62,63,163] In these, the pattern of frontal and temporal cortical atrophy observed on pathology was observed on CT, usually in association with ventricular enlargement. A relative sparing of parietal and occipital cortex was noted.

Although groups of patients with primary degenerative dementias consistently show more cerebral atrophy than their controls, diagnosis of dementia from CT is still problematic. Inspection of distributions of atrophy measures in the demented and control groups almost always reveals overlap between the groups. A recent pilot study by Brinkman and Largen [16] suggests that repeat scanning of suspected Alzheimer's patients may increase the separation of the groups, but even in this study one of five patients did not show a striking change.

In no study has it been conclusively demonstrated that a particular pattern of abnormality on CT predicts specific clinical features in the course of the illness. Even the differential diagnosis of primary dementias is not possible with CT. Glatt and associates [54] recently showed that CT does not reliably discriminate vascular dementias from degenerative dementias, although their results did suggest that negative CT findings rarely occur in cases of vascular dementia. Although the lobar pattern of cortical atrophy is usually different in Pick's disease, cases with clinical courses much more typical of Alzheimer's disease sometimes present with disproportionate fronto-temporal atrophy. Finally, radiological investigators repeatedly observe that individuals with moderately severe atrophy may have no clinical signs of abnormal mental decline.

¶ Bibliography

1. ANDREASEN, N. C., et al. "Hemispheric Asymmetries and Schizophrenia," *American Journal of Psychiatry,* 139 (1982):427–430.

2. ANDREASEN, N. C., et al. "Ventricular Enlargement in Schizophrenia: Definition and Prevalence," *American Journal of Psychiatry,* 139 (1982):292–296.

3. ANDREASEN, N. C., et al. "Ventricular Enlargement in Schizophrenia: Relationship to Positive and Negative Symptoms," *American Journal of Psychiatry,* 139 (1982):297–301.

4. ANSINK, B. J. J., BUIS, C., and TOLSMA, F. J. "The Pneumencephalogram in Chronic Schizophrenics," *Psychiatria, Neurologia, Neurochirurgia,* 66 (1963):120–130.

5. ARAI, H., et al. "A Computed Tomography Study of Alzheimer's Disease," *Journal of Neurology,* 229 (1983):69–77.

6. BANNA, M. "The Ventriculo-Cephalic Ratio on Computed Tomography," *Journal of the Canadian Association of Radiology,* 28 (1977):205–210.

7. BARR, A. N., et al. "Bicaudate Index in Computerized Tomography of Huntington's Disease and Cerebral Atrophy," *Neurology,* 28 (1978):1196–1200.

8. BARRON, S. A., JACOBS, L., and KINKEL, W. R. "Changes in Size of Normal Lateral Ventricles During Aging Determined by Computerized Tomography," *Neurology,* 26 (1976):1011–1013.

9. BEHAR, D., et al. "Computerized Tomography and Neuropsychological Test Measures in Adolescents with Obsessive-Compulsive Disorder," *American Journal of Psychiatry,* 141 (1984):363–368.

10. BENES, F., et al. "Normal Ventricles in Young Schizophrenics," *British Journal of Psychiatry,* 141 (1982):90–93.

11. BIRD, J. M. "Computerized Tomography. Atrophy and Dementia: A Review," *Progress in Neurobiology,* 19 (1982):91–115.

12. BLESSED, G., TOMLINSON, B. E., and ROTH, M. "The Association Between Quantitative Measures of Dementia and of Senile Changes in the Cerebral

Grey Matter of Elderly Subjects," *British Journal of Psychiatry*, 114 (1968):-797–811.

13. BLINDERMAN, E. E., WEIDNER, W., and MARKHAM, C. H. "The Pneumo-Encephalogram in Huntington's Chorea," *Neurology*, 14 (1964):601–607.

14. BONDAREFF, W., BALDY, R., and LEVY, R. "Quantitative Computed Tomography in Dementia," *Archives of General Psychiatry*, 38 (1981):1365–1368.

15. BOTWINICK, J. *Cognitive Processes in Maturity and Old Age.* New York: Springer, 1967.

16. BRINKMAN, S. D., and LARGEN, J. W., JR. "Change in Brain Ventricular Size with Repeated CAT Scans in Suspected Alzheimer's Disease," *American Journal of Psychiatry*, 141 (1984):81–83.

17. BRINKMAN, S. D., et al. "Quantitative Indexes of Computed Tomography in Dementia and Normal Aging," *Radiology*, 138 (1981):89–92.

18. CALA, L. A., et al. "Brain Density and Cerebrospinal Fluid Space Size: CT of Normal Volunteers," *American Journal of Neuroradiology*, 2 (1981):41–47.

19. CAMPBELL, M., et al. "Computerized Axial Tomography in Young Autistic Children," *American Journal of Psychiatry*, 139 (1982):510–512.

20. CAMPBELL, R., et al. "CT Scan Variants and Genetic Heterogeneity in Schizophrenics," *American Journal of Psychiatry*, 136 (1979):722–723.

21. CAPARULO, B. K., et al. "Computed Tomographic Brain Scanning in Children with Developmental Neuropsychiatric Disorders," *Journal of the American Academy of Child Psychiatry*, 20 (1981):338–357.

22. CLAVIERA, L. E., MOSELEY, I. F., and STEVENSON, J. F. "The Clinical Significance of Cerebral Atrophy as shown on CAT," in G. H. Du Boulay and I. F. Moseley, eds., *Computerized Axial Tomography in Clinical Practice.* Berlin: Springer, Verlag 1977, pp. 213–217.

23. COFFMAN, J. A., et al. "Cerebellar Atrophy in Chronic Schizophrenia," *Lancet*, 1 (1981):666.

24. COHEN, J. and COHEN, P. "Statistical Inference Strategy in Multiple Regression/Correlation," in *Applied Multiple Regression/Correlation Analysis for the Behavioral Sciences*, 2nd ed. Hillsdale, N.J.: Lawrence Erlbaum Associates, 1983, pp. 166–177.

25. CRAIK, F.I.M. "Age Differences in Human Memory," in J. E. Birren and K. W. Schaie, eds., *Handbook of the Psychology of Aging.* New York: Van Nostrand Reinhold, 1977, pp. 384–430.

26. CROW, T. J. "The Biology of Schizophrenia," *Experientia*, 38 (1982):1275–1282.

27. ————. "Neurohumoural and Structural Changes in Schizophrenia: Two Dimensions of Pathology," *Progress in Brain Research*, 55 (1982):407–417.

28. CROW, T. J., et al. "Schizophrenia and Cerebral Atrophy," *Lancet*, 1 (1980):-1129–1130.

29. DAMASIO, H., et al. "Computerized Tomographic Scan Findings in Patients with Autistic Behavior," *Archives of Neurology*, 37 (1980):504–510.

30. DASTUR, D. K. "The Pathology of Schizophrenia," *A.M.A. Archives of Neurology and Psychiatry*, 81 (1959):601–614.

31. DE LEON, M. J., and GEORGE, A. E. "Computed Tomography in Aging and Senile Dementia of the Alzheimer Type," *Archives of Neurology*, 38 (1983):103–122.

32. DE LEON, M. J., et al. "Computed Tomography Evaluations of Brain-Behavior Relationships in Senile Dementia of the Alzheimer's Type," *Neurobiology of Aging*, 1 (1980):69–79.

33. DE LEON, M. J., et al. "Regional Correlation of PET and CT in Senile Dementia of the Alzheimer Type," *American Journal of Neuroradiology*, 4 (1983):553–556.

34. DELISI, L. E., et al. "Increased Whole Blood Serotonin Concentrations in Chronic Schizophrenic Patients," *Archives of General Psychiatry*, 38 (1981):-647–650.

35. DELISI, L. E., et al. "Ventricular Brain Enlargement and Outcome of Acute Schizophreniform Disorder," *Psychiatry Research*, 9 (1983):169–171.

36. DEWAN, M. J., et al. "Cerebellar Morphology in Chronic Schizophrenic Patients: A Controlled Computed Tomography Study," *Psychiatry Research*, 10 (1983):-97–103.

37. DEWAN, M. J., et al. "Central Brain Mor-

phology in Chronic Schizophrenic Patients: A Controlled CT Study," *Biological Psychiatry,* 18 (1983):1133–1140.

38. DiCHIRO, G., et al. "The Apical Artifact: Elevated Attenuation Values Toward the Apex of the Skull," *Journal of Computer Assisted Tomography,* 2 (1978):-65–70.

39. DONNELLY, E. F., et al. "Cognitive Impairment Associated with Morphological Brain Abnormalities on Computed Tomography in Chronic Schizophrenic Patients," *Journal of Nervous and Mental Disease,* 168 (1980):305–308.

40. EARNEST, M. P., et al. "Cortical Atrophy, Ventricular Enlargement, and Intellectual Impairment in the Aged," *Neurology,* 29 (1979):1138–1143.

41. FAMUYIWA, O. O., et al. "Tardive Dyskinesia and Dementia," *British Journal of Psychiatry,* 135 (1979):500–504.

42. FORD, C. V., and WINTER, J. "Computerized Axial Tomograms and Dementia in Elderly Patients," *Journal of Gerontology,* 36 (1980):164–169.

43. FOX, J. H., TOPEL, J. L., and HUCKMAN, M. S. "Use of Computerized Tomography in Senile Dementia," *Journal of Neurology, Neurosurgery, and Psychiatry,* 38 (1975):948–953.

44. FRANGOS, E., and ATHANASSENAS, G. "Differences in Lateral Brain Ventricular Size Among Various Types of Chronic Schizophrenics," *Acta Psychiatrica Scandinavica,* 66 (1982):459–463.

45. FRANGOS, E., et al. "HLA Antigens in Schizophrenia: No Difference Between Patients With and Without Evidence of Brain Atrophy," *British Journal of Psychiatry,* 140 (1982):607–610.

46. GADO, M., and HUGHES, C. P. "Computerized Tomography Scan in the Diagnosis and Management of Senile Dementia," in K. Nandy, ed., *Senile Dementia: A Biomedical Approach.* New York: Elsevier/North Holland Biomedical Press, 1978, pp. 223–235.

47. GADO, M., et al. "Aging, Dementia, and Brain Atrophy: A Longitudinal Computed Tomographic Study," *American Journal of Neuroradiology,* 4 (1983):-699–702.

48. GADO, M., et al. "Volumetric Measurements of the Cerebrospinal Fluid Spaces in Demented Subjects and Controls," *Radiology,* 144 (1982):535–538.

49. GADO, M., et al. "Brain Parenchymal Density Measurements by CT in Demented Subjects and Normal Controls," *Radiology,* 147 (1983):703–710.

50. GADO, M., et al. "Brain Atrophy in Dementia Judged by CT Scan Ranking," *American Journal of Neuroradiology,* 4 (1983):499–500.

51. GEORGE, A. E., et al. "Parenchymal CT Correlates of Senile Dementia (Alzheimer Disease): Loss of Gray-White Matter Discriminability," *American Journal of Neuroradiology,* 2 (1981):205–213.

52. GEORGE, A. E., et al. "Ventricular Volume and Cognitive Deficit: A Computed Tomographic Study," *Radiology,* 149 (1983):493–498.

53. GILBERT, J. G., and LEVEE, R. F. "Patterns of Declining Memory," *Journal of Gerontology,* 26 (1971):70–75.

54. GLATT, S. L., et al. "Efficacy of CT in the Diagnosis of Vascular Dementia," *American Journal of Neuroradiology,* 4 (1983):703–705.

55. GLUCK, E., et al. "A Computed Tomographic Prolective Trohoc Study of Chronic Schizophrenics," *Neuroradiology,* 20 (1980):167–171.

56. GOLDEN, C. J., et al. "Brain Density Deficits in Chronic Schizophrenia," *Psychiatry Research,* 3 (1980):179–184.

57. GOLDEN, C. J., et al. "Differentiation of Chronic Schizophrenics with and without Ventricular Enlargement by the Luria-Nebraska Neuropsychological Battery," *International Journal of Neuroscience,* 11 (1980):131–138.

58. GOLDEN, C. J., et al. "Cerebral Ventricular Size and Neuropsychological Impairment in Young Chronic Schizophrenics," *Archives of General Psychiatry,* 37 (1980):619–623.

59. GOLDEN, C. J., et al. "Structural Brain Deficits in Schizophrenia," *Archives of General Psychiatry,* 38 (1981):1014–1017.

60. GOLDEN, C. J., et al. "Cross-Validation of the Ability of the Luria-Nebraska Neuropsychological Battery to Differentiate Chronic Schizophrenics With and Without Ventricular Enlargement," *Journal*

of Consulting and Clinical Psychology, 50 (1982):87–95.

61. GONZALES, C. F., LANTIERI, R. L., and NATHAN, R. J. "The CT Scan Appearance of the Brain in the Normal Elderly Population: A Correlative Study," *Neuroradiology*, 16 (1978):120–122.

62. GROEN, J. J., and ENDTZ, L. J. "Hereditary Pick's Disease: Second R-Examination of a Large Family and Discussion of Other Hereditary Cases, with Particular Reference to Electroencephalography and Computerized Tomography," *Brain*, 105 (1982):443–459.

63. GROEN, J. J., and HEKSTER, R.E.M. "Computed Tomography in Pick's Disease: Findings in a Family Affected in Three Consecutive Generations." *Journal of Computer Assisted Tomography*, 6 (1982):907–911.

64. GROSS, G., HUBER, G., and SCHUTTLER, R. "Computerized Tomography Studies on Schizophrenic Diseases," *Archiv für Psychiatrie und Nervenkrankheiten*, 231 (1982):519–526.

65. GUTZMANN, H., and AVDALOFF, W. "Mental Impairment (Dementia) and Cerebral Atrophy in Geriatric Patients," *Mechanisms of Ageing and Development*, 14 (1980):459–468.

66. GYLDENSTED, C. "Measurements of the Normal Ventricular System and Hemispheric Sulci of 100 Adults with Computed Tomography," *Neuroradiology*, 14 (1977):183–192.

67. HAHN, F.J.Y., and RIM, K. "Frontal Ventricular Dimensions on Normal Computed Tomography," *American Journal of Radiology*, 126 (1976):593–596.

68. HASLAM, R.H.A., et al. "Cerebral Asymmetry in Developmental Dyslexia," *Archives of Neurology*, 38 (1981):679–682.

69. HAUG, J. O. "Pneumoencephalographic Studies in Mental Disease," *Acta Psychiatrica Scandinavica*, 38 (1962):1–114.

70. HEATH, R. G., et al. "Cerebellar Vermal Atrophy in Psychiatric Patients," *Biological Psychiatry*, 17 (1982):569–583.

71. HIER, D. B., LeMAY, M. and ROSENBERGER, P. B. "Autism and Unfavorable Left-Right Asymmetries of the Brain," *Journal of Autism and Developmental Disorders*, 9 (1979):153–159.

72. HIER, D. B., et al. "Developmental Dys-

lexia," *Archives of Neurology*, 35 (1978):90–92.

73. HORN, J. L. "Psychometric Studies of Aging and Intelligence," in S. Gershon and A. Raskin, eds., *Aging*, vol. 2. New York: Raven Press, 1975, pp. 19–23.

74. HUCKMAN, M. S., FOX, J., and TOPEL, J. "The Validity of Criteria for the Evaluation of Cerebral Atrophy by Computed Tomography," *Radiology*, 116 (1975):-85–92.

75. INSEL, T. R., et al. "Neurological and Neuropsychological Studies of Patients with Obsessive-Compulsive Disorder," *Biological Psychiatry*, 18 (1983):741–751.

76. JACOBS, L., et al. "Computerized Tomography in Dementia with Special Reference to Changes in the Size of Normal Ventricles During Aging and Normal Pressure Hydrocephalus," in R. Katzman, R. D. Terry, and K. L. Bick, eds., *Alzheimer's Disease: Senile Dementia and Related Disorders*. New York: Raven Press, 1978, pp. 241–260.

77. JACOBY, R. J. and LEVY, R. "Computed Tomography in the Elderly: 2. Senile Dementia: Diagnosis and Functional Impairment," *British Journal of Psychiatry*, 136 (1980):256–269.

78. ———. "CT Scanning and the Investigation of Dementia: A Review," *Journal of the Royal Society of Medicine*, 73 (1980):366–369.

79. JACOBY, R. J., LEVY, R., and DAWSON, J. M. "Computed Tomography in the Elderly: 1. The Normal Population," *British Journal of Psychiatry*, 36 (1980):-249–255.

80. JACOBY, R. J., et al. "Quantitative Computed Tomography in Elderly Depressed Patients," *British Journal of Psychiatry*, 143 (1983):124–127.

81. JERNIGAN, T. L. "Anatomical Validators: Issues in the Use of Computed Tomography," in L. W. Poon, ed., *Handbook of Clinical Memory Assessment of Older Adults*. Washington, D.C.: American Psychological Association, forthcoming.

82. JERNIGAN, T. L., ZATZ, L. M., and NAESER, M. A. "Semiautomated Methods for Quantitating CSF Volume on Cranial Computed Tomography," *Radiology*, 132 (1979):463–466.

83. JERNIGAN, T. L., et al. "Measurement of

Cerebral Atrophy in the Aged by Computed Tomography," in L. W. Poon, ed. *Aging in the 1980's: Psychological Issues.* Washington D.C.: American Psychological Association, 1980, pp. 86–94.

84. JERNIGAN, T. L., et al. "Computed Tomography in Schizophrenics and Normal Volunteers: I. Fluid Volume," *Archives of General Psychiatry,* 39 (1982):765–770.

85. JERNIGAN, T. L., et al. "Computed Tomography in Schizophrenics and Normal Volunteers: II. Cranial Asymmetry," *Archives of General Psychiatry,* 39 (1982):771–773.

86. JESTE, D. V., et al. "Ex Uno Multi: Subtyping the Schizophrenic Syndrome," *Biological Psychiatry,* 17 (1982):199–222.

87. JESTE, D. V., et al. "Apomorphine Response and Subtyping of Schizophrenia," *Progress in Neuro-Psychopharmacology and Biological Psychiatry,* 7 (1983):83–88.

88. JOHNSTONE, E. C., et al. "Cerebral Ventricular Size and Cognitive Impairment in Chronic Schizophrenia," *Lancet,* 2 (1976):924–926.

89. JOHNSTONE, E. C., et al. "The Dementia of Dementia Praecox," *Acta Psychiatrica Scandinavica,* 57 (1978):305–324.

90. KASZNIAK, A. W., GARRON, D. C., and FOX, J. "Differential Effects of Age and Cerebral Atrophy Upon Span of Immediate Recall and Paired Associate Learning in Older Patients Suspected of Dementia," *Cortex,* 15 (1979):285–295.

91. KASZNIAK, A. W., et al. "Cerebral Atrophy, EEG Slowing, Age, Education, and Cognitive Functioning in Suspected Dementia," *Neurology,* 29 (1979):1273–1279.

92. KELLNER, C. H., et al. "Relationship of Cortisol Hypersecretion to Brain CT Scan Alterations in Depressed Patients," *Psychiatry Research,* 8 (1983):-191–197.

93. KLEINMAN, J. E., et al. "Plasma Prolactin Concentrations and Psychopathology in Chronic Schizophrenia," *Archives of General Psychiatry,* 39 (1982):655–657.

94. KLING, A. S., et al. "CT Scans in Sub-Groups of Chronic Schizophrenics," *Journal of Psychiatric Research,* 17 (1983):375–384.

95. KOHLMEYER, K., and SHAMENA, A. R. "CT Assessment of CSF Spaces in the Brain in Demented and Nondemented Patients over 60 Years of Age," *American Journal of Neuroradiology,* 4 (1983):706–797.

96. KUHL, D. E., et al. "Cerebral Metabolism and Atrophy in Huntington's Disease Determined by 18-FDG and Computed Tomography Scan," *Annals of Neurology,* 12 (1982):425–434.

97. LARGEN, J. W., CALDERON, M., and SMITH, R. C. "Asymmetries in the Densities of White and Gray Matter in the Brains of Schizophrenic Patients," *American Journal of Psychiatry,* 140 (1983):1060–1062.

98. LEMAY, M. "Morphological Cerebral Asymmetries of Modern Man, Fossil Man, and Nonhuman Primates," *Annals of the New York Academy of Sciences,* 280 (1976):349–366.

99. LEVY, B., KURTZ, N., and KLING, A. S. "Association Between Cerebral Ventricular Enlargement and Suicide Attempts in Chronic Schizophrenia," *American Journal of Psychiatry,* 141 (1984):438–439.

100. LIPPMANN, S., et al. "Cerebellar Vermis Dimensions on Computerized Tomographic Scans of Schizophrenic and Bipolar Patients," *American Journal of Psychiatry,* 139 (1982):667–668.

101. LIPSEY, J. R., et al. "Mood Change Following Bilateral Hemisphere Brain Injury," *British Journal of Psychiatry,* 143 (1983):266–273.

102. LISHMAN, W. A. "The Apparatus of Mind: Brain Structure and Function in Mental Disorder," *Psychosomatics,* 24 (1982):-699–720.

103. LUCHINS, D. J. "Computed Tomography in Schizophrenia," *Archives of General Psychiatry,* 39 (1982):859–860.

104. LUCHINS, D. J., and MELTZER, H. Y. "A Blind, Controlled Study of Occipital Cerebral Asymmetry in Schizophrenia," *Psychiatry Research,* 10 (1983):87–95.

105. LUCHINS, D. J., LEWINE, R.R.J., and MELTZER, H. Y. "Lateral Ventricular Size, Psychopathology, and Medication Response in the Psychoses," *Society of Biological Psychiatry,* 19 (1984):29–44.

106. LUCHINS, D. J., WEINBERGER, D. R., and WYATT, R. J. "Schizophrenia: Evidence for a Subgroup with Reversed Cerebral Asymmetry," *Archives of General Psychiatry*, 36 (1979):1309–1311.

107. ———. "Schizophrenia and Cerebral Asymmetry Detected by Computed Tomography," *American Journal of Psychiatry*, 139 (1982):753–757.

108. LUCHINS, D. J. et al. "HLA Antigens and Schizophrenia: Differences Between Patients With and Without Evidence of Brain Atrophy," *British Journal of Psychiatry*, 136 (1980):243–248.

109. LUCHINS, D. J. et al. "HLA-A2 Antigen in Schizophrenic Patients with Reversed Cerebral Asymmetry," *British Journal of Psychiatry*, 138 (1981):240–243.

110. LYON, K., et al. "Effects of Long-term Neuroleptic Use on Brain Density," *Psychiatry Research*, 5 (1981):33–37.

111. MASER, J. D., and KEITH, S. J. "CT Scans and Schizophrenia—Report on a Workshop," *Schizophrenia Bulletin*, 9 (1983):265–283.

112. MEESE, W., et al. "CT Evaluation of the CSF Spaces of Healthy Persons," *Neuroradiology*, 19 (1980):131–136.

113. MELAMED, E., et al. "Correlation Between Regional Cerebral Blood Flow and Brain Atrophy in Dementia," *Journal of Neurology, Neurosurgery, and Psychiatry*, 41 (1978):894–899.

114. NAESER, M. A., GEBHARDT, C., and LEVINE, H. L. "Decreased Computerized Tomography Numbers in Patients with Presenile Dementia," *Archives of Neurology*, 37 (1980):401–409.

115. NAGUIB, M., and LEVY, R. "Prediction of Outcome in Senile Dementia—A Computed Tomography Study," *British Journal of Psychiatry*, 140 (1982):263–267.

116. ———. "CT Scanning in Senile Dementia: A Follow-up of Survivors," *British Journal of Psychiatry*, 141 (1982):618–620.

117. NASRALLAH, H. A., McCALLEY-WHITTERS, M., and JACOBY, C. G. "Cerebral Ventricular Enlargement in Young Manic Males: A Controlled CT Study," *Journal of Affective Disorders*, 4 (1982):15–19.

118. ———. "Cortical Atrophy in Schizophrenia and Mania: A Comparative CT Study," *Journal of Clinical Psychiatry*, 43 (1982):439–441.

119. NASRALLAH, H. A., et al. "Cerebral Ventricular Enlargement in Subtypes of Chronic Schizophrenia," *Archives of General Psychiatry*, 39 (1982):774–777.

120. NASRALLAH, H. A., et al. "Clinical Differences Between Schizophrenic Patients With and Without Large Cerebral Ventricles," *Journal of Clinical Psychiatry*, 44 (1983):407–409.

121. NASRALLAH, H. A., et al. "Clinical Correlates of Sulcal Widening in Chronic Schizophrenia," *Psychiatry Research*, 10 (1983):237–242.

122. NEOPHYTIDES, A. N., et al. "Computed Axial Tomography in Huntington's Disease and Persons At-Risk for Huntington's Disease," *Advances in Neurology*, 23 (1979):185–191.

123. NYBACK, H., et al. "Computed Tomography of the Brain in Patients with Acute Psychosis and in Healthy Volunteers," *Acta Psychiatrica Scandinavica*, 65 (1982):403–414.

124. OEPEN, G., and OSTERTAG, C. "Diagnostic Value of CT in Patients with Huntington's Chorea and Their Offspring," *Journal of Neurology*, 225 (1981):189–196.

125. OKASHA, A., and MADKOUR, O. "Cortical and Central Atrophy in Chronic Schizophrenia," *Acta Psychiatrica Scandinavica*, 65 (1982):29–34.

126. PANDURANGI, A. K., et al. "The Ventricular System in Chronic Schizophrenic Patients: A Controlled Computed Tomography Study," *British Journal of Psychiatry*, 144 (1984):172–176.

127. PEARLSON, G. D., and VEROFF, A. E. "Computerised Tomographic Scan Changes in Manic-Depressive Illness," *Lancet*, 2 (1981):470–474.

128. PEARLSON, G. D., VEROFF, A. E., and McHUGH, P. R. "The Use of Computed Tomography in Psychiatry: Recent Applications to Schizophrenia, Manic-Depressive Illness and Dementia Syndromes," *The Johns Hopkins Medical Journal*, 149 (1981):194–202.

129. PEARLSON, G. D., et al. "Clinical Corre-

lates of Lateral Ventricular Enlargement in Bipolar Affective Disorder," *American Journal of Psychiatry*, 141 (1984):253–256.

130. PENN, R. D., BELANGER, M. G., and YASNOFF, W. A. "Ventricular Volume in Man Computed from CAT Scans," *Annals of Neurology*, 3 (1978):216–223.

131. POTKIN, S. G., et al. "Low CSF 5-Hydroxyindoleacetic Acid in Schizophrenic Patients with Enlarged Cerebral Ventricles," *American Journal of Psychiatry*, 140 (1983):21–25.

132. REISS, D., et al. "Ventricular Enlargement in Child Psychiatric Patients: A Controlled Study with Planimetric Measurements," *American Journal of Psychiatry* 140 (1983):453–456.

133. REVELEY, A. M., et al. "Cerebral Ventricular Size in Twins Discordant for Schizophrenia," *Lancet*, 1 (1982):540–541.

134. RIEDER, R. O., et al. "Sulcal Prominence in Young Chronic Schizophrenic Patients: CT Scan Findings Associated with Impairment on Neuropsychological Tests," *Psychiatry Research*, 1 (1979):1–8.

135. RIEDER, R. O., et al. "Computed Tomographic Scans in Patients with Schizophrenia, Schizoaffective, and Bipolar Affective Disorder," *Archives of General Psychiatry*, 40 (1983):735–739.

136. ROBERTS, M. A., and CAIRD, F. I. "Computerized Tomography and Intellectual Impairment in the Elderly," *Journal of Neurology, Neurosurgery, and Psychiatry*, 39 (1976):986–989.

137. ROBINSON, R. G., et al. "A Two-Year Longitudinal Study of Post-stroke Mood Disorders: Findings During the Initial Evaluation," *Stroke*, 14 (1983):736–741.

138. ROSENBERGER, P. B., and HIER, D. B. "Cerebral Asymmetry and Verbal Intellectual Deficits," *Annals of Neurology*, 8 (1980):300–304.

139. ROTH, M., TOMLINSON, B. E., and BLESSED, G. "Psychiatry: Correlation Between Scores for Dementia and Counts of 'Senile Plaques' in Cerebral Grey Matter of Elderly Subjects," *Nature*, 209 (1966):109–110.

140. ROTHPEARL, A. B., MOHS, R. C., and DAVIS, K. L. "Statistical Power in Biological Psychiatry," *Psychiatry Research*, 5 (1981):257–266.

141. SAX, D. S., et al. "Computed Tomographic, Neurologic, and Neuro-Psychological Correlates of Huntington's Disease," *International Journal of Neuroscience*, 18 (1983):21–36.

142. SCHULZ, S. C., et al. "Abnormal Scans in Young Schizophrenics," *Psychopharmacology Bulletin*, 18 (1982):163–164.

143. SCHULZ, S. C., et al. "Ventricular Enlargements in Teenage Patients with Schizophrenic Spectrum Disorder," *American Journal of Psychiatry*, 140 (1983):1592–1595.

144. SCHULZ, S. C., et al. "Treatment Response and Ventricular Brain Enlargement in Young Schizophrenia Patients," *Psychopharmacology Bulletin* 19 (1983):510–512.

145. SCOTT, M. L., et al. "Ventricular Enlargement in Major Depression," *Psychiatry Research*, 8 (1983):91–93.

146. SMITH, R. C., et al. "CT Scans and Neuropsychological Tests as Predictors of Clinical Response in Schizophrenics," *Psychopharmacology Bulletin*, 19 (1983):505–509.

147. SNIDER, S. R. "Cerebellar Pathology in Schizophrenia—Cause or Consequence?" *Neuroscience & Biobehavioral Reviews*, 6 (1982):47–53.

148. SOININEN, H., et al. "EEG and Computed Tomography in the Investigation of Patients with Senile Dementia," *Journal of Neurology, Neurosurgery, and Psychiatry*, 45 (1982):711–714.

149. SROKA, H., et al. "Organic Mental Syndrome and Confusional States in Parkinson's Disease," *Archives of Neurology*, 38 (1981):339–342.

150. STANDISH-BARRY, H.M.A.S., et al. "Pneumo-Encephalographic and Computerized Axial Tomography Scan Changes in Affective Disorder," *British Journal of Psychiatry*, 141 (1982):614–617.

151. STEVENS, J. R. "Neuropathology of Schizophrenia," *Archives of General Psychiatry*, 39 (1982):1131–1139.

152. SYNEK, V., and REUBEN, J. R. "The Ventricular Brain Ratio Using Planimetric Measurement of EMI Scans," *British*

Journal of Radiology, 49 (1979):233–237.

153. TANAKA, Y., et al. "Computerized Tomography of the Brain in Schizophrenic Patients," *Acta Psychiatrica Scandinavica,* 63 (1981):191–197.

154. TARGUM, S. D., et al. "Cerebral Ventricular Size in Major Depressive Disorder: Association with Delusional Symptoms," *Biological Psychiatry,* 18 (1983):-329–336.

155. TERRENCE, C. F., DELANEY, J. F., and ALBERTS, M. C. "Computed Tomography for Huntington's Disease," *Neuroradiology,* 13 (1977):173–175.

156. TOMLINSON, B. E., BLESSED, G., and ROTH, M. "Observations on the Brains of Demented Old People," *Journal of the Neurological Sciences,* 11 (1970):205–242.

157. TRIMBLE, M., and KINGSLEY, D. "Cerebral Ventricular Size in Chronic Schizophrenia," *Lancet,* 1 (1978):278–279.

158. TSAI, L. Y., JACOBY, C. G., and STEWART, M. A. "Morphological Cerebral Asymmetries in Autistic Children," *Biological Psychiatry,* 18 (1983):317–326.

159. TSAI, L. Y., NASRALLAH, H. A., and JACOBY, C. G. "Hemispheric Asymmetries on Computed Tomographic Scans in Schizophrenia and Mania," *Archives of General Psychiatry,* 40 (1983):1286–1289.

160. TSAI, L. Y., et al. "Unfavourable Left-Right Asymmetries of the Brain and Autism: A Question of Methodology," *British Journal of Psychiatry,* 140 (1982):312–319.

161. VAN KAMMEN, D. P., et al. "Dopamine-β-Hydroxylase Activity and Homovanillic Acid in Spinal Fluid of Schizophrenics with Brain Atrophy," *Science,* 220 (1983):974–977.

162. WALSER, R. L., and ACKERMAN, L. V. "Determination of Volume from Computerized Tomograms: Finding the Volume of Fluid-filled Brain Cavities," *Journal of Computer Assisted Tomography,* 1 (1977):117–130.

163. WECHSLER, A. F., et al. "Pick's Disease: A Clinical, Computed Tomographic, and Histologic Study with Golgi Impregnation Observations," *Archives of Neurology,* 39 (1982):287–290.

164. WEINBERGER, D. R., TORREY, E. F., and WYATT, R. J. "Cerebellar Atrophy in Chronic Schizophrenia," *Lancet,* 1 (1979):718–719.

165. WEINBERGER, D. R., WAGNER, R. L., and WYATT, R. J. "Neuropathological Studies of Schizophrenia: A Selective Review," *Schizophrenia Bulletin,* 9 (1983):193–212.

166. WEINBERGER, D. R., et al. "Lateral Cerebral Ventricular Enlargement in Chronic Schizophrenia," *Archives of General Psychiatry,* 36 (1979):735–739.

167. WEINBERGER, D. R., et al. "Structural Abnormalities in the Cerebral Cortex of Chronic Schizophrenic Patients," *Archives of General Psychiatry,* 36 (1979):-935–939.

168. WEINBERGER, D. R., et al. "Cerebral Ventricular Enlargement in Chronic Schizophrenia," *Archives of General Psychiatry,* 37 (1980):11–13.

169. WEINBERGER, D. R., et al. "Poor Premorbid Adjustment and CT Scan Abnormalities in Chronic Schizophrenia," *American Journal of Psychiatry,* 137 (1980):1410–1413.

170. WEINBERGER, D. R., et al. "Familial Aspects of CT Scan Abnormalities in Chronic Schizophrenic Patients," *Psychiatry Research,* 4 (1981):65–71.

171. WEINBERGER, D. R., et al. "Cerebral Ventricular Size and Response to Neuroleptic Treatment." Presented at the Annual Meeting of the American College of Neuropsychopharmacology, San Juan, Puerto Rico, 1982.

172. WEINBERGER, D. R., et al. "Computed Tomography in Schizophreniform Disorder and Other Acute Psychiatric Disorders," *Archives of General Psychiatry,* 39 (1982):778–783.

173. WELLS, C. "Chronic Brain Disease: An Update on Alcoholism, Parkinson's Disease, and Dementia," *Hospital and Community Psychiatry,* 33 (1982):111–126.

174. WILSON, R. S., et al. "Computed Tomography in Dementia," *Neurology,* 32 (1982):1054–1057.

175. WOODS, B. T., and WOLF, J. "A Reconsideration of the Relation of Ventricular Enlargement to Duration of Illness in

Schizophrenia," *American Journal of Psychiatry*, 140 (1983):1564–1570.

176. WU, S., et al. "Cognitive Correlates of Diffuse Cerebral Atrophy Determined by Computed Tomography," *Neurology*, 31 (1981):1180–1184.

177. ZATZ, L. M., JERNIGAN, T. L., and AHUMADA, A. J., Jr. "Changes on Com-

puted Cranial Tomography with Aging: Intracranial Fluid Volume," *American Journal of Neuroradiology*, (1982):1–11.

178. ———. "White Matter Changes in Cerebral Computed Tomography Related to Aging," *Journal of Computer Assisted Tomography*, 6 (1982):19–23.

CHAPTER 10

FUNCTIONAL IMAGING OF THE BRAIN IN PSYCHIATRY: POSITRON EMISSION TOMOGRAPHY AND BLOOD FLOW STUDIES

Monte S. Buchsbaum

¶ Introduction

With the continuing expansion of biological knowledge, the old distinction between functional and organic psychoses becomes problematical (see Roth[41]). As pictures of the structures and neural activity of the brain sharpen with technological advance, the use of the functional/organic dichotomy blurs. These new scanning techniques can provide an image

not only of a physically altered structure like a shrunken gyrus but also of its loss of chemical activity or its dysfunction during specific psychological states. Because the various structures of the brain are interrelated functionally as well as anatomically, functional brain imaging can reveal organizational details of the brain only hypothesized or hidden until now. This chapter reviews the current status of this developing field for both normal cognitive and emotional activity as well as for disturbance in psychiatric disorder.

¶ Positron Emission Tomography

Scanner Technology

Scanner technology uses a ringlike arrangement of radiation detectors to produce slice-images of the distribution of radioisotopes within the human brain.[5,34,35] Current scanners allow, for example, the metabolic rates of structures from the outer cortical mantle to the caudate nucleus to be visualized and quantitatively assessed (see color plate 2).

Positron emission tomography (PET) takes advantage of two properties of radionuclides such as oxygen-15 (^{15}O), nitrogen-13 (^{13}N), carbon-11 (^{11}C), and fluorine-18 (^{18}F)—their suitability as labels for neurochemicals and their emission of positrons. The first three are common constituents of many biological molecules; fluorine is a small and chemically reactive atom that can be attached to molecules as a label, often with minimal alteration of biological function (see Sokoloff[46]). The positrons leaving from these isotopes interact with electrons in quite short distances (about 1 mm or less); an annihilation results and two 511,000 electron volt gamma are emitted, which travel in opposite directions —almost exactly 180 degrees apart. The simultaneous arrival of this radiation in two crystals on opposite sides of the ring of detectors is the feature that allows the great spatial precision in mathematically reconstructing the location of the original position. The two-dimensional Fourier algorithm for reconstruction of the image from the sets of emission coincidence counts gathered during the scan is similar to that used with x-ray transmission computed tomography (CT) (see Moran, et al.[32]).

As of 1985, the resolution of commercially available PET scanners is in the range of 8 to 16 mm, or about the size of the caudate nucleus. Resolution is typically reported as full-width-half-maximum (FWHM). A line source such as a long, small-diameter needle filled with radioactivity and scanned produces a cross-sectional image of a spot—intense in the center and falling off to 50 percent of the center value in the FWHM number of millimeters as a diameter. In the brain, it means that a structure as wide as the FWHM would have its measured value diluted by surrounding tissue by about 70 percent. Thus very small, sufficiently intense structures can be visualized, but their quantitative interpretation would be clouded by the surrounding brain structures. Structures such as the caudate and thalamus, with volumes of the order of 5 cc, are thus well measured with PET resolution of 10 mm; the internal capsule or globus pallidus in the 2 cm^3 range is fairly quantitated; and structures such as the substantia nigra, with less than 1 cm^3, may be seen but poorly quantitated.[26,30] This dilution or blurring is quite important in PET work, where differences in local concentration of isotopes may be 10 to 100 percent. In contrast, the x-ray transmission differences seen on CT scans between bone and air are more than a thousand-fold, allowing quite a sharp skull image to be produced. However, gray matter/white matter differences are in the range of 0.5 percent, accounting for the ability of intrinsically lower resolution PET to reveal brain structures so dramatically in comparison to routine clinical CT.

Medical Cyclotrons

A cyclotron and a radiochemistry laboratory are essential components of each PET scanning operation.[50] The isotopes used in PET studies have quite short half-lives (^{15}O, 2 minutes; ^{13}N, 10 minutes; ^{11}C, 20 minutes; and ^{18}F, 110 minutes); thus a PET scan begins with a cyclotron run. The cyclotron's large magnet and high-tension electrodes accelerate ions in a spiral path until they are finally deflected and extracted in a beam. This beam strikes a specially constructed target containing the precursor atoms. The isotope must be produced, attached to the tracer molecule, purified, checked for radiochemical and/or radionuclide purity, tested for pyrogenicity, and injected into the subject in quite a short space of time.

Some tracers require little preparation. The use of ^{15}O as a breathable tracer of cerebral oxygen uptake requires production in the cyclotron but no elaborate synthetic step —simplifying the radiochemical purity and pyrogenicity testing. However, cyclotron use and scanning must be scheduled together. The production of ^{11}C- or ^{18}F-labeled drugs and metabolic tracers is more complex and requires stringent and rapidly completed quality control. In a typical synthesis, the ^{18}F is produced by bombardment of a neon-filled target for one to two hours and the $^{18}Fluoro$-2-deoxyglucose (^{18}F–2DG) synthesis completed, followed by purification. With ^{18}F, which has a 110-minute half-life, compounds can be synthesized and then shipped by air to a scanner at a distant site. Quality control testing is typically done during the flight.

Patient Risks in PET

There are two hazards of PET scanning— radiotracer toxicity and radiation dosage. For radiopharmaceuticals in unmodified form—for example, $^{15}O_2$, compounds labeled with ^{11}C, or compounds normally containing fluorine, this is a problem addressed at the synthesis stage, and the use in PET at low levels presents little additional risk. Careful monitoring of synthesis is clearly necessary, since each batch is individually produced. The problem is more complex for compounds not normally containing the radioisotope label, but must be addressed in toxicity studies. Since dose is normally orders of magnitude below a pharmacologically active dose, safety is more easily achieved than with new compounds given in full dosage.

Radiation dosage is kept relatively low because of the very short half-lives of the compounds. For example, typical ^{18}F–2DG doses of 4 millicuries (mCi) provide whole-body doses in the 300 mR range. Most centers limit PET scans to three per person or less. Dosim-

etry for ^{18}F–2DG is reviewed by Jones and associates.[24]

Glucose Metabolic Rate

Glucose is the main energy source for the brain. Its use follows local neural activity and in normal tissue is closely coupled to oxygen consumption and blood flow.[45] Raichle and coworkers[36] used ^{11}C-labeled glucose to produce provocative pictures of a rhesus monkey brain, and Widen and associates[48] have used it in schizophrenia. However, glucose itself is metabolized to carbon dioxide (CO_2) and water (H_2O), and sufficient amounts of $^{11}CO_2$ would be produced even during the short period of PET scanning. An alternate technique is to use an analogue of glucose, 2-deoxyglucose.[45,46] The missing oxygen at the 2 position allows its metabolism in the first step of the glycolytic pathway (to 2-deoxyglucose-6-phosphate) but limits further metabolism. The cells are thus labeled in proportion to their glucose uptake; uptake is 70 to 90 percent complete over the forty minutes after intravenous administration. At this point, scanning for glucose metabolic rate images begins.

The alternate tracers, glucose and deoxyglucose, have advantages and disadvantages, summarized by Raichle.[37] ^{11}C-glucose is biochemically identical to the compound being traced,[36,38] and some simple syntheses using CO_2 and algae have been used successfully (see Widen, et al.[48]). The technique does, however, require rapid collection of data immediately following isotope administration and measurement of cerebral blood volume to collect scan data for ^{11}C-glucose in the blood vessels of the brain. Further, more precise knowledge of the parameters of the tracer model is required. Deoxyglucose is an artificial analogue, similar to glucose, but not identical in transport and enzyme affinities. This analogue model of glucose allows longer scanning for higher resolution and additional images and does not require blood volume measurement. Perhaps most important for psychiatry, it also permits the separation of the uptake period from actual scanning. The deoxyglucose can be injected in a psychologically controlled environment. While the subject does a specific task, is asleep, or reports symptoms (see color plate 2 (a, b, c), the uptake and conversion to 2-deoxyglucose-6-phosphate takes place and can be largely complete before the patient is moved to the scanner and the imaging begins. It should be stressed that metabolic imaging is a functional technique and that the scan reflects brain activity, not static structure; the results are no more precise than the behavioral controlled conditions.

In a typical scan procedure with [18]F–2DG, the patient or normal control arrives an hour before the scan. An intravenous line is inserted in each arm. A psychological task may be started at the moment of [18]F–2DG injection or just before. The tracer is injected into one arm and a series of small blood samples are withdrawn from the opposite arm at short intervals. These samples will be counted for [18]F–2DG and chemically assayed for glucose. After thirty to forty minutes, the brain uptake of [18]F–2DG is 70 to 90 percent complete. The scan can then begin (see figure 10–1). Each slice requires the scanner from two to eight minutes to acquire enough counts to produce a usable picture. Some scanners have two or more rings of detectors, allowing simultaneous acquisition of more than a single slice-image.

The raw radioactivity count images computed by PET are next transformed into actual quantitative measures of glucose metabolic rate, typically expressed in micromoles or milligrams of glucose per unit of brain weight per unit time. This requires a mathematical model of the plasma and brain tissue compartments, rate constants for tracer movements, and information about the time course of plasma levels of tracer and glucose following injection. This is obtained from the samples drawn at short intervals following tracer injection throughout uptake and scanning (see Huang, et al.[18] and Sokoloff[46]).

In monkey studies, autoradiographs of ^{14}C-deoxyglucose show extraordinary detail, with functional units as small as the ocular dominance columns in striate cortex clearly visible.[25] In man, the computed tomographic resolution is less, but the much larger dimensions of corresponding brain regions and ease of behavioral control partly compensate for this loss of resolution.

Effects of Psychological State

PET with [18]F–2DG provides a technique for assessing regional brain metabolic changes with psychological tasks or states. Stimulation of the right forearm with brief electrical shocks during [18]F–2DG uptake reveals higher uptake in left somatosensory cortex (see color plate 3).[7] A visual vigilance task such as counting flashes of light increases metabolism in the primary visual cortex (see color plate 4), whereas a subject with eyes closed receiving the electric shocks in the dark shows a PET scan with a low metabolic rate in the primary visual cortex. Similarly, increases in left frontal and temporal cortex have been seen with the verbal stimulation of listening to a Sherlock Holmes story,[31] and visual stimulation studies demonstrate the hemifield projection to the opposite calcarine cortex.[40] More detailed studies will continue to reveal the neuroanatomic substrates of many tasks in greater detail.

Schizophrenia Patient Studies with 2-Deoxyglucose

In the earliest study of cerebral metabolic correlates of schizophrenia, Kety and Schmidt[27] used their nitrous oxide technique for whole brain. While the outcome was negative for whole brain, they suggested that regional metabolic abnormalities in this disorder might be occurring. Subsequently, using regional cerebral blood flow measurement with xenon-133, Ingvar and coworkers[9,20] found relatively lower frontal blood flow in schizophrenics. PET studies have tended to replicate and extend the initial blood flow studies.

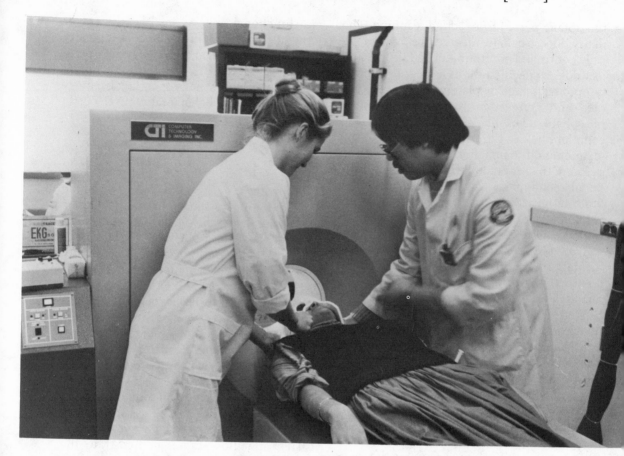

Figure 10–1. Subject is assisted into the PET scanner. A thermosetting plastic mask holds the patient's head still and allows accurate repositioning at a later date. The computer-controlled bed on which the subject lies advances the patient in steps into the PET scanner crystal ring.

The earliest report was by Farkas and associates,[15] who studied a forty-five-year-old patient with a twenty-nine-year history of schizophrenia. This patient had taken no neuroleptic medication before the scan. The patient showed a 40 percent depression in frontal glucose use in comparison to an unspecified control population. A second scan obtained when the patient was on phenothiazines showed an apparent return toward normal. They also noted a relative left hemisphere diminution in glucose use, especially in the temporal and motor cortices. The hypofrontal pattern of glucose seen in the case report by Farkas and associates[15] parallels the earlier blood flow findings of Ingvar and coworkers,[19,20] described later, and those found in subsequent studies.

In the first controlled report[6] local cerebral glucose uptake of $^{18}F–2DG$ use was measured by PET in eight medication-free patients with schizophrenia and six age-matched normal volunteers. Following injection of 3 to 5 mCi $^{18}F–2DG$, subjects rested with eyes closed in an acoustically treated, darkened room. Slices were treated digitally with a 2-cm-thick strip peeled off the periphery of each slice. Patients with schizophrenia showed lower ratios of frontal cortex to whole-slice activity than did normal controls. No systematic differences between left and right hemispheres were seen. In this initial exploration of glucose metabolism, Buchsbaum and coworkers chose the resting, eyes-closed condition for direct comparison with blood flow data.[19,20]

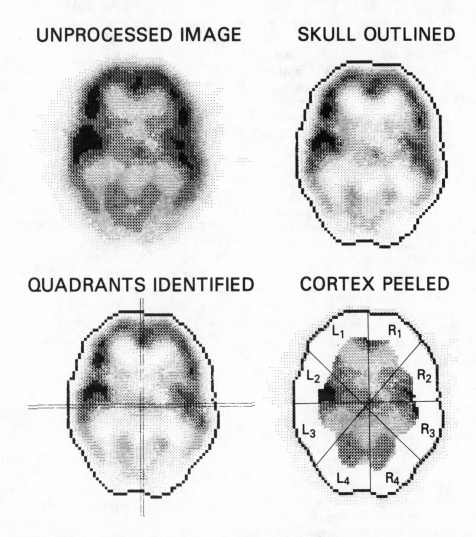

UNPROCESSED IMAGE   **SKULL OUTLINED**

QUADRANTS IDENTIFIED   **CORTEX PEELED**

Figure 10–2. PET scans show images of function, not structure. Thus quantitative regional assessment is important. Procedure for quantitative measurement of glucose use in tomographic slices: Unprocessed image is reconstructed by computer from coincidence count data. Next, boundary-finding algorithm outlines edge of brain. Vertical and horizontal meridians are calculated and slice center is located. Number of picture elements (pixels) within outline are counted, mean counts per pixel are calculated for each quadrant at bottom left, and ratio of quadrant/total slice is reported. Last, a 2.3 cm strip is peeled off, cut into four quadrants on each side; for each quadrant, the mean count per pixel is calculated, and glucose use is expressed as a ratio of quadrant/total slice.

In a second series of patients,[8] Buchsbaum and associates chose somatosensory stimulation of the right forearm as the condition. This was done because Ingvar and others[22,23] noted that frontal blood flow increased in subjects who inserted their hands in a bucket of ice water and observed a smaller increase in schizophrenic patients. This was consistent with the observations by ourselves and others (see Davis, et al.[11,12]) of diminished pain sensitivity in schizophrenia. Off-medication patients were administered the [18]F–2DG just before receiving a 34-minute series of unpleasant electrical stimuli to their right forearm while resting with their eyes closed in a darkened, psychophysiological testing chamber. Patients again showed a significantly lower anteroposterior gradient in glucose use. (See color plate 5 and figure 10–2.) The largest contribution to this gradient was the fact that the level above the ventricles had absolute glucose concentrations that were actually higher in posterior regions, rather than lower in frontal regions. (See figure 10–3.) Similar results were observed by others.[16,28,51] The anteroposterior ratios are largely similar from study to study (see table 10–1) and reveal similarities between blood flow and PET. No significant correlation was observed between front-to-back ratios and any of the following: length of time off neuroleptics, body weight, sex, or cerebral atrophy.

The finding of relative hypofrontality could reflect a trait marker of schizophrenia or be related to clinical state. One source of evidence on this issue is the studies of the identical Genain quadruplets, four adult women with schizophrenia. PET studies[9] found all four relatively hypofrontal (see color plate 6) despite great differences in overall severity, lifetime drug treatment, and current symptoms. The finding of a relative paucity of clinical correlates of the extent of hypofrontality[13] is also consistent with a trait variable status. To date, however, no reliability or follow-up studies have been completed.

Two studies using other tracers were only partially consistent. Wiesel and associates[49] used ^{11}C-glucose and found decreased left frontal glucose metabolism in patients, but a ratio of Brodmann's areas 6 and 8 (superior frontal) to areas 39 and 40 (parietal) was higher in patients (1.05) than in normals (1.00). Table 10–1 ratios are largely derived from Brodmann's area 8 compared to areas 17 and 18 (occipital cortex) rather than parietal areas and this, together with tracer and task differences, may explain disparities. Sheppard and coworkers[44] used ^{15}O as a tracer in patients with mixed medication status. Direct comparison with other researchers' data is difficult since data are presented with only one place after the decimal.

Affective Illness

Patients with bipolar affective illness (mainly depressed) were found to have relatively hypofrontal patterns of glucose metabolism,[8] similar to patients with schizophrenia. A similar pattern of reduced frontal lobe metabolic decreases in depressed bipolar patients was observed by Baxter[3] and associates. Relative decreases in basal ganglia metabolism, especially in unipolar patients, were also observed. Whole-brain metabolic rates increased with mania and decreased with depression in cycling patients. Exploratory data on drug effects similarly suggest the sensitivity of brain metabolism to behavioral and chemical change.

Autism

Adult men with well-documented histories of infantile autism had generally elevated levels of glucose metabolism when studied in a resting state.[42] However, normals had relatively higher metabolic rates in the superior frontal gyrus. Anteroposterior ratios were 1.14 in normals and 0.98 in patients with autism (left superior frontal gyrus/calcarine region; left side calculated from Rumsey and associates' table 2 to be analogous to other authors' reports). Thus relative hypofrontality may be found in autism as well as in schizophrenia.

Blood Flow

Blood flow can be measured with a number of tracers, including krypton-77, oxygen-15-labeled water, ^{13}NH$_3$, and molecules labeled with ^{18}F (see Phelps[35]). The short half-life of ^{15}O and ^{13}N (2 minutes and 10 minutes, respectively) makes them suitable for behavioral studies in which a series of scan studies can be used to compare different

PET Supraventricular Slice

Normal Controls

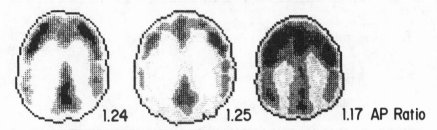

1.24   1.25   1.17 AP Ratio

Affective Disorder

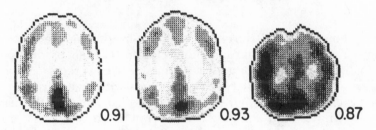

0.91   0.93   0.87

Schizophrenia

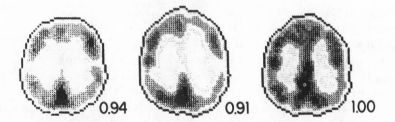

0.94   0.91   1.00

Figure 10–3. PET images in horizontal plane (parallel to and about 8 cm above the canthomeatal line) at supraventricular level. Three scans typical of normal controls, patients with affective disorder, and patients with schizophrenia are shown. A ratio of anterior to posterior cortex glucose use was calculated for each slice (see Buchsbaum et al.[6]) and is shown to the lower right of each slice.

TABLE 10–1

Anteroposterior Ratios of [18]F-2DG and Blood Flow in Schizophrenic Subjects and Normal Controls

Study	Date	Normals	Schizophrenics
PET with [18]F-2DG[a]			
Buchsbaum et al.[6]	1982	1.14	1.05
Buchsbaum et al.[8]	1984	1.08	1.02
Farkas et al.[16]	1984	1.14[b,c]	1.07[b,c]
Brodie et al.[4]	1985	1.03[d]	0.94[d]
Wolkin et al.[51]	1985	1.11[e]	0.98[e]
Blood Flow[a]			
Ingvar and Franzen[20]	1974	1.10[c]	1.04[c]
Ariel et al.[1]	1983	1.10	1.05

[a]Reports from which anteroposterior ratios cannot be calculated are not included.
[b]Calculated from semioval center slice for comparability.
[c]Calculated, see Buchsbaum et al.[6]
[d]See Brodie et al.,[4] color plate 3.
[e]Calculated in Wolkin et al., table 2, left frontal cortex/left occipital cortex.

psychological tasks within a space of thirty minutes to two hours. The studies of Ingvar and coworkers emphasize not only the large changes in blood flow with mental activity, with many brain areas changing flow more than 50 percent (e.g., Ingvar and Philipson[21]), but also the possibility of schizophrenia differences in these dynamic shifts. (See color plates 7 to 11.)

The rigorous testing of any of the major psychological theories of schizophrenia, such as a selective attentional deficit, requires at least two scans on a patient, one while the patient is doing the attentional task and a contrasting control. Since most tasks used in schizophrenia research involve motor, perceptual, and cognitive phases, many scan studies comparing isolated components of the task in normal controls will be necessary to characterize the nature of the deficit. One possible disadvantage of the very short half-life flow studies with [15]O and ^{13}N is that the entire isotope administration and scan process takes place in less than ten minutes; the psychological task must take place in the scanner room and the subject must do the task, then be positioned and scanned. With some kinetic models, scanning must actually be done during the task (see discussion in Phelps, et al.[35]), making complete sensory control and stimulus administration difficult.

These short-lived isotopes also require an on-site cyclotron for their production.

Reiman and coworkers[39] have reported that patients with panic disorder may have diminished blood flow in the left parahippocampal gyrus in comparison to the right using ^{15}O-H_2O and PET. The blood-flow method seems especially appropriate for following the course of panic attacks.

Receptor Imaging

The first published clinical PET study in psychiatry was by Comar and coworkers,[10] who used ^{11}C-chlorpromazine in twenty-two schizophrenic patients who had not been treated with neuroleptics for several months prior to the study. Neuroleptics have a higher binding affinity for the dopaminergic receptors in the brain than for other receptors. Thus a positron-emitting labeled drug such as chlorpromazine might reveal the location and density of dopamine (DA) receptors. The PET scan values could reflect the number of receptors per unit volume, receptor affinity for the labeled compound, and the concentrations of natural receptor agonists available. Thus it is a dynamic experiment reflecting the neurochemical status of the DA system at the time of the scan.

Unfortunately, other factors would also affect labeling. Neuroleptic ligands bind to receptors other than the DA receptor. Multiple DA receptors with different affinities complicate the direct interpretation of the quantitative image. Metabolic products of neuroleptics that retained the positron-emitting isotope would appear, although perhaps with a time course slower than the half-life of the isotope (see Comar, et al.[10]). In addition, these drugs are lipid-soluble and enter myelin and fatty material. The resultant image reflects all of these influences on radiolabel distribution. Comar and coworkers' images of schizophrenic brains show the gray matter labeled more strongly than the white matter. The cerebellum, where DA receptors are not thought to occur, appears clearly. Thus this tracer is not as specific a tool for receptor display as hoped.

Recently Wagner and associates[47] have used ^{11}C-labeled methyl-spiperone in PET studies. This tracer bound more selectively to the caudate than cerebellum with a 4.4 to 1 ratio at 70 to 130 minutes. This method may prove powerful in demonstrating receptor abnormalities in schizophrenia. Arnett and colleagues[2] have used ^{11}C-spiroperidol to image neuroleptic receptors in baboons, and they suggest the utility of pretreatment with drugs with high specific receptor binding to generate a second scan; image differences can then reveal specific binding patterns.

More specific binding with new compounds for visualization of D-2 DA receptors (e.g., Farde, et al.[14] and Sedvall, et al.[43]) may further extend clinical applications. In normal subjects, this binding is quite specific to the caudate and putamen and rapidly displaced by administration of haloperidol. Garnett and associates[17] used ^{18}F-labeled levodopa and showed caudate and frontal cortex concentration, demonstrating the versatility of PET approaches to DA neurochemistry in man.

Brain images of benzodiazepines have also been used in man[29,33] to produce PET images; the range of potential receptor/drug studies in psychiatry includes all of the current drug classes used in treatment.

¶ Conclusion: PET Diagnostic Specificity Versus Anatomical Specificity

Functional brain images reveal changes in particular brain structures. It is well known from neuropsychological studies of brain trauma that it is exceedingly difficult to relate specific neuropsychological deficits to lesions in single cortical or subcortical structures. While PET does not suffer the disadvantage of making interpretations from the irregular and often uncertainly known natural lesion, the other problems of localization remain. These include the complex interrelatedness of frontal and posterior structures and the vast individual differences in information processing and behavioral strategies. The "red spot" of schizophrenia on a PET scan will likely be elusive, both because of the just-mentioned factors and because of the often touted but more often ignored heterogeneity of the disease. The grouping of patients by anatomically related patterns of brain dysfunction may provide the most powerful tool yet for understanding the diversity of behavior and drug response in the psychiatrically ill.

¶ Bibliography

1. ARIEL, R. N., et al. "Regional Cerebral Blood Flow in Schizophrenics," *Archives of General Psychiatry*, 40 (1983):258–263.
2. ARNETT, C. D., et al. "Mapping Brain Neuroleptic Receptors in the Live Baboon," *Biological Psychiatry*, 19 (1984): 1365–1375.
3. BAXTER, L. R., Jr., et al. "Cerebral Metabolic Rates for Glucose in Mood Disorders," *Archives of General Psychiatry*, 42 (1985):441–447.
4. BRODIE, J. D., et al. "Analysis of Positron Emission Transaxial Tomography Images in Psychiatric Disorders," in T. Greitz et al., eds., *Metabolism of the Human Brain Studied with Positron Emission Tomography*. New York: Raven Press, 1985, pp. 441–451.

5. BROWNELL, G. L., et al. "Positron Emission Tomography and Nuclear Magnetic Resonance Imaging," *Science,* 215 (1982):619–626.

6. BUCHSBAUM, M. S., et al. "Cerebral Glucography with Positron Tomography," *Archives of General Psychiatry,* 39 (1982):251–259.

7. BUCHSBAUM, M. S., et al. "Cerebral Metabolic Consequences of Electrical Cutaneous Stimulation in Normal Individuals," *Human Neurobiology,* 2 (1983):35–38.

8. BUCHSBAUM, M. S., et al. "Anteroposterior Gradients in Cerebral Glucose Use in Schizophrenia and Affective Disorders," *Archives of General Psychiatry,* 41 (1984):1159–1166.

9. BUCHSBAUM, M. S., et al. "The Genain Quadruplets: Electrophysiological, Positron Emission and X-Ray Tomographic Studies," *Psychiatry Research,* 13 (1984):95–108.

10. COMAR, D., et al. "Brain Distribution and Kinetics of ^{11}C-Chlorpromazine in Schizophrenics: Positron Emission Tomography Studies," *Psychiatry Research,* 1 (1979):23–29.

11. DAVIS, G. C., et al. "Research in Endorphins and Schizophrenia," *Schizophrenia Bulletin* 5 (1979):244–250.

12. DAVIS, G. C., et al. "Analgesia to Pain Stimuli in Schizophrenics and Its Reversal by Naltrexone," *Psychiatry Research,* 1 (1979):61–69.

13. DeLISI, L. E., et al. "Clinical Correlates of Decreased Anteroposterior Metabolic Gradients in Positron Emission Tomography (PET) in Schizophrenic Patients," *American Journal of Psychiatry,* 142 (1985):78–81.

14. FARDE, L., et al. "Substituted Benzamides as Ligands for Visualization of Dopamine Receptor Binding in the Human Brain by Positron Emission Tomography," *Proceedings of the National Academy of Science,* 82 (1985):3863–3867.

15. FARKAS, T., et al. "The Application of [^{18}F]2-Deoxy-2-Fluoro-D-Glucose and Positron Emission Tomography in the Study of Psychiatric Conditions," in J. V. Passonneau et al., eds., *Cerebral Metabolism and Neural Function.* Bal-timore: Williams & Wilkins, 1980, pp. 403–408.

16. FARKAS, T., et al. "Regional Brain Glucose Metabolism in Chronic Schizophrenia," *Archives of General Psychiatry,* 41 (1984):293–300.

17. GARNETT, E. S., et al. "Dopamine Visualized in the Basal Ganglia of Living Man," *Nature,* 305 (1983):137–138.

18. HUANG, S. C., et al. "Non-invasive Determination of Local Cerebral Metabolic Rate of Glucose in Man," *American Journal of Physiology,* 238 (Supplement) (1980):69–82.

19. INGVAR, D. "Abnormal Distribution of Cerebral Activity in Chronic Schizophrenia: A Neurophysiological Interpretation," in C. F. Baxter and T. Melnechuck, eds., *Perspectives in Schizophrenia Research.* New York: Raven Press, 1980, pp. 107–125.

20. INGVAR, D., and FRANZEN, G. "Abnormalities of Cerebral Blood Flow Distribution in Patients with Chronic Schizophrenia," *Acta Psychiatrica Scandinavica,* 50 (1974):425–462.

21. INGVAR, D., and PHILIPSON, L. "Distribution of Cerebral Blood Flow in the Dominant Hemisphere During Motor Ideation and Motor Performance," *Annals of Neurology,* 2 (1977):230–237.

22. INGVAR, D., et al. "Effects of Somatosensory Stimulation Upon Rest," in M. Harper et al., eds., *Blood Flow and Metabolism in the Brain,* Proceedings of the 7th International Symposium on Cerebral Blood Flow and Metabolism. New York: Churchill Livingston, 1975, pp. 1429–1432.

23. INGVAR, D., et al. "Activation Patterns Induced in the Dominant Hemisphere by Skin Stimulation," in Y. Zotterman et al., eds., *Sensory Functions of the Skin.* London: Pergamon Press, 1976, pp. 549–559.

24. JONES, S. C., et al. "The Radiation Dosimetry of 2-[F-18]-Fluoro-2-Deoxyglucose in Man," *Journal of Nuclear Medicine,* 23 (1982):613–617.

25. KENNEDY, M., et al. "Metabolic Mapping of the Primary Visual System of the Monkey by Means of the Autoradiographic [^{14}C] Deoxyglucose Technique," *Proceedings of the National*

Academy of Science, 73 (1976):4230–4234.

26. KESSLER, R. M., et al. "Analysis of Emission Tomographic Scan Data: Limitations Imposed by Resolution and Background," *Journal of Computer Assisted Tomography,* in press.

27. KETY, S. S., and SCHMIDT, C. F. "The Nitrous Oxide Method for the Quantitative Determination of Cerebral Blood Flow in Man: Theory, Procedure and Normal Values," *Journal of Clinical Investigation,* 27 (1948):476–492.

28. KISIMOTO, H. "Studies in Brain Function in Schizophrenic Patients Using Positron CT." Paper presented at the 38th Annual Convention and Scientific Program of the Society of Biological Psychiatry, New York, April/May, 1983.

29. MAZIERE, M., et al. "Positron Tomography. A New Method for In Vivo Brain Studies of Benzodiazepine, in Animal and in Man," in E. Costa et al., eds. *GABA and Benzodiazepine Receptors.* New York: Raven Press, 1981, pp. 273–286.

30. MAZZIOTTA, J. C., et al., "Quantitation in Positron Emission Computed Tomography: 5. Physical-Anatomical Effects," *Journal of Computer Assisted Tomography,* 5 (1981):734–643.

31. MAZZIOTTA, J. C. et al. "Tomographic Mapping of Human Cerebral Metabolism: Auditory Stimulation," *Neurology,* 32 (1982):921–937.

32. MORAN, P. R. et al. "The Physics of Medical Imaging," *Physics Today,* July 1983, pp. 36–42.

33. PERSSON, A., et al. "Imaging of ^{11}C-Labeled RO 15–1788 Binding to Benzodiazepine Receptors in the Human Brain by Positron Emission Tomography," *Journal of Psychiatric Research,* in press.

34. PHELPS, M. E., and MAZZIOTTA, J. C. "Positron Emission Tomography: Human Brain Funtion and Biochemistry," *Science,* 228 (1985):799–809.

35. PHELPS, M. E., et al. "Study of Cerebral Function with Positron Computed Tomography," *Journal of Cerebral Blood Flow and Metabolism,* 2 (1982): 113–162.

36. RAICHLE, M. "Measurement of Regional Substrate Utilization Rates by Emission Tomography," *Science,* 199 (1978):986–987.

37. ———. "Positron Emission Tomography Tracer Techniques," in J. W. Root and K. A. Krohn, eds., *Advances in Chemistry Series,* no. 197, *Short-Lived Radio-Nuclides in Chemistry and Biology.* New York: American Chemical Society, 1981, pp. 420–436.

38. ———. "Positron Emission Tomography," *Annual Review of Neurology,* 6 (1983): 249–267.

39. REIMAN, E. M., et al. "A Focal Brain Abnormality in Panic Disorder, a Severe Form of Anxiety," *Nature,* 310 (1984): 683–685.

40. REIVICH, M., et al. "Positron Emission Tomographic Studies of Sensory Stimuli, Cognitive Processes and Anxiety," *Human Neurobiology,* 2 (1983):25–33.

41. ROTH, M. "Psychiatric Diagnosis in Clinical and Scientific Settings," in H. S. Akiskal and W. L. Webb, eds., *Psychiatric Diagnosis: Exploration of Biological Predictors.* New York: Spectrum Publications, 1978, pp. 9–47.

42. RUMSEY, J. M., et al. "Brain Metabolism in Autism," *Archives of General Psychiatry,* 42 (1985):448–457.

43. SEDVALL, G., et al. "PET Studies on Brain Energy Metabolism and Dopamine Receptors in Schizophrenic Patients and Monkeys," in P. Pichot et al., eds., *Psychiatry: The State of the Art.* New York: Plenum Press, 1984, pp. 305–312.

44. SHEPPARD, G., et al. "[15]O Positron Emission Tomographic Scanning in Predominantly Never-Treated Acute Schizophrenic Patients," *Lancet,* 2 (1983):1448–1452.

45. SOKOLOFF, L. "Relation Between Physiological Function and Energy Metabolism in the Central Nervous System," *Journal of Neurochemistry,* 29 (1977): 13–26.

46. ———. "The Radioactive Deoxyglucose Method: Theory, Procedure, and Applications for the Measurement of Local Glucose Utilization in the Central Nervous System," in B. W. Agranoff and M. H. Aprison, eds., *Advances in Neurochemistry,* vol. 4, New York: Plenum Press, 1982, pp. 1–82.

47. WAGNER, H. N., et al. "Imaging Dopamine Receptors in the Human Brain by Positron Tomography," *Science*, 221 (1983):1262–1264.

48. WIDEN, L., et al. "PET Studies of Glucose Metabolism in Patients with Schizophrenia," *American Journal of Neuroradiology*, 4 (1983):550–552.

49. WIESEL, F.-A., et al. "Brain Energy Metabolism in Schizophrenia Studied with ^{11}C-Glucose," in T. Greitz et al., eds., *The Metabolism of the Human Brain Studied with Positron Emission Tomography*. New York: Raven Press, 1985, pp. 485–493.

50. WOLF, A. P. "Cyclotrons, Radionuclides, Precursors, and Demands for Routine versus Research Compounds," *Annals of Neurology*, 15 (Supplement) (1984): 19–24.

51. WOLKIN, A., et al. "Persistence of Cerebral Metabolic Abnormalities in Chronic Schizophrenia as Determined by Positron Emission Tomography," *American Journal of Psychiatry*, 142 (1985):564–571.

CHAPTER 11

MAGNETIC RESONANCE AND *IN VIVO* STUDIES OF THE HUMAN BRAIN

Glen R. Elliott

¶ Introduction

Progress in understanding how the brain works often occurs in close conjunction with technological advances in monitoring aspects of its functions. Thus, as reviewed elsewhere in this volume (see chapter 2), many of the exciting discoveries about the brain that took place in the 1950s and 1960s grew out of applications of newly developed fluorometric and gas chromatographic assays for biogenic amines such as the catecholamines and serotonin. In the 1970s, with the development of mass spectroscopic, high-performance liquid chromatographic, radio-immunologic, and radioreceptor assays that pushed sensitivity and specificity even further, concepts about brain function became increasingly rich, as investigators continued to discover previously unsuspected neuroregulators.

A continuing frustration for biologically oriented investigators of mental disorders has been the limited extent to which such technological advances can be applied to studies of brain function in human beings. Certainly, progress has been made, as attested by many chapters in this volume. Improvements in analytical techniques have enabled researchers to go from studies of neuroregulator metabolites found in urine to research on changes in the much lower concentrations of neuroregulators and metabolites in blood and cerebrospinal fluid (CSF). However, such measures are still far from satisfying, because at best, they are only indirect indicators of events of interest at the level of the neuron; even compounds measured in lumbar CSF often have been processed so thoroughly that they in no way reflect actual neuronal activity in the brain.

One of the exciting developments of the 1980s has been the introduction of several techniques that yield much more direct information about brain function. Several of those methods, including computed axial tomography (CT; see chapter 9), positron emission tomography (PET; see chapter 10), and computer-analyzed electroencephalograms (EEGs; see chapter 8), are discussed in this volume. This chapter describes magnetic resonance (MR), one of the newest additions to this emerging research armamentarium. Medical applications of MR have attracted an enormous amount of attention over the past few years, and a number of excellent reviews are available.[31,51,63,70] Reviews of applications of MR specific to psychiatric problems have been much slower to appear.[29]

¶ Historical Aspects of Magnetic Resonance

Although MR has only recently attracted the intense interest of medical researchers, it has been an invaluable tool for physicists and chemists for many years. The phenomenon was first discovered independently in 1945 by two groups of physicists. Felix Bloch and his colleagues at Stanford[15] and Edward Purcell and his colleagues at Harvard[53] were working on quite different aspects of the phenomenon of nuclear magnetization; both groups discovered that a solid substance in a magnetic field will absorb and release energy at discrete radiofrequencies. This discovery, nuclear magnetic resonance (NMR), and its subsequent applications were of such major importance that Bloch and Purcell shared the 1952 Nobel Prize for Physics for their work.

The term nuclear magnetic resonance is still used widely in chemistry and physics. However, within medical circles, it is being supplanted with increasing frequency by the term magnetic resonance. In large part, this change has occurred because of concerns that patients might mistakenly assume that

"nuclear" implies the use of potentially harmful ionizing radiation. It also leads to euphonious acronyms for magnetic resonance imaging (MRI) and magnetic resonance spectroscopy (MRS).

The first specialties to make use of MR were physics and chemistry.[3] Physicists used it to measure nuclear magnetic moments precisely and as magnetometers for measuring variations in the earth's magnetic field. They quickly identified the fundamental principles and major parameters of MR and used them to gain insights into molecular interactions in a wide range of substances.[16,17,18,60]

Chemists became enamored of MR with the discovery that the observed MR frequency of a given nucleus was a function not only of the external magnetic field strength but also of its own electronic environment.[5] This slight effect of the electronic environment on the observed frequency, called a chemical shift, suggested the possibility that MR could be used to gain information about electronic environments and thus molecular structure. The further discovery that nearby nuclei interacted with each other to cause additional splitting of the signals (spin-spin coupling) further enhanced its utility as a molecular probe.[34,43] The difficult technological hurdle was creating high-strength magnetic fields of sufficient homogeneity throughout the sampling volume to permit detection of the markedly weaker variations in frequency caused by chemical shift and spin-spin coupling. Such changes, measured in parts per million, can be detected only with field uniformity of about one part per hundred million.[3] Once such requirements were met, high-resolution NMR spectrometers became and remain essential pieces of equipment in every chemistry research facility.

Technological advances continue to play a key role in the extension of MR applications into new areas. Especially important for the medical field has been the development of magnets that have an inner bore large enough to admit the human body and that also have the required field strength and ho-

TABLE 11–1
Magnetic Resonance Properties of Some Diagnostically Relevant Nucleotides

Nucleotide (spin)	Relative Atomic		Typical Observed Systems	Typical Concentrations (moles/liter)	Relative Actual Sensitivity
	Abundance	Sensitivity			
^{1}H (1/2)	99.9	1	Water	110	10,000
			Tissue	.010	1
^{13}C (1/2)	1.1	0.02	Natural	< 0.010	0.0001
			Enriched	< 0.050	0.001
^{19}F (1/2)	100	0.83	Tagged	< 0.070	3
^{7}Li (3/2)	81	0.29	Administered	0.1	2
^{23}Na (3/2)	100	0.09	CSF	0.160	1
			Tissue	0.040	0.3
^{31}P (1/2)	100	0.01	Tissue	< 0.010	0.06

SOURCE: A. A. Maudsley, "Technical Demands of Other Nuclei," Paper presented at the Third Annual Meeting of the Society of Magnetic Resonance in Medicine, New York, August 13–17, 1984, pp. 510–512; and O. Jardetzky and G.C.K. Roberts, *NMR in Molecular Biology* (New York: Academic Press, 1981), pp. 18–19.

mogeneity.[35] One of the impressive changes in the past few years has been the steady increase in the magnetic field strengths. For example, only ten years ago magnets large enough for the human body were quite rare, and magnetic field strengths for early clinical instruments were low; now hospitals across the United States and throughout the world are purchasing whole-body instruments that commonly have magnetic field strengths that are twenty times greater than the first instruments.

¶ Principles of Magnetic Resonance

As noted earlier, the fundamental principles underlying MR have been well known for a number of years. They have been enunciated in precise mathematical formulations that are extremely valuable for researchers but much less informative for those with a more casual interest in the topic. Thus the following description is greatly simplified, using no mathematical expressions. Those wanting slightly more mathematical detail can refer to Young[70] or Hendee and Morgan[36]; even more rigorous treatments also are readily available.[40,49,60]

The key to MR lies in the subatomic particles from which nuclei are constructed—protons and neutrons, both of which possess the quality of "spin," which creates a minute amount of electromagnetic energy. Nuclei that contain an even number of protons plus neutrons have no net spin, so they do not exhibit MR. Nuclei with an odd number of protons plus neutrons do have a net spin that can be detected as MR. Table 11–1 lists the nuclei that display MR and that are of most interest to medical researchers and clinicians.

Under usual conditions, the extremely weak magnetic fields of odd-numbered nuclei are readily overcome by other forces, so collections of such nuclei are randomly oriented, producing an overall magnetic force of zero (see figure 11–1*a*). The imposition of a strong, static magnetic field imposes order on the system, with the nuclei tending to line up with (parallel to) or against (antiparallel to) the field (see figure 11–1*b*). This has the effect of creating two energy states that the nuclei can occupy. However, the nuclei do not point exactly along the axis defined by the magnetic field; instead they gyrate—precess —about that axis, much as a top wobbles about its axis as gravity exerts an effect on it. For each nucleotide, the frequency of precession is a constant called the Larmor frequency.

If energy is introduced into the system with a radiofrequency at exactly the Larmor frequency, the nuclei begin to resonate and

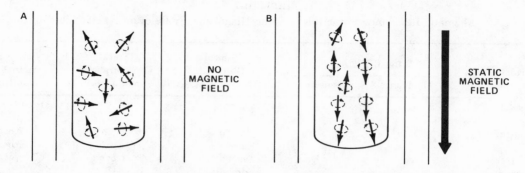

Figure 11–1. Schematic representation of the effects of a static magnetic field on ¹H protons. *a.* In the absence of a magnetic field, orientation of the nuclei are random and the net magnetic moment for the solution is zero. *b.* Introduction of a magnetic field creates a preferential orientation with (parallel) or against (antiparallel) the field. More protons occupy the parallel than the antiparallel state.

can absorb a quantum of energy, flipping from the lower-energy parallel state to the higher energy antiparallel state (see figure 11–2). The Larmor frequency, which is specific for each nucleotide, is directly proportional to the static magnetic field strength. In fact, this mathematical relationship has resulted in two equivalent methods of identifying the strength of an MR instrument. Chem-

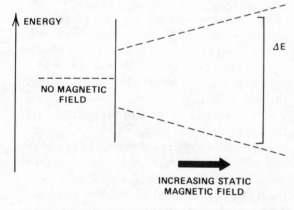

Figure 11–2. The effect of a static magnetic field on nuclei with observable spins. In the absence of a magnetic field, nuclei occupy the same energy state. Imposition of a static magnetic field creates two energy states; the energy difference between them is directly proportional to the strength of the magnetic field times a specific constant for each nucleotide, the Larmor frequency.

ists, who initially were interested almost exclusively in proton NMR, typically think of the field strength in terms of the Larmor frequency for hydrogen-1 (¹H); for example, 100 megahertz (MHz) instruments are fairly common. In contrast, medical researchers have adopted the convention of identifying the actual magnetic field strength in kilogauss or Tesla (10,000 kilogauss). For ¹H, the Larmor frequency is 42.58 MHz per Tesla, so a 100-MHz instrument has a 2.3 Tesla magnet.

As already noted, if radiofrequency energy at the Larmor frequency is applied to nuclei aligned in a static magnetic field, some will flip from the lower to the higher energy state. When the energy source is removed, they gradually return to their previous state, emitting a quantum of energy at the Larmor frequency, which can be detected with a radiofrequency receiver coil. The time that it takes to return to the original alignment along the axis of the static magnetic field is called T_1, or longitudinal relaxation time; T_1 reflects the rate at which energy is dissipated into structures around the nuclei. Neighboring nuclei that have the same spin can also interact, further dispersing energy over a time T_2, called transverse or spin-spin relaxation time; the magnitude of T_2 reflects the relative tendency of nuclei to resonate together. A large number of factors affect the observed T_1 and T_2 in tissues, most of them understood only in broad detail.[41] Empirically, differences between tissues in either or both of these relaxation times can be used to good advantage, as discussed in the next section.

Actual data collection is done by repeatedly exposing the sample to an appropriate radiofrequency and then monitoring how long it takes for the system to return to equilibrium. A variety of standard sequences are being developed, including saturation recovery, inversion recovery, and spin-echo. The utility of a particular sequence depends on the tissue being studied and the question being asked.[29,69] For example, inversion recovery sequences, which are especially sensitive to T_1 differences, provide excellent contrast between gray and white matter in the brain. In general, data collection is relatively time-consuming, often requiring thirty to sixty minutes or more, but a variety of efforts are underway to reduce the time required.

¶ Magnetic Resonance Imaging

Although there were some antecedents,[3] the suggestion of using MR for imaging of solids such as tissue typically is credited to Lauterbur.[42] In his 1973 letter to *Nature,* he propounded the idea of using a gradient magnetic field to generate topographical information about nuclei. Knowing the Larmor frequency of a nucleus and determining where it resonates in a ramped magnetic field, one can calculate where it is along one dimension; by using orthogonal gradients, one can generate a precise two-dimensional map. Lauterbur demonstrated the practical feasibility of his suggestion with reconstructed images of two tubes of water. Since then a number of imaging methods have been devised, several of which generate true three-dimensional information about a structure such as the head. Because protons are by far the most abundant nuclei in the body, an overwhelming proportion of attention has been given to ^{1}H MR images.[31,39,62]

In a little over a decade, MRI has gone from a demonstration project to big business. The state-of-the-art instrument already has image resolution comparable to CT under most conditions and is superior to it in some settings, especially for imaging the brain.[26,28] Whereas the skull is a major obstacle to obtaining good CT images, bone contains little water and thus does not contribute much to ^{1}H MR scans. The resulting images have an astounding clarity, crispness, and detail (see color plate 12).

Few studies have been published yet that compare MR images of brain in subjects having a defined mental disorder with images of healthy controls. Such research is of considerable interest, so data will undoubtedly be forthcoming over the next few years. MRI is certainly relevant for efforts to clarify the conflicting CT studies suggesting ventricular enlargement and other anatomical abnormalities found in some patients with severe mental disorders such as schizophrenia (cf. chapter 9).

In a small pilot study, Smith and colleagues[61] compared nine young patients meeting Research Diagnostic Criteria (RDC) for schizophrenia with five nonpsychotic, healthy controls whose mean age was nearly eleven years greater than that of the patients. Using a 0.3 Tesla instrument, they reported good visualization of brain tissue and structures, but found no differences between patients and controls. Because of the small sample size and many unresolved issues about comparability of CT and MR techniques, this report adds little to the controversy about possible anatomical changes in individuals with schizophrenia. However, larger studies making use of better resolution available with 1.5 Tesla instruments and taking advantage of the true three-dimensional data base possible with MRI should be enormously helpful.

Another approach in MR studies of patients with mental disorders involves measures of regional T_1 values. So far, the few reports in the literature raise more questions than they answer. In the first reported study of this type, Besson and colleagues[10] measured T_1 in the cerebral gray and white matter of six chronic alcoholic patients and six nonalcoholic controls; alcoholic patients were studied during intoxication, during withdrawal, and six weeks after abstinence. In both gray and white matter, the T_1 for alcoholic patients was lower than that for controls during intoxication but higher than control values during withdrawal and after sustained abstinence. As noted earlier, many factors influence relaxation times,[41] and the exact meaning or even reliability of this change in T_1 remains unclear. Furthermore, this study and the others cited all calculate T_1 values from relatively limited areas of the brain, and not nearly enough is known yet about how T_1 changes across brain regions in healthy and pathological conditions.

Rangel-Guerra and colleagues[55] studied twenty patients who met the RDC diagnosis of bipolar affective disorder and eighteen controls; patients were studied on and off lithium carbonate. The authors measured T_1 in both the frontal cortex and temporal lobe but reported results only for the temporal lobe. T_1 for the untreated patients was 277 ± 11 milliseconds (msec); T_1 for controls was 210 ± 8 msec. After treatment, the mean T_1 for patients decreased to 209 ± 7 msec—not different from controls. The authors suggest, with no direct evidence, that the increased T_1 in untreated patients reflects an excess of intracellular free water and that reversal of this presumed excess may explain lithium's therapeutic action. Many other possible explanations, including direct effects of lithium on ^1H relaxation times, have yet to be studied.

Two groups have reported on the use of MRI for diagnosing dementia. Besson and colleagues[11] studied thirteen patients with Alzheimer-type senile dementia and twelve patients with multi-infarct dementia, all between sixty-five and eighty-five years of age. They measured proton density and T_1 in the left and right frontal, parietal, and occipital cortex. Both types of dementia were associated with elevated relaxation times when compared with control values; but T_1 did not distinguish between the dementias themselves. Patients with Alzheimer-type senile dementia had decreased proton densities in white matter when compared with either control subjects or patients with multi-infarct dementia; however, there was substantial overlap between the two dementias. Using a clinical/descriptive approach in studying thirteen patients with various forms of dementia, Erkinjuntti and colleagues[30] concluded that MR was potentially of value in distinguishing among some but not all dementias, without suggesting any specific diagnostic criteria.

In a preliminary report Besson and colleagues[13] described results on twenty-three patients who met the RDC diagnosis of schizophrenia and fifteen control subjects of comparable age. They calculated T_1 values for parts of the corpus callosum and thalamus, the temporal lobe, and various regions of the cerebral cortex. Compared with controls, schizophrenic patients had an elevated T_1 in the right basal ganglia but in no other brain area measured; also T_1 values in the right basal ganglia had a correlation of 0.53 with scores for tardive dyskinesia. Again, these findings must be replicated.[29]

Much remains to be learned about the full potential of MRI of the brain for psychiatric research. At present, considerable effort is still being expended on such issues as the appropriate strength of the magnetic field.[14,27,69] The relative merits of such factors as cost, ease of use, sensitivity, resolution, and speed are proving to be difficult to balance, especially with the field evolving as rapidly as it has over the past decade. Also important are basic studies to establish the extent and causes of intra- and interindividual variability of T_1 and T_2 in various tissues and physiological states, as well as over time. Furthermore, relatively little is known yet about how to translate observed changes in relaxation times into alterations in neuroregulatory mechanisms that may help to clarify the etiology or pathology of severe mental disorders.

¶ Magnetic Resonance Spectroscopy

The extension of high-resolution MRS to *in vivo* studies of human beings has become feasible only recently, because the requirements for magnetic field strength and homogeneity are substantially greater than those for imaging.[3] To date, MRS has not shared the glamour and popular acclaim of MRI; yet there are good reasons to believe that spectroscopy ultimately will be even more valuable to psychiatric research than high-resolution imaging.

In principle, *in vivo* MRS is analogous to the NMR spectroscopy that chemists have used for years. Basically, a sample is irradiated with the Larmor frequency of the nucleotide of interest; chemical shifts are monitored in the resulting signal emission and used to infer information about substances within the sample. Much of the *in vivo* work has been done with phosphorus-31 (^{31}P), both because of its natural abundance (see table 11–1) and because it is present in a number of key compounds in cellular systems that store and supply energy, including adenosine triphosphate (ATP) and phosphocreatine. George Radda pioneered in using ^{31}P spectroscopy to monitor muscle, and he and his colleagues have made impressive progress in demonstrating its clinical utility.[4,54,63]

Studies of ^{31}P spectra of brain have proceeded somewhat more slowly, in part because of difficulties in distinguishing brain signals from those that originate in overlying skin, muscle, and bone. Even so, reports are appearing of animal research on the effects on brain function of such conditions as hypoxia,[52,65,68] status epilepticus,[52] and aging.[33] Robert Shulman and his coworkers at Yale have been especially vigorous in pursuing such applications.[7,52,56] Their efforts and those of others have established the feasibility of using MRS as a probe for monitoring important aspects of brain function.

Work of Jardetzky and colleagues with the diving turtle offers a good illustration of the potential power of this technique.[68] They constructed an apparatus within the bore of a 2.3 Tesla MR instrument that enables them to immobilize the turtle's head within the field and to submerge it underwater at will. Figure 11–3 is a typical ^{31}P spectrum of a turtle while breathing air. The general configuration of peaks resembles that for other tissues and animals, with prominent peaks from the three phosphates of ATP, a single major peak from phosphocreatine, and another peak reflecting the contribution of inorganic phosphates. Figure 11–4 depicts the effects over time of submerging the turtle's head: The phosphocreatine peak intensity decreases and the inorganic phosphate peak both increases and shifts position. The peak shift in inorganic phosphate reflects changes in the relative abundance of its various ionic forms,[48] which are sensitive to changes in pH. As a result, it is possible to calculate pH *in vivo* from the distance of the inorganic phosphate peak from some other "standard," typically phosphocreatine. This is only one example of the rich information contained in an MR spectrum. Figure 11–5 graphically dis-

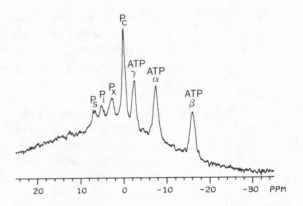

Figure 11–3. A ^{31}P magnetic resonance spectrum of a turtle head. The spectrum, generated in a 2.3 T Varian XL-100 spectrometer, was taken while the turtle was breathing air.

NOTE: Reprinted, by permission of the authors, from D. Wemmer et al., "Changes in Phosphorus Metabolism of a Diving Turtle Observed by ^{31}P-NMR," *Biochimica et Biophysica Acta* 720 (1982):282.

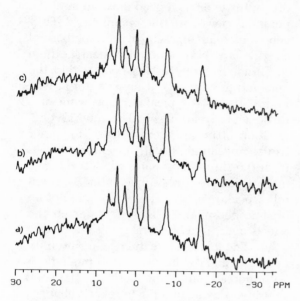

Figure 11–4. Sequential ^{31}P spectra of a turtle head submerged in water. The spectra were taken at the following times after the submersion: (a) 20–40 minutes; (b) 40 to 60 minutes; and (c) 60 to 80 minutes.

NOTE: Reprinted, by permission of the authors, from D. Wemmer et al., "Changes in Phosphorus Metabolism of a Diving Turtle Observed by ^{31}P-NMR," *Biochimica et Biophysica Acta* 720 (1982):283.

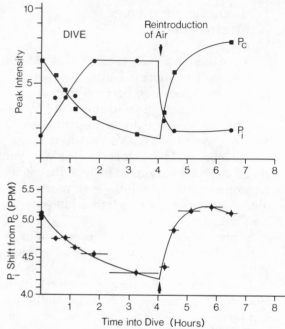

Figure 11–5. The effects of submersion and recovery on phosphocreatine and inorganic phosphate in the turtle head. Pi = inorganic phosphate; Pc = phosphocreatine.

NOTE: Reprinted, by permission of the authors, from D. Wemmer et al. "Changes in Phosphorus Metabolism of a Diving Turtle Observed by ^{31}P-NMR," *Biochimica et Biophysica Acta* 720 (1982):284.

plays changes in inorganic phosphate, phosphocreatine, and pH in the turtle brain as a function of time during and after a "dive." It is difficult to imagine obtaining such data any other way, especially without harming the animal.

The first MRS studies of brain function in human beings were done several years ago in neonates at the University College London Hospital. Newborn infants were used partly because they fit within the thirty-centimeter-bore of the only high-field-strength instruments that were available for such *in vivo* studies at the time and also because of interest in studying the effects of neonatal insults on brain function.[23,38] These studies have shown, for example, that the ^{31}P spectra of infants suffering from asphyxia at birth display no differences from controls on the first day; but, over two to nine days, an inversion occurs in the peak intensities of phos-

phocreatine and inorganic phosphate. This finding led the investigators to hypothesize that very early intervention, before irreversible metabolic changes occur, may be of some help. Furthermore, they noted that ^{31}P MR may be useful clinically, because a marked inversion of the phosphocreatine/inorganic phosphate ratio carried with it a bad prognosis for survival.

The use of other nucleotides for MR studies of brain function should enhance the power of the technique substantially. As noted earlier (see table 11–1), ^{1}H has a much more favorable combination of abundance and sensitivity than any of the other odd-number nucleotides, including ^{31}P. However, under usual conditions, the water peak is such an overwhelming component of *in vivo* spectra that all other peaks are essentially lost as background noise. Fortunately, methods now exist for suppressing the water peak, greatly enhancing the feasibility of monitoring other parts of the spectra, and evidence is accumulating from animal studies that it will be possible to detect at least some putative neuroregulators, including gamma-aminobutyric acid (GABA), in ^{1}H spectra of brain.[6,7]

Researchers wanting to obtain routine MR spectra of the human brain still have a number of hurdles to overcome. One difficulty on which a great deal of work is being done relates to gaining greater control over selecting the tissue that is generating the signal. For several years the most popular method of doing *in vivo* spectroscopy has entailed the use of a surface coil—a loop of copper tubing that can be placed over the area of interest and serve as a radiofrequency antenna, receiver, or both.[1] With simple signal sequences, the coil picks up signals from all of the tissue beneath, with the nearest tissue contributing the most. Thus signals from scalp and muscle predominate when such coils are used on the head, and it is virtually impossible to look at spectra from brain structures deep in the brain. For animal work, many investigators circumvent this problem by removing scalp and skull and placing the coil directly on the brain tissue; however, this greatly diminishes any claims about the noninvasiveness of the technique and is not practical for human studies. Ingenious techniques now are being introduced that will enable investigators to select and define the size and location of the area from which spectra are obtained.*

Another difficulty with *in vivo* MRS is its relatively poor specificity. In many ways, the issues of specificity are analogous to those for gas chromatography. One must constantly ask whether changes in observed peaks are solely the result of concentration changes in the substance of interest. Even in the ^{31}P spectrum, only a few major peaks have been identified definitively, and additional basic work is needed to identify important peaks unambiguously. However, even with this

vital information, artifacts may arise in studies of new conditions or pathological states because an unsuspected substance is contributing to the intensity of what appears to be a single peak.

Selective decoupling and spectral subtraction techniques can help with positive identification of compounds of interest[7,8] and almost certainly will become standard tools for the MR spectroscopist. These techniques take advantage of spin-spin coupling. For example, an apparent single peak A actually may be the sum of a large number of spectra. Selective irradiation of a nucleus in the same compound that is coupled with the nucleus contributing to peak A can establish just how much that nucleus contributes to the total intensity of the peak. The proportionality between spectral resolution and magnetic field strength also spurs the continuing interest of spectroscopists in stronger and stronger magnets.

¶ Safety and Feasibility of Magnetic Resonance

The remarkable safety of MR has been one of its especially attractive features for medical researchers and clinicians alike.[2,32,36,57] The technique requires no ionizing radiation and typically is done without the use of any exogenous agents, making it one of the least invasive diagnostic methods in medicine, especially considering the amount of data it can provide. The magnetic fields themselves have not been linked to any problems for otherwise healthy adults working in the area. There are concerns about placing people in the instrument if they have metal implants of any type, especially new ones, for which even minor movement might be damaging. People with metal fillings report that their teeth tingle, but this does not pose any risk. Patients with pacemakers are not studied, and the possibility of adverse effects of electrical and magnetic field gradients on individuals with compromised cardiac conduction systems has been raised; however, the

*See references 9, 20, 44, 58, and 66.

clinical importance of such effects has yet to be established.

Some issues of safety simply have yet to be addressed adequately. For instance, no teratogenic effects of MR have been shown or even suggested, but MR studies of pregnant women are discouraged until definitive data are available to rule out adverse effects on the fetus. Essentially no work has been done either in animals or in human beings to assess possible behavioral or cognitive effects of MR. In possibly the first such studies in human subjects, Besson and colleagues[12] found no adverse effects on several measures of cognitive function in volunteers who underwent brain MRI.

Probably the biggest health-related concern, especially for researchers interested in studying the brain, involves the heating effects of prolonged radiofrequency irradiation. At least within the current feasible magnetic field strength of 1.5 Tesla, it is possible to keep exposure well within the conservative federal guidelines; however, as magnetic field strengths continue to increase rapidly, additional research is needed to provide information about the actual degree of risk and ways of reducing that risk. Researchers are quite aware of this potential hazard and continually seek signal sequencing methods that minimize subjects' total exposure to radiofrequency.

At present, MR systems large enough for human studies are quite expensive: Whole-body, 1.5 Tesla imaging instruments cost from $1 million to $2 million. Furthermore, the instruments produce large magnetic fringe fields, and ferromagnetic materials within those fields can adversely affect instrument performance, so expensive new building sites often are needed. This latter problem is of great interest to manufacturers, because it limits their potential market; it seems likely that changes in instrument design and methods of shielding will be forthcoming shortly to help minimize requirements for large amounts of specially designed space.

From a practical standpoint, obtaining an MR image or spectrum is a slow process, during which the subject must be cooperative enough to at least hold still. For example, Smith and associates[61] noted that most of their subjects with schizophrenia were able to tolerate testing times of up to ninety minutes, if given occasional breaks, but doubted if many of these patients could tolerate the substantially longer testing of up to four hours needed to collect some types of desirable spectroscopic information. Also, subjects must insert their head and upper torso into a relatively small space during the testing, and the radiofrequencies used produce loud, frequent thumpings, which some people find quite annoying. Patients with claustrophobia, paranoid fears, or frank psychosis may find it impossible to tolerate the testing conditions. Again, advances in instrument design, including possible development of an instrument specifically for studying the head, may alleviate some of these difficulties.

¶ Future Directions

MRI and MRS promise to offer unprecedented access to the human brain. Valuable as these techniques should be for research on and clinical care of adults with mental disorders, their use with children and adolescents may be even more exciting. Even the relatively few measures used in adult psychiatric research typically cannot be applied to youth because the techniques carry with them too much risk. MR promises to be a probe that can be used safely through the entire age range.

The preceding discussion mainly describes applications of MR that already have demonstrated some level of clinical utility. An astonishing aspect of this field is the ever-growing array of potential additional uses. For example, relatively little attention has been given yet to nucleotides other than ^1H and ^{31}P. Some reports suggest that sodium-23 (^{23}Na) imaging not only is technically feasible but may have marked advantages over ^1H imaging in selected circumstances because of the sharp demarcation between intra- and extracellular sodium concentrations.[37,46] Sodium

TABLE 11–2

Desirable Applications of *In Vivo* Monitoring Techniques for Psychiatric Research

Application	Cerebral Blood Flow	CT	PET	MRI	MRS	Computer-assisted EEG
Anatomical pathology	+	+ +	+	+ + +	+	−
Ventricular size	−	+ +	−	+ + +	−	−
Receptor distribution	−	−	+ + +	?	−	−
Blood flow	+ + +	−	+ + +	+?	−	−
Metabolic status	+	−	+	−	+ + +	−
Glucose utilization	−	−	+ + +	−	?	−
Regional activity	+ + +	−	+ + +	−	?	+ + +
Functional abnormality	+ +	−	+ +	+	+ +	+ + +
Neuroregulator quantitation	−	−	−	−	+ +	−
Neuroregulator turnover	−	−	+ +	−	+ +	−

NOTE: These assessments reflect the best judgment of the author, based on existing literature. Evaluations range from not useful (−) to already or potentially extremely valuable (+ + +). In several instances, promising applications have been suggested but remain unproven (?).

imaging may be especially useful for definitively assessing the accuracy of reports that some patients with chronic mental disorders have increased ventricular size. Also, lithium exhibits MR, and comparisons of its brain distribution in patients with bipolar affective disorder who are lithium-responsive or nonresponsive and in healthy controls could be of great interest.

In addition, efforts are underway to devise methods for using MR to image blood vessels and blood flow.[25,59,67] At least in theory, such techniques may offer a noninvasive alternative to current methods of assessing regional cerebral blood flow. Also, there are nascent efforts[19,21,47] to wed imaging and spectroscopy. Such attempts have sparked hot debates within the field about the feasibility and ultimate resolution these methods can achieve, and the controversy can be resolved only with empirical data; but, to the extent that this approach is successful, it will become increasingly feasible to create maps of compounds of interest in living animals and human beings and to monitor changes in the distributions of those substances over time and with specific interventions.

Even the most obvious applications of MRS to psychiatric research remain to be done. Cortical ^{31}P spectroscopy of patients with different forms of dementia may provide unique information about changes in important brain substances, including choline, that accompany those disorders. If so, such information might be useful in distinguishing major depression from dementia in the elderly. In addition, ^{31}P and ^{1}H spectra of major childhood and adult psychiatric disorders, including autism, affective disorders, and schizophrenia, may reveal previously unsuspected characteristic features in brain constituents. Such research must be done with great care to ensure that any identified substances are real; an array of additional analytical skills will be required to permit unequivocal identification of any unusual peaks that may be found.

The potential use of carbon-13 (^{13}C) as a nonradioactive tag for systems of interest also needs further exploration. To date, most research has involved studies of energy metabolism in the liver[24] and heart,[50] using ^{13}C-labeled glucose. The poor sensitivity of ^{13}C to MR means that relatively long sample-collection times are needed, limiting the frequency with which a system can be monitored. However, because ^{13}C and ^{1}H are coupled, it is possible to observe ^{13}C compounds indirectly through the much more powerful ^{1}H signal.[56] At least in animals and possibly in humans, this approach might make possible some exciting new methods of monitoring aspects of brain function.

Table 11–2 attempts to put the realized and

potential uses of MRI and MRS into the larger context of psychiatric research. It demonstrates quite clearly that investigators are suddenly acquiring a powerful array of probes into the brain but also suggests that no single technique or approach is likely to fill all of their needs. Rather, what seems to be emerging are techniques that will be useful not only in isolation but even more in conjunction with other methods. As these new techniques become more firmly established and researchers learn the strengths and limitations of each, the field is going to witness an unprecedented explosion of data that explore human brain function much more directly than ever before.

¶ Bibliography

1. ACKERMAN, J.J.H., et al. "Mapping of Metabolites in Whole Animals by ^{31}P NMR Using Surface Coils," *Nature*, 283 (1980):167–170.

2. ANDREW, E. R. "Perspectives in NMR Imaging," in C. L. Partain, et al., eds., *Nuclear Magnetic Resonance (NMR) Imaging.* Philadelphia: W. B. Saunders, 1983, pp. 26–41.

3. ———. "A Historical Review of NMR and Its Clinical Applications," *British Medical Bulletin*, 40 (1984):115–119.

4. ARNOLD, D. L., et al. "Excessive Intracellular Acidosis on Skeletal Muscle on Exercise in a Patient with a Post-viral Exhaustion/Fatigue Syndrome. A ^{31}P Magnetic Resonance Study," *Lancet*, 1 (1984):1367–1369.

5. ARNOLD, J. T., DHARMATTI, S. S., and PACKARD, M. E. "Chemical Effects on Nuclear Induction Signals from Organic Compounds," *Journal of Chemistry and Physics*, 19 (1951):507.

6. BEHAR, K. L., et al. "High-resolution 1H Nuclear Magnetic Resonance Study of Cerebral Hypoxia in Vivo," *Proceedings of the National Academy of Sciences* (USA), 80 (1983):4945–4948.

7. BEHAR, K. L., et al. "Homonuclear ^{1}H Double-resonance Difference Spectroscopy of the Rat Brain in vivo," *Proceed-ings of the National Academy of Sciences* (USA), 81 (1984):6330–6334.

8. BEHAR, K. L., et al. "Effect of Hypoglycemia Encephalopathy upon Amino Acids, High-energy Phosphates, and pH$_i$ in the Rat Brain in vivo: Detection by Sequential ^{1}H and ^{31}P NMR Spectroscopy," *Journal of Neurochemistry*, 44 (1985):1045–1055.

9. BENDAL, M. R., and PEGG, D. T. "DEPT at Depth. Polarization Transfer and Sample Localization Combined Using Surface Coils," *Journal of Magnetic Resonance*, 57 (1984):337–343.

10. BESSON, J.A.O., et al. "Nuclear Magnetic Resonance Observations in Alcoholic Cerebral Disorder and the Role of Vasopressin," *Lancet*, 2 (1981):923–924.

11. BESSON, J.A.O., et al. "Differentiating Senile Dementia of Alzheimer Type and Multi-infarct Dementia by Proton NMR Imaging," *Lancet*, 2 (1983):789.

12. BESSON, J.A.O., et al. "Cognitive Evaluation Following NMR Imaging of the Brain," *Journal of Neurology, Neurosurgery, and Psychiatry*, 47 (1984):314–316.

13. BESSON, J.A.O., et al. "T1 Changes in Schizophrenic Disorders Measured by Proton NMR," Paper presented at the Third Annual Meeting of the Society of Magnetic Resonance in Medicine in New York, August 13–17, 1984.

14. BILANIUK, L. T., et al. "Cerebral Magnetic Resonance: Comparison of High and Low Field Strength Imaging," *Radiology*, 153 (1984):409–414.

15. BLOCH, F. "Nuclear Induction," *Physical Review*, 70 (1946):460–474.

16. BLOCH, F., HANSEN, W. W., and PACKARD, M. E. "Nuclear Induction," *Physical Review*, 69 (1946):127.

17. ———. "The Nuclear Induction Experiment," *Physical Review*, 70 (1946):474–485.

18. BLOEMBERGEN, N., PURCELL, E. M., and POUND, R. V. "Relaxation Effects in Nuclear Magnetic Resonance Absorption," *Physical Review*, 73 (1948):679–712.

19. BOTTOMLEY, P. A., FOSTER, T. H., and LEUE, W. M. "Chemical Imaging of the Brain by NMR," *Lancet*, 1 (1984):1120.

20. BOTTOMLEY, P. A., et al. "NMR Imaging/

Spectroscopy System to Study Both Anatomy and Metabolism," *Lancet*, 2 (1983):273–274.

21. BOTTOMLEY, P. A., et al. *"In vivo* Solvent-suppressed Localized Hydrogen Nuclear Magnetic Resonance Spectroscopy: A Window to Metabolism," *Proceedings of the National Academy of Sciences* (USA), 82 (1985):2148–2152.

22. BRINDLE, K. M., et al. "Spectral Editing in ^{31}P NMR Spectra of Human Brain," *Journal of Magnetic Resonance*, 61 (1985):559–563.

23. CADY, E. B., et al. "Non-invasive Investigation of Cerebral Metabolism in Newborn Infants by Phosphorus Nuclear Magnetic Resonance Spectroscopy," *Lancet*, 1 (1983):1059–1062.

24. COHEN, S. M. "Simultaneous ^{13}C and ^{31}P NMR Studies of Perfused Rat Liver. Effects of Insulin and Glucagon and a ^{13}C NMR Assay of Free Mg^{+2}," *Journal of Biological Chemistry*, 258 (1983):14294–14308.

25. CROOKS, L. E., and KAUFMAN, L. "NMR Imaging of Blood Flow," *British Medical Bulletin*, 40 (1984):167–169.

26. CROOKS, L. E., et al. "Clinical Efficiency of Nuclear Magnetic Resonance Imaging," *Radiology*, 146 (1983):123–128.

27. CROOKS, L. E., et al. "Magnetic Resonance Imaging: Effects of Magnetic Field Strength," *Radiology*, 151 (1984):127–133.

28. DAVIS, P. L., et al. "Nuclear Magnetic Resonance Imaging: Current Capabilities," *Western Journal of Medicine*, 137 (1982):290–293.

29. DEMYER, M. K., et al. "Magnetic Resonance Imaging in Psychiatry," *Psychiatric Annals*, 15 (1985):262–267.

30. ERKINJUNTTI, T., et al. "Cerebral NMR and CT Imaging in Dementia," *Journal of Computer Assisted Tomography*, 8 (1984):614–618.

31. FOSTER, M. A. *Magnetic Resonance in Medicine and Biology.* Oxford: Pergamon Press, 1984.

32. GADIAN, D. G. *Nuclear Magnetic Resonance and Its Application to Living Systems.* Oxford: Clarendon Press, 1982.

33. GOLCZEWSKI, J., NG, T. C., and HIRAMOTO, R. N. "In vivo Measurement of ^{31}P Nuclear Magnetic Resonance Spectrum of Aging Mouse Brain," *Physiological Chemistry and Physics and Medical NMR*, 15 (1983):13–17.

34. HAHN, E. L., and MAXWELL, D. E. "Chemical Shift and Field Independent Frequency Modulation of the Spin Echo Envelope," *Physical Review*, 84 (1951):1246–1247.

35. HANLEY, P. "Magnets for Medical Applications of NMR," *British Medical Bulletin*, 40 (1984):125–131.

36. HENDEE, W. R., and MORGAN, C. J. "Magnetic Resonance Imaging. Part I—Physical Principles," *Western Journal of Medicine*, 141 (1984):491–500.

37. HILAL, S. K. "The Clinical Application of Sodium Imaging," Paper presented at the Third Annual Meeting of the Society of Magnetic Resonance in Medicine, New York, August 13–17, 1984.

38. HOPE, P. L., et al. "Cerebral Energy Metabolism Studied with Phosphorus NMR Spectroscopy in Normal and Birth-asphyxiated Infants," *Lancet*, 2 (1984):366–370.

39. HOULT, D. I. "NMR Imaging Techniques," *British Medical Bulletin*, 40 (1984):132–138.

40. JARDETZKY, O., and ROBERTS, G.C.K. *NMR in Molecular Biology.* New York: Academic Press, 1981.

41. KING, R., and JARDETZKY, O. "A General Formalism for the Analysis of NMR Relaxation Measurements on Systems with Multiple Degrees of Freedom," *Chemical Physics Letters*, 55 (1978):15.

42. LAUTERBUR, P. C. "Image Formation by Induced Local Interactions: Examples Employing Nuclear Magnetic Resonance," *Nature*, 242 (1973):190–191.

43. MCCONNEL, H. M. "Theory of Nuclear Magnetic Shielding in Molecules. I. Long-range Dipolar Shielding of Protons," *Journal of Chemistry and Physics*, 27 (1957):226–229.

44. MANSFIELD, P. "Spatial Mapping of the Chemical Shift in NMR," *Magnetic Resonance in Medicine*, 1 (1984):370–386.

45. MAUDSLEY, A. A. "Technical Demands of Other Nuclei," Paper presented at the Third Annual Meeting of the Society of

Magnetic Resonance in Medicine, New York, August 13–17, 1984.

46. MAUDSLEY, A. A., and HILAL, S. K. "Biological Aspects of Sodium-23 Imaging," *British Medical Bulletin,* 40 (1984):165–166.

47. MAUDSLEY, A. A., et al. *"In vivo* MR Spectroscopic Imaging with P-31," *Radiology,* 153 (1984):745–750.

48. MOON, R. B., and RICHARDS, J. H. "Determination of Intracellular pH by ^{31}P Magnetic Resonance," *Journal of Biological Chemistry,* 248 (1973):7276–7278.

49. MOORE, W. S. "Basic Physics and Relaxation Mechanisms," *British Medical Bulletin,* 40 (1984):120–124.

50. NEUROHR, K. J. "Carbon-13 Nuclear Magnetic Resonance Studies of Myocardial Glycogen Metabolism in Live Guinea Pigs," *Biochemistry,* 23 (1984):5029–5035.

51. NEWMAN, R. J. "Clinical Applications of Nuclear Magnetic Resonance Spectroscopy: A Review," *Journal of the Royal Society of Medicine,* 77 (1984):774–779.

52. PRICHARD, J. W., et al. "Cerebral Metabolic Studies *in vivo* by ^{31}P NMR," *Proceedings of the National Academy of Sciences* (USA), 80 (1983):2748–2751.

53. PURCELL, E. M., TORREY, H. C., and POUND, R. V. "Resonance Absorption by Nuclear Magnetic Moments in a Solid," *Physical Review,* 69 (1946):37–38.

54. RADDA, G. K., BORE, P. J., and RAJAGOPALAN, B. "Clinical Aspects of ^{31}P NMR Spectroscopy," *British Medical Bulletin,* 40 (1984):155–159.

55. RANGEL-GUERRA, R., et al. "Nuclear Magnetic Resonance in Bipolar Affective Disorders," *American Journal of Nuclear Radiology,* 4 (1983):229–231.

56. ROTHMAN, D. L., et al. "^{1}H-Observe ^{13}C-Decouple Spectroscopic Measurements of Lactiat and Glutamate in the Rat Brain in vivo," Paper presented at the Third Annual Meeting of the Society of Magnetic Resonance in Medicine, New York, August 13–17, 1984.

57. SAUNDERS, R. D., and SMITH, H. "Safety Aspects of NMR Clinical Imaging," *British Medical Bulletin,* 40 (1984):148–154.

58. SHAKA, A. J., and FREEMAN, R. "Spatially Selective Radio Frequency Pulses," *Journal of Magnetic Resonance,* 59 (1984):169–176.

59. SINGER, J. R., and CROOKS, L. E. "Nuclear Magnetic Resonance Blood Flow Measurements in Human Brain," *Science,* 221 (1983):654–656.

60. SLICHTER, C. P. *Principles of Magnetic Resonance,* 2nd ed. Berlin: Springer-Verlag, 1978.

61. SMITH, R. C., et al. "Nuclear Magnetic Resonance in Schizophrenia: A Preliminary Study," *Psychiatry Research,* 12 (1984):137–147.

62. SMITH, S. L. "Nuclear magnetic resonance imaging," *Analytical Chemistry,* 57 (1985):595A–680A.

63. STEINER, R. E., and RADDA, G. K. "Nuclear Magnetic Resonance and Its Applications," *British Medical Bulletin,* 40 (1984):113–201.

64. TAYLOR, D. J., et al. "Bioenergetics of Intact Human Muscle: A ^{31}P Nuclear Magnetic Resonance Study," *Molecular Biology and Medicine,* 1 (1983):77–94.

65. THULBORN, K. R., et al. "A ^{31}P Nuclear Magnetic Resonance in vivo Study of Cerebral Ischaemia in the Gerbil," *Journal of Cerebral Blood Flow and Metabolism,* 2 (1982):299–306.

66. TOFTS, P. S., et al. "Surface Coil NMR Spectroscopy of Brain," *Lancet,* 1 (1984):459.

67. VAN AS, H., et al. "Flow Imaging by Nuclear Magnetic Resonance," *Annales de Radiologie,* 27 (1984):405–413.

68. WEMMER, D., et al. "Changes in the Phosphorus Metabolism of a Diving Turtle Observed by ^{31}P-NMR," *Biochimica et Biophysica Acta,* 720 (1982):281–287.

69. YOUNG, I. R. "Considerations Affecting Signal and Contrast in NMR Imaging," *British Medical Bulletin,* 40 (1984):139–147.

70. YOUNG, S. W. *Nuclear Magnetic Resonance Imaging. Basic Principles.* New York: Raven Press, 1984.

PART THREE

The Biology and Treatment

of Specific Psychiatric

Disorders

CHAPTER 12

BIOLOGICAL HYPOTHESES OF AFFECTIVE DISORDERS

Robert H. Gerner and William E. Bunney, Jr.

¶ Introduction

Most biological hypotheses of affective illness rely on the assumption that a genetic factor is responsible for abnormal brain biochemical functioning. Such a dysfunction might be present but not express itself until other events (either endogenous, such as hormonal changes, or exogenous, such as stress) require normal function of this "weak link," or vulnerability. It is also possible that the dysfunction might express itself independently of other parameters.

It is now accepted that bipolar, unipolar, and schizo-affective disorders have major genetic contributions.[110,111] Several possibilities exist for the mode of genetic transmission. If a unitary mode of inheritance exists, it is likely that a single factor is responsible for the disorder (similar to Down's syndrome). On the other hand, if multifactorial transmission occurs, heterogenous factors in several combinations might provide the basic vulnerability for the illnesses. If the latter is true, the study of large groups of patients with the same phenomenological disorder is likely to demonstrate a large variance for any single factor studied, and the chance that the average value of the factor in the affectively ill group would differ from normal controls would be small.

Additionally, either mode of inheritance could be associated with a final common pathway that could produce at some point the phenomena of affective illness. If some final common pathway was present, regardless of initial cause, the chances of finding such a common abnormality would be relatively greater, although the abnormality would only be the distal cause of affective illness. Such genetic issues are important, since they may partially explain the heterogeneity of biological findings in affective disorders. Gershon[111] reexamined several studies using a multifactorial model of inheritance and concluded that there are more biological abnormalities to be found in bipolar or schizo-affective than in unipolar patients. Thus, although it may be easier to delineate an abnormality in the first two disorders, this does not suggest that the heritability of some factor is not intrinsic to the etiology of unipolar depression.

Historically, the paradigms used to develop data on biological factors in affective illness have (1) examined behavioral changes following drug administration (either producing or alleviating affective symptoms) and developed hypotheses based on the drug's known effects in animals or man; and/or (2) compared biological fluid or physiologic measures in affectively ill subjects with controls, subsequently developing hypotheses relating observed alterations of specific factors to the mood disorder. Subsequently, hypotheses based on altered neurotransmitter receptor function and anatomical alterations have also emerged. However, one must consider whether any abnormality has sensitivity and specificity for a disorder or whether it occurs among a wide number of disorders. If the latter is the case, the hypothesis of a direct association between the abnormality and a specific disorder is considerably weakened.

Such considerations are relevant to all medical tests. For example, individuals with syphilis should have a positive Venereal Disease Research Laboratory test (VDRL), and individuals with a positive VDRL test should have syphilis. The former statement reflects sensitivity of a test and the latter the specificity. Neither of the conditions are met 100 percent by the VDRL test, since there are both false negative and false positive tests respectively. Similarly, if most depressed patients have abnormal levels of x compared to normals, and patients with schizophrenia, or dementia, or anorexia have similar levels of x, one cannot specifically link x to depression without more evidence. If no one has low levels of y except depressed patients, the y test would be very specific for depression. However, if only 15 percent of depressed patients have low levels of y, the sensitivity would be so low that one cannot argue that y is linked to all depression. However, it may suggest that a subgroup of depressed patients with abnormal levels of y exists.

The presence of biological abnormalities in a disorder does not always require the creation of a specific biological hypothesis. For example, neuroendocrine abnormalities (see chapter 4) on the dexamethasone suppression test manifested by hypercortisol excretion and blunting of thyroid stimulating hormone (TSH) response to thyrotropin-releasing hormone (TRH) have been noted in depression and in other diagnostic groups. It has been suggested that these tests reflect a phenomenon intrinsic to the depressed state. Could the hypercorticoid state play an etiological role in depression? Cerebrospinal fluid (CSF) levels of cortisol are elevated in depression,[104] and depression is one of the psychiatric manifestations of Cushing's syndrome. However, because CSF levels are also elevated in anorexia nervosa with or without depression and in mania, it is unlikely that the levels of cortisol found in depression are primary to the disorder.

At this time no biological abnormality found in those studies based on biological hypotheses of affective illness can absolutely discriminate individual affective patients from normal controls or patients with other psychiatric disorders. However, significant findings have been made for groups of affective patients, relevant both for the state of illness (i.e., when depression or mania is present) as well as for traits that are present regardless of whether the patient is well or ill. Unfortunately, most studies of individual hypotheses have not yet been able to examine the relationship of the hypothesis under consideration to other major ones.

Most of the studies cited and the theories based on them have multiple weaknesses of methodology that leave important questions unanswered. These areas of incompleteness commonly involve imprecise or inconsistent specification of the diagnostic groups making up the sample, low numbers of subjects for statistical questions, and narrowness of comparison-group diagnoses. Furthermore, there is variance among studies due to differences in patient recruitment and diagnostic procedures, biological sample collection methods, drug dosage, rating instruments, and assay methods. However, it would be unfair to go beyond calling attention to these methodological issues, since these inquiries are exploratory in nature and variations that occur in these complex areas may even provide an advantage in discovering better methods to prevent and treat these disabling illnesses.

¶ Neurotransmitter Hypotheses of Affective Disorders

Norepinephrine and Affective Disorders

The first major biochemical hypothesis of affective disorders was related to the catecholamines,[41,261] dopamine (DA) and, in particular, norepinephrine (NE) (see figure 12–1). The precursor of the catecholamines is the dietary amino acid tyrosine, which competes with other amino acids for uptake into the central nervous system (CNS). The rate-limiting step in catecholamine biosynthesis is generally accepted to be the enzyme tyrosine hydroxylase, which forms DOPA, although there is some evidence that increasing dietary tyrosine can increase catecholamine levels.[100,345] DOPA is decarboxylated to form DA, which is a neurotransmitter itself in some neurons and functions as a precursor in others for formation of NE by the enzyme dopamine beta-hydroxylase (DBH). Both DA and NE are catabolized by the enzymes monoamine oxidase (MAO) and catechol-O-methyltransferase (COMT) to produce their respective metabolites, homovanillic acid (HVA) and 3-methoxy-4-hydroxyphenyl-glycol (MHPG) (major central NE metabolite) or vanillylmandelic acid (VMA) (major peripheral NE metabolite).

One of the bases for the catecholamine theory of affective disorders was the appreci-

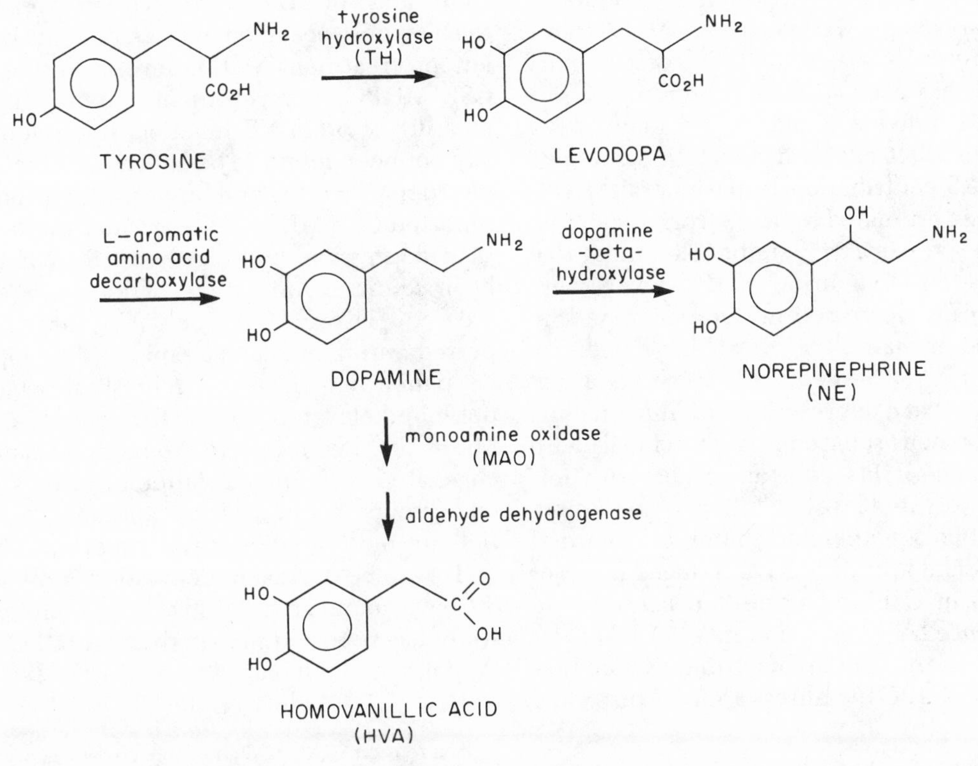

Figure 12–1. Synthesis and metabolism of dopamine.

ation that the antihypertensive drug reserpine, which can cause depression, was associated with the depletion of catecholamines in presynaptic neurons. Although reserpine depletes NE, DA, and serotonin (5HT), the initial theory centered on NE and its possible relationship to depression. This theory was supported by initial studies with tricyclic antidepressants revealing that they inhibited NE reuptake into the presynaptic neuron and functionally increased NE within the synapse.[263] Further, stimulants such as amphetamines, which produce an acute antidepressive effect, also released NE. Additional support for such a theory is based on findings that the beta-NE receptor blocker propranolol hydrochloride can produce depression in susceptible individuals.[213] Subsequently it was found that reserpine does not appear to cause depression ubiquitously but rather preferentially in individuals who have a genetic depressive diathesis.[110]

The investigation of NE's relationship to affective disorders has included sampling CSF for NE and MHPG, urinary MHPG, and, more recently, plasma MHPG levels. Urinary MHPG has been studied in hundreds of depressed individuals and is the main metabolic product of NE in the CNS. Although the CNS contribution to peripheral MHPG has been estimated to range from 20 percent to 60 percent,[28,123] initial findings that twenty-four-hour urine MHPG levels were specifically decreased in depression and increased in mania[123,264,265,329] have been revised.[41,42,44,45] Subsequently it has been suggested that depressed patients include heterogenous subgroups of individuals with decreased MHPG levels and others with normal or elevated levels.[270] Bipolar and unipolar patients with endogenous or retarded depressions appear to have reduced levels of MHPG in CSF and urine.* In contrast, no difference has been found in VMA levels.[140] However, the overlap of normals is such that urinary MHPG measures cannot be used as a

reliable test for the diagnosis of depression.[271]

Results of MHPG investigations in unipolar depression have been much less consistent. Patients with primary depression have been reported to have reduced levels by some,[47,71,166,314] while others have reported no difference from normals,[21,120] or even increased levels.[97] One explanation offered for these discrepant findings is the heterogeneity of unipolar depression. In any case, the group of depressions has a very wide range of urinary MHPG.[260,270,297] This led to a hypothesis that antidepressant responsivity may be correlated with low, high, or normal urinary MHPG levels. Several studies have reported[177,263,328] an association of low urinary MHPG with antidepressant responses to relatively specific noradrenergic heterocyclic antidepressants such as maprotiline hydrochloride, desipramine hydrochloride, nortriptyline hydrochloride, or imipramine hydrochloride. When imipramine or desipramine was given to depressed patients with a wide range of urinary MHPG, a more positive response occurred in those patients with low pretreatment MHPG levels.* Although CSF MHPG may represent a more direct measure of brain NE function, it has generally not been found to be altered in affective disorders.[11,227] Several investigators† have reported CSF MHPG to be greater in mania than depression, and elevated CSF NE has been found in one study of mania.[228] Increased plasma MHPG has also been reported during mania in a rapid-cycling bipolar patient.[217] However, four studies have not found elevated CSF MHPG in mania.[227] MHPG has been reported to be significantly correlated with mania symptom ratings by one group[306] but not by another.[109] Although most studies have reported CSF MHPG to be normal in depression, a minority have found it to be low.[11,227] Only one study has reported elevated CSF MHPG in unipolar and bipolar depression.[148] When

---

*See references 22, 71, 81, 97, 120, 121, 168, 267, 268, and 269.

*See references 22, 51, 85, 165, 169, 171, 250, 260, 272, and 299.
†See references 7, 109, 148, 306, and 331.

plasma MHPG levels are examined,[154,306] morning mean MHPG levels in depression are similar to those of normal subjects. However, in contrast to normals, depressed individuals do not show an increase in plasma MHPG from 8:00 A.M. to noon, suggesting a decrease in the amplitude of the diurnal increase in MHPG.

While there is variance from study to study, these findings are consistent with a relationship of NE to depression and mania; however, the association appears to be more complex than simple under- or oversecretion of NE. Additional indirect measures of NE and its relationship to depression have been investigated through the use of alpha-methylparatyrosine (AMPT), which is an inhibitor of tyrosine hydroxylase, the rate-limiting step in the conversion of tyrosine to DOPA, and subsequently to DA and NE. AMPT increases sedation and decreases motor activity when given to animals. Monkeys receiving AMPT also have marked decreases in social interaction and appear to become withdrawn.[148] AMPT has been reported to improve mania[37] and worsen depression in already depressed patients and produce depressive symptoms in normals.[42] However, depressed patients who have improved following tricyclic treatment do not show vulnerability to recurrence of depression when given AMPT. Although nonspecifically increasing both NE and DA, their precursor, tyrosine, may have antidepressant effects.[101] These precursor studies are generally supportive of an association between decreased catecholamine activity and depression, although it would be imprudent to argue that all depressive illness is a result of decreased catecholamine activity.

Dopamine and Affective Disorders

The DA hypothesis[106] of affective disorders has been less extensively investigated than either the 5HT or NE hypotheses. DA is a well-localized neurotransmitter. Most DA-containing cell bodies are in the brain stem and project either to the striatum (extrapyramidal system) or to limbic structures (mesolimbic system). Because some of the effects of stimulants are dopaminergic in addition to noradrenergic, it was hypothesized that stimulants might produce antidepressant effects via dopaminergic systems. Similarly, reserpine-associated depression could involve DA, since reserpine depletes both DA and NE. The simplistic form of this hypothesis is that the maniclike behavior of individuals receiving high doses of amphetamine is associated with dopaminergic stimulation. Additionally, some individuals with Parkinson's disease who were treated with the DA precursor levodopa developed hypomanic symptomatology. The pathophysiologic decrease in dopaminergic neurons in Parkinson's disease might also be a cause of the very substantial incidence of concomitant depression in that disease.[184,315] Thus there is a rationale for considering DA to be specifically associated with affective disorders.[85]

The possible relationship of dopamine to affective disorders has been investigated by measuring the CSF DA metabolite HVA and through the use of DA agonists and antagonists. HVA has been reported to be decreased in bipolar depression,[16] in retarded depression,[219,314] in unipolar depression,[11,14] in a combined group[144] of depressive patients, and in depressed women.[148] In contrast, Vestergaard, Sorensen, and Hoppe[326] reported HVA to be higher in depressed neurological subjects. However, some studies[109] have found no differences of HVA in depression or in depressed subgroups compared to normals. Manic patients have been reported to have higher HVA than controls by Sjostrom and Roos,[293] Banki,[16] Vestergaard, Sorensen, and Hoppe,[326] and Gerner and associates,[109] but not by others.[138,231,306] Swann and associates[306] reported that manic women, but not men, had elevated HVA. Most investigators, however, have not found significant HVA differences between patients with affective disorders and healthy controls.[227]

Two DA receptor agonists (bromocriptine mesylate and piribedil) have been shown in several studies to have antidepressant effects.[58,211,327] However, levodopa, the immediate precursor of DA, has not been found to be an effective antidepressant, although hypomania was induced in a significant number of bipolar patients who received it.[202] One study examined the correlation of CSF HVA level to response by the DA agonist piribedil and found a negative correlation, with the greatest degree of improvement being found in individuals who had the lowest levels of HVA and presumably the least amount of CNS DA.[229] Some arguments for the DA hypothesis of affective disorders are nonspecific and would also apply to the NE hypothesis. This would be true for the catecholamine-depleting action of AMPT and reserpine, which decrease both DA and NE. Similarly, amphetamine and methylphenidate increase the release of both NE and DA.

When CSF studies have been conducted using probenecid to inhibit the egress of the metabolite HVA from the spinal fluid, CSF HVA levels have typically been decreased in individuals with depression.* The difference was more robust for patients with psychomotor retardation, whereas agitated depressed patients did not have decreased HVA levels.† In some studies a decrease in HVA concentration has been found in bipolar but not in unipolar patients.[29] Further, it has been reported in some, but not all, studies that among depressed patients, those with psychotic features had higher probenecid HVA levels than normals,[16,308] as did patients with agitation.[325] This is consistent with clinical observations that psychotic depressed and agitated patients tend to improve with neuroleptic compounds.

One of the major arguments against the DA hypothesis of depression is that neuroleptic medications that block DA receptors are not usually associated with the induction of classical depression. One study[253] investigated the relationship of depression to neuroleptic treatment in schizophrenia. This study did not support an induction of depression associated with neuroleptic use in schiz-

ophrenia, and the results are consistent with other reports.[147,194] Of course, tests for depression in schizophrenia cannot necessarily be generalized to nonschizophrenic patients.

The use of neuroleptics for depression has been thoroughly reviewed[249,341]; neuroleptics were superior to placebo in 90 percent of studies, superior to tricyclic antidepressants in 21 percent of studies, equally effective in 63 percent, and inferior in 16 percent. Part of the reason for efficacy of neuroleptics in depression may be the heterogeneity of subgroups of depressed individuals. Tricyclics were superior to neuroleptics for retarded, withdrawn patients, who may be the group with decreased HVA, while neuroleptics were superior to tricyclics for anxious, agitated patients,[129,218,241] who may have normal levels of HVA. Thus there is support from pharmacological and CSF studies for an involvement of DA in affective illness, with more consistent findings in bipolar disorder. However, many questions relating to correlations with symptomatic features remain.

Serotonin and Affective Disorders

Because the indoleamine hypothesis of affective disorders spans all aspects of 5HT metabolism, a basic knowledge of its synthesis and degradation is important (see figure 12–2). The precursor of 5HT is L-tryptophan, an essential amino acid obtained from the diet. Its transport into the CNS is proportional to the ratio of plasma-free tryptophan (the nonprotein-bound fraction in blood) to certain other amino acids. Tryptophan is taken up into serotonergic neurons and hydroxylated by the rate-limiting enzyme tryptophan-hydroxylase and then decarboxylated to 5HT. The cell bodies of virtually all 5HT neurons that project into the cerebrum originate in the raphe nuclei, located in the lower midbrain and upper pons. Serotonergic axons ascend in the medial forebrain bundle into all brain regions, with high concentrations of terminals in the hypothalamus, thalamus, limbic areas, and striatum. After release from presynaptic nerve endings into the synapse, 5HT undergoes reuptake into

*See references 29, 292, 293, 323, 324, and 341.
†See references 16, 18, 219, 323, and 337.

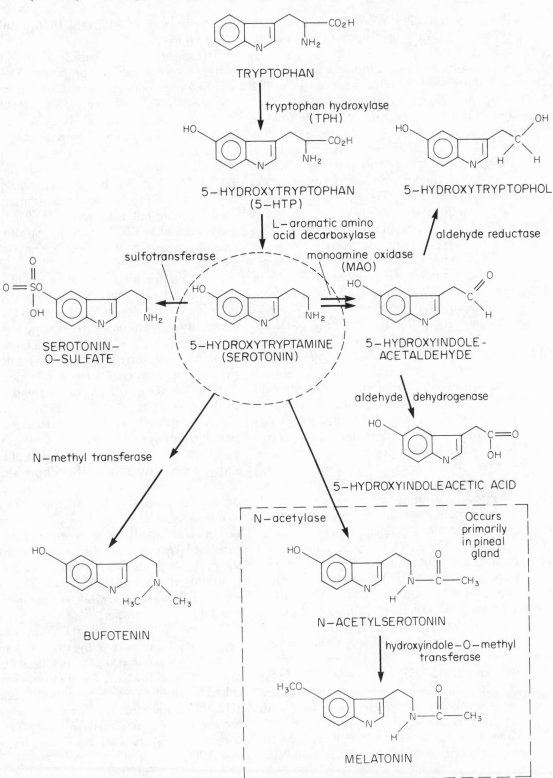

Figure 12–2. Synthesis and metabolism of serotonin.

the presynaptic nerve endings and is metabolized by MAO to 5-hydroxyindoleacetic acid (5-HIAA).

There are two major indoleamine hypotheses postulated for affective disorders. The simplest hypothesis suggests there is a reduction in functional 5HT during the depressive phase of unipolar or bipolar illness.[201] If true, there should be evidence of changes in levels of 5HT, 5HT precursors, and/or 5-HIAA. The second hypothesis is a permissive one that suggests that 5HT is the vulnerability factor in affective disorders and is reduced in individuals who are predisposed to such disorders.[235] In this case, depression would be manifest when NE is decreased, and mania would occur when NE is increased. Levels of 5HT would be decreased during depression, mania, and euthymic periods.

Levels of 5HT or its metabolite, 5-HIAA, have been measured in the CSF and in the brains of suicide victims. CSF 5-HIAA has been reported to be low in depression.* However, recent large and well-controlled studies are not consistent with one another. One report found 5-HIAA greater in depressed compared to manic and control females, with no differences in depressed compared to manic and control males.[148] However, Asberg and coworkers[11] reported lower concentrations of CSF 5-HIAA in melancholic patients than in normal controls, and Gerner and associates[109] found no differences in CSF 5-HIAA in manic patients and depressed groups compared to normal controls or among subgroups of depression. Only one study[16] has reported CSF 5-HIAA to be decreased during mania. Some,[11] but not all,[61] investigators report higher CSF 5-HIAA in women than in men. Others report higher CSF 5-HIAA in depressed women than in nondepressed women.[109,148] Six groups of investigators have determined 5HT levels in suicide victims who had depression compared to controls.[11,19,275,321] However, only three of the six groups reported decreased levels in brain serotonergic

areas such as the hindbrain, brain stem, and raphe nuclei.[19,321]

The heterogeneity of these findings led to a hypothesis based on a proposed biochemical heterogeneity of depression, supported by the finding that low 5-HIAA in CSF is associated with suicidal behavior in depressed* and nondepressed patients.† It has been hypothesized that there is a bimodal distribution of CSF 5-HIAA, with the low CSF 5-HIAA group being particularly vulnerable to suicide,[8,173] while phenomenologically similar but less anxious[17,256] patients have normal levels. However, not all investigators have found such a bimodal distribution.[109,148] Unfortunately, such findings may be confounded by the possibility that CSF 5-HIAA may reflect spinal cord levels in addition to brain levels.[344] However, the vulnerability hypothesis is further supported by preliminary studies of van Praag and de Haan,[322] suggesting that treatment with the 5HT precursor 5-hydroxytryptophan (5-HTP) significantly reduces the relapse rate in depressed patients who have low CSF 5-HIAA compared to those who do not. Additionally, patients who have low CSF 5-HIAA and their relatives have more frequent episodes of depression than other depressed patients.[321] Further, an increased frequency of depression among family members of normal healthy volunteers who had low baseline CSF 5-HIAA levels has been reported.[275] Because 5-HIAA is under genetic control, as shown by twin studies,[274] there is indeed a possibility that low 5-HIAA levels, reflecting low 5HT turnover, may define a genetic vulnerability to depression.[19]

The possibility of a low 5HT state during depression is supported by studies demonstrating decreased 5HT effects following administration of the drug fenfluramine hydrochloride, which releases presynaptic stores of 5HT.[285] The mechanism for the postulated occurrence of functionally low 5HT is not known. One possibility is decreased levels of the 5HT precursor.[59]

---

*See references 8, 12, 13, 17, 33, 61, 172, 206, 310, and 321.

*See references 2, 9, 17, 18, 136, and 215.
†See references 38, 39, 163, 218.

Few double-blind controlled studies have been carried out giving oral L-tryptophan or another 5HT precursor, 5-HTP, for depression, and the results are inconsistent both when precursors are given alone or in combination with tricyclics, MAO inhibitors (MAOIs), or lithium.[43] The well-controlled studies are contrasted to open studies where more frequent antidepressant responses have been reported.[36,62,146,175] While it is likely that these discrepancies are due to rater bias in open trials, the discrepancies also occur in double-blind studies. They may reflect a difference in responsivity of the postulated subgroup of depressed patients who have low 5HT levels. Several studies have suggested[52,57,93,322] that patients who respond to 5HT precursors have low CSF 5-HIAA. Precursor studies are complicated by the possibility that the large amounts of the compound ingested may not be metabolized in a normal manner. Thus large doses of tryptophan may be metabolized in nonserotonergic neurons.[1,93]

If low 5HT levels were associated with depression, the use of parachlorophenylalanine (PCPA), which is an inhibitor of tryptophan hydroxylase (the rate-limiting step for conversion of L-tryptophan to 5HT), might be associated with the onset or worsening of a depression. In the few studies reported, PCPA has been noted to reverse the antidepressant effects of imipramine.[278]

The hypothesis that chronic low 5HT levels are associated with vulnerability to depression is further supported by a two-year double-blind, placebo-controlled crossover study conducted by van Praag and de Haan,[322] in which the 5HT precursor 5-HTP was given to twenty depressed patients receiving clomipramine hydrochloride, thirteen of whom had low CSF 5-HIAA levels. Relapses were significantly greater during placebo periods than when patients were also receiving 5-HTP (seventeen versus six respectively) and the depressive episodes on placebo were longer.

A significant correlation exists between plasma and brain tryptophan levels, suggesting that increasing peripheral tryptophan does cause changes in the brain. This has been confirmed by CSF studies demonstrating that CSF 5-HIAA levels increase following oral tryptophan loading.[120] Thus it is possible that low central 5HT might be secondary to decreased levels of its precursor. Initial studies reported that when free and total bound plasma tryptophan were measured in depressed patients and groups of recovered patients (both drug-free and on lithium), the depressed group had lower free plasma tryptophan values than controls.[60] Most subsequent investigations, however, have been unable to replicate these findings,[43] and no differences in CSF tryptophan have been found.[18,109,113] Thus, even if peripheral levels were decreased in depressed individuals, it appears that levels in the CNS may not be significantly affected.

There is a substantial amount of evidence linking 5HT to depression, but relatively less suggesting its role in mania. The studies to date cannot address whether 5HT has a primary or secondary role in the etiology of affective disorders.

Biogenic Amine Metabolic Enzymes and Affective Disorders

MONOAMINE OXIDASE AND CATECHOL-O-METHYLTRANSFERASE

The enzymes responsible for metabolizing catecholamines and indoleamines have been considered for possible relevance to affective illness. Two enzymes are responsible for the initial metabolism of NE and DA, MAO and COMT (see figure 12–1). MAO is also involved in 5HT metabolism (see figure 12–2). Elevated levels of these enzymes might deplete presynaptic stores of NE, DA, and/or 5HT.

COMT is present in the extracellular fluid of the synapse in the brain and is also found in other tissues, including blood, where it is commonly measured in erythrocytes. Investigations in depressed patients have found it to be low,[34,54,76] normal,[77,78,182,338] or elevated[112,237,279] compared to control subjects.

Effects of gender are also conflicting. COMT has been reported to be greater[84,237] or lower[54,77] in depressed females, elevated in depressed males,[279] and higher in normal males than in females.[237] In summary, COMT has not been found to have a consistent relationship to affective disorders, and no studies have been published of its relationship to MHPG or HVA levels in affective disorders.

MAO enzymes are membrane-bound and therefore found intracellularly. They are the main presynaptic metabolizers of catecholamines and the only metabolizing enzymes of 5HT. The enzyme exists in two forms, MAO-A and MAO-B. The platelet contains the B form exclusively, while the brain also contains a proportion of MAO-A.[74,200,204] Platelet MAO activity is the usual method for determining MAO levels. Because MAO activity is heritable,[92,208,333] it might function as a trait vulnerability factor to affective and other mental illnesses.[196,199,200]

It has been postulated that high levels of MAO might be associated with depression because of increased metabolism of presynaptic neurotransmitters. In contrast to this hypothesized expectation, several investigators have reported MAO activity to be reduced in depression, particularly in bipolar patients.* Most, although not all, studies have found normal levels in unipolar depression.† Skeletal muscle MAO activity has also been reported to be decreased in bipolar and unipolar affective disorder patients.[186] Increased MAO activity has been reported in some studies of depression,‡ and some authors have reported increased MAO activity in nonendogenous depressions,[339] while finding normal levels in patients with bipolar and unipolar illness. Such a wide range of reports may reflect heterogeneity of the subgroups that were investigated, differences in techniques of measurement, or random effects. Females have been reported to have higher levels[199,239,247] and some,[247] but not all,[150,205] studies have reported increases in MAO activity with age.

A relationship between the phenomenological features of depression and MAO activity has been suggested in several studies. Robinson and associates[248] reported patients who were depressed and had high MAO levels were more ill and had less response to treatment; and others[150] found patients who had unipolar depression and elevated MAO levels to have increased levels of anxiety. The higher levels of MAO reported for females could be related to their increased incidence of depression.

Haier and coworkers[125] reported differences in college students by evaluating personality and family history characteristics and MAO levels. Students with low MAO activity had more instability in job and schooling over a two-year follow-up period. However, in contrast to the major MAO hypothesis of affective illness, the low-MAO nondepressed males reported more mental health problems in their families, especially depression, alcoholism, and suicide attempts.

In contrast to the varied results in studies of MAO levels, pharmacological effects are generally supportive of an MAO hypothesis. Drugs that inhibit MAO have been found to be useful antidepressants, and these MAOIs have been associated with the induction of mania in bipolar patients.[158] It is not clear whether the type of MAO is significant for affective illness. Drugs that inhibit MAO-A (clorgyline) and MAO-B (pargyline hydrochloride) are associated equally with induction of hypomania,[196,224] although they affect neurotransmitters differentially. MAO-A inhibitors are relatively more effective for inhibiting 5HT metabolism, while MAO-B inhibitors are more effective as inhibitors of phenylethylamine metabolism. Although there are suggestions that MAO-A inhibitors are more effective as antidepressants than MAO-B inhibitors,[163] the common MAO inhibitors in current use are all nonspecific, inhibiting both A and B forms of MAO.

---

*See references 110, 113, 150, 200, 216, 302, and 303.
†See references 23, 80, 113, 150, and 183.
‡See references 23, 100, 101, 108, 132, and 145.

DOPAMINE BETA-HYDROXYLASE

One of the mechanisms that could decrease NE levels in depressed patients would be low levels of the enzyme responsible for converting DA to NE, DBH (figure 12–1). DBH is present in plasma, brain, adrenals, and sympathetically innervated areas. DBH activity is a highly heritable trait and stable within an individual over time.[159,252,333] No age or male-female differences have been found* except in one study, which found females to have greater levels.[133]

Studies of DBH levels measured in blood have generally not found differences between affective disorder patients and controls.[119,326] However, three recent studies have reported decreased DBH levels: in psychotic unipolar depressions, with a trend for decreased levels in bipolar depression[187]; in endogenously depressed patients, especially those with bipolar disorder[238]; and in depressed patients, particularly bipolar patients compared to unipolars.[300]

If DBH were decreased, one might expect decreased levels of NE and its metabolites (MHPG and VMA) and increased levels of DA or its metabolite (HVA). Unfortunately, a relationship of CSF DBH to CSF MHPG, VMA, or HVA has not been published. The three significant plasma DBH studies are consistent with decreased NE in bipolar depression and increased DA and decreased NE in unipolar psychotic depressions.[187,238,300]

If increased levels of NE were associated with mania, then fusaric acid (which inhibits DBH, thus decreasing the conversion of DA to NE) might treat mania effectively by diminishing NE levels and might provoke a depression. Fusaric acid has been studied in one trial in manic patients and found not to be associated with a switch from mania to depression; nor was it an effective antimanic agent.[258] Rather it was found to increase the severity of mania. This is consistent with a DA theory of mania and unsupportive of NE involvement in mania and depression.

*See references 91, 212, 252, 324, 325, and 326.

Studies of CSF are also disparate. Lerner and associates[155] found no difference in DBH in CSF of bipolar and unipolar patients compared to controls. However, Post, Ballenger, and Goodwin[227] evaluated normals and depressed and recovered affectively ill patients and found CSF DBH to be significantly decreased in manic patients and elevated in bipolar depressed patients. This is also consistent with a dopaminergic theory of mania, since decreased DBH is hypothesized to increase DA levels by preventing its conversion to NE. It is also consistent with decreased DA and increased NE in bipolar depression. Thus, even if one restricts consideration to only the significant studies, a disparity between blood and CSF data will be found. Last, the range for depressive patients, manic patients, and normals in these plasma and CSF studies overlaps considerably, suggesting that a discrete DBH defect is not specific to affective disorders.

In summary, there is only inconsistent evidence to support a DBH or COMT hypothesis of affective disorder. The significant data from studies of MAO are opposite to the initial hypothesis. MAO levels have more consistently been reported to be decreased in bipolar depression, while low values in "normals" may reflect vulnerability to mental disorders. These data suggest that MAO inhibitors might be less effective in bipolar depression (low MAO levels to begin with) compared to unipolar anxious depression, especially in females. Studies to date have not yet fully explored this therapeutic issue, although clinical hypotheses similar to this have been made.[162]

Acetylcholine and Affective Disorders

Acetylcholine (ACh) was the first neurotransmitter to be discovered. Studies of its possible involvement in neuropsychiatric disorders have been hampered because of the difficulty in measuring ACh and because of its lability. The metabolism of ACh is well understood (see figure 12–3). Its precursors are choline and acetylcoenzyme A (acetyl-

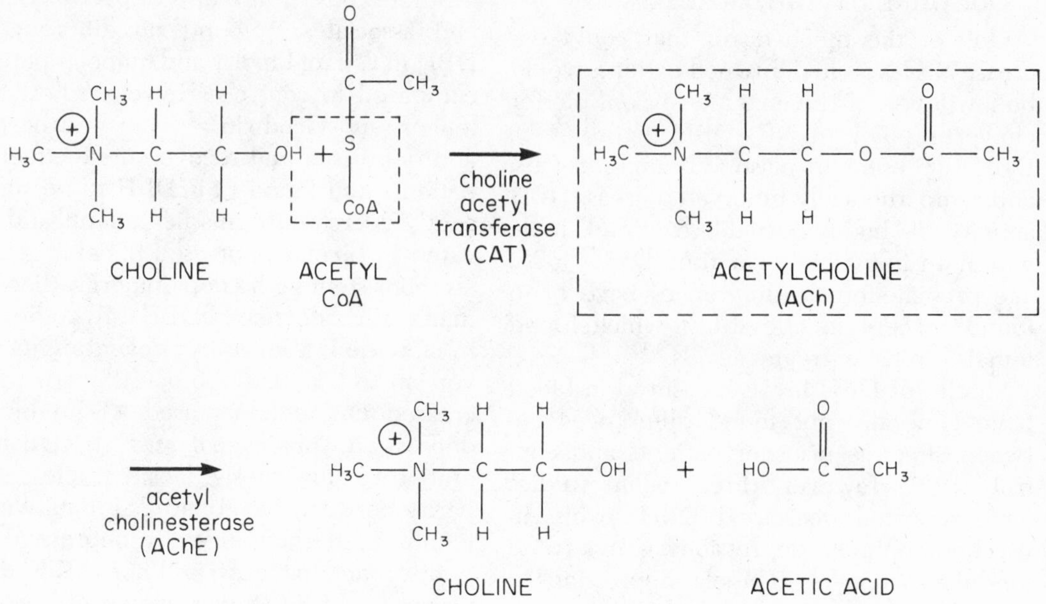

Figure 12–3. Synthesis and metabolism of acetylcholine.

CoA). Dietary choline in the plasma is taken into nerve endings by an active transport system. Acetyl-CoA is synthesized from pyruvate. Acetyl-CoA and choline are combined into ACh in nerve endings by the enzyme choline acetyltransferase (CAT). After release into the synapse, ACh is not taken back up into presynaptic neurons like NE, DA, or 5HT, but rather is split by acetylcholinesterase into choline and acetic acid and water.

A hypothesized relationship of ACh to affective illness may have originally been based on the effects of anticholinergic compounds on behavior.[130] Anticholinergic toxicity is associated with a euphoric state not unlike mania,[116] while the effects of cholinergic agents in animals produce a syndrome of lethargy and decreased motor movements similar to retarded depression.[45,137] Individuals who are exposed to cholinesterase inhibitors in industry develop elevated brain ACh levels and have been reported to display depressive symptomatology not unlike that of idiopathic depression.[30,115,138]

Janowsky and associates[139] carried out systematic double-blind trials utilizing intrave-nous physostigmine, a centrally active cholinesterase inhibitor. When administered to euthymic or mildly depressed individuals, a syndrome emerges characterized by lethargy, flattened facies, social withdrawal, psychomotor retardation, and depressed thoughts.[69,138,139] A noncentrally active cholinesterase inhibitor (neostigmine) has no such effects. Further, the physostigmine-induced depression can be blocked by anticholinergic drugs such as atropine. However, only a subgroup of a normal volunteer control group was found to become depressed or to have a complete depressive symptomatic profile[244,245] in addition to the anergic inhibitory syndrome that typically occurs with physostigmine infusion.

Manic patients given physostigmine[70] or the ACh precursors choline or lecithin[53,205] have an acute antimanic response often associated with depressive symptomatology. The antimanic effect of physostigmine has been demonstrated in several studies,* but not all manic symptoms are reversed by phy-

*See references 70, 131, 191, 192, and 215.

sostigmine. In particular, grandiosity may continue to occur even though other manic symptoms have been attenuated.[46,278] Some individuals become depressed when given the precursors of ACh such as deanol, acetamidobenzoate, choline, or lecithin for nonaffective disorders such as tardive dyskinesia or dementia. Passive symptomatology increased in schizophrenic patients treated with choline[68,192,312] and in some, but not the majority of, individuals receiving choline or lecithin for Alzheimer's disease.[68]

Increasing cholinergic tone through the use of arecoline during sleep has been associated with the induction of rapid-eye-movement (REM) sleep.[290] REM sleep is induced more easily in depressed patients.[291] This sensitivity to REM sleep induction is consistent with the polysomnographic finding that depression is characterized by a shortened REM latency. REM latency is significantly shorter following the administration of cholinomimetic compounds in individuals who have a history of primary affective illness than in normals.[291] This also suggests that there may be a trait sensitivity to cholinergic effects in affectively vulnerable patients.[289]

Further support relevant to a mechanism for cholinergic sensitivity in affective disorders comes from the report that patients with depression and their euthymic relatives who had a history of affective illness have an increased number of ACh muscarinic receptors on cultured skin fibroblasts compared to controls or to relatives without a history of affective illness.[205]

ACh may also play a role in the hypersecretion of cortisol found in individuals with affective disordered states. Corticotropin-releasing factor (CRF) release is stimulated by ACh.[31,82,127] Further, the release is inhibited by NE,[141] suggesting that there might be a cholinergic-noradrenergic balance associated with depression, with depressed states having increased ACh and decreased NE and manic states having decreased ACh and increased NE.[243] In conclusion, the available data strongly support an important

role for ACh in the pathophysiology of affective illnesses.

Gamma-amino Butyric Acid and Affective Disorders

The metabolism of gamma-amino butyric acid (GABA) is less specific than that of the biogenic amines or ACh (see figure 12–4). GABA is synthesized by the enzyme glutamic acid decarboxylase from the ubiquitous amino acid, glutamate, which can be synthesized from a number of sources in the brain. GABA is metabolized by several pathways, the main one using the enzyme GABA-α-ketoglutarate transaminase (GABA-T). Reviews of several clinical studies suggest that GABA may be decreased in the CSF and plasma of patients with depression during the depressed state. Three studies report decreased CSF GABA[102,117,144] obtained from the first 12 ml of CSF collected, and one study of a rapid-cycling bipolar patient has reported lower GABA levels in depressed compared to manic phases.[24] However, two studies[102,230] reported no difference in depressive patients and controls when more cephalad CSF from the sixteenth to the twenty-seventh ml was analyzed, suggesting that the lower GABA levels may reflect GABA levels in the spinal cord rather than in the brain.

GABA plasma levels have been reported as reduced in euthymic bipolar patients compared to normals, while for bipolar patients who were receiving lithium, plasma GABA levels were equivalent to those of normals.[24,25] Altered GABA metabolism may be a trait marker for bipolar disorder since bipolar patients who are euthymic have decreased levels of the catabolic enzyme GABA-T in platelets. Normals or lithium-treated bipolar patients do not.[24] If this represents a trait phenomenon in certain patients (bipolar) with affective disorder, it is of interest because the hypothesized defect is normalized by treatment with lithium. However, such a trait hypothesis is complicated by the CSF findings in mania. If CSF GABA

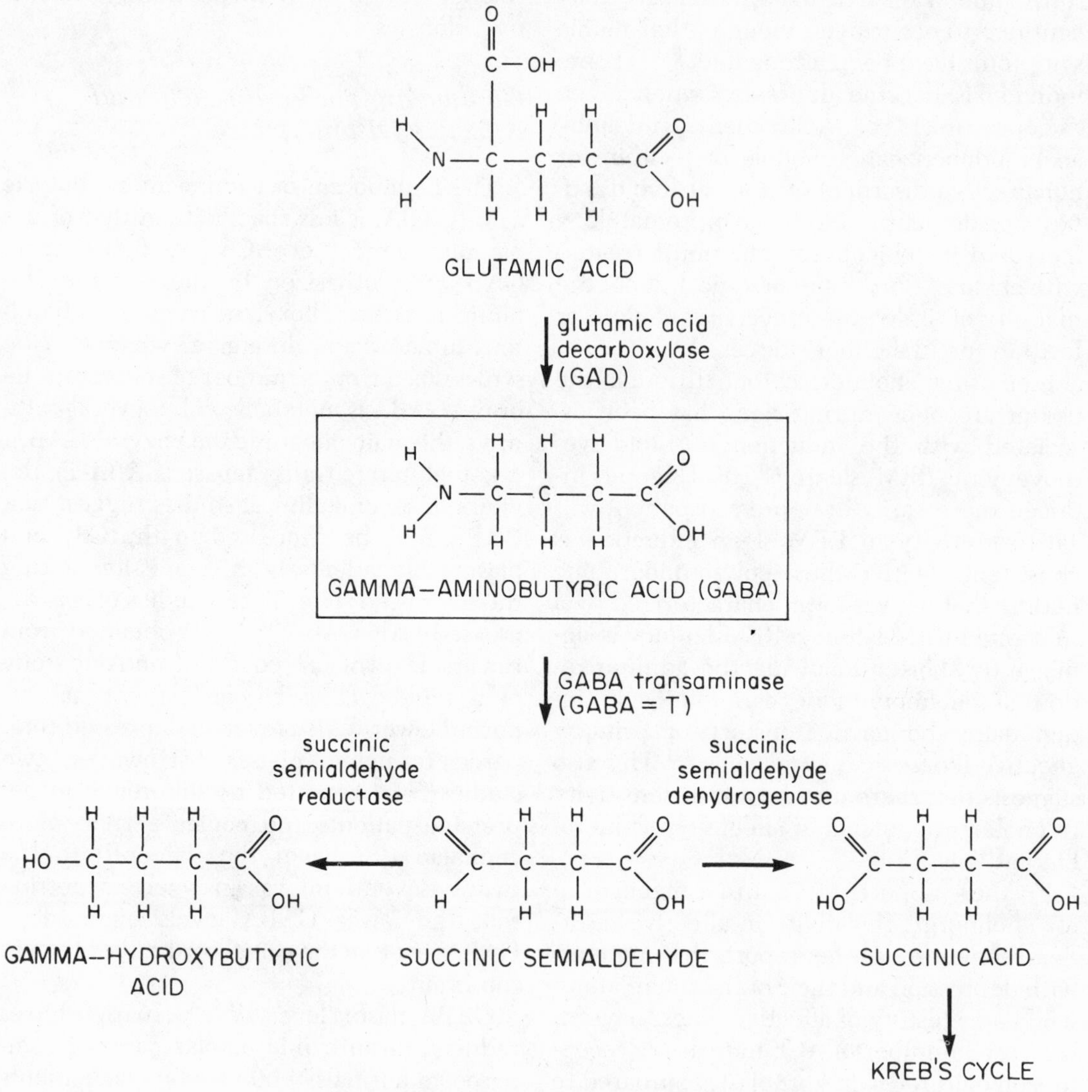

GLUTAMIC ACID

glutamic acid
decarboxylase
(GAD)

GAMMA—AMINOBUTYRIC ACID (GABA)

GABA transaminase
(GABA = T)

succinic
semialdehyde
reductase

succinic
semialdehyde
dehydrogenase

GAMMA—HYDROXYBUTYRIC
ACID

SUCCINIC SEMIALDEHYDE

SUCCINIC ACID

KREB'S CYCLE

Figure 12–4. Synthesis and metabolism of GABA.

is decreased in depression, one might expect it to be altered in mania. This does not appear to be the case. CSF GABA from manic patients is found to have levels equivalent to normals.[24,102]

Only one GABA agonist, progabide,[195] has been studied in affective illness. This agonist appears to have antidepressant properties, although a correlation of clinical response with CSF or plasma GABA was not carried out.

Other possible relationships of GABA to affective illness have been proposed on the basis of pharmacological considerations. GABA is a major inhibitory neurotransmitter in all mammalian brains, is ubiquitous, and may be the neurotransmitter at the plurality of all synapses in the CNS.[246,273] Many compounds that have an effect on mood and brain function also have some effect on GABA. Antidepressants might be hypothesized to functionally affect GABA by some mechanism. Inhibition of the catabolic enzyme GABA-T results in decreased GABA turnover and increased GABA levels. Carbamazapine, which has mood-stabilizing effects in addition to anticonvulsant activity,[233] decreases GABA turnover, as does the somatic treatment electroconvulsive therapy (ECT).

One antidepressant that has been evaluated with regard to GABA, desipramine,[277] mimics the action of GABA in the learned helplessness model of depression.[190] In contrast to antidepressants, neuroleptic agents[180] increase GABA turnover, thus decreasing GABA levels; and lithium[176] decreases the number of GABA receptors.

Animal studies suggest that low GABA may be associated with decreased firing and synthesis at DA and 5HT neurons, as well as decreased release of NE.[3,27] Thus the finding of decreased GABA in depression is also consistent with the more traditional biogenic amine hypothesis of decreased 5HT or catecholamines, which in a GABA model might function as final pathway mechanisms for affective illness. However, the CSF studies of GABA have not shown a correlation in affective disorder patients with GABA and the metabolites of NE, DA, or 5HT.

GABA may also be involved with the hypercorticoid state seen in affective disorders. CRF secretion is stimulated by 5HT or ACh and is inhibited by GABA and NE. Thus CRF release might be increased as a result of decreased levels of GABA at critical hypothalamic areas.

Because GABA is ubiquitous in the CNS, definition of specific anatomic areas where GABA may be abnormal is critical. Thus, if GABA metabolism were altered in the hypothalamus, some of the phenomena of depression, such as anorexia, biorhythm disturbances, cortisol hypersecretion, and mood disturbances, might be explicable. Frontal cortex areas depleted of GABA might be associated with some of the animal study models of depression, such as the learned helplessness paradigm. Unfortunately, anatomic localization of areas critical to mood has not been possible. Further, clinical studies of GABA are limited by the lack of nontoxic, specific inhibitors of GABA-T and by the many pathways of GABA synthesis. Therefore, the results of CSF and plasma levels and pharmacological interventions only provide support consistent with, but not specifically for, a GABAergic relationship to affective illness.

Neurotransmitter Receptors and Affective Disorders

While most investigations have focused on altered levels of neurotransmitters associated with mood, another series of hypotheses has been developed based on receptor function. The receptor hypotheses propose that amounts of critical neurotransmitters might be unaltered during mood changes; however, functional activity in neuronal systems could be altered if the receptor of the neurotransmitter became more or less sensitive, causing an increased or decreased physiological effect. In fact, most basic studies suggest that the sensitivity of the receptors does not change, but instead there is an increase or decrease in their concentration at nerve terminals.[42,295,296] There are three well-developed receptor hypotheses: (1) the tritiated-imipramine (^{3}H-IMI) receptor hypothesis; (2) the presynaptic alpha-2 NE receptor hypothesis; and (3) the postsynaptic beta-NE receptor hypothesis.

The relationship of affective disorders to 5HT and to receptor sites has been partially explored by the use of ^{3}H-IMI binding to blood platelets. It is of special interest that ^{3}H-IMI binding is highly associated with, although not identical to, the 5HT receptor sites in the brain.[152] Evidence from pharmacological studies[151,153] suggests an association of these binding sites with the presynaptic reuptake process for 5HT.[135,220] The first studies of platelet binding found that ^{3}H-IMI binding was lower in depressed patients than in normal controls.[6,35,220,305] The affinity for ^{3}H-IMI at these binding sites was not changed in these patients, suggesting that the number of receptor sites is decreased in depression, regardless of subtype, since no difference was found between unipolar and bipolar depressed patients.[35] Further, the number of ^{3}H-IMI binding sites in the brain of suicide victims was reduced compared to controls.[179,222,298] It is now considered less likely that this is a trait marker,[222,240] since several investigations have found no differences between normals and recovered depressed patients.[26,305,337] This conclusion remains controversial.[222] However, decreased ^{3}H-IMI binding may be relatively specific for affective disorder, since significantly lower levels have not been found in other major mental illnesses such as schizophrenia or schizo-affective illness.[305] Unfortunately, manic patients have not yet been studied. While these initial findings are provocative and potentially informative, several groups of investigators have not replicated them,[185] and they must, therefore, be interpreted judiciously.

Antidepressant agents initially were not thought to have an effect on the binding sites[220,240,305]; however, several animal studies have reported that antidepressant treatment alters ^{3}H-IMI binding in the brain. Some treatments, such as MAOIs, increase the number of binding sites,[305] whereas other antidepressant therapies, such as ECT or sleep deprivation, apparently decrease binding.[151,193] Chronic amitriptyline,[32] and nortriptyline but not mianserin,[134] treatment increases the number of binding sites that return to baseline levels when treatment is discontinued. If these studies are confirmed, they would suggest that a significant decrease in maximal uptake of 5HT may be specifically associated with depressive states and that an inherited or acquired deficiency of the protein-transport systems for 5HT might be an integral part of the pathophysiology of depressive illness in some patients. Presumably a chronic low uptake of 5HT would lead to a 5HT-deficient state consistent with an indoleamine hypothesis of affective illness.

The relationship of depression to the postsynaptic beta-receptor has been based on response to antidepressant treatments. Virtually all antidepressants or antidepressant treatments, including ECT, produce a reduced sensitivity of postsynaptic beta-receptors[15,48,304] that occurs gradually over time similar to clinically observable antidepressant effects. This phenomenon is thought to be an adaptive response secondary to the increased synaptic concentration of NE[343] that occurs immediately after tricyclic-type antidepressants reach the synapse, inhibiting the reuptake of NE back into the presynaptic neuron. This so-called downregulation of beta-receptors associated with most, and possibly all, antidepressant treatments suggests that these receptors might be "supersensitive" during the depressed state because of a decrease in presynaptic secretion of NE. It is unclear, however, whether this can be reconciled with the non-NE neurotransmitter specificity of several newer antidepressants, such as trazodone.

The relationship of the presynaptic noradrenergeric alpha-2 receptor, which inhibits the release of NE, has been studied recently in relationship to depression. Five studies have measured alpha-2 receptors in platelets of affectively ill patients compared to normal controls. Platelet alpha-2 receptors are thought to have similar characteristics to presynaptic alpha-2 receptors in the brain. Three of these studies found that the number of alpha-2 receptors is increased in unipolar and bipolar depression,[95,143,284] while two did not.[66,226]

Another method used for assessment of alpha-2 receptor number and function *in vivo* is the administration of medication that specifically acts on the receptor. Several human investigations of growth hormone (GH) response to clonidine[48,96,280] suggest that chronic treatment with antidepressants decreases the sensitivity of the alpha-2 receptor.

This led to the development of a hypothesis that some antidepressant agents have a therapeutic mechanism modulated by changes in receptor activity.* These studies suggest that some depressed patients may have increased sensitivity (or number) of these presynaptic alpha-2 receptors. This could result in decreased release of

*See references 48, 64, 96, 174, 280, 294, and 309.

NE,[56,280,294] since increased presynaptic sensitivity would mean that NE in the synapse would have a greater effect on presynaptic nerve functioning, inhibiting the synthesis and release of more NE.

The etiology of an increased number of alpha-2 receptors in depression is not fully known, but an interaction of genetic predisposition and stress is possible. Stress induced in rats by immobilization produces an acute and chronic increase in alpha-2 receptors in the cortex, midbrain, and brain stem.[317,319] This stress effect may be relatively specific to alpha-2 receptors, since no change was found in alpha-1 or DA receptors. If confirmed in human studies, this may provide a link between stress and biochemical pathophysiology in affective disorders.

There are, however, other reports regarding alpha-2 receptors that suggest caution in associating depression with presynaptic alpha-2 NE receptor abnormalities. The effect of clonidine on stimulation of GH release appears to be due to stimulating postsynaptic alpha-2 receptors,[79,181,189,320] while MHPG and blood pressure are both decreased by clonidine's effect on the presynaptic alpha-2 receptors. Charney and associates[49] reported no difference in the MHPG or blood pressure effect of clonidine between depressed and healthy patients, suggesting normal alpha-2 presynaptic receptors in depressed patients. However, other groups found GH response to clonidine to be blunted in depression.[282] This suggests that presynaptic receptors are normal during depression while there is a decreased sensitivity (or density) of the postsynaptic alpha-2 NE receptor.

Similar tests using insulin-induced hypoglycemia in children have shown decreased GH secretion, suggesting both that depression in children may be similar to that of adults and that the postsynaptic alpha-2 NE receptors may be hyposensitive in this population.[236]

A decrease in postsynaptic alpha-2 receptors would presumably represent a pathophysiological response to increased NE activity in depression. Increased NE activity is, of course, inconsistent with the original catecholamine hypothesis. If true, one would expect to find a subgroup of depressed patients who had elevated levels of the NE metabolite MHPG and who had a particularly blunted GH response to clonidine. Siever and associates[283] reported on two groups of patients for whom this appeared to be the case. Increased plasma NE was associated with a blunted GH response to clonidine, and, conversely patients with low MHPG had a larger GH response to clonidine.[286]

In a more definitive study,[281] plasma MHPG concentrations, blood pressure, heart rate, and plasma NE decreased significantly in normal subjects following clonidine infusions but not in individuals who were depressed. These measures are associated with presynaptic alpha-2 activity and suggest that presynaptic alpha-2 receptors are less responsive (fewer in number) in depressed subjects than in normal subjects. The subgroup examined in this study appears to have been treatment-refractory patients with unipolar depression. This suggests that such a subgroup of patients may have increased NE, decreased presynaptic, and increased postsynaptic alpha-2 receptors. Such a group would be consistent with the elevated urinary MHPG subgroup postulated by Schildkraut.[271]

In summary, receptor changes in affective illness are relatively well documented in depression but not in mania. The possibility of decreased ^{3}H-IMI receptors may be consistent with other studies implicating 5HT in depression. Beta-receptor down-regulation during antidepressant treatment in animal models of depression is consistent with the catecholamine hypothesis, although levels of beta-receptors cannot yet be measured in the brains of humans. Studies of alpha-2 receptor activity measured in platelets and measured indirectly by challenge tests produce inconsistent results that can be reconciled with other hypotheses of depression only with complicated reasoning. Clearly, a more parsimonious explanation of this entire area is desirable for the development of an internally consistent hypothesis.

Brain Peptides and Affective Disorders

Peptides are now recognized as potent neuromodulators affecting all levels of brain function. Many peptides have characteristics of neurotransmitters and are controlled by, and themselves control, neurotransmitters. Since peptides are composed of long chains of amino acids, virtually an endless combination of naturally occuring sequences is possible. By the same token, there is an enormous potential for abnormal peptide metabolism to occur, as we know from the multitude of congenital disorders of protein metabolism already described. Only a few of the major brain peptides have been evaluated in mental illness, although this is an area of exploding knowledge.

OPIOIDS

An opioid hypothesis for affective illness is based on the observation of euphoric effects of exogenously administered opioids and the discovery of endogenous opioids.[223] Few studies have been carried out to test such a hypothesis. One of the endogenous opioids, beta-endorphin, has been administered intravenously to patients with depression.[108] An antidepressant response tended to occur for most of the patients, although the effect typically lasted less than twenty-four hours.

If endorphins were intrinsically antidepressant agents, one might also expect to find that the opiate antagonist, naloxone hydrochloride, would have had antimanic effects. A recent World Health Organization Project failed to demonstrate any such antimanic effects.[225] Further, most studies have found no effect of naloxone on normals[124,142] or in depression,[67,83,315] although one high-dose study suggests naloxone may worsen preexisting depression.[55]

Other studies have measured opioid activity in individuals with affective disorder, with the expectation that opioid levels would be higher in mania and lower in depression. The earlier studies examining CSF for opioids have been questioned because of the complexity of carrying out an accurate assay of these compounds. Two similar well-controlled studies did not find any differences among normals or manic or depressed (unipolar or bipolar)[103,234] patients in CSF beta-endorphin or total opioid binding. One group[234] reported a positive correlation of anxiety to CSF opioid levels, suggesting that higher opioid levels were associated with higher levels of anxiety in depressed patients, but neither found correlations with depression or mania ratings. These studies suggest that a specific endorphin hypothesis of affective disorders is relatively unsupported.

SOMATOSTATIN AND VASOPRESSIN

The other peptides that have been implicated in affective disorders are somatostatin and vasopressin. Somatostatin is an active neuromodulator associated with increased turnover of NE, DA, ACh, and 5HT. The relationship of these neurotransmitters to somatostatin is complex, however, because somatostatin itself is regulated in part by these neurotransmitters and additionally by GABA. Thus it is possible that altered somatostatin could result in observed secondary changes in the major neurotransmitter systems implicated in affective disorders. The reverse could also be true. Gerner and Yamada[105] and Rubinow and associates[254] have reported decreased CSF somatostatin levels in unipolar and bipolar depressed patients compared to normals. Manic and euthymic affectively disordered patients were not different from normals.

CSF vasopressin levels have been investigated[118] in drug-free unipolar and bipolar depression, mania, and normal controls. Both unipolar and bipolar depressed patients had significantly lower CSF vasopressin levels compared to controls and to manic patients, the latters' levels being slightly, but not significantly, higher than controls.

Both the peripheral and the central nervous system utilize vasopressin as a neuromodulator, where its central effect is discretely different from its effect on osmolarity regulation in the periphery. Since vasopressin has been associated with improvement in memory and cognitive processes after acute administration, it has been hypothesized that the cognitive disturbance in depression may be associated with the observed decrease in vasopressin levels. Vasopressin is also involved in a variety of other functions besides memory, including biological rhythms, REM sleep, pain perception, and neuroendocrine regulation, as well as fluid and electrolyte balance. Administration of the vasopressin analogue 1-Desamino-8-D-arginine vasopressin (DDAVP) was shown to produce significant functional improvement in the specific components of cognition known to be impaired in the depressed state. DDAVP has also been reported to reverse ECT-induced retrograde amnesia. However, DDAVP itself has not been shown to possess general antidepressant effects in studies to date.[118]

In summary, the three peptides most associated with affective illness each have tenuous support based on biochemical levels and/or a single pharmacological study. Much more confirming data must be produced before specific hypotheses can be established.

¶ Biorhythms and Affective Disorders

Sophisticated investigations of the relationship of biorhythms to affective disorders are relatively recent. Several biorhythm abnormalities have been described, especially in patients who have bipolar disorder:[332] (1) blunting of the amplitude of circadian rhythms, (2) advancing position of circadian rhythm phases, and (3) occasional doubling of the length of the sleep-wake cycle preceeding mood switches.

A basis for biorhythm alteration in affective disorders can be found in clinical as well as experimental data. Depressive symptoms are often more severe in the morning immediately after awakening and improve during the day. Thus this particular phenomenon of depression itself exhibits a daily rhythm. Similarly, the early-morning awakening typically found in affective disorders may represent a phase shift advance of some

circadian rhythm clock to an earlier time.[65] Sophisticated studies have shown that compared to normals, bipolar patients exhibit a blunting (loss of amplitude) of cortisol[257] and thyrotropin[330] diurnal secretions. Further, urine MHPG excretion may exhibit a phase shift to an earlier peak in bipolar patients compared to controls.[332]

Intentionally manipulating biorhythms may be associated with changes in mood. Altering diurnal rhythms by one night of total sleep deprivation can be associated with temporary remission of depressive symptoms[107] and may also be associated with switches from depression into mania in bipolar patients. A single night of total sleep deprivation is similar to the forty-eight-hour sleep cycle that often occurs in manic-depressive patients when they spontaneously switch from depression to mania.[331]

Depressive symptomatology has a relationship to seasons of the year in some patients.[251] This appears to be more common in individuals with bipolar disorder.[251] There is a consistency of these seasonal mood changes in affective patients, with depressions most frequently having an onset between October and December and spontaneous remission of symptoms usually occurring in March.[251] Depressions have been reported to be alleviated in some patients by altering the day-night cycle artificially to mimic summer daylight hours.[160] The sensitivity of these patients to light suggests that they may be a unique subgroup of bipolar disorder. Most of these patients had a family history of major affective disorder and met diagnostic criteria for bipolar I or II disorder. However, they showed no changes throughout the year on parameters associated with affective illness (altered REM latency, dexamethasone suppression test, and TRH-TSH challenge test). The relationship of light to these individuals' mood may be mediated in some way through biochemical phenomena.[159] For example, light signals on the retina are transmitted through a complex neurological system into the pineal gland, inhibiting NE release and thus preventing secretion of melatonin.

The nocturnal rise of melatonin has been used as a phase marker in bipolar disorder. During depression, and particularly when manic, patients have an earlier onset of melatonin secretion consistent with a phase-advance hypothesis of affective illness. Because NE mediates melatonin release, this is also consistent with increased functional NE during mania relative to depression. Additional work has demonstrated that euthymic bipolar patients may be more sensitive to light than normals, suppressing the melatonin response to light at much lower intensity than do normals. Circa-annual changes have also been identified for several biochemical parameters associated with affective pathophysiology. ^{3}H-IMI platelet uptake is significantly higher in the fall and winter in controls, but in depressed patients, the uptake is lower than in controls throughout the year, with lowest levels in December.[5] CSF 5-HIAA,[10] MHPG,[11] and brain monoamines[44] all exhibit systematic seasonal changes. Thus there is strong evidence for biorhythm abnormalities in affective illness, although several critical areas are yet to be delineated, including subgroups of patients so affected and the pathophysiology of the relationship of mood to the many biorhythms.

¶ Anatomical Hypotheses of Affective Disorders

One of the early anatomical hypotheses of affective disorders was based on the observation that an anesthetic agent injected into either the right or left carotid artery differentially affected mood.[131] Injection into the right carotid artery put the right brain to sleep and produced a more talkative state (presumably the left brain was awake), whereas injection into the left carotid artery produced a state that was associated with symptomatology of depression (right brain dominating).

Evidence from a variety of techniques has suggested that during depressive phases of illness, there may be abnormally increased right-hemisphere activity,[86,87,288] abnormally decreased[77,99] left-hemisphere activity, or pathology[73,90,99,276] of the right hemisphere. The evidence from many of these studies suggests that the balance between the right and left hemispheres shifts toward the right during depressive phases and toward the left during mania.[88,336] Additional work[288] has shown that whereas normal subjects show overall right visual field advantage for recognition (a left-brain function), depressed individuals have a trend toward a left visual field advantage. Similarly, Shaffer and associates[276] found greater right frontal deviation in depressed patients compared to nondepressed controls, utilizing computer-averaged electroencephalogram (EEG). They also found a trend for the right frontal area to be correlated with the Beck Depression Inventory Scales, suggesting that more depressed individuals had a more deviant asymmetry.

However, the shift to the right may not be unique to depression. Flor-Henry[87] reported that a shift to the right hemisphere utilizing EEG measures occurred in both depression and mania. Unfortunately, the exact site or source of the EEG-reported effects has not been identified. Additionally, the determination of left or right activation depends greatly on the method of measurement,[88] with the result that mania has also been associated with right dominance[89] and depression with left dominance.[90]

It is generally accepted that asymmetry from normal is common in mania and depression. Flor-Henry[88] has conceptualized that manic symptoms occur when the nondominant hemisphere loses control of the dominant, and depression when the nondominant is no longer controlled by the dominant. Asymmetry of electrophysiological function in mood disorders is of additional interest since it has become clear that the biochemistry of the brain is not symmetrical.[178,242,287,349]

Recently positron emission tomography has been carried out in individuals with affective disorder in depressed, euthymic, and manic states.[20] No differences were reported in unipolar or manic patients compared to normals. However, bipolar depressed patients had a significantly reduced glucose metabolic rate in the whole brain, with no regional specificity. No left-right differences were seen in the depressed, manic, or euthymic state or in normals. This decrease in glucose metabolic rate in bipolar depressed patients appears to be state-dependent, since case studies of rapid-cycling patients have shown a normalization of glucose metabolic rate as the patient switches from depression into mania or euthymia.

¶ Conclusion

In conclusion, it is manifest that over the past decade there has been an expanding number of hypotheses about the pathophysiology of affective disorders. The older hypotheses relevant to catecholamines, 5HT, and MAO have been extended by new studies and continue to be of scientific and heuristic use. Newer hypotheses have arisen as new physiological abnormalities in affective disorders have been discovered. The data base of many of the new hypotheses is less broad, however, and therefore they might better be viewed in the context of an emerging set of hypotheses that will continue to be refined. It is unlikely that any current single hypothesis will explain all of the biological abnormalities in affective illnesses, much less the etiology. Because there is not enough information to integrate into an overall theory, it is necessary to pursue the lines of inquiry suggested by the individual hypotheses, developing enough information to define their limits and their relationship to one another and to specific affective disorders.

¶ Bibliography

1. AGHAJANIAN, G. K., and ASHER, I. M. "Histochemical Fluorescence of Raphe Neurons: Selective Enhancement by Tryptophan," *Science*, 172 (1971):1150–1161.

2. AGREN, H. "Symptom Patterns in Unipolar and Bipolar Depression Correlating with Monoamine Metabolites in the Cerebrospinal Fluid. II. Suicide," *Psychiatry Research*, 2 (1980):225–236.

3. ARBILLA, S., and LANGER, S. Z., "Facilitation by GABA of the Potassium Evoked Release of 3H-Noradrenaline from the Rat Occipital Cortex," *Nauyn-Schmiedebergs Archives of Pharmacology*, 306 (1979):161–168.

4. ARORA, R. C., KREGEL, L., and MELTZER, H. Y., "Seasonal Variation of Serotonin Uptake in Normal Controls and Depressed Patients," *Biological Psychiatry*, 19 (1984):795–804.

5. ARORA, R. C., et al. "Serotonin Uptake and Imipramine Binding in Blood Platelets and Brain of Fawn-hooded and Sprague Dawley Rats," *Life Science*, 33 (1983):437–442.

6. ASARCH, K. B., SHIH, J. C., and KULESAR, A. "Decreased ^{3}H-Imipramine Binding in Depressed Males and Females," *Communication in Psychopharmacology*, 4 (1980):425–442.

7. ASBERG, M., BERTILSSON, L., and THOREN, P. "CSF Monoamine Metabolites in Depressive Illness," in S. Garatini, ed., *Depressive Disorders*. New York: Stuttgart Schattauer, 1978, pp. 293–305.

8. ASBERG, M., THOREN, P., and TRASKMAN, L., "Serotonin Depression—A Biochemical Subgroup Within Affective Disorders," *Science*, 191 (1976):478–479.

9. ASBERG, M., TRASKMAN, L., and THOREN, P. "5-HIAA in the Cerebrospinal Fluid —A Biochemical Suicide Predictor?" *Archives of General Psychiatry*, 33 (1976):1193–1197.

10. ASBERG, M., et al. "Monoamine Metabolites in Cerebrospinal Fluid in Relation to Depressive Illness, Suicidal Behavior and Personality," in B. Angrist et al., eds., *Recent Advances in Neuropharmacology*. New York: Pergamon Press, 1981, pp. 257–271.

11. ASBERG, M., et al. "CSF Monoamine Metabolites in Melancholia," *Acta Psychiatrica Scandinavica*, 69 (1984):201–219.

12. ASHCROFT, G. W., and GLEN, A.I.M. "Mood and Neuronal Function: A Modified Amine Hypothesis for the Eti-

ology of Affective Illness," *Advances in Biochemical Psychopharmacology,* 11 (1974):335–339.

13. ASHCROFT, G. W., CRAWFORD, T.T.B., and ECCLESTON, D. "5-Hydroxyindole Compounds in the Cerebrospinal Fluid of Patients with Psychiatric or Neurological Diseases," *Lancet,* 2 (1966):1049–1050.

14. ASHCROFT, G. W., et al. "Significance of Lumbar CSF Metabolite Measures in Affective Illness," in J. Tuomisto and M. K. Paasonen, eds., *CNS and Behavioral Pharmacology,* vol. 3. Helsinki, Finland: University of Helsinki, 1976, pp. 277–284.

15. BANERJEE, S. P., et al. "Development of Beta-adrenergic Subsensitivity by Antidepressants," *Nature,* 268 (1977):455–456.

16. BANKI, C. M. "Correlation Between Cerebrospinal Fluid Amine Metabolites and Psychomotor Activity in Affective Disorders," *Journal of Neurochemistry,* 28 (1977):255–257.

17. BANKI, C. M., and MOLNAR, G. "Cerebrospinal Fluid 5-HIAA as an Index of Central Serotonergic Processes," *Psychiatry Research,* 5 (1981):77–83.

18. BANKI, C. M., MOLNAR, G., and VOJNIK, M. "Cerebrospinal Fluid Amine Metabolites, Tryptophan and Clinical Parameters in Depresion II," *Journal of Affective Disorders,* 3 (1981):91–99.

19. BARON, M., KLOTZ, J., and MENDLEWICZ, J. "Multiple-threshold Transmission of Affective Disorders," *Archives of General Psychiatry,* 38 (1981):79–84.

20. BAXTER, L., et al. "Cerebral Metabolic Rate for Glucose in Mood Disorders Studied with Positron Emission Tomography," *Archives of General Psychiatry,* in press.

21. BECKMANN, H., and GOODWIN, F. K. "Antidepressant Response to Tricyclics and Urinary MHPG in Unipolar Patients," *Archives of General Psychiatry,* 32 (1975):17–21.

22. ———. "Urinary MHPG in Subgroups of Depressed Patients and Normal Controls," *Neuropsychobiology,* 6 (1980):91–100.

23. BELMAKER, R. H., et al. "Platelet Monoamine Oxidase in Schizophrenia and Manic-depressive Illness," *British Journal of Psychiatry,* 129 (1976):227–232.

24. BERRETTINI, W. H., and POST, R. M. "GABA in Affective Illness," in R. M. Post and J. C. Ballenger, eds., *Neurobiology of Mood Disorders.* Baltimore: Williams & Wilkins, 1984, pp. 673–685.

25. BERRETTINI, W. H., et al. "Plasma and CSF GABA in Affective Illness," *British Journal of Psychiatry,* 141 (1982):483–487.

26. BERRETTINI, W. H., et al. "Platelet ^{3}H-Imipramine Binding in Euthymic Bipolar Patients," *Psychiatry Research,* 7 (1982):215–219.

27. BISWAS, B., and CARLSSON, A. "The Effect of Intracerebroventricularly Administered GABA on Brain Monoamine Metabolism," *Nauyn-Schmiedebergs Archives of Pharmacology,* 299 (1977):41–46.

28. BLOMBERY, P. A., et al. "Conversion of MHPG to Vanillylmandelic Acid," *Archives of General Psychiatry,* 37 (1980):1095–1098.

29. BOWERS, M. B. "Cerebrospinal Fluid 5-Hydroxyindoleacetic Acid (5-HIAA) and Homovanillic Acid (HVA) Following Probenecid in Unipolar Depressives Treated with Amitriptyline," *Psychopharmacology,* 23 (1972):26–33.

30. BOWERS, M. B., GOODMAN, E., and SIM, V. M. "Some Behavioral Changes in Man Following Anticholinesterase Administration," *Journal of Nervous and Mental Disorders,* 138 (1964):383–389.

31. BRADBURY, M.W.B., et al. "Stimulation Electrically and by Acetylcholine of the Rat Hypothalamus in Vitro," *Journal of Physiology (London),* 239 (1974):269–283.

32. BRADDOCK, L. E., et al. "Changes in the Binding to Platelets of 3H-Imipramine and 3H-Yohimbine in Normal Subjects Taking Amitriptyline," *Neuropharmacology,* 23 (1984):285–286.

33. BRIDGER, P. K., et al. "Precursors and Metabolites of 5-Hydroxytryptamine and Dopamine in the Ventricular Cerebrospinal Fluid of Psychiatric Patients," *Psychological Medicine,* 6 (1976):399–405.

34. BRIGGS, H. M., and BRIGGS, M. "Hormonal Influences on Erythrocyte Cate-

chol-O-methyltransferase Activity in Humans," *Experientia,* 29 (1973):279–280.

35. BRILEY, M. S., et al. "Tritiated Imipramine Binding Sites Are Decreased in Platelets of Untreated Depressed Patients," *Science,* 209 (1980):303–395.

36. BROADHURST, A. D. "L-tryptophan versus ECT," *Lancet,* 1 (1970):1392–1393.

37. BRODIE, H.K.H., et al. "Catecholamines and Mania: The Effect of Alpha-methyl-paratyrosine on Manic Behavior and Catecholamine Metabolism," *Clinical Pharmacology Therapy,* 12 (1971):218–224.

38. BROWN, G. L., GOODWIN, F. K., and BALLENGER, J. C. "Aggression in Humans Correlates with Cerebrospinal Fluid Amines Metabolites," *Psychiatric Research,* 1 (1979):131–139.

39. BROWN, G. L., et al. "Aggression, Suicide, and Serotonin: Relationships to CSF Monoamine Metabolites," *American Journal of Psychiatry,* 139 (1982):741–746.

40. BUNNEY, W. E., Jr. "The Current Status of Research in the Catecholamine Theories of Affective Disorders," *Psychopharmacology Communication,* 1 (1975):599–609.

41. BUNNEY, W. E., Jr., and DAVIS, J. M. "Norepinephrine in Depressive Reactions," *Archives of General Psychiatry,* 13 (1965):483–494.

42. BUNNEY, W. E., Jr., and GARLAND, B. L. "Lithium and Its Possible Mode of Action," in R. M. Post and J. C. Ballenger, eds., *Neurobiology of Mood Disorders.* Baltimore: Williams & Wilkins, 1984, pp. 731–743.

43. BURNS, D., and MENDELS, J. "Biogenic Amine Precursors and Affective Illnesses," in W. E. Fann, et al., eds., *Phenomenology and Treatment of Depression.* New York: Spectrum, 1977, pp. 33–67.

44. CARLSSON, A., SVENNERHOLM, L., and WINBLAD, B. "Seasonal and Circadian Monoamine Variations in Human Brains Examined Post Mortem," *Acta Psychiatrica Scandanavica* 280 (Supplement) (1980):75–83.

45. CARLTON, P. L. "Cholinergic Mechanisms in the Control of Behavior by the Brain," *Psychology Review,* 70 (1963):19–39.

46. CARROLL, B. J., et al. "Cholinergic Reversal of Manic Symptoms," *Lancet,* 1 (1973):427.

47. CASPER, R. C., et al. "Neuroendocrine and Amine Studies in Affective Illness," *Psychoneuroendocrinology,* 2 (1977):105–113.

48. CHARNEY, D. S., et al. "Presynaptic Adrenergic Receptor Sensitivity in Depression: The Effect of Chronic Desipramine Treatment," *Archives of General Psychiatry,* 38 (1981):1334–1340.

49. CHARNEY, D. S., et al. "Adrenergic Receptor Sensitivity in Depression," *Archives of General Psychiatry,* 39 (1982):290–294.

50. CHECKLEY, S. A., and CRAMMER, J. L. "Hormonal Responses to Methylamphetamine in Depression: A New Approach to the Noradrenaline Depletion Hypothesis," *British Journal of Psychiatry,* 131 (1977):582–586.

51. COBBIN, D. M., et al. "Urinary MHPG Levels and Tricyclic Antidepressant Drug Selection," *Archives of General Psychiatry,* 36 (1979):1111–1115.

52. COHEN, B. M., LIPINSKI, J. F., and ALTESMAN, R. I. "Lecithin in the Treatment of Mania: Double-blind Placebo-controlled Trials," *American Journal of Psychiatry,* 139 (1982):1162–1164.

53. COHEN, B. M., et al. "Lecithin in Mania: A Preliminary Report," *American Journal of Psychiatry,* 137 (1980):242–243.

54. COHEN, C. K., DUNNER, D. L., and AXELROD, J. "Reduced Catechol-O-methyltransferase Activity in Red Blood Cells of Women with Primary Affective Disorders," *Science,* 170 (1970):1323–1324.

55. COHEN, M. R., et al. "High Dose Naloxone in Depression," *Biological Psychiatry,* 19 (1984):825–832.

56. COHEN, R. M., and CAMPBELL, I. C. "Receptor Adaptation in Animal Models of Mood Disorders: A State Change Approach to Psychiatric Illness," in R. M. Post and J. C. Ballenger, eds., *Neurobiology of Mood Disorders.* Baltimore: Williams & Wilkins, 1984, pp. 572–586.

57. COHEN, R. M., et al. "Presynaptic Noradrenergic Regulation During Depression and Antidepressant Drug Treat-

ment," *Psychiatry Research,* 3 (1980):
93–106.

58. COLONNA, L., PETIT, M., and LEPINE, J. P.
"Bromocriptine in Affective Disorders:
A Pilot Study," *Journal of Affective Disorders,* 1 (1979):173–177.

59. COPPEN, A. J., and WOOD, K. "5-Hydroxytryptamine in the Pathogenesis of
Affective Disorders," in B. T. Ho, J. C.
Schoolar, and E. Usdin, eds., *Serotonin
in Biological Psychiatry.* New York:
Raven Press, 1982, pp. 249–258.

60. COPPEN, A. J., ECCELESTON, E. G., and
PEET, M. "Total and Free Tryptophan
Concentration in the Plasma of Depressive Patients," *Lancet,* 2 (1973):60–63.

61. COPPEN, A. J., PRANGE, A. J., and WHYBROW, P. C. "Abnormalities of Indoleamines in Affective Disorders," *Archives
of General Psychiatry,* 26 (1972):474–
478.

62. COPPEN, A. J., et al. "Tryptophan in the
Treatment of Depression," *Lancet,* 2
(1967):731–734.

63. CREWS, F. T., and SMITH, C. B., "Presynaptic α-receptor Subsensitivity After
Long-term Antidepressant Treatment,"
Science, 202 (1978):322–423.

64. ———. "Potentiation of Responses to Adrenergic Nerve Stimulation in Isolated
Rat Atria During Chronic Tricyclic Antidepressant Administration," *Journal
of Pharmacology and Experimental
Therapy,* 214 (1980):143–149.

65. CZEISLER, C. A., et al. "Timing of REM
Sleep Is Coupled to the Circadian
Rhythm of Body Temperature in Man,
Sleep, 2 (1980):329.

66. DAIGUJI, M., et al. "α-2-Adrenergic Receptor Labeling with 3H-Yohimbine, A
Selective Agonist Ligand," *Life
Sciences,* 28 (1981):2705–2717.

67. DAVIS, G. C., et al. "Intravenous Naloxone
Administration in Schizophrenia and
Affective Illness," *Science,* 197 (1977):-
74–76.

68. DAVIS, K. L., HOLLISTER, L. E., and
BERGER, P. A. "Choline Chloride in
Schizophrenia," *American Journal of
Psychiatry,* 136 (1979):1581–1584.

69. DAVIS, K. L., et al. "Physostigmine Effects
on Cognition and Affect in Normal Subjects," *Psychopharmacology,* 51 (1976):-
23–27.

70. DAVIS, K. L., et al. "Physostigmine in
Mania," *Archives of General Psychiatry,* 35 (1978):119–122.

71. DeLEON-JONES, R., et al. "Diagnostic Subgroups of Affective Disorders and Their
Urinary Excretion of Catecholamine
Metabolites," *American Journal of Psychiatry,* 132 (1975):1140–1148.

72. D'ELIA, G., and PERRIS, C., "Cerebral
Functional Dominance and Depression:
An Analysis of EEG Amplitude in Depressed Patients," *Acta Psychiatrica
Scandinavica,* 49 (1973):191–197.

73. DOBROKHOTOVA, T. A., and BRAPHINA,
N. N. "Functional Asymmetry of the
Cerebral Hemispheres in Psychopathological Cases Due to Brain Lesions,"
Psychology Abstracts, 53 (1975):9932–
9939.

74. DONNELLY, C. H., and MURPHY, D. L.
"Substrate- and Inhibitor-related Characteristics of Human Platelet Monoamine Oxidase," *Biochemical Pharmacology,* 26 (1977):853–858.

75. DUNNER, D. L., and GOODWIN, F. K.
"Effect of L-tryptophan on Brain
Serotonin Metabolism in Depressed Patients," *Archives of General Psychiatry,*
26 (1972):364–366.

76. DUNNER, D. L., et al. "Differential Catechol-O-methyltransferase Activity in
Unipolar and Bipolar Affective Illness,"
Archives of General Psychiatry, 25
(1971):348–353.

77. DUNNER, D. L., et al. "Erythrocyte Catechol methyltransferase Activity in Primary Affective Disorder," *Biological
Psychiatry,* 12 (1976):237–245.

78. EBSTEIN, R., et al. "Electrophoretic Pattern of Red Blood Cell Catechol-O-methyltransferase in Schizophrenia and
Manic-depressive Illness," *Biological
Psychiatry,* 11 (1976):613–623.

79. EDEN, S., et al. "Evidence for a Growth
Hormone Releasing Factor Moderating
Alpha-adrenergic Influence on
Growth Hormone Secretion in the
Rat," *Neuroendocrinology,* 33 (1981):-
24–27.

80. EDWARDS, D. J., et al. "Platelet Monoamine Oxidase in Affective Disorders,"
Archives of General Psychiatry, 35
(1978):1443–1446.

81. EDWARDS, D. J., et al. "MHPG Excretion

in Depression," *Psychiatry Research*, 2 (1980):295–305.

82. EDWARDSON, J. A., and BENNETT, G. W. "Modulation of Corticotropin-releasing Factor Release from Hypothalamic Synaptosomes," *Nature*, 251 (1974):425–427.

83. EMRICH, H., CORDING, C., and PIREE, S "Action of Naloxone in Different Types of Psychosis," in E. Usdin, W. E. Bunney, Jr., and N. S. Kline, eds., *Endorphins in Mental Health Research.* New York: Oxford University Press, 1979, pp. 452–460.

84. FAHNDRICH E., et al. "Erythrocyte COMT-activity in Patients with Affective Disorders," *Acta Psychiatrica Scandinavica*, 61 (1980):427–437.

85. FAWCETT, J., MAAS, J. W., and DEKIRMENJIAN, H. "Depression and MHPG Excretion—Response to Dextroamphetamine and Tricyclic Antidepressants," *Archives of General Psychiatry*, 26 (1972):246–251.

86. FLOR-HENRY, P. "Lateralized Temporallimbic Dysfunctions and Psychopathology," *Annals of the New York Academy of Science*, 280 (1976):777–795.

87. ———. "On Certain Aspects of the Localization of the Cerebral Systems Regulating and Determining Emotion," *Biological Psychiatry*, 14 (1979):677–698.

88. ———. "Hemispheric Laterality and Disorders of Affect," in R. M. Post and J. C. Ballenger, eds., *Neurobiology of Mood Disorders.* Baltimore: Williams & Wilkins, 1984, pp. 467–480.

89. FLOR-HENRY, P., and KOLES, Z. J. "EEG Studies in Depression, Mania and Normals: Evidence for Partial Shifts of Laterality in the Affective Psychoses," *Advances in Biological Psychiatry*, 4 (1980):21–43.

90. FOLSTEIN, M. F., MAIBERGER, R., and MCHUGH, P. R. "Mood Disorder as a Specific Complication of Stroke," *Journal of Neurology, Neurosurgery and Psychiatry*, 40 (1977):1018–1020.

91. FREEDMAN, L. S., et al. "Changes in Serum Dopamine-β-hydroxylase with Age," *Nature*, 236 (1972):310–311.

92. FRIEDL, W., KRUGER, J., and PROPPING, P. "Intraindividual Stability and Extent of Genetic Determination of Platelet

Monoamine Oxidase Activity," *Pharmacopsychiatry*, 14 (1981):82–86.

93. FUXE, K., BUTCHER, L. L., and ENGEL, J. "DL-5-Hydroxytryptophan-induced Changes in Central Monoamine Neurons After Peripheral Decarboxylase Inhibition," *Journal of Pharmacy and Pharmacology*, 23 (1971):420–424.

94. GAINOTTI, G. "Emotional Behavior and Hemispheric Side of the Lesion," *Cortex*, 8 (1972):41–55.

95. GARCIA-SEVILLA, J. A., et al. "Platelet α -2-Adrenergic Receptors in Major Depressive Disorder," *Archives of General Psychiatry*, 38 (1981):1327.

96. GARCIA-SEVILLA, J. A., et al. "Tricyclic Drug Treatment Decreases α-2-adrenoceptors on Human Platelet Membranes," *European Journal of Pharmacology*, 69 (1981):121–123.

97. GARFINKEL, P. E., WARSH, J. J., and STANCER, H. C. "Depression: New Evidence in Support of Biological Differentiation," *American Journal of Psychiatry*, 136 (1979):535–539.

98. GARFINKEL, P. E., et al. "CNS Monoamine Metabolism in Bipolar Affective Disorders," *Archives of General Psychiatry*, 34 (1977):35–73.

99. GASPARINI, W. G., et al. "Hemispheric Asymmetries of Affective Processing as Determined by the Minnesota Multiphasic Personality Inventory," *Journal of Neurology, Neurosurgery and Psychiatry*, 41 (1978):470–473.

100. GELENBERG, A. J., et al. "Tyrosine for the Treatment of Depression," *American Journal of Psychiatry*, 137 (1980):622–623.

101. GELENBERG, A. J., et al. "Tyrosine for Depression," *Journal of Psychiatric Research*, 17 (1983):175–180.

102. GERNER, R. H., and HARE, T. A. "CSF GABA in Normals, Depression, Schizophrenia, Mania, and Anorexia Nervosa," *American Journal of Psychiatry*, 138 (1981):1098–1101.

103. GERNER, R. H., and SHARP, B., "CSF β -Endorphin Immunoreactivity in Normal, Schizophrenic, Depressed, Manic and Anorexic Subjects," *Brain Research*, 237 (1982):244–247.

104. GERNER, R. H., and WILKINS, J. N. "Elevated CSF Cortisol in Depression,

Mania, and Anorexia Nervosa Compared to Normals," *American Journal of Psychiatry,* 140 (1983):92–94.

105. GERNER, R. H., and YAMADA, T. "Altered Neuropeptide Concentrations in Cerebrospinal Fluid of Psychiatric Patients," *Brain Research,* 238 (1982):298–302.

106. GERNER, R. H., POST, R. M., and BUNNEY, W. E., Jr. "A Dopaminergic Mechanism in Mania," *American Journal of Psychiatry,* 133 (1976):1177–1180.

107. GERNER, R. H., et al. "Biological and Behavioral Effects of One Night's Sleep Deprivation in Depressed Patients and Normals," *Journal of Psychiatry Research,* 15 (1979):21–40.

108. GERNER, R. H., et al. "Beta-endorphin: Intravenous Infusion Causes Behavioral Changes in Psychiatric Patients," *Archives of General Psychiatry,* 37 (1980):642–647.

109. GERNER, R. H., et al. "Cerebrospinal Fluid Neurochemistry in Depressed, Manic, and Schizophrenic Patients Compared to Normal Controls," *American Journal of Psychiatry,* 141 (1984):1533–1547.

110. GERSHON, E. S. "The Search for Genetic Markers in Affective Disorders," in M. A. Lipton, A. DiMascio, and K. F. Killam, eds., *Psychopharmacology: A Generation of Progress.* New York: Raven Press, 1978, pp. 1197–1212.

111. GERSHON, E. S., "The Genetics of Affective Disorders," in L. Grinspoon, ed., *Psychiatry Update,* vol. 2. Washington, D.C.: American Psychiatry Press, 1983, pp. 434–457.

112. GERSHON, E. S., and JONAS, W. Z. "Erythrocyte Soluble Catechol-O-methyltransferase Activity in Primary Affective Disorder," *Archives of General Psychiatry,* 32 (1975):1351–1356.

113. GERSHON, E. S., TARGUM, S. D., and LECKMAN, J. F. "Platelet Monoamine Oxidase (MAO) Activity and Genetic Vulnerability to Bipolar (BP) Affective Illness," *Psychopharmacology Bulletin,* 15 (1979):27–30.

114. GERSHON, E. S., et al. "Genetic Studies and Biologic Strategies in the Affective Disorders," in A. G. Steinberg, ed., *Progress in Medical Genetics,* vol. 2.

Philadelphia: W. B. Saunders Co., 1977, pp. 101–164.

115. GERSHON, S., and SHAW, F. H. "Psychiatric Sequelae of Chronic Exposure to Organophosphorus Insecticides," *Lancet,* 1 (1961):1371–1374.

116. GISSELMANN, A., MARIN, A., and SIMON, P. "Etude Pilot des Effets d'un Antiparkinsonian Anticholinergique au Cours d'Etats Depressifs," *Encephale,* 1 (1975):363–366.

117. GOLD, B. I., et al. "GABA Levels in CSF of Patients with Psychiatric Disorders," *American Journal of Psychiatry,* 137 (1980):362–364.

118. GOLD, P. W., et al. "Vasopressin in Affective Illness: Direct Measurement, Clinical Trials, and Response to Hypertonic Saline," in R. M. Post and J. C. Ballenger, eds., *Neurobiology of Mood Disorders.* Baltimore: Williams & Wilkins, 1984, pp. 323–339.

119. GOLDSTEIN, M., et al. "Studies on Dopamine-β-hydroxylase in Mental Disorders," *Journal of Psychiatric Research,* 11 (1974):205–210.

120. GOODWIN, F. K., and Post, R. M. "Studies of Amine Metabolites in Affective Illness and Schizophrenia: A Comparative Analysis," in D. X. Freedman, ed., *Biology of the Major Psychoses.* New York: Raven Press, 1975, pp. 299–332.

121. GOODWIN, F. K., and POTTER, W. Z. "Norepinephrine Metabolite Studies in Affective Illness," in E. Usdin, I. Kopin, and J. Barchas, eds., *Catecholamines: Basic and Clinical Frontiers,* vol. 2. New York: Pergamon Press, 1973, pp. 1863–1965.

122. GOWER, A. J., and MARRIOTT, A. S. "The Inhibition of Clonidine-Induced Sedation in the Mouse by Antidepressant Drugs," *British Journal of Pharmacology,* 69 (1980):287.

123. GREENSPAN, K., et al. "Catecholamine Metabolism in Affective Disorders. III. MHPG and Other Catecholamine Metabolites in Patients Treated with Lithium Carbonate," *Journal of Psychiatry Research,* 7 (1970):171–183.

124. GREVART, P., and GOLDSTEIN, A. "Endorphins: Naloxone Fails to Alter Experimental Pain or Mood in Humans," *Science,* 199 (1978):1093–1095.

125. HAIER, R. J., et al. "Psychiatric Vulnerability, Monoamine Oxidase, and the Average Evoked Potential," *Archives of General Psychiatry*, 37 (1980):340–345.

126. HALBREICH, U., et al. "Growth Hormone Response to Dextroamphetamine in Depressed Patients and Normal Subjects," *Archives of General Psychiatry*, 39 (1982):189–192.

127. HILLHOUSE, E. W., BURDEN, J., and JONES, M. T. "The Effect of Various Putative Neurotransmitters on the Release of Corticotropin Releasing Hormone from the Hypothalamus of the Rat in Vitro. I. The Effect of Acetylcholine and Noradrenaline," *Neuroendocrinology*, 17 (1975):1–11.

128. HOEHN-SARIC, R., and MASEK, B. J. "Effects of Naloxone on Normals and Chronically Anxious Patients," *Biological Psychiatry*, 16 (1981):1041–1050.

129. HOLLISTER, L. E., and OVERALL, J. E. "Reflections on the Specificity of Action of Antidepressants," *Psychosomatics*, 6 (1965):361–365.

130. HOLLISTER, L. E., et al. "Drug Therapy of Depression. Amitriptyline, Perphenazine, and Their Combinations in Different Syndromes," *Archives of General Psychiatry*, 17 (1967):486–493.

131. HOMMES, O. R., and PANHUYSSEN, L.H.H.M. "Bilateral Intracarotid Amytal Injection," *Psychiatry, Neurology and Neurosurgery*, 73 (1970):447–459.

132. HONECKER, H., et al. "Serum DBH and Platelet MAO in Patients with Depressive Disorders," *Pharmacopsychiatry*, 14 (1981):10–14.

133. HORWITZ, D., et al. "Human Serum Dopamine-β-hydroxylase: Relationship to Hypertension and Sympathetic Activity," *Circulatory Research*, 32 (1973):594–599.

134. HRDINA, P. D. "^{3}-H-imipramine Binding Sites in Brain Down-Regulated by Chronic Nortiptyline and Haloperidol but Not Mianserin Treatment," *Psychiatry Research*, 11 (1984):271–278.

135. HRDINA, P. D., et al. "Regulation of [^{3}-H] Imipramine Binding Sites in Rat Brain Regions: Effect of Neonatal 5, 7-Dihydroxytryptamine Treatment," *European Journal of Pharmacology*, 83 (1982):343–344.

136. JAKUPCEVIC, M., LACKOVIC, Z., and STEFOSKI, D. "Nonhomogenous Distribution of 5-Hydroxyindoleacetic Acid and Homovanillic Acid in the Lumbar Cerebrospinal Fluid of Man," *Journal of Neurological Science*, 31 (1977):165–171.

137. JANOWSKY, D. S., et al. "A Cholinergic-adrenergic Hypothesis of Mania and Depression," *Lancet*, 2 (1972):6732–6735.

138. JANOWSKY, D. S., et al. "Acetylcholine and Depression," *Psychosomatic Medicine*, 35 (1973):459.

139. JANOWSKY, D. S., et al. "Parasympathetic Suppression of Manic Symptoms by Physostigmine," *Archives of General Psychiatry*, 28 (1973):542–547.

140. JIMERSON, D. C., et al. "Central Noradrenergic Function in Man: Vanillylmandelic Acid in CSF," *Brain Research*, 99 (1975):434–439.

141. JONES, M., HILLHOUSE, E., and BURDEN, J. "The Secretion of Corticotropin-releasing Hormone in Vitro," in L. Martini and W. F. Ganong, eds., *Frontiers of Neuroendocrinology*, vol. 4. New York: Raven Press, 1969, pp. 195–226.

142. JONES, R. T., and HERNING, R. "Naloxone-induced Mood and Physiologic Changes in Normal Volunteers," in E. Usdin, W. E. Bunney, Jr., and N. S. Kline, eds., *Endorphins in Mental Health Research*. New York: Oxford University Press, 1979, pp. 484–491.

143. KAFKA, M. S., et al. "Alpha-adrenergic Receptor Function in Schizophrenia, Affective Disorder and Some Neurological Diseases," *Communications in Psychopharmacology*, 4 (1980):477.

144. KASA, K., et al. "CSF GABA and HVA in Depressive Disorders," *Biological Psychiatry*, 17 (1982):877–883.

145. KLAIBER, E. L., et al. "Effects of Estrogen Therapy on Plasma MAO Activity and EEG Driving Response of Depressed Women," *American Journal of Psychiatry*, 128 (1972):1492–1498.

146. KLINE, N. S., and SHAW, B. K. "Comparable Therapeutic Efficacy of Tryptophan and Imipramine: Average Therapeutic Ratings Versus 'True' Prevalence: An Important Difference," *Current Therapeutic Research*, 15 (1973):484–487.

147. KNIGHTS, A., and HIRSCH, S. "Revealed

Depression and Drug Treatment for Schizophrenia," *Archives of General Psychiatry*, 38 (1981):806–811.

148. KOSLOW, S. H., et al. "CSF and Urinary Biogenic Amines and Metabolites in Depression and Mania," *Archives of General Psychiatry*, 40 (1983):999–1010.

149. KRAEMER, G. W., and MCKINNEY, W. T. "Interaction of Pharmacological Agents Which Alter Biogenic Amine Metabolism and Depression: An Analysis of Contributing Factors Within a Primate Model of Depression," *Journal of Affective Disorders*, 1 (1979):33–54.

150. LANDOWSKI, J., LYSIAK, W., and ANGIELSKI, S. "Monoamine Oxidase Activity in Blood Platelets from Patients with Cyclophrenic Depressive Syndromes," *Biochemical Medicine*, 14 (1975):347–354.

151. LANGER, S. Z., and BRILEY, M. "High Affinity [3H] Imipramine Binding: A New Biological Tool for Studies in Depression," *Trends in Neuroscience*, 4 (1981):28–31.

152. LANGER, S. Z., and RAISMAN, R. "Binding of 3H-imipramine and 3H-desipramine as Biochemical Tools for Studies in Depression," *Neuropharmacology*, 22 (1983):407–413.

153. LANGER, S. Z., et al. "High Affinity 3H-imipramine Binding in Rat Hypothalamus: Association with Uptake of Serotonin but Not of Norepinephrine," *Science*, 210 (1980):1133–1135.

154. LECKMAN, J. F., MAAS, J. W., and HENINGER, G. R. "Covariance of Plasma Free 3-Methoxy-4-hydroxyphenethylene Glycol and Diastolic Blood Pressure," *European Journal of Pharmacology*, 70 (1981):111–120.

155. LERNER, P., et al. "Dopamine-β-hydroxylase in the Cerebrospinal Fluid of Psychiatric Patients," *Biological Psychiatry*, 13 (1978):685–694.

156. LEVITT, M., et al. "Serum Dopamine-β-hydroxylase Activity in Affective Psychoses and Schizophrenia," *Archives of General Psychiatry*, 33 (1976):585–591.

157. LEWIS, J. L., and WINOKUR, G. "The Induction of Mania: A Natural History Study with Controls," *Archives of General Psychiatry*, 39 (1982):303–306.

158. LEWITT, M., and MENDLEWICZ, J. "A Genetic Study of Plasma Dopamine-β-

hydroxylase in Affective Disorder. Genetic and Pharmacopsychiatry," *Modern Problems in Pharmacopsychiatry*, 10 (1975):89–98.

159. LEWY, A. J. "Human Melatonin Secretion (II): A Marker for the Circadian System and the Effect of Light," in R. M. Post and J. C. Ballenger, eds., *Neurobiology of Mood Disorders*. Baltimore: Williams & Wilkins, 1984, pp. 215–226.

160. LEWY, A. J., et al. "Bright Artificial Light Treatment of a Manic-depressive Patient with a Seasonal Mood Cycle," *American Journal of Psychiatry*, 139 (1982):1496–1498.

161. LIEBOWITZ, M. R., and KLEIN, D. F. "Hysteroid Dysphoria," in H. S. Akiskal, ed., *Affective Disorders: Special Clinical Forms. Psychiatric Clinics of North America*. Philadelphia: W. B. Saunders, 1979, pp. 555–576.

162. LIPPER, S., et al. "Comparative Behavioral Effects of Clorgyline and Pargyline in Man: A Preliminary Evaluation," *Psychopharmacology*, 62 (1979):123–127.

163. LLOYD, K. G., et al. "Serotonin and 5-Hydroxy-indoleacetic Acid in Discrete Areas of the Brainstems of Suicide Victims and Control Patients," *Advanced Biochemical Psychopharmacology*, 11 (1974):387–397.

164. LOSCHER, W., and FREY, W. H. "Effect of Convulsant and Anticonvulsant Agents on Level and Metabolism of GABA in Mouse Brain," *Naunyn-Schmiedebergs Archives of Pharmacology*, 296 (1977):263–267.

165. MAAS, J. W. "Biogenic Amines and Depression: Biochemical and Pharmacological Separation of Two Types of Depression," *Archives of General Psychiatry*, 32 (1975):1357–1361.

166. ———. "Clinical and Biochemical Heterogeneity of Depressive Disorders," *Annual International Medicine*, 88 (1978):556–563.

167. ———. "Neurotransmitters and Depression. Too Much, Too Little, or Too Unstable," *Trends in Neuroscience*, 2 (1979):306–310.

168. MAAS, J. W., DEKIRMENJIAN, H., and DELEON-JONES, F. "The Identification of Depressed Patients Who Have Disorders of Norepinephrine Metabolism

and Disposition," in E. Usdin and S. Snyder, eds., *Frontiers in Catecholamine Research.* New York: Pergamon Press, 1973, pp. 1091–1096.

169. MAAS, J. W., FAWCETT, J. A., and DEKIRMENJIAN, H. "Catecholamine Metabolism, Depressive Illness and Drug Response," *Archives of General Psychiatry,* 26 (1972):252–260.

170. MAAS, J. W., et al. "3-Methoxy-4-hydroxyphenethyleneglycol Production by Human Brain in Vivo," *Science,* 205 (1979):1025–1027.

171. MAAS, J., et al. "Neurotransmitter Metabolites and the Therapeutic Response to Antidepressant Drugs," Paper presented at the 12th Congress of the College of Internationale Neuropsychopharmacologicum, Goteborg, Sweden, June 22–26, 1980.

172. MCLEOD, W., and MCLEOD, M. "Indoleamines and the Cerebrospinal Fluid," in B. M. Davies, B. J. Carroll, and R. M. Mowbray, eds., *Depressive Illness: Some Research Studies.* Springfield, Ill.: Charles C Thomas, 1972, pp. 209–225.

173. MCMANUS, I. C. "Bimodality of 5-HIAA Concentrations in the CSF of Depressed Patients: A Statistical Re-analysis," *British Journal of Psychiatry,* in press.

174. MCMILLEN, B. A., WARNACK, W., and GERMAN, D. C. "Effects of Chronic Desipramine Treatment on Rat Brain Noradrenergic Responses to α-adrenergic Drugs," *European Journal of Pharmacology,* 61 (1980):239–246.

175. MACSWEENEY, D. A., "Treatment of Unipolar Depression (letter)," *Lancet,* 2 (1975):510–511.

176. MAGGI, A., and ENNA, S. J. "Regional Alterations in Rat Brain Neurotransmitter Systems Following Chronic Lithium Treatment," *Journal of Neurochemistry,* 34 (1980):888–892.

177. MAITRE, L., et al. "Maprotiline—Its Position as an Antidepressant in the Light of Recent Neuropharmacological and Neurobiochemical Findings," *Journal of International Medical Research,* 3 (Supplement 2) (1975):2–15.

178. MANDELL, A. J., and KNAPP, S. "Asymmetry and Mood, Emergent Properties of Serotonin Regulation," *Archives of General Psychiatry,* 36 (1979):909–916.

179. MANN, J. J., and STANLEY, M. "Postmortem Monoamine Oxidase Enzyme Kinetics in the Frontal Cortex of Suicide Victims and Controls," *Acta Psychiatrica Scandinavica,* 69 (1984):135–139.

180. MAO, C. C., et al. "Antipsychotics and GABA Turnover in Mammalian Brain Nuclei," in S. Garattini, J. F. Pujol, and R. Samanin, eds., *Interactions Between Putative Neurotransmitters in the Brain.* New York: Raven Press, 1978, pp. 151–160.

181. MARTIN, J. B. "Neural Regulation of Growth Hormone Secretion," *New England Journal of Medicine,* 288 (1973):-1384–1393.

182. MATTSON, B., et al. "Catechol-O-methyltransferase and Plasma Monoamine Oxidase in Patients with Affective Disorders," *Acta Psychiatrica Scandinavica,* 255 (Supplement) (1974):187–197.

183. MAUBACH, M., et al. "Platelet MAO Activity in Patients with Affective Psychosis and Their First-degree Relatives," *Pharmacopsychiatry,* 14 (1981):87–93.

184. MAYEUX, R., et al. "Depression, Intellectual Impairment, and Parkinson Disease," *Neurology,* 31 (1981):645–650.

185. MELLERUP, E. T., PLENGE, P., and ROSENBERG, R. "^{3}-H-Imipramine Binding Sites in Platelets from Psychiatric Patients," *Psychiatry Research,* 7 (1982):-221–227.

186. MELTZER, H. Y., and ARORA, R. C. "Skeletal Muscle MAO Activity in the Major Psychoses," *Archives of General Psychiatry,* 37 (1980):333–339.

187. MELTZER, H. Y., et al. "Serum Dopamine-β-hydroxylase Activity in the Affective Psychoses and Schizophrenia," *Archives of General Psychiatry,* 33 (1976):585–591.

188. MENDLEWICZ, J., LEVITT, M., and PLEISS, J. L. "A Genetic Study of Plasma Dopamine-β-hydroxylase Activity in Man," *Acta Genetica Medicale Gemmellol* (Rome), 24 (1975):105–110.

189. MIECH, P. J., DAUSEE, J. P., and MEYER, P. "Direct Biochemical Demonstration of Two Types of Alpha-adrenoreceptor in Rat Brain," *Nature,* 274 (1978):492–494.

190. MILLER, W. R., and SELIGMAN, M.E.P.

"Depression and Learned Helplessness in Man," *Journal of Abnormal Psychology*, 84 (1975):228–238.

191. MODESTIN, J. J., HUNGER, J., and SCHWARTZ, R. B. "Uber Die Depressogene Wirkung von Physostigmim," *Archivfuer Psychiatrie und Nervenkrankheiten*, 218 (1973):67.

192. MODESTIN, J. J., SCHWARTZ, R. B., and HUNGER, J. "Zur Frage der Beeinflussung Schizophrener Symptom Physostigmin," *Pharmakopsychiatrie*, 9 (1973):300–304.

193. MOGILNICKA, E., and PILC, A. "Rapid-eye-movement Sleep Deprivation Inhibits Clonidine-induced Sedation in Rats," *European Journal of Pharmacology*, 71 (1981):123–126.

194. MOLLER, H. J., and VON ZERSSEN, D. "Depressive Symptomatik in Stationaren Behandlungsverlauf von 280 Schizophrenen Patienten," *Pharmacopsychiatria*, 14 (1981):172–179.

195. MORSELLI, P. L., et al. "On the Therapeutic Action of SL 76 002, a New GABA-mimetic Agent," *Brain Research Bulletin*, 5 (Supplement 2) (1980):411–415.

196. MURPHY, D. L. "The Behavioral Toxicity of Monoamine Oxidase Inhibiting Antidepressants," *Advances in Pharmacology and Chemotherapy*, 81 (1976):178–202.

197. MURPHY, D. L. "Clinical, Genetic, Hormonal and Drug Influences on the Activity of Human Platelet Monoamine Oxidase," in G.E.W. Wolstenholme and J. Knight, eds., *Monoamine Oxidase and Its Inhibition*. Amsterdam: Elsevier (Ciba Foundation Symposium 39), 1976, pp. 341–351.

198. MURPHY, D. L., and BUCHSBAUM, M. D. "Neurotransmitter-related Enzymes and Psychiatric Diagnostic Entities," in R. L. Spitzer and D. F. Klein, eds., *Critical Issues in Psychiatric Diagnosis*. New York: Raven Press, 1978, pp. 305–321.

199. MURPHY, D. L., and WEISS, R. "Reduced Monoamine Oxidase Activity in Blood Platelets from Bipolar Depressed Patients," *American Journal of Psychiatry*, 128 (1972):1351–1357.

200. MURPHY, D. L., BELMAKER, R., and WYATT, R. J. "Monoamine Oxidase in Schizophrenia and Other Behavioral Disorders," *Journal of Psychiatry Research*, 11 (1974):221–247.

201. MURPHY, D. L., CAMPBELL, I., and COSTA, J. L. "Current Status of the Indoleamine Hypothesis of the Affective Disorders," in M. A. Lipton, A. DiMascio, and K. F. Killam, eds., *Psychopharmacology: A Generation of Progress*. New York: Raven Press, 1978, pp. 1235–1247.

202. MURPHY, D. L., et al. "L-DOPA: Regular Induction of Hypomania in 'Bipolar' Manic-Depressive Patients," *Nature*, 229 (1971):135–136.

203. MURPHY, D. L., et al. "Platelet and Plasma Monoamine Oxidase Activity in 680 Normals: Sex and Age Differences and Stability Over Time," *Biochemistry Medicine*, 16 (1976):254–265.

204. MURPHY, D. L., et al. "Selectivity of Clorgyline and Pargyline as Inhibitors of Monoamine Oxidases A and B in Vivo in Man," *Psychopharmacology*, 62 (1979):129–132.

205. NADI, N. S., NURNBERGER, J. I., and GERSHON, E. S. "Muscarinic Cholinergic Receptors on Skin Fibroblasts in Familial Affective Disorder," *New England Journal of Medicine*, 311 (1984):225–230.

206. NAIR, M. C., and RAO, B.S.S.R. "Tryptophan Metabolites in Cerebrospinal Fluid and Urine of Patients with Affective Disorders," *Indian Journal of Medical Research*, 75 (1982):274–276.

207. NIES, A., et al. "Amines and Monoamine Oxidase in Relation to Aging and Depression in Man," *Psychosomatic Medicine*, 33 (1971):470.

208. NIES, A., et al. "Genetic Control of Platelet and Plasma Monoamine Oxidase Activity," *Archives of General Psychiatry*, 28 (1973):834–838.

209. NIES, A., et al. "Comparison of Monoamine Oxidase Substrate Activities in Twins, Schizophrenics, Depressives and Controls," in E. Usdin, ed., *Neuropsychopharmacology of Monoamines and Their Regulatory Enzymes: Advances in Biochemistry Psychopharmacology*, vol. 12. New York: Raven Press, 1974, pp. 59–79.

210. NIHAN, P. I., et al. "CSF 5-Hydroxyindoleacetic Acid Levels in Suicidal Schiz-

ophrenic Patients," *American Journal of Psychiatry*, 141 (1983):566–579.

211. NORDIN, C., SIWERS, B., and BERTILSSON, L., "Bromocriptine Treatment of Depressive Disorders: Clinical and Biochemical Effects," *Acta Psychiatrica Scandinavica*, 64 (1981):25–33.

212. OGIHARA, T., et al. "Serum Dopamine-β-hydroxylase Activity in Parents and Children," *Journal of Laboratory and Clinical Medicine*, 85 (1975):566–573.

213. OPPENHEIM, G. "Propranolol-induced Depression: Mechanism and Management," *Australian and New Zealand Journal of Psychiatry*, 17 (1983):400–402.

214. OPPENHEIMER, G., EBSTEIN, R., and BELMAKER, R. "Effects of Lithium on the Physostigmine-induced Behavioral Syndrome and Plasma Cyclic GMP," *Journal of Psychiatry Research*, 14 (1979):133–138.

215. ORELAND, L., et al. "Platelet MAO Activity and Monoamine Metabolites in Cerebrospinal Fluid in Depressed and Suicidal Patients and in Healthy Controls," *Psychiatry Research*, 4 (1981):21–29.

216. ORSULAK, P. J., et al. "Differences in Platelet Monoamine Oxidase Activity in Subgroups of Schizophrenic and Depressive Disorders," *Biological Psychiatry*, 13 (1978):637–647.

217. OSTROW, D., et al. "State Dependence of Noradrenergic Activity in a Rapid Cycling Bipolar Patient," *Journal of Clinical Psychiatry*, 45 (1984):306–309.

218. OVERALL, J. E., et al., "Nosology of Depression and Differential Response to Drugs," *Journal of the American Medical Association*, 195 (1966):946–948.

219. PAPESCHI, R., and MCCLURE, D. J. "Homovanillic Acid and 5-Hydroxyindoleacetic Acid in Cerebrospinal Fluid of Depressed Patients," *Archives of General Psychiatry*, 25 (1971):354–358.

220. PAUL, S. M., et al. "Depressed Patients Have Decreased Binding of Tritiated Imipramine to Platelet Serotonin 'Transporter,'" *Archives of General Psychiatry*, 38 (1981):1315–1317.

221. PAUL, S. M., et al. "Does High Affinity ^{3}H-Imipramine Binding Label Serotonin Reuptake Sites in Brain and Platelet?" *Life Science*, 28 (1981):2753–2760.

222. PAUL, S. M., et al. "High Affinity Binding of Antidepressants to Biogenic Amine Transport Sites in Human Brain and Platelet: Studies in Depression," in R. M. Post and J. C. Ballenger, eds., *Neurobiology of Mood Disorders*. Baltimore: Williams & Wilkins, 1984, pp. 846–853.

223. PERT, C., and SNYDER, S. "Opiate Receptor: Demonstration in Nervous Tissue," *Science*, 179 (1973):1011–1014.

224. PICKAR, D., et al. "Selective and Nonselective Monoamine Oxidase Inhibitors," *Archives of General Psychiatry*, 39 (1982):535–540.

225. PICKAR, D., et al. "Short-term Naloxone Administration in Schizophrenic and Manic Patients: A Project of the Biological Psychiatry Collaborative Program of the World Health Organization," *Archives of General Psychiatry*, 39 (1982):313–323.

226. PIMOULE, C., et al. "^{3}H-Rauwolscine Binding in Platelets from Depressed Patients and Healthy Volunteers," *Psychopharmacology*, 79 (1983):308.

227. POST, R. M., BALLENGER, J. C., and GOODWIN, F. K. "Cerebrospinal Fluid Studies of Neurotransmitter Function in Manic and Depressive Illness," in J. H. Wood, ed., *Neurobiology of Cerebrospinal Fluid I*. New York: Plenum Press, 1980, pp. 685–718.

228. POST, R. M., et al. "Cerebrospinal Fluid Norepinephrine in Affective Illness," *American Journal of Psychiatry*, 135 (1976):907–912.

229. POST, R. M., et al. "Effects of a Dopamine Agonist Piribedil in Depressed Patients," *Archives of General Psychiatry*, 35 (1978):609–615.

230. POST, R. M., et al. "CSF GABA in Normals and Patients with Affective Disorder," *Brain Research Bulletin*, 5 (Supplement 2) (1980):755–759.

231. POST, R. M., et al. "Dopamine and Mania: Behavioral and Biochemical Effects of the DA Receptor Blocker Pimozide," *Psychopharmacology*, 67 (1980):297–305.

232. POST, R. M., et al. "Dopaminergic Mechanisms in Affective Illness," in B. Angrist, et al., eds., *Recent Advances in Neuropsycho-Pharmacology*, vol. 31.

New York: Pergamon Press, 1981, pp. 55–61.

233. POST, R. M., et al. "Efficacy of Carbamazepine in Manic-Depressive Illness: Implications for Underlying Mechanisms," in R. M. Post and J. C. Ballenger, eds., *Neurobiology of Mood Disorders.* Baltimore: Williams & Wilkins, 1984, pp. 777–816.

234. POST, R. M., et al. "Endogenous Opiates in Cerebrospinal Fluid: Relationship to Mood and Anxiety," in R. M. Post and J. C. Ballenger, eds., *Neurobiology of Mood Disorders.* Baltimore: Williams & Wilkins, 1984, pp. 356–368.

235. PRANGE, A. J., JR., et al. "L-tryptophan in Mania: Contribution to a Permissive Hypothesis of Affective Disorders," *Archives of General Psychiatry,* 30 (1974):- 56–62.

236. PUIG-ANTICH, J., et al. "Growth Hormone Secretion in Prepubertal Children with Major Depression," *Archives of General Psychiatry,* 41 (1984):455–460.

237. PUZYNSKI, S., HAUPTMANN, M., and ZALUSKA, M. "Studies on Biogenic Amine Metabolizing Enzymes (DBH, COMT, MAO) and Pathogenesis of Affective Illness. II," *Acta Psychiatrica Scandinavica,* 67 (1983):101–108.

238. PUZYNSKI, S., RODE, A., and ZALUSKA, M., "Studies on Biogenic Amine Metabolizing Enzymes (DBH, COMT, MAO) and Pathogenesis of Affective Illness. I," *Acta Psychiatrica Scandinavica,* 67 (1983):89–95.

239. PUZYNSKI, S., et al. "Studies on Biogenic Amine Metabolizing Enzymes (DBH, COMT, MAO) and Pathogenesis of Affective Illness. III," *Acta Psychiatrica Scandinavica,* 67 (1983):96–100.

240. RAISMAN, R., et al. "High-affinity ^{3}H-imipramine Binding in Platelets from Untreated and Treated Depressed Patients Compared to Healthy Volunteers," *Psychopharmacology,* 75 (1981): 368–371.

241. RASKIN, A., and CROOK, T. H. "The Endogenous-neurotic Distinction as a Predictor of Response to Antidepressant Drugs," *Psychological Medicine,* 6 (1976):59–70.

242. REUS, V. I., BUCHSBAUM, M. S., and POST, R. M. "D-Amphetamine: Differential

Effects on Right and Left Hemispheres," in J. J. Gruzelier and P. Flor-Henry, eds., *Hemisphere Asymmetries of Function in Psychopathology.* New York: Elsevier/North Holland, 1979, pp. 329–338.

243. RISCH, S. C., and JANOWSKY, D. S. "Cholinergic-Adrenergic Balance in Affective Illness," in R. M. Post and J. C. Ballenger, eds., *Neurobiology of Mood Disorders.* Baltimore: Williams & Wilkins, 1984, pp. 652–663.

244. RISCH, S. C., KALIN, H. J., and JANOWSKY, D. S. "Cholinergic Challenges in Affective Illness: Behavioral and Neuroendocrine Correlates," *Journal of Clinical Psychopharmacology,* 1 (1981): 186–192.

245. RISCH, S. C., et al. "Physostigmine Induction of Depressive Symptomatology in Normal Volunteer Subjects," *Journal of Psychiatric Research,* 4 (1981):89–94.

246. ROBERTS, E., CHASE, T. N., and TOWER, D. B., eds. *GABA in Nervous System Function.* New York: Raven Press, 1976.

247. ROBERTSON, M. M., and TRIMBLE, M. R. "Major Tranquilizers Used as Antidepressants: A Review," *Journal of Affective Disorders,* 4 (1982):173–193.

248. ROBINSON, D. S., et al. "Relation of Sex and Aging to Monoamine Oxidase Activity of Human Brain, Plasma, and Platelets," *Archives of General Psychiatry,* 24 (1971):536–539.

249. ROEMER, R. A., et al. "Pattern Evoked Potential Measurements Suggesting Lateralized Hemispheric Dysfunction in Chronic Schizophrenics," *Biological Psychiatry,* 13 (1978):185–202.

250. ROSENBAUM, A. H., et al. "MHPG as a Predictor of Antidepressant Response to Imipramine and Maprotiline," *American Journal of Psychiatry,* 137 (1980):- 1090–1092.

251. ROSENTHAL, N. E., et al. "Seasonal Affective Disorder," *Archives of General Psychiatry,* 41 (1984):72–80.

252. ROSS, S. B., WETTERBERG, L., and MYRHED, M. "Genetic Control of Plasma Dopamine-β-hydroxylase," *Life Science,* 12 (1973):529–532.

253. ROY, A. "Do Neuroleptics Cause Depression?" *Biological Psychiatry,* 19 (1984):- 777–781.

254. RUBINOW, D. R., et al. "Somatostatin in

Patients with Affective Illness and in Normal Volunteers," in R. M. Post and J. C. Ballenger, eds., *Neurobiology of Mood Disorders.* Baltimore: Williams & Wilkins, 1984, pp. 369–387.

255. RUDOLPH, C. D., KAPLAN, S. L., and GANONG, W. F. "Sites at Which Clonidine Acts to Affect Blood Pressure and the Secretion of Renin, Growth Hormone, and ACTH," *Neuroendocrinology,* 31 (1980):121–128.

256. RYDIN, E., SHALLING, D., and ASBERG, M. "Rorschach Ratings in Depressed and Suicidal Patients with Low Levels of 5-Hydroxyindole Acetic Acid in Cerebrospinal Fluid," *Psychiatry Research,* 7 (1982):229–243.

257. SACHAR, E. J., et al. "Disrupted 24-Hour Patterns of Cortisol Secretion in Psychotic Depression," *Archives of General Psychiatry,* 28 (1973):19–24.

258. SACK, R. L., and GOODWIN, F. K. "Inhibition of Dopamine-beta-hydroxylase in Manic Patients," *Archives of General Psychiatry,* 31 (1974):649–654.

259. SCHAFFER, C. E., DAVIDSON, R. J., and SARON, C. "Frontal and Parietal Electroencephalogram Asymmetry in Depressed and Non-Depressed Subjects," *Biological Psychiatry,* 18 (1983):753–762.

260. SCHATZBERG, A. F., et al. "Toward a Biochemical Classification of Depressive Disorders. IV. Pretreatment Urinary MHPG Levels as Predictors of Antidepressant Response to Imipramine," *Communication in Psychopharmacology,* 4 (1980–1981):441–445.

261. SCHILDKRAUT, J. J. "The Catecholamine Hypothesis of Affective Disorders: A Review of Supporting Evidence," *American Journal of Psychiatry,* 122 (1965):509–522.

262. ———. "The Current Status of the Catecholamine Hypothesis of Affective Disorders," in M. Lipton, A. DiMascio, and K. F. Killam, eds., *Psychopharmacology: A Generation of Progress.* New York: Raven Press, 1978, pp. 1223–1234.

263. SCHILDKRAUT, J. J., DODGE, G. A., and LOGUE, M. A. "Effects of Tricyclic Antidepressants on the Uptake and Metabolism of Intracisternally Administered Norepinephrine-3H in Rat Brain," *Journal of Psychiatric Research,* 7 (1969):29–34.

264. SCHILDKRAUT, J. J., et al. "Amphetamine Withdrawal: Depression and MHPG Excretion," *Lancet,* 2 (1971):485–486.

265. SCHILDKRAUT, J. J., et al. "Catecholamine Metabolism in Affective Disorders: A Longitudinal Study of a Patient Treated with Amitriptyline and ECT," *Psychosomatic Medicine,* 34 (1972):470; plus erratum *Psychosomatic Medicine,* 35 (1973):274.

266. SCHILDKRAUT, J. J., et al. "MHPG Excretion and Clinical Classification in Depressive Disorders," *Lancet,* 1 (1973):1251–1252.

267. SCHILDKRAUT, J. J., et al. "MHPG Excretion in Depressive Disorders: Relation to Clinical Subtypes and Desynchronized Sleep," *Science,* 181 (1973):762–764.

268. SCHILDKRAUT, J. J., et al. "Toward a Biochemical Classification of Depressive Disorders. I. Differences in Urinary MHPG and Other Catecholamine Metabolites in Clinically Defined Subtypes of Depressions," *Archives of General Psychiatry,* 35 (1978):1427–1433.

269. SCHILDKRAUT, J. J., et al. "Toward a Biochemical Classification of Depressive Disorders. II. Application of Multivariate Discriminant Function Analysis to Data on Urinary Catecholamines and Metabolites," *Archives of General Psychiatry,* 35 (1978):1436–1439.

270. SCHILDKRAUT, J. J., et al. "Possible Pathophysiological Mechanisms in Subtypes of Unipolar Depressive Disorders Based on Differences in Urinary MHPG Levels," *Psychopharmacology Bulletin,* 17 (1981):90–91.

271. SCHILDKRAUT, J. J., et al. "Urinary MHPG in Affective Disorders," in R. M. Post and J. C. Ballenger, eds., *Neurobiology of Mood Disorders.* Baltimore: Williams & Wilkins, 1984, pp. 519–528.

272. SCHILDKRAUT, J. J., et al. "The Role of Norepinephrine in Depressive Disorders," in E. Friedman, ed., *Depression and Antidepressants.* New York: Raven Press, forthcoming.

273. SCHON, F. E., and IVERSEN, L. L. "GABA Synapses in the Central Nervous System," *Life Science,* 15 (1974):157–166.

274. SEDVALL, G., and OXENSTIERNA, G. "Genetic and Environmental Influences on Central Monoaminergic Mechanisms in Man," in B. Jansson and C. Perris, eds., *Biological Psychiatry 1981*. Amsterdam: Elsevier/North Holland, 1981, pp. 163–171.

275. SEDVALL, G., et al. "Relationships in Healthy Volunteers Between Concentrations of Monoamine Metabolites in Cerebrospinal Fluid and Family History of Psychiatric Morbidity," *British Journal of Psychiatry*, 136 (1980):366–374.

276. SHAFFER, D., et al. "Localized Cortical Injury and Psychiatric Symptoms in Childhood," cited in M. Rutter, ed., "Psychological Sequelae of Brain Damage in Children," *American Journal of Psychiatry*, 138 (1981):1533–1544.

277. SHERMAN, A. D., and PETTY, F. "Neurochemical Basis of the Action of Antidepressants on Learned Helplessness," *Behavioral and Neural Biology*, 30 (1980):119–134.

278. SHOPSIN, B., et al. "Rebound Phenomena in Mania Patients Following Physostigmine," *Neuropsychobiology*, 1 (1975):180–187.

279. SHULMAN, R., GRIFFITHS, J., and DIEWOLD, P. "Catechol-O-methyltransferase Activity in Patients with Depressive Illness and Anxiety States," *British Journal of Psychiatry*, 132 (19789):133–138.

280. SIEVER, L. J., COHEN, R. M., and MURPHY, D. L. "Antidepressants and α-2 Adrenergic Autoreceptor Desensitization," *American Journal of Psychiatry*, 138 (1981):681–682.

281. SIEVER, L. J., UHDE, T. W., and MURPHY, D. L. "Strategies for Assessment of Noradrenergic Receptor Function in Patients with Affective Disorders," in R. M. Post and J. C. Ballenger, eds., *Neurobiology of Mood Disorders*. Baltimore: Williams & Wilkins, 1984, pp. 502–518.

282. SIEVER, L. J., et al. "Growth Hormone Response to Clonidine as a Probe of Noradrenergic Receptor Responsiveness in Affective Disorder Patients and Controls," *Psychiatry Research*, 6 (1982):171–183.

283. SIEVER, L. J., et al. "Extreme Elevations in Plasma Norepinephrine Associated with Decreased α-Adrenergic Responsivity in Major Depressive Disorder: Two Case Reports," *Journal of Clinical Psychopharmacology*, 3 (1983):39–41.

284. SIEVER, L. J., et al. "Differential Inhibitory Noradrenergic Response to Clonidine in 25 Depressed Patients and 25 Normal Control Subjects," *American Journal of Psychiatry*, 141 (1984):733–741.

285. SIEVER, L. J., et al. "Plasma Prolactin Changes Following Fenfluramine in Depressed Patients Compared to Controls: An Evaluation of Central Serotonergic Responsibility in Depression," *Life Sciences*, 34 (1984):1029–1039.

286. SIEVER, L. J., et al. "Platelet Alpha-Adrenergic Binding and Biochemical Responsiveness in Depressed Patients and Controls," *Psychiatry Research*, 11 (1984):287–302.

287. SILBERMAN, E. K., et al. "Heterogeneity of Amphetamine Response in Depressed Patients," *American Journal of Psychiatry*, 138 (1981):1302–1307.

288. SILBERMAN, E. K., et al. "Altered Lateralization of Cognitive Processes in Depressed Women," *American Journal of Psychiatry*, 140 (1983):1340–1344.

289. SITARAM, N., and GILLIN, J. C. "Development and Use of Pharmacological Probes of the CNS in Man: Evidence of Cholinergic Abnormality in Primary Affective Illness," *Biological Psychiatry*, 15 (1980):925–955.

290. SITARAM, N., MOORE, A. M., and GILLIN, J. C. "Induction and Resetting of REM Sleep Rhythm in Normal Man by Arecoline: Blockade by Scopolamine," *Sleep*, 1 (1978):83–90.

291. SITARAM, N., et al. "Faster REM Sleep Induction in Remitted Patients with Primary Affective Illness," *Science*, 208 (1980):200–202.

292. SJOSTROM, R. "5-Hydroxyindoleacetic Acid and Homovanillic Acid in Cerebrospinal Fluid in Manic-depressive Psychosis and the Effect of Probenecid Treatment," *European Journal of Clinical Pharmacology*, 6 (1973):75–80.

293. SJOSTROM, R., and ROOS, B. E. "5-Hydroxyindoleacetic Acid and Homovanillic Acid in Cerebrospinal Fluid in Manic-depressive Psychosis," *European Jour-*

nal of Clinical Pharmacology, 4 (1972):-170–176.

294. SMITH, C. B., GARCIA SEVILLA, J. A., and HOLLINGSWORTH, P. J., "α-2 Adrenoceptors in Rat Brain Are Decreased After Long-term Tricyclic Antidepressant Drug Treatment," *Brain Research*, 210 (1981):413–418.

295. SNYDER, S. H., and PEROUTKA, S. J. *Antidepressants and Neurotransmitter Receptors in Neurobiology of Mood Disorders*. Baltimore: Williams & Wilkins, 1984, pp. 686–697.

296. ———. "The Treatment of Affective Illness: Relationship to Underlying Mechanisms," in R. M. Post and J. C. Ballenger, eds., *Neurobiology of Mood Disorders*. Baltimore: Williams & Wilkins, 1984, pp. 686–697.

297. SPITZER, R. L., ENDICOTT, J., and ROBINS, E. "Research Diagnostic Criteria. Rationale and Reliability," *Archives of General Psychiatry*, 35 (1978):773–782.

298. STANLEY, M., VIRGILIO, J., and GERSHON, S. "Tritiated Imipramine Binding Sites Are Decreased in the Frontal Cortex of Suicides," *Science*, 216 (1982):1337–1339.

299. STEINBOOK, R. M., et al. "Amoxapine, Imipramine and Placebo: A Double-blind Study with Pretherapy Urinary 3-Methoxy-4-hydroxyphenylglycol Levels," *Current Therapy Research*, 26 (1979):490–496.

300. STRANDMAN, E., et al. "Serum Dopamine-beta-hydroxylase in Affective Disorders," *Neuropsychobiology*, 4 (1978): 248–255.

301. SUGRUE, M. F. "Effects of Acutely and Chronically Administered Antidepressants on the Clonidine-induced Decrease in Rat Brain 3-Methoxy-4-hydroxyphenethyleneglycol Sulphate," *Life Science*, 28 (1980):377–384.

302. SULLIVAN, J. L., DACKIS, C., and STANFIELD, C. "In Vivo Inhibition of Platelet MAO Activity by Tricyclic Antidepressants," *American Journal of Psychiatry*, 134 (1977):188–190.

303. SULLIVAN, J. L., et al. "Platelet MAO Activity Predicts Response to Lithium in Manic-depressive Illness," *Lancet*, 2 (1977):1325–1327.

304. SULSER, F. "New Perspectives on the Mode of Action of Antidepressant Drugs," *Trends in Neuroscience* 2 (1979):92–94.

305. SURANYI CADOTTE, B. E., et al. "Normalization of Platelet [3H] Imipramine Binding in Depressed Patients," *European Journal of Pharmacology*, 85 (1983):351–358.

306. SWANN, A., et al. "Catecholamine Metabolites in Human Function: Effects of Debrisoquin," *Life Science*, 27 (1980):1857–1862.

307. SWANN, A., et al. "CSF Monoamine Metabolites in Mania," *American Journal of Psychiatry*, 140 (1983):396–400.

308. SWEENEY, D., et al. "Delusional Versus Non-delusional Depression: Neurochemical Differences," *Lancet*, 2 (1978):100–101.

309. SYPRAKI, C., and FIBIGER, H. C. "Functional Evidence for Subsensitivity of Noradrenergic α-2-Receptors After Chronic Desipramine Treatment," *Life Science*, 27 (1980):1863–1867.

310. TAKAHASHI, S., et al. "CSF Monoamine Metabolites in Alcoholism: A Comparative Study with Depression," *Folia Psychiatrica et Neurologica Japanica*, 28 (1974):347–354.

311. TAMMINGA, C., et al. "Depression Associated with Oral Choline," *Lancet*, 2 (1976):905.

312. TANG, S. W., HELMESTE, D. M., and STANCER, H. C. "The Effect of Acute and Chronic Desipramine and Amitriptyline Treatment on Rat Brain Total 3-Methoxy-4-hydroxyphenylglycol," *Naunyn-Schmiedebergs Archives of Pharmacology*, 305 (1978):207–211.

313. ———. "Interaction of Antidepressants with Clonidine on Rat Brain Total 3-Methoxy-4-hydroxyphenylglycol," *Canadian Journal of Physiology and Pharmacology*, 57 (1979):435–437.

314. TAUBE, S. L., et al. "Urinary 3-Methoxy-4-hydroxyphenylglycol and Psychiatric Diagnosis," *American Journal of Psychiatry*, 135 (1978):78–82.

315. TERENIUS, L., WAHLSTROM, A., and AGREN, H. "Naloxone Treatment in Depression: Clinical Observations and Effects on CSF Endorphins and Monoamine Metabolites," *Psychopharmacology*, 54 (1977):31–33.

316. TERRY, L. C., and MARTIN, J. B. "Evidence for α-Adrenergic Regulation of Episodic Growth Hormone and Prolactin Secretion in the Undisturbed Male Rat," *Endocrinology*, 108 (1981):1869–1973.

317. TORDA, T., et al. "Mepacrine Treatment Prevents Immobilization-induced Desensitization of Beta-adrenergic Receptors in Rat Hypothalamus and Brainstem," *Brain Research*, 205 (1981):441–444.

318. TRASKMAN, L., et al. "Monoamine Metabolites in Cerebrospinal Fluid and Suicidal Behavior," *Archives of General Psychiatry*, 38 (1981):631–636.

319. U'PRICHARD, D. C., and KVETNANSKY, R. "Central and Peripheral Adrenergic Receptors in Acute and Repeated Immobilization Stress," in E. Usdin, R. Kvetnansky, and I. J. Kopin, eds., *Catecholamines and Stress: Recent Advances*. New York: Elsevier/North Holland, 1980, pp. 299–308.

320. U'PRICHARD, D. C., GREENBERG, D. A., and SNYDER, S. H. "Binding Characteristics of a Radiolabeled Agonist and Antagonist at Central Nervous System Alpha Noradrenergic Receptors," *Molecular Pharmacology*, 13 (1977):454–473.

321. VAN PRAAG, H. M., and DE HAAN, S. "Central Serotonin Metabolism and the Frequency of Depression," *Psychiatry Research*, 1 (1979):219–224.

322. ———. "Depression Vulnerability and 5-Hydroxytryptophan Prophylaxis," *Psychiatry Research*, 3 (1980):75–83.

323. VAN PRAAG, H. M., and KORF, J. "Retarded Depression and the Dopamine Metabolism," *Psychopharmacology* (Berlin), 19 (1971):199–203.

324. VAN PRAAG, H. M., KORF, J., and SCHUT, T. "Cerebral Monoamines and Depression. An Investigation with the Probenecid Technique," *Archives of General Psychiatry*, 28 (1973):827–831.

325. VAN PRAAG, H. M., et al. "Dopamine Metabolism in Depressions, Psychoses, and Parkinson's Disease: The Problem of the Specificity of Biological Variables in Behavior Disorders," *Psychological Medicine*, 5 (1975):138–146.

326. VESTERGAARD, P., SORENSEN, T., and HOPPE, E. "Biogenic Amine Metabolites in Cerebrospinal Fluid of Patients with Affective Disorders," *Acta Psychiatrica Scandinavica*, 58 (1978):88–96.

327. WAEHRENS, J., and GERLACH, J. "Bromocriptine and Imipramine in Endogenous Depression: A Double-blind Controlled Trial in Outpatients," *Journal of Affective Disorders*, 3 (1981):193–202.

328. WALDMEIER, P. C., et al. "Effects of Clomipramine and Other Tricyclic Antidepressants on Biogenic Amine Uptake and Turnover," *Postgraduate Medical Journal*, 52 (Supplement 3):33–39.

329. WATSON, R., HARTMANN, E., and SCHILDKRAUT, J. J. "Amphetamine Withdrawal: Affective State, Sleep Patterns and MHPG Excretion," *American Journal of Psychiatry*, 129 (1972):263–269.

330. WEEKE, A., and WEEKE, J. "The 24-Hour Pattern of Serum TSH in Patients with Endogenous Depression," *Acta Psychiatrica Scandinavica*, 62 (1980):69–74.

331. WEHR, T. A., and GOODWIN, F. K. "Rapid Cycling in Manic-depressives Induced by Tricyclic Antidepressants," *Archives of General Psychiatry*, 36 (1979):555–559.

332. WEHR, T. A., et al. "Circadian Rhythm Disturbances in Manic-Depressive Illness," *Federation Proceedings*, 42 (1983):2809–2814.

333. WEINSHILBOUM, R. M., and AXELROD, J., "Reduced Plasma DBH Activity in Familial Dysautonomia," *New England Journal of Medicine*, 285 (1971):938–942.

334. WEINSHILBOUM, R. M., et al. "Serum Dopamine-β-hydroxylase Activity: Sibling-sibling Correlation," *Science*, 181 (1973):943–945.

335. WETTERBERG, L., et al. "Plasma Dopamine-B-hydroxylase Activity in Hypertension and Various Neuropsychiatric Disorders," *Scandinavian Clinical Laboratory Investigations*, 30 (1972):283–289.

336. WEXLER, B. E. "Cerebral Laterality and Psychiatry: A Review of the Literature," *American Journal of Psychiatry*, 137 (1980):279–291.

337. WHITAKER, P. M., et al. "Seasonal Variations in Platelet ^{3}H-imipramine Bind-

ing: Comparable Values in Control and Depressed Populations," *Psychiatry Research*, 11 (1984):127–131.

338. WHITE, H. L., MCLEOD, M. N., and DA-VIDSON, J.R.T. "Catechol-O-methyl-transferase in Red Blood Cells of Schizo-phrenic Depressed and Normal Human Subjects," *British Journal of Psychiatry*, 128 (1976):184–187.

339. WHITE, K., et al. "Elevated Plasma Mono-amine Oxidase Activity in Patients with Non-endogenous Depression," *American Journal of Psychiatry*, 137 (1980):-1258–1259.

340. WILK, S., et al., "Cerebrospinal Fluid Lev-els of MHPG in Affective Disorders," *Nature*, 235 (1972):440–441.

341. WILLNER, P. "Dopamine and Depression. A Review of Recent Evidence I. Empir-ical Studies," *Brain Research News*, 6 (1983):211–224.

342. WINTER, H., et al. "A Twin Study of Three Enzymes (DBH, COMT, MAO) of Cate-cholamine Metabolism," *Psycho-pharmacologia*, 57 (1978):63–69.

343. WOLFE, B. B., et al. "Presynaptic Modula-tion of Beta-adrenergic Receptors in Rat Cerebral Cortex After Treatment with Antidepressants," *Journal of Phar-macology and Experimental Therapy*, 207 (1978):446–457.

344. WOOD, J. H. "Sites of Origin and Cerebro-spinal Fluid Concentration Gradients: Neurotransmitters, Their Precursors and Metabolites, and Cyclic Nucleo-tides," in H. J. Wood, ed., *Neurobiology of Cerebrospinal Fluid I*. New York: Plenum Press, 1980, pp. 53–69.

345. WURTMAN, R. J., and FERNSTROM, J. D. "Control of Brain Monoamine Synthesis by Diet and Plasma Amino Acids," *American Journal of Clinical Nutrition*, 28 (1975):638–647.

346. YOZEWITZ, A., et al., "Dichotic Percep-tion: Evidence for Right Hemisphere Dysfunction in Affective Psychosis," *British Journal of Psychiatry*, 135 (1979):224–227.

347. YU, P. H., et al. "Dopamine-β-hydroxylase and Its Apparent Endogenous Inhibi-tory Activity in the Plasma of Some Psy-chiatric Patients," *Psychiatry Research*, 3 (1980):205–210.

348. ZALUSKA, M., PUZYNSKI, S., and RODE, A. "Studies on Biogenic Amine Metaboliz-ing Enzymes (DBH, COMT, MAO) and Pathogenesis of Affective Illness. I," *Acta Psychiatrica Scandinavica*, 67 (1983):89–95.

349. ZIMMERBERG, B., GLICK, S. D., and JERUSSI, T. P. "Neurochemical Corre-late of a Spatial Preference in Rats," *Science*, 185 (1974):623.

350. ZSILLA, G., et al. "(−)-Deprenyl, a Selec-tive MAO 'B' Inhibitor, Increases [^{3}H]imipramine Binding and Decreases β-adrenergic Receptor Function," *Euro-pean Journal of Pharmacology*, 83 (1983):111–117.

CHAPTER 13

BIOLOGICAL TREATMENT OF AFFECTIVE DISORDERS

John M. Davis and Rajiv P. Sharma

¶ **Introduction**

Once clinicians reported dramatic success with tricyclic antidepressants and the monoamine oxidase inhibitors (MAOIs), these drugs were widely used throughout the world for the treatment of depression. This use preceded controlled studies to prove efficacy. Nonetheless, the most convincing evidence of efficacy comes from controlled clinical trials rather than from open studies. The term open refers to a nonblind study (open label) in which clinicians report their experience with a given number of patients treated with a new agent. Open studies of antidepressants are of limited value because depression is a self-limiting disorder. Some patients have transitory depressions that may improve in a few weeks, while others have long-lasting depressions that may last for several years. Many

We wish to gratefully acknowledge the support of the MacArthur Foundation.

depressed patients will have spontaneous remissions. For a patient with a brief depressive episode, specific treatment may not be necessary because the depression may lift in a short period of time.

We evaluated the placebo-controlled studies of antidepressant efficacy and would estimate that approximately 40 percent of the 4,000 depressed patients studied do improve, albeit to a partial degree, in three or four weeks on placebo treatment. [257,491] Many of those patients who did not improve by three to six weeks would have protracted depression lasting anywhere from six months to five years (or more). Percentage improvement figures, while helpful for understanding that some spontaneous partial improvement takes place, are not that helpful in evaluating efficacy. If a group of depressed patients with a high percentage of spontaneous remissions is studied in an open trial, an ineffective drug could falsely look good because the patients would have recovered anyway. Similarly, treatment-resistant populations may have only a modest improvement rate with a drug, but this could be a substantial increment over what would have occurred spontaneously. Placebo-controlled double-blind clinical trials are necessary for the most precise evaluation of efficacy of any new antidepressants.

The percent of patients improving on placebo reflects (1) the spontaneous recovery with a passage of three to six weeks of time, (2) improvement produced by various internal or external environmental reasons, (3) the improvement caused by the suggestive effects of receiving a placebo (dummy) tablet, (4) an improvement caused by the psychological-social therapies and other non-drug aspects of the treatment, and/or (5) rater bias, in that the rater who knows a patient is receiving a drug may falsely read into the patient's clinical picture a degree of improvement. (The most important of these reasons is the spontaneous remission rate and the evaluating clinician's bias in either wishing to see improvement or anticipating improvement.) The use of a placebo control addresses all these types of bias. The best evidence for efficacy is the demonstration that drug produces a better response than placebo.

The comparison of a new antidepressant to a standard one is a less useful design for this particular purpose. Comparisons of this sort can lead to artifactual results when there is a large error of measurement and when a treatment-resistant population is studied. If the standard drug is ineffective in a treatment-resistant population and if the new drug is also ineffective, then the new drug must equal the standard drug, because both are ineffective. In addition, assuming a large error of measurement, both drugs could prove equal to each other not because they were equally effective, but rather because there was so much error of measurement that all differences in efficacy would be obscured. Of course, if the new drug is clearly superior to a standard, these particular problems do not arise.

Once a new drug is shown to be superior to placebo, then it is useful to have some comparison to standard drugs to show that the new drug is at least as effective as the standard one. If a sample size large enough to support a three-group design (new drug, standard drug, and placebo) is available, then it is possible to demonstrate simultaneously that the new drug and the standard drug are both better than placebo and the new drug is at least equal to the standard drug. The use of placebo in the design strengthens the comparison of the new drug to the standard one because superiority over placebo means that the test system is valid. In addition, a single clinical study cannot necessarily be considered definitive. Individual studies may contradict each other. With the availability of numerous studies on a given question, how we combine the evidence from all of them to arrive at a conclusion then becomes important.

¶ Antidepressant Efficacy: Combining Evidence from Several Studies

In 1965 we summarized the data from a large sample of double-blind studies listing the number of studies in which the drug was superior to placebo, not statistically different from placebo, and inferior to placebo.[110,256] Nine years later Morris and Beck[336] reviewed our material and more recent studies and did not disagree with our results. The method used is referred to as the box score method, as it gives, for example, a tabulation of the number of studies in which a given drug is statistically superior to a standard drug (or placebo), is equal to the standard (i.e., not statistically different from the standard), or is inferior to the standard.

We feel we can now go beyond the box score method because this method is insensitive. Certainly the fact that all of a large number of well-controlled studies found the drug more effective than placebo provides a consistency of results. Problems arise when only a small number of studies have been done and when they have conflicting results. Consider several examples. Five studies, of which three find a massive and very significant drug effect and the other two show a trend in that direction but just miss the 0.05 level of significance, provide far more evidence for efficacy than five studies that are just barely statistically significant to the 0.05 level. There is a substantial difference in meaning between two studies with findings in a similar direction, such as that a new drug is better than placebo, and that just miss statistical significance versus two studies that just miss statistical significance and have findings in opposite directions. In the first case, the studies support each other, indicating a trend for drugs to be better than placebo, while in the second case, the studies do not confirm each other and, in fact, their averaged mean effect might show no difference between drug and placebo. Much information is discarded when a table summarizes a number of studies that find a drug more effective than placebo and a number of studies that find it equal to placebo, meaning, by "equal," that no statistically significant difference was found. Information that is discarded is the size effect and information about consistency of results. There is a need to combine data from different drug studies in more sophisticated ways than just listing the number of studies where the drug is better than placebo, not statistically different from placebo, and so on. Thus we believe that the box score method is excessively conservative and misses important differences.

Drug effectiveness is usually expressed in one of two ways. Some investigators prefer to note the percentage of patients who improve with a drug or placebo, and others favor a rating scale that demonstrates the mean change in a patient population. Among the forty-four controlled studies comparing imipramine hydrochloride with a placebo, thirty provided data on the percentage of improvement associated with a drug or placebo. Occasionally British or Australian literature states that tricyclic drugs are not clinically effective. To respond to this, a method of combining data was proposed by one of the authors (J.M.D.) based on the number of patients who have a good or poor response to drugs and the number of patients who have a good or poor response to placebo.[111,112] Parenthetically, some years later analogous statistical methods were used by others to analyze psychotherapy data, and this procedure has come to be called meta-analysis.

There are a variety of data-combination methods. Data can be combined by the use of parametric statistics, such as means and standard deviation, or by combining probabilities that the drug is better than placebo. Although some authors will present means and standard deviations, many do not. Some present covariate adjusted means but no measure of standard deviations. In addition, since different rating scales are used, there is the problem of combining means and standard deviations of different scales. Also, some authors give final scores, but others give changed scores (prevalues minus postvalues). Furthermore, even if the same scale is used, there are different versions to be considered (e.g., the seventeen- versus the twenty-one-item Hamilton Depression Scale). All these factors make it difficult to combine data based on means and standard deviations. The most common metric, therefore, is the basic fourfold table of percent good and poor responders referred to earlier, and this is the one we have used.

Imipramine

Collectively, the data from thirty studies yield a total of 1,334 patients treated with imipramine or placebo (see table 13–1). Approximately 65 percent of the subjects treated with imipramine showed significant improvement, compared to 30 percent on the placebo.[113] None of the studies in this group demonstrated a clearly greater therapeutic effect from the placebo. The average drug-placebo difference of 35 percent was obtained after subtracting the percentage of improvement with a placebo from the percentage of improvement with imipramine. It is not surprising to note that since imipramine so consistently predicted more favorable improvement than did placebo, there is only an infinitesimal statistical probability

TABLE 13–1

Summary of Controlled Double-blind Evaluations of the Antidepressant Drugs[a]

Treatment		Number of Studies in Which Effect Was				
Generic name	Trade name	Greater than placebo	Equal to placebo	Greater than imipramine	Equal to imipramine	Less than imipramine
Tricyclic Drugs						
Imipramine	Tofranil	30	14	–	–	–
Amitriptyline	Elavil	9	2	2	5	0
Desipramine	Norpramin Pertofrane	3	2	0	6	1
Nortriptyline	Aventyl	4	0	0	0	0
Protriptyline	Vivactil	2	0	0	2	0
Opipramol	Insidon	4	0	0	0	0
Trimipramine	Surmontil	1	0	2	0	0
Maprotiline	Ludiomil	2	2	0	10[b]	0
MAOIs						
Tranylcypromine	Parnate	2	1	0	3	0
Iproniazid	Marsilid	4	3	0	0	1
Isocarboxazid	Marplan	2	4	0	2	2
Nialamide	Niamid	0	3	0	0	1
Pheniprazine	Caitron	1	1	0	1	1
Phenelzine	Nardil	11	4	0	4	3
Pargyline	Eutonyl	2	0	0	0	0
Etryptamine	Monase	1	0	0	0	0
Other Treatments						
Electroshock therapy		7	1	4	3	0
Chlorpromazine	Thorazine	3	0	0	3	0
Thioridazine	Mellaril	0	0	0	1	0
Chlorprothixene	Taractan	0	0	0	1	0

[a]The figures include controlled studies only. A drug was not considered better than another drug unless a statistically significant difference existed between the two drugs in their relative effectiveness. Nortriptyline = amitriptyline in three studies.
[b]Also twelve studies showing equivalence to amitriptyline.

that chance alone could lead to these results. The probability of these results, which favor imipramine over placebo, being obtained by chance is 10^{-31}.[159] With large sample sizes, however, one can achieve a highly statistically significant result in a drug that is otherwise of only moderate effectiveness.

We might add parenthetically that most of the studies on imipramine were done shortly after the drug was discovered and used doses of 75 to 150 mg per day. Our current opinion is that the therapeutic dose of imipramine is closer to 150 to 300 mg per day. We believe that some of these patients were treated with lower than optimal dose, and the drug-placebo difference would have been slightly larger had more adequate doses been given.

There remains an urgent need for more effective treatment methods since approximately 30 percent of the depressed patients did not respond to the medication. Clinical experience indicates that some patients will respond to a second antidepressant after having failed to respond to the first one. The drug-placebo difference would be greater if responders to the first or the second drug could be compared to placebo.

Amitriptyline

Most comparative studies of amitriptyline hydrochloride and imipramine have found the drugs about equal in efficacy (see table 13–1). No studies have shown amitriptyline to be less effective than imipramine. Two double-blind studies by the same research group showed 200 mg amitriptyline to be superior to imipramine in the same dosage, although that finding may be a dosage artifact.[222] When the drugs were administered in different dose ratios by Sandifer, Wilson, and Gambill[436] (maximum dose of amitriptyline 240 mg per day and imipramine 300 mg per day), they were found to be equally effective. The findings indicated that the two drugs were generally similar in their therapeutic efficacy.

Desipramine, Nortriptyline, Protriptyline

The desmethyl derivatives of imipramine and amitriptyline, desipramine hydrochloride and nortriptyline hydrochloride, are similar in many pharmacological parameters to their parent compounds but appear to be less sedating. Since they are active metabolites and have clearly established antidepressant efficacy, it is argued that administration of desipramine and nortriptyline might lead to a more rapid and enhanced antidepressant effect. However, controlled comparisons have failed to confirm a faster onset of action. On the basis of comparisons to imipramine or amitriptyline, desipramine and nortriptyline show no practical differences in therapeutic efficacy.

Protriptyline hydrochloride is an imipramine-type drug. Because of its single methyl group, it is referred to as a secondary amine, along with the other desmethyl derivatives, desipramine and nortriptyline. Its therapeutic potency is comparable to amitriptyline or imipramine using functionally equivalent dosages,[480] although it is more potent on a milligram-per-kilogram basis. It has minimal sedating properties and is, indeed, at times even slightly stimulatory. Protriptyline has an unusually long half-life, approximately 54 to 124 hours after a single oral dose of 30 mg.

Doxepin

In the treatment of depressed patients, doxepin hydrochloride has been found to be superior to placebo and about equal to tricyclic antidepressants and to an amitriptyline-

perphenazine combination.[419] There is also significant evidence that doxepin is useful in outpatient anxiety. Three studies comparing doxepin and imipramine showed the two drugs to be about equal (see table 13–2). Milligram-for-milligram, doxepin may be slightly less potent than imipramine, and, if a slightly higher dose of doxepin had been used, doxepin might have been shown to be equal in efficacy to imipramine.

Virtually all studies of doxepin involve outpatients with mixed anxiety-depression rather than inpatients with endogenous depression.[215] It is difficult to interpret the specificity of studies using subjects with mixed anxiety-depression, because the beneficial effect observed could be either the result of an antianxiety agent without any antidepressant properties or of an antidepressant agent with no specific antianxiety properties. Such studies can demonstrate that a drug is more effective than a placebo, but fail to answer these questions: Effective for what diagnosis? Effective with which mechanism: true antidepressant or true anxiolytic?

This methodological limitation notwithstanding, it would seem reasonable to conclude that doxepin has true antidepressant properties. Doxepin bears a structural resemblance to the tricyclic antidepressants and inhibits the membrane pump for biogenic amines, which, we have found, consequently interferes with the antihypertensive actions of guanethidine. For mixed outpatient anxiety-depression, the usual dose of

TABLE 13–2

Doxepin Versus Placebo or Standard Drug in Treatment of Depression

	Number of Studies in Which DOXEPIN Was:		
	Superior	Equal	Inferior
Placebo	2	0	0
Imipramine	0	3	0
Amitriptyline	0	8	0
Amitriptyline-Perphenazine	0	1	0

doxepin ranges from 100 to 300 mg per day, with slightly lower doses for anxiety. The authors recommend any of the conventional tricyclic and tricycliclike drugs, including doxepin and the MAOIs, for the treatment of depression with anxiety. When it is difficult to decide whether the patient has primarily a depressive syndrome or an anxiety disorder, doxepin is useful because of its broad-spectrum quality.

Trimipramine

Trimipramine maleate is structurally very similar to imipramine and differs only by the presence of an additional methyl group attached to the aliphatic side chain. Clinical studies including both open and double-blind trials have for the most part found trimipramine to be an effective antidepressant. Comparisons between trimipramine and a standard tricyclic have been evaluated in a variety of depressed populations, such as inpatients, outpatients, and geriatric patients (see table 13–3). These studies have reported trimipramine to have similar therapeutic efficacy or a trend for superior efficacy to standard antidepressants and an almost similar side-effect profile.[65,176,277] In a large, well-controlled trial of amitriptyline, trimipramine, and placebo, both active drugs were shown to be effective antidepressants. In this study, amitriptyline was slightly but nonsignificantly superior[416] (see table 13–4). This perhaps counteracts a trend set up in several other smaller studies reporting a modest superiority of trimipramine over the standard tricyclic. On balance, we consider trimipra-

TABLE 13–3
Trimipramine Versus Standard Tricyclic

Study	N	Percentage Good Result		
		Trimipramine (%)	Standard Tricyclic (%)	Difference (%)
Evans[139]	68	42	40	+ 2
Lean and Sidhu[277]	40	65	30	+35
Salzman[435]	27	62	29	+33
Burke, Sainsbury, and Meyo[64]	26	69	54	+15
Rifkin et al.[422]	38	84	58	+26
Overall	199	60	42	+18

TABLE 13–4
**Trimipramine and Amitriptyline in Neurotic Depressed Outpatients:
Summary of the Rickels Study[416] [a]**

Results[b]	Covariate Adjusted Group Mean			Trend Favorite
	Trimipramine	Amitriptyline	Placebo	
Hamilton Depression Scale	0.48	0.36	0.67	amitriptyline
Physicians' Questionnaire	1.97	1.84	2.33	amitriptyline
Zung Depression Scale	2.13	2.07	2.37	amitriptyline
Global Estimate of Psychopathology	2.75	2.62	3.28	Amitriptyline
Global End Point (Physicians)	5.27	5.22	4.65	Trimipramine
Global End Point (Patients)	3.6	3.29	2.63	Amitriptyline

[a]The sample consisted of 122 depressed patients. Data are from week 4.
[b]In the first four items, a low number indicates a good response; in the last two items, a high number means a good response.

TABLE 13-5
Amoxapine Versus Placebo

		Percentage Good Result		
Study	N	Amoxapine (%)	Placebo (%)	Difference (%)
Steinbook et al.[477]	14	90	100	−10
Wilson et al.[508]	13	75	40	+35
Gallant et al.[170]	24	83	67	+16
Smith[467]	50	69	42	+27
Kiev and Okerson[253]	47	88	83	+ 5
Fabre et al.[145]	38	83	35	+48
Overall	186	81	57	+24

TABLE 13-6
Amoxapine Versus Standard Antidepressant

		Percentage Good Result		
Study	N	Amoxapine (%)	Standard Tricyclic (%)	Difference (%)
Steinbook et al.[477]	19	90	89	+ 1
Wilson et al.[508]	17	75	56	+19
Smith[467]	50	69	58	+11
Kiev and Okerson[253]	48	88	79	+ 9
Fabre et al.[145]	41	83	70	+13
Sethi et al.[453]	50	76	80	− 4
Bagadia et al.[40]	48	59	62	− 3
Sathananthan et al.[438]	20	80	70	+10
Takahashi, Sakuma, and Hoh[486]	102	81	68	+13
Paprocki et al.[362]	38	86	82	+ 4
de Souza Campos et al.[122]	44	90	71	+19
Fruensgaard et al.[168]	34	91	91	0
Yamhure and Villalobos[516]	53	82	100	−18
Aberg and Holmberg[1]	58	83	97	−14
de Paula et al.[121]	46	63	45	+18
Kaumeier and Haase[244]	48	83	50	+23
Holden, Kerry, and Orme[219]	21	90	64	+26
Burrows, Norman, and Davies[68]	16	88	75	+13
Donlon, Biertuemphel, and Willenbring[126]	31	71	65	+ 6
Overall	784	79	73	+ 6

TABLE 13-7
Chlorimipramine Versus Standard Tricyclic

		Percentage Good Result		
Study	N	Chlorimipramine (%)	Standard Tricyclic (%)	Difference (%)
Gore[192]	45	87	82	+ 5
Kampman, Ummikko-Pelkonen, and Kuha[241]	53	71	52	+19
Rickels et al.[418]	121	53	69	−16
Arfwidsson et al.[29]	40	39	59	−20
Mulgirigama et al.[337]	34	83	44	+39
Poldinger et al.[389]	57	47	48	− 1
Overall	350	61	62	− 1

mine about equally effective as the standard tricyclics.

Amoxapine

Amoxapine is another drug that a large number of double-blind studies has shown to be safe and effective (see tables 13–5 and 13–6). Its efficacy and safety have been demonstrated in a number of double-blind studies comparing it to standard antidepressants.* Amoxapine is a dibenzoxazepine derivative that is both a norepinephrine (NE)- and serotonin (5HT)- reuptake inhibitor, and it has a chemical structure similar to that of the antipsychotic agent loxapine succinate. Amoxapine's effects are partially similar to those of neuroleptics in that it produces dopamine (DA) blockade, extrapyramidal side effects, elevated prolactin, transitory suppression of avoidance reaction, and inhibition of stereotyped behavior induced by amphetamines.[80] Since one of amoxapine's active metabolites, 7-hydroxyamoxadine, has considerable DA-blocking properties that are similar to high-potency neuroleptics, long-term use might produce tardive dyskinesia. It has been shown, using the plasma radioreceptor assay for dopamine studies, that patients on amoxapine have plasma neuroleptic levels similar to those of patients taking antipsychotics.

Chlorimipramine

Chlorimipramine hydrochloride has been used in Europe, Canada, and England for a number of years.† Chlorimipramine blocks 5HT reuptake *in vitro,* and its metabolite, desmethylchlorimipramine, blocks the reuptake of NE.[290,406] Plasma-level studies indicate that after chlorimipramine administration, there are substantial levels of desmethylchlorimipramine present in plasma. Furthermore, a drug-induced decrease in 3-methoxy-4-hydroxy-phenylglycol (MHPG) indicates that in humans, sufficient

amounts of desmethylchlorimipramine are formed so that chlorimipramine can also be considered to affect the noradrenergic system. Six random-assignment double-blind studies demonstrate that chlorimipramine is almost equal in efficacy to the standard tricyclics (see table 13–7). Placebo-controlled studies of chlorimipramine demonstrate a trend for the drug to have both an anti-obsessive effect[17,74,487,518] and an antiphobic effect.[76,137,313,499]

Tandamine

Tandamine hydrochloride is a thiopyranoindole compound that inhibits the reuptake of NE. There is some evidence for efficacy, but the drug was never marketed.

Oxaprotiline

Oxaprotiline hydrochloride is an NE-uptake inhibitor that a collaborative study has shown to be more effective than placebo and at least equal to amitriptyline in efficacy. Oxaprotiline has fewer anticholinergic properties than amitriptyline and only minimal sedative properties.

Nomifensine

Nomifensine maleate inhibits both NE and DA reuptake but not 5HT uptake.[226,440] While in theory it is postulated to have amphetaminelike properties, whether it indeed has clinical properties (paranoid psychosis at overdose, abuse of the amphetamine type, etc.) similar to amphetamine remains to be determined. Nomifensine is a mild stimulatory drug and can cause agitation as a side effect. It is excreted by the kidney and its active metabolites have a short half-life. Numerous studies of nomifensine have been conducted in Europe and South America.* Three double-blind studies showed it to be more effective than placebo (see table 13–8). Its antidepressant activity resembles that of the standard tricyclics (see table 13–9). It is

*See references 125, 126, 165, 174, 214, 230, 420, and 438.
†See references 47, 210, 227, 304, 306, and 483.

*See references 2, 164, 283, 301, 302, 358, 484, and 511.

TABLE 13-8
Nomifensine Versus Placebo

		Percentage Good Result		
Study	N	Nomifensine (%)	Placebo (%)	Difference (%)
Eckmann 1[133]	60	90	7	+83
Eckmann 2[133]	64	80	23	+57
Kroeger and Eckmann[268]	31	90	67	+23
Overall	155	80	24	+62

TABLE 13-9
Nomifensine Versus Standard Tricyclic

		Percentage Good Result		
Study	N	Nomifensine (%)	Standard Tricyclic (%)	Difference (%)
Sharma[456]	35	44	32	+12
Ananth and Von Der Steen[18]	26	92	92	0
Amin, Ban, and Pecknold[13]	26	33	91	−58
Amin, Ban and Lehmann[12]	19	60	67	− 7
Angst et al.[23]	30	47	47	0
Poldinger and Gommel[388]	40	70	55	+15
Van Scheyen, Van Praag, and Korf[495]	20	45	33	+12
Grof, Saxena, and Daigle[199]	24	42	33	+ 9
Overall	220	54	55	− 1

both a safe and nonsedating agent[18,163,204] and is associated with a relatively reduced incidence of anticholinergic side effects and a relatively low propensity for causing convulsions. Nomifensine has been extensively investigated and is, at present, under serious consideration by the Federal Drug Administration (FDA) for release.

Opipramol

Although it contains a tricyclic nucleus, opipramol hydrochloride has a piperazine side chain similar to that present in some phenothiazine neuroleptic drugs. Despite this chemical similarity, opipramol's pharmacological effects are similar to those of the other tricyclic drugs.

In the treatment of depression, opipramol has been shown to be superior[33,77,472] to placebo and clearly comparable to the other

tricyclic antidepressants, namely imipramine[340] and desipramine.[428] A double-blind comparison of opipramol with the combined effects of phenelzine and chlordiazepoxide showed no advantage to either regimen at the end of six weeks.[75]

Numerous studies have evaluated the relative effectiveness of opipramol in the treatment of anxiety. Results have varied, including statistically insignificant superiority to placebo,[67] equivalent efficacy to chlordiazepoxide,[233] and inferiority to diazepam.[28] From the available evidence, it can be concluded that opipramol has similar antidepressant properties to the other tricyclics and its anxiolytic effects, at best, equal those of the benzodiazepines.

Lofepramine

Lofepramine hydrochloride is a NE-uptake inhibitor that is an analogue of imipramine and is metabolized to the desmethyl derivative of imipramine, desipramine. It is not surprising, therefore, that studies should show it to be similar to imipramine in antidepressant effect (see table 13–10).[464]

Viloxazine

Viloxazine hydrochloride inhibits the uptake of NE.[23,381] A number of double-blind studies have shown viloxazine to be essentially equal in efficacy to the standard tricyclics (see table 13–11).* Viloxazine is a bicyclic compound and differs in its side-effect profile from the standard tricyclics in that, although producing less anticholinergic effects, it increases the convulsive threshold.[384]

Mianserin

Mianserin hydrochloride is a tetracyclic compound with some interesting properties.[93] It is not a DA-, NE-, or 5HT-uptake inhibitor, nor is it an MAOI. Mianserin appears to act via a presynaptic mechanism to increase NE turnover. Thus mianserin's efficacy is consistent with the NE theory, even though its mechanisms of action are quite different from those of the standard antidepressants. Mianserin has been shown to be clearly superior to placebo (see table 13–12) and has also been intensively compared to standard tricyclics.† Combined evidence from nine double-blind studies revealed mianserin to be 10 percent less effective than standard tricyclics, which is a statistically significant difference (see table 13–13). While if too low a dose was used, this may be a dose artifact, on the other hand, it could represent a real difference.

It is reasonable to expect that all NE-uptake inhibitors would be equally effective since they share a common mechanism of action. Mianserin is the prototype of a different class of antidepressant and has a different mechanism of action. It may thus have a different efficacy from other tricyclics. In other words, we believe that although it is unlikely that drugs which act through the same mechanism have different efficacy, drugs which act through different mechanisms could potentially have different overall efficacy.

Novel Antidepressants

Novel antidepressants may potentiate NE, but differential evidence is lacking. Our research has provided some evidence that drugs in this group down-regulate NE receptors and hence probably potentiate NE transmission in some fashion. The tentative evidence implicating NE notwithstanding, the involvement of NE in the action of these drugs is best described as nonproven.

BUPROPION

Bupropion hydrochloride has been well studied in a number of double-blind studies that have shown it to be an effective antidepressant that is superior to placebo and equal to a standard antidepressant.* It is neither a tricyclic nor an MAOI, and it demonstrates none of the cardiovascular, anticholinergic, or sedative side effects common to those drugs.

Feighner, Meredith, and Cleghorn[152] studied forty-nine hospitalized patients on bupropion (N = 34) and placebo (N = 15) in a random assignment double-blind study. Seventy-nine percent, or twenty-seven, patients on bupropion and 13 percent, or two, patients on placebo were rated as at least much improved on "end-point analysis." When more stringent criteria of a final Hamilton Depression score of 9 or less was used, 53 percent, or eighteen, bupropion patients and no placebo patients were recovered. Goode and Manning,[189] in an open, random-assignment study of schizo-affective patients, found that bupropion plus haloperidol produced better effects than bupropion alone. Three out of nine patients on bupropion experienced an exacerbation of

---

*See references 16, 44, 45, 46, 354, 489, and 506.
†See references 155, 221, 231, 401, 433, and 498.

*See references 143, 146, 367, 470, and 478.

TABLE 13–10
Lofepramine Versus Standard Tricyclic

		Percentage Good Results		
Study	N	Lofepramine (%)	Tricyclic (%)	Standard Difference (%)
d'Elia et al.[118]	49	58	78	−20
McClelland et al.[303]	41	86	85	+ 1
Wright and Hermann[515]	40	15	35	−20
Goncalves and Wegener[188]	30	60	33	+27
Overall	160	55	60	− 5

TABLE 13–11
Viloxazine Versus Standard Tricyclic

		Percentage Good Result		
Study	N	Viloxazine (%)	Standard Tricyclic (%)	Difference (%)
Floru and Tegeler[160]	50	76	60	+16
Santonastaso, Maistrello, and Battistin[437]	26	54	69	−15
Pichot, Guelt and Dreyfus[381]	119	64	56	+ 8
Kiloh et al.[254]	57	30	58	−28
Peet[370]	23	54	60	− 6
Elwan[136]	51	83	67	+16
McEvoy et al.[305]	22	90	67	+23
Lennox[282]	29	88	92	− 4
Davies et al.[109]	22	55	45	+10
Overall	399	64	62	+ 2

TABLE 13–12
Mianserin Versus Placebo

		Percentage Improvement		
Study	N	Mianserin (%)	Placebo (%)	Difference (%)
Hamouz et al.[208]	80	63	20	+43
Perry et al.[377]	28	60	69	− 9
Russell et al.[432]	48	79	8	+71
Overall	156	67	25	+42

TABLE 13-13
Mianserin Versus Standard Tricyclic

| Study | N | Percentage Improvement | | |
		Mianserin (%)	Standard Tricyclic (%)	Difference (%)
Blaha, Pinder, and Stolemeijer[54]	48	57	60	− 3
DeBuck[116]	32	76	80	− 4
Murphy and Bridgman[343]	84	44	37	+ 7
Kretschmar[266]	36	55	19	+36
Conti et al.[88]	137	51	66	−15
Pinder et al.[385]	65	68	71	− 3
Pinder et al.[385]	62	43	71	−28
Perry et al.[377]	28	60	77	−17
Svestka et al.[484]	82	55	88	−33
Overall	574	54	64	−10

psychotic symptoms, and only one of the nine was moderately improved. Nine of eleven on the combination were at least moderately improved, one slightly improved, and one had an episode of violent acting out.

Bupropion appears to exert virtually no inhibition of the reuptake of 5HT or NE. However, Pandey, in our laboratory, found that high doses of the drug in rodents will produce a significant reduction of noradrenergic beta-receptor density; in other words, there is a down-regulation of the noradrenergic receptor sites.[360] Unlike most psychotropic drugs, bupropion is nonsedative, which is very important to a patient who values optimal mental functions. Bupropion is not a stimulant or euphoriant (i.e., it is not self-administered in animal studies using the paradigm in which amphetaminelike drugs are self-administered). It does not cause weight gain, is not cardiotoxic, and is safe in the overdose situation. Further, it does not cause dysphoria and exhibits minimal anticholinergic side effects.

IPRINDOLE

Iprindole hydrochloride is neither an NE- nor a 5HT-reuptake inhibitor, nor is it an MAOI. Its efficacy has been demonstrated in double-blind studies.[235,478,483] Iprindole has been shown to down-regulate the noradrenergic receptor sites in the brain.[429]

ALPRAZOLAM

Alprazolam is a triazalobenzodiazepine and is characterized by the incorporation of a triazole ring in its basic benzodiazepine structure. Benzodiazepines have a clearly established role in the treatment of anxiety and insomnia. In a review of the use of benzodiazepines in depressive disorders, it has been suggested that these agents may be of some nonspecific value in combating symptoms of anxiety.[441] Alprazolam has been the focus of some recent interest, in that it has demonstrated clinical effectiveness as an antidepressant that is unexplained by its anxiolytic action alone (see table 13-14).

In addition to several positive case reports, alprazolam has been evaluated in a six-week, double-blind, multicenter comparison with imipramine and placebo.[151] Subjects were 906 outpatients suffering from a unipolar major depressive disorder of at least one month's duration. Alprazolam was reported to have a more rapid onset of action than imipramine (average daily dose of imipramine was 132 mg) with equivalent antidepressant effect on all major parameters and was significantly superior to placebo (see table 13-15). In addition, it had the advantage of fewer side effects. Further support for this unique antidepressant action is provided by sleep studies that have shown that alprazolam had an effect similar to the tricyclic and MAOI varieties of antidepressant on rapid-eye-movement sleep in depressed patients.[149] Although the mechanism of its antidepressant action is unclear, recent animal work suggests that alprazolam reverses reserpine-induced changes on beta-adrenergic receptors.[454] In our laboratory, Pandey has shown that alprazolam down-regulates beta-adrenergic receptors.[360]

TRAZODONE

Trazodone hydrochloride, a triazolopyridine derivative, is structurally unrelated to any other psychotropics and represents a new class of antidepressant. It is a selective inhibitor of 5HT reuptake and also down-regulates beta-adrenergic receptor sites. Although the precise mechanism of the phenomenon of down-regulation has not been elucidated, it may index a functional increase of NE available at the receptor site caused by the drug. Trazodone has been extensively compared to placebo and standard tricyclics.[309,330,342,427] In a review of thirty random-assignment double-blind studies, it proved to be 32 percent more effective than placebo (see table 13–16) and 4 percent more effective than a standard tricyclic, the latter difference being nonsignificant (see table 13–17).

Conceivably, trazodone's most valuable therapeutic asset is its lack of any anticholinergic properties. In a multicenter placebo-controlled study of 379 patients comparing imipramine and trazodone, the incidence of the four main anticholinergic effects—dry mouth, blurred vision, bowel movement disturbance, and delayed urine flow—was no different between the trazodone and the placebo groups.[178] Trazodone has been used in patients with glaucoma and was not found to affect conditions adversely.[106] In addition, trazodone has not been proven to cause seizures. However, it does have sedative properties, and although sedation can be used advantageously, patients should be carefully cautioned.

MAPROTILINE

Although marketed rather ingeniously as a "tetracyclic" antidepressant, maprotiline

hydrochloride resembles the tricyclic antidepressants in many of its pharmacological properties.[383] Unlike standard tricyclics, maprotiline is a highly selective inhibitor of NE uptake and has barely appreciable actions on 5HT uptake.[43] Controlled double-blind studies have shown it to be superior to placebo and as effective as the standard antidepressants, amitriptyline, imipramine, and doxepin (see table 13–18).* Maprotiline was compared to a standard tricyclic preparation (usually amitriptyline or imipramine) by means of the random assignment of 2,-078 patients to one of these drugs. Examination of the number and percentage of individuals according to outcome, as well as an analysis of the data by means of the Fleiss method,[159] revealed no difference in efficacy among the groups. Six hundred sixty patients (73.6 percent) who had received maprotiline did well,—that is, showed moderate improvement or better—compared to 640 (72.6 percent) on standard drug. Maprotiline's side-effect profile is similar to that of the tricyclics, except that in overdose it shows central nervous system (CNS) toxicity and can also induce seizures. The cardiac toxicity that standard tricyclics rarely cause at therapeutic dosages, but can cause when an overdose is taken, is less of a problem with maprotiline.[26,250]

Serotonin-Uptake Inhibitors

FLUOXETINE

Fluoxetine hydrochloride is a specific 5HT-uptake inhibitor with no known effect on noradrenergic systems.[280] A substantial body of evidence indicates that it is at least equal in efficacy to standard antidepressants and clearly superior to placebo. Using a cut-off point requiring a substantial degree of improvement for classification as an improver, placebo produced improvement in 26 percent, while fluoxetine produced an improve-

*See references 30, 32, 103, 287, 331, 333, 344, and 413.

TABLE 13–14
Alprazolam Versus Placebo

Study	N	Percentage Good Result		
		Alprazolam (%)	Placebo (%)	Difference (%)
Feighner[149]	344	75	49	+26
Upjohn[492]	164	70	62	+ 8
Overall	508	73	53	+20

TABLE 13–15
Alprazolam Versus Standard Tricyclic

Study	N	Percentage Good Result		
		Alprazolam (%)	Standard Tricyclic (%)	Difference (%)
Feighner, Aden, and Fabre[151]	382	75	72	+3
Upjohn[492]	282	70	77	−7
Overall	664	73	74	−1

TABLE 13–16
Trazodone Versus Placebo

Non-U.S. Studies	N	Percentage Good Result		
		Trazodone (%)	Placebo (%)	Difference (%)
Vinci[497]	48	73	6	+67
Cianchetti and Gainotti[81]	58	51	24	+27
Antonelli et al.[26]	53	72	14	+58
Eckmann et al.[134]	90	69	33	+36
Eckmann et al.[134]	90	76	29	+47
Escobar et al.[138]	25	62	50	+12
Subtotal	364	68	27	+41
U.S. Studies				
Goldberg and Finnerty[186]	80	81	58	+23
Kellams, Klapper, and Small[247]	18	56	0	+56
Feighner[148]	27	53	0	+53
Fabre, McClendon, and Gainey[144]	18	56	11	+45
Gerner et al.[177]	25	42	23	+19
Gershon et al.[181]	173	42	30	+12
Subtotal	341	54	31	+23
Overall	705	61	29	+32

TABLE 13–17
Trazodone Versus Standard Antidepressant

| Non-U.S. Studies | N | Percentage Improvement | | |
		Trazodone (%)	Standard Tricyclic (%)	Difference (%)
DeGregorio and Dionisio[117]	74	57	62	− 5
Vinci[497]	49	73	75	− 2
Cianchetti and Gainotti[81]	59	51	36	+15
Cioffi et al.[82]	24	42	25	+17
Peterova[380]	20	80	60	+20
Eckmann, et al.[134]	90	69	49	+20
Pariante[363]	34	71	59	+12
Agnoli et al.[6]	82	78	76	+ 2
Mazzei, Marri, and Fabiani[318]	39	84	75	+ 9
Al-Yassiri and Bridges[9]	25	92	54	+38
Escobar et al.[138]	28	62	93	−31
Pierce (single-blind)[382]	35	62	63	− 1
Subtotal	559	67	61	+ 6
U.S. Studies				
Goldberg and Finnerty[186]	76	81	71	+10
Kellams, Klapper, and Small[247]	19	56	20	+36
Feighner[148]	35	53	28	+25
Fabre, McClendon, and Gainey[144]	19	56	60	− 4
Gerner et al.[177]	21	42	33	+ 9
Gershon et al.[181]	184	42	55	−13
Subtotal	354	54	53	+ 1
Overall	913	62	58	+ 4

ment in 49 percent of patients, a drug-placebo difference of 23 percent. Standard antidepressants produced improvement in 48 percent, which, in comparison to fluoxetine, showed the new drug to be slightly (1 percent) better than the standard. We emphasize that the absolute improvement rate is meaningless. It is the comparative improvement rate to that of standard drug or placebo that is meaningful. If patients who improve minimally are classified as improved, there will be a high improvement rate; if only those patients with substantial improvement are classified as improved, a low absolute rate is seen. We favor the former. Fluoxetine does not cause weight gain. In general, it has a favorable side-effect profile and causes fewer side effects overall than standard antidepressants. So far, there have been four cases of overdose, and none of these produced serious medical consequences.

OTHER SEROTONIN-UPTAKE INHIBITORS

A limited number of clinical trials of other presumably specific 5HT-uptake inhibitors, such as fluvoxamine maleate, have provided evidence of their clinical efficacy.* A number of drugs, such as chlorimipramine or zimelidine hydrochloride, have been suggested to be specific serotonergic drugs,[273] but more recent research has suggested the presence of a noradrenergic metabolite. Zimelidine is metabolized to norzimelidine, which may cause Guillain-Barré syndrome and, therefore, will perhaps not be marketed. It is entirely possible that new research may find a noradrenergic component to the drugs cur-

*See references 83, 98, 228, 430, and 514.

TABLE 13–18
Maprotiline Versus Standard Tricyclic

Study	N	Percentage Improvement with Drugs		
		Maprotiline (%)	Standard Tricyclic (%)	Difference (%)
Trick[489]	21	83	89	− 6
Mathur[315]	30	80	60	+20
Murphy[341]	61	56	41	+15
Liebling[288]	19	70	89	−19
Forrest[161]	184	89	82	+ 7
Weissman et al.[502]	66	77	81	− 4
Amin et al.[14]	20	40	70	−30
Scandinavian Collaborative Study (8 hospitals)[276]	208	62	64	− 2
Marais[310]	24	100	83	+17
Collaborative vs. Outpt.[252]	124	90	87	+ 3
Levin[286]	44	91	64	+27
International Collaborative[252]	417	66	74	− 8
Jones[239]	32	75	88	−13
Middleton[326]	26	64	75	−11
Kessell and Holt[249]	73	72	73	− 1
Guz[202]	57	75	62	+13
Angst et al.[22]	22	67	64	+ 3
Collaborative Outpatient Studies[297]	99	73	77	− 4
Collaborative Inpatient Studies[327]	71	81	60	+21
Lehmann et al.[278]	39	68	55	+13
Overall	1,638	73	73	0

rently thought to be 5HT-specific. Since it has no known NE effect, fluoxetine represents a theoretically important drug in that a specific 5HT-uptake inhibitor can benefit depression.

¶ Drug Maintenance in Affective Disorders

A major therapeutic decision facing the clinician once the patient is discharged from the hospital, contingent on a good response to treatment with tricyclic medications, is when to discontinue the antidepressant drug. Considering that depression is a recurrent disorder, one often wonders whether continued treatment with tricyclic drugs will truly prevent relapse.

Patients frequently relapse months after receiving electroconvulsive therapy (ECT) and recovering from their depression. Two groups decided to investigate whether post-ECT relapse could be prevented by maintenance treatment with tricyclic drugs. Seager and Bird[452] used a random-assignment, double-blind method to follow patients who received either placebo or imipramine for six months or until relapse occurred. Maintenance imipramine had an impressive prophylactic effect: 69 percent of the placebo patients relapsed in contrast to only 17 percent of the imipramine maintenance patients (see table 13–26 in the lithium section).

Kay, Fahy, and Garside[245] performed a similar study. Patients were assigned to receive amitriptyline or diazepam randomly, using the double-blind design at the start of ECT. Diazepam was included as an active placebo, as previous research had demonstrated its lack of antidepressant properties.[101] Kay found that a substantially greater number of diazepam patients were considered treatment failures than were amitriptyline patients (see table 13–26). In this study, failure to improve, patients who needed further ECT, and suicide victims were considered failures. Although neither of these post-ECT studies involved large samples, the results of the two were consistent in demonstrating the tricyclics' prophylactic properties.

There have also been three large collaborative studies on maintenance tricyclics in patients initially treated with tricyclics. Klerman and coworkers[258] and Paykel and coworkers[366] performed a collaborative study in the United States comparing maintenance amitriptyline therapy, maintenance psychotherapy, and placebo therapy. Patients were initially treated with amitriptyline; those patients who improved were then assigned to the maintenance study using double-blind, placebo-controlled methods. The groups receiving the placebo and psychotherapy had virtually identical results with respect to prevention of relapse. Therefore, both can be considered control groups for comparison with the drug group. The tricyclic drugs demonstrated a substantial prophylactic effect (see table 13–26). Psychotherapy, although not effective in preventing depressive relapse, did improve social adjustment.

Mindham, Howland, and Shepherd[328] completed a collaborative study that included thirty-four psychiatrists in Great Britain. Patients who had suffered a depressive illness and had responded to treatment with either imipramine or amitriptyline in doses of at least 150 mg per day were studied. These patients were classified as follows: One group was continued on treatment with tricyclic drugs in doses of 75 to 100 mg per day, while the other was placed on a placebo for a period of fifteen months. When this period ended, relapse was observed among 22 percent of the tricyclic maintenance group, compared to 50 percent of the group treated with a placebo.

The relapse rate appears to be constant over time, given that the appropriate correction is made (see chapter 18 for discussion of relapse rate). Data are not yet available for predicting which patients need tricyclic drugs to prevent relapse, but those with a

history of many relapses or incomplete remissions are known clinically to do so with greater regularity. The time course of the relapses with tricyclics and placebo (see table 13–26) in Mindham's[328] and Schou's[447] studies is shown in Figure 13–1. In the veterans' administration (VA) collaborative study, Prien and associates[398,399] also compared imipramine with placebo and found that imipramine had prophylactic properties in unipolar depression (see table 13–26). In this study, placebo or maintenance tricyclics were administered in a double-blind, random-assignment design. Upon pooling the data from these various studies, there remains no real doubt that maintenance tricyclics are able to successfully prevent relapse. The results of these studies might have been slightly more dramatic had the investigators restricted their samples to patients with unipolar depression. Nevertheless, when the data from all of these studies is combined, the probability that these prophylactic effects would occur by chance alone would be 1.6×10^{-8} (Fleiss chi-square association = 31.9, $df = 1$).

In patients who are prone to multiple relapses, maintenance tricyclics should be considered for the prevention of recurrence. Some patients will experience only a single depressive episode in their lifetime. Maintenance tricyclics are not necessarily recommended for such cases. The decision for prophylaxis should be based on clinical indications, such as the frequency of depres-

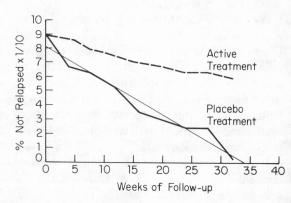

Figure 13–1.   Time course of relapse of patients taking tricyclics or placebo.

sion, the severity of depression, risk of suicide, and the social consequences of the behavioral impairment produced by the depression.

As tricyclic drugs do not prevent and, indeed, can precipitate the manic phase of bipolar illness,[112] lithium carbonate is clearly the prophylactic agent of choice in bipolar disease. It is interesting to note that maintenance lithium is also used to prevent relapses in patients with recurrent unipolar depression (see table 13–24 in the lithium section).[99] There is not yet enough evidence comparing the effects of lithium versus tricyclics in the prevention of unipolar disease to determine which of these two prophylactic agents is preferable (see table 13–29 in the lithium section). The literature, though, suggests that the magnitude of the drug-placebo difference in prophylactic effect is greater with lithium than with tricyclics. Prien and associates verified this opinion when they studied bipolar patients[399,400] and were unable to demonstrate that tricyclics were useful in maintenance treatment. However, the lithium and tricyclic trials have studied mostly different populations of patients. Controlled trials comparing lithium and maintenance tricyclics are needed to decide this question. In this connection, the VA Collaborative Study[393,395,396,397] is important as the first of these trials.

Klerman and associates[258] examined the role of psychotherapy and maintenance treatment. Psychotherapy was not effective in preventing relapse, yet it did improve the adjustment at the social level. Again, this research describes a qualitatively important role for drugs in the treatment of depressed patients. In sum, both psychological therapies and drug treatment should be seriously considered.

Selection of Patients

Several recent studies have focused on identifying a group of patients for whom imipramine has proven to be particularly effective. The clinical characteristics associated with good drug response were those indica-tive of endogenous depression—that is, depression different in quality from a general state of sadness and characterized by severe psychomotor retardation or agitation, feelings of severe guilt and unworthiness, and symptoms such as early-morning awakening, decrease in appetite, or weight loss.[48,349] Other studies have found that retarded patients tend to do well with tricyclic drugs. Conversely, patients with neurotic depressions whose premorbid personalities showed self-pity, irritability, and/or hysterical and hypochondriacal features did not demonstrate as clear-cut favorable response to the drug.

In 1975 Glassman, Kantor, and Shostak[183] noted that delusional patients did not do well on imipramine alone but did respond to ECT. The researchers were able to rule out low plasma levels as an explanation. A review of the literature on that point revealed that several other investigators observed the same thing and that a reinterpretation of Horndern's data[222] also lends support to that finding.[403,408] Although some delusional depressive patients do respond to imipramine, a fair amount of evidence indicates that they may be less responsive to that drug than are nondelusional depressives. Delusional depressive patients often respond to antipsychotic drugs plus tricyclics or ECT. Furthermore, 50 percent of nonresponders to tricyclics do recover with ECT.

Role of Psychotherapy

Weissman and associates[124,501,503] reported on a series of well-controlled outpatient depression studies comparing tricyclics, psychotherapy, tricyclics plus psychotherapy, and a control group. The control group was composed of patients who called for emergency appointments only when they needed help; this demand-only psychotherapy group was used as an alternative to waiting-list controls. The research demonstrated that both tricyclics and regular psychotherapy had a greater antidepressant effect than demand-only psychotherapy. However, both treatments together (tricyclics plus psychotherapy) produced a more favorable clinical response than either treatment by itself. The two treatments augmented each other. Covi and coworkers[101] detected a significant therapeutic effect from imipramine, but were unable to show that group therapy was beneficial.

In the future we expect to see an effort toward evaluating nondrug forms of therapy. With this in mind, it is important to consider what constitutes an adequate "placebo" for psychotherapy. A methodological problem encountered in such studies is that a nonspecific placebolike effect is poorly controlled for; patients on a waiting list or in a demand-only control group know that they are not receiving routine psychotherapy. The demand characteristics of these control situations are substantially different from routine, specific treatment. Therefore, it cannot be said that such studies are truly placebo controlled. A highly suitable control experiment would be to compare a given type of standard acceptable "specific" psychotherapy against a "nonspecific nontherapeutic" type of psychological support, based on an equal number of hours. This control experience would lack the ingredients seen as specific to psychotherapy and would perhaps arrange for approximately the same demand characteristics. Adequate control necessitates that the demand characteristics be roughly the same in both the control and the experimental groups. Another key consideration in this type of investigation is that blind assessment may not be blind in actuality. Some patients may be cognizant of their particular psychological intervention and may inadvertently communicate to the blind assessors the "demand characteristics." In other words, all comparison groups are not necessarily control groups.

A large body of clinical opinion favors psychological interventions for depressed patients, and certainly those patients who can benefit from psychotherapy should not be neglected. Nearly all studies, however, have demonstrated the beneficial effects of drugs. The weight of the evidence is such that the clinician should not neglect physical treatment for depression. Furthermore, psychotherapy and drugs are not an either/or proposition. Patients can receive both.

¶ Plasma Levels of Tricyclic Antidepressants

Antidepressant drugs have been shown to benefit at least 70 percent of depressed patients. Certainly some percentage of the patients who have not benefited are suffering from a type of depression that does not respond to this class of drugs. However, others may not respond as a function of pharmacological factors—that is, too little or too much drug reaching the brain. Patients have large interindividual differences in the plasma level. This raises the question of whether the lack of response can be attributed to an abnormality in the metabolic rate of the tricyclic drug (see tables 13–19 and 13–20; figures 13–2, 13–3, 13–4, and 13–5). Certain individuals might metabolize the drug quite quickly, fail to build up a sufficient blood level, and subsequently show low brain levels and poor clinical response. Other patients may have a defective metabolism, such that high plasma and brain levels may accumulate. Patients may, therefore, fail to improve clinically either because they are the recipients of toxic doses or because the drug may lose efficacy at increased levels. Even though it has been fifteen years since the thirty- to forty-fold interindividual variability of steady-state tricyclic antidepressant plasma concentrations was first measured, we still do not know the relationship between steady-state plasma concentrations and clinical response for most antidepressants.[196,207]

In this section, we summarize the empirical evidence on plasma levels, making an effort to combine the data from multiple studies to see if the results are consistent. For authors who did not publish data tables but did present graphs, we obtained the data from the graph by visual inspection. If an investigator reports amitriptyline and nortriptyline data, or imipramine and desipramine data, on two separate graphs, and a

TABLE 13–19

Desipramine Plasma Level and Clinical Response

Study		Plasma level (ng/ml)		
		0–92	82–115	115+
Amin et al.[16]	R[a]	0	0	2
	NR	1	0	2
Hrdina and Lapierre[223]	R	0	0	3
	NR	3	0	1
Nelson et al.[348]	R	2	1	8
	NR	13	5	1
Total		0–115	115+	
	R	3	13	
	NR	22	4	
Percent Response (%)		12	76	

[a]R = Responder; NR = Nonresponder.

TABLE 13–20

Plasma Levels versus Clinical Response in Patients Treated with Imipramine

		Plasma Levels (ng/ml)		
		0–180	180–240	+240
Glassman, et al.[184]	R[a]	8	22[b]	
Perel, Stiller, and Glassman[372]	NR	21	8[b]	
Matuzas, et al.[316]	R	1	1	0
	NR	6	2	0
Matuzas, et al.[317]	R	5	1	2
	NR	5	2	1
Reisbey, et al.[414]	R	11	4	18
	NR	23	5	5
Olivier-Martin, et al.[357]	R	0	2	4
	NR	3	1	4
Simpson, et al.[462]	R	8	3	7
	NR	6	1	2
Total	R	33	11	53[c]
	NR	64	11	20
Percent Response (%)		34	50	73

[a]R = Responder; NR = Nonresponder.
[b]Author gave plasma levels only as below or above 180.
[c]The 22 responders and 8 nonresponders were put in the 240 ng/ml category. If these are not counted, there are 31 responders and 12 nonresponders with a response rate of 72 percent.

given data point matches up uniquely to a given improvement score, we can obtain the total amitriptyline plus nortriptyline level or the total imipramine plus desipramine level. (When two or more patients have an identical improvement score, we cannot recover data.) Some investigators presented the number of patients above or below a certain cut-off point, and we combined this data as best we could. The empirical investigations on the relationship between antidepressant plasma level and therapeutic response are summarized in tables 13–19, 13–20, and 13–21, and in figures 13–2 and 13–3. Where an inves-

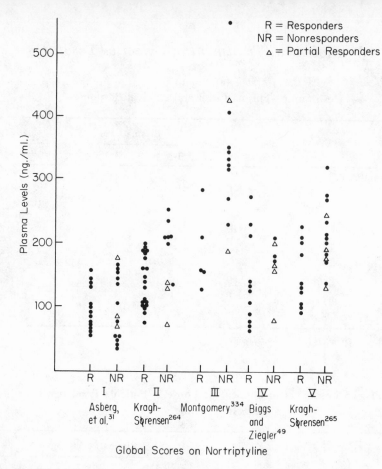

Figure 13–2. Nortriptyline plasma levels and clinical response.

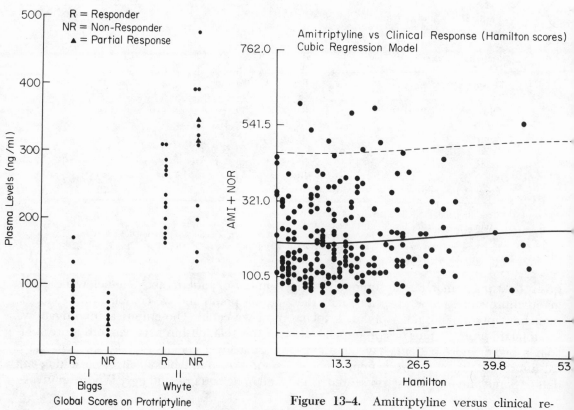

Figure 13–3. Protriptyline plasma levels and clinical response.

Figure 13–4. Amitriptyline versus response (Hamilton scores).

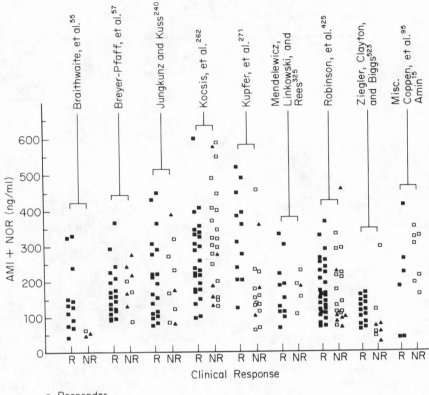

Figure 13–5. Amitriptyline plus nortriptyline plasma levels and clinical response.

tigator reported a preliminary trial and later extended the trial to a large number of patients, and if we found identical values in the larger series to those that occurred in the preliminary report, we assumed that the preliminary data was included in the larger series and counted this data only once. When investigators reported plasma levels drawn on several different weeks, we averaged those plasma levels to obtain a mean plasma level and related this to a measure of clinical response available.

Asberg and associates[31] examined associations between plasma nortriptyline concentrations and therapeutic response. It was found that some patients who failed to respond had notably reduced levels of blood nortriptyline, while other such patients had relatively higher levels of nortriptyline. Predictably, there must be a lower limit to the therapeutic window with virtually all drugs. In other words, if a sufficiently low dose was given, an insufficient quantity of the drug would be available to the receptor site to produce a therapeutic response. It was reported that the lower level of the therapeutic window was approximately 50 ng per ml since five patients who had levels below this had failed to respond.[31] It is of interest that the precise location of the "low window" derives principally from data from these five patients. This same study further reported that patients who had plasma levels that exceeded 140 ng per ml tended to display an unfavorable clinical response. This did not appear to be due to CNS toxicity; rather, the

TABLE 13-21
Result of Rickel's Study Compared with Other Studies

Study	Clinical Results	Plasma Level	
		Low (< 100 ng/ml)	High (> 100 ng/ml)
Rickel's study	Good	0	4 (20%)
	Moderate	8 (67%)	15 (75%)
	Poor	4 (33%)	1 (5%)
Combined data	Good	12 (34%)	106 (50%)
from other studies	Moderate-Poor	23 (66%)	104 (50%)
All data combined	Good	12 (26%)	110 (48%)
	Moderate-Poor	35 (74%)	120 (52%)

drug seemed to lose its therapeutic effectiveness when plasma levels were elevated (see figure 13–2).

In view of the tremendous theoretical interest generated by the paradoxical property of nortriptyline—namely, that it seemed to diminish in efficacy at high plasma levels—it was studied closely by several investigators. Kragh-Sorensen and associates [263,264,265] and Montgomery, Braithwaite, and Crammer [332] confirmed this result, noting poor responses with plasma levels above 175 ng per ml and 200 ng per ml, respectively. Montgomery and coworkers [334] noted that from among a group of sixteen patients with high plasma levels who had had their clinical doses reduced, twelve improved within approximately a week. Kragh-Sorensen and associates [263,264,265] examined patients whose doses had been adjusted to either above 180 ng per ml or below 150 ng per ml and reported that a disproportionately large number of subjects in the first group showed a poor clinical response. This study progressed to a second phase in which a subgroup of the original sample was selected at random and the subgroup of the original high-plasma-level group (180+ ng/ml) had their dose lowered to the therapeutic range. Five out of five patients improved. In contrast, six patients who continued to have high plasma levels had a poor response.

The upper end of the therapeutic window varies substantially from study to study; hence, on examination of the pooled data, it cannot be precisely defined. Note that the 140 ng per ml upper limit, so widely quoted in secondary sources, is actually well within the range of the therapeutic window reported by most of the studies (see figure 13–2).

Two fixed-dose studies have failed to find a significant relationship between nortriptyline plasma levels and clinical response. Burrows and his associates [66,69] treated patients with a fixed dose of nortriptyline for four weeks. Using the criterion of a 50 percent decrease on the Hamilton scale at four weeks for a responder, we noted that there were sixteen responders and sixteen nonresponders. Six patients had a plasma level below 50 ng per ml at either two or four weeks. Five of these six were nonresponders. Of the twenty-six with levels above 50 ng per ml at both two and four weeks, eleven were nonresponders ($p = 0.09$ on Fisher's Exact Test, one-tailed). This trend did not reach the 5 percent confidence level.

Davies, Burrows, and Scoggins [66,108] made an interesting clinical observation in another study of patients who had had a history of good response to tricyclics. Each patient underwent dosage reduction and all patients deteriorated when plasma levels were decreased and then improved when levels were raised again. The doctor rating the depression was unaware of the dose change. Although the plasma levels associated with this deterioration differed widely, it seemed that there was a critical plasma level for each patient below which the patient became worse.

Burrows, Maguire, and Scoggins[67] did a subsequent study where patients were treated with a moderate dose of nortriptyline for two weeks and then randomly assigned to receive either a low dose (50 mg/day) or a high dose (200 mg/day) during the third week. In week 4, patients who received the low dose in week 3 crossed over to the high dose and vice versa. A patient who had an increase of three or more points on the Hamilton scale during the week the low dose received was classified as worsening. Of the six patients who showed a worsening, three showed plasma levels at or below 50 ng per ml. Of the patients whose plasma levels were above 50 ng per ml during the trial low dose, three out of sixteen showed a worsening ($p = 0.18$ on Fisher's Exact Test, one-tailed). In none of Burrows's studies was there evidence for an upper end of the therapeutic window.

Data from two protriptyline studies are presented in figure 13–3. Whyte and coworkers[507] reported several nonresponders who had high plasma levels and two nonresponders who had low plasma levels. In the other study, Biggs and Ziegler[49] found that almost all nonresponders had low plasma levels. What is particularly striking is that overall, Whyte's patients had higher plasma levels than Biggs's. Whyte and associates[507] suggested an inverted U-shaped relationship, with a lower limit to the therapeutic window of below 140 ng per ml and upper above 260 ng per ml, using a 40 mg dose. Biggs and Ziegler,[49] using a 20 mg dose, found poor responses in patients with plasma levels under 70 ng per ml. This group used a 50 percent lower dose than did Whyte and coworkers, but observed disproportionately lower plasma levels. From this data it is incorrect to state the location of the therapeutic window limits for protriptyline, as these studies disagree with each other as to absolute plasma levels. When determinations using a specific laboratory method are made on patients at steady-state dose, plasma levels should prove identical from study to study and in that sense provide an absolute level. Since protriptyline has an unusually long half-life, patients in protriptyline studies may not necessarily be at steady-state in the first two weeks. In addition, not all assay techniques are completely specific. Fluorometric methods, for example, may be less specific than mass spectroscopic methods.

Several studies of amitriptyline[55,270,271,523] find a lower limit to the therapeutic window but disagree where it is—that is, at 90 ng per ml, 200 ng per ml, or 75 ng per ml, respectively (see figure 13–5). Rickels and his coworkers found that all four good responders had plasma levels above 100 ng per ml and that four out of five nonresponders had plasma levels below 100 ng per ml.[421] When we tabulated the findings from a further ten amitriptyline studies* (see table 13–21), we found more good responders had levels above 100 ng per ml and more moderate or poor responders had levels below 100 ng per ml.

Total amitriptyline plus nortriptyline plasma levels and final Hamilton scores for the ten studies were evaluated using a cubic regression model (see figure 13–4), and no systematic relationship between plasma levels and clinical response could be found ($r^2 = 0.006$). We classified patients into responder or nonresponder categories and constructed a scatter graph of amitriptyline plus nortriptyline plasma levels and clinical response (see figure 13–5). No relationship between plasma level and clinical response appeared. Inspection of the figure shows that most of the responders have about the same plasma levels as the nonresponders. There is no obvious upper end of the therapeutic window where the drug loses effectiveness. At the doses used in this study, nonresponders occur at almost all plasma levels. Only when plasma levels fall below 100 ng per ml does the relative number of nonresponders increase. Thus there seems to be only a very crude relationship between response and plasma levels. The reason for this is unclear.

Three studies (see table 13–19) examine desipramine plasma levels. Summation of

*See references 15, 55, 57, 95, 240, 262, 271, 325, 426, and 523.

the data indicates that the percent of response is low when plasma levels are below 115 ng per ml.

In the well-controlled studies of Glassman and associates[184] and Reisby and coworkers,[414] patients were administered a fixed dose of imipramine yielding plasma levels from 50 ng per ml to 1,000 ng per ml (see table 13–20). These studies, plus more recent work, reported poor clinical responses with low plasma levels (under 180 ng per ml or under 240 ng per ml). They did not find an upper limit for the therapeutic window in the sense that they did not find a loss of efficacy at high plasma levels. They did, of course, find toxicity in some patients with very high plasma levels, but this defines a different type of upper limit to the therapeutic window. When summated, patients with plasma levels below 180 ng per ml responded at a rate of 30 percent, which is about the placebo response rate. About 70 percent of those above 240 ng per ml responded. These findings illustrate a somewhat indeterminate therapeutic range of 180 to 250 ng per ml.

Most reviews place absolute limits on the upper and lower limits of the therapeutic window. This is misleading. Therapeutic windows are not written in stone. For example, if they were absolute and if the limit of the therapeutic window was from 100 to 200, then a patient with 99 ng per ml would be below and a patient with 201 would be above the window. From inspection of figures 13–2, 13–3, and 13–5, it would appear that such an absolute interpretation of the therapeutic window is not supported. Most nonresponders are within the therapeutic window. We believe that the best way to get a feel for plasma levels is not through arbitrarily selected numbers defining the upper or lower end to the therapeutic window, but by placing a given plasma level in the context of the data base on that drug presented graphically. Furthermore, patients within the therapeutic window in one study would be clearly below the therapeutic window in another study. For example, many review articles give the upper limit of the nortriptyline ther-

apeutic window at 140 ng per ml, yet inspection of figure 13–2 shows that many responders have levels above 140 ng per ml.

If patients are at steady-state, a given plasma level should be an absolute number, since it represents the physical presence of a substance in plasma. A plasma level should relate absolutely to another plasma level. These are not arbitrarily defined scores on a rating scale, which are only relative to another rating score on that same scale. Some of this variability can be explained by the fact that different authors measure the tricyclics at different points in time, as all patients are not at steady-state by the fourteenth day of treatment. For example, Asberg measured tricyclics during the first two weeks, while Kragh-Sorensen made his determinations at the fourth week. Perhaps correcting observed levels from the first few weeks to a predicted steady-state would help clarify the difference in normative data from study to study. Plasma levels should be proportioned to doses[7,8] based on what is known of their pharmacokinetics. If we want to change from a plasma level obtained under steady-state conditions from a given dose to a different plasma level, we can adjust dose by simple proportion. A relatively low dose can be adjusted upward or a high dose can be adjusted downward, if this makes clinical sense. The most important data for dose adjustment are side effects and clinical response, and plasma levels in the relative sense can sometimes help in this endeavor.

More work is needed to define the therapeutic window so that the plasma levels can be clinically useful. Not only must the existence of the therapeutic window be firmly established, but it is also necessary for laboratories to agree on its exact location. These figures will help the reader place a given plasma level into perspective. Plasma levels differ widely among individuals due in part to differences in the rate of metabolism, as in the liver. Hence the clinician must adjust the dose for each patient individually to achieve maximum benefit with minimal side effects. Accurately determined plasma levels have the potential to aid in dose adjustment when the literature provides enough data to establish a therapeutic window.

¶ Monoamine Oxidase Inhibitors

A considerable resurgence of interest in the MAOI antidepressants is underway in present-day psychopharmacology. Although numerous factors may contribute to this occurrence, a particularly important one has been the increased safety of their clinical use secondary to the elucidation of the mechanism of hypertensive reactions.[51] The first MAOI widely prescribed as an antidepressant was iproniazid. Iproniazid bears a close relationship to isoniazid, which is a well-established antituberculosis drug; iproniazid itself had originally been developed as an antituberculous agent. Its use for this purpose was discontinued after it was noted to produce euphoria in some tuberculous patients.

Iproniazid's MAO-enzyme-inhibiting properties were discovered in 1952,[522] but only after the first positive reports of its antidepressant effect[102,259,298] were its MAO-inhibiting properties reconsidered and integrated into what has become an important concept in the biogenic amine hypothesis of depression.[62,172,442,444] Unfortunately, iproniazid had to be removed from the market after reports of drug-induced hepatotoxicity causing fatalities in some cases. The hydrazine component of the molecule was held responsible for this adverse reaction, and this stimulated the development of nonhydrazine compounds, of which the only member in clinical use is tranylcypromine sulfate. With the advent of tricyclic antidepressants, which proved to be effective over a wider spectrum of depressive patients, and reports at that time of severe and poorly understood hypertensive reactions associated with the MAOIs, these agents gradually fell into disrepute. MAOIs have entered another more positive phase in their checkered history amid recent advances in technology; better definition of various subcategories of depres-

sion, some of which may respond to MAOIs; and the overall need for a larger armamentarium of effective antidepressants.

Classification and Pharmacological Considerations

Clinically relevant MAOIs are classified into two basic groups, the hydrazine and the nonhydrazine compounds, depending on the presence or absence of a hydrazine moiety. The hydrazine group includes phenelzine sulfate, isocarboxazid, nialamide, and iproniazid phosphate, while the nonhydrazine compounds include tranylcypromine sulfate, pargyline hydrochloride, and the selective MAOIs deprenyl hydrochloride and clorgyline hydrochloride. A substantial portion of the evidence supporting clinical efficacy has been for phenelzine, which also has been the most often prescribed. Although it has been suggested that the hydrazine compounds may be the more effective antidepressants among the two groups, they have the disadvantage of being associated with severe adverse reactions such as hepatotoxicity and, very rarely, a lupuslike syndrome.

Tranylcypromine, the only nonhydrazine MAOI in clinical use as an antidepressant, is an interesting compound in that it is metabolized to amphetamine in the body. Furthermore, it inhibits NE reuptake and in a sense acts like a combination of amphetamine, tricyclic, and MAOI. Its side-effect profile differs from that of the hydrazine group because, although lacking hepatotoxic effects, it may induce a more severe hypertensive reaction.

The definition of the MAOI class of antidepressants indicates a common property of these drugs: the inhibition of the MAO enzyme that is responsible for the inactivation of catecholamines such as DA, 5HT, and NE. The most prominent and earliest consequence of MAO inhibition is a rapid increase of brain monoamine concentration.[471] Upon continued administration, adaptive changes secondary to these elevated monoamine levels begins to occur. These include a reduction in amine synthesis via a feedback mechanism[289,346] resulting in a gradual decline of monoamine concentration toward normal levels. Other dynamic readjustments include a deacceleration of neuronal firing rates that has been demonstrated in 5HT- and NE-containing neurons,[4,73] perhaps reflecting a presynaptic autoreceptor feedback mechanism. After several weeks of treatment, a reduction in the number of alpha-2 and beta-adrenergic receptors as well as the number of 5HT receptors occurs.[85,374,439,481] Beta-receptor functional activity is also decreased as measured by NE-stimulated cyclic adenosine monophosphate (AMP) formation.

Possible correlations between the neurochemical alterations described and the behavioral responses observed with MAOIs have been explored in a number of ways. Using platelet MAO inhibition as a quantitative measure of drug activity, it has been shown that phenelzine (dose approximately 1 mg/kg) produces 80 to 85 percent enzyme inhibition.[425] This level of inhibition or more is required to obtain significantly greater antidepressant or antianxiety activity as compared to lesser degrees of inhibition.[107] No connection between response to phenelzine and pretreatment levels of platelet MAO activity has been reported.

The existence of two functional forms or subtypes of the enzyme, MAO-A and MAO-B,[236] each with a tendency toward substrate specificity[519] and different distributions in various tissues in the body, has been defined. MAO-A selectively deaminates 5HT and NE,[169,193,236,339] while MAO-B preferentially degrades benzylamine and phenylethylamine.[261,517] There is some speculation that human brain has a modest predominance of MAO-A activity and, in further speculation, it follows that a selective inhibitor of MAO-A would have a more focused site of action, thereby bypassing other tissues and consequently having fewer side effects.[356] The comparative efficacy and safety of these so-called selective inhibitors are currently topics of investigation. It has been suggested that clinical antidepressant effects follow from inhibition of

MAO-A, and this has been supported by clinical studies showing some antidepressant efficacy of the selective MAO-A inhibitor, clorgyline hydrochloride. However, other studies suggest MAO-B inhibitors to be effective.[405]

These suppositions are simplistic and need further clarification, as the selective action of these agents established *in vitro* in acute experiments may dissipate during chronic treatment with loss of MAO selectivity and limitation of clinical advantage.[72,294] Currently prescribed MAOI antidepressants inhibit both MAO-A and MAO-B. Furthermore, MAO-A inhibitors may, along with their antidepressant effects, display the characteristic adverse reaction associated with the more routinely prescribed MAOIs. This is unlike the MAO-B inhibitor deprenyl, which has not been reported to have any significant adverse effect with its clinical use as an antiparkinsonian agent. Thus the predicted advantage of clinical efficacy with fewer side effects has yet to be confirmed for any individual drug.

PHARMACOKINETICS

MAOIs are, as a rule, rapidly absorbed through the gut and are widely distributed through all parts of the body. Acetylation has been postulated to be the major biotransformation pathway, and patients can be separated into slow or fast acetylators by the rate with which they acetylate a sulfonamide drug.[139] Initial reports have supported this relationship between acetylator phenotype and clinical response with greater improvement[237] and more severe side effects[140] described among the slow acetylators, but later investigations have been unable to confirm these findings.[107,312] A study that defined patients by the rate of acetylation of a loading dose of sulfapyridine used adequate dosages of phenelzine (60 mg/day), achieved platelet MAO inhibition of 86 percent after six weeks, and found no differences between fast and slow acetylators in either clinical or pharmacological measures.[425] A recent placebo-controlled double-blind study using phenelzine showed slow acetylators to have a more rapid therapeutic response, evident after two weeks of treatment.[365] However, there was no difference in improvement after six weeks of treatment between the slow and fast acetylators. Acetylation has not yet been proven to be the primary metabolic pathways of phenelzine, and there is currently insufficient evidence to support the pretreatment routine estimation of acetylator phenotype.

Clinical Applications

Tables 13–1 and 13–22 list a number of controlled studies demonstrating the efficacy of MAOIs compared to a placebo and also to imipramine, which provides a good standard. There is evidence from well-controlled studies that iproniazid, tranylcypromine, phenelzine, and pargyline are all therapeutically effective, although pargyline is marketed only as an antihypertensive. On the basis of the evidence, one may rank the efficacy of the MAOIs as follows: Iproniazid appears to be most effective, nialamide and isocarboxazid the least effective, and phenelzine and tranylcypromine occupy an intermediate position.

Substantial controversy still exists over the clinical indications for MAOIs. As a class, the MAOIs seem very slightly less effective than the tricyclic drugs, particularly in the treatment of depression with endogenous features. The combined data from a number of studies on the imipramine-phenelzine comparison yielded an improvement rate of 71 percent for imipramine (138 of 196 patients) versus 62 percent (101 of 164 patients) for phenelzine. In view of this fact and considering the sufficiently dangerous side effects associated with the currently prescribed MAOIs, it is improbable that they will be found more useful than the tricyclic antidepressants in the routine treatment of endogenous depression. However, there is suggestive evidence to support a role for MAOIs in the treatment of nonendogenous or atypical varieties of depression. Perhaps the earliest such evidence was found in patients described as having a mixture of phobic, hysterical, and anxiety symptoms together with a lack of energy and diurnal mood swings.[505] Similar depressive symptoms reported to be responsive to MAOI treatment have been delineated by cluster analysis and described as an admixture of anxiety and minor neurotic symptoms, such as fatigue, obsessional symptoms, and depersonalization.[364] In general, depression associated with a strong anxiety component, rapid changes in mood, overreactivity, and somatization has been shown to have a better chance of improvement with MAOIs than depression associated with the typical endogenous features of insomnia, weight loss, and guilt.[410,424,490]

Recognizing the clinical heterogeneity of depressive symptoms, particularly those that have a potential response to MAOIs, it is important to place patients along a continuum, identifying them as having a predominantly endogenous or nonendogenous depression. In a double-blind, placebo-controlled experiment, eighty-seven outpatient depressives were thus identified and assigned to six weeks of phenelzine treatment or placebo.[424] The phenelzine-treated patients showed significantly greater improvement in composite ratings of total depression, total anxiety, somatic anxiety, hypochondriasis-agitation, and psychomotor change. Furthermore, responders had complaints with more typically nonendogenous content, such as fatigue, phobias, somatic complaints, anxiety, and chronic depression. These findings were replicated in a later study by the same authors[410] and more recently by Leibowitz and associates.[279] Panic attacks and related symptomatology (endogenous anxiety or phobic anxiety syndrome) have been shown to respond to phenelzine treatment, and this has been documented in numerous reports.[295,469]

Several hospitalized populations that included schizo-affective and chronic anergic schizophrenic patients failed to improve with MAOI treatment. Clinical reports indicate that some patients who fail to respond to tricyclics or ECT will respond to MAOIs.

TABLE 13–22

Studies Comparing Phenelzine and Placebo

Study	Patients	Dosage/Duration	Type of Improvement	Results — Phenelzine	Results — Placebo	Significance
Rees and Davies[411]	20 patients.	90 mg/day for 3 weeks before crossover	Complete to moderate	14	7	0.006
			Slight change to moderately worse	6	13	
Schildkraut et al.[443]	Severely depressed middle-aged patients with vegetative signs.	45–60 mg, 3 weeks	Improvement	5	0	0.01
			No improvement	1	5	
Robinson et al.[424]	44 phenelzine, 43 placebo. Moderately depressed with associated features of anxiety, phobia, and somatic concerns.	45–75 mg (58.5 mg mean) for 6 weeks	Definite improvement	21	10	0.02
			Possible improvement to worse	19	26	
Ravaris et al.[410]	49 of 62 completed: 14 phenelzine—06 mg, 16 phenelzine—30 mg, 19 placebo.	30 mg and 60 mg for 6 weeks	Definitely to possibly improved	11	10	0.03
			No change to worse	5	11	
	Matched groups, age 23–81 years. Depressed mood associated with anxiety, phobia, somatic concerns, coping problems.		Phenelzine (30 mg) = placebo			
Johnstone and Marsh[238]	Completed: 39 slow acetylators, 33 fast acetylators. Neurotic depression.	45–90 mg/day for 3 weeks before crossover	Improvement on weekly severity ratings			
			Slow acetylators	Phenelzine > placebo		0.0018
			Fast acetylators	Phenelzine ≥ placebo		0.077[a]
Lascelles[272]	40 atypical anxious depressives: 20 phenelzine, 20 placebo.	45 mg/day for 4 weeks before crossover	Marked to moderate improvement	6	7	
			No change to worse	5	13	
Leibowitz et al.[279]	Patients met Research Diagnostic Criteria for major, minor, or intermittent depression—associated with mood reactivity, rejection, sensitivity, and atypical vegetative features.	60 mg/day for 4 weeks	Improvement	10	7	0.02
			No improvement	5	17	
	24 placebo, 15 phenelzine.		No improvement	5	17	

TABLE 13-22 (Continued)

			Type of Improvement	Results Phenelzine	Results Placebo	Significance
Study	Patients	Dosage/Duration				
Rowan, Paykel, and Parker[430]	Mild to moderate depressives or mixed anxiety depression (severe endogenous or bipolar types excluded). 42 phenelzine, 45 placebo.	60 mg (+15 mg optional) for 6 weeks	Marked improvement Some improvement to worsening	41 59	18[b] 82	0.05
Raft et al.[407]	Patients attending pain clinic with definite primary major depression according to Feighner criteria. 10 phenelzine, 6 placebo.	1.5 mg/kg/day for 5 weeks	Phenelzine > placebo[c] at week 5			0.05
Raskin et al.[409]	Completed: 110 phenelzine, 111 placebo. 36% psychotic, 17% schizophrenic, 51% neurotic. Significant placebo dropout rate.	45 mg/day for 5 weeks	Phenelzine = placebo			NS
Hare, Dominian, and Sharpe[211]	43 predominantly day-hospital patients with primary depressive illness.	30 mg/day for 2 weeks	Phenelzine > placebo on anxiety Phenelzine = placebo on depression			NS
Shephard[459]	61 phenelzine, 61 placebo.	60 mg/day for 4 weeks	Improved No improvement	19 23	31 28	NS
Greenblatt, Grosser, and Wechsler[197]	Severely depressed (includes schizophrenics [20%] and character disorders)	60 mg/day (+15 mg optional) for 8 weeks	Improved No improvement	23 25	40 27	0.14
Agnew et al.[5]	Depressed schizophrenics and schizoid personality disorders. 4 phenelzine, 5 placebo.	45 mg/day for 3 weeks	Much improved Slight improvement to worse	2 2	0 4	0.12

[a]Trend toward improvement with drug slightly short of significance.
[b]Percent improved on total depression ratings.
[c]Improvement on weekly severity ratings.

Therapeutic improvement with MAOIs often occurs from four to six weeks after the initiation of therapy, and its onset is frequently quite dramatic.

In summary, there is sufficient evidence to support a role for MAOIs in outpatient depressives with a predominance of nonendogenous symptomatology. Although in one well-done study[411] the MAOIs have been shown to be effective in endogenous patients, they have little or no advantage over tricyclics in the average severe endogenous-type depressions. Clinical evidence indicates that some patients who do not respond to tricyclics may respond to MAOIs, so a trial period on MAOIs for tricyclic nonresponders may be useful. In addition, MAOIs may have a role in panic attack syndrome (phobic anxiety syndrome or endogenous anxiety syndrome). As a practical consideration, the clinician should review the patient's capacity to follow the dietary restrictions required by MAOIs.

¶ Psychomotor Stimulants

The psychomotor stimulants include amphetamine, dextroamphetamine, methylphenidate hydrochloride, deanol acetamidobenzoate, and pipradrol hydrochloride. The British General Practitioner Research Group[175] found amphetamine to be less effective than placebo in the treatment of depressed outpatients. In another British study, amphetamine proved less effective than phenelzine and no better than a placebo in the treatment of depression.[211] In a VA study, dextroamphetamine was found to be no more effective than placebo in treating hospitalized depressed patients.[359] Indeed, amphetamine given in combination with chlorpromazine produced a less favorable response in chronic schizophrenic patients than did phenothiazine alone.

Uncontrolled clinical evidence suggests that amphetamine may have some value for a rare outpatient with mild depression, but there is no evidence of its effectiveness in moderate to severe depression. Methylphenidate and pemoline have been suggested to be of value in treating outpatients with mild depression, particularly those patients who drink three or more cups of coffee a day. Patients who complain of fatigue may not necessarily have true biological depressions, and we must limit generalization from one type of patient to another. Any antidepressant effect has been documented in only a very few controlled studies, and hence these findings cannot be considered proven. Additional investigation is needed to identify clearly the subtype of patient who may be benefited by such treatment. As with amphetamines, there is no evidence indicating that methylphenidate is beneficial in cases of moderate to severe depression. Except for the hint that a subgroup of mildly depressed patients may be helped, there is as yet inadequate evidence to support the efficacy of methylphenidate in depression.

The amphetaminelike drugs have been known to cause palpitations, jitteriness, paranoid psychoses, and other toxic effects. Dextroamphetamine may produce psychic dependence, and depression can occur after drug discontinuance. High doses of amphetamine can produce a florid psychosis that resembles paranoid schizophrenia. Even small doses of amphetamine have been known to induce psychotic episodes in patients with active, prodromal, or residual (or in remission) schizophrenic diseases.

The evidence for the efficacy of the other drugs generally classified with the stimulants in the treatment of depression is even weaker than the evidence just presented. However, there is considerable evidence that methylphenidate, pemoline, and amphetamines are effective in the reduction and control of hyperkinetic behavior in children, a pharmacological paradox of considerable clinical significance. The stimulants can also postpone the deterioration in psychomotor performance often concomitant with fatigue, a property that may be useful in carefully selected instances.

¶ Benzodiazepines as Antidepressants

Since anxiety is often associated with depression, a reasonable question that comes to mind is: Are benzodiazepines effective antidepressants? In a thoughtful, comprehensive literature review, Schatzberg and Cole[441] failed to find any study that indicated benzodiazepines were significantly better than antidepressants. On the other hand, benzodiazepines were significantly inferior to the antidepressants in ten studies, and there were no significant differences in the other nine studies. For example, Ives and associates[229] divided depressed patients into several groups and treated them with phenelzine plus chlordiazepoxide hydrochloride, phenelzine alone, a placebo alone, and a placebo plus chlordiazepoxide. Chlordiazepoxide did not alleviate depression with the placebo or with the phenelzine.

In separate studies, Kay, Fahy, and Garside,[245] Lipman and associates,[293] and Covi and coworkers[101] found that diazepam was inferior to imipramine in treating depression. The majority of studies show that benzodiazepines are virtually ineffective in the treatment of depression. Some investigations, however, show that minor tranquilizers may temporarily and presumably nonspecifically relieve some symptoms of depression. Alprazolam may be unique in this regard, in that recent reports indicate it may have antidepressant properties unexplained by its anxiolytic actions. More work is needed in this area to understand the exact role of anxiety in depression, but minor tranquilizers have only a minor role in treating true depression.

Anxiolytic-tricyclic Combinations

Roche has introduced a fixed-dose preparation that combines chlordiazepoxide and amitriptyline for the treatment of mixed anxiety-depression outpatients. They demonstrate effectiveness of this combination by the results from a double-blind, multicenter collaborative study of 279 outpatients that compared the drug (trade name Limbitrol, 10 mg chlordiazepoxide plus 25 mg amitriptyline) to amitriptyline alone, chlordiazepoxide alone, and placebo.[154] Chlordiazepoxide and amitriptyline are both sedative drugs that possess antianxiety properties and are beneficial to insomnia and psychic and somatic anxiety. Due to their combined sedative-anxiolytic properties, it is not surprising that they exert an additive effect on anxiety symptoms. In one week of treatment, the combination clearly produced greater improvement on items from the Hamilton Depression Rating Scale such as insomnia, agitation, and somatic and psychic anxiety. This effect is also reflected in overall scores on the Global Hamilton Depression Scale, and the Beck Inventory demonstrated that the combination was superior to either of the individual drugs at the end of the first week. After several weeks amitriptyline alone was equally as effective as the combination on many of the measures and slightly, but not significantly, exceeded the combination on certain measures, such as the depression factor of the Hopkins Symptom Checklist and the Beck Depression Inventory. Unfortunately, the authors present selected findings rather than a more systematic portrayal of the data.

Rickels and associates[417] conducted a comparable study of 243 mild to moderately depressed outpatients suffering from either a reactive neurotic depression or a mixed anxiety-depressive reaction. Owing to the fact that patients were first evaluated at the end of two weeks, it is impossible to determine if the week 1 effect observed by the Roche collaborative study occurred here as well. This study demonstrated that an overall drug effect was statistically significant both for the combination and for each of the individual components, in comparison to the placebo. However, it is difficult to interpret this study due to the investigators' failure to present statistics on the comparisons between the combination versus each drug separately.

Hare[212] completed two studies that used

twenty outpatients with mixed anxiety-depression. He compared the drug combination against amitriptyline given alone. In the first study, the former appeared superior after one week. By the third week, this difference had been equalized. In the second study, the effects of the combination were similar to those from the amitriptyline alone. Haider[205] examined seriously depressed inpatients. While he only assessed results at the end of a three-week period, he noted that the combination was superior to amitryptiline alone.

While the combination may help at one week, after three weeks it is difficult to conclude that it clearly has proved to be superior. Another methodological problem is diagnostic homogeneity. Some method is needed to separate out the two populations of patients: one with pure depression and only mild secondary anxiety, and the other with pure anxiety accompanied by only mild secondary depression. Also, note the nonspecific nature of these rating scales: for example, depression scales have anxiety items and vice versa. Some symptoms are entirely nonspecific. Furthermore, improvement in anxiety may artificially improve depression due to a sort of halo effect. The addition of an antianxiety agent, however, in the first week of antidepressant therapy would do no harm and might possibly have some beneficial effect.

¶ Dihydro-ergotoxine Mesylate

Many well-controlled double-blind scientific studies found that dihydro-ergotoxine mesylate (Hydergine) is somewhat effective in treating impaired CNS function in the elderly. However, it is doubtful that alleviation of symptoms such as confusion, disorientation, poor self-care, depression, anxiety, agitation, and irritability results from the drug's vasodilating action. Improvement with dihydro-ergotoxine mesylate is noted to be slow in onset (about three to six months), and further research is essential to determine the mechanism by which the drug accomplishes

clinical improvement. It is clear that elderly patients do slightly but progressively better over time compared to what they would have done on placebo, but how this is accomplished is unknown. Some have speculated that the drug has mild antidepressant properties, but the mode of action is unknown.

¶ Lithium

The recognition that lithium, a simple cation, can have such an impressive effect on behavior constitutes one of the more remarkable chapters in modern therapeutics. Lithium's first medicinal use was as a solvent for bladder calculi.[493] Thus the first reported use of lithium in the treatment of an affective disorder was under the premise that it increased the secretion of uric acid, thereby causing an amelioration of the uric acid diathesis that was responsible for the depression.[206] In the 1940s lithium chloride was developed as a salt substitute for cardiac patients. With the knowledge now available, it is not surprising that the ensuing salt depletion in these patients precipitated a vicious cycle that resulted in lithium toxicity. Lithium was hastily removed from the market by the FDA in 1949 after reports of several fatalities.

That same year Cade[70] published the first report on the use of lithium in the manic phase of bipolar illness. In an attempt to alter the postulated toxic effects of uric acid obtained from the urine of manic patients, Cade used its most soluble form, lithium urate. Upon injection into guinea pigs, the substance not only failed to show the expected toxicity of the urates, but made the normally excitable animals placid and lethargic. Upon determining that the calming effect was due to lithium, Cade confirmed this serendipitous finding in ten manic patients, all of whom showed marked improvement in their manic symptoms.[70] Although these findings were replicated in uncontrolled trials with small samples,[352] reactions from the scientific community remained modest. The first major double-blind controlled trial was conducted by Schou and associates.[450] Subsequent investigations established these findings and culminated in the approval by the FDA in 1970 for its use in the acute treatment of mania and in 1974 for the prophylaxis of bipolar affective disorder. The history of its development illustrates perhaps only too well the unfortunate moratorium that sometimes occurs between discovery and application.

Mode of Action

Lithium is present as a trace element in normal human tissue, but its physiological function, if any, is unknown. It is the lightest known metal; other members of its periodic group are sodium and potassium.

Lithium has varying effects on monoamine activity depending on its acute or chronic administration. When given for longer periods, lithium stimulates turnover of 5HT, possibly by inducing tryptophan hydroxylase activity.[308,373] It also increases NE reuptake across synaptosomal membranes.[86] Reports on its action on dopaminergic systems are complex, including a decrease in DA synthesis[166] and DA receptor binding[379] and the prevention of DA receptor supersensitivity.[255] Other effects, such as a decrease in acetylcholine synthesis, have also been reported.[14] The relevance of these neurochemical findings to the observed clinical actions and side effects of the drug is unclear.

Lithium has been shown to inhibit hormone-stimulated adenylate cyclase in many organs throughout the body, including the brain. The action of many neurotransmitters, neuromodulators, and hormones are mediated in part by the production of cyclic AMP in the target cell. Cyclic AMP is involved in neuronal transmission, and it is not inconceivable that the therapeutic actions of lithium may be to some extent dependent on cyclic AMP's decreased production.[132] More specifically, adenylate cyclase inhibition may explain some of the side effects of lithium. Lithium reduces release of thyroxine from the thyroid gland and inhibits the effect of antidiuretic hormone (ADH) on the distal renal tubule. Both these actions can quite possibly be due to the inability of the hormones to express their full activity because of the lack of cyclic AMP.

Pharmacokinetics

Lithium is absorbed more rapidly from the gastrointestinal tract than it can be distributed in the tissues. This gives rise to a peak concentration that occurs within one to four hours of an oral dose, and this peak is often two to three times the trough value. Lithium is neither metabolized nor bound to plasma proteins and passes readily into every fluid compartment. Its distribution across cellular membranes differs in different cell groups. Its concentration in the red blood cell (RBC) is, however, lower than in plasma, and the ratio of RBC to plasma lithium has been the focus of much interest. This ratio is under genetic control.[127] Experiments demonstrate the existence of a lithium-sodium exchange diffusion countertransport at the cell membrane that serves to expel lithium from the RBC[361] and presumably from tissue in general. Patients with low lithium exchange diffusion countertransport, and hence with high RBC lithium, may have an inherent deficit in cell membrane function that has been postulated to render them susceptible to the development of an affective disorder.

Clinical Applications of Lithium in Affective Disorders

TREATMENT OF ACUTE MANIA

There is today a large body of literature supporting the efficacy of lithium carbonate in the treatment of acute mania. Prior to the surge of interest in lithium in the mid-1960s, very few controlled trials described pharmacological interventions in this disorder. Due to the practical difficulties in managing excited manic patients, a biasing of the sample occurred when severely disturbed patients could not complete the trial because of the need for more acute management. After the initial discovery of the antimanic effects of lithium,[70] these findings were replicated by Noack and Trautner[352] and in numerous other uncontrolled, small-sample studies. The first major double-blind, placebo-controlled trial was conducted by Schou and associates.[450] The sample consisted of thirty "typical" and eight "atypical" patients, all treated with either lithium or placebo. The dose of lithium ranged from 900 mg to 1,800 mg daily. As prevention constituted one of the four outcome criteria, this may have confused the results somewhat. Nevertheless, there was an improvement rate of 90 percent for the "typical" and 62 percent for the "atypical" group.

In the double-blind crossover study by Maags,[300] a fixed dose of lithium (1,500 mg) was alternated with placebo. Twenty-eight manic patients were randomly assigned to two groups, one of which received lithium for two weeks followed by a two-week drug-free period and ending with a two-week placebo period. The other group followed the same schedule but received the placebo first. Lithium was significantly superior to placebo in the eighteen patients who completed the trial.

Stokes and associates[480] studied the effects of lithium and placebo in a double-blind trial conducted with thirty-eight manic patients. Active and placebo treatments were given in four alternate periods of seven to ten days each, all patients starting with lithium. Symptom resolution was significantly better during periods of lithium administration.

Lithium and chlorpromazine were evaluated in a comparative trial in 255 manic patients who were divided into "highly active" or "mildly active" groups.[394] This categorization was particularly informative because prior studies, although establishing the efficacy of lithium in mild and moderately severe manic patients, had not dealt with severely ill subjects. Chlorpromazine (200–3,000 mg/day) was significantly superior to lithium (1,800 mg/day) in the "highly active" group, and the magnitude of this effect was evident in a number of ways. Chlorproma-

zine was superior in its speed of action and in the magnitude of its effect upon the reduction of psychotic disorganization and manic symptoms. There was no difference between the two drugs in the "mildly active" group. Two other comparative studies[235,485] report the superiority of lithium over chlorpromazine, although in one,[485] dosages of medication used were too low and, in the other,[235] the difference was not significant.

In a three-week comparative trial of active medication, manic patients were randomly assigned to lithium, chlorpromazine, or haloperidol treatment.[461] There was no significant difference in ratings between the lithium and haloperidol groups, and both of these were superior to chlorpromazine. However, a substantially higher proportion of patients on lithium were considered ready for discharge than were patients on either neuroleptic. The authors concluded that while neuroleptics may help suppress the active symptoms in the acute phase, lithium was better able to qualitatively change the underlying manic process, thereby resulting in greater subjective improvement.

Numerous studies done all over the world uniformly support the therapeutic efficacy of lithium in acute mania.* These reports are perhaps more conclusive for mild to moderately severe symptomatology. In patients who are severely ill, the period between initiation of treatment and therapeutic response to lithium may be too long, usually about ten days. Such cases can be treated initially with neuroleptics. Once the illness is under a reasonable degree of control, lithium can be added to the regimen and the neuroleptic tapered off and discontinued.

TREATMENT OF DEPRESSION

The efficacy of lithium in the management of various components of the major affective disorders is now firmly established. Enough evidence supports its use in the treatment of the acutely manic state and in the prophy-

*See references 21, 34, 63, 190, 201, 213, 217, 347, 448, 455, and 496.

laxis of both mania and depression in bipolar and unipolar illness. Its most debatable role, however, is probably as an antidepressant in the management of an acute depressive episode. Although some open and some controlled studies conclude that lithium does have an antidepressant action,* other investigators have refuted this claim. [157,446,479]

Interpretation of some of these studies is difficult, as not all differentiate between unipolar and bipolar patients. In the ones that do, data suggest that lithium may have a differential and more efficacious effect in bipolar patients presenting with depression than in unipolar patients. Evidence to support an effect in unipolar patients may be diluted by the fact that 10 to 20 percent of any group of patients with unipolar disorder will eventually have a manic episode and be reclassified. Others have bipolar II disease or have mild hypomania, which may not be seen as abnormal. In other words, a fraction of all unipolar patients are actually bipolar patients.

A comparative study of lithium and imipramine in depression was done in twenty-nine patients randomly assigned to either treatment. [157] Imipramine was reported to be closely superior, although statistical significance was not reported, nor were lithium levels or the proportion of bipolar to unipolar patients. Mendels, [322] in a placebo-controlled lithium trial, reported lithium to have an active antidepressant effect. Seventy-five to 85 percent of bipolar and 30 to 50 percent of unipolar patients showed improvement. The response rate in unipolar patients in general does not seem to be very different to that seen with placebo. A recent well-controlled study by Worrall and associates [513] reports superiority of lithium over imipramine in sixty-three unipolar and bipolar depressed patients. Lithium's antidepressant response did not appear until the second or third week. Stokes and associates [480] reported no significant difference between lithium and placebo. Similarly, in the overall study by Lingjaerde and coworkers, [292] there was a slight,

but not overwhelming, statistically significant difference between a combination of lithium and tricyclic and tricyclic alone. The combination treatment can be safely and effectively used. Thus, although unequivocal conclusions cannot be drawn, there is some evidence that lithium has acute antidepressant properties in some depressive patients, particularly bipolars.

Clinical Application of Lithium in Other Conditions

TREATMENT OF AGGRESSIVE BEHAVIOR

A number of studies report an antiaggressive effect of lithium. In a double-blind, placebo-controlled trial conducted in sixty-six male prisoners with a history of poor impulse control and episodic assaultive behavior, lithium was administered for up to three months, preceded and followed by a drug-free period of one month. [457] Lithium had a significant antiaggressive effect compared with placebo, and a relapse of aggressive behavior occurred during the drug-free month at the end of the study. This antiaggressive property has been reported in different populations, including epileptic patients, [311] mentally retarded patients, [105,512] and children and adolescents. [281] Dostal [128] reported a lithium trial in fourteen mentally retarded adolescents displaying aggressive and hyperkinetic features. His observation was that patients with such behavior who lacked an accompanying affective component demonstrated practically no therapeutic response. However, in those patients who did demonstrate an affective component, there was a 65 percent reduction in the total incidence of acute aggressive outbursts.

TREATMENT OF DISORDERS OF CHILDHOOD AND ADOLESCENCE

Although typical presentations of bipolar illness are rare before puberty, the few case reports that are available indicate that these children respond very well to treatment with

*See references 42, 191, 234, 322, 323, and 353

lithium.[520] In addition, lithium has been found to be effective in selected cases of numerous other psychiatric syndromes. What appears to be predictive of a treatment response is the concomitant occurrence of either an affective symptom or a positive family history of affective disorder.[520] Thus individual patients with symptoms of childhood schizophrenia, hyperactive behavior, poor impulse control, and unsocialized aggressive behavior have all been noted to respond to treatment.[25] The affective component does not necessarily have to be the major psychiatric symptom and can be associated with a wide spectrum of other symptoms including anorexia, auditory hallucinations, and epilepsy. It is noteworthy that a number of patients who showed improvement had positive indicators of CNS dysfunctioning, such as abnormal electroencephalograms and neuropsychological testing.

TREATMENT OF OTHER CONDITIONS

There have been claims that lithium may be effective in decreasing drinking behavior in alcoholic patients.[147,260,415] This has been questioned by Pond and associates.[390] A VA collaborative trial of lithium in alcoholic patients is underway. This is a very important area in which clinical trials are needed.

Lithium has been used in research trials for a number of nonpsychiatric conditions such as hyperthyroidism, neutropenia, cluster headache, and the pancreatic cholera syndrome. Its mode of action in the latter affliction has been linked with its ability to block adenylate cyclase, thereby preventing the action of the vasoactive intestinal peptide that is secreted by the pancreatic tumor.

Adjustment of Lithium Dosage

In mild to moderately severe mania, lithium can be initiated as the primary medication. The disadvantage is its slow onset of action with a lag period of two to three weeks before full effects are seen. This is offset by its relatively mellow, more pleasant, and more specific effect on the patient.

In more severely manic patients, where the threat of violence or the catastrophic results of poor judgment coupled with poor impulse control are omnipresent, lithium's slow onset of action is a decided disadvantage. In such cases, acute management can be done with a neuroleptic, the neuroleptic being discontinued after lithium has been instituted once reasonable control begins to be achieved.

If indicated in any given patient, therapeutic use of lithium leads directly into prophylactic use. However, prophylactic use may be started during a depression or a normothymic interval between the two phases. Ongoing tricyclic antidepressant medication is not a contraindication to the starting of lithium during a depressive episode, as the tricyclic may actually enhance the antidepressant effects of lithium or vice versa.[291,292]

The starting dose of lithium in healthy young adults being treated for mania or depression as inpatients is 900 mg per day. This is increased fairly rapidly over the next few days with frequent measurements of serum lithium. In older patients or those with some compromising factors that may increase lithium levels, such as the concomitant use of diuretics, lithium can be started at a lower dose. The lithium level should be titrated and maintained within the range of 0.6 to 1.0 milliequivalent per liter (meq/l) in the treatment of mania and within a range of 0.5 to 1.0 meq/l during prophylaxis. Furthermore, the level should always be raised above 1.0 meq/l, up to as much as 1.6 meq/l, in patients who have not previously responded.

The use of a test to determine lithium dose requirements has been reported.[89,473] The dosage required to achieve a therapeutic level can then be estimated and the patient started directly on that dose.

In an attempt to standardize the interval between the last dose of lithium and withdrawal of blood for serum lithium concentration, a twelve-hour period has been accepted as standard.[10] This is known as the standardized twelve-hour lithium concentration and is normally assumed of any level reported unless otherwise stated.

Prophylactic Uses of Lithium

In his original report in 1949, Cade noted that a patient treated with lithium relapsed when medication was discontinued.[70,71] Gershon and Trautner,[179] Noack and Trautner,[352] and others began to use lithium to maintain remission in patients who experienced frequent relapses and who had previously required maintenance shock treatment.

The relapse observation was later reported and extended in Denmark by Schou and associates[450] and Baastrup[34,35] and in the United States by Gershon and Yuwiler,[180] and was also noted independently by Hartigan,[213] who clearly expounded its prophylactic use. The term normothymic was proposed by Schou[445] to describe drugs that acted specifically against affective disease.

To test this hypothesis, Baastrup and Schou analyzed[36,37,448] a naturalistic study (which has become a psychiatric "classic") on eighty-eight patients who had experienced recurrent manic-depressive illnesses. They compared the frequency of episodes of illness during a period after lithium treatment with their frequency during an equivalent period before lithium treatment. Prior to lithium treatment, the patients spent an average of thirteen weeks a year in a manic or depressed state; after lithium treatment, they spent less than two weeks a year in this state. Similarly, relapses occurred on an average of every eight months before treatment; during lithium maintenance, relapses occurred on the average of once every sixty to eighty-five months.

Lithium prevents the recurrence of both manic and depressive episodes in bipolar patients and the recurrence of depressive episodes in unipolar patients. Patients respond better to lithium after they have received this treatment for some months or years. This may be due in part to the fact that a physician will find the most effective individual dose after experience with a particular patient. In addition, a long normothymic period may lead to stabilization of the patient's social and vocational functioning, which may in turn reinforce his overall stability.

STUDIES OF LITHIUM PROPHYLAXIS IN AFFECTIVE DISORDERS

The best hypothesis-confirmation data on lithium prophylaxis come from carefully executed random-assignment, double-blind studies comparing the effects of lithium and placebo. This section will review the evidence for the fact that lithium does exert prophylactic effects in affective illness and develop information as to whether it is prophylactic in both bipolar and unipolar illness and whether it is equally prophylactic for manic and depressive states in bipolar illness. Twelve studies are presented comparing placebo with lithium using a random-assignment and blind-evaluation method. In addition to these, Persson's study,[378] which uses matched patients and provides further confirmatory evidence, is included in table 13–23.

Baastrup, Poulson, and Schou dramatically demonstrated lithium's effects on patients in Denmark who had been maintained on lithium for at least one year and therefore were well stabilized.[39] This ensured that these particular patients had the type of illness that responds to lithium. Random-assignment, double-blind methods were used. None of the patients who received lithium for five months relapsed, compared with relapses in 55 percent of the bipolar patients and 53 percent of the unipolar patients taking placebo (see table 13–24).

A collaborative study conducted by Coppen and associates[90,91] at four separate centers in Great Britain randomly assigned patients to lithium or placebo for periods of up to two years. Lithium clearly demonstrated prophylactic properties. Similar results were obtained by Mendlewicz, Fieve, and Stallone[324] in New York City. In two studies, Prien, Caffey, and Klett[393,395,396,397] followed manic and depressed patients in VA hospitals and public and private hospitals to assess a two-year lithium prophylactic maintenance therapy program. Their reports, along with

TABLE 13-23
Effectiveness of Lithium Versus Placebo in Preventing Relapse[a]

Investigators[b]	N	Patients in lithium group		N	Patients in placebo group	
		Relapsed N (%)	Not relapsed N (%)		Relapsed N (%)	Not relapsed N (%)
Baastrup, Poulsen, and Schou[39]	45	0 (0)	45 (100)	39	21 (54)	18 (46)
Coppen et al.[90, 91]	28	4 (14)	24 (86)	36	33 (92)	3 (8)
Hullen, McDonald, and Allsopp[224, 225]	18	1 (6)	17 (94)	18	6 (33)	12 (67)
Mendelwicz et al.[324, 474]	36	12 (33)	24 (67)	36	27 (75)	9 (25)
Prien, Caffey, and Klett[393, 395-397]	97	48 (49)	49 (51)	102	91 (89)	11 (11)
Prien, Caffey, and Klett[393, 395-397]	37	18 (49)	19 (51)	31	28 (90)	3 (10)
Cundall, Brooks, and Murray[104]	16	7 (44)	9 (56)	16	13 (81)	3 (19)
Persson et al.[378]	33	11 (33)	22 (67)	33	25 (76)	8 (24)
Fieve et al.[130, 156, 158]	29	8 (28)	22 (72)	31	26 (84)	5 (16)
Fieve, Platman, and Plutchik[157]	7	1 (14)	6 (86)	11	7 (64)	4 (36)
Kane et al.[243]	11	3 (27)	8 (73)	13	11 (85)	2 (15)
Glen, Johnson, and Shepherd[185]	12	5 (42)	7 (58)	9	8 (89)	1 (11)
Prien et al.[400]	37	21 (57)	16 (43)	34	24 (71)	10 (29)

[a]By the Fisher Exact Test. Overall significance $p = 2 \times 10^{-34}$.
[b]Most of the studies used a noncrossover design with random assignment and blind evaluation; however, the study of Cundall, Brooks, and Murray used an open crossover design, and Persson's study used a matched design (control patients were matched with lithium patients).

studies by Cundall, Brooks, and Murray[104] in the United Kingdom and Persson[378] in Scandinavia, are also consistent with the results in tables 13-23 and 13-24.

In some studies, many patients who had not previously received lithium and who were atypical manic or schizoaffective began taking the drug on a prophylactic basis. In these studies, there was a higher base rate of relapse with lithium than in other studies that used atypical manics or patients who had a good lithium effect. However, even in the studies with a higher base rate of relapse, a greater percentage of patients in the placebo groups than in the lithium groups relapsed. In both types of studies, there was a difference between drug and placebo groups of about 40 to 50 percent, although the base rate for relapse differed from study to study. Studies in several countries all confirm the prophylactic value of lithium. In the thirteen studies summarized in table 13-23, 66 percent of patients on lithium did not relapse. This contrasts sharply with the results for patients on placebo. In this group, only 22 percent did not relapse. Lithium clearly demonstrates efficacy in prophylaxis.

The statistical significance of the difference in effect between lithium and placebo in each of the studies can be calculated by the Fisher Exact Test. When data from these studies are combined according to the method of Fleiss,[159] the superiority of lithium over placebo is highly significant ($p = 2 \times 10^{-39}$). (A more detailed discussion of the methodology can be found in Cochran.[84]) Although this probability value appears dramatic and infinitesimal, it is a valid reflection of a powerful effect demonstrated repeatedly and homogeneously in a series of studies.

DOES LITHIUM PREVENT UNIPOLAR AS WELL AS BIPOLAR DEPRESSION?

A growing body of evidence from clinical drug response and genetic data indicates that bipolar affective disease may be a separate entity from unipolar depression.* The two disorders may be distinguished genetically, by drug responsivity, and in terms of their psychopathology. Therefore, lithium should be examined in both unipolar and

*See references 19, 20, 224, 284, 285, 376, 423, and 510.

TABLE 13–24
Lithium Prevention of Relapse

Investigators	N	Bipolar Patients (I & II)		N	Unipolar Depressions	
		Relapsed N (%)	Well N (%)		Relapsed N (%)	Well N (%)
Baastrup, Poulsen, and Schou[39]						
Placebo	22	12 (55)	10 (45)	17	9 (53)	8 (47)
Lithium	28	0 (0)	28 (100)	17	0 (0)	17 (100)
Prien, Caffey, and Klett[393]						
Placebo	10	9 (90)	1 (10)	21	19 (90)	2 (10)
Lithium	14	5 (31)	9 (69)	23	13 (57)	10 (43)
Prien, Caffey, and Klett[395]						
Placebo	102	91 (89)	11 (11)	—		
Lithium	97	48 (49)	49 (51)	—		
Persson[378]						
Placebo	12	11 (92)	1 (8)	21	14 (67)	7 (33)
Lithium	12	5 (42)	7 (58)	21	6 (29)	15 (71)
Coppen et al.[90]						
Placebo	21	21 (100)	0 (0)	15	12 (80)	3 (20)
Lithium	17	3 (18)	14 (82)	11	1 (9)	10 (91)
Fieve, Platman, and Plutchik[157]						
Placebo	11	7[a] (64)	4 (36)	—		
Lithium	7	1 (14)	6 (86)	—		
Fieve et al.[130, 158]						
Placebo	17	17[b] (100)	0 (0)	14	9 (64)	5 (36)
Lithium	15	0 (0)	15 (100)	14	8 (57)	6 (43)
Kane et al.[243]						
Placebo	7	5 (71)	2 (29)	6	6 (100)	0 (0)
Lithium	4	1 (25)	3 (75)	7	2 (29)	5 (71)
Glen, Johnson, and Shepherd[185]						
Placebo	—			9	8 (89)	1 (11)
Lithium	—			12	5 (42)	7 (58)
Prien et al.[399]						
Placebo	—			34	24 (71)	10 (29)
Lithium	—			37	21 (57)	16 (43)

[a]Bipolar II patients.
[b]Bipolar I patients.

bipolar depression. Those studies that evaluated these two populations separately are summarized in table 13–24. A collaborative longitudinal study conducted in three European countries[21,200,451] provides evidence on a larger number of patients and supplements the evidence from double-blind comparisons, although longitudinal naturalistic studies are not as well controlled as conventional random-assignment, blind-evaluation studies.

For purposes of analysis, it is necessary to distinguish statistical significance from magnitude of association (size effect). A high correlation involving four or five subjects may just barely be statistically significant, while a low correlation involving thousands of subjects may be highly significant. Most of the studies noted here had more bipolar subjects than unipolar subjects; therefore, it is important to distinguish the overall findings from the degree of prophylaxis (size effect) exer-

TABLE 13–25
Lithium Versus Placebo (Prophylaxis). Phi Coefficients for Individual Studies and Average
Weighted Correlation

Study	Bipolars Phi coefficient	(N)	Unipolars Phi coefficient	(N)
Baastrup, Poulsen, and Schou[39]	0.63	(50)	0.60	(34)
Prien, Caffey, and Klett[393]	0.54	(24)	0.38	(44)
Prien, Caffey, and Klett[395]	0.43	(199)	–	–
Persson[378]	0.53	(24)	0.38	(42)
Coppen et al.[90]	0.85	(38)	0.70	(26)
Fieve, Platman, and Plutchnik[157]	0.48	(18)	–	–
Fieve et al.[130, 158]	1.00	(32)	0.07	(28)
Kane et al.[243]	0.45	(11)	0.73	(13)
Glen, Johnson, and Shepherd[185]	–	–	0.48	(21)
Prien et al.[399]	–	–	0.14	(71)
International Collaborative Study[a] [21, 200, 451]	0.44	(450)	0.54	(196)
Average Weighted Correlation	0.49		0.44	

[a] Regression coefficient.

cised by lithium in each subgroup of patients. This can be expressed as the correlation coefficient between degree of prophylaxis and lithium administration in unipolar versus bipolar patients when quantitative data are available, or as the phi coefficient when categorical data are available. The phi coefficient is the correlation between relapsed versus nonrelapsed states and lithium versus placebo treatment; each category is assigned a numerical score of 1 or 0. Table 13–25 illustrates the degree of association as measured by the average weighted correlation between lithium treatment and prophylaxis in bipolar and unipolar depression.

Does lithium prevent relapse in a larger proportion of bipolar patients than unipolar patients? The reader can quantitatively compare the phi coefficients for the bipolar patients and the unipolar patients. In addition, the raw numbers given for each study in table 13–24 can give the reader an intuitive impression of the magnitude of the prophylactic effect. Each study is summarized by the number and percentage of patients who relapsed or remained well.

The International Collaborative Study compared the effect of lithium treatment on the course of recurrent unipolar or bipolar illness with the course of the disease in the same patients prior to receiving lithium.[21,200,451] The design was much like that used in Baastrup and Schou's classic naturalistic study.[36,448] The size effect of the prophylactic properties of lithium compared to the historical control period can be measured in the multiple regression analysis in unipolar or bipolar groups. This is not strictly comparable to the drug versus placebo differences in table 13–24. Since it represents episodes and not individual patients, it is intended here only as a rough approximation. It does represent a quantitative comparison of differential efficacy of lithium in preventing relapse in both unipolars and bipolars. The same design was applied to both groups, so the contrast between groups is valid. The statistical significance of the lithium prophylactic effect was greater in the bipolar group because more patients with bipolar disease than with unipolar disease were studied. However, the magnitude of the association of a good response to lithium treatment reveals that in comparison with their course before receiving lithium, unipolar patients had a very slightly better prophylactic effect with lithium ($d = 0.54$) than did bipolar patients ($d = 0.44$). Table 13–25 concludes with an average weighted correlation for either group based on all the studies cited therein.

Table 13–30 attempts to compare the overall prophylactic effects of lithium, antidepressants, and the combination of lithium and antidepressants in both unipolar and bipolar patients separately. Probability values and the homogeneity of studies have been calculated by summarizing the relevant studies presented in tables 13–23, 13–24, 13–26, 13–27, and 13–28 according to the method of Fleiss.[159] Lithium proves to be clearly efficacious prophylactically in both bipolar and unipolar disease. Antidepressants similarly have a strong action in unipolar disease. Although there appears to be no difference between lithium and antidepressants in the prevention of unipolar disease, there is a clear loss of homogeneity between the studies evaluated, which are presented in table 13–29. Lithium is superior to antidepressants in the prophylaxis of bipolar disease. The combination of lithium and imipramine is no more effective than lithium alone in bipolar disease. In unipolar disease the very same comparison demonstrates an interesting trend: The combination is marginally superior. Although this result is by no means definitive, future evaluations should perhaps focus on this combination, and perhaps even on other combinations, to further improve prophylaxis.

EFFICACY OF LITHIUM PROPHYLAXIS IN MANIC VERSUS DEPRESSIVE PHASES

It is important to maintain the conceptual distinction between lithium's effect in preventing the depression in unipolar illness and its relative prophylactic action against either the manic phase only or the depressive phase only in bipolar illness. Prien, Caffey, and Klett [393,395,396,397] and Cundall, Brooks, and Murray[104] found that lithium had a larger quantitative effect in preventing the manic phase of bipolar illness than it did in preventing the depressive phase of bipolar illness. In contrast, Baastrup, Poulsen, and Schou[39] and Coppen and associates[90] found

essentially similar prophylactic effects against the manic and the depressive phases of bipolar illness. Whether the differences among these studies lie in definitional problems, represent random variation within the small samples used, or represent substantial differences cannot be ascertained at this time.

TIME COURSE OF RELAPSE IN BIPOLAR PATIENTS

Schou, Thomsen, and Baastrup[449] examined the time course of relapse among bipolar patients. These results, along with those of Mindham and associates,[328,329] are summarized in figure 13–1. When plotted semilogarithmically, the rate of relapse for manic-depressive patients maintained on placebo indicates an exponential curve, that is, a straight line representing the number of logged relapses over time. Based on Schou's data, approximately 15 percent of the patients relapsed each month (i.e., the constant rate for relapse = 0.15); therefore, the "half-life" of untreated patients in remission is approximately four and one-half months. This figure of 15 percent for relapses per month gives an indication of what would have happened to patients who had not been treated with lithium. Although the relapse rate may not seem very noteworthy at first, the number of relapses becomes impressive when they occur at this rate month after month (see figure 13–1).

Schou and Baastrup also compared the relapse rate of patients studied in their double-blind clinical trial[449] with those studied during their naturalistic open study[36] and found the relapse rates in both studies to be essentially equal. Incidentally, the controlled study supports the methodology of the naturalistic study insofar as it indicates that the therapist's attitude is not sufficient to effectively prevent relapses in recurrent affective disorders. It would appear, then, that this source of variation is not major when dealing with a severe disorder like bipolar depression.

TABLE 13–26
Placebo Versus Tricyclics for Prevention of Relapse of Recurrent Depression

Investigators	N	Relapsed N (%)	Well N (%)
Prien, Caffey, and Klett[393]			
Placebo	21	19 (90)	2 (10)
Drug	19	11 (58)	8 (42)
Mindham, Howland, and Shepherd[328, 329]			
Placebo	42	21 (50)	21 (50)
Drug	50	11 (22)	39 (78)
Klerman and Cole[257]			
Placebo	67	27 (40)	40 (60)
Drug	39	6 (15)	33 (85)
Coppen et al.[96]			
Placebo	16	5 (31)	11 (69)
Drug	13	0 (0)	13 (100)
Kane et al.[243]			
Placebo	6	6 (100)	0 (0)
Drug	8	5 (83)	1 (17)
Seager and Bird[452]			
Placebo	16	11 (69)	5 (31)
Drug	12	2 (17)	10 (83)
Kay, Fahy, and Garside[245]			
Placebo	51	24 (47)	27 (53)
Drug	34	8 (24)	26 (76)
Stein, Rickels, and Weise[476]			
Placebo	26	18 (69)	8 (31)
Drug	29	8 (28)	21 (72)
Glen, Johnson, and Shepherd[185]			
Placebo	9	8 (89)	1 (11)
Drug	7	4 (57)	3 (43)
Prien et al.[399]			
Placebo	34	24 (71)	10 (29)
Drug	38	16 (42)	22 (58)

TABLE 13–27
Lithium/Imipramine Combination in the Prevention of Depression

Investigators	Unipolar			Bipolar		
	N	Relapsed N (%)	Well N (%)	N	Relapsed N (%)	Well N (%)
Kane et al.[242]						
Imipramine/Lithium				37	12 (32)	25 (68)
Lithium				38	8 (21)	30 (79)
Kane et al.[243]						
Imipramine/Lithium	8	1 (13)	7 (87)	6	1 (17)	5 (83)
Imipramine	6	5 (83)	1 (17)	5	3 (60)	2 (40)
Lithium	7	2 (29)	5 (71)	4	1 (25)	3 (75)
Placebo	6	6 (100)	0 (0)	7	5 (71)	2 (29)
Prien et al.[399]						
Imipramine/Lithium	37	12 (32)	25 (65)	35	18 (51)	17 (49)
Imipramine	38	16 (42)	22 (58)	36	29 (81)	7 (19)
Lithium	37	21 (57)	16 (43)	42	23 (55)	19 (45)

TABLE 13–28
Lithium Versus Antidepressants in the Prevention of Recurrent Affective Diseases

	Unipolar			Bipolar		
Investigators	N	Relapsed N (%)	Well N (%)	N	Relapsed N (%)	Well N (%)
Coppen et al.[94, 97]						
Mianserin	13	7 (54)	6 (46)	—		
Lithium	15	0 (0)	15 (100)	—		
Coppen et al.[92]						
Maprotiline	8	6 (75)	2 (25)	1	1 (100)	0 (0)
Lithium	12	3 (25)	9 (75)	4	1 (25)	3 (75)
Kane et al.[243]						
Imipramine	6	5 (83)	1 (17)	5	3 (60)	2 (40)
Lithium	7	2 (29)	5 (71)	4	1 (25)	3 (75)
Glen, Johnson, and Shepherd[185]						
Amitriptyline	47	32 (68)	15 (32)	—		
Lithium	56	39 (70)	17 (30)	—		
Prien, Caffey, and Klett[393]						
Imipramine	25	12 (48)	13 (52)	13	10 (77)	3 (23)
Lithium	27	13 (52)	14 (48)	18	5 (28)	13 (72)
Prien et al.[399]						
Imipramine	38	16 (42)	22 (58)	36	29 (81)	7 (19)
Lithium	37	21 (57)	16 (43)	42	23 (55)	19 (45)

TABLE 13–29
Lithium Versus Antidepressants in the Prevention of Bipolar and Unipolar Recurrent Affective Disorder

	Relapse %	Well %	p	HOM[a]
Bipolar				
Lithium	32	68	2×10^{-28}	NS[b]
Placebo	86	14		
Lithium	44	56	0.002	NS
Antidepressants	78	22		
Lithium/Imipramine	40	60	NS	NS
Lithium	38	62		
Unipolar				
Lithium	39	61	1×10^{-9}	NS
Placebo	74	26		
Antidepressant	29	71	5×10^{-13}	NS
Placebo	57	43		
Lithium	51	49	NS	0.002
Antidepressants	57	43		
Lithium/Imipramine	29	71	0.03	NS
Lithium	52	48		

[a]Homogeneity of studies calculated using the method of Fleiss.[159]
[b]Nonsignificant.

OTHER EVIDENCE FOR EFFICACY OF LITHIUM

Different investigators reporting a large number of uncontrolled case reports or open or single-blind studies have also noted the prophylactic effect of lithium.* When placebo was substituted for lithium in these reports and studies, patients relapsed. While these studies were excluded from the tables herein because they did not employ the crossover or uncrossed double-blind, random-assignment design, their findings are consistent with those from the controlled studies.

LITHIUM PROPHYLAXIS IN ATYPICAL AFFECTIVE SYNDROMES

The success of lithium prophylaxis in typical affective syndromes prompted physicians to investigate whether the indication for lithium could be extended to atypical affective syndromes. These studies have investigated recurrent disease with affective features in children[24,131,167,195] and schizo-affective psychosis or similar diagnostic labels in other nomenclatures (atypical mania, cycloid psychosis, etc.) in adults.[375,468] In a controlled study, Hanna and associates[209] demonstrated lithium's effectiveness in patients with a forty-eight-hour periodic psychosis. In a classic study of lithium prophylaxis, Baastrup and Schou[36] reported that atypical manic patients responded to lithium less well than did typical manic patients, but did show a substantial reduction in episodes per year (1.22 without lithium and 0.35 with lithium). This study has been the subject of some discussion in the literature.[52,53] Similarly, although the European collaborative study found statistically significant lithium prophylaxis in schizo-affective patients, the results[21,200,451] were less impressive than those found in typical unipolar and bipolar patients.

Smulevitch[468] and Gardner[171] conducted open studies that provide clinical evidence in support of lithium's efficacy in schizo-affective or atypical manic patients. Perris[375]

*See references 157, 198, 274, 386, 387, and 465.

performed extensive clinical studies on a syndrome referred to as "cycloid," which resembles schizo-affective psychosis in the standard DSM-III nomenclature. Eighteen subjects took lithium regularly, and Perris compared the mean number of affective episodes before and after receiving lithium (both before and after periods are equivalent in length). The patients experienced a mean of 2.06 episodes during the pretreatment period, in contrast to only 0.5 episodes after receiving lithium treatment ($p < 0.01$). Perris also calculated the average number of months patients spent in hospitals during equivalent periods before and during lithium treatment. Patients spent an average of 2.34 months in the hospital during the period before lithium treatment; during lithium treatment patients were hospitalized for only 0.2 months ($p < 0.01$). It should be noted that some schizophrenic patients displayed a CNS toxicity syndrome (confusion, etc.) on acute lithium treatment.[460] Because of this vulnerability to lithium-induced CNS toxicity, treatment of schizophrenic patients should be undertaken with caution (e.g., less rapid dose increments and alertness to CNS toxicity).

In summary, recurrent affective disease with predominantly manic and some schizophrenic features may indeed benefit from acute lithium treatment and also from lithium prophylaxis. Further research is needed to establish clinical indications for lithium in atypical cases, but at this time there is some empirical basis for proposing lithium prophylaxis as a reasonable strategy for certain atypical manic or schizo-affective patients. Assuming good clinical response, lithium prophylaxis may well be a better long-term treatment than antipsychotic medication, which carries the risk of tardive dyskinesia.

Dyson and Barcai,[131] Annell,[24] and Frommer[167] have used lithium to treat episodic affective disorders in children. Gram and Rafaelsen[195] performed a twelve-month randomized, double-blind crossover study, in which they administered lithium or placebo to eighteen patients who were pupils at a special school for psychotic children. Eleven of the patients were rated as responding better during the lithium period.

Because some patients with mental deficiency can have coexisting manic-depressive disease [371,412] and because there is clinical evidence that manic-depressive mentally defective patients respond to lithium,[3] Naylor and associates [345] conducted a two-year random-assignment, double-blind crossover trial of lithium versus placebo in the treatment of mental defectives with bipolar disorder. They found that lithium had a moderately beneficial effect for this population.

CLINICAL ISSUES WITH LITHIUM PROPHYLAXIS

A common problem facing the clinician is whether to institute prophylactic lithium in patients who have had only a relatively small number of manic and/or depressive attacks. Most lithium maintenance studies have used patients with documented recurrent manic-depressive illness consisting of several episodes in the last two to four years. Because it is difficult to do research on patients who have had infrequent episodes (a very large sample is required for purposes of statistical analysis), there is presently no clinically useful research evidence concerning how severe the affective disease must be to justify maintenance medication. Using existing knowledge, the clinician must generalize to the particular patient, taking into account the nature of the affective disorder (i.e., the severity of the illness, suicidal or foolish behavioral risks, and whether it is bipolar or unipolar disease, typical or atypical, and primarily affective or schizo-affective). Consultation between the patient and physician is the best way to decide about lithium treatment after the patient has been fully informed as to the advantages and the disadvantages of such treatment. An alternate approach would be to observe the patient closely for early signs of relapse and initiate treatment immediately if symptoms present.

In deciding whether lithium is indicated for a particular patient, the physician should bear in mind that lithium does not protect patients against or ameliorate normal feelings of sadness or unhappiness that come from, and are unfortunately a part of, everyday life. The physician must also consider the patient's reliability; patients must take their medication regularly, blood levels must be monitored, and other medical precautions need to be taken (i.e., avoidance of thiazide diuretics and low-salt diets). For various reasons (e.g., lack of intelligence or conscientiousness), patients may occasionally be unable to take their lithium reliably. Sometimes enlisting the aid of family members can help with patient reliability issues.

Drug Combinations with Lithium

If a patient develops a depressive episode during lithium maintenance, the physician must decide whether other forms of treatment should be initiated; therefore, drug interaction must be considered. If MAOIs, tricyclics, or ECT are indicated, can these be added to the lithium or must it be stopped? Most clinical observations indicate that tricyclics and MAOIs can be used with lithium without adverse interactions and with good therapeutic effect.* Lingjaerde and associates [291,292] studied the effect of lithium plus tricyclics versus tricyclics alone in treating depression and found that the combination produced somewhat better results than tricyclics alone. This difference was significant in only one hospital out of the network studied, but the general trend was consistent for all facilities. The main point here, however, is not that lithium plus tricyclics may be more effective than tricyclics alone, but that it is a reasonable strategy to treat depressive relapses with tricyclics. Then, typically, after the depressive episode has abated, the tricyclics can be gradually tapered off and the maintenance lithium continued.

An open study of MAOIs in conjunction with lithium by Zall [521] reported good results in three treatment-resistant patients. Similarly, Himmelhoch and associates [218] described a series of patients successfully

---

*See references 216, 232, 291, 292, and 355.

TABLE 13–30
Percentage of Patients Who Do Well on Various Treatments

		% Good Response	% Poor Response	Phi Coefficient
Antipsychotic for treatment of	Drug	70	25	0.45
acute schizophrenia	Placebo	30	75	
Maintenance antipsychotic for	Drug	80	20	0.34
prophylaxis	Placebo	47	53	
Imipramine for treatment	Drug	65	35	0.33
of acute depression	Placebo	32	68	
Tricyclic prophylaxis of	Drug	73	27	0.26
depression	Placebo	48	52	
Lithium for treatment	Drug	73	28	0.38
of acute mania	Placebo	34	66	
Lithium prophylaxis of manic-	Drug	63	37	0.43
depression	Placebo	21	79	
Streptomycin for tuberculosis	Drug	69	33	0.36
	Standard	31	67	
Penicillin for pneumococcal	Penicillin	93	6	0.10
pneumonia	Sulfanilamide	88	11	
Drugs in surgery, 1964–72	New	63	37	0.06
	Old	57	43	

treated with lithium and tranylcypromine in an open design. This is positive evidence, but more carefully controlled investigations will be needed.

Rapid Cyclers

Dunner and Fieve[129] and Stancer, Furling, and Godse[475] have described a subtype of manic-depressive patients who undergo a very rapid cycle (four or more affective episodes per year). They note that these patients seem to respond very poorly to lithium. Whether these rapid cyclers represent a diagnostically different subtype of manic-depressive illness or just a particularly severe form of the disease is not known.

Discussion of Lithium Treatment

It is not known whether lithium prevents manic-depressive illness in a fundamental sense. Current data are insufficient to permit a definitive answer to this question; indeed, the question may be unanswerable. Descriptively, however, it is definitely true that once an adequate dose of lithium is determined,

some patients never have another episode of mania or depression, or the intensity of the manic and/or depressive phase is reduced. It is unfortunate that the qualitative nature of lithium's effect has not been investigated in more detail because, now that lithium's efficacy is well established, there are ethical questions about conducting further placebo-controlled trials in order to elucidate the qualitative nature of the change produced by lithium prophylaxis or acute treatment.

¶ Conclusion: The Power of Psychoactive Drugs

The drug-placebo difference is a meaningful measurement of the overall efficacy of a specific drug administered to patients with a specific disease. In terms of drug-placebo differences, the advance in psychotropic drugs is comparable to major innovations in chemotherapy.

Table 13–30 summarizes data from the National Institute of Mental Health Collaborative Study Number 1 on the efficacy of the treatment of acute schizophrenia with drugs and placebo and all controlled maintenance studies of antipsychotics versus placebo[87] and from studies by the British Medical Research Council on the efficacy of treatment for tuberculosis with streptomycin.[319] Data on the treatment of pneumococcal pneumonia with penicillin and sulfonilamide is also included. In addition, a summation of the double-blind studies that compare (1) imipramine versus placebo in acute depression, (2) tricyclics versus placebo in prevention of depression, and (3) lithium versus placebo in the prevention of affective illness has been provided. The drug-placebo difference is expressed as a phi coefficient in which the higher the correlation, the bigger the difference.

Although we would caution against an overly concrete interpretation of such data, it appears that the discovery of effective psychotropic drugs is as much a breakthrough for psychiatry as the discovery of antibiotics was for medicine. Of course, no quantitative comparison can be made on the efficacy of different drugs for different disorders. However, the fourfold drug-placebo differences presented here facilitate qualitative comparisons between diseases treated and drug effects.

¶ Bibliography

1. ABERG, A., and HOLMBERG, G. "Controlled Trial of a New Antidepressant, Amoxapine, in Comparison with Amitriptyline," *Current Therapeutic Research*, 22 (1977):304–315.

2. ACEBAL, E., et al. "A Double-Blind Comparative Trial of Nomifensin and Desimipramine in Depression," *European Journal of Clinical Pharmacology*, 10 (1976):109–113.

3. ADAMS, G. L., KIVOWITZ, J., and ZISKIND, E. "Manic-Depressive Psychosis, Mental Retardation, and Chromosomal Rearrangement," *Archives of General Psychiatry*, 23 (1970):305–309.

4. AGHAJANIAN, G. K. "Influences of Drugs on the Firing of Serotonin-Containing Neurons in Brain," *Federal Proceedings*

of the American Society for Experimental Biology, 31 (1972):91–96.

5. AGNEW, P. C., et al. "A Clinical Evaluation of Four Antidepressant Drugs (Nardil, Tofranil, Marplan, and Deprol)," *American Journal of Psychiatry*, 118 (1961):160.

6. AGNOLI, A., et al. "Psychopharmacological Effects of Trazodone," *Journal de Pharmacologie Clinique*, 2 (1973):219–225.

7. ALEXANDERSON, B. "Pharmacokinetics of Nortriptyline in Man After Single and Multiple Oral Doses," *European Journal of Clinical Pharmacology*, 4 (1972): 82.

8. ———. "Predictions of Steady State Plasma Levels of Nortriptyline From Single Oral Dose Kinetics, Studied in Twins," *European Journal of Clinical Pharmacology*, 6 (1973):44–53.

9. AL-YASSIRI, M. M., and BRIDGES, P. K. "Trazodone Efficacy and Safety in Endogenous Depression: A Double-blind Comparison with Imipramine," *Neuropharmacology*, 19 (1980):1191–1193.

10. AMDISEN, A. "Sustained Release Preparation of Lithium," in F. N. Johnson, ed., *Lithium Research and Therapy*. London: Academic Press, 1975, pp. 197–210.

11. AMERICAN PSYCHIATRIC ASSOCIATION. "Efficacy of ECT; Schizophrenia" in *Task Force Report 14—Electroconvulsive Therapy*, (September 1978):23–30.

12. AMIN, M. M., BAN, T. A., and LEHMANN, H. E. "Nomifensine in the Treatment of Depression: A Report on the Canadian Part of a Transcultural Study," *Psychopharmacology Bulletin*, 14 (1978):35–37.

13. AMIN, M. M., BAN, T. A. and PECKNOLD, J. C. "Nomifensine in the Treatment of Depression: A Standard-Controlled Clinical Study," *Psychopharmacology Bulletin*, 14 (1978):37–39.

14. AMIN, M., et al. "A Double-blind Comparative Clinical Study with Ludiomil (CIBA 34,276-Ba) and Amitriptyline in Newly Admitted Depressed Patients," *Current Therapeutic Research*, 15 (1973):691–699.

15. AMIN, M., et al. "A Comparison of Desipramine and Amitriptyline Plasma Levels and Therapeutic Response," *Psycho-*

pharmacology Bulletin, 14 (1978): 45–46.

16. AMIN, M. M., et al. "Viloxazine in the Treatment of Depression: Psychophysical Measures and Clinical Response," *Psychopharmacology Bulletin,* 14 (1978):33–35.

17. ANANTH, J. "Chlorimipramine in Obsessive-Compulsive Disorder. A Review," *Psychosomatics,* 24 (1983):723.

18. ANANTH, J., and VON DER STEEN, N. "A Double-blind Controlled Comparative Study of Nomifensine in Depression," *Current Therapeutic Research,* 23 (1978):213–221.

19. ANGST, J., and WEISS, P. "Periodicity of Depressive Psychoses," Paper presented at the Fifth Collegium Internationale Neuro-Psychopharmacologicum, Washington, D.C., March 28–31, 1966.

20. ———. "Zum Verlauf Depressiver Psychosen," in W. Schulte and W. Mende, eds., *Melancholie in Forschung, Klinik und Behandlung.* Stuttgart: Thieme, 1969, pp. 2–9.

21. ANGST, T., et al. "Lithium Prophylaxis in Recurrent Affective Disorders," *British Journal of Psychiatry,* 116 (1970):604–614.

22. ANGST, J., et al. "A Double-blind Comparative Study on the Effectiveness of Maprotiline (Ludiomil) and Imipramine (Tofranil) in Endogenous Depression," in P. Kielholz, ed., *Depressive Illness. Diagnosis, Assessment, Treatment.* Berne: Hans Huber, 1972, pp. 245–252.

23. ANGST, J., et al. "Ergebnisse eines Offenen und eines Doppelblind-versuches von Nomifensin Imvergleich zu Imipramine," *Archiv für Psychiatrie und Nervenkrankheiten,* 219 (1974):265–276.

24. ANNELL, A. L. "Manic-depressive Illness in Children and Effect of Treatment with Lithium Carbonate," *Acta Paedopsychiatrica* (Basel), 36 (1959):282–301.

25. ———. "Lithium in the Treatment of Children and Adolescents," *Acta Psychiatrica Scandinavica,* 207 (Supplement) (1969):19–30.

26. ANTONELLI, F., et al. "Trazodone in the Treatment of Neurosis," in T. A. Ban and B. Silvestrini, eds., *Modern Problems of Pharmacopsychiatry,* vol. 9.

Rome: Karger, Basel, 1974, pp. 127–139.

27. APPLETON, W. S., and DAVIS, J. M. *Practical Clinical Psychopharmacology,* 4th ed. New York: Medcomb, 1980.

28. ARFWIDSSON, L., et al. "A Comparison Between Diazepam, Dixyrazine, Opipramol and Placebo in Anxiety States," *Acta Psychiatrica Scandinavica,* 221 (Supplement) (1971):19–32.

29. ARFWIDSSON, L., et al. "Comparison of Chlorimipramine and Imipramine in Ambulatory Treatment of Depression," *Acta Psychiatrica Scandinavica,* 48 (1972):367–376.

30. ARVIN, M., et al. "A Double-blind Comparative Clinical Trial with Ludiomil (Ciba 34, 276-Ba) and Amitriptyline in Newly-admitted Depressed Patients," *Current Therapeutic Research,* 15 (1973):691–699.

31. ASBERG, M., et al. "Relationship Between Plasma Levels and Therapeutic Effect of Nortriptyline," *British Medical Journal,* 3 (1971):331.

32. AYD, F. "Maprotiline: An Effective Tetracyclic Antidepressant," *International Drug Therapy Newsletter,* 8 (1973):17–24.

33. AZIMA, H., SILVER, A., and ARTHURS, D. "The Effects of G-33040 in Depressive States. A Multi-blind Study," *American Journal of Psychiatry,* 119 (1962):465–466.

34. BAASTRUP, P. C. "The Use of Lithium in Manic-Depressive Psychosis," *Comprehensive Psychiatry,* 5 (1964):396–408.

35. ———. "Lithium—Behandling of Maniodepressiv Psykose: En Psykoseforebyggendo Behandlings Made (Lithium Treatment of Manic Depressive Psychosis: A Procedure for Preventing Psychotic Relapses)," *Nordisk Psykiatrisk Tiddskrift,* 20 (1966):441–450.

36. BAASTRUP, P. C., and SCHOU, M. "Lithium as a Prophylactic Agent Against Recurrent Depressions and Manic-Depressive Psychosis," *Archives of General Psychiatry,* 16 (1967):162–172.

37. ———. "Prophylactic Lithium," *Lancet,* 1 (1968):1419–1422.

38. ———. "Prophylactic Lithium," *Lancet,* 2 (1968):349–350.

39. BAASTRUP, P., POULSEN, K. S., and

SCHOU, M. "Prophylactic Lithium: Double-blind Discontinuation in Manic-Depressive and Recurrent-Depressive Disorders," *Lancet*, 2 (1970):326–330.

40. BAGADIA, V. N., et al. "A Double-Blind Controlled Study of Amoxapine and Imipramine in Cases of Depression," *Current Therapeutic Research*, 26 (1979):417–429.

41. BALESTRIERI, A., et al. "Clinical Comparative Evaluation of Maprotiline, a New Antidepressant Drug. A Multicentre Study," *International Pharmacopsychiatry*, 6 (1971):236–248.

42. BARON, M., et al. "Lithium Carbonate Response in Depression," *Archives of General Psychiatry*, 32 (1975):1107–1111.

43. BAUMANN, P. A., and MAITRE, L. "Neurobiochemical Aspects of Maprotiline (Ludiomil) Action," *Journal of International Medical Research*, 7 (1979): 391–400.

44. BAYLISS, P.F.C., and DUNCAN, S. M. "The Clinical Pharmacology of Viloxazine Hydrochloride—A New Antidepressant of Novel Chemical Structure," *British Journal of Clinical Pharmacology*, 1 (1974):431–437.

45. BAYLISS, P.F.C., et al. "A Double-blind Controlled Trial of 'Vivalan' (Viloxazine Hydrochloride) and Imipramine Hydrochloride in the Treatment of Depression in General Practice," *Journal of International Medical Research*, 2 (1974):260–264.

46. BAYLISS, P.F.C., et al. "An Open Study of Two Dose Levels of 'Vivalan' (Viloxazine Hydrochloride ici 58-834) in Depression General Practice," *Journal of International Medical Research*, 2 (1974):253–259.

47. BIEBER, H., and KUGLER, J. "Die Behandlung von Depressiven Kranken mit Chlorimipramin Infusionen," *Archiv für Psychiatrie und Nervenkrankheiten*, 219 (1969):329–338.

48. BIELSKI, R. J., and FRIEDEL, R. O. "Prediction of Tricyclic Antidepressant Response: A Critical Review," *Archives of General Psychiatry*, 33 (1976):1479–1489.

49. BIGGS, J. T., and ZIEGLER, V. E. "Protriptyline Plasma Levels and Antidepressant Response," *Clinical Pharmacology and Therapeutics*, 22 (1977):269–273.

50. BLACKBURN, T. P., et al. "Effects of Viloxazine, Its Major Metabolites, on Biogenic Amine Uptake Mechanisms In Vitro and In Vivo," *European Journal of Pharmacology*, 52 (1978):367–374.

51. BLACKWELL, B. "Hypertensive Crisis Due to Monoamine Oxidase Inhibitors," *Lancet*, 2 (1963):849–851.

52. BLACKWELL, B. "Need for Careful Evaluation of Lithium (letter to the editor)," *American Journal of Psychiatry*, 125 (1969):1131.

53. BLACKWELL, B., and SHEPHERD, M. "Prophylactic Lithium: Another Therapeutic Myth? An Examination of the Evidence to Date," *Lancet*, 1 (1968):968–971.

54. BLAHA, L., PINDER, R. M., and STOLEMEIJER, S. M. "Double-blind Comparative Trial of Mianserin Versus Chlorimipramine," *Current Medical Research and Opinion*, 6 (Supplement) (1980):99–106.

55. BRAITHWAITE, R. A., et al. "Plasma Concentration of Amitriptyline and Clinical Response," *Lancet*, 1 (1972):1297–1300.

56. BRANCONNIER, R. J., et al. "Treating the Depressed Elderly Patient: The Comparative Behavioral Pharmacology of Mianserin and Amitriptyline," in E. Costa and G. Racagni, eds., *Typical and Atypical Antidepressants: Clinical Practice*. New York: Raven Press, 1982, pp. 195–212.

57. BREYER-PFAFF U., et al. "Antidepressive Effect and Pharmacokinetics of Amitriptyline with Consideration of Unbound Drug and 10-Hydroxynortriptyline Plasma Levels," *Psychopharmacology*, 76 (1982):240–244.

58. BRODIE, H. "Clinical Investigator's Manual (Wellbatrin)." Unpublished manuscript, Burroughs Wellcome Company, 1976.

59. BRUCKNER, G. W., and JANSEN, W. "Nomifensin: Anwendung bei Altersdepressionen," in *Alival Symposium uber Ergebnisse der Experimentellen und Klinischen Prufung* (1976). Stuttgart: F.K. Schattauer, 1977.

60. BRUNNER, H., et al. "Cardiovascular Effects of Preparation CIBA 34,276-Ba

and Imipramine," *Agents and Actions*, 2 (1971):69–82.

61. BUNNEY, W. E., JR. "Psychopharmacology of the Switch Process in Affective Illness," in M. A. Lipton, A. DiMascio, and K. F. Killam, eds., *Psychopharmacology: A Generation of Progress.* New York: Raven Press, 1978, pp. 1249–1260.

62. BUNNEY W. E., JR., and DAVIS, J. M. "Norepinephrine in Depressive Reactions," *Archives of General Psychiatry*, 13 (1965):483–494.

63. BUNNEY, W. E., et al. "A Behavioral Biochemical Study of Lithium in Therapy," *American Journal of Psychiatry*, 125 (1968):91–103.

64. BURKE, B. V., SAINSBURY, M., and MEYO, B. A. "A Comparative Trial of Amitriptyline and Trimipramine in Therapy of Depression," *Medical Journal of Australia*, 1 (1967):1216–1218.

65. BURNS, B. H. "Preliminary Evaluation of a New Antidepressant, Trimipramine, by a Sequential Method," *British Journal of Psychiatry*, 111 (1965):1155–1157.

66. BURROWS, G. D., DAVIES, B., and SCOGGINS, B. A. "Plasma Concentration of Nortriptyline and Clinical Response in Depressive Illness," *Lancet*, 2 (1972):619–623.

67. BURROWS, G. D., MAGUIRE, K. P., and SCOGGINS, B. A. "Plasma Nortriptyline and Clinical Response—A Study Using Changing Plasma Levels," *Psychiatric Medicine*, 7 (1977):87–91.

68. BURROWS, G. D., NORMAN, T. R., and DAVIES, B. M. "A Comparative Study of Amoxapine and Amitriptyline for Depressive Illness," *Australian Family Physician*, 9 (1980):763–766.

69. BURROWS, G. D., et al. "A Sequential Trial Comparing Plasma Levels of Nortriptyline," *Australian and New Zealand Journal of Psychiatry*, 8 (1974):21–23.

70. CADE, J. F. J. "Lithium Salts in the Treatment of Psychotic Excitement," *Medical Journal of Australia*, 2 (1949):349–352.

71. ———. "The Story of Lithium," in F. J. Ayd, Jr., and B. Blackwell, eds., *Discoveries in Biological Psychiatry.* Philadelphia: J. B. Lippincott, 1970, pp. 218–229.

72. CAMPBELL, I. C., et al. "The Effects of Chronic Regimens of Clorgyline and Pargyline on Monoamine Metabolism in the Rat Brain," *Journal of Neurochemistry*, 32 (1979):49–55.

73. CAMPBELL, I. C., et al. "Neurotransmitter-related Adaptation in the Central Nervous System Following Chronic Monoamine Oxidase Inhibition," in T. P. Singer, R. W. Vonkorff, and D. L. Murphy, eds., *Monoamine Oxidase: Structure, Function, and Altered Functions.* New York: Academic Press, 1979, pp. 517–530.

74. CAPSTICK, N. "Chlorimipramine in Obsessional States," *Psychosomatics*, 12 (1971):332–335.

75. CAPSTICK, N., and ROOKE, K. C. "A Comparative Kind of Opipramal with Phenelzine and Chlordiazepoxide in the Treatment of Depression," *Journal of Internal Medical Research*, 2 (1974):293–297.

76. CAREY, M. S., et al. "The Use of Chlorimipramine in Phobic Patients," *Current Therapeutic Research*, 17 (1975):107–110.

77. CARNEY, M. W. P. "Investigations of the Clinical Effects of Opipramol," *Proceedings of the Fourth World Congress of Psychiatry*, 3 (1968):1904–1908.

78. CARNEY, M.W.P., and MAXWELL, C. "Sequential Double-blind Controlled Trial of Opipramol in Anxiety Neurosis," *International Journal of Neuropsychiatry*, 3 (1967):491–493.

79. CHANG, S. S., et al. "Pharmacokinetics of Lithium: Predicting Optimal Dosage," in T. B. Cooper et al., eds., *Lithium—Controversies and Unresolved Issues.* Amsterdam: Excerpta Medica, 1979, pp. 419–426.

80. CHERMAT, R., SIMON, P., and BOISSIER, J. R. "Amoxapine in Experimental Psychopharmacology: A Neuroleptic or an Antidepressant?" *Arzneimittel-Forschung*, 29 (1979):814–820.

81. CIANCHETTI, C., and GAINOTTI, G. "Studio Clinico Controllato Dell'Attivita Antidepressiva e Ansiolitica di un Nuovo Psicofarmaco L'AF-1161," *Gazzetta Internazionale di Medicina e Chirurgia*, 72 (1968):1–10.

82. CIOFFI, F., et al. "Ulteriori Dati Sull'azione Antidepressiva di un Nuovo Psicofarmaco L'A.F.-1161," *Rassegna Interna-*

zionale di Clinica e Terapia, 49 (1969): 1483–1487.

83. CLAASSEN, V., et al. "Fluvoxamine, a Specific 5-HT Uptake Inhibitor," *British Journal of Pharmacology,* 60 (1977): 505–516.

84. COCHRAN, W. G. "Some Methods of Strengthening the Common Chi-Square Tests," *Biometrics,* 10 (1954):417–451.

85. COHEN, R. M., et al. "Changes in alpha- and beta-Receptor Density in Rat Brain as a Result of Treatment with Monoamine Oxidase Inhibiting Antidepressants," *Neuropharmacology,* 21 (1982): 293–298.

86. COLBURN, R. W., GOODWIN, F. L., and BUNNEY, W. E. "Effect of Lithium on the Uptake of Noradrenaline by Synaptosomes," *Nature,* 215 (1967):1395–1397.

87. COLE, J. O., GOLDBERG, S. C., and KLERMAN, G. L. "Phenothiazine Treatment in Chronic Schizophrenia," *Archives of General Psychiatry,* 27 (1972):479.

88. CONTI, L., et al. "Clinical Experience with Mianserin," in G. Drykonnigen et al., eds., *Progress with the Pharmacotherapy of Depression: Mianserin HCl.* (Symposium Proceedings, Barcelona, 1978). Amsterdam: Excerpta Medica, 1979, pp. 65–73.

89. COOPER, T. B., and SIMPSON, G. M. "The 24-Hour Lithium Level as a Prognosticator of Dosage Requirement. A 2-Year Follow-up," *American Journal of Psychiatry,* 133 (1976):440–443.

90. COPPEN, A., et al. "Double-blind and Open Prospective Studies of Lithium Prophylaxis in Affective Disorders," *Neurologia, Neurochirurgia, Psychiatria,* 76 (1963):500–513.

91. COPPEN, A., et al. "Prophylactic Lithium in Affective Disorders," *Lancet,* 2 (1971):275–279.

92. COPPEN, A., et al. "A Double-blind Comparison of Lithium Carbonate and Maprotiline in the Prophylaxis of the Affective Disorders," *British Journal of Psychiatry,* 128 (1976):479–485.

93. COPPEN, A., et al. "Mianserin Hydrochloride: A Novel Antidepressant," *British Journal of Psychiatry,* 129 (1976):342–345.

94. COPPEN, A., et al. "Mianserin in the Pro-

phylactic Treatment of Bipolar Affective Illness," *Journal of Pharmacopsychiatry,* 12 (1977):95–99.

95. COPPEN, A., et al. "Amitriptyline Plasma-Concentration and Clinical Effect: A World Health Organization Collaborative Study," *Lancet,* 1 (1978):63–66.

96. COPPEN, A., et al. "Continuation Therapy with Amitriptyline in Depression," *British Journal of Psychiatry,* 133 (1978):28–33.

97. COPPEN, A., et al. "Mianserin and Lithium in the Prophylaxis of Depression," *British Journal of Psychiatry,* 133 (1978): 206–210.

98. COPPEN, A., et al. "Inhibition of 5-HT Reuptake by Amitriptyline and Zimelidine and Its Relationship to Their Therapeutic Action," *Psychopharmacology,* 63 (1979):125–129.

99. COPPEN, A., et al. "Lithium Continuation Therapy Following Electroconvulsive Therapy," *British Journal of Psychiatry,* 139 (1981):284–287.

100. CORONA, G. L., et al. "Amitriptyline, Nortriptyline Plasma Levels and Clinical Response in Women with Affective Disorders," *Pharmacopsychiatry,* 13 (1980):102–110.

101. COVI, L., et al. "Drugs and Group Psychotherapy in Neurotic Depression," *American Journal of Psychiatry,* 131 (1974):191–198.

102. CRANE, G. E. "Iproniazid (Marsilid) Phosphate, a Therapeutic Agent for Mental Disorders and Debilitating Diseases," *Psychiatric Research Reports,* 8 (1957): 142–152.

103. CRAWFORD, R., et al. "A Clinical Trial of Maprotiline (Ludiomil) in the Treatment of Depressive Patients in General Practice and the Psychiatric Clinic," *Journal of International Medical Research,* 3 (Supplement) (1975):89.

104. CUNDALL, R. L., BROOKS, P. W., and MURRAY, L. S. "A Controlled Evaluation of Lithium Prophylaxis in Affective Disorders," *Psychological Medicine,* 2 (1972):308–311.

105. DALE, P. G. "Lithium Therapy in Aggressive Mentally Subnormal Patients," *British Journal of Psychiatry,* 137 (1980):469–474.

106. DANIELLE, S., and FIORE, C. "Hypoten-

sive Effect on Intraocular Tension by AF-1161 (Trazodone)," *Annals di Ottalmologia et Clinica Oculistica*, 98 (1972):1–6.

107. DAVIDSON, J., McLEOD, M. N., and BLUM, R. "Acetylation Phenotype, Platelet Monoamine Oxidase Inhibition, and the Effectiveness of Phenelzine in Depression,"*American Journal of Psychiatry*, 135 (1978):467–469.

108. DAVIES, B., BURROWS, G. D., and SCOGGINS, B. "Plasma Nortriptyline and Clinical Response," *Australian and New Zealand Journal of Psychiatry*, 9 (1975):249–253.

109. DAVIES, B., et al. "A Sequential Trial of Viloxazine (Vivalon) and Imipramine in Moderately Depressed Patients," *Medical Journal of Australia*, 1 (1977):521–22.

110. DAVIS, J. M. "Efficacy of Tranquilizing and Antidepressant Drugs," *Archives of General Psychiatry*, 13 (1965):552–572.

111. ———. "Maintenance Therapy in Psychiatry: I. Schizophrenia," *American Journal of Psychiatry*, 132 (1975):1237–1245.

112. ———. "Overview: Maintenance Therapy and Psychiatry: II. Affective Disorders," *American Journal of Psychiatry*, 133 (1976):1–13.

113. DAVIS, J. M., and ERICKSEN, S. E. "Controlled Trials of Imipramine," *British Journal of Psychiatry*, 129 (1976):192.

114. DAVIS, J. M., and GREENBLATT, D. *Psychopharmacology Update: New and Neglected Areas.* New York: Grune & Stratton, 1979.

115. DAVIS, J. M. "Antidepressant Drugs," in H. I. Kaplan and B. J. Sadock, eds., *Comprehensive Textbook of Psychiatry*, 4th ed. Baltimore: William & Wilkins, 1985, pp. 1513–1536.

116. DEBUCK, R. "A Comparison of the Efficacy and Side Effects of Mianserin and Chlorimipramine in Primary Depression: A Double-blind Randomized Trial," *Current Medical Research and Opinion*, 6 (Supplement) (1980):88–98.

117. DEGREGORIO M., and DIONISIO, A. "A Controlled Clinical Study of a New Antidepressant (Trazodone)," *Panminerva Medica*, 13 (1971):27–30.

118. D'ELIA, G., et al. "Comparative Clinical Evaluation of Lofepramine and Imipramine," *Acta Psychiatrica Scandinavica*, 55 (1977):10–20.

119. DELL, A. J. "A Comparison of Maprotiline (Ludiomil) and Amitriptyline (1)," *Journal of International Medical Research*, 5 (Supplement) (1977):22–24.

120. DEMONTIGNY, C., et al. "Lithium Carbonate Addition in Tricyclic Antidepressant-resistant Unipolar Depression," *Archives of General Psychiatry*, 40 (1983):1327.

121. DE PAULA, J., HECKERT, V., and ABIZAID, W. "Amoxapine and Amitriptyline: A Double-blind Study in Depressed Patients," *A Folha Medica*, (Rio de Janeiro) 75 (1977):165–169.

122. DE SOUZA CAMPOS, J., DELGADO, J., and VERSIANA, M. "A Double-blind Comparative Study Between Amoxapine and Imipramine in the Treatment of Depression," *A Folha Medica*, (Rio de Janeiro) Vol 75, No 2. (1977).

123. DEWILDE, J. "Double-blind Controlled Trial of Viloxazine and Imipramine in the Treatment of Hospital Depressed Patients," *Acta Therapeutica*, 3 (1977): 49–56.

124. DIMASCIO, A., et al. "Differential Symptom Reduction by Drugs and Psychotherapy in Acute Depression," *Archives of General Psychiatry*, 36 (1979):1450–1456.

125. DOMINGUEZ, R. A., et al. "A Placebo-controlled Comparison of Amoxapine and Imipramine in the Treatment of Depressed Outpatients," *Current Therapeutic Research*, 29 (1981):714–727.

126. DONLON, P. T., BIERTUEMPHEL, H., and WILLENBRING, M. "Amoxapine and Amitriptyline in the Outpatient Treatment of Endogenous Depression,"*Journal of Clinical Psychiatry*, 42 (1981):11–15.

127. DORUS, E., et al. "Genetic Determinant of Lithium Ion Distribution. I. An in vitro Monozygotic–Dizygotic Twin Study," *Archives of General Psychiatry*, 31 (1974):463–465.

128. DOSTAL, T. "Antiaggressive Effects of Lithium Salts in Mentally Retarded Adolescents," in A. Annell, ed., *Depressive States in Childhood and Adolescence.* Stockholm: Almquist and Wiksell, 1972, pp. 66–81.

129. DUNNER, D. L., and FIEVE, R. R. "Clinical Factors in Lithium Carbonate Prophylaxis Failure," *Archives of General Psychiatry,* 30 (1974):229–233.

130. DUNNER, D. L., STALLONE, F., and FIEVE, R. R. "Lithium Carbonate and Affective Disorders: V. A Double-blind Study of Prophylaxis of Depression in Bipolar Illness," *Archives of General Psychiatry,* 33 (1976):117–120.

131. DYSON, W. L., and BARCAI, A. "Treatment of Children of Lithium-responding Parents," *Current Therapeutic Research,* 12 (1970):286–290.

132. EBSTEIN, R. P., and BELMAKER, R. H. "Lithium and Brain Adenylate Cyclase," in T. B. Cooper et al., eds., *Lithium—Controversies and Unresolved Issues.* Amsterdam: Excerpta Medica, 1979, pp. 703–729.

133. ECKMANN, F. "Klinische Untersuchungen mit dem Antidepressivum Nomifensin," in W. Walcher, ed., *Systematization, Provocation and Therapy of Depressive Psychoses,* Second International Symposium, Brazil, April 1973. Vienna: Hollinek, 1974, pp. 199–204.

134. ECKMANN, F., et al. "Clinical Trials with Thombrance: Results of Double-blind Studies," in S. Gershon et al., eds., *Trazodone, A New Broad-Spectrum Antidepressant.* Amsterdam: Excerpta Medica, 1980, pp. 69–74.

135. EDWARDS, J. G., and GOLDIE, A. "Placebo-Controlled Trial of Mianserin and Maprotiline in Primary Depressive Illness: A Preliminary Report," *British Journal of Clinical Pharmacology,* 15 (1983):239S–248S.

136. ELWAN, O. "A Comparative Study of Viloxazine and Imipramine in the Treatment of Depressive States," *Journal of International Medical Research,* 8 (1980):7–17.

137. ESCOBAR, J. I., and LANDBLOOM, R. P. "Treatment of Phobic Neurosis with Chlorimipramine: A Controlled Clinical Trial," *Current Therapeutic Research,* 20 (1976):680–685.

138. ESCOBAR, J. I., et al. "Controlled Clinical Trial with Trazodone, a Novel Antidepressant. A South American Experience," *Journal of Clinical Pharmacology,* 20 (1980):124–130.

139. EVANS, D. A. P. "An Improved and Simplified Method of Detecting the Acetylator Phenotype," *Journal of Medical Genetics,* 6 (1969):405–407.

140. EVANS, D. A. P., DAVIDSON, K., and PRATT, R.T.C. "The Influence of Acetylator Phenotype on the Effects of Treating Depression with Phenelzine," *Clinical Pharmacology and Therapeutics,* 6 (1965):430–435.

141. EVANS, J. I. "General Practitioner Clinical Trials: Two New Psychotropic Drugs," *Practitioner,* 198 (1967):135–139.

142. FABRE, L. "Pilot Open-Label Study with Alprazolam in Outpatients with Neurotic Depression," *Current Therapeutic Research,* 19 (1976):661–668.

143. FABRE, L., and McCLENDON, D. "A Double-blind Placebo Controlled Study of Bupropion (Wellbatrin) in the Treatment of Depressed Inpatients," *Current Therapeutic Research,* 23 (1978):393–402.

144. FABRE, L., McCLENDON, D., and GAINEY, A. "Trazodone Efficacy in Depression: A Double-blind Comparison with Imipramine and Placebo in Day-hospital Type Patients," *Current Therapeutic Research,* 25 (1979):827–834.

145. FABRE, L., et al. "Double-blind Placebo-controlled Comparison of Amoxapine and Imipramine in Depressed Outpatients," *Current Therapeutic Research,* 22 (1977):611–619.

146. FANN, W. E., et al. "Clinical Trial of Bupropion HCL in Treatment of Depression," *Current Therapeutic Research,* 23 (1978):222–229.

147. FAWCETT, J. Unpublished data.

148. FEIGHNER, J. P. "Trazodone, a Triazolopyridine Derivative, in Primary Depressive Disorder," *Journal of Clinical Psychiatry,* 41 (1980):250–255.

149. FEIGHNER, J. P. "Benzodiazepines as Antidepressants. A Triazolobenzodiazepine Used to Treat Depression," in T. A. Ban, F. A. Freyhan, and W. Poldinger, eds., *Modern Problems of Pharmacopsychiatry.* New York: S. Karser, 1982, pp. 196–212.

150. FEIGHNER, J. P. Unpublished data.

151. FEIGHNER, J. P., ADEN, G. C., and FABRE, F. L. "Comparison of Alprazolam, Imipramine and Placebo in the Treatment

of Depression," *Journal of the American Medical Association,* 269 (1983): 3057.

152. FEIGHNER, J. P., MEREDITH, C. R., and KLAGHORN, J. "Multi-centered Placebo-controlled Evaluation of Nomifensine Treatment in Depressed Outpatients," *Journal of Clinical Psychiatry,* 45 (1984):47–51.

153. FEIGHNER, J. P., MERIDETH, C. H., and HENDRICKSON, G. "Maintenance Antidepressant Therapy: A Double-blind Comparison of Trazodone and Imipramine," *Journal of Clinical Psychopharmacology,* 1 (1981):45S–48S.

154. FEIGHNER, J., et al. "A Placebo-controlled Multicenter Trial of Limbitrol Versus Its Components (Amitriptyline and Chlordiazepoxide) in the Symptomatic Treatment of Depressive Illness," *Psychopharmacology,* 61 (1979):217.

155. FEIGHNER, J. P., et al. "A Double-blind Comparative Trial with Mianserin and Amitriptyline in Outpatients with Major Depressive Disorders," *British Journal of Clinical Pharmacology,* 15 (Supplement) (1983):227–237.

156. FIEVE, R., KUMBARACI, T., and DUNNER, D. L. "Lithium Prophylaxis of Depression in Bipolar I, Bipolar II, and Unipolar Patients," *American Journal of Psychiatry,* 133 (1976):925–929.

157. FIEVE, R. R., PLATMAN, S. R., and PLUTCHIK, R. R. "The Use of Lithium in Affective Disorders: II. Prophylaxis of Depression in Chronic Recurrent Affective Disorders," *American Journal of Psychiatry,* 125 (1968):492–498.

158. FIEVE, R., et al. "Lithium Carbonate Prophylaxis of Depression in Three Subtypes of Primary Affective Disorders," *Pharmacopsychiatry,* 9 (1976):100–107.

159. FLEISS, J. L. *Statistical Methods for Rates and Proportions.* New York: John Wiley & Sons, 1973.

160. FLORU, L., and TEGELER, J. "Eine Vergleichende Untersuchung der Beiden Antidepressiva Viloxazin und Imipramin," *Pharmakopsychiatrie,* 12 (1979):313–320.

161. FORREST, W. A. "A Comparison Between Daily and Nightly Dose Regimen of Amitriptyline and Maprotiline (Ludi-omil) in the Treatment of Reactive Depression in General Practice," *Journal of International Medical Research,* 3 (Supplement) (1975):120.

162. FORREST, W. A. "Maprotiline (Ludiomil) in Depression: A Report on a Hospital-Monitored Release Study," in J. E. Murphy, ed., *Research and Clinical Investigation in Depression.* Northampton, England: Cambridge Medical Publications, 1976, p. 77.

163. FORREST, A., HEWETT, A., and NICHOLSON, P. "Controlled Randomized Group Comparison of Nomifensine and Imipramine in Depressive Illness," *British Journal of Clinical Pharmacology,* 4 (Supplement) (1977):215–220.

164. FRANCHIN, E. A. "Ensaio Clinico em 30 Pacientes de una Nova Medicaio Antidepressiva: Nomifensin," *Revista Brasiliera Clinica Terapeutica,* 2 (1973): 317–322.

165. FRANZCP, B. J. A Double-blind Comparative Clinical Study of Amoxapine and Amitriptyline in Depressed, Hospitalized Patients," *New Zealand Medical Journal.* 9 June 1982, pp. 391–393.

166. FRIEDMAN, E., and GERSHON, S. "Effect of Lithium on Brain Dopamine," *Nature,* 243 (1973):520–521.

167. FROMMER, E. "Depressive Illness in Childhood," in A. Coppen and A. Walk, eds., *Recent Developments in Affective Disorders.* British Journal of Psychiatry Special Publication 2. London: London Royal Medico-Psychological Association, 1968, pp. 117–136.

168. FRUENSGAARD, K., et al. "Amoxapine Versus Amitriptyline in Endogenous Depression: A Double-blind Study," *Acta Psychiatrica Scandinavica,* 59 (1979):502–508.

169. FULLER, R. W. "Influence of Substrate in the Inhibition of Rat Liver and Brain Monoamine Oxidase," *Archives Internationales de Pharmacodynamie et de Therapie,* 174 (1968):32–37.

170. GALLANT, D. M., et al. "Amoxapine: A Double-blind Evaluation of Antidepression Activity," *Current Therapeutic Research,* 15 (1973):56–59.

171. GARDNER, R. "Lithium Prophylaxis." Paper presented at the World Psychiatric Association Symposium on Aspects

of Schizophrenia, Yerevan-Tibilisi, USSR, October 1973.

172. GARVER, D. L., and DAVIS, J. M. "Biogenic Amine Hypothesis of Affective Disorders," *Life Science*, 24 (1979):383–394.

173. GELENBERG, A. J., and KLERMAN, G. L. "Antidepressants: Their Use in Clinical Practice," *Rationalization of Drug Therapy*, 12 (1978):1.

174. GELENBERG, A. J., et al. "Double-blind Comparison of Amoxapine and Imipramine in the Treatment of Depressed Patients," *Journal of Clinical Psychiatry*, 45 (1984):54–59.

175. General Practitioner Research Group, Report no. 51. "Dexamphetamine Compared with an Inactive Placebo in Depression," *Practitioner*, 192 (1964):151.

176. General Practitioner Research Group. "Two New Psychotropic Drugs: (1) A New Antidepressant," *Practitioner*, 198 (1967):135–141.

177. GERNER, R., et al. "Treatment of Geriatric Depression with Trazodone, Imipramine, and Placebo: A Double-blind Study,"*Journal of Clinical Psychiatry*, 41 (1980):216–220.

178. GERSHON, S., and NEWTON, R. "Lack of Anticholinergic Side Effects with a New Antidepressant—Trazodone," *Journal of Clinical Psychiatry*, 41 (1980):100–104.

179. GERSHON, S., and TRAUTNER, E. M. "Treatment of Shock Dependency by Pharmacological Agents," *Medical Journal of Australia*, 1 (1956):783–787.

180. GERSHON, S., and YUWILER, A. "Lithium Ion: A Specific Psychopharmacological Approach to the Treatment of Mania," *Journal of Neuropsychiatry*, 1 (1960):229–241.

181. GERSHON, S., et al. "Evaluation of Trazodone in the Treatment of Endogenous Depression: Results of a Multi-Centre Double-blind Study," *Journal of Clinical Psychopharmacology*, 1 (1981):39–44.

182. GLASSMAN, A. H., and PEREL, J. M. "Plasma Levels and Tricyclic Antidepressants," *Clinical Pharmacology Therapy*, 16 (1974):198.

183. GLASSMAN, A., KANTOR, S., and SHOSTAK, M. "Depression, Delusions, and Drug Response," *American Journal of Psychiatry*, 132 (1975):716.

184. GLASSMAN, A. H., et al. "Clinical Implications of Imipramine Plasma Levels for Depressive Illness," *Archives of General Psychiatry*, 34 (1977):197–204.

185. GLEN, A.I.M., JOHNSON, A. L., and SHEPHERD, M. "Continuation Therapy with Lithium and Amitriptyline in Unipolar Depressive Illness: A Randomized, Double-blind, Controlled Trial," *Psychological Medicine*, 14 (1984):37–50.

186. GOLDBERG, H., and FINNERTY, R. "Trazodone in the Treatment of Neurotic Depression," *Journal of Clinical Psychiatry*, 41 (1980):430–434.

187. GOLDBERG, H. L., RICKELS, K., and FINNERTY, R. "Treatment of Neurotic Depression with a New Antidepressant," *Journal of Clinical Psychopharmacology*, 1 (1981):35S–38S.

188. GONCALVES, N., and WEGENER, G. "Wirkungsvergleich von Lofepramin und Mianserin an Depressiven Patienten und Doppelblind," *International Pharmacopsychiatry*, 14 (1979):312–318.

189. GOODE, D. J., and MANNING, A. A. "Comparison of Bupropion Alone and with Haloperidol in Schizo-Affective Disorder, Depressed Type," *Journal of Clinical Psychiatry*, 44 (1983):253–255.

190. GOODWIN, F. K., MURPHY, D. L., and BUNNEY, W. E. "Lithium Carbonate Treatment in Depression and Mania," *Archives of General Psychiatry*, 21 (1969):486–496.

191. GOODWIN, F. K., et al. "Lithium Response of Unipolar Versus Bipolar Depression," *American Journal of Psychiatry*, 129 (1972):44–47.

192. GORE, C. P. "Clomipramine (Anafranil), Tofranil (Imipramine) and Placebo: A Comparative Study in Relation to Electroconvulsive Therapy," *Journal of International Medical Research*, 1 (1973):347–351.

193. GORIDIS, C., and NEFF, N. H. "Evidence for a Specific Monoamine Oxidase Associated with Sympathetic Nerves," *Neuropharmacology*, 10 (1971):557–564.

194. GRAM, L. F., and OVERO, K. F. "Drug Interaction: Inhibitory Effect of Neuroleptics on Metabolism of Tricyclic Antidepressants in Man," *British Medical Journal*, 1 (1972):463–465.

195. GRAM, L. F., and RAFAELSEN, O. J. "Lith-

ium Treatment of Psychotic Children and Adolescents: A Controlled Clinical Trial," *Acta Psychiatrica Scandinavica*, 48 (1962):253–260.

196. GRAM, L. F., et al. "Steady-state Kinetics of Imipramine in Patients," *Psychopharmacology*, 54 (1977):255–261.

197. GREENBLATT, M., GROSSER, G. H., and WECHSLER, H. "Differential Response of Hospitalized Depressed Patients to Somatic Therapy," *American Journal of Psychiatry*, 120 (1964):935–943.

198. GROF, P., CAKULS, P., and DOSTAL, T. "Lithium Drop-outs: A Follow-up Study of Patients Who Discontinued Prophylactic Treatment," *International Pharmacopsychiatry*, 5 (1970):162–169.

199. GROF, P., SAXENA, B., and DAIGLE, L. "Dopaminergic Agonist Nomifensine Compared with Amitriptyline: A Double-blind Clinical Trial in Acute Primary Depressions," *British Journal of Clinical Pharmacology*, 4 (Supplement) (1977):221–225.

200. GROF, P., et al. "Methodological Problems of Prophylactic Trials in Recurrent Affective Disorders," *British Journal of Psychiatry*, 116 (1970):599–603.

201. GROMSKA, J. "Treatment of Manic States with Lithium Salts," *Neurologia, Neurolchirurgia Polska*, 12 (1962):575–581.

202. GUZ, H. "A Controlled Double-blind Patient Trial Comparing CIBA 34.276-Ba with Imipramine in Depressive State," in P. Kielholz, ed., *Depressive Illness. Diagnosis, Assessment, Treatment.* Berne: Hans Huber, 1972, pp. 234–244.

203. GUZ, I. "A Controlled, Double-blind, Between-patient Trial Comparing CIBA 34.276-Ba and Imipramine in Depressive States," *New Zealand Medical Journal*, June (1982):391–393.

204. HABERMAN, W. "A Review of Controlled Studies with Nomifensine Performed Outside the U.K.," *British Journal of Clinical Pharmacology*, 4 (Supplement 2) (1977):237–241.

205. HAIDER, I. "A Comparative Trial of Ro 4–6270 and Amitriptyline in Depressive Illness," *British Journal of Psychiatry*, 113 (1967):993.

206. HAIG, A. *Uric Acid as a Factor in the Causation of Disease.* London: Churchill, 1892.

207. HAMMER, W., and SJOQVIST, F., "Plasma Levels of Monomethylated Tricyclic Antidepressants During Treatment with Imipramine-like Compounds," *Life Science*, 6 (1967):1895–1903.

208. HAMOUZ, W., et al. "A Double-blind Group Comparative Trial of Mianserin and Diazepam in Depressed Outpatients," *Pharmakopsychiatrie*, 13 (1980):79–83.

209. HANNA, S. M., et al. "The Therapeutic Effect of Lithium Carbonate on a Patient with a Forty-eight-hour Periodic Psychosis," *British Journal of Psychiatry*, 121 (1972):271–280.

210. HARDING, M. B. "A Comparative Clinical Trial of Oral Chlorimipramine (Anafranil) Against Amitriptyline," *Journal of International Medical Research*, 1 (1973):353–356.

211. HARE, E. H., DOMINIAN, J., and SHARPE, L. "Phenelzine and Dexamphetamine in Depressive Illness. A Comparative Trial," *British Medical Journal*, 1 (1962):9.

212. HARE, H. P., JR. "Comparison of Chlordiazepoxide-Amitriptyline Combination with Amitriptyline Alone in Depressive States," *Journal of Clinical Pharmacology*, 11 (1971):456–460.

213. HARTIGAN, G. P. "The Use of Lithium Salts in Affective Disorders," *British Journal of Psychiatry*, 109 (1963):810–814.

214. HEKIMIAN, L., FRIEDHOFF, A. J., and DEEVER, E. "A Comparison of the Onset of Action and Therapeutic Efficacy of Amoxapine and Amitriptyline," *Journal of Clinical Psychiatry*, 39 (1978):633–637.

215. HEKIMIAN, L. J., WEISE, C. C., and FRIEDHOFF, A. J. "Onset of Action of Amoxapine and Doxepin in Outpatients with Mixed Anxiety/Depression," *Journal of Clinical Psychiatry*, 44 (1983):248–252.

216. HENINGER, G. R., CHARNEY, D. S., and STERNBERG, D. E. "Lithium Carbonate Augmentation of Antidepressant Treatment," *Archives of General Psychiatry*, 40 (1983):1335.

217. HERLOFSEN, H. R. "Litumbehandling und Mannisk-Depressin Sinnslidese," Paper presented at the annual meeting

of the Norwegian Psychiatric Society, Oslo, Norway, September 1965.

218. HIMMELHOCH, J. M., et al. "Treatment of Previously Intractable Depression with Tranylcypromine and Lithium," *Journal of Nervous and Mental Disease*, 155 (1972):216–220.

219. HOLDEN, J. M., KERRY, R. J., and ORME, J. E. "Amoxapine in Depressive Illness," *Current Medical Research and Opinion*, 6 (1979):338–341.

220. HOLLISTER, L. E. "Tricyclic Antidepressants," *New England Journal of Medicine*, 299 (1978):1106–1168.

221. HOPMAN, H. "Mianserin, in Out-patients with Depressive Illness, in Dosage Up to 130 mg Daily," *Current Medical Research and Opinion*, 6 (Supplement 7) (1980):107–114.

222. HORNDERN, A., et al. "Amitriptyline in Depressive States. Six-Month Treatment Results," *British Journal of Psychiatry*, 110 (1964):641–647.

223. HRDINA, P., and LAPIERRE, Y. "Clinical Response, Plasma Levels and Pharmacokinetics of Desipramine in Depressed Patients," *Progress in Neuro-Psychopharmacology*, 4 (1981):591–601.

224. HULLEN, R. P., MCDONALD, R., and ALLSOPP, M. "Prophylactic Lithium in Recurrent Affective Disorders," *Lancet*, 1 (1972):1044–1046.

225. ———. "Further Report on Prophylactic Lithium in Recurrent Affective Disorders," *British Journal of Psychiatry*, 126 (1975):281–284.

226. HUNT, P., et al. "Nomifensine, a New Potent Inhibitor of Dopamine Uptake into Synaptosomes from Rat Brain Corpus Striatum," *Journal of Pharmacy and Pharmacology*, 26 (1974):370–371.

227. HYNES, M. V. "A Comparative Clinical Trial of Oral Chlorimipramine (Anafranil) Against Amitriptyline," *Journal of International Medical Research*, 1 (1973):338–342.

228. ITIL, T. M., et al. "Fluvoxamine, a New Antidepressant," *Progress in Neuro-Psychopharmacology*, 1 (1977):309–322.

229. IVES, J., et al. "The Ineffectiveness of Chlordiazepoxide in Depression Disorders," *Psychiatric Journal of the University of Ottawa*, 3 (1978):115.

230. JASKARI, M. O., et al. "Zur Behandlung der depression. Vergliechende Untersuchung der Wirkung von Mianserin (Tolvin) und Amitriptylin," *Therapie der Gegenwart* (Munich), 118 (1979):806–818.

231. JEFFERSON, J. W., and AYD, F. J., JR. "Combining Lithium and Antidepressants," *Journal of Clinical Psychopharmacology*, 3 (1983):303.

232. JEPSON, K., and BEAUMONT, G. A. "A Comparative Trial of Opipramol and Chlordiazepoxide in the Treatment of Anxiety," *Journal of Internal Medical Research*, 1 (1973):145–150.

233. JOHNSON, G. "Antidepressant Effects of Lithium," *Comprehensive Psychiatry*, 15 (1974):43–47.

234. JOHNSON, G., et al. "Comparative Effects of Lithium and Chlorpromazine in the Treatment of Acute Manic States," *British Journal of Psychiatry*, 119 (1971):267–276.

235. JOHNSON, J., and MADEN, J. G. "A New Antidepressant—Pramindole—A Double-blind Controlled Trial," *Clinical Trials Journal*, 4 (1967):787–790.

236. JOHNSTON, J. P. "Some Observations on a New Inhibitor of Monoamine Oxidase in Brain Tissue," *Biochemical Pharmacology*, 17 (1968):1285–1297.

237. JOHNSTONE, E. C. "The Relationship Between Acetylator Status and Inhibition of Monoamine Oxidase Excretion of Free Drug and Antidepressant Response in Depressed Patients on Phenelzine," *Psychopharmacologia*, 46 (1976):289–294.

238. JOHNSTONE, E. C., and MARSH, W. "Acetylator Status and Response to Phenelzine in Depressed Patients," *Lancet*, 1 (1973):567–570.

239. JONES, F. Unpublished data.

240. JUNGKUNZ, G., and KUSS, H. J. "On the Relationship of Nortriptyline/Amitriptyline Ratio to Clinical Improvement of Amitriptyline-treated Depressive Patients," *Pharmakopsychiatrie—Neuro-Psychopharmakologie*, 13 (1980):111–116.

241. KAMPMAN, R., UMMIKKO-PELKONEN, A., and KUHA, S. "Tricyclic Antidepressants in the Treatment of Depressions: A Double-blind Comparison of Chlorimipramine (Anafranil) and Amitripty-

line," *Acta Psychiatrica Scandinavica*, 58 (1978):142–148.

242. KANE, J. M., et al. "Prophylactic Lithium With and Without Imipramine for Bipolar I Patients: A Double-blind Study," *Psychopharmacology Bulletin*, 17 (1981):144–145.

243. KANE, J. M., et al. "Lithium Carbonate and Imipramine in the Prophylaxis of Unipolar and Bipolar II Illness," *Archives of General Psychiatry*, 39 (1982): 1065–1069.

244. KAUMEIER, H. S., and HAASE, H. J. J. "A Double-blind Comparison Between Amoxapine and Amitriptyline in Depressed In-patients," *International Journal of Clinical Pharmacology, Therapy, and Toxicology*, 18 (1980):177–184.

245. KAY, D. W. K., FAHY, T., and GARSIDE, R. F. "A Seven-Month Double-blind Trial of Amitriptyline and Diazepam in ECT-Treated Depressed Patients," *British Journal of Psychiatry*, 117 (1970):667–671.

246. KAY, N. E., and DAVIES, B. "A Controlled Trial of Maprotiline (Ludiomil) and Amitriptyline in General Practice," *Medical Journal of Australia*, 1 (1974): 704.

247. KELLAMS, J., KLAPPER, M., and SMALL, J. "Trazodone, a New Antidepressant: Efficacy and Safety in Endogenous Depression," *Journal of Clinical Psychiatry*, 40 (1979):390–395.

248. KELLY, D., et al. "Treatment of Phobic States with Antidepressants. A Retrospective Study of 246 Patients," *British Journal of Psychiatry*, 116 (1970):387–398.

249. KESSELL, A., and HOLT, N. F. "A Controlled Study of a Tetracyclic Antidepressant—Maprotiline (Ludiomil)," *Medical Journal of Australia*, 1 (1975): 773.

250. KHAN, M.C.A. "A Review of Cardiac Condition Effects of Maprotiline and Mianserin," *British Journal of Clinical Practice*, 5 (Supplement) (1980):29–34.

251. KHAN, M.C.A., and MOSLEHUDDIN, K. "A Double-blind Comparative Trial of Mianserin and Maprotiline in the Treatment of Depression," *Current Medical Research and Opinion*, 6 (Supplement) (1980):63–71.

252. KIELHOLZ, P. *Depressive Illness: Diagnosis, Assessment, Treatment.* Baltimore: Williams & Wilkins, 1972.

253. KIEV, A., and OKERSON, L. "Comparison of the Therapeutic Efficacy of Amoxapine with That of Imipramine," *Clinical Trials Journal*, 16 (1979):68–72.

254. KILOH, L. G., et al. "Double-blind Comparative Trial of Viloxazine and Amitriptyline in Depressed Geriatric Patients," *Clinical Trials Journal*, 6 (1979):13–17.

255. KLAWANS, H. L., WEINER, W. S., and NAUSIEDA, P. A. "The Effect of Lithium on an Animal Model of Tardive Dyskinesia: Progress," *Neuropsychopharmacology*, 1 (1977):53–60.

256. KLEIN, D. F., and DAVIS, J. M. *Diagnosis and Drug Treatment of Psychiatric Disorders.* Baltimore: Williams & Wilkins, 1969.

257. KLERMAN, G. L., and COLE, J. O. "Clinical Pharmacology of Imipramine and Related Compounds," *Pharmacology Review*, 17 (1965):101.

258. KLERMAN, G. L., et al. "Treatment of Depression by Drugs and Psychotherapy," *American Journal of Psychiatry*, 131 (1974):186–191.

259. KLINE, N. S. "Clinical Experience with Iproniazid (Marsilid)," *Journal of Clinical and Experimental Psychopathology*, 19 (Supplement 1) (1958):72–78.

260. KLINE, N. S., et al. "Evaluation of Lithium Therapy in Chronic and Periodic Alcoholism," *American Journal of Medical Sciences*, 268 (1974):15–22.

261. KNOLL, J., and MACYAR, K. "Some Puzzling Pharmacological Effects of Monoamine Oxidase Inhibitors," in E. Costa and M. Sandler, eds., *Advances in Biochemical Psychopharmacology.* New York: Raven Press, 1972, pp. 393–408.

262. KOCSIS, J., et al. "Tricyclic Plasma Levels and Clinical Response," *Syllabus and Scientific Proceedings of the American Psychiatric Association*, 136 (1983):128.

263. KRAGH-SORENSEN, P., ASBERG, M., and EGGERT-HANSEN, C. "Plasma Nortriptyline Levels in Endogenous Depression," *Lancet*, 1 (1973):113.

264. KRAGH-SORENSEN, P., HANSEN, I. E., and

ASBERG, M. "Plasma Levels of Nortriptyline in the Treatment of Endogenous Depression," *Acta Psychiatrica Scandinavica*, 49 (1973):445–456.

265. KRAGH-SORENSEN, P., et al. "Self-inhibiting Action of Nortriptyline Antidepressive Effect at High Plasma Levels," *Psychopharmacologia*, 45 (1976):305–312.

266. KRETSCHMAR, J. H. "Mianserin and Amitriptyline in Elderly Hospitalized Patients with Depressive Illness: A Double-blind Trial," *Current Medical Research and Opinion*, 6 (Supplement) (1980):144–151.

267. KRISTOF, F. E., LEHMANN, H. E., and BAN, T. A. "Systematic Studies with Trimipramine—A New Antidepressant Drug," *Canadian Psychiatric Association Journal*, 12 (1967):17–20.

268. KROEGER, R., and ECKMANN, F. "Klinische Untersuchungen mit Nomifensin. Bericht uber Einen Doppelblindvergleich Zwischen Nomifensin und Placebo: Wirkungsnachweis bei Endogenen und Involutiven Depressionen," in *Alival Symposium uber Ergebnisse der Experimentellen und Klinischen Prufung* (1976). Stuttgart: F. K. Schattauer, 1977.

269. KUHN, R. "The Treatment of Depressive States with G 22355 (Imipramine Hydrochloride)," *American Journal of Psychiatry*, 115 (1958):459–464.

270. KUPFER, D. J., et al. "Amitriptyline Plasma Levels and Clinical Response: II," *Communications in Psychopharmacology*, 2 (1975):441–450.

271. KUPFER, D. J., et al. "Amitriptyline Plasma Levels and Clinical Response in Primary Depression," *Clinical Pharmacology Therapy*, 22 (1977):904–911.

272. LASCELLES, R. G. "Atypical Facial Pain and Depression," *British Journal of Psychiatry*, 112 (1966):651.

273. LASSEN, J. B., et al. "Inhibition of 5-HT Uptake into Neurons and Platelets in Mice Treated Chronically with Chlorimipramine and Femoxetine," *Psychopharmacology*, 64 (1979):149–153.

274. LAURELL, B., and OTTOSSON, J. O. "Prophylactic Lithium?" *Lancet*, 2 (1968):1245–1246.

275. LAURITSEN, B. "Continental Hospital Studies with Maprotiline (Ludiomil),"

Journal of International Medical Research, 3 (Supplement) (1975):61.

276. LAURITSEN, B., and MADSEN, H. "A Multinational Double-blind Trial with a New Antidepressant (Ludiomil) and Amitriptyline," *Acta Psychiatrica Scandinavica*, 50 (1974):192.

277. LEAN, T. H., and SIDHU, M. S. "Comparative Study of Imipramine (Tofranil) and Trimipramine (Surmontil) in Depression Associated with Gynaecological Conditions," *Proceedings of the Society for Obstetrics and Gynecology*, 3(1978):222–228.

278. LEHMANN, H. E., et al. "A Double-blind Comparative Clinical Trial with Maprotiline (Ludiomil) and Imipramine in Newly-admitted Depressed Patients," *Current Therapeutic Research*, 19 (1976):463.

279. LEIBOWITZ, M. R., et al. "Phenelzine vs. Imipramine in Atypical Depression," *Archives of General Psychiatry*, 41 (1984):669–677.

280. LEMBERGER, L., et al. "Fluoxetine, a Selective Serotonin Uptake Inhibitor," *Clinical Pharmacology and Therapeutics*, 23 (1978):421–429.

281. LENA, B. "Lithium in Child and Adolescent Psychiatry," *Archives of General Psychiatry*, 36 (1979):854–855.

282. LENNOX, I. G. "Viloxazine and Amitriptyline in Depressive Illness," *The Practitioner* 216 (1976):153–156.

283. LEON, P., and OSORIO, M. "Efficacy and Tolerance of a New Psychotherapeutic Antidepressant—Nomifensine," *Acta Medica Peruana*, 3 (1974):202–206.

284. LEONHARD, K. *Aufteilung der Endogenen Psychosen*, 2nd ed. Berlin: Akademie-Veriag, 1959.

285. LEONHARD, K., KORFF, I. and SCHULZ, H. "Temperament in Families with Unipolar and Bipolar Phasic Psychoses," *Psychiatric Neurology*, 143 (1962):416–434.

286. LEVIN, A. "Maprotiline and Amitriptyline in the Treatment of Depressive Illness. A Double-blind Comparison," *South African Medical Journal*, 48 (1974):47.

287. LEVINE, S. "A Controlled Comparison of Maprotiline (Ludiomil) with Imipramine Avoiding Observer Bias," *Journal of International Medical Research*, 3 (Supplement) (1975):75.

288. LIEBLING, L. I. "Once-daily Dosage Study with Maprotiline (Ludiomil)," *Journal of International Medical Research,* 3 (Supplement) (1975):109.

289. LIN, R. C., et al. "Turnover Rates of Serotonin and Norepinephrine in Brain of Normal and Pargyline Treated Rats," *Life Sciences,* 8 (1969):1077–1084.

290. LINGJAERDE, O. "Inhibition of Platelet Uptake of Serotonin in Plasma from Patients Treated with Chlorimipramine and Amitriptyline," *European Journal of Clinical Pharmacology,* 15 (1979):335–340.

291. LINGJAERDE, O. "Synergistic Effect of Tricyclic Antidepressants and Lithium Carbonate in Endogenous Depression (letter to the editor)," *Lancet,* 2 (1973): 1260.

292. LINGJAERDE, O., et al. "The Effect of Lithium Carbonate in Combination with Tricyclic Antidepressant in Endogenous Depression," *Acta Psychiatrica Scandinavica,* 50 (1974):233–242.

293. LIPMAN, R. S., et al. "Medication, Anxiety Reduction and Patient Report of Significant Life Situation Events," *Diseases of the Nervous System,* 32 (1971):240–244.

294. LIPPER, S., et al. "Comparative Behavioral Effects of Clorgyline and Pargyline in Man. Preliminary Evaluation," *Psychopharmacology,* 62 (1979):123–128.

295. LIPSEDGE, M. S., et al., "The Management of Severe Agoraphobia: A Comparison of Iproniazid and Systematic Desensitization," *Psychopharmacologia,* 32 (1973):67–80.

296. LOGUE, J. N., SACHAIS, B. A., and FEIGHNER, J. P. "Comparisons of Maprotiline with Imipramine in Severe Depression: A Multicenter Controlled Trial," *Journal of Clinical Pharmacology,* 19 (1979):64–74.

297. LOMAN, D. H. "A Comparative Study of Maprotiline (Ludiomil) and Viloxazine in the Management of Depressed Patients in General Practice," *Journal of International Medical Research,* 5 (Supplement 4) (1977):39–45.

298. LOOMER, H. P., SAUNDERS, J. C., and KLINE, N. S. "A Clinical and Pharmacodynamic Evaluation of Iproniazid as a Psychic Energizer," *Psychiatric Research Reports,* 8 (1957):129–141.

299. LOUDON, J. B. Personal communication, 1980.

300. MAAGS, R. "Treatment of Manic Illness with Lithium Carbonate," *British Journal of Psychiatry,* 109 (1963):56–65.

301. MCCAWLEY, A. "A Double-blind Evaluation of Nomifensine and Imipramine in Depressed Outpatients," *American Journal of Psychiatry,* 136 (1979):841–842.

302. MCCLELLAND, H. A., KERR, T. A., and LITTLE, J. C. "A Clinical Comparison of Nomifensine and Amitriptyline," *British Journal of Pharmacology,* 4 (Supplement) (1977):233–236.

303. MCCLELLAND, H. A., et al. "The Comparative Antidepressant Value of Lofepramine and Amitriptyline," *Acta Psychiatrica Scandinavica,* 60 (1979):190–198.

304. MCCLURE, D. J., LOW, G. L, and GANT, M. "Chlorimipramine HCl—A Double-blind Study of a New Antidepressant Drug," *Canadian Psychiatric Association Journal,* 18 (1973):403–408.

305. MCEVOY, J., et al. "Viloxazine in the Treatment of Depressive Neurosis: A Controlled Clinical Study with Doxepin and Placebo," *British Journal of Psychiatry,* 137 (1980):440–443.

306. MADALENA, J. C. "The Treatment of Depressive States with Monochlorimipramine in Slow Intravenous Perfusion and by the Oral Route," *Hospital* (Rio de Janiero), 74 (1968):147.

307. MAGNUS, R. V. "A Placebo-Controlled Trial of Viloxazine With and Without Tranquilizers in Depressive Illness," *Journal of International Medical Research,* 3 (1975):207–213.

308. MANDELL, A. J., and KNAPP, S. "Asymmetry and Mood. Emergent Properties of Serotonin Regulation," *Archives of General Psychiatry,* 36 (1979):909–916.

309. MANN, J. J., et al. "A Controlled Study of Trazodone, Imipramine, and Placebo in Outpatients with Endogenous Depression," *Journal of Clinical Psychopharmacology,* 1 (1981):75–80.

310. MARAIS, G.F.T. "Clinical Evaluation of the Antidepressants Maprotiline and Amitriptyline. A Double-blind Controlled Trial," *South African Medical Journal,* 48 (1974):1530.

311. MARINI, J. L., and SHEARD, N. H. "Anti-

aggressive Effect of Lithium Ion in Man," *Acta Psychiatrica Scandinavica*, 55 (1977):267–286.

312. MARSHALL, E. F., et al. "The Influence of Acetylator Phenotype on the Outcome of Treatment with Phenelzine in a Clinical Trial," *British Journal of Clinical Pharmacology*, 6 (1978):247–254.

313. MARSHALL, W. K. "Chlorimipramine (Anafranil) in the Treatment of Phobic States: A Psychiatrist's View," *Journal of International Medical Research*, 3 (Supplement) (1975):89–93.

314. MARTIN, L., BAKER, G., and MITCHELL, P. "The Effects of Viloxazine HCl on the Transport of Noradrenaline, Dopamine and 5-Hydroxytryptamine and Aminobuteric Acid in Rat Brain Tissue," *Neuropharmacology*, 17 (1978):421.

315. MATHUR, G. N. "A Double-blind Comparative Clinical Trial with Maprotiline (Ludiomil) and Amitriptyline," *Journal of International Medical Research*, 3 (Supplement) (1975):71.

316. MATUZAS, W., et al. "Plasma Concentrations of Imipramine and Clinical Response Among Depressed Outpatients," *Journal of Clinical Psychopharmacology*, 2(1982):140–142.

317. MATUZAS, W., et al. "Plasma and Red Blood Cell Concentrations of Imipramine and Clinical Response Among Depressed Outpatients," paper presented at the annual meeting of the American Psychiatric Association, 1983.

318. MAZZEI, M., MARRI, F. M., and FABIANI, F. "Relazione Clinica su uno Studio Sperimentale con un Nuovo Pisofarmaco: L'A.F.-1161 (Trazodone)," *Rivista Neurobiologia*, 17 (1971):238–260.

319. Medical Research Council. "Streptomycin Treatment of Pulmonary Tuberculosis," *British Medical Journal*, 2 (1948): 769.

320. Medical Research Council Drug Trials Subcommittee Report. "Continuation Therapy with Lithium and Amitriptyline in Unipolar Depressive Illness: A Controlled Clinical Trial," *Psychological Medicine*, 11 (1981):409–416.

321. MELIA, P. L. "Prophylactic Lithium: A Double-blind Trial in Recurrent Affective Disorders," *British Journal of Psychiatry*, 116 (1970):621–624.

322. MENDELS, J. "Lithium in the Treatment of Depression," *American Journal of Psychiatry*, 133 (1976):373–378.

323. MENDELS, J., SECUNDA, S., and DYSON, W. L. A. "A Controlled Study of the Antidepressant Effects of Lithium," *Archives of General Psychiatry*, 26 (1972): 154–157.

324. MENDELWICZ, J., FIEVE, R., and STALLONE, F. "Relationship Between Effectiveness of Lithium Therapy and Family History," *American Journal of Psychiatry*, 130 (1973):1011–1013.

325. MENDELWICZ, J., LINKOWSKI, P., and REES, J. A. "A Double-blind Comparison of Dothiepin and Amitriptyline in Patients with Primary Affective Disorder: Serum Levels and Clinical Response," *British Journal of Psychiatry*, 136 (1980):154–160.

326. MIDDLETON, R. S. W. "A Comparison Between Maprotiline (Ludiomil) and Imipramine in the Treatment of Depressive Illness in the Elderly," *Journal of International Medical Research*, 3 (Supplement) (1975):79.

327. MINDHAM, B. A. E. "A Comparison of Maprotiline (Ludiomil) and Amitriptyline (2)," *Journal of International Medical Research*, 5 (Supplement) (1977):25–33.

328. MINDHAM, R. H. S., HOWLAND, C., and SHEPHERD, M. "Continuation Therapy with Tricyclic Antidepressants in Depressive Illness," *Lancet*, 2 (1972):854–855.

329. ———. "An Evaluation of Continuation Therapy with Tricyclic Antidepressants in Depressive Illness," *Psychological Medicine*, 3 (1973):5–17.

330. MOISES, H. W., KASPER, S., and BECKMANN, H. "Trazodone and Amitriptyline in Treatment of Depressed Inpatients: A Double-blind Study," *Pharmakopsychiatrie*, 14 (1981):167–171.

331. MOLNAR, G. "Maprotiline—A Double-blind Study of a New Tetracyclic Antidepressant in Severe Depression," *Canadian Psychiatric Association Journal*, 22 (1977):19–23.

332. MONTGOMERY, S. A., BRAITHWAITE, R. A., and CRAMMER, J. L. "Routine Nortriptyline Levels in Treatment of Depression," *British Medical Journal*, 2 (1977): 166.

333. MONTGOMERY, S. A. et al. "Differential Effects on Suicidal Ideation of Mianserin, Maprotiline and Amitriptyline," *British Journal of Clinical Pharmacology,* 5 (1978):775–805.

334. MONTGOMERY, S. A., et al. "High Plasma Nortriptyline Levels in the Treatment of Depression. I," *Clinical Pharmacology Therapeutics,* 23 (1978):309–314.

335. MONTGOMERY, S. A., et al. "Pharmacokinetics and Efficacy of Maprotiline and Amitriptyline in Endogenous Depression: A Double-blind Controlled Trial," *Clinical Therapeutics,* 3 (1980):292–310.

336. MORRIS, J. B., and BECK, A. T. "The Efficacy of Antidepressant Drugs: A Review of Research (1958–1972)," *Archives of General Psychiatry,* 30 (1974):667–674.

337. MULGIRIGAMA, L. D., et al. "An Assessment of Uptake Inhibition of 5-Hydroxytryptamine, Dopamine, and Noradrenaline in a Double-blind Clinical Trial of Chlorimipramine and Maprotiline in Depressed Outpatients." Unpublished manuscript.

338. MURPHY, D. L., et al. "Biochemical Indices of the Effects of Selective MAO Inhibitors (Clorgyline, Pargyline, Deprenyl) in Man," in E. Usdin, et al., eds., *Clinical Pharmacology in Psychiatry.* London: Macmillan, 1981, pp. 307–316.

339. MURPHY, E. J., DONALD, J. F., and MOLLA, A. L. "Mianserin in the Treatment of Depression in General Practice," *Practitioner,* 217 (1976):135–138.

340. MURPHY, J. E. "A Comparative Trial of Drug GB94 and Imipramine in the Treatment of Depression in General Practice," *Journal of International Medical Research,* 3 (1975):251–260.

341. MURPHY, J. E. "A Double-blind General Practice Trial of Maprotiline (Ludiomil) Against Amitriptyline in the Treatment of Reactive Depression," *Journal of International Medical Research,* 3 (Supplement) (1975):97.

342. MURPHY, J. E., and ANKIER, S. I. "An Evaluation of Trazodone in the Treatment of Depression," *Neuropharmacology,* 19 (1980):1217–1218.

343. MURPHY, J. E., and BRIDGMAN, K. M. "A Comparative Clinical Trial of Mianserin (Normal) and Amitriptyline in the Treatment of Depression in General Practice," *Journal of International Medical Research,* 6 (1978):199–206.

344. MURPHY, J. E., and FORREST, W. A. "A Comparison Between Maprotiline (Ludiomil) and Amitriptyline in the Treatment of Depressive Reaction in General Practice," *Journal of International Medical Research,* 3 (Supplement) (1975):108.

345. NAYLOR, G. J., et al. "A Double-blind Trial of Long-Term Lithium Therapy in Mental Defectives," *British Journal of Psychiatry,* 124 (1974):52–57.

346. NEFF, N. H., and COSTA, E. "The Influence of Monoamine Oxidase Inhibition on Catecholamine Synthesis," *Life Sciences,* 5 (1966):951–958.

347. NEITO, D. "Treatment of Maniacal States with Lithium Carbonate," *Revista de Investigacion Clinica,* 4 (1965):81–85.

348. NELSON, J. C., et al. "Desipramine Plasma Concentration and Antidepressant Response," *Archives of General Psychiatry,* 39 (1982):1419–1422.

349. NELSON, J. C., et al. "Drug-response Symptoms in Melancholia," *Archives of General Psychiatry,* 41 (1984):663–668.

350. NIES, A., et al. "The Efficacy of the Monoamine Oxidase Inhibitor Phenelzine: Dose Effects and Prediction of Response," in J. R. Boissier, H. Hipptus, and P. Pichot, eds., *Neuropsychopharmacology,* vol. 39. Amsterdam: Excerpta Medica, 1975, p. 47.

351. NIMH Research Branch Collaborative Study Group. "Short-term Improvement in Schizophrenia: The Contribution of Background Factors," *American Journal of Psychiatry,* 124 (1968):900–909.

352. NOACK, C. H., and TRAUTNER, E. M. "The Lithium Treatment of Maniacal Psychosis," *Medical Journal of Australia,* 2 (1951):219–222.

353. NOYES, R., et al. "Lithium Treatment of Depression," *Comprehensive Psychiatry,* 15 (1974):187–193.

354. NUGENT, D. "A Double-blind Study of Viloxazine (Vivalan) and Amitriptyline in Depressed Geriatric Patients," *Clinical Trials Journal,* 6 (1979):13–17.

400. PRIEN, R. F., et al. "Drug Therapy in the Prevention of Recurrences in Unipolar and Bipolar Affective Disorders," *Archives of General Psychiatry*, 41 (1984): 1096–1104.

401. PULL, C. B., et al. "Double-blind Multi-center Trial Comparing Mianserin and Imipramine," *Acta Psychiatrica Belgica*, 78 (1978):827–832.

402. QUITKIN, F., RIFKIN, A., and KLEIN, D. F. "Prophylaxis of Affective Disorders," *Archives of General Psychiatry*, 33 (1976):337–341.

403. ———. "Imipramine Response in Deluded Depressive Patients," *American Journal of Psychiatry*, 135 (1978): 806–811.

404. QUITKIN, F. M., et al. "Lithium and Imipramine in the Prophylaxis of Unipolar and Bipolar II Depression: A Prospective, Placebo-controlled Comparison," *Psychopharmacology Bulletin*, 17 (1981):142–144.

405. QUITKIN, F. M., et al. "Duration of Antidepressant Drug Treatment," *Archives of General Psychiatry*, 41 (1984): 238–245.

406. RACK, P. H. "A Comparative Clinical Trial of Oral Chlorimipramine (Anafranil) Against Imipramine," *Journal of International Medical Research*, 1 (1973): 332–337.

407. RAFT, D., et al. "Relationship Between Response to Phenelzine and MAO Inhibition in a Clinical Trial of Phenelzine, Amitriptyline, and Placebo," *Neuropsychobiology*, 7 (1981):122–126.

408. RASKIN, A., et al. "Differential Response to Chlorpromazine, Imipramine and a Placebo: A Study of Hospitalized Depressed Patients," *Archives of General Psychiatry*, 23 (1970):165–173.

409. RASKIN, A., et al. "Depression Subtypes and Response to Phenelzine, Diazepam and Placebo," *Archives of General Psychiatry*, 30 (1974):66–75.

410. RAVARIS, C. L., et al. "A Multiple-Dose, Controlled Study of Phenelzine in Depression-Anxiety States," *Archives of General Psychiatry*, 33 (1976):347–350.

411. REES, L., and DAVIES, B. "A Controlled Trial of Phenelzine (Nardil) in the Treatment of Severe Depressive Illness," *Journal of Mental Science*, 107 (1961):560–566.

412. REID, A. H. "Psychoses in Adult Mental Defectives: I. Manic-Depressive Psychosis," *British Journal of Psychiatry*, 120 (1972):205–212.

413. REIGER, W., et al. "Maprotiline (Ludiomil) and Imipramine in Depressed Inpatients. A Controlled Study," *Journal of International Medical Research*, 3 (1975):413.

414. REISBY, N., et al. "Imipramine: Clinical Effects and Pharmacokinetic Variability," *Psychopharmacology*, 54 (1977): 263–272.

415. REYNOLDS, C. M., et al. "A Double-blind Trial of Lithium in Alcoholism," in F. S. Johnson, and S. Johnson, eds., *Lithium in Medical Practice*. Baltimore: University Park Press, 1978, pp. 53–60.

416. RICKELS, K., et al. "Amitriptyline and Trimipramine in Neurotic Depressed Patients: A Collaborative Study," *American Journal of Psychiatry*, 127 (1970):208–218.

417. RICKELS, K., et al. "Doxepin and Amitriptyline-Perphenazine in Mixed Anxious-Depressed Neurotic Outpatients: A Collaborative Controlled Study," *Psychopharmacologia*, 23 (1972):305–318.

418. RICKELS, K., et al. "Chlorimipramine and Amitriptyline in Depressed Outpatients," *Psychopharmacologia*, 34 (1974):361–376.

419. RICKELS, K., et al. "Doxepin and Amitriptyline-Perphenazine in Mixed Anxious-Depressed Neurotic Outpatients: A Collaborative Controlled Study," *Psychopharmacologia*, 18 (1977):239.

420. RICKELS, K., et al. "Amoxapine and Imipramine in the Treatment of Depressed Outpatients: A Controlled Study," *American Journal of Psychiatry*, 138 (1981):20–24.

421. RICKELS, K., et al. "Tricyclic Plasma Levels in Depressed Outpatients Treated with Amitriptyline," *Psychopharmacology*, 80 (1983):14–18.

422. RIFKIN, A., et al. "Comparison of Trimipramine and Imipramine: A Controlled Study," *Journal of Clinical Psychiatry*, 41 (1980):124–129.

423. ROBINS, E., and GUZE, S. B. "Classification

of Affective Disorders: The Primary-Secondary, the Endogenous-Reactive and the Neurotic-Psychotic Concepts," in T. A. Williams, M. M. Katz, and J. A. Shield, Jr., eds., *Recent Advances in the Psychobiology of the Depressive Illnesses,* U.S. Department of Health, Education and Welfare Publication 70–9053. Washington, D.C.: U.S. Government Printing Office, 1972, pp. 283–293.

424. ROBINSON, D.S., et al. "The Monoamine Oxidase Inhibitor Phenelzine in the Treatment of Depressive-Anxiety States: A Controlled Clinical Trial," *Archives of General Psychiatry* 29 (1973): 407–413.

425. ROBINSON, D. S., et al. "Clinical Pharmacology of Phenelzine," *Archives of General Psychiatry,* 35 (1978):629–635.

426. ROBINSON, D. S., et al. "Plasma Tricyclic Drug Levels in Amitriptyline-treated Depressed Patients," *Psychopharmacology* (Berlin), 63 (1979):223–231.

427. ROBINSON, D. S., et al. "A Comparison of Trazodone, Amoxapine and Maprotiline in the Treatment of Endogenous Depression: Results of a Multicenter Study," *Current Therapeutic Research,* 35 (1984):549–560.

428. ROGERS, S.C., DAVIES, I. J., and GALBRAITH, A.W. "A Study of Depression in Two General Practices. A Double-blind Comparison of Desipramine and Opipramol," *Clinical Trials Journal,* 6 (1969):5–11.

429. ROSLOFF, B. N., and DAVIS, J. M. "Effects of Iprindole on Norepinephrine Turnover and Transport," *Psychopharmacologia,* 40 (1974):53–64.

430. ROWAN, P. R., PAYKEL, E. S., and PARKER, R. R. "Phenelzine and Amitriptyline: Effects on Symptoms of Neurotic Depression," *British Journal of Psychiatry,* 140 (1982):475–483.

431. ROY, J. Y., et al. "Evaluation Comparative de la Dibencycladine (Ludiomil) et de l'Imipramine Chez le Deprime Psychotique," *International Journal of Clinical Pharmacology,* 7 (1973):54.

432. RUSSELL, G.F.M., et al. "Comparative Double-blind Trial of Mianserin Hydrochloride (Organon GB94) and Diazepam in Patients with Depressive Ill-

ness," *British Journal of Clinical Pharmacology,* 5 (Supplement) (1978): 57–65.

433. SALETU, B., and GUENBERGER, J. "Changes in Clinical Symptomatology and Psychometric Assessments in Depressed Patients During Mianserin and Combined Amitriptyline/Chlordiazepoxide Therapy: A Double-blind Comparison," *Current Medical Research and Opinion,* 6 (Supplement) (1980):52–62.

434. SALETU, B., et al. "Fluvoxamine—A New Serotonin Reuptake Inhibitor: First Clinical and Psychometric Experiences in Depressed Patients," *Journal of Neural Transmission,* 41 (1977):17–36.

435. SALZMAN, M. M. "A Controlled Trial of Triimipramine, a New Antidepressant Drug," *British Journal of Psychiatry,* 111 (1965):1105–1106.

436. SANDIFER, M. G., WILSON, I. C., and GAMBILL, J. M. "The Influence of Case Selection and Dosage in Antidepressant Drug Trial," *British Journal of Psychiatry,* 111 (1965):142–148.

437. SANTONASTASO, P., MAISTRELLO, I., and BATTISTIN, L. "Comparison of Vivalan (Viloxazine Hydrochloride) with Imipramine in the Treatment of Depression," *Acta Psychiatrica Scandinavica,* 60 (1979):137–143.

438. SATHANANTHAN, G. L., et al. "Amoxapine and Imipramine: A Double-blind Study in Depressed Patients," *Current Therapeutic Research,* 15 (1973):919–922.

439. SAVAGE, D. J., MENDELS, J., and FRAZER, A. "Monoamine Oxidase Inhibitors and Serotonin Uptake Inhibitors: Differential Effects on (^{3}H) Serotonin Binding Sites in Rat Brains," *Journal of Pharmacological and Experimental Therapeutics,* 212 (1980):259–263.

440. SCHACHT, R., and HEPTNER, W. "Effect of Nomifensine, a New Antidepressant, on the Uptake of Noradrenaline and Serotonin and on Release of Noradrenaline in Rat Brain Synaptosomes," *Biochemical Pharmacology,* 23 (1974): 3413–3422.

441. SCHATZBERG, A. F., and COLE, J. O. "Benzodiazepines in Depressive Disorders," *Archives of General Psychiatry,* 35 (1978):1359–1365.

442. SCHILDKRAUT, J. J. "The Catecholamine Hypothesis of Affective Disorders (A Review of Supporting Evidence)," *American Journal of Psychiatry*, 122 (1965):509.

443. SCHILDKRAUT, J. J., et al. "Excretion of 3-Methoxy-4-Hydroxy-Mandelic Acid in Depressed Patients Treated with Antidepressant Drugs," *Journal of Psychiatric Research*, 2 (1964):257–266.

444. SCHILDKRAUT, J. J., et al. "Norepinephrine Metabolism and Drugs Used in the Affective Disorders: A Possible Mechanism of Action," *American Journal of Psychiatry*, 124 (1967):600–608.

445. SCHOU, M. "Normythymics 'Mood Normalizers' Are Lithium and the Imipramine Drugs Specific for Affective Disorders," *British Journal of Psychiatry*, 109 (1963):803–804.

446. ———. "Lithium in Psychiatric Therapy and Prophylaxis," *Journal of Psychiatric Research*, 6 (1968):67–95.

447. ———. "Prophylactic and Maintenance Therapy in Recurrent Affective Disorders," in D. M. Gallant, and G. M Simpson, eds., *Depression: Behavioral, Biochemical, Diagnostic, and Treatment Considerations*. New York: Spectrum Publications, 1976, pp. 309–334.

448. SCHOU, M., and BAASTRUP, P. C. "Lithium and Manic-Depressive Psychosis," *Sandorama*, 17 (special issue) (1966):48–49.

449. SCHOU, M., THOMSEN, K., and BAASTRUP, P. C. "Studies on the Course of Recurrent Endogenous Affective Disorders," *International Pharmacopsychiatry*, 5 (1970):100–106.

450. SCHOU, M., et al. "The Treatment of Manic Psychoses by the Administration of Lithium Salts," *Journal of Neurology, Neurosurgery and Psychiatry*, 17 (1954):250–260.

451. SCHOU, M., et al. "Pharmacological and Clinical Problems of Lithium Prophylaxis," *British Journal of Psychiatry*, 116 (1970):615–619.

452. SEAGER, C. P., and BIRD, R. L. "Imipramine with Electrical Treatment in Depression: A Controlled Trial," *Journal of Mental Science*, 108 (1962):704–707.

453. SETHI, B. B., et al. "Amoxapine and Amitriptyline: A Double-blind Study in Depressed Patients," *Current Therapeutic Research*, 25 (1979):726–737.

454. SETHY, V. H., and HODGES, D. H. "Role of β-Adrenergic Receptors in the Antidepressant Activity of Alprazolam," paper read before the Benzodiazepine Symposium, National Institute of Mental Health, April 1982.

455. SHAIUSUPOVA, A. V. "Treatment of Manic Symptoms with Lithium Salts," *Meditsinskaia Zhurnal Uzbek*, 11 (1962):36–37.

456. SHARMA, S. D. "A Double-blind Clinical Evaluation of Nomifensine," *Current Therapeutic Research*, 27 (1980):157–163.

457. SHEARD, M. H., et al. "The Effect of Lithium on the Impulsive Aggressive Behavior in Man," *American Journal of Psychiatry*, 133 (1976):1409–1413.

458. SHEEHY, L. M., and MAXMEN, J. "Phenelzine Induced Psychosis," *American Journal of Psychiatry*, 135 (1978):1422.

459. SHEPHARD, M. "Report to the Medical Research Council by Its Clinical Psychiatry Committee: Clinical Trial of the Treatment of Depressive Illness," *British Medical Journal*, 1 (1965):881.

460. SHOPSIN, B., and GERSHON, S. "Pharmacology-Toxicology of the Lithium Ion," in S. Gershon and B. Shopsin, eds., *Lithium: Its Role in Psychiatric Research and Treatment*. New York: Plenum Press, 1973, pp. 107–146.

461. SHOPSIN, B., GERSHON, S., and THOMPSON, H. "Psychoactive Drugs in Mania," *Archives of General Psychiatry*, 32 (1975):34–35.

462. SIMPSON, G., et al. "Relationship Between Plasma Antidepressant Levels and Clinical Outcome for Inpatients Receiving Imipramine," *American Journal of Psychiatry*, 139 (1982):358–360.

463. SINGH, A. N., et al. "Maprotiline (Ludiomil, CIBA 34:276 Ba) and Imipramine in Depressed Outpatients: A Double-blind Clinical Study," *Current Therapeutic Research*, 19 (1976):451.

464. SIVERS, B., et al. "Comparative Clinical Evaluation of Lofepramine and Imipramine," *Acta Psychiatrica Scandinavica*, 55 (1974):21–31.

465. SMALL, J. G., SMALL, I. F., and MOORE, D. F. "Experimental Withdrawal of Lith-

ium in Recovered Manic-Depressive Patients: A Report of Five Cases," *American Journal of Psychiatry,* 127 (1971):1555–1558.

466. SMITH, A.H.W., NAYLOR, G. S., and MOODY, J. P. "Placebo-Controlled Double-blind Trial of Mianserin Hydrochloride," *British Journal of Clinical Pharmacology,* 5 (1978):675–705.

467. SMITH, R. C. "Amoxapine, Imipramine and Placebo in Depressive Illness," *Current Therapeutic Research,* 18 (1975): 346.

468. SMULEVITCH, A. "The Treatment and Prevention of Affective and Schizoaffective Psychoses," paper presented at the World Psychiatric Association Symposium on Aspects of Schizophrenia, October 1973.

469. SOLYOM, L., et al. "Behavior Therapy Versus Drug Therapy in the Treatment of Phobic Neurosis," *Canadian Psychiatric Association Journal,* 18 (1973):25–32.

470. SOROKO, F. E., et al. "Bupropion Hydrochloride ([+/−] Alpha-t-Butylamino-3-chloropiophenone HCL): A Novel Antidepressant," *Journal of Pharmacy and Pharmacology,* 29 (1977):767–770.

471. SPECTOR, S., HIRSCH, C. W., and BRODIE, B. B. "Association of Behavioral Effects of Pargyline, a Non-Hydrazine MAO Inhibitor, with Increase in Brain Norepinephrine," *International Journal of Neuropharmacology,* 2 (1963):81–93.

472. SPLITTER, S. R. "Comprehensive Treatment of Office Patients with the Aid of a New Psychophysiologic Agent: Opipramol," *Psychosomatics,* 4 (1963):283–289.

473. SRINIVASAN, D. P., and HULLIN, R. P. "Current Concepts of Lithium Therapy," *British Journal of Hospital Medicine,* (1980):466–475.

474. STALLONE, F., et al. "The Use of Lithium in Affective Disorders. III. A Double-blind Study of Prophylaxis in Bipolar Illness," *American Journal of Psychiatry,* 130 (1973):1006–1010.

475. STANCER, H. C., FURLING, F. W., and GODSE, D. D. "A Longitudinal Investigation of Lithium as a Prophylactic Agent for Recurrent Depression," *Canadian Psychiatric Association Journal,* 15 (1970):29–40.

476. STEIN, M. K., RICKELS, K., and WEISE, C. C. "Maintenance Therapy with Amitriptyline: A Controlled Trial," *American Journal of Psychiatry,* 137 (1980): 370–371.

477. STEINBOOK, R. M., et al. "Amoxapine, Imipramine, and Placebo: A Double-blind Study with Pretherapy Urinary 3-Methoxy-4-Hydroxy-Phenylglycol Levels," *Current Therapeutic Research,* 26 (1979):490–496.

478. STERLIN, C., et al. "A Preliminary Investigation of WY-3263 Versus Amitriptyline in Depressions," *Current Therapeutic Research,* 10 (1968):576–582.

479. STERN, W. C., and HARTO-TRUAX, N. "Two Multicenter Studies of the Antidepressant Effects of Bupropion HCl Versus Placebo," *Psychopharmacology Bulletin,* 16 (1980):43–46.

480. STOKES, P. E., et al. "Efficacy of Lithium as Acute Treatment of Manic-Depressive Illness," *Lancet,* 1 (1971):1319–1325.

481. STRAKER, M., DAVANLOO, H., and MOLL, A. A. "A Double-blind Comparison of a New Antidepressant, Protriptyline, with Imipramine and Amitriptyline," *American Medical Association Journal,* 94 (1966):1220–1222.

482. SULSER, F., VETULANI, J., and MOBLEY, P. "Mode of Action of Antidepressant Drugs," *Biochemical Pharmacology,* 27 (1978):257–261.

483. SUTHERLAND, M. S., et al. "Comparison of Effects of Pramindole and Imipramine," *Clinical Trials Journal,* 4 (1967): 857–860.

484. SVESTKA, J., et al. "Controlled Comparison of Mianserin with Imipramine in Endogenous Depressions," *Activitas Nervosa Superior,* 21 (1979):147–148.

485. TAEUBER, K. "Comparison of Nomifensine and Placebo," *British Journal of Clinical Pharmacology,* 4 (Supplement) (1977):209–213.

486. TAKAHASHI, R., SAKUMA, A., and HOH, K. "Comparison of Efficacy of Lithium Carbonate and Chlorpromazine in Mania," *Archives of General Psychiatry,* 32 (1975):1310–1318.

487. TAKAHASHI, R., et al. "Comparison of Efficacy of Amoxapine and Imipramine in a Multi-Clinic Double-blind Study Using the WHO Schedule for a Standard As-

sessment of Patients with Depressive Disorders," *Journal of International Medical Research,* 7 (1979):7–18.

488. THOREN, P., et al. "Chlorimipramine Treatment of Obsessive-Compulsive Disorder," *Archives of General Psychiatry,* 37 (1980):1281–1285.

489. TRICK, K. S. "Double-blind Comparison of Maprotiline with Amitriptyline in the Treatment of Depressive Illness," *International Pharmacopsychiatry,* 10 (1975):193–198.

490. TYRER, P. "Towards Rational Therapy with Monoamine Oxidase Inhibitors," *British Journal of Psychiatry,* 128 (1976):354–360.

491. UHLENHUTH, E. H., and PARK, L. C. "The Influence of Medication (Imipramine) and Doctor in Relieving Depressed Psychoneurotic Outpatients," *Journal of Psychiatric Research,* 2 (1964):101.

492. Upjohn Labs, Alprazolam in the Treatment of Depression. Data on file, 1985.

493. URE, A. "Observation and Researches Upon a New Solvent for Stone in the Bladder," *Pharmaceutical Journal,* 5 (1843):71–74.

494. VAISANEN, E., et al. "Maprotiline and Doxepin in the Treatment of Depression. A Double-blind Multicentre Comparison," *Acta Psychiatrica Scandinavica,* 57 (1978):193–201.

495. VAN SCHEYEN, J. D., VAN PRAAG, H. M., and KORF, J. "Controlled Study Comparing Nomifensine and Chlorimipramine in Unipolar Depression, Using the Probenecid Technique," *British Journal of Clinical Pharmacology,* 4 (1977): 1795–1845.

496. VARTANYAN, M. Y. "Result of Lithium Carbonate Therapy in Agitation States," *Zhurnal Neuropatologii i Psikhiatrii,* 59 (1959):581–589.

497. VINCI, M. "Contributo Clinico alla Terapia delle Depressioni Endogene con un Derivato della Triazolpiridina," *L'Ospedale Psichiatrica,* 39 (1971):416–433.

498. VOGEL, H. P., BENTE, D., and FEDER, J. "Mianserin Versus Amitriptyline: A Double-blind Trial Evaluated by the AMP System," *International Pharmacopsychiatry,* 11 (1976):25–31.

499. WASMAN, D. "An Investigation into the Use of Anafranil in Phobic and Obsessional Disorders," *Scottish Medical Journal,* 20 (Supplement) (1975):61–66.

500. WATANABE, S., ISHINO, H, and OTSUKI, S. "Double-blind Comparison of Lithium Carbonate and Imipramine in Treatment of Depression," *Archives of General Psychiatry,* 32 (1975):659–668.

501. WEISSMAN, M. M. "Psychotherapy and Its Relevance to the Pharmacotherapy of the Affective Disorders: From Ideology to Evidence," in M. A. Lipton, A. DiMascio, and K. F. Killam, eds., *Psychopharmacology: A Generation of Progress.* New York: Raven Press, 1978, pp. 1313–1321

502. WEISSMAN, M. M., et al. "A Double-blind Trial of Maprotiline (Ludiomil) and Amitriptyline in Depressed Outpatients," *Acta Psychiatrica Scandinavica,* 52 (1975):225.

503. WEISSMAN, M. M., et al. "The Efficacy of Drugs and Psychotherapy in the Treatment of Acute Depressive Episodes," *American Journal of Psychiatry,* 136 (1979):555.

504. WELNER, J. "A Multinational, Multi-Centre, Double-blind Trial of a New Antidepressant (CIBA 34, 276 – Ba)," in P. Kielholz, ed., *Depressive Illness: Diagnosis, Assessment, Treatment.* Baltimore: Williams & Wilkins, 1972, pp. 209–219.

505. WEST, E. D., and DALLY, P. J. "Effects of Iproniazid in Depressive Syndromes," *British Medical Journal,* 1 (1959):1491–1494.

506. WHEATLEY, D. "Viloxazine—A New Antidepressant," *Current Therapeutic Research,* 16 (1974):821–828.

507. WHYTE, S. F, et al. "Plasma Concentrations of Protriptyline and Clinical Effects in Depressed Women," *British Journal of Psychiatry,* 128 (1976):384–390.

508. WILSON, C., et al. "A Double-blind Clinical Comparison of Amoxapine, Imipramine and Placebo in the Treatment of Depression," *Current Therapeutic Research,* 22 (1977):620–627.

509. WINER, B. J. *Statistical Principles in Experimental Design.* New York: McGraw-Hill, 1971.

510. WINOKUR, G. S., CLAYTON, P. J., and

REICH, T. *Manic-Depressive Illness.* St. Louis: C. V. Mosby, 1969.

511. WISTEDT, B., et al. "Nomifensine and Amitriptyline in the Treatment of Depression: A Multicentre Double-blind Comparison," *Acta Psychiatrica Scandinavica,* 68 (1983):212–220.

512. WORRALL, E. P., MOODY, J. P., and NAYLOR, G. J. "Lithium in Non-Manic Depressives. Antiaggressive Effect and Red Blood Cell Lithium Values," *British Journal of Psychiatry,* 126 (1975): 464–468.

513. WORRALL, E. P., et al. "Controlled Studies of the Acute Antidepressant Effects of Lithium," *British Journal of Psychiatry,* 135 (1979):255–262.

514. WRIGHT, J. H., and DENBER, H.C.B. "Clinical Trial of Fluvoxamine: A New Serotonergic Antidepressant," *Current Therapeutic Research,* 23 (1978):83–89.

515. WRIGHT, V. S., and HERMANN, L. "A Double-blind Comparative Study on the Effects of Lofepramine and Amitriptyline in Depressive Outpatients," *Drug Research,* 26 (1976):1167–1169.

516. YAMHURE, A., and VILLALOBOS, A. "Amoxapine—A Double-blind Comparative Clinical Study on Amitriptyline in Depressed, Hospitalized Patients," *Current Therapeutic Research,* 21 (1977): 502–506.

517. YANG, H., and NEFF, N. H. "The Monoamine Oxidase of Brain. Selective Inhibition with Drugs and the Consequences for the Metabolism of Biogenic Amines," *Journal of Pharmacology and Experimental Therapeutics,* 189 (1974): 733–740.

518. YARYURA-TOBIAS, J. A., NEZIROGLU, M. A., and BERGMAN, L. "Chlorimipramine for Obsessive-Compulsive Neurosis: An Organic Approach," *Current Therapeutic Research,* 20 (1976):541–548.

519. YOUDIM, M.D.H., et al. "Human Brain Monoamine Oxidase, Multiple Forms and Selective Inhibition," *Nature,* 236 (1972):225–228.

520. YOUNGERMAN, J., and CANINO, I. "Lithium Carbonate Used in Children and Adolescents: A Survey of the Literature," *Archives of General Psychiatry,* 35 (1978):210–224.

521. ZALL, H. "Lithium Carbonate and Isocarboxazid: An Effective Drug Approach in Severe Depression," *American Journal of Psychiatry,* 127 (1971):1400–1403.

522. ZELLER, E. A., BARKSY, J., and FOUTS, J. R. "Influence of Isonicotinic Acid Hydrazid (INH) and 1-Isonicotinyl-2-Isopropyl hydrazid (IIH) on Bacterial and Mammalian Enzymes," *Experientia,* 8 (1952):349–350.

523. ZIEGLER, V. E., CLAYTON, P. J., and BIGGS, J. T. "A Comparison Study of Amitriptyline and Nortriptyline with Plasma Levels," *Archives of General Psychiatry,* 34 (1977):607–612.

524. ZIEGLER, V. E., et al. "Amitriptyline Plasma Levels and Therapeutic Response," *Clinical Pharmacology and Therapeutics,* 19 (1976):795–801.

525. ZIS, A. P., and GOODWIN, F. K. "Novel Antidepressants and the Biogenic Amine Hypothesis of Depression—The Case for Iprindole and Mianserin," *Archives of General Psychiatry,* 36 (1979): 1097–1107.

TRICYCLIC ANTIDEPRESSANTS: BLOOD LEVEL MEASUREMENTS AND CLINICAL RESPONSE

Alexander H. Glassman, Joseph J. Schildkraut, Thomas B. Cooper, and Paul J. Orsulak

¶ Introduction

The tricyclic antidepressants (TCAs) are extremely lipid-soluble drugs and, as such, are markedly dependent on hepatic metabolism for their elimination from the body.[24] In such cases, the liver adds polar molecular groups, usually hydroxyl groups, which serve, in essence, as detergents to increase the aqueous solubility of these compounds and allow them to pass more readily from the lipid areas of the body into the plasma and urine. By the mid-1960s, it was apparent that drugs with a dependence on this hepatic metabolism were subject to large interindividual differences in their steady-state plasma levels, because the liver's ability to metabolize drugs is a characteristic that varies remarkably from one individual to an-

other. This process is, in addition, subject to influence by environmental factors and a patient's medical condition.

The TCAs' unusually low steady-state plasma levels made them difficult to measure and delayed studies on the relation between plasma levels and clinical effect. For this reason, in the early 1970s there was a much better understanding of the impact of these metabolic differences on compounds in other fields of medicine than there was knowledge of the implications these differences would have for depressed psychiatric patients. However, over the last ten to fifteen years, there has been significant progress in our ability to measure the low levels of antidepressant drugs characteristically found in the plasma of patients and in our understanding of the meaning of these plasma-level measurements.[64]

¶ Clinical Studies

The relationship between plasma-level measurements and clinical outcome is clearest and most straightforward with imipramine hydrochloride. Here large studies by Glassman and associates[26] and Reisby and coworkers[55] both show a linear or sigmoid relationship between plasma level and clinical outcome. Both groups of investigators measured imipramine and its demethylated metabolite, and both found that when the combined level of these two compounds exceeded 200 ng per ml of plasma, the percentage of patients responding favorably was higher than it was with lower levels. Two smaller studies,[50,66] although not convincing by themselves because of sample size and certain methodological problems, are, nevertheless, in agreement with the two larger studies. Puig-Antich and associates* have found similar results in children. Recently Preskorn, Weller, and Weller[54] also demonstrated a relationship between plasma level and outcome in children, although their data suggested that higher levels of desipramine hydrochloride might impair response.

Thus all six studies of imipramine agree that: (1) interindividual metabolic differences do influence outcome, (2) the percentage of patients responding favorably increases as plasma levels are increased up to 200 to 250 ng per ml (although some patients may show favorable clinical response at lower plasma levels), and (3) higher levels (more than 250 ng per ml) can produce more side effects, but in five of the six studies, no change in antidepressant response was seen. The effect of unusually high plasma levels (more than 750 ng per ml) has not been systematically studied; and although they occasionally occur, their effect on therapeutic response is not well understood.

It is worthwhile to note that the single study that varies at all from the other five is one of the two studies in children; all adult inpatient studies showed the same results.

Although this chapter will not examine the relationship between TCA plasma levels and response in children specifically, it is interesting to note that a number of exceptions to the results of clinical pharmacological studies with TCA drugs in adults have been found in children. In addition to Preskorn's study suggesting that desipramine may have a curvilinear blood-level response characteristic in children, Greenberg and Yellin[28] and Lake and coworkers[38] have demonstrated that children show diastolic hypertension with imipramine and desmethylimipramine, something that is rarely seen in adults.

The situation with nortriptyline hydrochloride is somewhat more complex. This complexity comes not from a lack of agreement about the relationship between plasma levels and clinical response but from the nature of that relationship. Unlike imipramine, nortriptyline appears to have a specific therapeutic window between 50 and 150 ng per ml within which favorable antidepressant responses occur.[6,34,36] However, both above and below this specific plasma-level range (therapeutic window), there is a poor clinical response. Why this window effect exists is still unclear, but it is not related to toxicity.

There are now nine published studies of the relationship between nortriptyline plasma levels and clinical outcome, and six of these studies found a relationship between plasma level and outcome.* The two that did not find a relationship and the third that is equivocal were all done early in the 1970s by the same group working in Australia.[14,15,16] The former studies are flawed by very large variations in the reported plasma levels within the same patient. Either compliance or analytic methodological problems could cause such fluctuation. Certainly the bulk of the evidence available does point to a significant relationship between plasma levels and clinical outcome with nortriptyline, and suggests that the nature of that relationship is curvilinear.

There are less extensive data available ex-

---

*J. Puig-Antich, personal communication, April 1985.

*See references 6, 10, 14, 15, 16, 34, 36, 42, and 70.

amining the relationship between plasma concentration of desmethylimipramine and clinical outcome when the drug is administered as the parent drug. To date, six such studies have been published,* but one of these[2] describes only five patients. Of the other five, both Khalid, Amin, and Ban[31] and the studies of Nelson and coworkers[46,49] describe a linear relationship between drug concentration and outcome. The number of patients in the Khalid paper is also small, but the two Nelson studies are large and well designed. In their original study in a group of thirty-two unipolar, melancholic, nondelusional patients, Nelson and associates[49] found that plasma concentrations above 125 ng per ml were significantly more effective than lower levels.

In a more recent study, Nelson and co-workers[46] looked at the relationship of desmethylimipramine in a group of older patients. They found exactly the same plasma-level–response relationship in twenty-five unipolar nondelusional patients. Patients got better at approximately 135 ng per ml of desipramine, even though the average age was some twenty-five years older than the average age in Nelson's earlier study. This served both to replicate his earlier study and to show that in a hospitalized group of seriously depressed patients, the plasma levels necessary for a therapeutic response do not change with increasing age. Recently, Amsterdam and others[4] published results from an outpatient study of fifty-nine depressed patients, and, as has been characteristic of outpatient studies, they found no consistent relationship of response to plasma levels of desipramine or its 2-hydroxy metabolite.

The absence of any curvilinear response is strongly supported by two studies that were not primarily concerned with plasma-level measurements but did find higher oral doses increasingly effective.[62,67] This would be a very unlikely response pattern if desmethylimipramine had a therapeutic window like nortriptyline. As with imipramine, there are no systematic data available on the effect

*See references 2, 4, 22, 31, 46, and 49.

of unusually high (greater than 750 ng/ml) concentrations of the drug.

At present, the most controversy surrounds amitriptyline hydrochloride. Here at least ten different studies have given three different answers. Three studies showed a linear relationship like that found with imipramine[11,37,69]; three studies revealed a curvilinear (windowlike) relationship similar to that seen with nortriptyline,[43,45,65]; and four studies found no relationship at all between plasma level and outcome.[20,39,41,56]

Recent studies by the National Institute of Mental Health Collaborative Studies on the biology of depression[33] looked at the relationship between plasma levels and clinical outcome with amitriptyline. Although these were not set up as plasma-level studies, the data do suggest that high levels of amitriptyline do not inhibit an antidepressant response.[33] The reason for the discrepancies between the various amitriptyline studies remains obscure. However, the best guess would be that plasma levels below 50 ng per ml of amitriptyline and its desmethylated metabolite are not efficacious and that higher levels, at least those levels usually seen, do not inhibit antidepressant response. However, such a statement is hardly specific and is still open to significant question.

Only very limited information is available concerning maprotiline,[41,44] doxepin hydrochloride,[21,32] and protriptyline hydrochloride[9,68]; even less is known about the other antidepressant drugs marketed in this country. However, even with drugs such as imipramine and nortriptyline, for which there are clear relationships between plasma-level measurements and clinical outcome, there are still significant gaps in our understanding. It is important to remember that even large-scale controlled studies provide information over a limited range of plasma concentrations of any given drug. As a result we can discuss with confidence the effect of plasma concentrations only within the range studied. Systematic studies of patients in whom chronic oral administration of normal doses produces unusually high plasma levels are not available, but the few case reports available suggest that atypical response relationships may exist with unusually high plasma levels (see section entitled "Case Observations"). In a similar way, these studies have been conducted in patients who represent only a limited portion of the spectrum of patients commonly given these drugs in general medical practice.

¶ Methodological Problems with Plasma-level Studies

To assess the state of our knowledge, it is important to review critically the methods used in plasma-level studies and to consider how these methods may have influenced the information currently available. First, it is important to recognize that TCAs are present in the plasma in very low concentrations, and because of this, their measurement involves sophisticated technology (see section entitled "Analytical Methods"). Although these methods have improved greatly over the last decade, in the early 1970s the difficulties in the methods of plasma-level measurement limited their availability.

Another critical issue in the plasma-level studies cited involves the patient populations examined. To find a relationship between plasma level and outcome—if such a relationship exists—one must examine a population in which a drug is efficacious. If part of an experimental population suffers from a condition not responsive to TCAs, that part of the population would obscure any relationship between the plasma concentration of the drug and the patient's clinical response. Among patients with endogenous unipolar depression, it is now unequivocally clear that delusional patients are far less responsive to tricyclic drugs than their nondelusional counterparts.[25,47,61]

This issue of differences within depressive subtypes might also be important with melancholic depressions. Most studies that have found a relationship between clinical response and plasma level have examined depressed inpatients. It is probable that there is a higher percentage of endogenous (melancholic or endogenomorphic) depressions among hospitalized inpatients than would be found in an outpatient clinic. Large studies by both Reisby and associates[55] and Robinson and coworkers[56] suggested a stronger relationship between plasma levels and clinical outcome in the endogenously, rather than nonendogenously, depressed portion of their samples. If patients with nonendogenous depression simply had a higher placebo response rate, this would serve as a source of additional "noise" in the system. As a result, even if there were a relationship between plasma level and outcome in the nonendogenous patients, a significantly larger sample of patients could be required to demonstrate that relationship.

This same kind of difficulty could arise even among a group of patients who all had endogenous depression if the placebo response rate varied with severity. Evidence already exists that very mild endogenous depressions have a higher spontaneous response rate.[63] In the same way, patients recently described as having "double depression" (major depressive disorder with preexisting chronic minor depression of at least two years' duration or dysthymia), could easily obscure the relationship between plasma concentration and clinical response because their response to antidepressant drugs appears to be less complete than that of patients with more typical major affective disorder.[30]

Issues of this type could relate to the current confusion with amitriptyline. Almost all of the early studies of both imipramine and nortriptyline were inpatient studies. However, because of both the enormous cost involved in five-to-seven-week inpatient studies (one to two weeks of placebo and four to five weeks of active drug treatment) and the difficulties in collecting such population samples, investigators have increasingly used outpatient samples. This may serve to alter the population being studied and potentially increase the difficulty in observing a relationship between plasma levels and clinical response, if it exists. Unfortunately, the delay in studying amitriptyline together with the difficulty in developing reliable methods has resulted in a situation where most studies with amitriptyline have been done with outpatients.

Thus it would be ideal to establish the existence of any relationship between antidepressant plasma level and response in a sample of depressed patients who are most likely to respond to antidepressants. This can best be done under inpatient conditions. Because the patients are under observation for a longer time, an inpatient study can better control for variance due to noncompliance or ingestion of other drugs and increase diagnostic accuracy. Inpatient studies also decrease the chance of obtaining patients with nonendogenous or milder depression. This is not to say that outpatient studies are not valuable, but they may yield somewhat different information. Early studies of the application of plasma-level measurements to anticonvulsant drugs in clinical populations of epileptic patients showed that the greatest improvement resulted from marked improvements in patient compliance.[52] In this way, outpatient studies can show differences in outcome from sources other than metabolic variance.

Another issue that remains to be resolved concerns the measurement of the metabolites of these antidepressant drugs. The initial studies in this area made the assumption that only the secondary and tertiary tricyclic compounds were active antidepressants and that the hydroxy metabolites of these compounds did not penetrate the brain. It is now clear that this is not the case. Most TCAs have hydroxy metabolites that are pharmacologically active and that do penetrate the brain.[7,53] The role these compounds play and the need to measure them in clinical practice are at present unclear. It would seem likely that if the measurements of these hydroxy metabolites are meaningful, they are most likely to be so for amitriptyline or nortriptyline. The 10-hydroxy metabolites associated with these compounds frequently occur at levels exceeding those of the parent compounds; the ratios of hydroxy metabolites

that are usually associated with either imipramine or desmethylimipramine are considerably lower.[48]

¶ Case Observations

As the number of patients in whom plasma levels of TCAs have been measured grows, we have gradually accumulated a series of case reports of atypical effects. It has become apparent that a small percentage of patients are extraordinarily poor metabolizers of these drugs.[8] These patients may have plasma levels as high as 2,000 and even 3,000 ng per ml, in spite of usual oral doses. The magnitude of these levels becomes apparent when one realizes not only that usual levels are closer to 200 ng per ml, but also that patients who have overdosed and are comatose may have plasma levels of 1,500 ng per ml.

Some patients with very high levels are actually asymptomatic, but serious cardiac toxicity has been seen. Interestingly, some of these patients who felt well at very high levels experience a return of their depression if their levels are lowered to more usual ones and will again improve when plasma levels are raised to a level intermediate between their extraordinary and more usual levels.[23] This may occur because these patients' whole pattern of metabolites is disrupted and, although the parent compound is high, the hydroxy metabolites are very low and usual plasma-level–response relationships may not hold. However, at present, this is all at the level of speculation. In addition, some of these patients may have unusual protein binding, which can alter plasma levels without altering clinical efficacy.[35] This could produce apparently high plasma levels of the drug while, in fact, the unbound or active fraction of the drug could be entirely within a normal range.

Several case reports have appeared describing patients receiving modest doses of imipramine who developed plasma concentrations of imipramine plus desipramine close to 1,000 ng per ml without evident antidepressant effect. However, the patients' depressions seemed to improve when the plasma level was reduced, and this improvement was not related to a decrease in side effects.[5] Whether such cases represent unusual binding or unusual receptor sensitivity is not easily established, and because the rate of such cases is so low, they cannot be studied prospectively. Routine use will fortuitously uncover such cases and facilitate their more careful study. However, the clinician must be careful, because such case reports frequently do not distinguish between the effects of changing plasma levels and passage of time. The report of an unusual case should be examined critically; the data from such observations are much more difficult to interpret than those obtained from systematic prospective studies.

Another related situation in which case report information seems to indicate that an unusual relationship exists between plasma levels and clinical response is in patients who have inflammatory reactions. Kragh-Sorensen, Gram, and Larsen[35] reported a case history of a patient with inflammatory disease in which tricyclic plasma levels rose dramatically in association with a rise in alpha-1 acid glycoproteins. These proteins have been reported to rise in patients experiencing infectious processes, malignancies, and stress reactions. It is unclear at present if this rise in drug plasma levels is associated with an increase in active drug (that is, drug available to interact with receptors). It is conceivable, and perhaps likely, that in this situation the amount of free drug in the plasma remains unchanged, even though the total level of the drug increases. The increased plasma concentration observed could represent an increase in drug bound to alpha-1 acid glycoprotein, while the free drug concentration remains unchanged.[29] In this situation the measured total concentration (bound plus free) of the drug during an inflammatory process would lead to an overestimation of the active drug (free drug) available to the patient. Drug binding is not readily studied in clinical laboratories; the physician would have to depend on his or her clinical judgment and not on the measured concentration of the drug. High plasma levels without concomitant conduction changes in the electrocardiogram would suggest unusual protein binding. Readers interested in the pharmacokinetic principles underlying plasma level measurements are referred to three recent review articles.[3,29,60]

¶ Analytical Methods

In the decade since the initial studies demonstrating the clinical applicability of monitoring TCA plasma levels, more than one hundred methods for the analysis of TCAs have been described. The low concentrations of these drugs found in plasma presented formidable technical difficulties during the early years. Many attempts were made to develop suitable methods involving spectrophotometry, spectrofluorometry, thin-layer chromatography, radioimmunoassay (RIA), and isotope derivative analysis.

Contemporary methods of analysis for TCAs include gas chromatography with a nitrogen-specific detector, high-pressure liquid chromatography, and RIA. Mass-fragmentographic methods are generally considered to be the most reliable and specific when appropriate deuterium-labeled internal standards are available, but these techniques require access to expensive mass spectrometry equipment. However, the introduction of standardized equipment and procedures is now providing methods that are robust enough to provide analytically valid data in the routine therapeutic drug monitoring laboratory, even though the TCAs are still among the most difficult drugs to analyze.[57,58]

In choosing a method for therapeutic monitoring of TCAs, several issues need to be considered. The method chosen must be specific—that is, capable of measuring the antidepressant drug (and active metabolites) individually without interference from other metabolites or other drugs that may be administered concurrently. Because both gas chromatography with nitrogen detection and liquid chromatography with suitably low wavelength ultraviolet detectors can meet most of these criteria, the choice of a particular method can be based on other factors, including availability or cost of equipment, the skill and experience of the laboratory staff, and the particular requirements of each laboratory.

Both gas chromatographic and liquid chromatographic techniques are suitable for the analysis of the TCAs and their desmethylated metabolites, but high-performance liquid chromatographic techniques are proving more suitable for the routine analysis of the TCAs. Chromatographic techniques, including gas and/or high-pressure liquid chromatography, will probably also be required in most laboratories because of the number of new antidepressants that are currently being investigated. The immunoassay techniques may eventually prove convenient and cost effective but will be limited to only the most frequently used TCAs. Laboratories engaged in therapeutic monitoring of antidepressant medications may have to use at least two different techniques to provide the full range of analyses with maximum cost effectiveness.

Although the U.S. Clinical Laboratory Improvement Act of 1972 states that proficiency testing should be used for educational purposes and improvement of clinical laboratories, until 1980 such testing for antidepressants was limited to internal quality-control systems and to local exchange of specimens among laboratories. In early 1980 both the American Association for Clinical Chemistry and the American Society of Clinical Pathology began active development of quality-control programs for analysis of antidepressants. In July 1981 the American Association for Clinical Chemistry Therapeutic Drug Monitoring Program began including TCAs in its monthly survey specimens. Laboratories engaged in the analysis of antidepressants should be encouraged to participate in such a program, since it provides an objective external assessment of laboratory performance.

The history of this program, based on reports from approximately one hundred laboratories reporting results for antidepressants included in the survey vials, shows that significant advances have been made in the performance and reliability of TCA assays, even though they are still less well-developed and controlled than the analysis of other drugs that are currently monitored for therapeutic purposes.

At present, there are no reference methods available for the TCAs, and no laboratories have been established to serve this purpose. Intermethod variability has improved in recent years.

Further attention to internal quality-control procedures and participation in the available external proficiency testing programs can serve to improve the reliability of antidepressant determinations, as they have for other drugs measured for therapeutic purposes.

¶ Sources of Variation in the Determination of Tricyclic Antidepressants

Error and variability in the analysis of TCAs can be introduced at several stages. The sources of these errors include method and time of collection, specimen containers and transport systems,[12,51] and inadequate or inappropriate quality control for the analytic procedures themselves. Errors in interpretation can also occur as the result of poor specificity or inadequate sensitivity of the method used to perform the analyses.

When plasma levels of TCAs are requested, attention must be paid to specimen collection and preparation, since large variations in results can be introduced at this point. At the present time, it is impossible to assume that all collection containers are sufficiently inert to use without qualification.[12,51] All collection containers used should be examined by the addition of known specimens, which are then analyzed to evaluate their performance under a variety of conditions.

Numerous studies have shown that large variations in plasma TCA levels can be introduced by the use of poorly selected vacuum blood collection systems. This variability stems from contamination of the specimen by tris-butoxyethyl phosphate (TBEP) in the tube stoppers and by absorption onto separation devices. Vacuum blood collection tubes with stoppers that are free of TBEP and other contaminants are available. However, the user should be certain that only those tubes are used. Tubes containing gel for separating cells from plasma are not suitable for determination of TCA levels.

Once the specimen has been collected in an appropriate container, it should be handled as expeditiously as possible to avoid contamination or decomposition. The suitability of transport containers should be verified by a reputable laboratory. The laboratory system should also ensure correct patient and specimen identification. TCAs are stable up to one year in frozen plasma and up to five days at ambient temperature.[18,51] With reasonable care, plasma or serum specimens (not whole blood) can also be mailed to laboratories. However, specimens should be centrifuged as soon as possible after collection.

Standardization of sampling time is important when comparing plasma levels of the TCAs to reported therapeutic ranges. In most of the more carefully done plasma-level studies, an evening dose of drug was given, and the blood sample was drawn early the next morning, before the administration of the morning dose. Thus study results relate approximately ten-hour postingestion plasma concentrations to clinical outcome. Kinetic studies also show that the optimal time for collection of specimens for determination of steady-state levels of plasma TCAs is between ten and fourteen hours after the last dose of medication for patients taking antidepressants once a day and just before the morning dose if patients are on a divided-dose schedule.[13,27]

¶ Clinical Indications

The clinical usefulness of obtaining plasma-level measurements of antidepressants varies with the clinical situation, the ability to evaluate laboratory accuracy, and the particular drug involved. As previously noted, the data available allow the clearest statements to be made concerning imipramine, nortriptyline, and desmethylimipramine. With these drugs, plasma-level measurements are unequivocally useful in problem patients who do not respond to usual oral doses; in high-risk patients who, because of age or medical illness, would be best treated with the lowest possible effective dose; or in patients on multiple drugs, where estimates of plasma levels would be nearly impossible because of the multiplicity of possible drug-drug interactions.

Another important clinical situation in which measurements of these drugs can undoubtedly be justified is where there is an urgency to the patient's treatment. This would involve potentially suicidal patients, either in or out of the hospital; inpatients whose hospital stay and the costs involved could be reduced by reducing the time to response; or patients whose illness jeopardizes their work or their ability to care for their family. Obviously, this argument can be extended to the point that any patient with a depression warranting drug treatment is worth treating in the most expedient way possible. Therefore, at least with imipramine and nortriptyline, obtaining plasma levels is worthwhile in any patient.

Certainly, many patients who are relatively slow metabolizers will easily develop adequate plasma levels and will respond to tricyclics in the same five or ten days, whether plasma-level measurements are obtained or not. In addition, it is now clear that the characteristic delay in response with antidepressant drugs has two components. One has to do with the time required for a patient to reach an adequate concentration of the drug and the other seems to be an inherent pharmacological characteristic of the way in which these drugs work. Only this first delay can be modified by obtaining plasma levels. However, this difficulty in obtaining an adequate plasma concentration of the drug is a major source of difficulty in a large number of patients.

Many patients are exposed to lengthy sub-therapeutic trials. Whether these low concentrations of drug result from poor patient compliance, genetic differences in metabolism, or a variety of drug-drug interactions, plasma-level measurements—especially with imipramine, desmethylimipramine, and nortriptyline—would eliminate these subtherapeutic trials. In addition, with drugs for which effective plasma concentrations have been established, determining plasma levels would be useful even in those patients who show a good clinical response, because plasma levels will occasionally identify slow metabolizers who would otherwise receive unnecessarily high oral doses.

Good estimates of whether a patient is a slow, normal, or fast metabolizer and of his or her eventual steady-state level can be obtained by drawing a blood sample five days after achieving a consistent dose regimen of either imipramine or nortriptyline. A number of investigators[1,19] have shown that a single measurement twenty-four or thirty-six hours after a single dose of a given tricyclic will usually predict an appropriate oral dose. However, this requires a laboratory that can dependably make precise measurements at very low plasma concentrations. There is also recent evidence that some patients will show nonlinear kinetics at relatively low oral doses.[17]

Most TCAs have half-lives of approximately twenty-four hours. This means that plasma levels obtained four or five days after reaching a constant oral dose will, in fact, represent values between 80 and 90 percent of the steady-state level of the drug. Although not entirely accurate, this gives very good estimates of eventual steady-state levels. If a patient has very low levels at four or five days, he or she is either noncompliant or is a rapid metabolizer and will need higher doses; if the patient's levels are already adequate, his or her current dose is probably appropriate; and if the patient's levels are already significantly above therapeutic levels, his or her rate of metabolism is very slow and the dose level can probably be reduced.

Recently, the first cost/benefit analysis related to blood-level measurements appeared. Although retrospective and not ideal in its design, it did show that empirically dosed depressed inpatients spent more days in the hospital (6.1) and took significantly longer to return to work than those patients whose therapy was guided by blood-level measurement.[59]

Recently reported studies[46,49] relating plasma levels of desmethylimipramine to outcome are consistent with clinical experience[62,67] and suggest that plasma-level measurements will be as useful with this drug as they are with imipramine and nortriptyline. The more controversial use of plasma-level measurements involves antidepressants other than imipramine, nortriptyline, or desmethylimipramine, for which the relationship between the measured plasma levels and clinical response is less clear. Some experts advocate the use of plasma-level measurements to identify unusually rapid metabolizers. Certainly, for compounds like amitriptyline, where enough data are available to describe the range of plasma levels seen with usual treatment regimens, it is possible to define certain levels as extremely low and as unlikely to be therapeutic. However, this limited statement is all that can actually be made from the data available, and for many of the newer or less commonly used antidepressants, even this type of information is not available.

Some experts have advocated measuring plasma levels of every patient treated with any antidepressant at the time of response, so that a record is obtained of the level at which that patient responds. Such data, they suggest, may be useful to assess compliance in patients who may relapse during maintenance drug treatment and to assist the physician in the treatment of subsequent episodes of recurrent depression. However, other experts have questioned the usefulness of plasma-level measurements in this situation; further studies, as well as additional clinical experience, will be required to resolve this issue.

It is important to recall that even with the best-studied drugs—imipramine and nortriptyline—the data available have been collected primarily from inpatients with endogenous major depressive disorder, and it remains to be proven that the same dose-response relationships apply for outpatients, patients with mild or nonendogenous depressions, or patients for whom these drugs are being used prophylactically. Very few data have been published on the relationship between plasma level and response with these drugs in patients with panic or anxiety disorders.[40] Many basic data remain to be scientifically gathered concerning plasma-level measurements and antidepressant drugs before the clinician can make an entirely rational use of these tests. In most instances these data are, at present, not even being gathered.

In spite of this, we believe that plasma-level measurements are already unequivocally useful clinically. However, this usefulness varies. For those apparently refractory patients with endogenous depression treated with imipramine or nortriptyline, it is unfortunate if the clinician does not have access to an experienced, reliable laboratory. For patients given a newer antidepressant, where even the usual range of plasma concentrations or the number of active metabolites may not be known, plasma level measurements are of uncertain value. It is perhaps relevant to recall that when plasma-level measurements of antiepileptic drugs were first introduced, their major impact was to reduce dramatically the rate of noncompliance. There is no question that these tests have introduced a more rational basis for our therapeutics and that their usefulness is very likely to grow. Despite their limitations, plasma-level measurements of the tricyclics are one of the most useful and yet underutilized of the biological tests in psychiatry.

¶ **Bibliography**

1. ALEXANDERSON, B. "Pharmacokinetics of Desmethylimipramine and Nortriptyline in Man After Single and Multiple Oral Doses—a Cross-over Study," *European Journal of Clinical Pharmacology,* 5 (1972):1–10.

2. AMIN, M. M., et al. "A Comparison of Desipramine and Amitriptyline Plasma Levels and Therapeutic Response," *Psychopharmacology Bulletin,* 14 (1978): 45–46.

3. AMSTERDAM, J. D., BRUNSWICK, D., and MENDELS, J. "The Clinical Application of Tricyclic Antidepressant Pharmacokinetics and Plasma Levels," *American Journal of Psychiatry,* 137 (1980):653–662.

4. AMSTERDAM, J. D., et al. "Desipramine and 2-hydroxydesipramine Plasma Levels in Endogenous Depressed Patients: Lack of Correlation with Therapeutic Response," *Archives of General Psychiatry,* 42 (1985):361–364.

5. APPELBAUM, P. S., et al. "Clinical Utility of Tricyclic Antidepressant Blood Levels: A Case Report," *American Journal of Psychiatry,* 136 (1979):339–341.

6. ASBERG, M., et al. "Relationship Between Plasma Level and Therapeutic Effect of Nortriptyline," *British Medical Journal,* 3 (1971):331–334.

7. BERTILSSON, L., MELLSTROM, B., and SJOQVIST, F. "Pronounced Inhibition of Noradrenaline Uptake by 10-hydroxy-metabolites of Nortriptyline," *Life Sciences,* 25 (1979): 1285–1292.

8. BERTILSSON, L., et al. "Pharmacogenetic Aspects of the Metabolism of Tricyclic Antidepressants," in S. Z. Langer, et al., eds., *New Vistas in Depression.* Elmsford, N.Y.: Pergamon Press, 1982, pp. 263–269.

9. BIGGS, J. T., and ZIEGLER, V. E. "Protriptyline Plasma Levels and Antidepressant Response," *Clinical Pharmacology and Therapeutics,* 22 (1977):269–273.

10. BRAITHWAITE, R. A., MONTGOMERY, S., and DAWLING, S. "Nortriptyline in Depressed Patients with High Plasma Levels," *Clinical Pharmacology and Therapeutics,* 23 (1978):303–314.

11. BRAITHWAITE, R. A., et al. "Plasma Concentration of Amitriptyline and Clinical Response," *Lancet,* 1 (1972):1297–1300.

12. BRUNSWICK, D. J., and MENDELS, J. "Reduced Levels of Tricyclic Antidepressants in Plasma from Vacutainers,"

Communications in Psychopharmacology, 1 (1977):131–134.

13. BURCH, J. E., et al. "Time Course of Plasma Drug Levels During Once-daily Oral Administration of Clomipramine," *Psychopharmacology,* 77 (1982):344–347.

14. BURROWS, G. D., DAVIES, B., and SCOGGINS, B. A. "Plasma Concentration of Nortriptyline and Clinical Response in Depressive Illness," *Lancet,* 2 (1972):619–623.

15. BURROWS, G. D., et al. "Plasma Nortriptyline and Clinical Response," *Clinical Pharmacology and Therapeutics,* 16 (1974):639–644.

16. BURROWS, G. D., et al. "Plasma Nortriptyline and Clinical Response—A Study Using Changing Plasma Levels," *Psychological Medicine,* 7 (1977):87–91.

17. COOKE, R. G., et al., "The Nonlinear Kinetics of Desipramine and 2-hydroxydesipramine in Plasma," *Clinical Pharmacology and Therapeutics,* 36 (1984):343–349.

18. COOPER, T. B. "Nitrogen Phosphorous Detector: Experiences in Psychotropic Drug Level Monitoring," in E. Usdin, ed., *Clinical Pharmacology in Psychiatry.* New York: Elsevier, 1981, pp. 35–42.

19. COOPER, T. B., and SIMPSON, G. M. "Prediction of Individual Dosage of Nortriptyline," *American Journal of Psychiatry,* 135 (1978):333–335.

20. COPPEN, A., et al. "Amitriptyline Plasma-Concentration and Clinical Effect. A World Health Organization Collaborative Study," *Lancet,* 1 (1978):63–66.

21. FRIEDEL, R. O., and RASKIND, M. A. "Relationship of Blood Levels of Sinequan to Clinical Effects in the Treatment of Depression in Aged Patients," in J. Mendels, ed., *Sinequan (Doxepin HCl): A Monograph of Recent Clinical Studies.* Amsterdam: Excerpta Medica ICS, 1975, pp. 51–53.

22. FRIEDEL, R. O., et al. "Desipramine Plasma Levels and Clinical Response in Depressed Outpatients," *Communications in Psychopharmacology,* 3 (1979):81–87.

23. GARVEY, M. J., et al. "Elevated Plasma Tricyclic Levels with Therapeutic Doses of Imipramine," *American Journal of Psychiatry,* 141 (1984):853–856.

24. GLASSMAN, A. H. and PEREL, J. M. "The Clinical Pharmacology of Imipramine," *Archives of General Psychiatry,* 28 (1973):649–653.

25. GLASSMAN, A. H., and ROOSE, S. P. "Delusional Depression: A Distinct Clinical Entity?" *Archives of General Psychiatry,* 38 (1981):424–427.

26. GLASSMAN, A. H. et al. "Clinical Implications of Imipramine Plasma Levels for Depressive Illness," *Archives of General Psychiatry,* 34 (1977):197–204.

27. GRAM, L. F., et al. "Steady-state Kinetics of Imipramine in Patients," *Psychopharmacology,* 54 (1977):255–261.

28. GREENBERG, L. M., and YELLIN, A. M. "Blood Pressure and Pulse Changes in Hyperactive Children Treated with Imipramine and Methylphenidate," *American Journal of Psychiatry,* 132 (1975):1325–1326.

29. GREENBLATT, D. J., SELLERS, E. M., and KOCH-WESER, J. "Importance of Protein Binding for the Interpretation of Serum of Plasma Drug Concentrations," *Journal of Clinical Pharmacology,* 22 (1982):259–263.

30. KELLER, M. B., et al. "'Double Depression': Two-year Follow-up," *American Journal of Psychiatry,* 140 (1983):689–694.

31. KHALID, R., AMIN, M. M., and BAN, T. A. "Desipramine Plasma Levels and Therapeutic Response," *Psychopharmacology Bulletin,* 14 (1978):43–44.

32. KLINE, N. S., COOPER, T., and JOHNSTON, B. "Doxepin and Desmethyldoxepin Serum Levels and Clinical Response," in L. A. Gottschalk and S. Merlis, eds., *Pharmacokinetics of Psychoactive Drugs: Blood Levels and Clinical Response.* New York: Spectrum Publications, 1976, pp. 221–228.

33. KOCSIS, J. H., et al. "Imipramine and Amitriptyline Plasma Concentrations and Clinical Response," *British Journal of Psychiatry,* in press.

34. KRAGH-SORENSEN, P., ASBERG, M., and EGGERT-HANSEN, C. "Plasma-nortriptyline Levels in Endogenous Depression," *Lancet,* 1 (1973):113–115.

35. KRAGH-SORENSEN, P., GRAM, L. F., and

LARSEN, N. E. "Routine Use of Plasma Concentration Measurement of Tricyclic Antidepressant Drugs: Indications and Limitations," in E. Usdin, ed., *Clinical Pharmacology in Psychiatry.* New York: Elsevier North Holland, 1981, pp. 287–300.

36. KRAGH-SORENSEN, P., et al. "Self-inhibiting Action of Nortriptyline's Antidepressive Effect at High Plasma Levels," *Psychopharmacologia,* 45 (1976): 305–312.

37. KUPFER, D. J., et al. "Amitriptyline Plasma Levels and Clinical Response in Primary Depression," *Clinical Pharmacology and Therapeutics,* 22 (1977): 904–911.

38. LAKE, C. R., et al. "Effect of Imipramine on Norepinephrine and Blood Pressure in Enuretic Boys," *Clinical Pharmacology and Therapeutics,* 26 (1979): 647–653.

39. LIISBERG, P., et al. "A Clinical Trial Comparing Sustained Release Amitriptyline (Saroten Retard) and Conventional Amitriptyline Tablets (Saroten) in Endogenously Depressed Patients with Simultaneous Determination of Serum Levels of Amitriptyline and Nortriptyline," *Acta Psychiatrica Scandinavica,* 57 (1978):426–435.

40. MAVISSAKALIAN, M., PEREL, J. M., and MICHELSON, L. "The Relationship of Plasma Imipramine and N-desmethylimipramine to Improvement in Agoraphobia," *Journal of Clinical Psychopharmacology,* 4 (1984):36–40.

41. MENDLEWICZ, J., LINKOWSKI, P., and REES, J. A. "A Double-blind Comparison of Dothiepin and Amitriptyline in Patients with Primary Affective Disorder: Serum Levels and Clinical Response," *British Journal of Psychiatry,* 136 (1980):154–160.

42. MONTGOMERY, S. A., et al. "High Plasma Nortriptyline Levels in the Treatment of Depression, I," *Clinical Pharmacology and Therapeutics,* 23 (1978): 309–314.

43. MONTGOMERY, S. A., et al. "Amitriptyline Plasma Concentration and Clinical Response," *British Medical Journal,* 1 (1979):230–231.

44. MONTGOMERY, S. A., et al. "Pharmacokinetics and Efficacy of Maprotiline and Amitriptyline in Endogenous Depression: A Double-blind Controlled Trial," *Clinical Therapeutics,* 3 (1980):292–310.

45. MOYES, I.C.A., RAY, R. L., and MOYES, R. B. "Plasma Levels and Clinical Improvement—A Comparative Study of Clomipramine and Amitriptyline in Depression," *Postgraduate Medical Journal,* 56 (Supplement 1) (1980):127–129.

46. NELSON, J. C. JATLOW P., and MAZURE, C. "Desipramine Plasma Levels and Response in Elderly Melancholic Patients," *Journal of Clinical Psychopharmacology,* 5 (1985):217–220.

47. NELSON, J. C., and BOWERS, M. B., Jr. "Delusional Unipolar Depression: Description and Drug Response," *Archives of General Psychiatry,* 35 (1978):1321–1328.

48. NELSON, J. C., BOCK, J. L., and JATLOW, P. I. "Clinical Implications of 2-hydroxy-desipramine Plasma Concentrations," *Clinical Pharmacology and Therapeutics,* 33 (1983):183–189.

49. NELSON, J. C. et al. "Desipramine Plasma Concentration and Antidepressant Response," *Archives of General Psychiatry,* 39 (1982):1419–1422.

50. OLIVIER-MARTIN, R., et al. "Concentrations Plasmatiques de l'Imipramine et de la Desmethylimipramine et Effet Anti-depresseur au Cours d'un Traitement Controlé," *Psychopharmacologia,* 41 (1975):187–195.

51. ORSULAK, P. J., SINK, M., and WEED, J. "Blood Collection Tubes for Tricyclic Antidepressant Drugs: A Reevaluation," *Therapeutic Drug Monitoring,* 6 (1984):444–448.

52. PENRY, J. K. Paper presented at the Annual Meeting of the American College of Neuropsychopharmacology, New Orleans, 1976.

53. POTTER, W. Z., et al. "Active Metabolites of Imipramine and Desipramine in Man," *Clinical Pharmacology and Therapeutics,* 31 (1982):393–401.

54. PRESKORN, S. H., WELLER, E. B., and WELLER, R. A. "Depression in Children: Relationship Between Plasma Imipramine Levels and Response," *Journal of Clinical Psychiatry,* 43 (1982):450–453.

55. REISBY, N., et al. "Imipramine: Clinical Effects and Pharmacokinetic Variability," *Psychopharmacology,* 54 (1977): 263–272.

56. ROBINSON, D. S., et al. "Plasma Tricyclic Drug Levels in Amitriptyline-treated Depressed Patients," *Psychopharmacology,* 63 (1979):223–231.

57. SCOGGINS, B. A., et al. "Measurement of Tricyclic Antidepressants. Part I. A Review of Methodology," *Clinical Chemistry,* 26 (1980):5–17.

58. ———. "Measurement of Tricyclic Antidepressants, Part II. Applications in Methodology," *Clinical Chemistry,* 26 (1980):805–815.

59. SIMMONS, S. A., et al. "Cost-benefit Analysis of Prospective Pharmacokinetic Dosing of Nortriptyline in Depressed Patients," *Journal of Affective Disorders,* 8 (1985):47–53.

60. SJOQVIST, F., and BERTILSSON, L. "Clinical Pharmacology of Tricyclic Antidepressants: Facts, Controversies, and Future Challenges," in E. Usdin, ed., *Clinical Pharmacology in Psychiatry.* New York: Elsevier, 1981, pp. 141–153.

61. SPIKER, D. G., et al. "The Pharmacological Treatment of Delusional Depression," *American Journal of Psychiatry,* 142 (1985):430–436.

62. STEWART, J. W., et al. "Efficacy of Desipramine in Endogenomorphically Depressed Patients," *Journal of Affective Disorders,* 2 (1980):165–176.

63. STEWART, J. W., et al. "Efficacy of Desipramine in Mildly Depressed Patients: A Double-blind, Placebo-controlled Trial," *Psychopharmacology Bulletin,* 17 (1981):136–138.

64. Task Force on the Use of Laboratory Tests in Psychiatry. "Tricyclic Antidepressants—Blood Level Measurements and Clinical Outcome: An APA Task Force Report," *American Journal of Psychiatry,* 142 (1985):155–162.

65. VANDEL, S., et al. "Clinical Response and Plasma Concentration of Amitriptyline and Its Metabolite Nortriptyline," *European Journal of Clinical Pharmacology,* 14 (1978):185–190.

66. WALTER, C.J.S. "Clinical Significance of Plasma Imipramine Levels," *Proceedings of the Royal Society of Medicine,* 64 (1971):282–285.

67. WATT, D. C., Crammer, J. L., and Elkes, A. "Metabolism, Anticholinergic Effects, and Therapeutic Outcome of Desmethylimipramine in Depressive Illness," *Psychological Medicine,* 2 (1972):397–405.

68. WHYTE, S. F., et al. "Plasma Concentrations of Protriptyline and Clinical Effects in Depressed Women," *British Journal of Psychiatry,* 128 (1976):384–390.

69. ZIEGLER, V. E., et al. "Amitriptyline Plasma Levels and Therapeutic Response," *Clinical Pharmacology and Therapeutics,* 19 (1976):795–801.

70. ZIEGLER, V. E., et al. "Nortriptyline Plasma Levels and Therapeutic Response," *Clinical Pharmacology and Therapeutics,* 20 (1976):458–463.

CHAPTER 15

EXPERIMENTAL TREATMENTS FOR AFFECTIVE DISORDERS

Russell T. Joffe and Robert M. Post

¶ Introduction

Despite the established efficacy and extensive clinical use of tricyclic antidepressants, monoamine oxidase inhibitors, and lithium, 20 to 30 percent of episodes of mania and depression are unresponsive to these conventional treatments. Consequently, a large number of new therapies have been proposed and tested as primary or adjunctive treatments for manic-depressive illness, based on their ability to alter various biological systems that have been implicated in the pathophysiology of affective illness. The experimental treatments for affective disorders will be reviewed by consideration of each biological system and its role in affective disorder.

¶ Biogenic Amines

Norepinephrine

The biogenic amine hypothesis of affective illness, based on indirect pharmacological evidence, proposes that there is a functional deficiency in depression and excess in mania of norepinephrine (NE) at brain neuronal synapses.[148] Although many direct studies of NE and its metabolites in a variety of body fluids have been inconclusive,[180] experimental treatments have been studied that act by decreasing noradrenergic function in mania or that have the opposite effect in depression.

Clonidine hydrochloride reduces noradrenergic transmission by a direct agonist action on the inhibitory presynaptic alpha-2 adrenergic receptor, thus being a potent inhibitor of firing of noradrenergic cells in the locus coeruleus. Jouvent and associates[81] reported antimanic effects in six of eight patients in an open trial of clonidine, whereas Uhde and coworkers[160] found that depressed patients as a group demonstrated no overall mood response to clonidine treatment, although individual patients had notable antidepressant responses.[77,160] Furthermore, there are two reports of abrupt onset of mania with rapid withdrawal of clonidine in both affectively ill[77] and psychiatrically normal subjects.[158] Reintroduction of clonidine improved the mood disturbance. These collective data suggest that clonidine, by altering brain NE, affects mood state so that further double-blind, placebo-controlled clinical trials may be indicated.

Propranolol hydrochloride, a beta-adrenergic blocker, has been reported to be effective in preliminary studies of patients with acute mania or maniclike illness.[5,179] The doses used in these studies were large, up to 2,400 mg per day, so that it is uncertain whether the beta-adrenergic blocking effects of propranolol account for the clinical change or whether its other local anesthetic and membrane-stabilizing effects are operative. In this regard, Emrich and colleagues[39] have shown that d-propranolol, which is practically devoid of beta-blocking activity, is effective in mania.

There are no studies of alpha-adrenergic blockers in depression and mania.

Salbutamol is a direct beta-2 receptor agonist, and it is, therefore, feasible that it would be useful in the treatment of depression. In various animal models it has been found to have antidepressant properties.[95] The majority of clinical studies have involved intravenous infusions as the drug is reported to have poor bioavailability. In two open studies[94,152] involving in excess of fifty patients, 6 mg salbutamol per day, for six to ten days, was found to be an effective antidepressant with an onset of action within two to three days. The drug was reported to be effective in both unipolar and bipolar depression, and there was only one case of drug-induced hypomania. These findings were confirmed in a controlled study[95] where 6 mg intravenous salbutamol per day for fifteen days was found to be superior to chlorimipramine in twenty patients. Unfortunately, the short duration of these trials and the lack of follow-up preclude definitive conclusions about the use of salbutamol as an antidepressant. In an open study, seventeen patients with treatment-resistant depression were given salbutamol alone or in combination with lithium carbonate in doses up to 16 mg per day orally for twenty-one days.[9] Only three of seventeen patients failed to improve. However, in many, response was incomplete and its onset of action was similar to typical antidepressants. Nonetheless, these preliminary findings are highly suggestive of antidepressant efficacy and require further investigation.

L-tyrosine is the amino acid precursor of the catecholamines dopamine (DA) and NE. Administration of L-tyrosine elevates brain tyrosine concentration and causes parallel increases in brain catecholamine synthesis with increased brain NE release but has little effect on cerebral DA.[53] Despite an initial negative report,[15] a subsequent open study[64] involving two patients and a double-blind, placebo-controlled study with six patients[53] have shown that 100 mg per kilogram of body weight of L-tyrosine has a noticeable antidepressant effect. These preliminary findings require replication in a larger study.

Dopamine

The biogenic amine theory suggests that, like NE, the neurotransmitter DA is functionally deficient in depression and increased in mania. Therefore, several compounds that affect specific aspects of DA metabolism have been utilized in the treatment of affective illness.

Alpha-methylparatyrosine (AMPT), an inhibitor of tyrosine hydroxylase, the rate-limiting enzyme in the synthesis of DA and NE, has been reported to have antimanic effects in five of seven patients.[12] In the same study three of four depressed patients experienced an exacerbation of their condition when treated with AMPT, suggesting that a decrease in brain catecholamines is associated with worsening of depression. In contrast, fusaric acid, a specific inhibitor of dopamine beta-hydroxylase, which, therefore, decreases NE but not DA, did not have substantial antimanic effects.[146]

Both levodopa and piribedil (ET 495) enhance brain DA function. However, their clinical profiles differ, probably as a result of their different mechanism of action on cerebral DA metabolism.

Levodopa is a catecholamine precursor that, unlike DA and NE, readily crosses the blood-brain barrier and is then rapidly decarboxylated to DA.[13] However, levodopa is also transported into serotonergic neurons where it interferes with normal indoleamine metabolism.[114] Therefore, levodopa leads to increased brain DA and decreased brain serotonin, (5HT), while NE remains relatively unaffected.[65] Several trials of levodopa, with or without a peripheral decarboxylase inhibitor, have been carried out for the treatment of depression. Results have been consistently negative* although levodopa appears to have a nonspecific activating effect, especially in retarded depression. Van Praag and Korf reported that in patients with retarded depression, low cerebrospinal fluid (CSF) homovanillic acid (HVA), the major metabolite of DA, predicted response to levodopa.[169] Furthermore, levodopa may induce hypomania in bipolar but not unipolar depressed patients[108] and may aggravate psychotic symptoms.[65]

Piribedil is a relatively specific DA receptor agonist.[133] At lower doses, it may act predominantly at the presynaptic DA receptor to decrease functional dopaminergic activity; in larger doses it may enhance DA function by stimulation of the postsynaptic DA receptor.[133]

Two studies have reported antimanic effects of piribedil.[4,132] In the first study[132] involving two patients, low doses of 60 mg per day were used; dose-response relationships were not specified in the second study.[4]

In larger doses, up to 240 mg per day, piribedil has been reported to have a transient antidepressant effect in one open, uncontrolled study[149] and partial antidepressant effects in a double-blind, placebo-controlled trial.[32] In depressed patients, piribedil rarely induces mania.[169] Those with low CSF HVA showed a better antidepressant response.[133]

Bromocriptine mesylate is a DA agonist

*See references 32, 65, 103, 108, and 123.

with a pharmacological effect on DA receptors similar to that of piribedil.[22] Preliminary studies have shown that bromocriptine has limited effects in both mania and depression.[22,153] In one study, the drug's antidepressant effects were similar to those of imipramine.[22]

Serotonin

Based on the serotonin-deficiency hypothesis of both mania and depression, various pharmacological agents that enhance brain 5HT function have been tested in acutely manic and depressed patients.

Both L-tryptophan and 5-hydroxytryptophan (5-HTP) are amino acid precursors that, when administered orally, will increase levels of brain 5HT as reflected by 5-hydoxyindoleacetic acid (5-HIAA) levels in CSF.[33,167] However, neither of these substances has effects confined to serotonergic neurons. L-tryptophan loading in animals decreases brain DA and NE concentrations[154] probably by competition with tyrosine for transport mechanisms into brain,[45] whereas decarboxylation of 5-HTP is not restricted to 5HT neurons and may, therefore, decrease brain catecholamine function.[97]

Despite several studies, the antimanic and antidepressant effect of L-tryptophan remains uncertain (see table 15–1). Several factors have been suggested as possible reasons for these inconclusive data. First, L-tryptophan may only be effective in a subgroup of affective disorders characterized by 5HT deficiency as evidenced by low post-probenecid CSF 5-HIAA, the major metabolite of 5-HT.[33] There is no experimental evidence for this hypothesis although there is for 5-HTP.[33] Second, a subgroup of patients with a low plasma ratio of total tryptophan to competing neutral amino acids may better utilize and, therefore, respond to L-tryptophan treatment.[105] Last, it is possible that L-tryptophan may have a "therapeutic window" that varies with diagnosis and mood state so that overdosage or underdosage may account for treatment failures.[19] Doses up to 6 mg per day for unipolar depression and in excess of this for bipolar depression are recommended for L-tryptophan alone, and less is required if it is used together with nicotinamide and pyridoxine, both of which enhance plasma tryptophan levels.[33]

The majority of studies have reported that 5HTP, with or without a peripheral decarboxylase inhibitor, has antidepressant effects.[2,101,165,168] Few studies have been negative.[11,156] Furthermore, van Praag has shown that 5-HTP may be effective not only in the acute treatment but also in the prophylaxis of recurrent depression.[168]

It is unclear why 5-HTP and L-tryptophan appear to differ in their antidepressant efficacy although the greater effect of 5-HTP on catecholamines may be important in this regard.

Side effects with 5HT precursors are rare. L-tryptophan may cause nausea, tremor, and dizziness, whereas gastrointestinal symptoms are most common with 5-HTP.

Fenfluramine hydrochloride, a 5HT agonist, has been reported by Murphy and associates,[110] in a single hypomanic patient, and by Pearce,[122] in a study of four acutely manic subjects, to have possible antimanic effects. On the other hand, a study of seven manic patients reported that fenfluramine had therapeutic effects on motor activity but not on altered mood and ideation.[23]

Inhibitors of 5HT would be expected to exacerbate mania or aggravate depression. Parochlorphenylalanine (PCPA), a partial tryptophan hydroxylase inhibitor, reverses the antidepressant effect of imipramine[107] and the monoamine oxidase inhibitor (MAOI) tranylcypromine,[150] but is not associated with alteration in either mood phase in bipolar patients when used alone.[107] Methysergide, a probable 5HT antagonist, has been reported, in controlled trials, to aggravate mania[25,27,102] although earlier poorly controlled studies reported it to have an antimanic effect.[31,171]

Acetylcholine

Early reports[10,56] that cholinomimetics induced a syndrome of depression, anergia, and apathy, common features of depressive illness, preceded the suggestion by Janowsky and associates[73] that depression is a disorder of cholinergic predominance, whereas mania is characterized by a deficiency of acetylcholine (ACh) relative to NE.

All double-blind studies to date report that the cholinomimetic agent physostigmine has antimanic effects when given intravenously as a single dose up to 6 mg.[17,73,74,151] Furthermore, precipitation of depression is a common feature of physostigmine treatment of mania.[73,74] However, physostigmine seems to have a predominant effect in slowing psychomotor activity in both normal and affectively ill subjects,[73] so that the specificity of its antimanic effects requires clarification. Lecithin, the dietary precursor of choline, increases brain ACh levels[70] when given orally and, therefore, may be a useful treatment for mania since it would be impractical for physostigmine, which has to be given parenterally and has a very short half-life, to be given over an extended period of time. In a preliminary study[21] lecithin, in conjunction with lithium, was reported to have possible antimanic effects. Further systematic study is required.

Centrally active anticholinergic agents may induce a maniclike state[147] and have been reported to have antidepressant activity both in an open[58] and a preliminary, double-blind trial with trihexyphenidyl hydrochloride.[78]

¶ Neuropeptides

Opiates

The discovery[124] of specific opiate receptors and of endogenous opiate peptides[71] has led to the investigation of the role of the opioid system in the mediation of normal and abnormal behavior and emotions.

The notion that the endogenous opiates are implicated in the pathogenesis of mania and depression is based on several factors. First, opiate alkaloids have long been ob-

TABLE 15–1

Studies of L-Tryptophan in Depression and Mania

Study	Date	N	Diagnosis	Design	Dose of L-tryptophan (g/day)	Other Drugs	Duration (days)	Results
Coppen et al.[24]	1967	41	Severe depression	Nonblind: compared patients previously given ECT	5–6	Pyridoxine 100 mg/day	28	L-tryptophan as effective as ECT.
Glassman and Platman[59]	1969	20	Depression	Double-blind, placebo-controlled	12–18	Phenelzine 30 mg/day	21	L-tryptophan enhanced effects of MAOI.
Carroll et al.[16]	1970	12	Primary depression	Nonblind: compared to ECT in sequential randomized trial	7	Pyridoxine 100 mg/day	21	L-tryptophan inferior to ECT.
Bunney et al.[12]	1971	8	Manic-depressive and psychotic depression	Double-blind, placebo-controlled	8		16	No responders to L-tryptophan.
Coppen et al.[26]	1972	15	Primary depression	Double-blind	9	Imipramine 150 mg/day; pyridoxine 100 mg/day; ascorbic acid 100 mg/day	28	L-tryptophan as effective as imipramine.
Herrington et al.[68]	1974	22	Primary depression	Nonblind, compared to ECT	6–8	Pyridoxine 100 mg/day	28	Equal improvement at 2 weeks; greater improvement thereafter with ECT.
Murphy et al.[109]	1974	34	24 primary depression (16 unipolar, 8 bipolar) 10 acute mania	Double-blind, placebo-controlled	9.6	Ascorbic acid 100 mg/day; pyridoxine 50 mg/day	20	1/16 unipolar and 5/8 bipolar depressions improved. 7/10 manias improved.
Prange et al.[142]	1974	10	Mania	Double-blind, placebo-controlled crossover with chlorpromazine	6	Chlorpromazine 400 mg/day	14	L-tryptophan slightly superior to chlorpromazine.
Jensen et al.[76]	1975	22	Endogenous depression	Double-blind	3–6	Imipramine 150 mg/day	21	L-tryptophan as effective as imipramine.
Herrington et al.[69]	1976	20	Primary depression	Double-blind	6–8	Amitriptyline 150 mg/day; pyridoxine 100 mg/day	28	L-tryptophan as effective as amitriptyline.
Chambers and Naylor[18]	1976	10	Acute mania	Double-blind, placebo-controlled	6	Pyridoxine 60 mg/day; ascorbic acid 120 mg/day	14	No significant difference between L-tryptophan and placebo.
Farkas, Dunner, and Fieve[43]	1976	16	Primary affective disorder (10 unipolar, 6 bipolar)	Double-blind, placebo-controlled	6–9	Ascorbic acid 100 mg/day; pyridoxine 100 mg/day	10–18	1/10 unipolar and 3/6 bipolar depressives responded.
Walinder et al.[173]	1978	24	Endogenous depression	Double-blind, placebo-controlled	3–4	Chlorimipramine	21	L-tryptophan potentiates antidepressant effect of chlorimipramine.
Chouinard et al.[20]	1979	17	Primary depression (10 unipolar, 7 bipolar)	Double-blind	4–6	Imipramine 150 mg/day; nicotinamide 1 g/day	28	L-tryptophan/nicotinamide as effective as imipramine.
Moller, Kirk, and Honore[105]	1980	32	Depression	Nonblind	3–4		21	12/32 responders to L-tryptophan. Low total tryptophan to competing amino acid ratio in plasma predicts response.

served to cause both euphoria and dysphoria,[89] and there are longstanding, largely anecdotal clinical reports that opioids have antidepressant effects.[36] Second, opiate receptors and peptides occur predominantly in brain areas associated with the regulation of behavior and emotion.[166] Third, opiate antagonists inhibit stimulant-induced hyperactivity in rats.[170] Last, opiates interact with neurotransmitters, particularly the catecholamines, thought to be involved in the pathogenesis of depression.[170]

From these data, it has been hypothesized that mania is associated with endogenous opiate hyperactivity, whereas depression is associated with diminished opiate function.[36] However, studies have reported no differences in plasma or CSF opioid activity between groups of manic, depressed, and control subjects, although mania is associated with higher CSF opioid activity compared to depression in the same patients.[112]

Nonetheless, trials of the opiate antagonist naloxone hydrochloride in mania have been undertaken. Janowsky and associates[75] reported significant decreases in euphoria and activation in twelve manic patients in a double-blind, placebo-controlled crossover study using 20 mg intravenous naloxone. These investigators were not able to replicate their own findings in a subsequent study using a similar design, although one-third of their subjects did show an antimanic response to the same dose of naloxone.[82] Two subsequent double-blind, placebo-controlled studies on a total of thirty-six patients also failed to show an antimanic effect of naloxone.[29,126] Differences in drug dose and length of rating periods may account for the different results of these studies, and further investigation is necessary before definite conclusions can be reached about the antimanic effects of naloxone.

In accordance with the hypothesis that depression is associated with endogenous opiate hypofunction, opiate peptides have been tested for their antidepressant efficacy. Two open studies have reported antidepressant effects, occasionally complicated by precipitation of mania, with up to 9 mg parenteral beta-endorphin treatment in a combined total of eight depressed patients.[3,88] This was confirmed in a subsequent double-blind, placebo-controlled study in ten depressed patients given up to 10 mg beta-endorphin.[55] However, another double-blind study in four depressed patients showed no significant antidepressant effect of up to 15 mg intravenous beta-endorphin.[125] The data on the effectiveness of beta-endorphin in the treatment of depression are inconclusive. This may be due to methodological difficulties in the studies to date, particularly the small sample sizes. Nonetheless, although inconclusive, the data are suggestive of some antidepressant effect of beta-endorphin, and this is further substantiated by a report of enhanced plasma beta-endorphin immunoreactivity with electroconvulsive therapy (ECT).[38] Furthermore, buprenorphine, an opiate mixed agonist-antagonist, has been reported to have antidepressant effects in a double-blind, placebo-controlled study of ten depressed subjects.[37] In an open study, the narcotic antagonist cyclazocine has also been reported to improve depression after four weeks in eight of ten subjects who received 1 to 3 mg per day.[47]

Other Peptides

Besides the opiate system, a large number of peptides have been measured in the CSF of man.[137] These peptides are postulated to be involved in the modulation of normal behavior and to be altered in psychiatric disorders.[137] To date, use of peptides for treatment of affective illness has been limited. Gold, Goodwin, and Reus[61] postulated that central vasopressin function was decreased in depressed as compared to normal or manic subjects. They subsequently reported that CSF arginine vasopressin was reduced in nonpsychotic bipolar depressed patients compared to normal subjects.[63] Furthermore, in a preliminary study, these researchers found that the arginine vasopressin analogue 1-deamino-8-D-arginine vasopressin improved both cognition and affect in depressed patients, although only two of seven showed significant improvement in affect.[62]

Melanocyte-stimulating hormone-release-inhibiting factor (MIF-1) is a hypothalamic tripeptide with the structure prolyl-leucyl-glycinamide.[63] It is identical to the C-terminal portion of oxytocin.[164]

In animal studies, MIF-1 increases the rate of synthesis of central DA but not NE or 5HT: the DA effect requires the presence of an intact pituitary gland.[127] MIF-1 is also effective in the pargyline dopa model, which is used to test compounds for possible antidepressant effects.[128]

In several double-blind studies, MIF-1 has been found to have antidepressant effects greater than placebo and similar to imipramine with short-term use of up to one to two weeks.[8,35,48] However, with more prolonged treatment trials, more than half the patients treated with MIF-1 relapsed, suggesting that its antidepressant effect is transient and of questionable clinical significance.[96,164]

Somatostatin has been reported to be reduced in the CSF of depressed patients.[54,145] No specific attempts have been made to manipulate this peptide system, although carbamazepine, which has antidepressant properties,[138] reduces somatostatin in CSF.

A recent study has reported that calcitonin reduces psychotic behavior and cycle length in a small number of rapid-cycling bipolar patients.[14] The clinical significance of these findings and their relationship to alterations in calcium metabolism are unclear.

¶ Hormones

Based on the observation, in both animals and man, that thyroid hormones enhanced the toxicity of tricyclic antidepressants, Prange and coworkers hypothesized that such hormones may also potentiate the therapeutic effect of these drugs.[143] In a subsequent double-blind study, they found that use of triiodothyronine (T_3) shortened the latency of the antidepressant effect of imipramine, particularly in women.[140] Further studies have confirmed their findings (see

table 15–2). Furthermore, T_3 appears to enhance the antidepressant effect of tricyclic antidepressants in treatment-resistant patients, regardless of sex.

The mechanism of action of T_3 is unknown although it does not appear to act by enhancing tricyclic plasma levels.[52] Its antidepressant efficacy, at first glance, appears consistent with the hypothesis that enhanced thyroid function favors recovery from depression.[143] However, T_3 supplementation suppresses T_4, which is critical for the intracellular production of T_3 in the brain. Thus T_3 may render the brain relatively hypothyroid, consistent with the recent observation that better responders to both lithium and carbamazepine have evidence of greater chemical hypothyroidism than nonresponders.[80]

The use of T_3 alone does not produce a clinically significant antidepressant effect.[143] However, earlier studies reported that the hypothalamic tripeptide thyroid-releasing hormone (TRH) had a rapid but brief antidepressant effect when administered alone under double-blind, placebo-controlled conditions.[139,141] Some studies have replicated these findings,[84] but by far the majority have been unable to demonstrate an antidepressant effect of TRH.[51,155,162,163]

¶ Sleep and Circadian Manipulations

Several manipulations of sleep have been reported to have antidepressant effects of varying duration.[57] These include rapid-eye-movement (REM) sleep deprivation, total sleep deprivation, partial sleep deprivation, and phase advance of the sleep-wake cycle.

Vogel and associates[172] have described the potential therapeutic benefit of REM sleep deprivation. Endogenous depressed patients require two to three weeks of treatment, which involves interruption of electroencephalogram (EEG)-monitored sleep at the onset of each REM period. Therapeutic benefit may last several months. REM sleep deprivation is, in effect, a form of REM sup-

TABLE 15–2

Studies of Triiodothyronine (T$_3$) in Depression

Study	Date	N	Diagnosis	Design	Dose of T$_3$ (μ/day)	Antidepressant	Duration (days)	Results
Prange et al.[14]	1969	20	Primary retarded depression	Randomized double-blind, placebo-controlled	25	Imipramine 150 mg/day	28	T$_3$ accelerates onset of action and may enhance efficacy of imipramine. More effect in females.
Earle[34]	1970	25	Treatment-resistant depression	Single-blind with T$_3$ added to unsuccessful antidepressant trial	25	Imipramine 150 mg/day, amitriptyline 150 mg/day, or protriptyline 40 mg/day	28	14/25 improved with T$_3$. No sex difference.
Coppen et al.[26]	1972	30	Primary, unipolar depression	Randomized, double-blind, placebo-controlled	25	Imipramine 150 mg/day or L-tryptophan 9 g/day	14	T$_3$ accelerates antidepressant effect of imipramine but not L-tryptophan.
Feighner et al.[44]	1972	21	Primary depression	Randomized, double-blind, placebo-controlled	25	Imipramine 200 mg/day	10	No effect of T$_3$ on treatment response to imipramine.
Wheatley[76]	1972	57	Depression	Randomized, double-blind, placebo-controlled	20–40	Amitriptyline 100 mg/day	21	T$_3$ accelerates efficacy of amitriptyline in females.
Ogura et al.[116]	1974	44	Resistant depression	Nonblind, T$_3$ added to unsuccessful antidepressant trial	25–30	Imipramine, amitriptyline, nortriptyline, or desipramine 75 mg/day	7–136	Improvement in 29 cases. No sex difference.
Tsutsui et al.[159]	1979	11	Prolonged depression	Nonblind, uncontrolled	5–25	Variety, mainly chlorimipramine in varying doses	14–56	T$_3$ enhances efficacy of various antidepressants.
Goodwin et al.[66]	1982	12	Major depressive illness	Open T$_3$ added to double-blind tricyclics	25–50	Imipramine or amitriptyline 150–300 mg/day	up to 28	9/12 enhanced antidepressant response with T$_3$.

pression, which is a feature common to a wide range of antidepressants.[172]

Numerous reports have confirmed that approximately 50 to 70 percent of patients will have an acute antidepressant effect to one night of total sleep deprivation.[144,172] Patients usually respond immediately, on the first day or even during the night of sleep deprivation.[144] However, the beneficial effect is transient and usually lasts only until the next night of sleep; occasionally, however, it may last a few days or even longer.[79,144] Some patients do not improve until the day after recovery sleep.[42] Fahndrich[42] noted that neurotic depressives typically show this pattern of response. Concomitant use of sleep deprivation and tricyclic antidepressants may decrease the rebound phenomenon and render the procedure more clinically useful.[177] Repeated sleep deprivation may be effective in some patients, but not in others.[144]

Total sleep deprivation is reported to be particularly effective in patients with endogenous depression[79] regardless of the bipolar-unipolar and primary-secondary distinction. Furthermore, diurnal variation in mood, but not age, sex, or sleep disturbance, appears to predict response to total sleep deprivation.[79]

The mechanism of the antidepressant effect of total sleep deprivation is unknown.[79,144] However, prevention of sleep during the second part of the night seems particularly important as partial sleep deprivation during the second half of the night appears to have similar clinical effects to total sleep deprivation.[57] Furthermore, van Bemmel and van den Hoofdakker[161] have shown that partial sleep deprivation on the recovery night after total sleep deprivation may augment the antidepressant effect and prevent relapse.

Goetz and Tolle[60] reported that partial sleep deprivation during the first half of the night had a limited antidepressant effect, certainly inferior to that of other types of sleep deprivation.

Sleep deprivation has also been reported to have other potential uses. First, Papadimitriou and associates[121] have suggested that once-a-week total sleep deprivation decreases the number of cycles in rapid-cycling bipolar patients. Second, sleep deprivation response has been reported to predict response to a variety of tricyclic antidepressants.[79,177]

Wehr and colleagues[175] have reported that, in a limited number of patients, advancing the sleep period approximately six hours for several days produces an antidepressant effect. This maneuver is an attempt to correct the hypothesized desynchronization between the sleep-wake and REM cycles due to phase advance of REM sleep, which is thought to be implicated in the pathogenesis of depression[174] (see chapter 16).

¶ Anticonvulsants

Carbamazepine is emerging as an experimental treatment of the affective disorders that has substantial clinical utility.[131,138,141] As summarized in table 15–3, its acute antimanic effects have been documented in several double-blind, placebo-controlled studies as well as in a number of open and uncontrolled investigations. It appears to have a rapidity of onset and a time course of effect not dissimilar to that of neuroleptics,[119,134] although it does not appear to act, as do classical neuroleptics, by blocking DA receptors.[129,131,138] Unequivocal antimanic responsivity to carbamazepine has also been documented in individual patients (many of whom were not responsive to lithium) by utilizing a double-blind "off-on-off-on" design.[138] In these instances patients repeatedly improved on carbamazepine, relapsed on placebo substitution, and again improved when active drug was readministered.[6,7,129]

The acute antidepressant effects of carbamazepine have also been described in approximately 50 percent of depressed patients.[129,135] These antidepressant responses were observed in fifteen of thirty-one patients who were initially more severely depressed during the placebo period than nonresponders. As with other agents, there was a typical lag in antidepressant response; improvement generally was not present until the second or third week of treatment. These preliminary data require further confirmation in other experimental designs, particularly those using randomized clinical trials and comparison with other agents. Parenthetically, the emerging clinical profile of efficacy of carbamazepine in affective illness appears to be similar to that established for lithium, where its acute antimanic efficacy is well accepted, while, even after more than a decade, controversy continues as to its acute antidepressant effects. However, it remains to be established whether carbamazepine and lithium responders will overlap, particularly in light of the early data that many patients who do not adequately respond to lithium may respond to carbamazepine.[138]

This also appears to be the case for carbamazepine prophylaxis (see table 15–4); 96 of 146 patients (66 percent) have been reported to respond to carbamazepine, most of whom were initially inadequately responsive to lithium carbonate. With the exception[136] of the National Institute of Mental Health study and Okuma's study,[120] all of the long-term studies have been of an uncontrolled nature and often with carbamazepine added to existing treatments. However, both the double-blind and open trials appear to show approximately the same rate of response, with adequate prophylaxis observed in both the depressed and manic phases of the illness.

Although there is accumulating evidence of carbamazepine's clinical utility in manic-depressive illness and now widespread clinical use in the United States and in many other countries, it is unlikely that it will achieve formal approval by the United States Food and Drug Administration (FDA) soon, as no drug company is currently interested in pursuing this option. Thus it would appear that this anticonvulsant will be in wide clinical use and be tested for many years before it is no longer classed as an "experimental" agent. It should be noted, however, that with appropriate informed consent and clinical monitoring,[129] the FDA sanctions, for individual patients on a physician-option basis, the use of drugs like carbamazepine that are commercially available for other approved uses.

Other anticonvulsants have been less extensively studied. The early uncontrolled trials of Kalinowsky and Putnam,[83] Freyhan,[50] and Kubanek and Rowell[90] have not provided convincing evidence of the efficacy of phenytoin in affective illness. One of the patients cited by Freyhan[50] did appear to respond multiple times to phenytoin and show exacerbations on drug withdrawal, however. Lambert and coworkers[93] and more recently Emrich and associates[40] have reported that the anticonvulsant valproic acid may be useful in the treatment of acute mania and in long-term prophylaxis when used in combination with lithium. Progabide, an anticonvulsant with direct gamma-aminobutyric acid (GABA) agonist activity, has also been reported to be effective in the treatment of acute depression.[100] Chouinard and coworkers[20] reported that the anticonvulsant clonazepam possessed antimanic effects equivalent to those of lithium, but was more sedating.

The mechanisms of action of the anticonvulsants in general, and of carbamazepine in particular, have not been adequately delineated either for their anticonvulsant efficacy or their effects on manic-depressive illness. Effects of carbamazepine on NE, DA, 5HT, GABA, adenosine, the so-called peripheral benzodiazepine system, vasopressin, somatostatin, and cyclic nucleotides have been identified; all of these are potential candidates for the therapeutic or side effects of this agent.[131,134,138] It is hoped that more systematic comparisons of the biological effects of carbamazepine to classical psychotropic agents and to anticonvulsants that are not effective in manic-depressive illness will yield further insights about the mode of action of anticonvulsants in affective illness.

It is of some interest that one of the first and best-documented effective treatments for depression and mania remains ECT, that is, the induction of major motor seizures.[46] (See chapter 33.) Post, Putnam, and Contel[130] have documented that the major sei-

TABLE 15-3

Studies of Carbamazepine in Acute Mania

Study	Date	N	Diagnosis	Design	Dose of CBZ (mg/day) (blood level)	Other Drugs	Duration	Results
Takezaki and Hanaoka[157]	1971	10	Manic-depressive psychosis	Open	200–600	Neuroleptics; tricyclics in some cases	1–11 mos.	6/10 improved in days to weeks.
Okuma et al.[117,118]	1973, 1975	64	Manic-depressive psychosis	Open	400–1,200	Neuroleptics	Variable	22/64 improved (marked to moderate).
Ballenger and Post[6,7]	1978, 1980	9	Manic-depressive psychosis	*Double-blind.* Placebo-controlled "off-on-off-on"	600–1,600 [7–15.5 ug/ml]	*None*	11–56 days	5/9 improved. 4 showed relapse on placebo and repeated improvement on CBZ.
Okuma et al.[119]	1979	32 CBZ 28 chlor.	Manic-depressive psychosis (ICD-9)	*Double-blind* comparison with chlorpromazine 150–450 mg	300–900 [2.7–11.7 ug/ml] [mean = 7.2 ± 3.4]	Bedtime hypnotics	3–5 weeks	21/32 improved on CBZ (marked to moderate). 15/28 improved on chlorpromazine.
Inoue et al.[72]	1981	5	Bipolar disorder	Open	400–800	Lithium, neuroleptics, tricyclics	Variable	3/5 improved
Folks et al.[49]	1982	10	4 bipolar, 3 schizo-affective, 3 organic affective	Open	600–1,600	Concomitant medications in 6/10	—	8/10 improved–CBZ may be especially effective for affective cases with CNS disorder.

Table 15-3 (Continued)

Study	Date	N	Diagnosis	Design	Dose of CBZ (mg/day) (blood level)	Other Drugs	Duration	Results
Kwamie, Persad, and Stancer[92]	1982	12	Manic-depressive	Open	–	Others	–	5/12 improved.
Lipinski and Pope[98]	1982	3	2 bipolar manic, 1 hexosaminidase A deficient	Open lithium discontinuation	Not specified [8.5–9.5 ug/ml]	Lithium and neuroleptics	Variable	3/3 improved, but all relapsed on lithium discontinuation, suggesting combination necessary.
Moss and James[106]	1982	1	Major affective disorder, manic	Open	600–800 [4.5–5.7 ug/ml]	Lithium	–	0/1 partial response only; partially improved but relapsed on combination of CBZ and lithium.
Post et al.[134,138]	1982, 1984	12	Manic-depressive psychosis	Double-blind	600–2,000 [7–15.5 ug/ml]	None	11–56 days	8/12 improved—time course similar to neuroleptics (update of Okuma et al.[117,118]).
Yassa[178]	1982	1	Manic-depressive	Open	600 [8 ug/ml]	Chlorpromazine	26 mos.	1/1 improved.
Enrich et al.[41]	1983	6	Maniform psychoses	Double-blind	1800–2,100 oxycarbamazepine	Not stated	Variable	5/6 (> 25% improvement on IMPS).
Keisling[85]	1983	3	1 Schizo-affective, 1 bipolar, 1 mania	Open	600–1,400	Lithium (all; tricyclics in one case	2–3 mos.	3/3 improved in combination with lithium.
Klein et al.[87]	1984	11	Excited mania or 3 excited schizo-affective	Blind	600–1,600 [6–18 ug/ml]	Haloperidol (15–45 mg/day) all patients	5 weeks	10/14 improved in CBZ and haloperidol. 7/13 improved on placebo and haloperidol.
Total								95/73 (55% moderate-marked improvement).

TABLE 15-4
Carbamazepine Prophylaxis in Manic-Depressive Illness

Study	Date	N	Diagnosis	Design	Dose of CBZ (mg/day) [blood level]	Other Drugs	Duration	Results
Takezaki and Hanaoka[157]	1971	10	Manic-depressive	Open	200-600	Neuroleptics, tricyclics in some cases	1-11 mos.	9/10 improved.
Okuma et al.[117,118]	1973, 1975	51	Manic-depressive	Open	400-1,200	Neuroleptics, lithium, tricyclics	Approx. 25 weeks	34/51 improved.
Ballenger and Post[6,7]; Post et al.[136]	1978	7	6 manic-depressive, 1 confirmed psychosis	4 blind, 3 open	800-2,000 [11.3 ug/ml]	None for 3 patients	6-51 mos.	6/7 improved, especially lithium-nonresponsive rapid cyclers.
Inoue et al.[72]	1981	3	Manic-depressive	Open	400-600	Lithium	18-32 mos.	2/3 improved.
Okuma et al.[120]	1981	12 CBZ 10 placebo	Manic-depressive	Open CBZ vs. placebo, blind, random assignment	400-600 [5.6 ± 2.0 ug/ml]	Acute treatments added during episode breakthroughs	12 mos. either Rx	6/10 improved on CBZ. 2/9 improved on placebo.
Kwiamie, Persad, and Stancer[92]	1982	12	Manic-depressive	Open	—	Others	—	5/12 improved (lithium-resistant).
Lipinski and Pope[98]	1982	3	2 manic-depressive, 1 hexosaminidase A deficient	Open	Not specified [8.5-9.5 ug/ml]	Lithium and neuroleptics in one case	3-8 mos.	3/3 improved but relapsed on lithium discontinuation—combination—combination necessary?
Yassa[78]	1982	1	Manic-depressive	Open	600 [8 ug/ml]	Chlorpromazine; decreasing doses from 1,700 mg/day	26 mos.	1/1 improved.
Keisling[85]	1983	3	1 schizo-affective, 1 bipolar, 1 manic	Open	600-1,400 [8-9 ug/ml]	Lithium (all); 1 tricyclic	2-8 mos.	3/3 improved on lithium combination.
Kishimoto[96]	1983	32	Manic-depressive	Open	100-1,200 [6-10 ug/ml]	Lithium and others	2-11 years.	24/32 improved, especially early onset and continuous cyclers.
Nolen[115]	1983	8	Manic-depressive	Open	400 [6-12 ug/ml]	Lithium, neuroleptics, antidepressants	6-36 mos.	4/8 improved (all lithium-resistant).
Total								97/140 improved (69% moderate-marked improvement).

zures of electroconvulsive shock in the rat are potent anticonvulsants to the development of amygdala kindling or to its persistence. Thus it remains a possibility that the biochemical effects associated with the ability of both electroconvulsive seizures and the anticonvulsants to inhibit paroxysmal neuronal activity could be related to their psychotropic effects. It is worth highlighting, however, that carbamazepine is a highly effective agent in treating paroxysmal pain syndromes such as trigeminal neuralgia, which do not appear to be associated with a seizure process. Similarly, the anticonvulsants are associated with some useful properties in certain cardiac arrhythmias. Therefore, it is clearly not a tenable proposition to conclude that the efficacy of anticonvulsant agents in manic-depressive illness indicates that an epileptic process (even a covert one in deep structures of the brain) underlies the pathophysiological disturbance of manic-depressive illness. Thus use of the category anticonvulsant may be a misnomer, even though biochemical and physiological mechanisms related to the anticonvulsant action of selected agents in this class may also be related to their psychotropic effects.

¶ Other Mechanistic Approaches

S-Adenosyl-L-methionine (SAMe) is a methyl donor that occurs naturally in the central nervous system.[111] Animal studies show that parenteral administration of SAMe increases turnover of brain serotonin and norepinephrine.[111] Furthermore, SAMe increases CSF 5-HIAA in depressed patients, probably by its effects on melatonin synthesis.[28]

In several double-blind studies, parenteral SAMe, in doses ranging from 45 to 150 mg per day for up to eighteen days, was found to be more effective than placebo and equal to standard antidepressants such as imipramine and chlorimipramine.[1,30,104] These studies were limited by heterogeneous groups of poorly defined depressed patients. Two later studies,[91,111] however, with homogeneous

samples, confirmed these earlier reports. A recent open study is also consistent with an antidepressant effect of SAMe, as seven of nine patients had a good response.[99] Therefore, SAMe appears to have antidepressant effects with a rapid onset of action—within four to seven days—and minimal side effects.

Membrane transport of sodium is thought to be increased in mania. However, in a randomized double-blind study, digoxin, an inhibitor of Na-K ATPase and, therefore, sodium transport, was found to be ineffective in the treatment of mania.[113] Spironolactone, another drug with probable effects on electrolyte transport, has been reported to be effective in the prophylaxis of patients with manic-depressive illness.[67]

¶ Conclusions

The experimental treatments we have outlined and briefly reviewed fall into several different categories. Promising, although the least well documented, are the specific strategies of dissecting possible neurotransmitter alterations in affective illness by using relatively selective antagonists or agonists of these systems. While preliminary data exist that implicate possible noradrenergic, dopaminergic, serotonergic, or GABAergic mechanisms in the affective disorders based on these clinical trials, none has received substantial enough study or convincing enough results to gain wide clinical use even on an experimental basis.

On the other hand, treatments such as sleep deprivation have been extensively documented. However, because of their transient clinical effects they have not been widely employed, except perhaps as an adjunct to other therapies. Moreover, their mechanism of action also remains elusive. Supplementation of tricyclic antidepressants with thyroid hormone also appears to be another treatment strategy that is moderately well established in the literature (see table 15-2), utilized in clinical practice, but unlikely to be taken out of the "experimental" mode for many years.

Finally, the recent introduction of such agents as carbamazepine for manic-depressive illness (based on a variety of empirical and theoretical rationales)[138] appears to be a practical clinical treatment option (particularly for lithium nonresponders) even in this early phase of their experimental use. As such, anticonvulsants such as carbamazepine may represent the first new class of psychopharmacological agents introduced in the last decade. A number of the agents reviewed in this chapter have considerable clinical and/or theoretical promise, and further clinical research investigations should prove to be rewarding both from the standpoint of support or repudiation of existing theories and from a clinical perspective.

¶ Bibliography

1. AGNOLI, A., et al. "Effect of S-adenosyl-L-methionine (SAMe) upon Depressive Symptoms," *Journal of Psychiatric Research*, 3 (1976):43–54.

2. ANGST, J., WOGGON, B., and SCHOEPF, J. "The Treatment of Depression with L-5-hydroxytryptophan versus Imipramine," *Archiv fuer Psychiatrie und Nervenkrankheiten*, 224 (1977):175–186.

3. ANGST, J., et al. "Preliminary Results of Treatment with Beta-endorphin in Depression," in E. Usdin, W. E. Bunney, Jr., and N. S. Kline, eds., *Endorphins in Mental Health Research*. London: Macmillan, 1979, pp. 518–528.

4. ARBUTHNOTT, G. W., and MURRAY, L. G. "Dopamine Receptor Agonists in Psychiatric Disease," in D. B. Calne, T. N., Chase, and A. Barbeau, eds., *Advances in Neurology*, vol. 9. New York: Raven Press, 1975, pp. 345–348.

5. ATSMON, A., et al. "The Short-term Effects of Adrenergic Blocking Agents in a Small Group of Psychotic Patients," *Psychiatry, Neurology, Neurochirurgie*, 74 (1971):251–258.

6. BALLENGER, J. C., and POST, R. M. "Therapeutic Effects of Carbamazepine in Affective Illness: A Preliminary Report," *Community Psychopharmacology*, 2 (1978):159–178.

7. ———. "Carbamazepine (Tegretol) in Manic-depressive Illness: A New Treatment," *American Journal of Psychiatry*, 137 (1980):782–790.

8. BARBEAU, A. "Potentiation of Levodopa Effect by Intravenous 1-Prolyl-1-lecyl-glycine Amide in Man," *Lancet*, 2 (1975):683–684.

9. BELMAKER, R. H., LERER, B., and ZOHAR, J. "Salbutamol Treatment of Depression," in E. Costa, and G. Racagni, eds., *Typical and Atypical Antidepressants*. New York: Raven Press, 1982, pp. 181–193.

10. BOWERS, M. B., GOODMAN, E., and SIM, V. M. "Some Behavioral Changes in Man Following Anticholinesterase Administration," *Journal of Nervous and Mental Disease*, 138 (1964):383–389.

11. BRODIE, H.K.H., SACK, R., and SIEVER, L. "Clinical Studies of L-5-hydroxytryptophan in Depression," in J. Barchas, and E. Usdin, eds., *Serotonin and Behavior*. New York: Academic Press, 1973, pp. 549–559.

12. BUNNEY, W. E., JR., et al. "Studies of Alpha-methyl-para-tyrosine, L-dopa and L-tryptophan in Depression and Mania," *American Journal of Psychiatry*, 127 (1971):872–881.

13. CARLSSON, A., and LINDQVIST, M. "Dependence of 5-HT and Catecholamine Synthesis of Concentrations of Precursor Amino Acids in Rat Brain," *Nauyn-Schmiedesbergs Archives of Pharmacology*, 303 (1978):157–164.

14. CARMAN, J., and WYATT, R. J. "The Use of Calcitonin in Psychiatric Agitation or Mania," *Archives of General Psychiatry*, 36 (1979):72–75.

15. CARROLL, B. J. "Monoamine Precursors in the Treatment of Depression," *Clinical Pharmacology and Therapeutics*, 12 (1978):743–761.

16. CARROLL, B. J., MOWBRAY, R. M., and DAVIES, B. M. "Sequential Comparison of L-tryptophan with E.C.T. in Severe Depression," *Lancet*, 1 (1970):967–969.

17. CARROLL, B. J., et al. "Cholinergic Reversal of Manic Symptoms," *Lancet*, 1 (1973):427–428.

18. CHAMBERS, C. A., and NAYLOR, G. J. "A Controlled Trial of L-tryptophan in

Mania," *British Journal of Psychiatry*, 132 (1978):555–559.

19. CHOUINARD, G., et al. "Tryptophan-nicotinamide, Imipramine and Their Combination in Depression," *Acta Psychiatrica Scandinavica*, 59 (1979):395–414.

20. CHOUINARD, G., et al. "Antimanic Effects of Clonazepam," *Biological Psychiatry*, 18 (1983):451–466.

21. COHEN, B. M., et al. "Lecithin in Mania: A Preliminary Report," *American Journal of Psychiatry*, 137 (1980):242–243.

22. COLONNA, L., PETIT, M., and LEPINE, J. P. "Bromocriptine in Affective Disorders. A Pilot Study," *Journal of Affective Disorders*, 1 (1979):173–177.

23. COOKSON, J., and SILVERSTONE, T. "5-Hydroxytryptamine and Dopamine Pathways in Mania: A Pilot Study of Fenfluramine and Pimozide," *British Journal of Clinical Pharmacology*, 3 (1976):942–947.

24. COPPEN, A., et al. "Tryptophan in the Treatment of Depression," *Lancet*, 2 (1967):1178–1180.

25. COPPEN, A., et al. "Methylsergide in Mania. A Controlled Trial," *Lancet*, 2 (1969):338–340.

26. COPPEN, A., et al. "The Comparative Antidepressant Value of L-tryptophan and Imipramine With and Without Attempted Potentiation by Liothyronine," *Archives of General Psychiatry*, 26 (1972):234–241.

27. COURT, J. M., and MAI, F. M. "A Double-blind Intensive Crossover Design Trial of Methylsergide in Mania," *Medical Journal of Australia*, 2 (1970):526–529.

28. CURCIO, M., et al. "Effect of S-adenosyl-L-methionine on Serotonin Metabolism in Rat Brain," *Progress in Neuropsychopharmacology*, 2 (1978):65–71.

29. DAVIS, G. C., et al. "Failure of Naloxone to Reduce Manic Symptoms," *American Journal of Psychiatry*, 137 (1980):583–585.

30. DEL VECCHIO, M., et al. "Has SAMe (Ado Met) an Antidepressant Effect? A Preliminary Trial Versus Chlorimipramine," *Rivista Sperimentale di Freniatria*, 102 (1978):344–358.

31. DEWHURST, W. G. "Methylsergide in Mania," *Nature*, 219 (1968):506–507.

32. DUNNER, D. L., and FIEVE, R. R. "Affective Disorder: Studies with Amine Precursors," *American Journal of Psychiatry*, 132 (1975):180–183.

33. DUNNER, D. L., and GOODWIN, F. K. "Effect of L-tryptophan on Brain Serotonin Metabolism in Depressed Patients," *Archives of General Psychiatry*, 26 (1972):364–366.

34. EARLE, B. V. "Thyroid Hormone and Tricyclic Antidepressants in Resistant Depressions," *American Journal of Psychiatry*, 126 (1970):1667–1669.

35. EHRENSING, R. H., and KASTIN, A. J. "Melanocyte-stimulating Hormone Release Inhibiting Hormone as an Antidepressant. A Pilot Study," *Archives of General Psychiatry*, 30 (1974):63–65.

36. EMRICH, H. M. "A Possible Role of Opioid Substances in Depression," in E. Costa and G. Racagni, eds., *Typical and Atypical Antidepressants: Clinical Practice*. New York: Raven Press, 1982, pp. 77–94.

37. EMRICH, H. M., VOGT, P., and HERZ, A. "Possible Antidepressive Effects of Opioid: Action of Buprenorphine," in L. Verebey, ed., *Opioids in Mental Illness*. New York: The New York Academy of Science, 1982, pp. 108–113.

38. EMRICH, H. M., et al. "Beta-endorphin-like Immunoreactivity in Cerebrospinal Fluid and Plasma of Patients with Schizophrenia and Other Neuropsychiatric Disorders," *Pharmacopsychiatria* 12 (1979):269–276.

39. EMRICH, H. M., et al. "Action of Propranolol in Mania: Comparison of Effects of the d- and l-stereoisomer," *Pharmacopsychiatria* 12 (1979):295–304.

40. EMRICH, H. M., et al. "Effect of Sodium Valproate in Mania. The GABA-hypothesis of Affective Disorders," *Archiv fuer Psychiatrie und Nervenkrankheiten*, 229 (1980):1–16.

41. EMRICH, H. M., et al. "Antimanic Action of Propranolol and of Sodium Valproate," Paper presented at the 13th CINP Congress, Tel Aviv, 1982.

42. FAHNDRICH, E. "Effects of Sleep Deprivation on Depressed Patients of Different Nosological Groups," *Psychiatry Research*, 5 (1981):277–282.

43. FARKAS, T., DUNNER, D. L., and FIEVE, R.

R. "L-tryptophan in Depression," *Biological Psychiatry*, 11 (1976):295–302.

44. FEIGHNER, J. P., et al. "Hormonal Potentiation of Imipramine and ECT in Primary Depression," *American Journal of Psychiatry*, 128 (1972):1230–1238.

45. FERNSTROM, J. D., and WURTMAN, R. J. "Brain Serotonin Content: Physiological Dependence on Plasma Tryptophan Levels," *Science*, 173 (1971):49–51.

46. FINK, M. *Convulsive Therapy: Theory and Practice.* New York: Raven Press, 1979.

47. FINK, M., et al. "Clinical Antidepressant Activity of Cyclazocine—a Narcotic Antagonist," *Clinical Pharmacology Therapeutics*, 11 (1970):41–48.

48. FISCHER, P. A., et al. "Effect of Melanocyte-stimulating Hormone Release Inhibiting Factor (MIF) in Parkinson's Syndrome," *European Neurology*, 12 (1974):360–368.

49. FOLKS, D. G., et al. "Carbamazepine Treatment of Selected Affectively Disordered Patients," *American Journal of Psychiatry*, 139 (1982):115–117.

50. FREYHAN, F. A. "Effectiveness of Diphenylhydantoin in Management of Non-epileptic Psychomotor Excitement States," *Archives of Neurology and Psychiatry*, 53 (1945):370–374.

51. FURLONG, F. W., BROWN, G. M., and BEECHING, M. F. "Thyrotropin-releasing Hormone: Differential Antidepressant and Endocrinological Effects," *American Journal of Psychiatry*, 133 (1976):1187–1190.

52. GARBUTT, J., et al. "Effects of Triiodothyronine on Drug Levels and Cardiac Function in Depressed Patients Treated with Imipramine," *American Journal of Psychiatry*, 136 (1979):980–982.

53. GELENBERG, A. J., et al. "Tyrosine for Depression, *Journal of Psychiatric Research*, 17 (1982/83):175–180.

54. GERNER, R. H., and YAMADA, T. "Altered Neuropeptide Concentrations in Cerebrospinal Fluid of Psychiatric Patients," *Brain Research*, 238 (1982):298–302.

55. GERNER, R. H., et al. "Beta-endorphin. Intravenous Infusion Causes Behavioral Change in Psychiatric Inpatients," *Archives of General Psychiatry*, 37 (1980):642–647.

56. GERSHON, S., and SHAW, F. H. "Psychiatric Sequelae of Chronic Exposure to Organophosphorous Insecticides," *Lancet*, 1 (1961):1371–1374.

57. GILLIN, J. C. "The Sleep Therapies of Depression," *Progress in Neuro-Psychopharmacology and Biological Psychiatry*, 7 (1983):351–364.

58. GISSELMAN, A., MARIN, A., and SIMON, P. "Etude Pilot des Effets d'un Antiparkinsonien Anticholinergique au Cours d'Etats Depressifs," *Encephale*, 1 (1975):363–367.

59. GLASSMAN, A. H., and PLATMAN, S. R. "Potentiation of a Monoamine Oxidase Inhibitor by Tryptophan," *Journal of Psychiatric Research*, 7 (1969):83–88.

60. GOETZE, U., and TOLLE, R. "Antidepressive Effect of Partial Sleep Deprivation During the First Half of the Night," *Psychiatrica Clinica* (Basel), 14 (1981):129–149.

61. GOLD, P. W., GOODWIN, F. K., and REUS, V. I. "Vasopressin in Affective Illness," *Lancet*, 1 (1978):1233–1236.

62. GOLD, P. W., et al. "Effects of 1-desamino-8-D-arginine Vasopressin on Behavior and Cognition in Primary Affective Disorder," *Lancet*, 2 (1979):992–994.

63. GOLD, P. W., et al. "Central Vasopressin Function in Affective Illness," in D. de Wied, ed., *The Brain as an Endocrine Target Organ in Health and Disease.* Belguim: MTP Press, 1981, pp. 241–252.

64. GOLDBERG, I. K. "L-tyrosine in Depression," *Lancet*, 2 (1980):364.

65. GOODWIN, F. K., et al. "L-dopa, Catecholamines and Behavior: A Clinical and Biochemical Study in Depressed Patients," *Biological Psychiatry*, 2 (1970):341–366.

66. GOODWIN, F. K., et al. "Potentiation of Antidepressant Effects by L-triiodothyronine in Tricyclic Nonresponders," *American Journal of Psychiatry*, 139 (1982):34–38.

67. HENDLER, N. H. "Spironolactone Prophylaxis in Manic-depressive Disease," *Journal of Nervous and Mental Disease*, 166 (1977):517–520.

68. HERRINGTON, R. N., et al. "Comparative Trial of L-tryptophan and ECT in Severe Depressive Illness," *Lancet*, 2 (1974):731.

69. HERRINGTON, R. N., et al. "Comparative Trial of L-tryptophan and Amitriptyline in Depressive Illness," *Psychological Medicine,* 6 (1976):673–678.

70. HIRSH, M. J., and WURTMAN, R. J. "Lecithin Consumption Increases Acetylcholine Concentrations in Rat Brain and Adrenal Gland," *Science,* 202 (1978):- 223–225.

71. HUGHES, J. "Opioid Peptides and Their Relatives," *Nature,* 278 (1979):394–395.

72. INOUE, K., et al. "A Lithium and Carbamazepine Combination in the Treatment of Bipolar Disorder: A Preliminary Report," *Folia Psychiatrica et Neurologica Japonica,* 35 (1981):465– 475.

73. JANOWSKY, D. S., EL-YOUSEF, M. K., and DAVIS, J. M. "Acetylcholine and Depression," *Psychosomatic Medicine,* 36 (1974):248–257.

74. JANOWSKY, D. S., et al. "Parasympathetic Suppression of Manic Symptoms by Physostigmine," *Archives of General Psychiatry,* 28 (1973):542–547.

75. JANOWSKY, D., et al. "Naloxone Effects on Manic Symptoms and Growth-hormone Levels," *Lancet,* 2 (1978):320.

76. JENSEN, K., et al. "Tryptophan-imipramine in Depression," *Lancet,* 2 (1975):- 920.

77. JIMERSON, D. C., et al. "Preliminary Trial of the Noradrenergic Agonist Clonidine in Psychiatric Patients," *Biological Psychiatry,* 15 (1980):45–57.

78. JIMERSON, D. C., et al. "Anticholinergic Treatment for Depression. Syllabus and Scientific Proceedings in Summary Form," Paper presented at the annual meeting of the American Psychiatric Association, Toronto, Canada, 1982.

79. JOFFE, R. T., and BROWN, P. "Clinical and Biological Effects of Sleep Deprivation in Depression," *Canadian Journal of Psychiatry,* 29 (1984):530–536.

80. JOFFE, R. T., et al. "Thyroid Function and Affective Illness: A Reappraisal," *Biological Psychiatry,* 19 (1984):1685–1691.

81. JOUVENT, R., et al. "Antimanic Effect of Clonidine," *American Journal of Psychiatry,* 137 (1980):1275–1276.

82. JUDD, L. L., et al. "Naloxone-induced Behavioral and Physiological Effects in Normal and Manic Subjects," *Archives of General Psychiatry,* 37 (1980):583– 586.

83. KALINOWSKY, L. B., and PUTNAM, T. J. "Attempts at Treatment of Schizophrenia and Other Non-epileptic Psychoses with Dilantin," *Archives of Neurology and Psychiatry,* 39 (1943):14–20.

84. KASTIN, A. J., et al. "Improvement in Mental Depression with Decreased Thyrotropin Response After Administration of TRH," *Lancet,* 2 (1972):740– 742.

85. KEISLING, R. "Carbamazepine and Lithium Carbonate in the Treatment of Refractory Affective Disorders," *Archives of General Psychiatry,* 40 (1983):223.

86. KISHIMOTO, A., et al. "Long-term Prophylactic Effects of Carbamazepine in Affective Disorder," *British Journal of Psychiatry,* 143 (1983):327–331.

87. KLEIN, E., et al. "Carbamazepine and Haloperidol Versus Placebo and Haloperidol in Excited Psychoses: A Controlled Study," *Archives of General Psychiatry,* 41 (1984):165–170.

88. KLINE, N. S., et al. "Beta-endorphin-induced Changes in Schizophrenic and Depressed Patients," *Archives of General Psychiatry,* 34 (1977):1111–1113.

89. KORNETSKY, C., et al. "Intracranial Self-stimulation Thresholds. A Model for the Hedonic Effects of Drugs of Abuse," *Archives of General Psychiatry,* 36 (1979):- 289–298.

90. KUBANEK, J. L., and ROWELL, R. C. "The Use of Dilantin on the Treatment of Psychotic Patients Unresponsive to Other Treatment," *Diseases of the Nervous System,* 7 (1946):47–50.

91. KUFFERTE, B., and GRUNBERGER, J. "Early Clinical Double-blind Study with S-adenosyl-L-methionine: A New Potential Antidepressant," in E. Costa and G. Racagni, eds., *Typical and Atypical Antidepressants: Clinical Practice.* New York: Raven Press, 1982, pp. 174– 180.

92. KWAMIE, Y., PERSAD, E., and STANCER, H. C. "The Use of Carbamazepine in the Management of Affective Disorders," Paper presented at the University of Toronto, Department of Psychiatry, Research Day, Toronto, Canada, 1982.

93. LAMBERT, P. A., et al. "Le Dipropylaceta-
mide dans l'etraitement de la Psychose
Maniaco-depressive," *Encephale*, 1
(1975):25–31.

94. LECRUBIER, Y., et al. "Effet Antidepress-
eur d'un Stimulant Beta Adrener-
gique," *Nouvelle Presse Medicale*, 6
(1977):2786.

95. LECRUBIER, Y., et al. "A Beta Adrenergic
Stimulant (Salbutamol) Versus Clomipramine in Depression: A Controlled
Study," *British Journal of Psychiatry*,
136 (1980):354–358.

96. LEVY, M. I., DE NIGRIS, Y., and DAVIS, K.
L. "Rapid Antidepressant Activity of
Melanocyte Inhibiting Factor: A Clinical Trial," *Biological Psychiatry*, 17
(1982):72–75.

97. LICHTENSTEIGER, W., MUTZNER, U., and
LANGEMANN, H. "Uptake of 5-Hydrox-
ytryptamine and S-hydroxytrytophan
by Neurons of the Central Nervous System Normally Containing Catecholamines," *Journal of Neurochemistry*, 14
(1967):489–497.

98. LIPINSKI, J. F., and POPE, H. G., JR. "Possible Synergistic Action Between Carbamazepine and Lithium Carbonate in
the Treatment of Three Acutely Manic
Patients," *American Journal of Psychiatry*, 139 (1982):948–949.

99. LIPINSKI, J. F., et al. "Open Trial of S-
adenosylmethionine for Treatment of
Depression," *American Journal of Psychiatry*, 141 (1984):448–450.

100. LLOYD, K. G., et al. "The Potential Use of
GABA Agonists in Psychiatric Disorders: Evidence from Studies with
Progabide in Animal Models and Clinical Trials," *Pharmacology, Biochemistry and Behavior*, 18 (1983):957–966.

101. LOPEZ-IBOR, J. J., GUTIERREZ, J.J.A., and
IGLESIAS, M.L.M.M. "5-Hydroxytrypto-
phan (5-HTP) and a MAOI (Nialamide)
in the Treatment of Depression. A Double-blind Controlled Study," *International Pharmacopsychiatry*, 11 (1976):8–
15.

102. MCNAMEE, H. B., LE POIDEVIN, D., and
NAYLOR, G. J. "Methylsergide in Mania:
A Double-blind Comparison with Thioridazine," *Psychological Medicine*, 2
(1972):66–69.

103. MENDELS, J., et al. "Amine Precursors and
Depression," *Archives of General Psychiatry*, 32 (1975):22–30.

104. MICCOLI, L., PORRO, V., and BERTOLINO,
A. "Comparison Between the Antidepressant Activity of S-adenosylmeth-
ionine (SAMe) and That of Some Tricyclic Drugs," *Acta Neurologica*, 33
(1978):243–255.

105. MOLLER, S. E., KIRK, L., and HONORE, P.
"Relationship Between Plasma Ratio of
Tryptophan to Competing Amino Acids
and the Response to L-tryptophan
Treatment in Endogenously Depressed
Patients," *Journal of Affective Disord-
ers*, 2 (1980):47–59.

106. MOSS, G. R., and JAMES, C. R. "Carbamazepine and Lithium Carbonate
Synergism in Mania," *Archives of General Psychiatry*, 40 (1983):588–589.

107. MURPHY, D. L., CAMPBELL, I., and
COSTA, J. L. "Current Status of the Indoleamine Hypothesis of the Affective
Disorders," in M. A. Lipton, A. Di
Mascio, and K. F. Killam, eds., *Psychopharmacology: A Generation in Progress.* New York: Raven Press, 1978, pp.
1235–1247.

108. MURPHY, D. L. et al. "L-dopa, Dopamine
and Hypomania," *American Journal of
Psychiatry*, 130 (1973):79–82.

109. MURPHY, D. L., et al. "L-tryptophan
in Affective Disorders: Indoleamine
Changes and Differential Clinical Effects," *Psychopharmacologia*, 34 (1974):-
11–20.

110. MURPHY, D. L., et al. "The Serotonergic
Neurotransmitter System in the Affective Disorders—a Preliminary Evaluation of the Antidepressant and Antimanic Effects of Fenfluramine," in P.
Deniker, C. Thomas-Raduoco, and A.
Villeneuve, eds., *Neuropsychopharmacology.* Oxford: Pergamon Press,
1978, pp. 675–683.

111. MUSCETTOLA, G., GALIZENATI, M., and
BALBI, A. "SAMe Versus Placebo: A
Double-blind Comparison in Major De-
pressive Disorders," in E. Costa and
Racagni, G. eds., *Typical and Atypical
Antidepressants: Clinical Practice.* New
York: Raven Press, 1982, pp. 151–156.

112. NABER, D., et al. "Endogenous Opioid
Activity and Beta-endorphin Immunoreactivity in CSF of Psychiatric

Patients and Normal Volunteers," *American Journal of Psychiatry*, 138 (1981):1457–1462.

113. NAYLOR, G. J., et al. "Trial of Digoxin in Mania," *Lancet*, 2 (1975):639–640.

114. NG, K. Y., et al. "L-dopa Induced Release of Cerebral Monoamines," *Science*, 170 (1970):76–77.

115. NOLEN, W. A. "Carbamazepine, a Possible Adjunct to or Alternative for Lithium in Bipolar Disorder," *Acta Psychiatrica Scandinavica*, 67 (1983):218–225.

116. OGURA, C., et al. "Combined Thyroid (Triiodothyronine)-tricyclic Antidepressant Treatment in Depressive States," *Folia Psychiatrica et Neurologica Japonica*, 28 (1974):179–186.

117. OKUMA, T., KISHIMOTO, A., and INOUE, K. "Anti-manic and Prophylactic Effects of Carbamazepine (Tegretol) on Manic-depressive Psychotic, [in Japanese] *Seishin Shinkeigaku Zasshi*, 17 (1975):617–630.

118. OKUMA, T., et al. "Anti-manic and Prophylactic Effects of Carbamazepine on Manic-depressive Psychosis," *Folia Psychatrica et Neurologica Japonica*, 27 (1973):283–297.

119. OKUMA, T., et al. "Comparison of the Antimanic Efficacy of Carbamazepine and Chlorpromazine: A Double-blind Controlled Study," *Psychopharmacology* (Berlin), 66 (1979):211–217.

120. OKUMA, T., et al. "A Preliminary Double-blind Study of the Efficacy of Carbamazepine in Prophylaxis of Manic-depressive Illness," *Psychopharmacology* (Berlin), 73 (1981):95.

121. PAPADIMITRIOU, G. V., et al. "Sleep Deprivation Psychoprophylaxis in Recurrent Affective Disorders," *Biblioteque Psychiatria*, 160 (1981):56–61.

122. PEARCE, J. B. "Fenfluramine in Mania," *Lancet*, 1 (1973):427.

123. PERSSON, T., and WALINDER, J. "L-dopa in the Treatment of Depressive Symptoms," *British Journal of Psychiatry*, 119 (1971):277–278.

124. PERT, C., and SNYDERS, S. "Opiate Receptor: Demonstration in Nervous Tissue," *Science*, 179 (1973):1011–1014.

125. PICKAR, D., et al. "Behavioral and Biological Effects of Acute Beta-endorphin Injection in Schizophrenic and Depressed Patients," *American Journal of Psychiatry*, 138 (1981):160–166.

126. PICKAR, D., et al. "Short-term Naloxone Administration in Schizophrenia and Manic Patients. A World Health Organization Collaborative Study," *Archives of General Psychiatry*, 39 (1982):313–319.

127. PLOTNIKOFF, N. P., MINARD, F. N., and KASTIN, A. J. "DOPA Potentiation in Ablated Animals and Brain Levels of Biogenic Amines in Intact Animals After Prolyl-leucyl-glycinamide," *Neuroendocrinology*, 14 (1974):271–279.

128. PLOTNIKOFF, N. P., et al. "DOPA Potentiation by a Hypothalamic Factor MSH-release Inhibiting Hormone (MIF)," *Life Sciences*, 10 (1971):1279–1283.

129. POST, R. M., and UHDE, T. W. "Carbamazepine as a Treatment for Depressive Illness: Lithium Non-responsive Rapid Cyclers," in J. Zohar and R. H. Belmaker, eds., *Special Treatments for Resistant Depression*. New York: Spectrum Press, forthcoming.

130. POST, R. M., PUTNAM, F. W., and CONTEL, N. R. "Electroconvulsive Shock Inhibits Amygdala Kindling," *Epilepsia*, 25 (1984):234–239.

131. POST, R. M., UHDE, T. W., and BALLENGER, J. C. "Efficacy of Carbamazepine in Affective Disorder: Implications for Underlying Biochemical and Physiological Substrates," in H. M. Emrich, T. Okuma, and A. A. Müller, eds., *Proceedings of the VII World Congress of Psychiatry*. Amsterdam: Elsevier Science Publishers, 1984, pp. 93–115.

132. POST, R. M., et al. "Effects of Low Doses of a Dopamine-receptor Stimulator in Mania," *Lancet*, 1 (1976):203–204.

133. POST, R. M., et al. "Effects of a Dopamine Agonist Piribedil in Depressed Patients," *Archives of General Psychiatry*, 35 (1978):609–615.

134. POST, R. M., et al. "Carbamazepine, Temporal Lobe Epilepsy, and Manic-depressive Illness," in M. Trimble and W. Koella, eds., *Temporal Lobe Epilepsy, Mania, Schizophrenia, and the Limbic System*. Basel: Karger 1982, pp. 117–156 (*Advances in Biological Psychiatry*, vol. 8).

135. POST, R. M., et al. "Carbamazepine and Its

-10,11-epoxide Metabolite in Plasma and CSF: Relationship to Antidepressant Response," *Archives of General Psychiatry*, 40 (1983):673–676.

136. POST, R. M., et al. "Prophylactic Efficacy of Carbamazepine in Manic-depressive Illness," *American Journal of Psychiatry*, 140 (1983):1602–1604.

137. POST, R. M., et al. "Cerebrospinal Fluid as Neuroregulatory Pathway. Peptides in Neuropsychiatric Illness," in J. H. Wood, ed., *Neurobiology of Cerebrospinal Fluid*, vol. 2. New York: Plenum Press, 1983, pp. 107–141.

138. POST, R. M., et al. "Efficacy of Carbamazepine in Manic Depressive Illness; Implications for Underlying Mechanisms," in R. M. Post and J. C. Ballenger, eds., *Neurobiology of Mood Disorders*. Baltimore: Williams & Wilkins, 1984, pp. 777–816.

139. PRANGE, A. J., JR., and WILSON, I. C. "Thyrotropin Releasing Hormone (TRH) for the Immediate Relief of Depression," *Psychopharmacologia*, 21 (1972):82.

140. PRANGE, A. J., JR., et al. "Enhancement of Imipramine Antidepressant Activity by Thyroid Hormone," *American Journal of Psychiatry*, 126 (1969):457–469.

141. PRANGE, A. J., JR., et al. "Effects of Thyrotropin Releasing Hormone in Depression," *Lancet*, 2 (1972):999–1002.

142. PRANGE, A. J., JR., et al. "L-tryptophan in Mania. Contribution to a Permissive Hypothesis of Affective Disorders. *Archives of General Psychiatry*, 30 (1974):56–62.

143. PRANGE, A. J., JR., et al. "Hormonal Alteration of Imipramine Response: A Review," in E. J. Sachar, ed., *Hormones, Behavior and Psychopathology*. New York: Raven Press, 1976, pp. 41–67.

144. ROY-BYRNE, P. P., UHDE, T. W., and POST, R. M. "Antidepressant Effects of One Night's Sleep Deprivation: Clinical and Theoretical Implications," in R. M. Post and J. C. Ballenger, eds., *Neurobiology of the Mood Disorders*. Baltimore: Williams & Wilkins, 1984, pp. 817–835.

145. RUBINOW, D. R., et al. "CSF Somatostatin in Affective Illness," *Archives of General Psychiatry*, 40 (1983):409–412.

146. SACK, R. L., and GOODWIN, F. K. "Inhibition of Dopamine-beta-hydroxylase in Manic Patients. A Clinical Trial of Fusaric Acid," *Archives of General Psychiatry*, 31 (1974):649–654.

147. SAFER, D. J., and ALLEN, R. P. "The Central Effects of Scopolamine in Man," *Biological Psychiatry*, 3 (1971):347–351.

148. SCHILDKRAUT, J. J. "Catecholamine Hypothesis of Affective Disorders: Review of Supporting Evidence," *American Journal of Psychiatry*, 122 (1965):509–522.

149. SHOPSIN, B., and GERSHON, S. "Dopamine Receptor Stimulation in the Treatment of Depression: Piribedil (ET-495)," *Neuropsychobiology*, 4 (1978):1–14.

150. SHOPSIN, B., FRIEDMAN, E., and GERSHON, S. "Parachlorophenylalanine Reversal of Tranylcypromine Effects in Depressed Patients," *Archives of General Psychiatry*, 33 (1976):811–819.

151. SHOPSIN, B., et al. "Use of Synthesis Inhibitors in Defining a Role for Biogenic Amines During Imipramine Treatment in Depressed Patients," *Psychopharmacology Communications*, 1 (1975):239–249.

152. SIMON, P., et al. "Experimental and Clinical Evidence of the Antidepressant Effect of a Beta-adrenergic Stimulant," *Psychological Medicine*, 8 (1978):335–338.

153. SMITH, A.H.W., CHAMBERS, C., and NAYLOR, G. J. "Bromocriptine in Mania—a Placebo-controlled Double-blind Trial," *British Medical Journal*, 1 (1980):86.

154. SOURKES, T. L., MURPHY, G. F., and CHAVEZ, B. "The Action of Some Alpha-methyl and Other Amino Acids on Cerebral Catecholamines," *Journal of Neurochemistry*, 8 (1961):109–115.

155. TAKAHASHI, S., et al. "Antidepressant Effects of Thyrotropin-releasing Hormone (TRH) and the Plasma Thyrotropin Levels in Depression," *Folia Psychiatrica et Neurologica Japonica*, 27 (1973):305–314.

156. TAKAHASHI, S., et al. "Measurement of 5-Hydroxyindole Compounds During 5-HTP Treatment in Depressed Patients," *Folia Psychiatrica et Neurologica Japonica*, 30 (1976):463–469.

157. TAKEZAKI, H., and HANAOKA, M. "The Use of Carbamazepine (Tegretol) in the Control of Manic-depressive Psychosis and Other Manic, Depressive States," *Clinical Psychiatry*, 13 (1971):173–183.

158. TOLLEFSON, G. D. "Hyperadrenergic Hypomania Consequent to the Abrupt Cessation of Clonidine," *Journal of Clinical Psychopharmacology*, 1 (1981):-93–95.

159. TSUTSUI, S., NAMBA, T., and TSUSHIMA, M. "Combined Therapy of T_3 and Antidepressants in Depression," *Journal of Internal Medicine Research*, 7 (1979):-138–146.

160. UHDE, T. W., et al. "Clonidine: Effect on Mood, Anxiety and Pain," *Psychopharmacology Bulletin*, 17 (1981):125–126.

161. VAN BEMMEL, A. L., and VAN DEN HOOF-DAKKER, R. H. "Maintenance of Therapeutic Effects of Total Sleep Deprivation by Limitation of Subsequent Sleep," *Acta Psychiatrica Scandinavica*, 63 (1981):453–462.

162. VAN DEN BURG, W., et al. "Thyrotropin Releasing Hormone (TRH) as a Possible Quick-acting but Short-lasting Antidepressant," *Psychological Medicine*, 5 (1975):404–412.

163. VAN DEN BURG, W., et al. "TRH by Slow Continuous Infusions: An Antidepressant?" *Psychological Medicine*, 6 (1976):393–397.

164. VAN DER VELDE, C. D. "Rapid Clinical Effectiveness of MIF-1 in the Treatment of Major Depressive Illness," *Peptides*, 4 (1983):297–300.

165. VAN HIELE, L. J. "L-5-hydroxytryptophan in Depression: The First Substitution Therapy in Psychiatry," *Neuropsychobiology*, 6 (1980):230–240.

166. VAN LOON, G. R., and KIM., C. "Beta Endorphin Induced Increases in Striated Dopamine Turnover," *Life Sciences*, 23 (1978):961–970.

167. VAN PRAAG, H. M. "Management of Depression with Serotonin Precursors," *Biological Psychiatry*, 16 (1981):291–310.

168. VAN PRAAG, H., and DE HAAN, S. "Depression Vulnerability and 5-Hydroxytryptophan Prophylaxis," *Psychiatry Research*, 3 (1980):75–83.

169. VAN PRAAG, H. M., and KORF, J. "Central Monoamine Deficiency in Depression: Causative or Secondary Phenomenon," *Pharmacopsychiatria*, 8 (1975):322–326.

170. VEREBEY, K., VOLAVKA, J., and CLOUET, D. "Endorphin in Psychiatry. An Overview and a Hypothesis," *Archives of General Psychiatry*, 35 (1978):877–888.

171. VESTER, J. P. "Preliminary Report on the Treatment of Mentally Disordered Patients," *South African Medical Journal*, 37 (1963):1086–1089.

172. VOGEL, G. W., et al. "Improvement of Depression by REM Sleep Deprivation. New Findings and a Theory," *Archives of General Psychiatry*, 37 (1980):247–253.

173. WALINDER, J., et al. "Potentiation of the Antidepressant Action of Clomipramine by Tryptophan," *Archives of General Psychiatry*, 33 (1976):1384–1389.

174. WEHR, T. A., and WIRZ-JUSTICE, A. "Circadian Rhythm Mechanisms in Affective Illness and in Antidepressant Drug Action," *Pharmacopsychiatria*, 15 (1982):31–39.

175. WEHR, T. A., et al. "Phase Advance of the Circadian Sleep-wake Cycle as an Antidepressant," *Science*, 206 (1979):710–713.

176. WHEATLEY, D. "Potentiation of Amitriptyline by Thyroid Hormone," *Archives of General Psychiatry*, 26 (1972):229–232.

177. WIRZ-JUSTICE, A., PURINGER, W., and HOLE, G. "Sleep Deprivation and Clomipramine in Endogenous Depression," *Lancet*, 2 (1976):912.

178. YASSA, R. "Carbamazepine: An Alternative to Lithium Therapy?" *Psychiatric Journal of the University of Ottawa*, 7 (1982):252–253.

179. ZERSSEN, D. V. "Beta-adrenergic Blocking Agents in the Treatment of Psychoses. A Report of 17 Cases," in C. Carlsson, ed., *Neuro-Psychiatric Effects of Adrenergic Beta Receptor Blocking Agents*. Munich: Urban Schwavzenberg, 1976, pp. 105–114.

180. ZIS, A. P., and GOODWIN, F. K. "The amine hypothesis," in E. S. Paykel, ed., *Handbook of Affective Disorders*. New York: Guilford Press, 1982, pp. 175–190.

CHAPTER 16

THE ROLE OF BIOLOGICAL RHYTHMS IN THE BIOLOGY AND TREATMENT OF INSOMNIA AND DEPRESSION

Thomas A. Wehr, David A. Sack,

Barbara L. Parry, and Norman E. Rosenthal

¶ Introduction

Rhythmic changes in behavior and physiology are ubiquitous in nature. The periods of such rhythms range from milliseconds (as on electroencephalograms) to years (as in predator-prey cycles). Of special interest are daily and seasonal biological rhythms, which are adaptations to cyclic changes in the external environment. Biological rhythms play prominent roles in certain psychiatric conditions, notably delayed sleep phase syndrome (a type of sleep disorder) and affective illness. These two disorders and their relationship to biological rhythms are the focus of this chapter.

¶ Delayed Sleep Phase Syndrome

Some people are unable to sleep during normal hours at night. If they retire at 11 or 12 P.M., they lie awake for hours in the dark. Finally at 2, 3, or 4 A.M., they fall asleep. From this point on, sleep proceeds normally and if conditions permit, they are able to obtain eight hours of uninterrupted sleep, arising at 10, 11, or 12 A.M. Thus the timing, not the quality, of sleep is abnormal. The clinical picture of this delayed sleep phase syndrome (DSPS)[10] is often complicated by chronic sleep deprivation, since ordinary work and social schedules interfere with the last hours of sleep. Patients therefore complain of daytime drowsiness and often sleep very late on weekends to compensate for lost sleep. The clinical picture is also often complicated by effects of chronic sedative use, such as drug dependence and tolerance, rebound insomnia, and impaired daytime functioning.

DSPS usually begins early in life, during childhood or adolescence. To diagnose DSPS, it is sometimes useful to obtain a sleep history from the period antedating the use of sedative-hypnotic drugs. It appears that DSPS is associated with a delay-shift of most physiological daily rhythms. The low ebb of daily rhythms in performance and alertness is shifted from its normal time of occurrence in the latter part of the night into the first part of the day, resulting in poor work and school functioning in the morning—a problem that is further exacerbated by the effects of chronic sleep deprivation. Often in the evaluation of such patients, it is useful to obtain a sleep log for two to three weeks. Characteristically, sleep onsets occur at 1 A.M. or later. Wake-up time is determined by work routines Monday through Friday and is quite late (e.g., 2 P.M.) on weekends (see figure 16–3). Lying in bed in the dark and being unable to fall asleep for several hours each night sometimes leads to psychological complications. This situation is somewhat comparable to sensory deprivation, and patients may be flooded by anxiety-producing internal stimuli. In fact, patients and their doctors may conclude that these stimuli cause the initial insomnia rather than vice versa.

Causes and Treatments of DSPS

In order to consider the possible causes of DSPS, it is necessary to review the basic physiology of the sleep-wake cycle. The timing of the sleep-wake cycle appears to be regulated by a pacemaker mechanism in the central nervous system. The existence of such a pacemaker has been inferred from the fact that near twenty-four-hour cycles of sleeping and waking persist when experimental subjects live in constant conditions without external time cues (zeitgebers).[70] In these circumstances, the period of sleep-wake cycles and other daily rhythms is slightly longer than twenty-four hours (e.g., twenty-five hours) (see figure 16–1). This deviation from a precise twenty-four-hour period confirms that the sleep-wake cycle is endogenous and not passively driven by an occult twenty-four-hour time cue (zeitgeber) in the experimental conditions. Since the intrinsic rhythm of the human circadian pacemaker is somewhat slower than one cycle per day,

most of us tend to shift our sleep periods later when we have the opportunity to do so (e.g., weekends and vacations) and have difficulty shifting it earlier (e.g., on Monday mornings). For the same reason, westward travel, which involves shifting sleep later, is more easily adjusted to than eastward travel. Advancing the time of sleep (shortening the sleep-wake cycle) goes against the tendency of the pacemaker to express its longer-than-twenty-four-hour period.

Obviously there must be a mechanism whereby the intrinsic period of the circadian pacemaker can be shortened to conform to the twenty-four-hour day-night cycle, otherwise our sleep period would drift gradually around the clock, making a full circuit in three to four weeks. The process of entrainment of the sleep-wake cycle to the day-night cycle is accomplished by daily phase shifts in its oscillations, which are induced by certain periodic stimuli in the environment that serve as time cues (zeitgebers). One important stimulus is light or light-dark transitions (e.g., dawn and dusk). Other stimuli such as alarm clocks, work schedules, or social activities may also be important in humans. The magnitude and direction of phase shifts induced by zeitgebers depends on the phase of the circadian cycle at which they are presented. Usually light pulses presented during subjective morning advance the pacemaker, during subjective evening delay it, and during subjective daytime have no effect at all. If the human pacemaker were controlled solely by light, then it is likely that morning light would play a critical role, since it is necessary to advance the twenty-five-hour pacemaker approximately one hour each day to maintain entrainment to the twenty-four-hour day-night cycle.

In experimental animals, neural substrates of the circadian system have been identified. The suprachiasmatic nuclei (SCN) of the hypothalamus appear to function as a master circadian pacemaker.[35] Zeitgeber effects of light and darkness are mediated by at least two pathways: the retinohypothalamic tract, going directly from the retina through the chiasm to the SCN, and a second connection

CIRCADIAN RHYTHMS:
I. ENDOGENOUS PACEMAKER
II. ENTRAINED TO DAY-NIGHT CYCLE

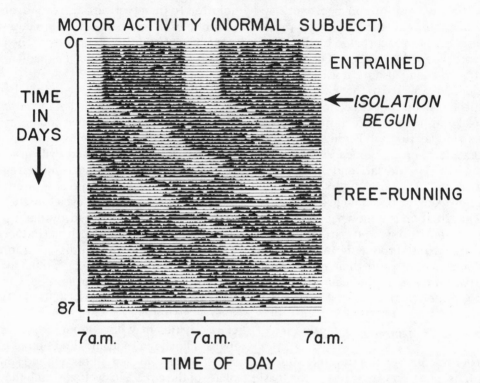

MOTOR ACTIVITY (NORMAL SUBJECT)

Figure 16–1. Human circadian rhythms persist with a near twenty-five-hour period in isolation from external time cues. Wrist activity was monitored using fifteen minute sampling intervals for several weeks in a normal subject entrained to a twenty-four-hour schedule (upper section of graph) and living in constant conditions (lower section of graph). Twenty-four-hour segments of data are plotted consecutively beneath one another. The data are double-plotted to the right to facilitate visual inspection of the courses of the activity-rest cycle. After temporal isolation, the longer-than-twenty-four-hour periodicity is responsible for the rightward drift of the activity-rest cycle pattern. SOURCE: Data obtained in collaboration with Elliott D. Weitzman, Janet Zimmerman, and Charles A. Czeisler.

from the retina to the intergeniculate leaflet of the lateral geniculate nucleus (LGN) and then via a second neuron to the SCN.[34] The neurochemical mediators of this circuitry have not been completely worked out. However, some effects of light on the SCN may be mediated by the neurotransmitter acetylcholine acting on a nicotinic receptor.[73] Some effects of darkness, possibly acting through the LGN, appear to be mediated by

the neurotransmitter neuropeptide Y (NPY) or a similar peptide, avian pancreatic peptide (APP), or both.[2] Administration of these substances to the SCN through cannulae can mimic the effects of light and darkness, respectively.

Compared with animals, the threshold for hypothalamic effects of light in humans appears to be rather high. Artificial light of ordinary intensity (100–500 lux) has little effect

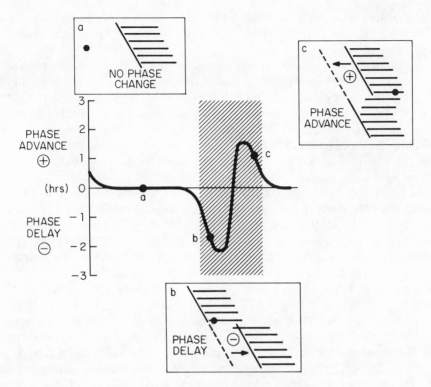

Figure 16–2.   Derivation of a phase-response curve (PRC). Light pulses induce phase shifts in free-running circadian rhythms. The magnitude and direction of shifts (advance or delays) depend on the circadian phase at which the pulse is administered. Animal activity data are plotted in a format similar to figure 16–1.

NOTE: Reprinted, by permission of the publisher, from M. C. Moore-Ede, C. A. Czeisler, and E. S. Richardson, "Circadian Timekeeping in Health and Disease: Part 1. Basic Properties of Circadian Pacemakers," *New England Journal of Medicine* 309(1983):474.

on the pacemaker. However, very bright light (3,000–4,000 lux, equivalent to sunlight observed through a window on a clear day) has powerful phase-shifting properties.[71] Because of this high threshold, artificial light that we use after sunset probably does little to "confuse" our biological clock.

In terms of phase-resetting effects of zeit-gebers, such as light, two opposite causes of DSPS are possible. Patients could be abnormally *insensitive* to light. In this case, the advancing effect of morning light would be abnormally weak, and the sleep-wake cycle would be insufficiently advanced each day. On the other hand, patients could be abnormally *sensitive* to light, so that artificial light used after sunset would exert a delaying effect each day. In the latter case, DSPS would be an artifact of civilization.

These two possibilities could be tested experimentally by devising a phase-response curve (PRC) for such patients. A PRC is simply a graph of the magnitude and direction of phase shifts of a circadian pacemaker free-running in constant conditions induced by a zeitgeber as a function of the circadian phase at which it is presented (see figure 16–2). If DSPS were shown to be caused by abnormal sensitivity or insensitivity to phase-shifting effects of light, it might be treated with pharmacological agents that mimic or antagonize these effects. In this type of treatment, the timing of drug administration could be critical, since it would determine the magnitude and direction of the phase response. Two relevant examples can be cited from animal pharmacology. The cholinergic agonist carbachol mimics phase-resetting effects of light pulses.[73] A drug of this type (e.g., nicotine) could be administered in the morning to advance patients' abnormally delayed sleep-wake cycle. Bicuculline, a gamma-aminobutyric acid (GABA) receptor antagonist, selectively blocks phase-delaying effects of light.[44] An analogous pharmacological intervention could be used to attenuate phase-delaying effects of evening light if DSPS is shown to arise from abnormal sensitivity to artificial light after sunset.

Theoretically, DSPS could be treated with manipulations of the light-dark cycle. Exposure to bright light early in the day and shielding from light late in the day should facilitate patients' attempts to advance their sleep period to a normal time. In an uncontrolled pilot study, we have had some success with this routine.

Another possible cause of DSPS is an abnormally slow circadian pacemaker. The phase position of a circadian rhythm (e.g., the sleep-wake cycle) relative to the entraining cycle (e.g., the day-night cycle) is partly determined by the intrinsic frequency of the rhythm. Slower pacemakers adopt later (more delayed) phase positions than faster ones. The period of the intrinsic rhythm of the circadian pacemaker in DSPS patients could be measured by placing them in conditions from which all twenty-four-hour zeitgebers had been removed. In this situation, the period of the sleep-wake cycle would be entirely governed by the rhythm of the free-running circadian pacemaker. Normally the period is close to twenty-five hours; in DSPS it might be longer. An abnormally slow rhythm could, in turn, result from chemical or metabolic changes, since certain hormones (estrogen, thyroid) have been shown to alter the intrinsic period of the circadian pacemaker in experimental animals.[3,37] Whether the intrinsic period in patients with DSPS is shortened or not, it might still be possible to treat the condition with agents that shorten the intrinsic period.

At present, the only documented form of treatment for DSPS is the "chronotherapy" developed by Czeisler and associates.[10] In this procedure, patients are asked to delay their sleep period by two to three hours per day until their sleep period is rotated to the desired bedtime (see figure 16–3). This approach is quite feasible since patients have little difficulty going to sleep *later* than usual.

Chronotherapy takes about ten days and, at certain stages, is disruptive to work and family life. In our experience, about fifty percent of patients respond favorably, as long as they adhere fairly rigidly to their new schedule. Sometimes patients discover that they have built an identity and a way of life around their abnormal sleep schedule and are unable to relinquish it. These patients eventually find that "circumstances" conspire to prevent them from adhering to their new sleep schedule.

An advanced sleep phase syndrome (ASPS) has not been systematically described, perhaps because the natural tendency of the twenty-five-hour human circadian pacemaker is to drift later each day. If such a syndrome exists, it could be treated with appropriate modifications of the approaches described for DSPS.

¶ Affective Disorders

Biological rhythms play an important role in affective illness. Because of its recurrent course with spontaneous relapses and remissions, which frequently occur at regular intervals, the illness appears to be inherently cyclic. In certain cases, the pattern of recurrences is periodic, resembling a true biological rhythm. Such cases led Falret, the co-discoverer of manic-depressive illness, to term it *la folie circulaire.*[15]

Periodic, circular forms of affective illness include seasonal, menstrual, and so-called rapid-cycling cases. In addition, many patients show daily cycles of intensification of symptoms during depressive episodes (diurnal variation in mood). In these examples, except for rapid cycling, affective episodes seem to be linked in some way to normal seasonal, menstrual, and daily biological rhythms. Recent research indicates that biological rhythms with periods similar to those

INSOMNIA AS A CIRCADIAN RHYTHM PHASE DISORDER: NON-PHARMACOLOGICAL TREATMENT

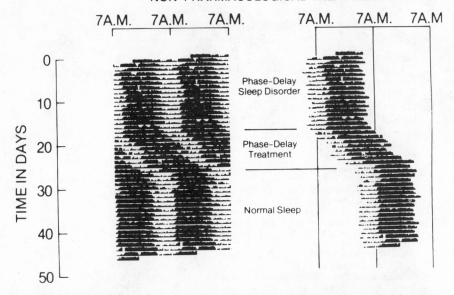

Figure 16–3. Chronotherapy of delayed sleep phase syndrome (DSPS). Motor activity data plotted as in figure 16–1. Sleep periods occur abnormally late in the night and early morning in this forty-six-year-old woman. Although she was unable to go to sleep earlier than usual, she was able to go to sleep progressively later and ultimately reached and maintained a normal bedtime.

of rapid-cycling cases may also occur in healthy persons.[13]

Thus it appears that certain phase intervals of normal biological rhythms influence the timing of affective episodes. A search for common features of winter, the late luteal phase, and the morning, all of which are associated with intensification of depressive symptoms, may help to identify biological factors that predispose to depression. For example, cortisol secretion, a focus of psychobiological investigations of depression, is maximal in winter[68] and in the morning hours. The cyclical forms of affective illness and their biological correlates are discussed individually below.

Seasonal Affective Disorder

Patients with seasonal affective disorder (SAD) experience depression in the fall and winter and become euthymic, hypomanic, or manic in the spring and summer.[45] Depressive episodes typically begin in November and end in March (see figure 16–4). They are characterized by many of the usual symptoms of depression, as well as by hypersomnia, anergia-fatigue, carbohydrate craving, and weight gain—symptoms characteristic of so-called atypical depression.[31] These symptoms are often worst in the midafternoon. Although an atypical depressive syndrome is most usual, SAD patients may present with more typical vegetative symptoms, insomnia, anorexia, and weight loss. SAD most commonly affects women and begins in the third decade. Patients frequently also suffer from premenstrual syndrome. However, men may be affected, and the condition also appears to affect children and adolescents. In these latter cases, the most common presenting symptoms are irritability, school difficulties, fatigue, and sadness in the winter months. Children are generally unaware that their problems originate from within and experience them instead as an unfair increase

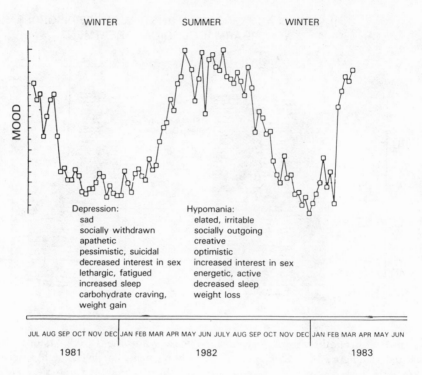

Figure 16–4. Symptoms and weekly averages of daily mood ratings in a patient with seasonal affective disorder (SAD).

in environmental demands. It is important to consider SAD in the differential diagnosis of school difficulties in the fall and winter months, especially since it is a reversible condition.

We have encountered other patterns of affective episodes occurring regularly in relation to the seasons—for example, spring depressions, spring-summer manias, spring and fall depressions, and even summer depressions. These patterns are less common than the SAD syndrome just outlined and have not been well characterized thus far.

Sleep changes reported in SAD have been confirmed by sleep electroencephalogram recordings.[45] In winter, patients sleep more but have reduced slow-wave sleep. The latter finding may correspond to their subjective assessment that winter sleep, though longer, is not refreshing. Rapid-eye-movement (REM) sleep abnormalities reported in other types of depression do not occur in SAD. So far, no other clear-cut biological correlates of the syndrome have been estab-

lished. Responses to dexamethasone administration or thyroid-releasing hormone infusion are generally normal.

The seasonal pattern of recurrences in SAD suggested to us that an environmental factor might play a role in the cause of the episodes. To examine this possibility, we turned to animal models. Seasonal rhythms in behavior and physiology are common in biology. Examples include hibernation, migration, reproduction, and coat-color changes. Many of these changes are triggered by seasonal changes in day length and are mediated by the pattern of secretion of the pineal hormone, melatonin.[5] The rhythmic secretion of melatonin at night is generated by the SCN and persists even if animals are isolated from time cues. However, light has a powerful influence on the secretion of melatonin and acts on the pineal via connections from the retina to the SCN of the hypothalamus, and then through sympathetic outflow to the pineal. Through this system, the changing duration of night is transduced into changing durations of melatonin secretion (melatonin secretion is inhibited during the daytime).

Thus melatonin in the internal environment is a chemical signal corresponding to darkness in the external environment. In certain animals, seasonal changes in behavior can be experimentally controlled by manipulating the duration of melatonin secretion. In these "photoperiodic" seasonal rhythms, the timing of light is a critical factor. If light is perceived sufficiently late in the evening and sufficiently early in the morning, a summer response occurs. Even brief flashes of light at the extremes of the day are sufficient to elicit a summer-type response (light in the middle of the day is unnecessary).[20,21] The SCN-circadian clock mechanism plays an important role in the detection of the time of occurrence of light. Lesioning of the SCN or the pineal abolishes many seasonal rhythms in animals.[20,21]

On the basis of animal models, we hypothesized that seasonal changes in day length triggered clinical changes in patients with SAD and that their winter depressions could be treated by extending the short winter day with bright artificial light in the morning and evening. Since we had previously shown that human nocturnal melatonin secretion could be suppressed with very bright artificial light, but not with light of ordinary intensity,[30] we further hypothesized that only very bright artificial light would be effective in treating SAD. The pineal's insensitivity to ordinary visible light suggested to us that this type of light might provide a suitable sham control treatment.

In a series of studies with a balanced randomization crossover design involving nearly fifty patients, five to six hours per day of phototherapy with bright artificial light proved to be an effective antidepressant in the majority of cases.[46,47] During the treatment procedure, patients sat one meter from a light source consisting of eight 40-watt, full-spectrum fluorescent bulbs behind a diffusing screen. Patients were instructed to glance at the lights every minute or so. The response was rapid; patients typically experienced complete remissions in three to four days. Relapses after withdrawal of treatment had similar latencies (see figure 16–5). With subsequent use, they did not seem to become tolerant to the treatment. Following their initial treatment, many patients have successfully used phototherapy as prophylaxis in the fall and winter. Recently other groups have found phototherapy to be effective in similar patients.*

We have carried out three experiments designed to test the hypothesis that the mechanism of action of phototherapy in SAD involves suppression of nocturnal pineal melatonin secretion. In the first experiment, we hypothesized that administration of melatonin during light treatments to patients who had responded to phototherapy would reverse the therapeutic effect of light and reproduce their depressive symptoms.

Patients took capsules of melatonin every hour while they were exposed to phototherapy. Subsequent analysis of half-hourly serum samples obtained during the treatment showed that supraphysiological serum levels of melatonin were achieved by this method of administration. The results of the experiment were equivocal.[48] Hamilton depression ratings, which had always been a sensitive indicator of responses to phototherapy, were unaffected by melatonin administration. On the other hand, supplemental rating items designed to measure characteristic atypical features of SAD, such as carbohydrate craving and hypersomnia—items not represented in the Hamilton ratings—suggested that melatonin might have partially antagonized the effects of phototherapy, as predicted by the hypothesis.

Pineal secretion of melatonin normally occurs in response to noradrenergic sympathetic stimulation of the gland. Therefore, melatonin secretion can be inhibited by beta-adrenergic antagonist drugs, such as atenolol. In this respect, atenolol mimics the suppressing effect of light on pineal melatonin secretion. Therefore, if phototherapy in

---

*A. J. Lewy, A. Wirz-Justice, and C. Hellekson each have unpublished data in support of phototherapy.

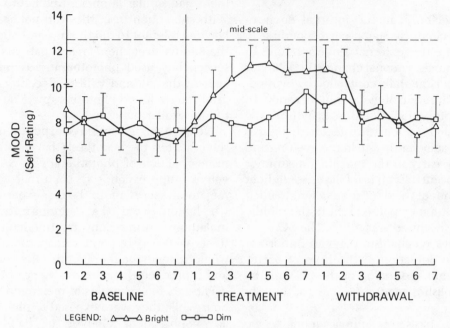

Figure 16–5. Modified 100-mm line self-ratings (mean ± standard error of mean) of mood for patients during baseline, dim- and bright-light treatment, and withdrawal from light treatment are shown for fifteen patients. Analysis of variance shows a significant mood effect of bright-light treatment ($p < 0.05$) and withdrawal from bright light ($p < 0.05$). Multiple t-tests reveal that days 1 and 2 of treatment differ significantly from days 3 through 7 (Duncan's multiple range t-test). Similarly, days 1 and 2 of withdrawal differ from days 3 through 7. The time course of the effects of treatment and withdrawal as seen in the figure agree with clinical observations that these effects generally take approximately three days to be clearly evident. There is no significant effect of dim light (treatment or withdrawal) on mood.

NOTE: Reprinted, by permission of the publisher, from N. E. Rosenthal et al., "Seasonal Affective Disorder and Phototherapy," *Annals of the New York Academy of Science*, 453 (1985):265.

SAD acts by suppressing melatonin secretion, it should be possible to mimic its beneficial effects with appropriately timed administration of atenolol. Cowen and coworkers showed that 100 mg atenolol administered orally in the late afternoon profoundly suppresses melatonin secretion during the subsequent night.[9] SAD patients were treated with atenolol or placebo in a double-blind, balanced-randomization crossover trial. Again, the results were equivocal.* Although there was no difference in efficacy between atenolol and placebo, some in-

*N. E. Rosenthal et al., unpublished data.

dividuals seemed to benefit greatly from atenolol, and this beneficial effect persisted throughout the winter months.

In a third experiment, SAD patients were exposed to light treatments at two very different times of day in a random-order, crossover trial. In one condition, they were exposed to a long (summer) skeleton photoperiod (7–10 A.M. and 8–11 P.M.); in another, to a short (winter) skeleton photoperiod (9–noon and 2–5 P.M.). The latter schedule had little effect on the secretion of the major urinary melatonin metabolite, 6-hydroxy-melatonin sulphate, which occurs mainly at night. If phototherapy acts through a photoperiodic mechanism and is mediated by changes in duration of melatonin secretion, the first schedule should be effective, the second one ineffective. Contrary to this prediction, patients responded equally well to both treatment schedules.[66]

While explanations can be advanced for why each of the three experiments just discussed failed to show a central role for melatonin in the symptomatology of SAD and for melatonin suppression as the mechanism of action of light therapy, the most parsimonious interpretation is that the case for the importance of melatonin in these processes is weak. Other possible mechanisms of action and different animal models must now be investigated. Ironically, on the basis of an animal model that, as it turns out, may not be entirely relevant, a powerful new treatment for depression, phototherapy, has been discovered and is already being used clinically.

Rapid-cycling Affective Disorder

Patients with regular alteration of depressive and euthymic or manic states occurring several times per year have been called "rapid cyclers." Most of these patients are bipolar, and most are women.* Typically, switches between depression and mania, or vice versa, are abrupt. Phenotypically, manias and depressions present essentially the same clinical picture as that seen in nonrapid-cycling forms of bipolar illness.

It was the rapid alternations between mania and depression in such cases that led to the nineteenth-century observation that mania and depression were separate manifestations of the same illness. Because of the rapidity and predictability of clinical changes in such patients, they have been the focus of intensive, prospective longitudinal investigations of manic-depressive illness over the years (see figure 16–6). For example, over fifty years ago Gjessing in Norway conducted a series of unprecedented investigations of metabolism and endocrine function in such patients.[17] Today few people realize that

*See references 8, 11, 12, 29, and 60.

Gjessing hypothesized on the basis of careful physical and biochemical observations that a shifting balance between noradrenergic and cholinergic systems was responsible for shifts between depression and mania in such patients. Research in recent decades has shown that many of the biological correlates of mania and depression in these cases are similar to those reported in nonrapid-cycling forms. Such patients fail to suppress cortisol secretion with dexamethasone[19] and exhibit short REM sleep latencies[43,62] during depressive phases.

CAUSES AND TREATMENTS OF RAPID-CYCLING AFFECTIVE ILLNESS

In contrast to daily, menstrual, and seasonal forms of affective illness, rapid-cycling forms have not been linked to any well-established physiological or environmental rhythm. The duration of rapid cycles ranges from a few days to many weeks. Careful analysis has revealed remarkably regular, albeit complex, patterns of recurrence of phases of the illness. For example, in one case we found that the occurrence of depressive episodes was governed by the precise interaction of two independent rhythms, a 43-day and a 35.5-day cycle, over a four-year period of observation[62] (see figure 16–7). It is possible that such cycles, like daily, menstrual, and seasonal ones, exist in the physiology and behavior of normal individuals.[13] In this case, rapid-cycling affective illness might be another instance of clinical state changes being driven by normal biological rhythms.

Altered thyroid axis functioning may play a role in the genesis of rapid mood cycles. Such patients have an increased incidence of thyroid disease and are unusually sensitive to thyroid axis perturbations induced by lithium carbonate.[6,8] Recent evidence from our laboratory suggests that basal secretion of thyroid-stimulating hormone (TSH), especially at night, is abnormally low in these patients. This defect is partially corrected by sleep deprivation, an intervention that also normalizes mood.[27,50] The increased incidence of rapid cycling in women may be

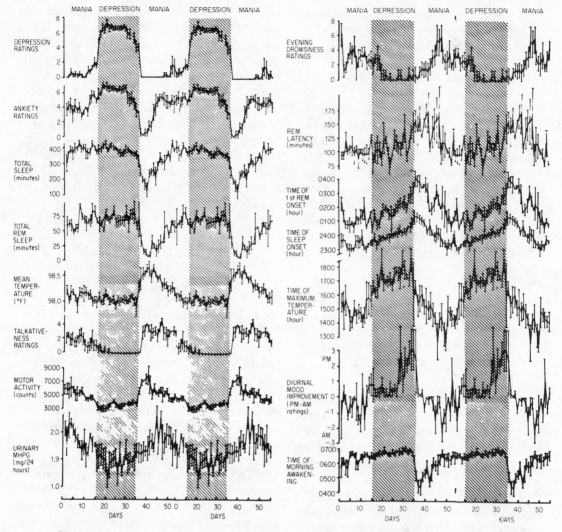

Figure 16–6. Mood cycle of forty-nine-year-old woman. Each variable was monitored longitudinally through four cycles. To construct an average cycle profile, all cycles were assumed to be replications of the same process; four depressive episodes of similar duration (20 $\pm$ 1 days) were used as a time reference to calculate daily means and standard errors for each variable. In contrast to longitudinal smoothing procedures, such as moving averages, this serial cross-sectional smoothing strategy removed random variation without blunting day-to-day changes. REM-rapid eye movement; MHPG-3methoxy-4-hydroxy-phenylglycol. The data have been plotted twice to facilitate inspection of the waveforms.

SOURCE: T. A. Wehr, "Phase and Biorhythm Studies of Affective Illness," *Annals of Internal Medicine*, 87 (1977):319–335.

partly related to the higher incidence of thyroid disease in women. Suppressive or hypermetabolic doses of thyroid hormone have been used successfully to treat refractory cases.[17,54]

In a significant percentage of cases, tricyclic or other antidepressants appear to be responsible for the induction of rapid cycles.[29,59,60] In these cases rapid cycling occurs when the drugs are maintained at a constant dose and therefore does not result from periodic administration of the drugs or

Frequency (Fourier) analysis of daily self-ratings of mood

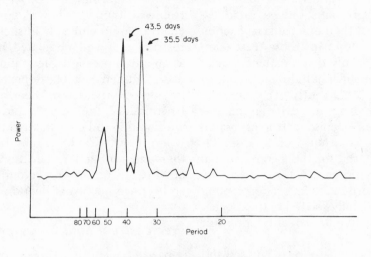

MANIC-DEPRESSIVE CYCLES

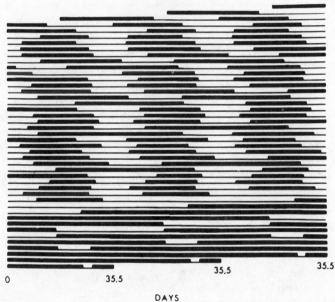

DAYS

Figure 16–7. Patterns of manic-depressive cycles in a forty-nine-year-old woman. Daily mood states (bars-mania, open spaces-depression) are shown in 35.5 day segments plotted consecutively beneath one another. Vertical alignment of phases indicates that manic-depressive cycle usually exhibits a 35.5-day period; every four to five cycles, however, the manic-depressive cycle lengthens dramatically for one cycle. Because of the repeated lengthening of its period, the average period of the cycle is approximately 43 days. The recurring tendency of the 43-day manic-depressive cycle to adhere to a 35.5-day period may indicate that it is coupled to an unidentified 35.5-day rhythm. According to this model, the oscillations of the manic-depressive cycle keep step with those of the faster 35.5-day rhythm except when every few cycles its slower intrinsic rhythm causes it to escape transiently from a one-to-one to a one-to-two mode of coupling to the 35.5-day rhythm. Spectral analysis (top) confirmed the presence of two rhythmic components in the data.

SOURCE: T. A. Wehr and F. K. Goodwin, "Biological Rhythms and Manic-depressive Illness," in T. A. Wehr and F. K. Goodwin, eds., *Biological Rhythms and Psychiatry,* Pacific Grove, Calif.: Boxwood Press, pp. 1983, 129–184.

the periodic increments of dose following repeated development of drug tolerance. The fact that antidepressants induce rapid cycling requires that their mechanism of action be reconceptualized. In these cases antidepressants not only drive patients out of depression into mania, but also out of mania into depression, recurrently. The time required for the drugs to drive a patient through a depressive episode, from its beginning to its end—two to four weeks—is similar to the time required for their conventional antidepressant response. Therefore, the mechanism of drug-induced rapid cycling may be fundamentally related to the mechanism of their conventional antidepressant effect.

Drug-induced cycles can be diagnosed and sometimes treated by withholding antidepressant medications for one or more cycles. Several outcomes are possible. Sometimes patients continue to cycle, but much more slowly. Sometimes they stop cycling and return to a euthymic state, or they may lapse into a protracted depression. In the first and third cases, treatment with lithium alone may be effective. Where the outcome is protracted depression, low-dose monoamine oxidase inhibitor (MAOI) treatment may be effective. Non-drug-induced rapid cyclers may respond to lithium alone, carbamazepine (Tegretol), low-dose MAOI, or thyroid hormone (see chapters 13 and 15).

Changes in the timing and duration of sleep are characteristic of bipolar illness and are particularly evident in rapid-cycling cases. Patients usually sleep more in depressive phases and less in mania (see figure 16–7). We found forty-eight-hour sleep-wake cycles (alternate nights of total insomnia) to occur in many cases in association with the depression-to-mania switch process.[64] A large body of experimental evidence indicates that changes in the timing and duration of sleep can profoundly affect clinical states in such patients (restriction of sleep alleviates depression and induces mania). Therefore a positive feedback loop exists between sleep and mood. When manic, patients sleep less, and reduced sleep induces mania. This relationship would tend to move patients away from equilibrium toward pathological extremes. It is unclear how sleep interventions could be used clinically in such cases. Sleep restriction, if well modulated, might be used as an antidepressant. Sleep induction might exert antimanic effects. Repeated prophylactic sleep deprivation has been advocated as a treatment for refractory rapid cyclers,[7] but we found it to be ineffective in three cases where it was tried.* It may be relevant to their mode of action that therapeutic doses of MAOI drugs often profoundly fragment and reduce nocturnal sleep in patients.

Premenstrual Syndromes

Premenstrual affective syndromes (PMS) are a form of a rapid-cycling mood disorder that occurs in association with the menstrual cycle. The diagnosis of PMS is based not only on the nature and severity of symptoms but also on the presence of a consistent pattern of remission and relapse of symptoms linked to specific phases of the menstrual cycle. It is desirable to base the diagnosis on prospective daily ratings over several cycles, since only 50 percent of retrospective reports of PMS are confirmed by daily ratings.

Symptoms of PMS generally include changes in mood (depression, anxiety); irritability; cognitive alterations (difficulty concentrating, negative self-perception); disturbances in sleep, appetite, and energy; and other somatic disturbances (weight gain, breast swelling and tenderness). Halbreich, Endicott, and Nee[24] suggest that premenstrual depressive features could be differentiated into three main subtypes characterized by (1) atypical depressive features (hypersomnia and increased appetite), (2) hostility, and (3) anxiety. These subtypes have not yet been validated.

The relation of PMS to other psychiatric syndromes is unclear. Many psychiatric illnesses (affective disorders, schizophrenia, eating disorders, anxiety disorders, and obsessive-compulsive disorders) and medical

*T. A. Wehr, unpublished data.

illnesses (migraine syndrome, seizures, allergies) can be exacerbated premenstrually. A link between PMS and major depressive disorder (MDD) is suggested by Halbreich and Endicott's finding[23] that 84 percent of women with premenstrual depressive syndrome also had a prior history of major depressive disorder and 57 percent of women with a lifetime diagnosis of MDD met criteria for premenstrual depressive syndrome. Comparable figures for normal subjects were 9 percent and 14 percent respectively.

The relation of PMS to SAD is suggested by the fact that the majority of women with SAD also have PMS. In some cases, PMS symptoms associated with SAD responded to phototherapy. We recently identified a patient with a seasonal form of PMS. She developed severe premenstrual depressions in the fall and winter, which remitted spontaneously in the spring and summer. Phototherapy in the winter alleviated her symptoms. Furthermore, the therapeutic effect of light could be blocked by simultaneous administration of melatonin. Propranolol hydrochloride and atenolol, which suppress melatonin secretion, had a therapeutic effect similar to that of light. Patients whose cyclic symptoms of PMS occur only in fall and winter are analogous to patients described by Gjessing,[17] whose cycles of periodic catatonia or rapid-cycling manic-depressive illness occurred only in fall and winter.

Affective illness occurs in association with other alterations in reproductive function, such as those induced by oral contraceptives, abortion, the postpartum period, and menopause. It may be that the clinical phenomenology and biological substrates of affective changes occurring in association with PMS are related to those associated with other aspects of reproductive function.

It is unclear whether the cyclicity of affective symptoms in PMS arises from a potentially independent mood cycle's having become synchronized or entrained by the menstrual cycle or is a direct expression of hormonal changes that are part of the menstrual cycle. The latter interpretation is supported by Muse and associates,[38] who report

alleviation of PMS symptoms by "medical ovariectomy." This procedure involves elimination of the pulsatile release of gonadatropins required for cyclic ovarian function by chronic administration of gonadotrophin-releasing hormone. However, there are anecdotal reports that PMS occurs even in anovulatory cycles, and oral contraceptives do not consistently eliminate PMS symptoms. There are also reports of cyclic disturbances of mood occurring after cessation of ovarian function (oophorectomy and menopause). Perhaps the cyclic programming of the hypothalamus rather than the ovary is responsible for the persistent cyclicity of affective changes.

There are several theories about the pathogenesis of PMS, none of which has been substantiated. For example, a decreased ratio of progesterone to estrogen has been postulated to cause PMS (exogenous estrogen was reported to induce symptoms of PMS). Also, many treatments have been proposed for PMS, but none has proven consistently effective. These treatments include diet (restriction of carbohydrates), vitamins (pyridoxine), diuretics, prostaglandin inhibitors, progesterone, bromocriptine, lithium, and other conventional antidepressant therapies.

In controlled studies, we have found that affective PMS patients respond to total and partial sleep deprivation.[41] This result strengthens the link between PMS and other affective syndromes and is consistent with the hypothesis that prolactin secretion is involved in the pathogenesis of PMS (sleep deprivation profoundly lowers prolactin levels, which are sleep-dependent and highest at night). Because PMS episodes are relatively short, total or partial sleep deprivation may prove clinically useful in their treatment.

Daily Rhythms in Affective Illness

In many cases, depressive patients exhibit daily cycles of intensification of their symptoms (diurnal variation in mood). The clinical pattern in endogenous depression involves morning worsening. Since many systems in the organism exhibit marked daily cycles in their levels of functioning (circadian rhythms), morning worsening of depression may result from normal circadian modulation of a system that is linked to depressive pathophysiology. For example, activity of the hypothalamic-pituitary-adrenal axis, previously linked to depression in other contexts, reaches the maximum of its circadian variation in the morning hours.

Morning worsening of depression may also be linked to the sleep phase of the daily sleep-wake cycle. There is considerable evidence that the timing of the sleep-wake cycle and the duration of the sleep phase powerfully affect clinical state in affective patients. Restriction of sleep (total or partial sleep deprivation) has antidepressant effects and can induce mania[64] (see figure 16–8). Usually the antidepressant effects of total sleep deprivation are reversed by recovery sleep. There is some evidence that the timing of the sleep-wake cycle is a critical factor in patients' responses to sleep interventions. Uncontrolled studies have shown that shifting the timing of sleep several hours earlier than usual, without restricting sleep (phase advance of the sleep-wake cycle), has sustained antidepressant effects in some patients.[51,63] Partial sleep deprivation in the second half but not the first half of the night induces temporary remissions in depression.[18,52,53] Thus the occurrence of sleep or wakefulness in the *second half of the night* appears to be the effective principle of sleep deprivation. This finding may indicate that biological processes responsible for depression are associated with a particular circadian interval and are sensitive to sleeping and waking.

Our existing knowledge of sleep-related processes is largely confined to neuroendocrine mechanisms. Growth hormone[55] and prolactin[40] secretion are inhibited and cortisol[69] and TSH[39] secretion are stimulated by sleep deprivation. In this regard, it is interesting that nocturnal TSH secretion is abnormally blunted in depressive patients[27,50] and (like mood) is normalized by sleep deprivation. In light of other research implicating

thyroid function in affective illness and its treatment, it is worth investigating the effects of sleep deprivation on hypothalamic-pituitary-thyroid function as possible mechanisms of its action.

REM sleep deprivation, in particular, may play a role in patients' response to sleep deprivation. REM sleep propensity exhibits a circadian rhythm (evident in nap studies), with REM sleep most likely to occur in the second half of the night and least likely to occur in the first half of the night.[33,67] Thus the superior antidepressant efficacy of sleep deprivation in the second half of the night compared with the first half of the night may depend on its differential effects on REM sleep. We found that the former treatment reduced REM sleep 50 percent, while the latter had no effect.[52] This interpretation is consistent with Vogel and coworkers' previous finding that selective REM sleep deprivation has antidepressant effects.[56]

Since changes in the timing and amount of sleep occur in the course of mood cycles and appear to have powerful effects on clinical state, mechanisms that regulate the sleep-wake cycle (discussed previously) deserve further investigation.

Circadian Rhythm Abnormalities in Affective Illness

In the past two decades, numerous reports of abnormalities in phase, amplitude, and waveform of circadian rhythms have appeared in the literature. These were the subject of a review in a previous volume of this *Handbook.*[61,62]

Halberg[22] proposed that cyclic (especially rapid-cycling) forms of affective illness might arise as a beat-phenomenon if one component of the circadian system were no longer entrained to the twenty-four-hour day-night cycle but free-ran according to its own intrinsic (e.g., twenty-five-hour) rhythm. In this case, the free-running component (e.g., the circadian temperature rhythm) would gradually go in and out of phase with other components (e.g., the sleep-wake cycle) still entrained to the twenty-four-hour day-night

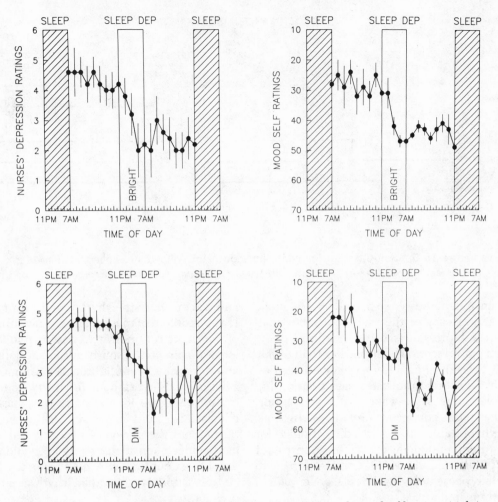

Figure 16–8. Two-hourly nurses' depression ratings (left) and mood self-ratings (right) (X ± standard error of mean) before, during and after one night's total sleep deprivation in bright light (top) and near total darkness (bottom) in five depressed patients. Antidepressant responses in both conditions were similar on the day after sleep deprivation, but may have differed during the sleep deprivation night when patients were exposed to the two different light conditions.

NOTE: Reprinted, by permission of the publisher, from T. A. Wehr et al., "Antidepressant Effects of Sleep Deprivation in Bright and Dim Light," *Acta Psychiatrica Scandinavica*, 72 (1985):161–165.

cycle. In support of the hypothesis, Kripke and coworkers reported what may be remarkable evidence[28] that is nevertheless weak because of shortcomings in the methods used for monitoring circadian rhythms. Other investigators have presented evidence interpreted to negate the hypothesis, but almost none have studied appropriate patients (rapid cyclers).

Over the years, many publications have reported that the timing of circadian rhythms seems to be shifted earlier in depressive patients compared with controls. These findings, exhaustively reviewed[61,62] elsewhere, led us to hypothesize that a phase advance of the dominant circadian oscillator may be responsible for certain sleep architectural abnormalities such as short REM latency, long first REM periods, and early-morning awakening, and for the abnormally early timing of other circadian rhythms influenced by this oscillator. The phase-

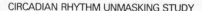

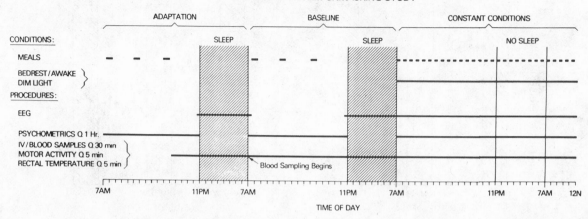

Figure 16–9. Study design for controlling distorting effects of evoked responses to meals, activity, and so on ("masking effects") in the measurement of circadian rhythms.

advance hypothesis also provided a rationale for the efficacy of the phase-advance treatment of depression (shifting the timing of the sleep period several hours earlier than usual). This procedure could be conceived to reestablish a normal internal phase relationship between the sleep-wake cycle and abnormally phase-advanced circadian rhythms. The hypothesis also provided a rationale for the therapeutic efficacy of antidepressant drugs (lithium and MAOI), which appear to exhibit phase-delaying effects on circadian rhythms in animals.[72]

The empirical data on which the phase-advance hypothesis rests is equivocal. While the results of many studies involving hundreds of patients show what appears to be a phase advance in circadian rhythms in depression (for a recent example, see Linkowski et al.[32]), some carefully done studies do not[57] or are equivocal.[49] The measurement of circadian rhythms and their phases is fraught with serious methodological problems. Most prominent is the problem of "masking"—distortions of the waveform of the endogenous rhythm by evoked responses to internal and external stimuli such as sleep, awakenings, meals, activity, light, and so on. In many instances effects of masking can obscure variance due to the endogenous rhythm, making it impossible to meaningfully describe the phase position, amplitude,

and waveform of the rhythm. One approach to the problem of masking is to study subjects on constant routines for a day or two. Subjects remain continuously awake, at bedrest, and in constant dim light, and consume isocaloric meals every hour for thirty hours or more (see figure 16–9). In this way masking effects are held more or less constant throughout the period of measurement. We have undertaken such a study in the hope of providing definitive information about phase and amplitude of circadian rhythms in depression.

¶ Conclusions

In this chapter we have reviewed the rhythmic manifestations of affective illness and the involvement of biological rhythms in its course, pathophysiology, and treatment. A comparative analysis of different rhythms involved in affective illness may yield clues to its pathogenesis. Two examples can be cited. There are many similarities between the oscillatory behavior of the human sleep-wake cycle and that of the manic-depressive cycle (see Wehr and Goodwin[62]). Both involve abrupt transitions between phases with marked changes in levels of activation; oscillations of either may dramatically change their period (often with period doubling) and may become entrained to other rhythms in the organism or environment. These parallels may indicate that biological processes underlying the rhythmic behavior of manic-depressive cycles and sleep-wake cycles are fundamentally similar, though their frequencies are very different.

As described, affective symptoms are strongly modulated by a variety of biological and environmental rhythms, ranging in period from one day to one year. Taken together, this spectrum of rhythms could provide an organizing principle for understanding biological factors predisposing to depression or mania. In the patients we have described, depression is intensified in winter, premenstrually, and in the morning. The consistent association of certain biological changes with these phases of annual, menstrual, and daily rhythms would provide a rationale for their inclusion in future hypotheses and investigations of the pathogenesis of affective illness.

¶ Bibliography

1. ADAMOPOULOS, D. A., et al. "Endocrine Profiles of Premenstrual Tension," *Clinical Endocrinology*, 1 (1972):283–292.

2. ALBERS, H. E., et al. "Avian Pancreatic Polypeptide Phase Shifts Hamster Circadian Rhythms When Microinjected into the Suprachiasmatic Region," *Science*, 223 (1984):833–835.

3. BEASLEY, L. J., and NELSON, R. J. "Thyroid Gland Influences the Period of Hamster Circadian Oscillations," *Experientia*, 38 (1982):870–871.

4. CARROLL, B. G., and STEINER, M. "The Psychobiology of Premenstrual Dysphoria: The Role of Prolactin," *Psychoneuroendocrinology*, 3 (1978):171–180.

5. CARTER, D. S., and GOLDMAN, B. D. "Antigonadal Effects of Timed Melatonin Infusion in Pinealectomized Male Djungarian Hamsters (Phodopus Sungorus Sungorus): Duration Is the Critical Parameter," *Endocrinology*, 113 (1983): 1261.

6. CHO, J. T., et al. "The Effect of Lithium Treatment on Thyroid Function in Patients with Primary Affective Disorder," *American Journal of Psychiatry*, 136 (1979):115–116.

7. CHRISTODOULOU, G. N., et al. "Possible Prophylactic Effect of Sleep Deprivation," *American Journal of Psychiatry*, 135 (1978):375–376.

8. COWDRY, R., et al. "Thyroid Abnormalities Associated with Rapid Cycling Bipolar Illness," *Archives of General Psychiatry*, 40 (1983):414–420.

9. COWEN, P. J., et al. "Atenolol Reduces Plasma Melatonin Concentration in Man," *British Journal of Clinical Pharmacology*, 15 (1983):579–581.

10. CZEISLER, C. A., et al. "Chronotherapy: Resetting the Circadian Clocks of Patients with Delayed Sleep Phase Insomnia." *Sleep*, 4 (1981):1–21.

11. DUNNER, D. L. "Rapid-Cycling Bipolar Manic-Depressive Illness," *Psychiatric Clinics of North America*, 2 (1979):461–467.

12. DUNNER, D. L., PATRICK, V., and FIEVE, R. R. "Rapid-Cycling Manic Depressive Patients," *Comprehensive Psychiatry*, 18 (1977):561–566.

13. EASTWOOD, M. R., et al. "Infradian Rhythms: A Comparison of Affective Disorders and Normal Persons," *Archives of General Psychiatry*, 42 (1985): 295–299.

14. ENDICOTT, G., and HALBREICH, U. "Retrospective Reports of Premenstrual Changes: Factor Affecting Confirmation by Daily Ratings," *Psychopharmacology Bulletin*, 18 (1982):109–112.

15. FALRET, J. P. "La Folie Circulaire," *Bulletin de l'Academie Nationale de Medicine*, 19 (1854):382.

16. GILLIN, J. C. "The Sleep Therapies of Depression," *Progress in Neuro-Psychopharmacology and Biological Psychiatry*, 7(2/3) (1983):351–364.

17. GJESSING, R. R. *Contribution to the Somatology of Periodic Catatonia*, edited by F. A. Jenner and L. R. Gjessing. Oxford: Pergamon Press, 1976.

18. GOETZE, U., and TOLLE, R. "Antidepressive Wirkung des Patiellen Schlafentzuges wahrend der 1. Halfte der Nacht," *Psychiatria Clinica*, 14 (1981):129.

19. GREDEN, J. F., et al. "Serial Dexamethasone Suppression Tests Among Rapidly Cycling Bipolar Patients," *Biological Psychiatry*, 17 (1982):455–462.

20. GWINNER, E. "Circannual Systems," in J. Aschoff, ed., *Handbook of Behavioral Neurobiology*. New York: Plenum Press, 1981, pp. 391–408.

21. ———. "Annual Rhythms: Perspective," in J. Aschoff, ed., *Handbook of Behavioral Neurobiology*. New York: Plenum Press, 1981, pp. 381–389.

22. HALBERG, F. "Physiologic Considerations Underlying Rhythmometry, with Special Reference to Emotional Illness," *Symposium Bel-Air III*. Geneva: Masson et Cie, 1968, p. 73.

23. HALBREICH, U., and ENDICOTT, J. "Relationship of Dysphoric Premenstrual Changes to Depressive Disorders," *Acta Psychiatrica Scandinavica*, 71 (1985):331–338.

24. HALBREICH, U., ENDICOTT, J., and NEE, G. "Premenstrual Depressive Changes," *Archives of General Psychiatry*, 40 (1983):535–542.

25. HAMILTON, J. A., et al. "Premenstrual Mood Changes: A Guide to Evaluation and Treatment," *Psychiatric Annals*, 14 (1984):426–435.

26. HOFFMAN, K. "Photoperiodism in Vertebrates," in J. Aschoff, ed., *Handbook of Behavioral Neurobiology*. New York: Plenum Press, 1981, pp. 449–473.

27. KJELLMAN, B. F., et al. "Twenty-Four Hour Serum Levels of TSH in Affective Disorders," *Acta Psychiatrica Scandinavica*, 69 (1984):491–502.

28. KRIPKE, D. F., et al. "Circadian Rhythm Disorders in Manic Depressives," *Biological Psychiatry*, 13 (1978):335.

29. KUKOPULOS, A., et al. "Course of the Manic-Depressive Cycle and Changes Caused by Treatments," *Pharmakopsychiatrie*, 13 (1980):156.

30. LEWY, A. J., et al. "Light Suppresses Melatonin Secretion in Human," *Science*, 210 (1980):1267–1269.

31. LIEBOWITZ, M. R., et al. "Phenelzine V. Imipramine in Atypical Depression. A Preliminary Report," *Archives of General Psychiatry*, 41 (1984):669–677.

32. LINKOWSKI, P., et al. "The 24-Hour Profile of ACTH and Cortisol in Unipolar and Bipolar Depression," *Journal of Endocrinology and Metabolism*, 61 (1965): 421–438.

33. MARON, L., RECHTSCHAFFEN, A., and WOLPERT, E. A. "Sleep Cycle During Napping," *Archives of General Psychiatry*, 11 (1964): 503–598.

34. MEIJER, J. H., RUSAK, B., and HARRINGTON, M. E. "Geniculate Stimulation Phase Shifts Hamster Circadian Rhythms," *Abstracts of the Society for Neuroscience*, 10 (1984):502.

35. MOORE, R. Y. "Central Neural Control of Circadian Rhythms," in W. F. Ganong and L. Martini, eds., *Frontiers in Neuroendocrinology*, vol. 5. New York: Raven Press, 1978, pp. 185–206.

36. MOORE-EDE, M. C., CZEISLER, C. A., and RICHARDSON, E. S. "Circadian Timekeeping in Health and Disease: Part 1. Basic Properties of Circadian Pacemakers," *New England Journal of Medicine*, 309 (1983):469–476.

37. MORIN, L. P., FITZGERALD, F. M., and ZUCKER, I. "Estradiol Shortens the Period of Hamster Circadian Rhythms," *Science*, 196 (1977):305–307.

38. MUSE, K. N., et al. "The Premenstrual Syndrome. Effects of Medical Ovariectomy," *New England Journal of Medicine*, 311 (1984):1345–1349.

39. PARKER, D. C., PEKARY, A. E., and HERSHMAN, J. M. "Effect of Normal and Reversed Sleep-Wake Cycles Upon Nyctohemeral Rhythmicity of Plasma Thyrotropin. Evidence Suggestive of an Inhibitory Influence in Sleep," *Journal of Clinical Endocrinology and Metabolism*, 43 (1976):318–329.

40. PARKER, D. C., ROSSMAN, L. G., and VANDERLAND, E. F. "Relation of Sleep-Entrained Human Prolactin Release to REM-non-REM cycles," *Journal of Clinical Endocrinology and Metabolism*, 38 (1974):646–651.

41. PARRY, B. L., and WEHR, T. A. "Antidepressant Effects of Total and Partial Sleep Deprivation in Premenstrual Affective Syndromes," submitted for publication.

42. PFLUG, B., and TOLLE, R. "Therapie Endogener Depressionen Durch

Schlafentzug. Praktische und Theoretische Konsequenzen," *Nervenarzt,* 42 (1971):117–124.

43. POST, R. M., et al. "Alterations in Motor Activity, Sleep, and Biochemistry in a Cycling Manic-Depressive Patient," *Archives of General Psychiatry,* 34 (1977): 470–477.

44. RALPH, M. R., and MENAKER, M. "Bicuculline Blocks Circadian Phase Delays but Not Advances," *Brain Research,* 325 (1985):362–365.

45. ROSENTHAL, N. E., et al. "Seasonal Affective Disorder. A Description of the Syndrome and Preliminary Findings with Light Therapy," *Archives of General Psychiatry,* 41(1984):72–80.

46. ROSENTHAL, N. E., et al. "Seasonal Affective Disorder and Phototherapy," *Annals of the New York Academy of Science,* 453 (1985):260–269.

47. ROSENTHAL, N. E., et al. "Antidepressant Effects of Light in Seasonal Affective Disorder," *American Journal of Psychiatry,* 142 (1985): 606–608.

48. ROSENTHAL, N. E., et al. "The Role of Melatonin in Seasonal Affective Disorder: A Preliminary Study," submitted for publication.

49. RUBIN, R. T., et al. "The Neuroendocrinology of Primary Endogenous Depression. I. Cortisol Secretory Dynamics in Patients and Control Subjects," submitted for publication.

50. SACK, D. A., ROSENTHAL, N. E., and WEHR, T. A. "Blunted Nocturnal TSH Secretion in Depressed Patients Normalized by Therapeutic Sleep Deprivation," submitted for publication.

51. SACK, D. A., et al. "The Potentiation of Antidepressant Medications by Phase-Advance of the Sleep-Wake Cycle," *American Journal of Psychiatry,* 142 (1985):606–608.

52. SACK, D. A., et al. "Early Versus Late Partial Sleep Deprivation Therapy of Depression," submitted for publication.

53. SCHILGEN, B., and TOLLE, R. "Partial Sleep Deprivation as Therapy for Depression," *Archives of General Psychiatry,* 37 (1980):261–271.

54. STANCER, H. C., and PERSAD, E. "Treatment of Intractable Rapid-Cycling Manic-Depressive Disorder with Levothyroxine," *Archives of General Psychiatry,* 39 (1982):311–312.

55. TAKAHASHI, Y., KIPNIS, D. M., and DAUGHADAY, W. H. "Growth Hormone Secretion During Sleep," *Journal of Clinical Investigation,* 47 (1968):2079–2090.

56. VOGEL, G. W., et al. "Improvement of Depression by REM Sleep Deprivation," *Archives of General Psychiatry,* 37 (1980):247–253.

57. VON ZERSSEN, D., et al. "Circadian Rhythms in Endogenous Depression," *Psychiatry Research,* in press.

58. WEHR, T. A. "Phase and Biorhythm Studies of Affective Illness," *Annals of Internal Medicine,* 87 (1977):319–335.

59. ———. "Rapid Cycling" (Letter to the Editor), *Archives of General Psychiatry,* 40 (1983):108.

60. WEHR, T. A., and GOODWIN, F. K. "Rapid Cycling in Manic-Depressives Induced by Tricyclic Antidepressants," *Archives of General Psychiatry,* 36 (1979):555–559.

61. ———. "Biological Rhythms and Psychiatry," in S. Arieti, and H.K.H. Brodie, eds., *American Handbook of Psychiatry,* vol. 7, 2nd ed. New York: Basic Books, 1981, pp. 46–74.

62. ———. "Biological Rhythms and Manic-Depressive Illness," in T. A. Wehr and F. K. Goodwin, eds., *Biological Rhythms and Psychiatry.* Pacific Grove, Calif.: Boxwood Press, 1983, pp. 129–184.

63. WEHR, T. A., et al. "Phase-Advance of the Circadian Sleep-Wake Cycle as an Antidepressant," *Science,* 206 (1979):710–713.

64. WEHR, T. A., et al. "48-Hour Sleep-Wake Cycles in Manic-Depressive Illness: Naturalistic Observations and Sleep Deprivation Experiments," *Archives of General Psychiatry,* 39 (1982):559–565.

65. WEHR, T.A., et al. "Antidepressant Effects of Sleep Deprivation in Bright and Dim Light," *Acta Psychiatrica Scandinavica,* 72(1985):161–165.

66. WEHR, T. A., et al. "Evidence for a Non-Photoperiodic Mechanism in the Antidepressant Effect of Light in Recur-

rent Winter Depression," submitted for publication.

67. WEITZMAN, E. D., et al. "Effects of a Prolonged 3-Hour Sleep-Wake Cycle on Sleep Stage, Plasma Cortisol, Growth Hormone and Body Temperature in Man," *Journal of Clinical Endocrinology and Metabolism,* 38 (1974): 1018–1070.

68. WEITZMAN, E. D., et al. "Seasonal Patterns of Sleep Stages and Secretion of Cortisol and Growth Hormone During 24 Hour Periods in Northern Norway," *Acta Endocrinologica,* 78 (1975):65–76.

69. WEITZMAN, E. D., et al. "The Sleep-Wake Pattern of Cortisol and Growth Hormone Secretion During Non-Entrained (Free-Running) Conditions in Man," in M. Nijhoff, ed., *Circadian and Ultradian Variations of Pituitary Hormones in Man.* Brussels: Elsevier, 1981.

70. WEVER, R. *The Circadian System of Man: Results of Experiments Under Temporal Isolation.* New York: Springer-Verlag, 1979.

71. WEVER, R. A., POLASEK, J., and WILDGRUBER, C. M. "Bright Light Affects Human Circadian Rhythms," *Pflugers Archives,* 396 (1983):85–87.

72. WIRZ-JUSTICE, A., GROOS, G., and WEHR, T. A. "The Neuropharmacology of Circadian Timekeeping," in J. Aschoff, S. Daan, and G. Groos, eds., *Vertebrate Circadian Systems: Structure and Physiology.* Heidelburg: Springer-Verlag, 1982, pp. 1–26.

73. ZATZ, M., and BROWNSTEIN, M. J. "Intraventricular Carbachol Mimics the Effects of Light on the Circadian Rhythm in the Rat Pineal Gland," *Science,* 203 (1979):358–361.

CHAPTER 17

BIOLOGICAL HYPOTHESES
OF SCHIZOPHRENIA

Michael Davidson, Miklos F. Losonczy, and Kenneth L. Davis

¶ Introduction

It has been the impression of neurologists and psychiatrists from Freud and Kraepelin to the present day that patients afflicted with the syndrome of schizophrenia are suffering from a physical illness originating in the central nervous system (CNS). This impression is based on the clinical similarities of schizophrenia with tertiary syphilis, some epileptic conditions, and other identified physical disorders known to cause chronic psychotic states. Subsequent investigations of the pathophysiology underlying the schizophrenic syndrome have not yet uncovered any specific etiologies, although current hypotheses have been rapidly increasing the areas under exploration. This chapter reviews some of the most important work in the genetics, neuropathology, and neurochemistry of schizophrenia.

¶ The Genetics of Schizophrenia

A considerable body of evidence has been established suggesting that at least some schizophrenic patients are suffering from an illness that has a component of heritability. This conclusion is based largely on epidemiology, family studies, twin studies, and adoption studies.

The lifetime risk for developing schizophrenia has variously been reported as between 0.35 and 2.85 percent throughout the world. [159] Because of changing definitions of the boundaries of this syndrome both over time and in different cultures, it is difficult to compare studies to assess if the prevalence of schizophrenia is relatively stable. Most studies suggest schizophrenia is found throughout the world at approximately the same rate of 1 to 2 percent in the general population. [111] This figure is generally used as a baseline comparison for assessing the increased familial incidence reported in all studies addressing this issue.

The risk of a relative of a schizophrenic patient developing this illness appears to be affected by the degree of genetic closeness and by the severity of the illness in the proband. Although a wide range has been reported for the prevalence of schizophrenia in first-degree relatives, approximately 10 percent of full siblings or children of an index case will develop the disorder at some point in life, while about 5 percent of parents of a schizophrenic proband will have a similar illness. When two schizophrenic individuals have children, up to 50 percent of these offspring may manifest this illness.[111,254] There is also evidence to suggest that those schizophrenic patients with the most severe form of the illness, institutionalized much of their lives, are more likely to have schizophrenic relatives than those probands with a milder form of the illness.

While the familial clustering of schizophrenia is well established and is consistent with a genetic vulnerability to the disease, the shared familial environment could be responsible for the increased risk in family members, by an infectious route, an environmental toxin, dietary factors, or learned patterns of behavior. Therefore, studies of twins have been important in providing strong evidence that a component of the vulnerability to schizophrenia is heritable.

The potential role of a common environment in the increased familial clustering in schizophrenia may be evaluated by comparing schizophrenic index cases who are members of a twin pair. Comparison of concordance rates for index cases who are members of a monozygotic (MZ) twin pair with index cases who have a same-sex, dizygotic (DZ) twin show dramatic increases in the MZ group. Reports of concordance for schizophrenia range from 33 to 78 percent in MZ twins, while DZ twins are generally reported as having the same concordance rate as siblings overall, approximately 10 percent. A comparison of the nine twin studies of schizophrenia that provided sufficient data for determination of concordance rates (given that one twin has schizophrenia) shows that though there is a large range in reported concordance for MZ twins, they are not significantly different from each other.* Assuming that MZ and DZ twins share etiologically relevant environmental factors, these studies together suggest that about 68 percent of the variance in liability to schizophrenia is due to genetic factors.[158] This figure is about the same or higher than that of various medical conditions commonly assumed to have a significant genetic component of vulnerability, such as diabetes, hypertension, and epilepsy.

It has been argued that the assumption of similar environmental factors for MZ and DZ twins in the development of schizophrenia is incorrect, based on the belief that the similarity in learned behavior in MZ twins is greater than in DZ twins.[180] Thus if the familial clustering of schizophrenia is due to a learned behavior in some families, MZ twins are more likely to share this risk factor. This argument is not supported by studies that examined the personalities of normal MZ twins reared apart. Those twins who grew up together in the same family unit actually had personalities that differed more from each other than personalities of MZ twins who were reared apart. It appears that the physical similarity experienced by MZ twins exerts a pressure to differentiate from each other, rather than to share similar patterns of behavior.[158]

Clearly, the difficult issue of separating the influence of postnatal environmental factors from genetic (and intrauterine) variables can be resolved definitively only by holding the genetic influence constant and varying the postnatal environment. Ideally, this would involve a large study of schizophrenic probands from MZ twin pairs reared apart from birth by biologically unrelated individuals, with no contact between twins. At this time such a study does not exist and in view of the low incidence of schizophrenia, monozygotic twinning, and separate adoption from birth of twins by unrelated individuals, a large series is unlikely to be developed in the near future. An alternate strategy—employing adoption to disentangle genetic from environmental influences without the use of twins—has yielded information suggesting a significant heritability for the development of schizophrenia.

This approach utilized the thorough rec-

*See references 6, 86, 93, 110, 135, 165, 172, 274, and 302.

ords of adoption and admission to mental hospitals in Denmark as a tool to identify schizophrenic probands who had been adopted at an early age. First- and second-degree relatives, both adoptive and biological, were identified and interviewed for evidence of schizophrenia or related behaviors.[160,255,335] As a control group, nonschizophrenic adoptees were also identified and similar assessments of their relatives were made. It was assumed that if schizophrenia is primarily a result of learned behaviors or other environmental influences, a larger number of schizophrenic individuals would be identified among the adoptive families of schizophrenic patients with whom they spent many years of their lives. On the other hand, if genetic influences are responsible for the increased risk of schizophrenia found in families of schizophrenic patients, one would expect an excess of schizophrenic individuals only in the biological relatives of schizophrenic adoptees. The latter hypothesis was preferentially supported by the results of this investigation.

The study group also included many half siblings, sharing a genetic component from only one parent. It was found that the biological paternal half siblings of schizophrenic probands were at increased risk to develop schizophreniclike behavior. This is significant, in that it suggests that the contribution of biological parents in increasing the risk of developing schizophrenia is not purely due to intrauterine factors, but from genetic influence. This interpretation is also supported by studies of children of a single schizophrenic biological parent, either mother or father, that found no difference in the risk to children for developing schizophrenia. This study is also noteworthy for identifying a group of diagnoses of aberrant behavior not sufficiently distinct to qualify as schizophrenia, but apparently genetically related to it. These diagnoses are collectively referred to as the schizophrenic spectrum disorders.[160,255,335]

A collateral investigation identified schizophrenic parents who either had children adopted away from them or who adopted children themselves, although often before exhibiting the illness. A control group of parents without psychiatric disease, who either had adopted away children or adopted them, was also located. The children of these subjects were interviewed for various degrees of psychopathology. Only those adoptees whose biological parents had schizophrenia showed increased psychopathology, even though they were raised by nonpsychotic adoptive parents. The children of nonschizophrenic biological parents reared by a parent who ultimately developed schizophrenia were no more likely to show psychopathology than other adoptive children.[336] These two approaches to separating the genetic from the postnatal environmental factors both give strong support for the heritability of risk to develop schizophrenia.

While there is strong evidence to implicate a genetic vulnerability for schizophrenia, its expression may be influenced by subsequent environmental factors. Prenatal complications may be associated with increased risk for the development of schizophrenia.[186] The Danish longitudinal study, following into adulthood the offspring of schizophrenic mothers, found a higher incidence of complications during pregnancy or birth in those offspring who ultimately became schizophrenic. Schizotypal offspring had the lowest incidence of such complications, and normal offspring had an intermediate incidence between schizophrenic and schizotypal subjects.[226] These results suggest that schizophrenic and schizotypal offspring may have shared the genetic predisposition for the illness, but its expression was modulated by the amount of stress experienced during the pregnancy or at birth.

Although most investigators are convinced that genetic factors are important influences on the subsequent development of schizophrenic symptoms, no single locus model of transmission is supported by the body of evidence. Several different analytic techniques have concluded that a polygenic model can be used to fit the data provided by twin studies.[111,158] It is also plausible that several different etiologies for schizophrenia may exist with differing genetic defects, complicating the interpretation of the available genetic data. Assuming that several different genetic forms of schizophrenia do exist, it is not yet possible to distinguish individuals with each form of the disorder.

The large body of evidence implicating an etiological role for genetics in at least some schizophrenic patients has been a major impetus for pursuing investigations of neuropathology and neurochemistry in this devastating syndrome. Whatever genetic factors exist in schizophrenia must be expressed by proteins that may be involved in maintaining the structural integrity of the CNS, or in the functional control of neurotransmission. The remainder of this chapter focuses on evidence that some schizophrenic subjects may differ from normals in neuroanatomy, neurophysiology, or neurochemistry.

¶ The Neuropathology of Schizophrenia

The search for a neuropathological basis of schizophrenia has resulted in hundreds of studies of histopathology in postmortem schizophrenic brains by many prominent investigators. Initially attention was focused on the cortical areas, as schizophrenia was theoretically viewed as a disturbance in higher mental functions. Although many studies reported significant differences in schizophrenic cortical areas, no clear pattern emerged. Interpretation of these inconsistent results was further confounded by major differences in diagnostic methods, selection of controls, and histopathological techniques. The likelihood that schizophrenia is etiologically a heterogeneous disorder also implies that no single finding is likely to emerge distinguishing schizophrenic subjects from normals, and that different populations studied are likely to have variable mixtures of etiology. The possibility that schizophrenic subjects may eventually be shown to be heterogeneous is underscored by the existence of a wide range of neurological and metabolic diseases that nevertheless can clinically present as similar to schizophrenia. The developing appreciation that various lesions disrupting limbic structures can produce psychotic symptoms has focused attention on these subcortical structures in recent neuropathological studies.

Histopathological Studies

Postmortem studies over the past twenty years, using blind assessments with improved methodological rigor, have consistently found evidence of brain pathology in schizophrenia, especially in the limbic structures. These findings have generally been nonspecific evidence of cell loss and gliosis, with disrupted intracellular structure. Pontine gliosis,[94] atrophy of the cerebellar vermis,[331] and disarray of hippocampal pyramidal cells[264] have also been described more often in schizophrenic brain tissue than in control tissue. In one large study almost 75 percent of schizophrenic brains showed gliosis confined to the basal forebrain or the periventricular and periaqueductal region, while other psychiatric and nonpsychiatric controls did not show such a regional distribution of gliosis.[292] This gliosis was interpreted as the residual effect of a previous inflammatory process. A recent postmortem study comparing brains of affective disorder patients with schizophrenic patients reported larger ventricles and thinning of the parahippocampal gyrus in schizophrenic patients, with the difference between the groups being greater on the left side of the brain.[68]

The microscopic approach to CNS pathology is severely limited by the relative lack of information about the clinical picture and course of the disease in the study subjects. *In vivo* imaging studies offer the capability of assessing neuropathology and neuropathophysiology in subjects whose history, course, and biological characteristics are open to close examination.

Neuroradiological Studies

The earliest neuroradiological studies involved pneumoencephalography (PEG), which makes possible a gross determination of brain atrophy by examining ventricular size. Several studies[17,116] reported larger ventricles, and presumably greater atrophy, in populations of schizophrenic patients relative to various nonnormal control groups. Within the groups of schizophrenic patients that were studied, a more severe form of the illness was often associated with larger ventricles. Cortical atrophy was also occasionally reported in PEG studies, at times even in the absence of ventricular enlargement.[213] The risks and inherent methodological difficulties of PEG inhibited systematic studies of these issues until the advent of the computerized tomography (CT) scan in the early 1970s.

Initial studies assessing ventricular size utilized various linear measures. However, it was shown that these linear measures did not correlate well with ventricular volume and, by extension, brain atrophy. The development of the ventricular brain ratio (VBR) offered a significant advance in the determination of central atrophy by imaging techniques.[297] The VBR is highly correlated with ventricular volume and is a fairly reliable measure when used by the same person on images from the same machine produced under similar conditions.

Using this measure, many well-controlled studies have found a significant increase in lateral ventricular size in schizophrenic subjects relative to age- and sex-matched normal controls.[150,214,330] Some studies have also reported the third and fourth ventricles to be enlarged.[224] However, a considerable range in the prevalence of ventricular enlargement in schizophrenia has been reported in various studies, with from 6 to 50 percent of subjects showing ventricles greater than 2 standard deviations above the appropriate normal mean. This range is probably a result of the widely disparate severity of illness in the populations studied, with the largest prevalence in chronically institutionalized patients.[151] Enlarged ventricles or signs of cortical atrophy are by no means limited to older patients with a long history of illness.[229,330] Even first-episode schizo-phreniform patients have shown enlarged ventricles on CT scan.[328] However, one well-controlled study of ventricular enlargement in schizophrenia reported no differences relative to controls.[147] Although this patient sample may have included schizophrenic patients capable of a higher level of social functioning than those of other studies, the disparity remains unexplained.

Of perhaps greater interest than the prevalence of ventricular enlargement is characterization of behavioral and biochemical differences in those schizophrenic subjects with enlarged ventricles compared to those without. Although a relationship between ventricular size and symptom complex has been hypothesized in schizophrenic subjects, this has received little support in well-controlled studies. Nonsignificant trends for an excess of negative symptoms in schizophrenic subjects with enlarged ventricles have been reported,[332] and a single study has reported significantly more positive symptoms in schizophrenic subjects with smaller ventricles.[10] This finding is difficult to interpret, however, since medicated groups were studied, confounding the issue by possible differential treatment responses in schizophrenic subjects with different degrees of central atrophy, as well as a significantly younger group in the smaller-ventricle population.

Ventricular size appears to be under genetic control, the correlation being significantly higher in normal MZ twins than in normal DZ twins, and, in general, ventricular size correlates in normal siblings. The high correlation observed in normal MZ twin pairs is not observed in MZ twins discordant for schizophrenia. The unaffected twin shows a ventricular volume above control, but smaller than the schizophrenic twin, suggesting a relationship between the disorder and ventricular enlargement.[247,333] The presence of enlarged ventricles in patients during their first schizophreniform episode suggests that the morphological impairment precedes the psychotic decompensation and cannot be explained by treatment or chronicity.[216,328] In the prospective Danish high-risk study that followed into adulthood individuals born to schizophrenic mothers, those who developed schizophrenia showed larger ventricles than schizotypal or mentally healthy individuals from the same high-risk group, again suggesting the relationship between the illness and ventricular dimensions.[329]

An association between ventricular enlargement and birth complications was found in only those schizophrenic patients without a family history of major psychiatric disorders. A recent study examining a group of schizophrenic patients of twin birth reported an association between normal ventricular volume and positive family history of major psychiatric disorders. Among those schizophrenic patients without such a family history, cerebral ventricular size was significantly increased and there was also evidence of birth complications. Enlarged ventricles were also found in normal control twins who reported complicated birth. These findings suggest that ventricular enlargement may be just one nonspecific indication of past or present cerebral pathology contributing to the genesis of a psychotic illness in those individuals with low genetic predisposition.[241]

Other CT observations in chronic schizophrenic patients have revealed cerebellar vermian atrophy with prevalences ranging from 5 to 40 percent.[329] This intriguing finding is not correlated with clinically expressed cerebellar signs. Cerebellar atrophy was not found in siblings of chronic schizophrenic patients or in patients at their first schizophrenic exacerbation.[334] Since the cerebellar cortex is believed to be particularly susceptible to toxic insults, vermian atrophy may be a secondary phenomenon. However, the existence of neural pathways between the vermian area and the limbic forebrain raises the interesting hypothesis that atrophy of the cerebellar vermis reduces the cerebellar inhibitory influence on the activity of the limbic forebrain.[278] This disinhibition may result in overactivity of the limbic regions and be the origin of psychotic symptoms in some individuals.

An apparently unrelated CT finding, re-ported by several groups, is the reversal of normal cerebral hemispheric asymmetry in some schizophrenic patients.[181] However, this finding is not specific for schizophrenia and appears to be unrelated to other CT abnormalities.[334] While ventricular enlargement and other nonspecific CT abnormalities are found in schizophrenic patients more frequently than in normal subjects, the majority of patients affected by this disorder appear to show no such abnormalities. Considering the probable heterogeneity of schizophrenia and the multiple etiological factors contributing to ventricular enlargement, it is unlikely that a specific pathological process will be associated with enlarged ventricles.

Abnormal lateral brain organization expressed by a defective pattern of dominance between hemispheres, abnormal integration of the two hemispheres across cerebral commissures, or abnormal structural asymmetries have all been postulated and studied in schizophrenia.[108,189,203,215]

Particular attention has been focused on possible left-hemisphere dysfunction following clinical observations associating schizophreniclike symptoms with epileptogenic foci of this hemisphere,[78] as well as the disturbed verbal function in schizophrenic patients believed to be associated with left-hemisphere dysfunction.[95]

Neuropathological, radiographic, electroencephalographic (EEG), regional blood flow, and cognitive tests have all been used to address the issue of abnormal cerebral laterality in schizophrenic subjects. Most of the studies reporting cortical atrophy in schizophrenia found it to be bilateral, with one exception reporting relatively more atrophy in the left frontal regions than in other brain areas.[108] Similarly, most EEG studies reported diffuse and bilateral abnormalities, with some exceptions suggesting increased left-hemisphere EEG variability in some subtype of schizophrenic subjects[87,252] or under evoked conditions.[253] Cerebral blood flow and cerebral glucography studies are consistent with bilateral frontal abnormalities showing a trend toward minor left frontal activation compared with the right lobe activation.

While the CT studies have explored the possibility of gross structural abnormalities in some patients with schizophrenia, other approaches were developed to assess potential disturbances in neuronal activity. Shifts in activity of the various brain regions have been the focus of cerebral blood flow studies and metabolic positron emission tomography (PET) scanning.

The determination of regional cerebral blood flow (rCBF) using the Xenon-133 (Xe-133) inhalation method has shown promise in uncovering abnormalities in schizophrenia. Neuronal activity is difficult to assess directly *in vivo;* however, indirect measures are available by virtue of the high correlation of activity with glucose metabolism, oxygen utilization, and local blood flow.[235,244] The Xe-133 inhalation method for determining rCBF has shown usefulness by its ability to determine decreases in blood flow following strokes and dementia, as well as increases in patients with epilepsy.[133,218,248] These findings have encouraged the utilization of rCBF techniques to assess brain dysfunction in psychopathological states.

PET has also been employed to address very similar issues. This technique uses a radiolabeled compound capable of emitting positrons, such as C-11, F-18, or O-15, and counting emissions using tomographic equipment quite similar in principal to that used in the CT scan. Most studies have used a glucose analogue, which is taken up by neurons at a rate proportional to their activity and enzymatically converted to a substance trapped within the cell.[283] The tomographic mapping of the brain produced by this technique is thought to represent the regional neuronal activity averaged over the long time scale necessary for adequate spatial resolution.

Several studies have reported evidence of differences in regional brain activities in schizophrenic patients compared to normal subjects,[41,42,46] although studies[109,115] not

finding such differences have also been reported. Lower whole brain activity, as reflected by blood flow, in schizophrenic patients has been reported by some studies[16]; while others, though not finding whole brain differences, reported shifts in rCBF in schizophrenic patients during quiet, resting conditions.[134] Most commonly, a relative decrease in blood flow to the frontal lobes has been found, both by Xe-133 inhalation techniques[16] and metabolic PET scanning.[90,115] Also reported are left-right hemispheric differences in blood flow of schizophrenic subjects relative to normal subjects under quiet, resting conditions, by both rCBF and PET scan methods.[271,337] Potentially more powerful techniques have recently been developed for assessing brain pathophysiology in schizophrenic subjects under conditions of cognitive arousal, when patterns of blood flow are typically shifted in normal subjects to brain regions thought to be involved in specific cognitive tasks.[109]

Electroencephalographic Studies

Regional brain activities can also be assessed using a recent methodological advance, brain electrical activity mapping (BEAM), which produces color-coded images of the topography of EEG amplitudes and can monitor the flow of electrical activity across the surface of the brain.[83] Additionally, BEAM maps can be made from composites of groups of subjects, allowing for regional comparison of EEG activity between groups.[82] This technique, when applied to schizophrenic patients, has suggested increased frontal delta waves compared to normal controls, just as other methodologies have suggested decreased neuronal activity in frontal lobes. In addition, fast beta-activity was observed in visually evoked potentials (EP) in the left parietal lobe of unmedicated schizophrenic patients, a fact consistent with increased left parietal irritability in schizophrenic patients.[207,208] This BEAM technique is an outgrowth of computerized analyses of standard EEG data, which have been often applied in the examination of pathophysiology in schizophrenia.

Nonspecific EEG abnormalities have been reported in schizophrenic patients.[45] The reported rate of EEG abnormalities ranges from 20 to 40 percent, compared to 0 to 10 percent in normal controls.[139,295] Chronic schizophrenic patients are found to have EEG wave patterns that are extremely regular,[269] diffusely abnormal,[92] and with poor response to stimulation and excessive slowing.[3] These very regular EEG recordings are often associated with poor prognosis.[230] In contrast, acute schizophrenic patients tend to show more paroxysmal activity,[75] with more alpha-rhythms and temporal lobe abnormalities.[92] Recordings from depth electrode implantation show random spike activity from the medio-basal frontal region in patients with normal scalp EEGs.[119,230]

A more sophisticated approach to the EEG is to record the effect of visual, auditory, or somatosensory stimuli, known as EPs. This technique provides the opportunity to compare the afferent and integrative neuronal processes of schizophrenic and normal subjects.[52] EPs can be divided in early, middle, and late phases. In normal controls, the early portion of the somatosensory EP, recorded at 50 milliseconds following the stimulus, has a maximum amplitude in the frontal regions, while in schizophrenic subjects the frontal signal is reduced and shifted centrally and postcentrally.[270] This finding is in agreement with dynamic studies (rCBF, PET, and BEAM) suggesting a frontal lobe disturbance in schizophrenia. The middle EP is reduced in schizophrenic subjects whether the stimulus is somatosensory, auditory, or visual.[44]

Contingent negative variation is an EP technique in which a subject is given two consecutive signals and asked to respond to the second one only. In normal subjects, but to a lesser extent in schizophrenic subjects, the first signal is extinguished by the following one as recorded on the EEG tracing.[257] This finding supports the clinical observation that schizophrenic patients may exhibit an attention deficit.

Neurological Studies

Evidence of regional neuronal dysfunction is also found in studies of the integrative mechanisms controlling fine eye muscle movements in schizophrenic subjects. Deviant eye tracking in schizophrenic subjects is believed to reflect low capacity to focus attention in tasks requiring continuous performance. Although part of eye tracking performance appears to be dependent on voluntary attention, an involuntary preattentive component may also be involved.[178]

Smooth pursuit eye movements (SPEMs) are the mechanism by which eye movements are matched to a moving target, thereby stabilizing moving images on the retina.[181,239] About half of the first-degree relatives of schizophrenic subjects demonstrate some qualitative disruption of SPEM, in comparison with 10 percent of the relatives of nonschizophrenic subjects.[123,178] There is also a significant concordance of this deficit among monozygotic twins concordant for schizophrenia.[124,140] These family studies suggest that psychosis per se is not responsible for the deficit and a related genetic predisposition for SPEM impairment and psychosis can be postulated. SPEM was observed to be impaired in a majority of schizophrenic patients.[178] Patients with structural brain diseases also demonstrated similar abnormalities.[63] Thus abnormal SPEMs may be a nonspecific marker of CNS dysfunction.[174]

Abnormal blink rate is another ocular abnormality observed in schizophrenic patients. Animal studies suggest that blink rate is at least partially under dopaminergic control. Blink rate was found to be increased by dopamine (DA) agonists and decreased by neuroleptics. Schizophrenic patients have generally an increased blink rate compared to normal subjects, and this rate is decreased by neuroleptic administration.[154,155,156] Further studies using provoked blinking and intraocular recordings are needed to clarify the relevance of this finding.

Other evidence of regional neuronal dysfunction in schizophrenia include peculiarity of gait, poor coordination, right-left disorientation, and poor graphesthetic ability, as well as nonaphasic speech disturbance. All of these are grouped together as a matter of convention as "neurological soft signs."[145] Neurological dysfunctions such as motor weakness, unilateral sensory impairment, pathological reflexes, and deficit disturbance of cranial nerves are grouped as "neurological hard signs."[305] The presence of the hard signs implies cerebral localization of the neurological deficit, while the pathophysiological mechanism involved in the presence of soft neurological signs is mostly unknown.

Multiple clinical studies have confirmed a higher frequency of soft neurological signs in schizophrenic patients compared with other psychiatric patients or controls.[305,311,312] This difference was found even in studies that accounted for age, sex, medication history, or chronicity.[233] The presence of soft neurological signs has been correlated by different researchers with low IQ, organicity on psychological tests, low birth weight and neonatal difficulties, severity of psychopathology, poor response to neuroleptics, and poor prognosis.[121,210,251] In spite of a persistently higher frequency of soft signs in schizophrenic patients and some possible clinical correlations, there is currently no generally accepted hypothesis relating this finding to the pathophysiology of schizophrenia.

These findings of nonspecific neuropathology and regional pathophysiology in schizophrenia are suggestive of disrupted cellular function in the CNS. Considerable effort has focused on identifying specific abnormalities, with special attention to potential abnormalities of neurotransmission. The next section describes the results of investigations based on several different hypotheses of neurochemical dysfunction.

¶ Neurotransmitters and Schizophrenia

Dopamine and Schizophrenia

The evidence that vulnerability to schizophrenia is genetically transmitted in some cases implies a biochemical defect in those patients. While there is no information on what genes or gene products may be involved in this process, considerable attention has been focused on the DA neuron in the CNS as a likely site of disturbance in schizophrenia.

The suggestion that some schizophrenic symptoms reflect central dopaminergic overactivity derives primarily from two complementary pharmacological pieces of evidence. Drugs that decrease dopaminergic activity can reduce schizophrenic symptoms,[55,193,238] while drugs that enhance or mimic dopaminergic activity worsen schizophrenic symptoms.[11,144,348] Basic research into the anatomy, physiology, and pharmacology of the dopaminergic system has accumulated some evidence in favor of the "dopaminergic hypothesis" in schizophrenia.[38,196] In addition, dopaminergic activity has been examined in clinical and postmortem studies in schizophrenic patients.

Although DA neurons perform diffuse neuroregulatory functions, they are also localized in a number of discrete pathways. Major DA pathways are nigrostriatal, tuberoinfundibular, mesolimbic, and mesocortical.[176] Nigrostriatal cell bodies are located in the substantia nigra, a pigmented nucleus in the midbrain. Axons projecting from those nerve cells terminate in the caudate and putamen of the neostriatum, synapsing with neurons containing receptors for DA.[314] Tuberoinfundibular dopaminergic pathways originate in neuronal cell bodies in the arcuate nucleus of the hypothalamus and terminate in the external layer of the median eminence.[101] The mesolimbic DA neuronal cell bodies are located in the ventral tegmental area of the midbrain, with axons projecting to the nucleus accumbens, septal nuclei, stria terminalis, and tuberculum olfactorium, structures composing the limbic forebrain.[314] These areas of the brain and other limbic nuclei are interconnected. The outflow of the limbic striatum is to the septum, hypothalamus, frontal lobe, and other cortical areas.[339] The mesocortical DA pathway originates in the mesencephalon and projects mainly into the frontal cortex.[24]

The nigrostriatal dopaminergic tract is involved in the regulation of extrapyramidal motor activity. Idiopathic Parkinson's disease is characterized by degeneration of dopaminergic neurons in the nigrostriatal tract,[126] resulting in DA deficiency and cholinergic predominance.[125] Clinically, Parkinson's disease is manifested by an extrapyramidal movement disorder very similar to that induced by antipsychotic drugs. Both idiopathic and neuroleptic-induced movement disorders are temporarily reversed by anticholinergic drugs, which should restore the DA-acetylcholine (Ach) balance.[161] These observations led to the hypothesis that neuroleptics block dopaminergic transmission and this blockade may be responsible for both the Parkinsonian and antipsychotic effects.[162]

Some discrepancies must be accounted for before such a conclusion can be reached, however. Clozapine and thioridazine hydrochloride are two antipsychotic drugs that infrequently produce Parkinsonian symptoms.[146] However, this may be due to their strong anticholinergic activity[204] and to the likelihood that DA-ACh balance is irrelevant in the brain area responsible for the antipsychotic effect.[26]

An additional problem with equating the antipsychotic and extrapyramidal effects originates from the screening method used to predict antipsychotic efficacy of new drugs. This method is based on the ability of the drug to block stereotypy in animals.[237] Stereotypy is a behavioral syndrome induced by DA agonists and regarded as the animal model of extrapyramidal symptoms.[236] By using the ability to block drug-induced stereotypy in animals as a predictor of antipsychotic effects, this screen makes it unlikely to uncover medications that do not produce extrapyramidal symptoms.

The tuberoinfundibular dopaminergic tract is involved in the neural control of prolactin and growth hormone secretion in the anterior pituitary lobe.[153,185,190] DA or agents enhancing DA release suppress prolactin and increase growth hormone secretion, and the reverse is true for agents that decrease dopaminergic activity, such as neuroleptics or reserpine.[202] Hence peripheral concentration of those two hormones could reflect, in part, central dopaminergic activity. If indeed schizophrenia is a consequence of generalized central DA hyperactivity that extends to the tuberoinfundibular dopaminergic neuron, one would expect that in unmedicated schizophrenic patients, prolactin levels would be reduced and growth hormone increased in comparison with controls. This is not borne out by clinical studies.* Any potential dopaminergic hyperactivity may be present in other brain areas relevant to the production of schizophrenia symptoms, but it does not seem to extend to the tuberoinfundibular system. In addition, multiple confounding factors can obliterate the difference between schizophrenic and normal subjects in neuroendocrine studies.[76]

The mesolimbic dopaminergic tract is believed to be involved in memory, learning, and affective symptoms.[136,145] The potential relevance of the mesolimbic system to schizophrenia mainly derives from the similarity between certain schizophrenic signs and symptoms resulting from experimental lesions or disease processes in this system. For example, hallucinations and disturbance in thinking have been reported after electrical stimulation of limbic structures.[129] Additionally, catatonia, paranoia, perceptual distortions, and mood changes have resulted from either stimulation or ablation of the limbic system in humans.[304] Viral encephalitis, neoplastic lesions, or epileptogenic foci located mainly in the temporal lobe may initially present as schizophrenic symptoms.[78,122,194]

Animal experiments further implicate the mesolimbic dopaminergic system in the pathophysiology of schizophrenic symptoms. Injection of DA intracerebrally into the tuberculum olfactorium or nucleus accumbens elicits an increase in the locomotor activity of the rat that is antagonized by neuroleptic

*See references 18, 88, 195, 198, 201, 258, and 323.

agents.[46] Thus reversal of this increase in locomotor activity by neuroleptics may be a reflection of their mesolimbic and perhaps antipsychotic action.

The mesocortical dopaminergic tract has been studied mainly through experimental destruction of the prefrontal cortex, the projection field of this tract.[23,43] In rodents and nonhuman primates, cortical ablation results in diminution of affective and social behavior, difficulty in suppressing irrelevant stimuli and consequent hyperactivity, and reduced performance in discrimination and delayed-response tasks.[99,100] An interesting hypothesis regarding the role of the mesocortical tract in schizophrenia is based on the observation that surgical or pharmacological induction of prefrontal dopaminergic hypoactivity may result in subcortical dopaminergic hyperactivity.[33,261] According to this hypothesis, if schizophrenia is etiologically related to frontal lobe dopaminergic hypoactivity, the subcortical or other cortical DA systems normally modulated by the prefrontal cortex might in turn be activated. The increased activity of these dopaminergic systems could account for some schizophrenic symptoms and for the therapeutic effect of the DA blocking agents in these systems.[21] Other schizophrenic symptoms related to frontal lobe dysfunction, such as cognitive and attention deficits—supposedly not mediated by subcortical dopaminergic hyperactivity, but perhaps by cortical hypoactivity—persist in schizophrenic patients on antipsychotic drugs when they attain partial remission.

Much of the evidence regarding the relation between the dopaminergic system and schizophrenia originates from the study of the antipsychotic drugs. When postsynaptic DA receptors are blocked by neuroleptic drugs, feedback mechanisms become involved in attempts to overcome the blockade. In the basal ganglia this feedback mechanism activates a short loop that consists of presynaptic DA receptors and a long loop that involves GABAergic and cholinergic neurons.[4,54,139] The increase in DA synthesis and turnover is reflected by an increase in homovanillic acid (HVA), the major DA metabolite.

Most neuroleptics with antipsychotic efficacy have a substantial effect on the production of HVA. Chemically related substances without antipsychotic action have negligible effects on HVA.[9] Thus the increase in DA turnover, as reflected by the HVA increase after the neuroleptic administration, has been proposed as relevant to their antipsychotic properties.[215] However, two neuroleptics, thioridazine and clozapine, do not have the predicted effect of increasing HVA production. Thioridazine, an antipsychotic agent generally regarded as equipotent with chlorpromazine, has a much lesser effect on HVA. Clozapine, an effective antipsychotic, also has less effect on HVA than would be expected based on its clinical potency.*

Another problem in associating increased DA turnover with antipsychotic activity arises from studies demonstrating that the increases seen in cerebrospinal fluid (CSF) HVA after acute neuroleptic administration return toward baseline with chronic neuroleptic exposure. Yet there is a lack of tolerance to the antipsychotic effects of neuroleptics. This is substantiated clinically by reported tolerance to neuroleptic-induced, striatal-mediated extrapyramidal reactions. A possible explanation for these discrepancies is that increased CSF HVA primarily reflects striatal DA neuron turnover. Hence mesolimbic and/or mesocortical DA systems, which develop tolerance more slowly, if at all, to neuroleptic-mediated increases in DA turnover, may be more likely loci of DA mediated psychotic symptoms.[39,196]

DA receptor binding has been demonstrated in brain membranes by labeling receptors both with the agonist tritiated DA and with the antagonist tritiated haloperidol, which seem to label specific agonist and antagonist sites respectively.[64,282] Antagonist binding has been proposed to be of more direct relevance to the clinical effects of antipsychotic drugs. The relative affinities of an

*See references 8, 105, 193, 285, and 338.

extensive series of antipsychotic agents, which include butyrophenones, phenothiazines, and other DA antagonists, in competing for tritiated haloperidol binding to the DA receptor correlate quite well with these drugs' clinical potencies in psychotic patients.[65] The close correlation between the clinical potencies of neuroleptics and their affinities in competing for the binding of tritiated haloperidol to DA postsynaptic receptors suggests that DA blockade is involved in the antipsychotic mechanism of these drugs.

Further evidence demonstrating a relationship between neuroleptic action and DA transmission is provided by recording the electrical activity of DA neurons after neuroleptic administration. These agents cause an increase in the firing rate of nigral DA neurons, corroborating the aforementioned feedback stimulation of DA neurons as evidenced by increased turnover following neuroleptic DA receptor blockade.[49] In contrast, the DA agonist amphetamine suppresses DA neuronal activity.[47] Antipsychotic agents reverse amphetamine-induced suppression of presynaptic DA neuronal activity.[49,50]

Neurotransmitters are believed to promote their physiological effect by interacting with receptors. The exact nature of the DA receptor is unclear, however; it has been suggested that DA may exert its effect postsynaptically at some sites through stimulation of a DA-sensitive membrane-bound enzyme, adenylate cyclase.[157] The activity of DA-sensitive adenylate cyclase is increased by DA, an effect blocked by neuroleptic drugs.[205] There is a rough correlation of clinical potency and the level of neuroleptic necessary to inhibit this enzyme. Inconsistencies, however, exist. Butyrophenones (e.g., haloperidol), indole derivatives (molindone), and the benzamide neuroleptics (metoclopramide and sulpiride) are all less potent inhibitors of DA-sensitive adenylate cylcase than might be predicted on the basis of their clinical potency.[64] One explanation for these exceptions is the existence of multiple DA receptors. Those coupled with adenylate cyclase activation by DA are termed D-1. That

clinically effective antipsychotics, like those mentioned, have little activity as antagonists of the adenylate cyclase system implicates the presence of a noncyclase-linked DA receptor, which has been labeled D-2 and may be particularly relevant in the etiology of schizophrenia.[279,280]

A second problem is that several tricyclic antidepressants, which lack antipsychotic activity, are as potent inhibitors of DA-sensitive adenylate cyclase as some clinically effective neuroleptics. Additionally, receptor supersensitivity to DA is not accompanied by an increase in DA-sensitive adenylate cyclase activity.[166] This may indicate that behavioral supersensitivity following the discontinuation of long-term antipsychotic drug treatment is mediated by a nonadenylate cyclase mechanism. Finally, no difference has been shown in DA-sensitive adenylate cyclase activity in the striatum between chronic schizophrenic and control autopsy brain tissue, and the use of selective DA agonists in binding studies have revealed in postmortem schizophrenic brain tissue an increase in D-2, but not D-1, receptor density.[53,279] Thus, taken together, the significance of D-2 receptors (DA receptors not coupled with adenylate cyclase) seems to be more relevant to the current treatment of schizophrenia than the D-1 receptors (DA receptors coupled with adenylate cyclase).

The DA hypothesis of schizophrenia has been lent further support by the examination of the clinical effect of both direct and indirect DA agonists. Levodopa, the precursor of DA, has been reported to worsen psychotic symptomatology in schizophrenic patients.[7,15,51] A psychosis resembling acute paranoid schizophrenia has been reported in human amphetamine users,[62] and, in clinical studies, amphetamine has produced a paranoid psychosis in normal volunteers.[11,12,15] Additionally, in some active schizophrenic patients, amphetamine[14,315] and methylphenidate[142,144] intensify preexisting psychotic symptoms. A dopaminergic mechanism is believed to underlie psychostimulant initiation and exacerbation of psychosis.

Recently this amphetamine-induced aggravation of psychosis has been shown to be state dependent. Schizophrenic patients whose symptoms worsened following amphetamine challenge were more psychotic at baseline than those patients who did not change. Additionally, patients treated with neuroleptics who worsened with amphetamine also had shown higher baseline psychotic ratings than those who remained stable. Thus chronic pretreatment with a DA receptor blocking agent did not consistently prevent amphetamine-induced increase in psychosis.[51,316,317,318] These data suggest that responsiveness to amphetamine reflects changes in clinical state, but that mechanisms underlying amphetamine activation of psychosis are not dependent solely on DA receptor actions. Furthermore, some schizophrenic patients improved when amphetamine was administered,[13] a fact that lends support to the syndromal heterogeneity theory of schizophrenia.

During the last two decades numerous attempts have been made to obtain direct clinical or postmortem evidence of DA hyperactivity in schizophrenic patients. CSF HVA concentration and dopaminergic-related enzyme activities in the periphery have been studied as possible markers for DA hyperactivity. HVA is the main DA metabolite in man and under many conditions reflects dopaminergic activity. Studies comparing CSF HVA in schizophrenic patients and normal controls have produced mainly negative findings.* However, differing CSF HVA concentrations have been found in subgroups of schizophrenic patients. Low CSF HVA was associated with poor prognosis[37] and the presence of first-rank Schneiderian symptoms,[36,231] while high CSF HVA was related to a positive family history of schizophrenia[267] and poor premorbid sexual adjustment.[170] These negative results may be explained by a multitude of factors. CSF HVA predominantly reflects DA activity in the nigrostriatum[284] and not in the limbic and cortical regions, which are more likely to be involved in schizophrenia.[201] Circadian and

*See references 28, 36, 58, 102, 231, and 267.

seasonal variations, physical activity, or factors related to the kinetics of CSF HVA accumulation can further cloud differences between patients and controls.[28] In addition, a state of DA hyperactivity mediated by receptor supersensitivity would have a paradoxical effect of lowering DA turnover and CSF HVA.

In addition to increased production, hyperdopaminergia could result from decreased inactivation of DA. Monoamine oxidase (MAO) is one of the enzymes involved in the conversion of DA into HVA in the brain and periphery. Low platelet MAO activity has been associated with paranoid symptoms and the presence of auditory hallucinations in schizophrenic patients.[265,266] However, long-term exposure to neuroleptics has also been shown to affect measurements of platelet MAO levels,[97] and a correlation between peripheral and brain MAO activity has not been established. Furthermore, the functional significance of any lowered MAO activity in schizophrenic patients is uncertain.[200] Current data suggest that an almost total inhibition of MAO activity would be required for functionally significant hyperdopaminergia to occur.[85] Furthermore, pharmacological inhibition of MAO activity with MAO inhibitors infrequently results in psychosis. Recent well-controlled postmortem studies comparing MAO activity in brain material from schizophrenic patients and control subjects have revealed no significant differences.[243]

Dopamine beta-hydroxylase (DBH) is the enzyme that catalyzes the conversion of DA to norepinephrine (NE) in noradrenergic neurons. Diminished activity of DBH in schizophrenic patients would involve the dopaminergic and the noradrenergic systems, producing an excessive accumulation of DA. In fact, drugs that inhibit DBH worsen schizophrenic symptoms.[120,260] Low CSF DBH levels were found to be of predictive value in acutely psychotic patients.[289] Nevertheless, the overwhelming majority of studies that compared DBH activity in the brain,[344] plasma,[84] or CSF[173] between schizophrenic patients and controls have not demonstrated any significant difference, although an inverse correlation has been reported between brain ventricular volume and CSF DBH concentration.[319]

Tyrosine hydroxylase (TH) is the initial and rate-limiting enzyme in the biosynthesis of catecholamine neurotransmitters. Thus the study of the regulation and pharmacological manipulation of its catalytic activity has been an obvious and intensive area of research. However, postmortem brain TH, like MAO, did not significantly differ between schizophrenic subjects and controls.[347]

Possible increased central DA activity has been sought in postmortem brain tissue by determining concentrations of DA and its major metabolite, HVA, in various brain regions. However, no consistent pattern has emerged in the several studies examining this issue, although there are some reports of increased DA in the caudate,[69,72] putamen,[71] and nucleus accumbens,[32] with elevations of HVA in the cingulate gyrus and frontal lobe.[20] These findings may reflect intrinsically more active DA neurons in some schizophrenic patients, or may simply be the result of increased activity in response to neuroleptic-induced blockade of postsynaptic receptors. These inconclusive findings on potential DA hyperactivity in schizophrenic patients have led to explorations of postsynaptic DA receptor activity.

Studies[171,183,223,240] of DA receptor densities in postmortem schizophrenic brains show strong evidence of increased neuroleptic binding sites relative to appropriate control tissue. This increase is limited to D-2 DA receptors. Interpretation of this finding, however, is confounded by the well-established ability of chronic neuroleptic administration to increase the number of DA receptors.[67,211] It is relatively rare to find postmortem tissue from schizophrenic patients who have never been exposed to neuroleptics, or even patients who were not exposed to the drug at least six months prior to death. Thus the finding of increased D-2 DA receptors in postmortem schizophrenic brain tissue may simply reflect prior medication use. Still, two studies have reported elevated D-2 DA receptor densities even in schizophrenic patients who were apparently drug-free,[66,223] but this finding could not be replicated by another group of investigators.[245]

A bimodal increase in DA receptor density in the caudate nucleus, putamen, and nucleus accumbens of schizophrenic patients has been reported. One mode occurred 25 percent above the control density, and the second mode occurred at a density 2.3 times that of controls for all three regions.[268] These results are suggestive of two different groups of schizophrenic patients, with one group having elevated DA receptors intrinsic to the disease process, and with a superimposition of neuroleptic-induced supersensitivity affecting both groups. Also plausible, however, is the existence of two modes of supersensitivity response to chronic antipsychotic use. Thus the potential etiological role of elevated postsynaptic D-2 DA receptor binding remains unresolved.

The recent development of *in vivo* receptor binding assays may be useful in addressing this issue. Positron-emitting neuroleptic analogues, which have similar pharmacological characteristics *in vitro* as neuroleptics, may produce PET scan images useful in the quantitative determination of D-2 DA receptor densities *in vivo*. To avoid the contamination of the issue with neuroleptic treatment effects, never-medicated individuals experiencing their first psychotic episodes would be ideal study candidates. Subsequently, clinical follow-up could establish which patients became truly schizophrenic, as reflected in their chronic course.

CRITIQUE OF THE DOPAMINE HYPOTHESIS

Although it is consistent with the pharmacological action of neuroleptics, major objections to the hyperdopaminergic hypothesis of schizophrenia have been raised.

1. No consistent evidence of DA hypersecretion has been found despite multiple postmortem and clinical studies.
2. Evidence for D-2 DA supersensitivity in postmortem schizophrenic brain tissue is

contaminated by the probable effects of neuroleptic on receptor number.

3. Neuroleptic drugs show no specificity for schizophrenia but rather have a general antipsychotic effect.

4. Some of the core symptoms in schizophrenia, such as anhedonia, negativism, and lack of motivation, are only partially affected by DA blocking agents.

5. DA agonists that would be expected to have a disastrous effect if administered to schizophrenic patients do not consistently worsen schizophrenic symptoms, particularly in the residual states of schizophrenia, and in certain instances prove to be therapeutic.

One of the limitations of the DA hypothesis may derive from the greatly simplified model of electrophysiology most often assumed, with a single population of homogenous DA neurons in simple feedback relations with their own firing rate and postsynaptic influences, maintaining a near-equilibrium homeostatic state. A nonlinear dynamic model of DA neuronal function has been developed that takes into account strong local dendrodendritic inhibitory feedback and long-loop striato-nigral feedback for neurons of the substantia nigra.[22] This model predicts that under perturbed conditions, populations of DA neurons may exist in two separate, quasi-stable states, one a relatively low steady firing rate and the other, more erratic and oscillating in behavior. The relative instability of the DA neuronal feedback loop may be associated in some way with the variable and chaotic clinical picture found in schizophrenia. The model predicts that increased effectiveness of DA postsynaptically, either through induced presynaptic activity or through postsynaptic receptor density or affinity, would shift DA neurons away from a simple homeostatic equilibrium toward a chaotic, abnormal domain, while neuroleptics would tend to return the system toward more stable behavior. While this model has yet to yield significant benefits for the treatment of schizophrenia, the development of even more realistic dynamic models of neuronal function may facilitate future research efforts in understanding the nature of this disease.

Alternatively, some of these inconsistencies may well prove to be the result of the etiological heterogeneity of the schizophrenic spectrum. An attempt to subdivide schizophrenia into the pathogenically distinct groups has received widespread attention. In this paradigm, the type I syndrome is associated with positive symptoms such as the presence of delusions, hallucinations, and thought disorder. Type II syndrome, or the "defect state," possesses negative symptoms such as affective flattening, poverty of speech, loss of drive, and intellectual impairment. It has been suggested that type I schizophrenia is etiologically related to a state of hyperdopaminergia, while type II schizophrenia is unrelated to DA or even represents a state of hypodopaminergia.[182]

Norepinephrine and Schizophrenia

Results from neurochemical, biochemical, and pharmacological investigations do not consistently support a dopaminergic hypothesis as the exclusive or primary lesion in the development of schizophrenia. Among alternative theories are those in which noradrenergic dysfunction is implied.

NE is extensively distributed in the brain of mammals.[206] The cell bodies are located in the lower brain stem, with dense projections into the limbic system. This neurotransmitter plays a part in numerous brain functions, including stress, rage, aggressiveness, locomotor behavior, arousal, reward, memory, sleep-wakefulness cycles, neuroendocrine regulation, and autonomic control.[138] Furthermore, NE may serve as a "gating" or "gain control" system for both inhibitory and excitatory inputs to a given neuronal system.[206]

Noradrenergic deficit[286] and excess[127] have both been hypothesized in the pathophysiology of schizophrenia. Noradrenergic deficit has been suggested on the basis of experimental work in reward/punishment paradigms and substantiated by postmortem enzyme measurements in human brain.[340] A noradrenergic deficit theory in schizophrenia has not, however, become universally accepted. The exclusive participation of NE in the reinforcement process has been challenged and appears untenable.[287,341] The CSF concentration of 3-methoxy-4-hydroxyphenylglycol (MHPG), the major metabolite of NE, is not altered appreciably during the active psychotic phase of schizophrenia, as compared to normal controls,[28,152,231] and the enzymatic deficit suggested has been disputed by investigations in the brain[346] and the periphery.[199] If a noradrenergic deficiency is a pathogenic trait in schizophrenia, then the noradrenergic blockade produced to some extent by all neuroleptics might be regarded as antitherapeutic.

In contrast to the noradrenergic deficit, an alternative hypothesis has been proposed based on experimental work in which an attentional deficit secondary to a hyperadrenergic state is postulated as the core deficit in schizophrenia.[164] This deficit is presumed to result from a dysfunction of brain regions concerned with attention, principally the reticular activation system (RS). In schizophrenia, there would be a general, non-specific arousal, resulting in a reduction of the filtering capacity of the RS and an overwhelming sensory load that gains access to consciousness. Since the activity of the reticular formation is affected by NE, increases in the level of activity of noradrenergic systems have been implied as a contributing factor in the generation of the schizophrenic symptomatology. This suggestion is consistent with the fact that compounds that, in part, increase noradrenergic brain activity (amphetamine, levodopa, tricyclic antidepressants) can activate patients and exacerbate schizophrenic symptomatology.[14,15,51,315] Furthermore, an elevated level of NE has been demonstrated in limbic system forebrain structures of schizophrenic patients and in their CSF.[31,91]

Although the correlation between NE-blockade and the clinical efficacy of neuroleptics is poor, an antinoradrenergic effect could complement the antipsychotic features mediated through DA-blockade. It also is important to recognize that blockade of postsynaptic DA receptors could indirectly reduce noradrenergic transmission.[9,29] Dopaminergic and noradrenergic pathways are anatomically close, and blockade of postsynaptic DA receptors increases the release of DA, increases its concentration within the synaptic cleft, and increases firing rates within the affected neuron. Should increased amounts of DA stimulate nearby DA receptors on noradrenergic presynaptic terminals, there could be an inhibition of NE release.[295]

Clinical attempts to refine a noradrenergic hypothesis of schizophrenia have been indirect and inconsistent. A larger fall in urinary MHPG in patients who showed complete remission of a schizophrenic process has been suggested,[153] implying an association between clinical improvement and reduced noradrenergic transmission. The possibility that beta-NE-blocking agents such as propranolol hydrochloride and iprindole reduce psychotic symptoms in schizophrenic patients also suggests that reduction in adrenergic transmission is a beneficial effect in schizophrenia.[19,104,113] However, the antipsychotic effect of beta-blockers may be based on a nonspecific membrane effect as well as beta-NE-blockade, and is not a universal finding. Clonidine hydrochloride, an alpha-NE-agonist that reduces noradrenergic transmission, has been investigated in clinical trials with either no effect or a deleterious effect on schizophrenic symptoms.[148] However, these data do not convincingly argue against a hypothesis of noradrenergic hyperactivity in schizophrenia, because doses that might adequately inhibit noradrenergic transmission could cause intolerable hypotension, as well as affect other neurotransmitter systems. The clinical examination of the hypernoradrenergic hypothesis in schizophrenia awaits the development of pharmacological agents with greater selectivity.

Alternatively, a modulatory function for NE is an attractive hypothesis, as it would unite the hyperdopaminergic hypothesis of schizophrenia with a hyperadrenergic hypothesis.[128] The projection system of noradrenergic neurons from the locus coeruleus in the rat brain suggests a unique capacity for NE to modify neuronal activity synchronously through a vast expanse of neocortex crossing both functional and architectural boundaries. Within the frontal cortex, these noradrenergic neurons are in close association with dopaminergic neurons—the latter, of course, being a proposed site of action of neuroleptics. Schizophrenia could readily involve multiple neurotransmitter abnormalities including NE, particularly in view of recent postmortem, urine, and CSF studies.[163,167,288]

Other Neurotransmitters and Schizophrenia

ACETYLCHOLINE

Like NE, ACh is another neurotransmitter that might interact with dopaminergic systems or independently influence schizophrenic symptoms. The initial suggestion that a cholinomimetic could improve the symptoms of schizophrenia was based on the effects of arecoline in patients with a diagnosis of catatonic schizophrenia. Arecoline was reported to produce a "brief lucid interval" in these patients.[98] The administration of another muscarinic agonist, oxotremorine, also produced short lucid intervals in otherwise withdrawn chronic schizophrenic patients.[60] Physostigmine, a reversible acetylcholinesterase inhibitor, has been given to schizophrenic patients refractory to antipsychotic medications. Neuroleptic agents were continued throughout physostigmine treatment. A marked reduction in schizophrenic symptoms coincident with the use of physostigmine has been seen. However, patients rapidly became tolerant to the effects of physostigmine and returned to their baseline level of psychopathology. Furthermore, physostigmine was found to reverse the aggravation in schizophrenic symptoms produced by methylphenidate hydrochloride.[143,144] This physostigmine-induced reversal of methylphenidate-induced exacerbation of schizo-

phrenia could in turn be antagonized by atropine.

These results suggest that there may be a balance between cholinergic and dopaminergic activity and that a relative overactivity of central dopaminergic neurotransmission or underactivity of cholinergic activity could contribute to schizophrenic symptoms. Attempts to find evidence of cholinergic activity in schizophrenic subjects by studying CSF acetylcholinesterase activity and postmortem brain examination of acetylcholinetransferase have resulted in equivocal findings. Although the cholinergic system may be involved to some degree in the psychotic process in some schizophrenic patients, whether its involvement is primary or only secondary to another disturbance in DA function remains to be clarified.

GAMMA-AMINOBUTYRIC ACID

The widespread inhibitory activity of gamma-aminobutyric acid (GABA) on many neuronal pathways in mammalian brain,[73] including DA, has led to the suggestion that GABA may be involved in the pathophysiology of schizophrenia.[249,251] *In vitro*, GABA inhibits the firing of DA neurons in the substantia nigra[335] and the ventral tegmental area,[343] which is the origin of the mesolimbic and mesocortical dopaminergic tract. If this inhibitory activity occurs physiologically, a reduction of GABAergic activity would be consistent with a state of dopaminergic hyperactivity. However, the precise relationship between the GABAergic and dopaminergic systems has not been clarified, GABA being reported to increase[112] or decrease* DA firing and turnover under different conditions.

At least some of the DA-mediated behaviors in animal studies, such as locomotor activity[30,61,262] and catalepsy,[220,263] are inhibited by GABA or GABA agonists. This relationship provides some support for the presumption that GABA is involved in schizophrenia. However, clinical studies in

*See references 35, 294, 325, 343.

which schizophrenic patients were treated with GABA agonists or GABA-related compounds in the hope that dopaminergic activity would be decreased have shown no therapeutic effect.[56,169,209,299] In an attempt to elucidate the GABAergic involvement in schizophrenia, CSF GABA concentrations and postmortem brain activity of the GABA-ergic system were measured in schizophrenic patients.* No conclusive evidence was obtained by either approach.[103] In spite of an attractive hypothesis of GABA deficiency inducing dopaminergic hyperactivity, no GABAergic involvement in schizophrenia can be established at present.

THE TRANSMETHYLATION HYPOTHESIS

Inspired by the observation that certain hallucinogenic agents like mescaline are structurally related to O-methylated derivatives of catecholamines,[222] the transmethylation hypothesis suggests that schizophrenia arises from the abnormal accumulation of a psychotogenic N- or O-methylated biogenic amine derivative. Incorrect methylation of catecholamines or indoleamines could produce "endogenous psychotogens" that structurally resemble hallucinogenic agents like mescaline, psilocybin, and LSD.[276] A related hypothesis suggests a deficit in the mechanism of the one-carbon cycle itself, which mediates all transmethylation reactions, rather than accumulation of any toxic product.[277]

Some circumstantial evidence supports the transmethylation hypothesis. The activity of methionine adenosyltransferase, an enzyme of the one-carbon cycle, was found to be reduced in some schizophrenic patients, and administration of methionine, a methyl donor, in combination with monoamines was found to produce abnormal behavioral symptoms.[35] However, most of the recent studies exploring different aspects of the transmethylation hypothesis do not support a role for the "endogenous psychotogens" in the etiology of schizophrenia.[187,191,275]

*See references 40, 70, 168, 227, and 320.

SEROTONIN

The serotonin (5HT) hypothesis of schizophrenia derives from the observation that LSD, a hallucinogenic compound, binds to 5HT receptors. However, the hallucinations following LSD administration are different and distinct from those spontaneously experienced by schizophrenic subjects.[281] An additional observation linking 5HT to schizophrenic symptoms is a similarity between this disorder and celiac disease, in which 5HT was found to be elevated.[57] These clinical observations prompted research aimed at obtaining direct evidence of 5HT excess or deficit.

Tryptophan, a dietary amino acid that can cross the blood-brain barrier and is the precursor of brain 5HT, was found decreased in acute schizophrenic subjects,[188] and its plasma concentration increased in parallel with clinical improvement.[107] Treatment with 5HT precursors had a mild therapeutic effect,[59,345] suggesting a 5HT deficit in schizophrenic subjects. However, other studies found a high level of platelet 5HT in schizophrenic subjects compared with controls.[96] Alternatively, it has been proposed that the involvement of 5HT in schizophrenia is not due to an excess or deficit, but to an abnormally methylated derivative of this neurotransmitter.

ENDORPHINS

The demonstration of stereoselective, saturable binding of radiolabeled opiate agonists and antagonists to membrane fractions prepared from specialized regions of CNS stimulated the discovery and isolation of endogenous morphine ligands.[176,177,272,301] Chemically these endogenous morphine ligands are a series of polypeptides referred to as endorphins. The isolation of endorphins was rapidly followed by the identification of a large series of diverse endorphin or enkephalinlike substances, as well as a host of other neuropeptides within the CNS.[114,176] Many of these compounds have highly specialized regional localizations, are released from either brain slices or synaptosomes upon electrical and potassium-induced depolarization, and have their release coupled to inward calcium ion conductance. Thus these neuropeptides are thought to share many common features with conventional neurotransmitters. Furthermore, the attribution of reproducible behavioral effects to certain neuropeptides, in addition to the known analgesic effects of endorphins, has opened a new area of biological investigation.[25,34,321]

An etiological role for endorphins in schizophrenia was suggested by early behavioral experiments in which a series of endogenous opioid peptides was administered to rats and mice.[34,141] In these experiments, opioid peptides were injected into the CSF or directly intracerebrally. The investigations showed that beta-endorphin was most potent in eliciting a long-lasting, naloxone-reversible cataleptic syndrome. The other peptide fragments examined included met-enkephalin, leu-enkephalin, alpha-endorphin, and gamma-endorphin. The cataleptic syndrome induced by beta-endorphin was characterized, in large part, by generalized muscular rigidity, absence of spontaneous movement, and the maintenance of awkward postures. The resemblance of this beta-endorphin–induced syndrome in rats to the catatonia and affective flattening seen in schizophrenia was consistent with an excess endorphinergic activity in schizophrenia.

However, an alternative interpretation suggested that the beta-endorphin–induced catalepsy resembled the syndrome induced by neuroleptics. Therefore, a possible deficiency or disturbance in availability of endorphins was proposed as an etiological mechanism. These preclinical data were used to support two diametrically opposed pharmacological approaches to treatment—administration of opiate antagonists and administration of exogenous opioid peptides. Despite the conflicting interpretations, the greater potency of beta-endorphin in the elicitation of the syndrome focused clinical attention upon this compound.[34,141]

The opioid antagonist naloxone has pro-duced improvement in the frequency of hallucinations and hallucinatory-related behavior experienced by schizophrenic patients. High doses of naloxone (10 mg) seem to result in a greater improvement, with neuroleptics exerting a synergistic effect, suggesting a relationship between the dopaminergic system and opioids.[229,324,327] In contrast, the effect of the opioid peptide beta-endorphin have been discouraging.[27,106,228]

In an attempt to obtain direct evidence of decreased or increased opioid activity in schizophrenia, patients' CSF was compared to normal controls.[212] Schizophrenic males, but not females, showed a lower opioid activity than controls. However, those findings do not extend to gamma-endorphins and raise issues regarding complicated endocrine-opioid interactions in schizophrenia.

The beta-endorphin fragment destyrosine-gamma-endorphin (DTγE, LPH$_{62\text{-}77}$) has been indentified in mammalian pituitary and may be an endogenous neuropeptide with antipsychotic efficacy. A potential antipsychotic effect of DTγE would be consistent with a variety of preclinical and human data.[77,322] The peptide has been shown to facilitate the extinction of conditioned avoidance task in the rat; displace *in vivo* radiolabeled spiroperidol from binding sites in rat hypothalamus, corpus striatum, and mesolimbic regions; and have effects similar to neuroleptics on the H-reflex, a monosynaptic spinal reflex, in human subjects. Furthermore, direct administration of DTγE into the rat nucleus accumbens inhibited the ability of methylphenidate to induce locomotor activity when injected directly into this mesolimbic nucleus.

However, DTγE had no effect on the increased locomotor activity induced by the direct injection of DA, a direct acting agonist, into the nucleus accumbens of rats. In addition, DTγE lacks other aspects of the pharmacological profile characteristic of and used to screen potential antipsychotic medications in preclinical studies. For example, DTγE fails to induce catalepsy, diminish exploration, or inhibit drug-induced stereotypy in rats. Moreover, *in vitro* studies suggest that it does not act directly at the DA receptor binding site.

Studies in which DTγE was administered to schizophrenic patients for short periods of time showed symptomatic improvement in some patients and no change in others. Furthermore, the antipsychotic effects of DTγE may not be mediated through direct DA receptor blockade. Serum prolactin elevation occurs following neuroleptic administration and is due to blockade of DA receptors in the pituitary. DTγE administration to schizophrenic patients does not result in elevation of serum prolactin levels.[197] Although a therapeutic role for DTγE in schizophrenia is unclear at this time,[298,300] the data are consistent with gamma-type endorphins possessing a possible neuroregulatory role in dopaminergic transmission. Future long-term clinical trials with this compound are awaited.

PROSTAGLANDINS

Prostaglandins are fatty acids present in most of the body tissues.[234,342] They play a variety of functions in inflammatory processes, fever, and pain sensitivity. Prostaglandin E_1 (PGE_1) was implicated in the pathophysiology of schizophrenia by a study reporting that adenosine diphosphate stimulates the release of this prostaglandin (PG) in platelets of normals and patients with affective disorders, but not in schizophrenic patients, suggesting a PGE_1 deficiency in schizophrenic patients.[1] This suggestion was supported by findings of low PGE_1-stimulated cyclic adenosine monophosphate accumulation in platelets of schizophrenic patients.[259] The PGE_1 deficiency in schizophrenia is also supported by observations that schizophrenic patients have a low incidence of rheumatoid arthritis, which is associated with PG excess.[130,131,132] Also, high doses of PGs may produce schizophrenialike symptoms.[303,313] Contrary to this hypothesis, at least one study reported high PGE_1 in schizophrenic patients[192]; however, treatment with prostaglandin E-suppressant drugs was not salutary.[89]

¶ Viral Abnormalities and Schizophrenia

Schizophrenialike symptoms are seen occasionally in association with influenzas, encephalitis, and other diseases caused by viruses.[304,306] Several epidemiological, biochemical, and clinical observations in schizophrenia are consistent with a viral etiology, including a preponderance of birth of schizophrenic subjects in winter and early spring,[74,117,118] unequal geographical distributions with pockets of relatively high distribution, antiviral or antibrain antibodies in serum or CSF, and abnormal leucocytes.[5,309,310]

The excess of births of schizophrenic subjects in the winter has proved to be a highly reproducible finding, especially accentuated in areas with severe winter climates.* This has been interpreted to reflect the increased likelihood of an intrauterine viral infection at a time of fetal CNS developmental susceptibility, during a period of peak maternal exposure. Alternatively, environmental influences that change through the seasons, such as maternal food intake, potential for dehydration, or physical activity level, may be responsible for the observed seasonality of schizophrenic births.

Other evidence consistent with a possible viral etiology for some schizophrenic subjects includes the cyclical clinical course of the illness, compatible with repeated reactivation and remission of an infectious agent or immunological process.[294] Herpes simplex virus and cytomegalovirus are known to preferentially invade limbic structures and thus have been suggested as potential causative agents in some schizophrenic subjects.[305] Reports of increased fibrillary gliosis, neuronal loss, or severe mineralization mainly in the limbic system of postmortem schizophrenic brain tissue[149,291,294] are compatible with a postviral inflammatory process. More directly, the CSF/serum ratio of IgG and CSF IgM level against cyto-

---

*See references 219, 225, 307, 308, and 322.

megalovirus were both found to be increased in a group of schizophrenic subjects compared with controls.[5] Similarly elevated levels of CSF IgG against herpes simplex virus were found in the CSF of schizophrenic subjects.[175] Other studies, however, have been unable to replicate this finding.[294]

A viral role in the etiology of schizophrenia may be compatible with neurochemical and genetic observations. Viruses may alter binding of other substances to the cell membrane and direct the cellular metabolic processes without destroying the host cell.[256] A viral genome, incorporated in the cell nucleus, can be transmitted with the genetic material of the host cell. Nonspecific factors like hospitalization, place of residence, and shared antigen reactivity with other viruses have to be considered before a clear relationship can be established between viral infection and schizophrenia. Current evidence is at best circumstantial for a possible role of viruses in chronic psychosis.

¶ Abnormal Reaction to Gluten and Schizophrenia

Epidemiological and some experimental evidence are consistent with the suggestion that the protein fraction of the cereal grains, gluten, may be a contributing factor in the production of schizophrenic symptoms in some individuals. Clinical observations have noted the coexistence of gluten enteropathy and schizophrenia. Furthermore, psychiatric symptoms have been noted in adult celiac disease patients consuming a gluten-containing diet. Worldwide epidemiologic studies have found a parallel reduction in first admissions for schizophrenia and per-capita consumption of gluten-rich foods.[80]

Initial studies that restricted schizophrenic patients to gluten-free diets showed symptomatic improvement in some, compared with patients placed on a regular diet.[81] Furthermore, when patients on the gluten-free diet were given foods containing gluten, there was significant worsening.[246,273] However, those findings were not replicated, and

symptomatic worsening was even reported by one study in patients on a gluten-free diet.[221,232,296] Thus the potential role of gluten in the pathophysiology of some schizophrenic subjects remains unresolved.

¶ Conclusion

In conclusion, studies of the biology of schizophrenia have produced many findings of CNS dysfunction, none specific for this disease and none shared by everyone with the diagnosis. Evidence is strong that some schizophrenic subjects have expressed a heritable vulnerability to the disorder. The clinical and preclinical evidence that neuroleptics reverse some symptoms of some schizophrenic subjects and interfere with neural transmission in specific regions supports the hypothesis of abnormal regional neuronal activities in some schizophrenic subjects. Direct evidence for a specific neurotransmitter or receptor abnormality is not yet available. One hopes that as knowledge of normal CNS anatomy and physiology expands and new methods for exploring aberrations from normal become available, new insights into the cause or causes of this very devastating illness will be possible.

¶ Bibliography

1. ABDULLA, Y. H., and HAMADAH, K. "Effect of ADP on PGE$_1$ Formation in Blood Platelets from Patients in Depression, Mania and Schizophrenia," *British Journal of Psychiatry*, 127 (1975):591–595.

2. ABENSON, M. H. "EEG's in Chronic Schizophrenia," *British Journal of Psychiatry*, 116 (1970):421–425.

3. ABRAMS, R., and TAYLOR, M. A. "Differential EEG Pattern in Affective Disorders and Schizophrenia," *Archives of General Psychiatry*, 38 (1979):1355–1358.

4. AGHAJANIAN, G. K., and BUNNEY, B. S. "Dopamine Autoreceptors: Pharmacological Characterization by Micro-ion-

tophoretic Single-cell Recording Studies," *Naunyn-Schmiedeberg's Archives of Pharmacology,* 297 (1977):1–7.

5. ALBRECHT, P., et al. "Raised Cytomegalovirus Antibody Levels in Cerebrospinal Fluid in Schizophrenia," *Lancet,* 2 (1980):769–772.

6. ALLEN, M. G., COREN, S., and POLLIN, W. "Schizophrenia in Veteran Twins: A Diagnostic Review," *American Journal of Psychiatry,* 128 (1972):939–945.

7. ALPERT, M., et al. "Paradoxical Reaction to L-DOPA in Schizophrenic Patients," *American Journal of Psychiatry,* 135 (1978):1329–1332.

8. ANDEN, N. E., and STOCK, G. "Effect of Clozapine on the Turnover of Dopamine in the Corpus Striatum and in the Limbic System," *Journal of Pharmacy and Pharmacology,* 25 (1973):396–398.

9. ANDEN, N. E., BUTCHER, S. G., and CORRODONI, H. "Receptor Activity and Turnover of Dopamine and Noradrenaline after Neuroleptics," *European Journal of Pharmacology,* 11 (1970):303–314.

10. ANDREASEN, N. C., et al. "Ventricular Enlargement in Schizophrenia: Relationship to Positive and Negative Symptoms," *American Journal of Psychiatry,* 139 (1982):297–302.

11. ANGRIST, B., and GERSHON, S. "Clinical Response to Several Dopamine Agonists in Schizophrenic and Nonschizophrenic Subjects," *Advances in Biochemical Psychopharmacology,* 16 (1977):667–680.

12. ANGRIST, B., LEE, H. K., and GERSHON, S. "The Antagonism of Amphetamine-Induced Symptomatology by Neuroleptics," *American Journal of Psychiatry,* 131 (1976):817–819.

13. ANGRIST, B., ROTROSEN, J., and GERSHON, S. "Differential Effects of Amphetamine and Neuroleptics on Negative vs. Positive Symptoms in Schizophrenia," *Psychopharmacology,* 72 (1980):17–19.

14. ———. "Responses to Apomorphine, Amphetamine and Neuroleptics in Schizophrenia Subjects," *Psychopharmacology,* 67 (1980):31–38.

15. ANGRIST, B., SATHANATHAN, G., and GERSHON, S. "Behavioral Effects of L-Dopa in Schizophrenic Patients," *Psychopharmacology,* 31 (1973):1–12.

16. ARIEL, R. N., et al. "Regional Cerebral Blood Flow in Schizophrenics: Tests Using the Xe 133 Inhalation Method," *Archives of General Psychiatry,* 40 (1983):258–263.

17. ASANO, N. "Pneumonoencephalographic Study of Schizophrenia," in H. Mitsuda, ed., *Clinical Genetics in Psychiatry: Problems in Nosological Classification.* Tokyo: Fgankashoin Ltd., 1967, pp. 209–219.

18. ASNIS, G. M., and RYAN, N. D. "The Psychoneuroendocrinology of Schizophrenia," in A. Rifkin, ed., *Schizophrenia and Affective Disorders, Biology and Drug Treatment.* Boston: John Wright, 1983, pp. 205–236.

19. ATSMON, A., BLUM, J., and STEINER, M. "Further Studies with Propranolol in Psychotic Patients; Relation to Initial Psychotic State, Urinary Catecholamines and 3-Methoxy 4-Hydroxyphenylglycol Excretion," *Psychopharmacology,* 27 (1972):249–252.

20. BACOPOLOUS, N., et al. "Antipsychotic Drug Action in Schizophrenic Patients: Effect on Cortical Dopamine Metabolism after Long-Term Treatment," *Science,* 205 (1979):1405–1407.

21. BANNON, M. J., and ROTH, R. H. "Pharmacology of Mesocortical Dopamine Neurons," *Psychopharmacology Review,* 1 (1983):53–68.

22. BARCHAS, J. D., KING, R., and BERGER, P. A. "Neuroregulators and Schizophrenia: A Look at the Dopamine and Endorphin Hypothesis," in H. C. Stancer, P. E. Garfinkel, and V. M. Rakoff, eds., *Guidelines for the Use of Psychotropic Drugs.* New York: Spectrum Publications, 1984, pp. 261–275.

23. BECKSTEAD, R. M. "Convergent Thalamic and Mesencephalic Projections to the Anterior Medial Cortex in Rat," *Journal of Comparative Neurology,* 166 (1976):403–416.

24. BERGER, B., et al. "Dopaminergic Innervation of the Rat Pre-frontal Cortex: A Fluorescent Histochemical Study," *Brain Research,* 106 (1976):133–145.

25. BERGER, P. A. "Investigating the Role of Endogenous Opioid Peptides and Be-

havior: A Critical Analysis of Research Strategies," *Neuroscience Research Progress Bulletin*, 16 (1978):585–599.

26. BERGER, P. A., ELLIOTT, G. R., and BARCHAS, J. D. "Neuroregulators in Schizophrenia," in M. A. Lipton, ed., *Pharmacology: A Generation of Progress*. New York: Raven Press, 1978, pp. 1071–1082.

27. BERGER, P. A., WATSON, S. G., and AKIL, H. "Beta Endorphin and Schizophrenia," *Archives of General Psychiatry*, 37 (1980):635–640.

28. BERGER, P. A., et al. "CSF Monoamine Metabolites in Depression and Schizophrenia," *American Journal of Psychiatry*, 137 (1980):174–180.

29. BERRIDGE, T. L., and SHARMA, D. F. "The Effect of Tranquilizing Drugs on the Concentration of the Sulfate Ester of 4-Hydroxy-3-Methoxyphenylethan-1,2-Diol in Rat Brain," *British Journal of Pharmacology*, 50 (1974):156–158.

30. BINAS, B., and CARLSSON, A. "Effect of Intraperitoneally Administered GABA on Locomotor Activity of Mice," *Psychopharmacology*, 59 (1978):91–94.

31. BIND, E. D., SPOKES, E. G., and IVERSEN, L. L. "Brain Norepinephrine and Dopamine in Schizophrenia," *Science*, 204 (1979):93–94.

32. BIND, E. D., et al. "Increased Brain Dopamine and Reduced Glutamic Acid Decarboxylase and Choline Acetyl-Transferase Activity in Schizophrenics and Related Psychoses," *Lancet*, 2 (1977):1157–1159.

33. BLANE, G., et al. "Response to Stress of Mesocortical Frontal Dopaminergic Neurons in Rats after Long-Term Isolation," *Nature* (London), 284 (1980): 265–267.

34. BLOOM, F., SEGAL, D., and LING, N. "Endorphins' Profound Behavioral Effects in Rats Suggest New Etiological Factors in Mental Illness," *Science*, 194 (1976): 630–632.

35. BOURDILLON, R. E., CLARKE, C. A., and RIDGES A. P. "Pink Spot in the Urine of Schizophrenics," *Nature*, 208 (1965): 453–455.

36. BOWERS, M. B., JR. "5-Hydroxyindoleacetic Acid (5-HIAA) and Homovanillic Acid (HVA) Following Probenecid in Acute Psychotic Patients Treated with Phenothiazines," *Psychopharmacology*, 28 (1973):309–318.

37. ———. "Central Dopamine Turnover in Schizophrenia Syndromes," *Archives of General Psychiatry*, 31 (1974):50–54.

38. ———. "Biochemical Processes in Schizophrenia Update," *Schizophrenia Bulletin*, 6 (1980):323–403.

39. BOWERS, M. B., JR. and ROSITIS, A. "Regional Differences in Homovanillic Acid: Concentration After Acute and Chronic Administration of Antipsychotic Drugs," *Journal of Pharmacy and Pharmacology*, 26 (1974):743–745.

40. BOWERS, M. B., JR., GOLD, B., and ROTH, R. "CSF—GABA in Psychotic Disorders." *Psychopharmacology*, 70 (1980): 279–282.

41. BRODIE, J. D., et al. "Evaluation of Regional Glucose Metabolism with Positron Emission Tomography in Normal and Psychiatric Populations," in W. D. Hess and M. E. Phelps, eds., *Positron Emission Tomography of the Brain*. Berlin: Springer-Verlag, 1983, pp. 201–206.

42. BRODIE, J. D., et al. "Patterns of Metabolic Activity in the Treatment of Schizophrenia," *Annals of Neurology* (Supplement), 15 (1984):5166–5169.

43. BROWN, R. M., CRANE, A. M., and GOLDMAN, P. S. "Regional Distribution of Monoamines in the Cerebral Cortex and Subcortical Structures in the Rhesus Monkey: Concentration and *in vivo* Synthesis Rates," *Brain Research*, 168 (1979):133–150.

44. BUCHSBAUM, M. S., "The Middle Evoked Response Components and Schizophrenia," *Schizophrenia Bulletin*, 3 (1977): 93–104.

45. ———. "Neuropsychological Syndrome," in L. Bellak, ed., *Disorders of the Schizophrenia Syndrome*. New York: Basic Books, 1978, pp. 152–180.

46. BUCHSBAUM, M. S., et al. "Cerebral Glucography with Positron Tomography: Use in Normal Subjects and in Patients with Schizophrenia," *Archives of General Psychiatry*, 39 (1982):251–259.

47. BUNNEY, B. S., and AGHAJANIAN, G. K. Evidence of Drug Actions on the Pre- and Postsynaptic Catecholamine

Receptors in CNS," in E. Udsin and W. E. Bunney, eds., *Pre- and Postsynaptic Receptors.* New York: Marcel Dekker, 1955, pp. 89–122.

48. ———. "Electrophysiological Effects of Amphetamine on Dopamine Neurons," in S. H. Snyder and E. Volsin, eds., *Frontiers in Catecholamines Research.* New York: Pergamon Press, 1973, pp. 957–963.

49. ———. "Mesolimbic and Mesocortical Dopaminergic System Physiology and Pharmacology," in M. A. Lipton, A. Dimascio, and K. F. Killam, eds., *Psychopharmacology: A Generation of Progress.* New York: Raven Press, 1978, pp. 159–167.

50. BUNNEY, B. S., et al. "Dopaminergic Neurons—Effects of Antipsychotic Drugs and Amphetamine on Single Cell Activity," *Journal of Pharmacological and Experimental Therapeutics,* 185 (1973): 560–571.

51. CAHIL, H. M., YESAVAGE, J. A., and HOLLISTER, L. E. "Low-dose Levadopa in Schizophrenia," *Communications in Psychopharmacology,* 1 (1977):593–596.

52. CALLOWAY, E. *Brain Electrical Potentials and Individual Psychological Differences.* New York: Grune & Stratton, 1975.

53. CARENSI, A., et al. "Dopamine-Sensitive Adenyl Cyclase in Human Caudate Nucleus: A Study in Control Subjects and Schizophrenic Patients," *Archives of General Psychiatry,* 38 (1978):1056–1059.

54. CARLSSON, A. "Mechanism of Action of Neuroleptics," in M. A. Lipton, A. Di-Mascio, and K. F. Killam, eds., *Pharmacology: A Generation of Progress.* New York: Raven Press, 1979, pp. 1057–1070.

55. CARLSSON, A., and LINDQUIST, M. "Effect of Chlorpromazine and Haloperidol on Formation of 3-Methoxytyramine and Normetanephrine in Mouse Brain," *Acta Pharmacologia et Toxologia,* 20 (1963):140–144.

56. CASSEY, D., GERLACH, J., and CHRISTENSSON, E. "Behavioral Aspects of GABA-dopamine Interrelationship in the Monkey," *Brain Research Bulletin,* 5 (Supplement 2) (1980):269–273.

57. CHALLACOMBE, D. N. "5-hydroxytryptamine Metabolism in Coeliac Disease," in G. Hemmings and W. A. Hemmings, eds., *Biological Basis of Schizophrenia.* Baltimore: University Park Press, 1978, pp. 209–212.

58. CHASE, T. N., cited in Schnur, J. A., and GORDON, E. K. "Cerebrospinal Fluid Catabolites in Drug-Induced Extrapyramidal Disorders," *Neuropharmacology,* 9 (1970):265–268.

59. CHOWINARD, G., ANNABEL, L., and YOUNG, S. N. "A Controlled Study of Trytophan-Benserazide in Schizophrenia," *Communications in Psychopharmacology,* 2 (1978):21–31.

60. COLLARD, J., LECOQ, R., and DEWARET, A. "Un Essai d'un Acetylcholinique: L'Oxotremorine," *Acta Neurologica Belgica,* 65 (1968):122.

61. COLTT, J., and ENGEL, J. "Suppression by GABA-ergic Drugs of the Locomotor Stimulation Induced by Morphine, Amphetamine, Apomorphine: Evidence for Both Pre- and Postsynaptic Inhibition of Catecholamine System," *Journal of Neural Transmission,* 40 (1977):253–268.

62. CONNELI, P. H. *Amphetamine Psychosis.* Mandsley Monograph 5. London: Oxford University Press, 1958.

63. CORVERA, J., TORRES-COURTNEY, G., and LOPEZ-RIOS, G. "The Neurological Significance of Alteration of Pursuit Eye Movements and Pendular Eye Tracking Test," *Annals of Otology and Laryngology,* 82 (1973):855–867.

64. CREESE, J., BURT, D. R., and SNYDER, S. H. "Dopamine Receptor Binding Predicts Clinical Pharmacological Potencies of Antischizophrenic Drugs," *Science,* 192 (1976):481–483.

65. ———. "Biochemical Actions of Neuroleptic Drugs—Focus on the Dopamine Receptor," in L. L. Iversen and S. H. Snyder, eds., *Handbook of Psychopharmacology.* New York: Plenum Press, 1978, pp. 37–89.

66. CROSS, A. J., CROW, T. J., and OWEN, F. "3H Fluphenthixol Binding in Postmortem Brains of Schizophrenics: Evidence for Selective Increase in Dopamine D_2 Receptors," *Psychopharmacology,* 74 (1981):122–126.

67. CROW, T. J. "Molecular Pathology Receptors of Schizophrenia: More than One Disease Process," *British Medical Journal,* 280 (1980):66–68.

68. ——. "Postmortem Evidence for Temporal Lobe Disturbance in Schizophrenia," Paper presented at the Biological Psychiatry Conference, Los Angeles, May 1983.

69. CROW, T. J. et al. "Dopaminergic Mechanisms in Schizophrenia: The Antipsychotic Effect and the Disease Process," *Life Science,* 23 (1978):563–568.

70. CROW, T. J., et al. "Letter," *Lancet,* 2 (1978):36–37.

71. CROW, T. J., et al. "Monoamine Mechanisms in Chronic Schizophrenia: Postmortem Neurochemical Findings," *British Journal of Psychiatry,* 134 (1979):249–256.

72. CROW, T. J., et al. "Time Course of the Antipsychotic Effect of Schizophrenia and Some Changes in Postmortem Brain and Their Relationship to Neuroleptic Medication," *Advances in Biochemical Psychopharmacology,* 24 (1980):495–503.

73. CURTIS, D. A. "GABA-ergic Transmissions in the Mammalian Central Nervous System," in P. Krogsgaard-Larsen, J. Schell-Kruger, and E. Koford, eds., *GABA Neurotransmitters: Pharmacochemical, Biochemical and Pharmacologic Aspects.* Copenhagen: Munksgaard, 1979.

74. DALEN, P. "Month of Birth in Schizophrenia," *Acta Psychiatrica Scandinavica* (Supplement) 203 (1968):55–60.

75. DAVIES, R. N., NEIL, J. F., and HIMMELHOCH, J. M. "Cerebral Dysrhythmias in Schizophrenics Receiving Phenothiazines: Clinical Correlates," *Chemical Electroencephalography,* 6 (1978):103–115.

76. DAVIS, B. M., et al. "Methodological Problems in Evaluating Prolactin Response to Dopamine Agonists in Schizophrenia," *Archives of General Psychiatry,* in press.

77. DAVIS, K. L., SAMUEL, A., and MATHÉ, A. A. "Intracerebral Des-tyrosine-gamma-endorphins Inhibits Methylphenidate-Induced Locomotor Activity," *Life Science,* 28 (1981):2421–2422.

78. DAVISON, K., and BUGLEY, C. R. "Schizophrenia-like Psychosis Associated with Organic Disorders of the CNS: A Review of the Literature," *British Journal of Psychiatry* (Special Publication) 4 (1969):113–184.

79. DICHIERA, G., et al. "Striato-Nigral and Nigro-talamic GABAergic Neurons as Output Pathways for Striatal Responses," in P. Korgsgaard-Larsen, J. Schell-Kruger, and H. Kofod, eds., *GABA Neurotransmitters Pharmacochemical, Biochemical and Pharmacological Aspects.* Copenhagen: Munksgaard, 1979, pp. 456–481.

80. DOHAN, F. C. "Schizophrenia: Are Some Food-Derived Polypeptides Pathogenic? Cardiac Disease as a Model," in G. Hemmings and W. A. Hemmings, eds., *Biological Basis of Schizophrenia.* Baltimore: University Park Press, 1978, pp. 167–178.

81. DOHAN, F. C., GRASBERGER, J. C., and LOWELL, F. M. "Relapsed Schizophrenics: More Rapid Improvement on Milk and Cereal-Free Diet," *British Journal of Psychiatry,* 115 (1969):595–596.

82. DUFFY, E. H., BARTELS, P. H., and BURCHFIELD, J. L. "Significance Probability Mapping: An Aid in the Topographic Analysis of Brain Electrical Activity," *Electroencephalography and Clinical Neurophysiology,* 51 (1981): 455–462.

83. DUFFY, F. H., BURCHFIELD, J. L., and LOMBROSCO, C. T. "Brain Electrical Activity Mapping (BEAM): A Method for Extending the Clinical Utility of EEG and Evoked Potential Data," *Annals of Neurology,* 5 (1979):309–332.

84. DUNNER, D. L., et al. "The Activity of Dopamine Hydroxylase and Methionine Activating Enzyme in Blood of Schizophrenic Patients," *Biological Psychiatry,* 6 (1973):215–220.

85. EDWARDS, D. J. "Molecular Properties of the Monoamine Oxidase," *Schizophrenia Bulletin,* 6 (1980):275–281.

86. ESSEN-MOLLER, E. "Psychiatrische Untersuchungen an Einer Seric von Zwillingen," *Acta Psychiatrica Scandinavica* (Supplement), 23 (1964):1–200.

87. ETEVENON, P., et al. "Intra- and Inter-

hemispheric EEG Differences Quantified by Spectral Analysis," *Acta Psychiatrica Scandinavica,* 60 (1979): 57–68.

88. ETTIGI, P., NEIR, N.V.P., and LAL, S. "Effect of Apomorphine on Growth Hormone and Prolactin Secretion in Schizophrenic Patients With and Without Oral Dyskinesia Withdrawn from Neuroleptic Therapy," *Journal of Neurology, Neurosurgery, and Psychiatry,* 39 (1976):870–876.

89. FALLON, I., WATT, D. C., and LUBE, K. "N-Acetyl-P-Amino-Phenol (Pariecetanol Acetminophen) in the Treatment of Acute Schizophrenia," *Psychological Medicine,* 8 (1978):495–499.

90. FARKAS, T., et al. "The Application of 18-F-2-Deoxy-2-Fluoro-d-glucose and Positron Emission Tomography in the Study of Psychiatric Conditions," in J. V. Passoneau, R. A. Hawkins, and W. D. Lust, eds., *Cerebral Metabolism and Neural Function.* Baltimore: Williams & Wilkins, 1980, pp. 403–408.

91. FARLEY, I. J., et al. "Norepinephrine in Chronic-paranoid Schizophrenia: Above-Normal Levels in Limbic Forebrain," *Science,* 200 (1978):456–458.

92. FENTON, G. W., et al. "EEG Spectral Analysis in Schizophrenia," *British Journal of Psychiatry,* 136 (1980):445–455.

93. FISCHER, M. "Genetic and Environmental Factors in Schizophrenia," *Acta Psychiatrica Scandinavica* (Supplement) 238 (1973):9–142.

94. FISHMAN, M. "The Brain Stem in Psychosis," *British Journal of Psychiatry,* 126 (1975):414–422.

95. FLOR-HENRY, P. *Cerebral Basis of Psychopathology.* Boston: John Wright, 1983.

96. FREEDMAN, D. Y., BELENDINK, K., and BELENDINK, G. W. "Blood Tryptophan Metabolism in Chronic Schizophrenics," *Archives of General Psychiatry,* 38 (1981):655–659.

97. FRIDEHOFF, A. J., MILLER, J. C., and WEISENFREUND, J. "Human Platelet MAO in Drug-free Medicated Schizophrenic Patients," *American Journal of Psychiatry,* 135 (1978):952–955.

98. FULCHER, J. H., GALLAGHER, W. J., and PFEIFER, C. C. "Comparative Lucid Interval After Amobarbital, CO_2 and Arecoline in the Chronic Schizophrenic," *Archives of Neurology and Psychology,* 78 (1957):392–395.

99. FUSTER, J. M. *The Prefrontal Cortex: Anatomy, Physiology and Neuropsychology of the Frontal Lobe.* New York: Raven Press, 1980.

100. ———. "Prefrontal Cortex in Motor Control," in V. B. Brooks, ed. *Handbook of Physiology,* vol. 2, *The Nervous System.* Washington, D.C.: American Physiological Society, 1981, pp. 1149–1178.

101. FUXE, K., and HOKFELDT, T. "Further Evidence for the Existence of Tuberoinfundibular Dopamine Neurons," *Acta Physiologica Scandinavica,* 66 (1966): 245–246.

102. FYRO, B., et al. "The Effect of Chlorpromazine on Homovanillic Acid Levels in Cerebrospinal Fluid of Schizophrenic Outpatients," *Psychopharmacology,* 35 (1974):287–294.

103. GARBUTT, J. C., and VAN KAMMEN, D. P. "The Interaction Between GABA and Dopamine: Implications for Schizophrenia," *Schizophrenia Bulletin,* 9 (1983):336–353.

104. GARDOS, G., COLE, J. O., and VOLICER, L. "A Dose-Response Study of Propranolol in Chronic Schizophrenics," *Current Therapeutics and Research* 15 (1973): 314–323.

105. GERLACH, J., THORSEN, K., and FOG, R. "Extrapyramidal Reactions and Amine Metabolites in Cerebrospinal Fluid During Haloperidol and Dopamine Treatment of Schizophrenic Patients," *Psychopharmacologia,* 40 (1975):341–350.

106. GERNER, R. H., CATLIN, D. H., and GOERLICK, D. A. "Beta-endorphins' Intravenous Infusion Causes Behavioral Changes in Psychiatric Patients," *Archives of General Psychiatry,* 37 (1980): 642–647.

107. GILMAR, D. G., MANOWITZ, P., and FROSCH, W. A. "Association of Plasma Tryptophan Levels with Clinical Change in Female Schizophrenic Patients," *Biological Psychiatry,* 6 (1973): 119–128.

108. GOLDEN, C. J., et al. "Structural Brain Deficits in Schizophrenia: Identification

by Computer Tomography Scan Density Measures," *Archives of General Psychiatry,* 38 (1981):1014–1017.

109. GORDAN, G. S., et al. "Cerebral Oxygen Intake in Chronic Schizophrenic Reactions," *Archives of Neurology,* 73 (1955):544–545.

110. GOTTESMAN, I. I., and SHIELDS, J. *Schizophrenia and Genetics: A Twin Study Vantage Point.* New York: New York University Press, 1972.

111. ———. *Schizophrenia: The Epigenetic Puzzle.* Cambridge: Cambridge University Press, 1982.

112. GRACE, A., HOMMER, D., and BUNNEY, C. B. "Peripheral and Striatal Influence on Nigral Dopamine Cells. Mediation by Reticulate Neurons," *Brain Research Bulletin,* 5 (Supplement 2) (1980):105–109.

113. GRUZELIER, J. H., and YORKSTON, N. J. "Propranolol and Schizophrenia: Objective Evidence of Efficacy," in G. Hemmings and W. A. Hemmings, eds. *Biological Basis of Schizophrenia.* Baltimore: University Park Press, 1978, pp. 127–146.

114. GUILLEMIN, R., VERGO, T., ROSSLER, J.B. "β-endorphins and Adrenocorticotropine Are Secreted by the Pituitary Gland," 197 (1977):1367–1369.

115. GUR, R. E., et al. "Brain Function in Psychiatric Disorders. I. Regional Cerebral Blood Flow in Medicated Schizophrenics," *Archives of General Psychiatry,* 40 (1983):1250–1254.

116. HANG, J. O. "Pneumoencephalographic Studies in Mental Disease," *Acta Psychiatrica Scandinavica,* 38 (1962):1–114.

117. HARE, E. H., and MORAN, P. "A Relationship Between Seasonal Temperature and the Birth Rate of Schizophrenia Patients," *Acta Psychiatrica Scandinavica,* 63 (1981):395–405.

118. HARE, E. H., PRICE, J. S., and SLATER, E. "Mental Disorder and Season of Birth," *Nature,* 241 (1973):480.

119. HEATH, R. G. "Subcortical Brain Function Correlates of Psychopathology and Epilepsy," in C. Shagass, S. Gershon, and A. J. FRIEDHOFF, eds., *Psychopathology and Brain Dysfunction,* New York: Raven Press, 1977, pp. 51–67.

120. HEATH, R. G., NESSELHOF, W., and

121. BISHOP, M. R. "Behavioral and Metabolic Changes Associated with Administration of Antabuse," *Diseases of the Nervous System,* 26 (1965):99–105.

121. HERZIG, M. E., and BIRCH, H. G. "Neurologic Organization in Psychotically Disturbed Adolescent Girls," *Archives of General Psychiatry,* 15 (1966):590–598.

122. HIMMELHOCH, J., et al. "Subacute Encephalitis: Behavioral and Neurochemical Aspects," *British Journal of Psychiatry,* 116 (1970):531–538.

123. HOLZMAN, P. S. "Smooth-pursuit Eye Movements in Schizophrenia. Recent Findings," in D. X. Freedman, ed., *Biology of Major Psychosis: A Comparative Analysis.* New York: Raven Press, 1978, pp. 217–228.

124. HOLZMAN, P. S., et al. "Deviant Eye Tracking in Twins Discordant for Psychosis: A Replication," *Archives of General Psychiatry,* 37 (1980):627–631.

125. HORNYKIEWICZ, O. "Neurochemistry of Parkinsonism," in A. Lajtha, ed., *Handbook of Neurochemistry,* vol. 7. New York: Plenum Press, 1972, pp. 465–501.

126. ———. "Parkinson Disease: From Brain Homogenate to Treatment," *Federation Proceedings,* 32 (1973):183–190.

127. ———. "Psychopharmacological Implications of Dopamine and Dopamine Agonists: A Critical Evaluation of Current Evidence," *Annual Review of Pharmacology and Toxicology,* 17 (1979): 545–559.

128. ———. "Brain Catecholamines in Schizophrenia: A Good Case for Noradrenaline," *Science,* 299 (1982):484–486.

129. HOROWITZ, M. J., and ADAMS, J. E. "Hallucinations on Brain Stimulations: Evidence for Revision of the Penfield Hypothesis," in W. Kemp, ed., *Origins and Mechanisms of Hallucinations.* New York: Plenum Press, 1970, pp. 13–22.

130. HORROBIN, D. F. "Indomethacin, Prostaglandins and Schizophrenia," *British Medical Journal,* 2 (1977):1357.

131. ———. "Schizophrenia As a Prostaglandin Deficiency Disease," *Lancet,* 1 (1977): 936–937.

132. HORROBIN, D. F., ALLY, A. P., and KARMALI, R.A. "Prostaglandins and Schizophrenia: Further Discussion of the Evi-

dence," *Psychological Medicine,* 8 (1978):43–48.

133.   HOUGAARD, K., et al. "Regional Cerebral Blood Flow in Focal Cortical Epilepsy," *Archives of Neurology,* 33 (1976):527–535.

134.   INGRAR, D. H. "Measurements of Regional Cerebral Blood Flow and Metabolism in Psychopathological States," *European Journal of Neurology,* 20 (1981):294–296.

135.   INOUYE, E. "A Search for Research Framework of Schizophrenia in Twins and Chromosomes," in A. R. Kaplan, ed., *Genetic Factors in Schizophrenia.* Springfield, Ill.: Charles C Thomas, 1972, pp. 495–503.

136.   ISAACSON, R. L. *The Limbic System.* New York: Plenum Press, 1974.

137.   ITIL, T. M. "Qualitative and Quantitative EEG Findings in Schizophrenia," *Schizophrenia Bulletin,* 3 (1977):61–79.

138.   IVERSON, L. L., IVERSON, S. D., and SNYDER, S. H. *Handbook of Psychopharmacology,* vol. 8. New York: Plenum Press, 1978.

139.   IVERSON, L. L., ROGAWSKI, M., and MILLER, R. J. "Comparison of the Effect of Neuroleptic Drug on Pre- and Postsynaptic Dopaminergic Mechanisms in the Rat Striatum," *Molecular Pharmacology,* 12 (1976):251–262.

140.   JACONO, W. G., and LYKKEN, D. J. "Electro-culographic Recording and Scoring of Smooth Pursuit and Saccadic Eye Tracking: A Parametric Study Using Monozygotic Twins," *Psychophysiology,* 16 (1974):94–107.

141.   JACQUET, Y. F., and MARKS, N. "The C-Fragment of B-lipoproteinine: An Endogenous Neuroleptic or Antipsychotogen?" *Science,* 194 (1976):632–635.

142.   JANOWSKY, D. S., and DAVIS, J. M. "Methylphenidate, Dextroamphetamine and Levoamphetamine Effects on Schizophrenic Symptoms," *Archives of General Psychiatry,* 33 (1976):304–308.

143.   JANOWSKY, D. S., El-Yousef, M. K., and Davis, J. M. "Antagonistic Effect of Physostigmine and Methylphenidate in Man," *American Journal of Psychiatry,* 130 (1973):1370–1376.

144.   JANOWSKY, D. S., et al. "Provocation of Schizophrenic Symptoms by Intravenous Administration of Methylphenidate," *Archives of General Psychiatry,* 28 (1973):185–191.

145.   JENKYN, L. R., et al. "Clinical Signs in Diffuse Cerebral Dysfunction," *Journal of Neurology, Neurosurgery and Psychiatry,* 40 (1977):956–966.

146.   JENNER, P., and MORDSEN, C. D. "Neuroleptics," in D. G. Graham Smith, H. Hippius, and G. Winokur, eds., *Psychopharmacology. I. A Biennial Critical Survey of the International Literature.* Amsterdam: Excerpta Medica, 1984, pp. 180–247.

147.   JERNIGAN, T. L., et al. "Computed Tomography in Schizophrenics and Normal Volunteers," *Archives of General Psychiatry,* 39 (1982):765–770.

148.   JOHNSON, R. T. "Selective Vulnerability of Neural Cells to Viral Infections," *Brain,* 103 (1980):447–472.

149.   JOHNSTONE, E. C., et al. "Cerebral Ventricular Size and Cognitive Impairment in Chronic Schizophrenics," *Lancet,* 2 (1976):924–926.

150.   JOHNSTONE, E. C., et al. "Act Study of Patients with Schizophrenia, Affective Psychosis and Neurotic Illness," in C. Purvis, G. Strune, and B. Jansson, eds., *Biological Psychiatry.* Amsterdam: Elsevier/North Holland Biomedical Press, 1981, pp. 237–240.

151.   JOSEPH, M. H., et al. "Determination of 3-Methoxy-4-Hydroxyphenylglycol Conjugates in Urine: Application to the Study of Central Noradrenaline Metabolism in Unmedicated Chronic Schizophrenic Patients," *Psychopharmacology,* 51 (1976):47–51.

152.   JOSEPH, M. H., et al. "3-Methoxy-4-Hydroxyphenylglycol Excretion in Acutely Schizophrenic Patients During Controlled Clinical Trial of the Isomer Flupenthixol," *Psychopharmacology* (Berlin), 64 (1979):35–40.

153.   KANEMATSU, S., and SAWYER, C. H. "Elevation of Plasma Prolactin after Hypophyseal Stalk Section in the Rat," *Endocrinology,* 93 (1973):238–241.

154.   KARSON, C. N. "Spontaneous Eye Blink Rate and Dopaminergic System," *Brain,* 106 (1983):643–653.

155.   KARSON, C. N., et al. "Drug Effect on

Blink Rate in Rhesus Monkey: Preliminary Studies," *Biological Psychiatry*, 16 (1981):150–154.

156. KARSON, C. N., et al. "Haloperidol-Induced Changes in Blink Rate Correlate with BPRS Score," *British Journal of Psychiatry*, 140 (1982):503–507.

157. KEBABIAN, J., PETZOLD, G. L., and GREENGARD, P. "Dopamine-Sensitive Adenylate Cyclase in Caudate Nucleus of Rat Brain: Its Similarity to the Dopamine Receptor," *Proceedings of the National Academy of Science, USA* 69 (1979):2145–2149.

158. KENDLER, K. S. "Overview: A Current Perspective on Twin Studies in Schizophrenia," *American Journal of Psychiatry*, 140 (1983):1413–1425.

159. KESSLER, S. "The Genetics of Schizophrenia: A Review," *Schizophrenia Bulletin*, 8 (1980):404–415.

160. KETY, S. S., et al. "The Types and Prevalence of Mental Illness in Biological and Adoptive Families of Adopted Schizophrenics," in D. Rosenthal and S. S. Kety, eds., *The Transmission of Schizophrenia*. Oxford: Pergamon Press, 1968, pp. 345–362.

161. KLAWANS, H. L. "The Pharmacology of Extrapyramidal Movement Disorders," in M. Cohen, ed., *Monograph in Neural Science*, vol. 2. Basel: Karger, 1973, pp. 1–136.

162. ———. "The Pharmacology of Tardive Dyskinesia," *American Journal of Psychiatry*, 130 (1973):82.

163. KLEINMAN, J. E., BRIDGE, P., and KAROUM, F. "Chronic Schizophrenia, Postmortem Studies," in C. Baxter and T. Melnechuk, eds., *Perspective in Schizophrenia Research*. New York: Raven Press, 1980, pp. 227–236.

164. KORNETSKY, C., and ELIASSON, M. "Reticular Stimulation and Chlorpromazine: An Animal Model for Schizophrenic Overarousal," *Science*, 165 (1969):1273–1274.

165. KRINGLER, E. "Twins—Still Our Best Method," *Schizophrenia Bulletin*, 12 (1976):429–433.

166. KRUGER, B. K., et al. "Stimulation by Dopamine of Adenosine Cyclic 3'5' Monophosphate Formation in Rat Caudate Nucleus: Effect of Lesions of the Nigro-Striatal Pathology," *Molecular Pharmacology*, 12 (1976):639–648.

167. LAKE, C. R., STERENBERG, D. E., and VAN KAMMEN, D. S. "Schizophrenia: Elevated Cerebrospinal Fluid Norepinephrine," *Science*, 207 (1980):331–333.

168. LANDER, K., et al. "Long-term Neuroleptic Treatment of Chronic Schizophrenia Patients: Clinical and Biochemical Effects of Withdrawal," *Psychopharmacology*, 73 (1981):43–47.

169. LAUTIN, A., et al. "Sodium Valproate in Schizophrenia: Some Biochemical Correlations," *British Journal of Psychiatry*, 137 (1980):240–244.

170. LECKMAN, D. F., Bowers, M. B. JR., and STURGES, J. S. "Relationship Between Estimated Premorbid Adjustment and CSF Homovanillic Acid and 5-Hydroxyindoleacetic Acid Levels," *American Journal of Psychiatry*, 138 (1981):472–477.

171. LEE, T., et al. "Binding of 3H Neuroleptics and 3H Apomorphine in Schizophrenic Brains," *Nature*, 274 (1978):897–900.

172. LEHONARD, K. *The Classification of Endogenous Psychoses*, R. Berman, transl. New York: Irvington Publishers, 1979.

173. LERNER, P., et al. "Dopamine Hydroxylase in the Cerebrospinal Fluid of Psychiatric Patients," *Biological Psychiatry*, 13 (1978):685–694.

174. LEVY, D. L., LIPTON, R. B., and HOLZMAN, P. S. "Smooth Pursuit Eye Movements in Schizophrenia: Recent Findings," in D. X. Friedman, ed., *Biology of Major Psychoses: A Comparative Analysis*. New York: Raven Press, 1975, pp. 217–228.

175. LIBIKO, H., et al. "Assay of Interferon and Viral Antibodies in Cerebrospinal Fluid in Clinical Neurology and Psychiatry," *Acta Biologica Medica Germanica*, 38 (1979):879–893.

176. LINDVALL, O., and BJORKLUND, A. "The Organization of the Ascending Catecholamine Neuron System in the Rat Brain as Revealed by the Glycoxide Acid Fluorescence Method," *Acta Physiologica Scandinavica*, 412 (Supplement), (1974):1–48.

177. LING, N., BURGER, R., and GUILLEMIN, N. "Isolation, Primary Structure, and Synthesis of Alpha-Enkephalin and Gam-

ma-Endorphin: Two Peptides of Hypothalamic Hypophyseal Origin with Morphinomimetic Activity," *Proceedings of the National Academy of Science, USA,* 73 (1976):3942–3946.

178. LIPTON, R. B., et al. "Eye Movement Dysfunction in Psychiatric Patients," *Schizophrenia Bulletin,* 8 (1983):13–32.

179. LUCHINS, D. J., WEINBERGER, D. R., and WYATT, R. J. "Cerebrospinal Asymmetry in Schizophrenia Determined by Computerized Tomography," *American Journal of Psychiatry,* 139 (1982): 753–757.

180. LYTTON, H. "Do Parents Create or Respond to Differences in Twins?" *Developmental Psychology,* 13 (1977):456–459.

181. MACK, A., FENDRICK, R., and PLEUNE, J. "Smooth Pursuit Eye Movements: Is Perceived Motion Necessary?" *Science,* 703 (1979):1361–1363.

182. MACKAY, A. V. P., and CROW, T. J. "Positive and Negative Schizophrenic Symptoms and the Role of Dopamine," *British Journal of Psychiatry,* 137 (1980):379–386.

183. MACKAY, A. V. P., et al. "Dopamine Receptors and Schizophrenia: Drug Effect or Illness?" *Lancet,* 2 (1980):915–916.

184. MACLEAN, P. D. "Some Psychiatric Implications of Physiological Studies on the Fronto-Temporal Portion of the Limbic System," *Electroencephalography and Clinical Neurophysiology,* 4 (1952):407–418.

185. MACLEOD, R. M. "Regulation of Prolactin Secretion," in L. Martini and W. F. Ganong, eds., *Frontiers of Neuroendocrinology.* New York: Raven Press, 1976, pp. 169–194.

186. MCNEIL, T. E., and KAIJ, L. "Obstetric Factors in the Development of Schizophrenia: Complications in the Birth of Preschizophrenics and in Reproduction by Schizophrenic Patients," in L. C. Wynne, R. L. Cromwell, and S. Matthysse, eds., *The Nature of Schizophrenia.* New York: John Wiley & Sons, 1978, pp. 401–429.

187. MAJ, M., LIZOLFI, S., and DELVECCHIO, M. "Blood Levels of S-adenosylmethanionine in Unmedicated Schizophrenic and Depressive Patients," *Neuropsychobiology,* 7 (1981):188–191.

188. MANOWITZ, P., GILMOR, D. G., and RACERVSKIS, J. "Low Plasma Tryptophan Levels in Recently Hospitalized Schizophrenics," *Biological Psychiatry,* 6 (1973):109–118.

189. MARIN, R. S., and TUCKER, G. J. "Psychopathology and Hemispheric Dysfunction," *Journal of Nervous and Mental Disease,* 169 (1981):546–557.

190. MARTIN, J. B. "Brain Regulation of Growth Hormone Secretion," in L. Martini and W. F. Ganong, eds., *Frontiers of Neuroendocrinology.* New York: Raven Press, 1976, pp. 129–168.

191. MASTERS, A. B. "The Pink Spot," *Lancet,* 1 (1980):16–17.

192. MATHE, A. A., SEDVALL, G., and WEISEL, F. A. "Increased Content of Immunoreactive Prostaglandin E in Cerebrospinal Fluid of Patients with Schizophrenia," *Lancet,* 1 (1980):16–17.

193. MATTHYSSE, S. "Antipsychotic Drug Actions: A Clue to the Neuropathology of Schizophrenia," *Federation Proceedings,* 32 (1973):200–208.

194. MELAMUD, N. "Psychiatric Disorders with Intracranial Tumors of the Limbic System," *Archives of Neurology,* 17 (1967): 113–124.

195. MELTZER, H. Y., and FANG, V. S. "The Effect of Neuroleptics on Serum Prolactin in Schizophrenic Patients," *Archives of General Psychiatry,* 33 (1976):279–286.

196. MELTZER, H. Y., and STAHL, S. M. "The Dopamine Hypothesis of Schizophrenia," *Schizophrenia Bulletin,* 2 (1976): 19–76.

197. MELTZER, H. Y., BUSCH, D. A., and SCHYVE, P. M. "Effect of Des-Tyr-Gamma Endorphin on Prolactin Secretion," *Archives of General Psychiatry,* 38 (1981):1138.

198. MELTZER, H. Y., BUSCH, D. A., and SO, R. "Neuroleptic-Induced Elevation in Serum Prolactin Levels: Etiology and Significance," in C. Baxter and T. Melnick, eds., *Perspectives in Schizophrenia Research.* New York: Raven Press, 1980, pp. 149–172.

199. MELTZER, H. Y., CHO, H. W., and CARROLL, B. J. "Serum Dopamine-Beta-

Hydroxylase Activity in the Affective Psychosis and Schizophrenia: Decreased Activity in Unipolar Psychotically Depressed Patients," *Archives of General Psychiatry,* 33 (1976):585–591.

200. MELTZER, H. Y., JACKMAN, H., and ARORA, R. C. "Brain and Skeletal Monoamine Oxidase Activity in Schizophrenia," *Schizophrenia Bulletin,* 6 (1980): 208–212.

201. MELTZER, H. Y., SACHAR, E. G., and FRANTS, A. G. "Serum Prolactin Levels in Unmedicated Schizophrenic Patients," *Archives of General Psychiatry,* 31 (1979):564–569.

202. MELTZER, H. Y., et al. "Dopamine and Schizophrenia," *Lancet,* 2 (1976):1142.

203. MERRIN, E. L. "Schizophrenia and Brain Asymmetry: An Evaluation of Evidence for Dominant Lobe Dysfunction," *Journal of Nervous and Mental Disease,* 169 (1981):405–416.

204. MILLER, R. J., and HILEY, R. "Anti-Muscarinic Properties of Neuroleptics and Drug-Induced Parkinsonism," *Nature* (London), 248 (1974):596–597.

205. MILLER, R. J., HORN, A., and IVERSEN, L. L. "The Action of Neuroleptic Drugs on Dopamine-Stimulated Adenosine Cyclic 3'5'-Monophosphate Production in Rat Neostriatum and Limbic Forebrain," *Molecular Pharmacology,* 10 (1974):759–766.

206. MOORE, R. Y., and BLOOM, F. E. "Central Catecholamine Neuron Systems: Anatomy and Physiology of the Dopamine System," *Annual Review of Neuroscience,* 1 (1978):129–169.

207. MORIHISIA, J. M., DUFFY, F. H., and WYATT, R. J. "Topographic Analysis of Computerized Processed Electroencephalography in Schizophrenia," in E. Usdin and J. Hanin, eds., *Biological Markers in Psychiatry and Neurology.* New York: Pergamon Press, 1982, pp. 495–504.

208. ——. "Brain Electrical Activity Mapping (BEAM) in Schizophrenic Patients," *Archives of General Psychiatry,* 40 (1983):719–728.

209. MORSSELLI, P., et al. "On the Therapeutic Action of SL-76-0002. A new GABAminergic Agent: Preliminary Observation in Neuropsychiatric Disorders,"

Brain Research Bulletin, 5 (Supplement 2) (1980):95–109.

210. MOSHER, L. R., POLLIN, W., and STOBENAU, J. R. "Identical Twins Discordant for Schizophrenia: Neurologic Findings," *Archives of General Psychiatry,* 24 (1971):422–430.

211. MULLER, P., and SEEMAN, P. "Dopaminergic Supersensitivity After Neuroleptics: Time Course and Specificity," *Psychopharmacology,* 60 (1978):1–11.

212. NABER, N., PICKAR, D., and POST, R. M. "Endogenous Opioid Activity and β-Endorphin Immunoreactivity in CSF of Psychiatric Patients and Normal Volunteers," *American Journal of Psychiatry,* 138 (1981):1457–1462.

213. NAGY, K. "Pneumoencephalographsche Befunole bei, Endogen Psychosen," *Nervenartz,* 34 (1963):543–548.

214. NASRALLAH, M. A., et al. "Cerebral Ventricular Enlargement in Subtypes of Chronic Schizophrenia," *Archives of General Psychiatry,* 319 (1982):774–777.

215. NEULIN, D. B., CARPENTER, B., and GOLDEN, C. J. "Hemispheric Asymmetries in Schizophrenia," *Biological Psychiatry,* 16 (1981):561–582.

216. NYBACK, H., BERGEN, B. M., and HINDMARSH, T. "Computed Tomography of the Brain in Patients with Acute Psychosis and in Healthy Volunteers," *Acta Psychiatrica Scandinavica,* 65 (1982): 403–414.

217. NYBACK, H., BORZECK, Z., and SEDVALL, G. "Accumulation and Disappearance of Catecholamine from Tryosine-^{14}C in Mouse Brain: Effect of Some Psychotropic Drugs," *European Journal of Pharmacology,* 4 (1968):395–403.

218. OBRIST, W. D., et al. "Regional Cerebral Blood Flow in Studies in Senile and Presenile Dementia," *Neurology,* 20 (1970):315–322.

219. ODEGARD, O. "Season of Birth in General Population and in Patients with Mental Disorder in Norway," *British Journal of Psychiatry,* 125 (1976):395–404.

220. OLIANAS, M., et al. "The Striatal Dopaminergic Function Is Mediated by the Inhibition of Nigral, Nondopaminergic Neuronal System via a Strionigral GABAergic Pathway," *European Journal of Pharmacology,* 49 (1978):233–241.

221. OSBORNE, M., CRAYTON, J. W., and JA-VAID, J. "Lack of Effect of a Gluten-Free Diet on Neuroleptic Blood Levels in Schizophrenic Patients," *Biological Psychiatry,* 17 (1982):627–629.

222. OSMOND, H., and SMYTHIES, J. "Schizophrenia: A New Approach," *Journal of Mental Science,* 98 (1952):309–315.

223. OWEN, F., et al. "Increased Dopamine Receptor Sensitivity in Schizophrenia," *Lancet,* 2 (1978):223–226.

224. PANDURANGI, A. K., et al. "The Ventricular System in Chronic Schizophrenic Patients: A Controlled Computed Tomography Study," *British Journal of Psychiatry,* 144 (1984):172–176.

225. PARKER, G., and NELSON, M. "Mental Disorder and Season of Birth: A Southern Hemisphere Study," *British Journal of Psychiatry,* 129 (1976):355–361.

226. PARNAS, J., SCHULSINGER, F., and TEAS-DALE, T. W. "Perinatal Complications and Clinical Outcome Within the Schizophrenia Spectrum," *British Journal of Psychiatry,* 140 (1982):416–420.

227. PERRY, E., et al. Letter, *Lancet,* 1 (1978): 35–36.

228. PICKAR, D., DAVIS, G. C., and SCHULTZ, C. "Behavioral and Biological Effects of Acute Endorphin Injection in Schizophrenic and Depressed Patients," *American Journal of Psychiatry,* 138 (1981):160–166.

229. PICKAR, D., VARTANIAN, F., and BUNNEY, W. E. "Short-Term Naloxone Administration in Schizophrenic and Manic Patients: A World Health Organization Collaborative Study," *Archives of General Psychiatry,* 39 (1982):313–319.

230. PINCUS, J. H., and TUCKER, G. I. *Behavioral Neurology.* New York: Oxford Press, 1978.

231. POST, R. M., CARPENTER, W. T., and GOODWIN, F. K. "Cerebrospinal Fluid Amine Metabolites in Acute Schizophrenia," *Archives of General Psychiatry,* 32 (1975):1063–1069.

232. POTKIN, S. G., WEINBERGER, D., and KLEINMAN, J. "Wheat Gluten Challenge in Schizophrenic Patients," *American Journal of Psychiatry,* 138 (1981):1208–1211.

233. QUITKIN, F., RIFKIN, A., and KLEIN, D. F. "Neurologic Soft Signs in Schizophrenia

and Character Disorders: Organicity in Schizophrenia with Premorbid Asociality and Emotionally Unstable Character Disorder," *Archives of General Psychiatry,* 33 (1976):845–853.

234. RAGHEB, M., and BON, T. A. "Prostaglandins and Schizophrenia: A Review," *Progress in Neuropsychopharmacology and Biological Psychiatry,* 6 (1982):87–93.

235. RAICHLE, M. E., et al. *"In vivo* Correlations Between Regional Cerebral Blood Flow and Oxygen Utilization in Man," *Acta Neurologica Scandinavica,* 56 (1977):240–241.

236. RANDRUP, A., and MUNKGAARD, J. "Behavioral Stereotypies Induced by Pharmacological Agents," *Pharmakopsychiatrie Und Neuro-Psychopharmakologie,* 1 (1968):1–26.

237. ———. "Biochemical, Anatomical and Psychological Investigation of Stereotyped Behavior Induced by Amphetamine," in E. Costa, and S. Garattini, eds., *Amphetamines and Related Compounds.* New York: Raven Press, 1970, pp. 695–713.

238. ———. "Evidence Indicating an Association Between Schizophrenia and Dopaminergic Activity in the Brain," *Orthomolecular Psychiatry,* 1 (1972): 2–7.

239. RASHBOSS, C. "The Relationship Between Saccadic and Smooth Tracking Eye Movement," *Journal of Physiology,* 159 (1961):326–338.

240. REISINE, T. D., et al. "Opiate and Neuroleptic Receptor Alterations in Human Schizophrenic Brain Tissue," *Advances in Biochemical Psychopharmacology,* 21 (1980):443–450.

241. REVELEY, A. M., REVELEY, M. A., and MURRAY, R. M. "Cerebral Ventricular Enlargement in Non-Genetic Schizophrenia: A Controlled Twin Study," *British Journal of Psychiatry,* 144 (1984):89–93.

242. REVELEY, A. M., et al. "Cerebral Ventricular Size in Twins Discordant for Schizophrenia," *Lancet,* 1 (1982):540–541.

243. REVELEY, M. A., GLOVER, V., and SANDLER, M. "Brain Monoamine Oxidase Activity in Schizophrenics and Controls,"

Archives of General Psychiatry, 38 (1981):663–665.

244. REVICH, M. "Blood Flow Metabolism Coupled in Brain," *Research Publication of the Association of Nervous and Mental Diseases,* 53 (1976):125.

245. REYNOLDS, G. B., et al. "Dopamine Receptors and Schizophrenia: Drug Effect or Illness?" *Lancet,* 2 (1980): 1251.

246. RICE, J. R., HAIN, C. H., and GORE, W. E. "Another Look at Gluten in Schizophrenia," *American Journal of Psychology,* 135 (1978):1417–1418.

247. RIDER, R. O., et al. "Sulcal Prominence in Young Chronic Schizophrenic Patients: CT Findings Associated with Impairment of Neuropsychological Tests," *Psychiatric Research,* 1 (1979):1–8.

248. RISBERG, J., et al. "Bilateral Measurements of the rCBF During Mental Activation in Normals and in Aphasic Patients," in A. N. Harper et al., eds., *Blood Flow and Metabolism in the Brain.* London: Churchill Livingstone, 1975, chap. 14.3–14.7.

249. ROBERTS, E. "An Hypothesis Suggesting That There Is a Deficiency in GABA System in Schizophrenia," *Neuroscience Research Program Bulletin,* 10 (1972):468–481.

250. ———. "Disinhibition as an Organizing Principle in the Nervous System: The Role of GABA System. Application to Neurologic and Psychiatric Disorders," in E. Roberts, T. Chase, and D. Tower, eds., *GABA in Nervous System Function.* New York: Raven Press, 1976, pp. 515–539.

251. ROCKFORD, J. M., et al. "Neuropsychological Impairment in Functional Psychiatric Diseases," *Archives of General Psychiatry,* 22 (1970):114–119.

252. ROCKFORD, J. M., et al. "Some Quantitative EEG Correlates of Psychopathology," *Research Communication in Psychology, Psychiatry and Behavior,* 1 (1976):211.

253. ROEMER, R. A., et al. "Somatosensory and Auditory Evoked Potential Studies of Functional Differences Between the Hemispheres in Psychosis," *Biological Psychiatry,* 14 (1979):354–374.

254. ROSENTHAL, D. *The Genetics of Psycho-pathology.* New York: McGraw-Hill, 1971.

255. ROSENTHAL, D., et al. "Schizophrenic Offspring Reared in Adoptive Homes," in D. Rosenthal and S. S. Kety, eds., *The Transmission of Schizophrenia.* Oxford: Pergamon Press, 1968, pp. 377–391.

256. ROSS, B. E. "Monoamine Metabolism and Viral Infection," Paper presented at the American College of Neuropsychopharmacology Meeting, San Juan, 1983.

257. ROTH, W. T. "Late Event-Related Potentials and Psychopathology," *Schizophrenia Bulletin,* 3 (1977):105–120.

258. ROTROSEN, J., Angrist, B., and GERSHON, S. "Neuroendocrine Effects of Apomorphine: Characterization of Response Patterns and Application to Schizophrenia Research," *British Journal of Psychiatry,* 135 (1979):444–456.

259. ROTROSEN, J., MILLER, A. D., and MANDIO, D. "Prostaglandins, Platelets and Schizophrenia," *Archives of General Psychiatry,* 37 (1980):1047–1054.

260. SACK, R. L., and GOODWIN, F. K. "Inhibition of Dopamine- β-Hydroxylase in Manic Patients: A Clinical Trial with Fusaric Acid," *Archives of General Psychiatry,* 31 (1974):649–654.

261. SCATTON, B., et al. "Cortical Modulation of Striatal Function," *Brain Research,* 232 (1982):331–343.

262. SCHECK-KRUGER, J., CHRISTENSEN, A., and AZUT, J. "Muscimol Differentially Facilitates Stereotypy but Antagonizes Motility Induced by Dopaminergic Drugs: A Complex GABA-Dopamine Interaction," *Life Science,* 22 (1978):75–84.

263. SCHECK-KRUGER, J., et al. "Behavioral Function of GABA in Basal Ganglia and Limbic System," *Brain Research Bulletin,* 5 (Supplement 2) (1980):261–267.

264. SCHEIBEL, A. B., and KORELMAN, J. A. "Disorientation of the Hippocampal Pyramidal Cell and Its Processes in the Schizophrenic Patient," *Biological Psychiatry,* 16 (1980):101–102.

265. SCHILDKRAUT, J. J., HERZOG, J. M., and ORSULAK, P. J. "Reduced Platelet Monoamine Oxidase Activity in a Subgroup of Schizophrenic Patients," *American*

Journal of Psychiatry, 133 (1976):438–440.

266. SCHILDKRAUT, J. J., ORSULAK, P. J., and SCHATZBERG, A. F. "Platelet Monoamine Oxidase Activity in a Subgroup of Schizophrenic Patients," *Schizophrenia Bulletin,* 6 (1980):220–225.

267. SEDVALL, G. C., and WODE-HELGODT, B. "Aberrant Monoamine Metabolite Levels in CSF and Family History of Schizophrenia: Their Relationship in Schizophrenic Patients," *Archives of General Psychiatry,* 37 (1980):1113–1116.

268. SEEMAN, P., et al. "Bimodal Distribution of Dopamine Receptor Density in Brains of Schizophrenics," *Science,* 225 (1984):728–731.

269. SHAGASS, C. "Twisted Thoughts, Twisted Brain Waves?" in C. Shagass, S. Gershon, and J. Friedhoff, eds., *Psychopathology and Brain Dysfunction.* New York: Raven Press, 1975, pp. 353–378.

270. SHAGASS, C., et al. "Evoked Potential Correlation of Psychosis," *Biological Psychiatry,* 13 (1974):168–184.

271. SHEPPARD, G., et al. "0–15 Positron Emission Tomographic Scans in Predominantly Never-Treated Acute Schizophrenic Patients," *Lancet,* 2 (1983): 1448–1452.

272. SIMON, E., MILLER, J. M., and EDELMAN, J. "Stereospecific Binding of the Potent Narcotic Analgesic (H^3) Ethorphine in the Rat Brain Homogenate," *Proceedings of the National Academy of Science USA,* 70 (1973):1947–1949.

273. SINGH, M. M., and KAY, S. R. "Wheat Gluten Schizophrenia Findings," *Science,* 194 (1976):449–450.

274. SLATER, E., and SHIELDS, J. "Psychotic and Neurotic Illness in Twins." Medical Research Council Special Report Series No. 278. London: Her Majesty's Stationery Office, 1953.

275. SMYTHIES, J. R. "The Pink Spot," *Lancet,* 1 (1966):367.

276. ———. "The Transmethylation and One-Carbon Cycle Hypotheses of Schizophrenia," *Psychological Medicine,* 13 (1983):711–717.

277. ———. "The Role of the One-Carbon Cycle in Neuropsychiatric Diseases," *Biological Psychiatry,* 9 (1984):755–758.

278. SNIDER, S. R. "Cerebellar Pathology in Schizophrenia: Cause or Consequence," *Neuroscience and Biobehavior Review,* 6 (1982):47–53.

279. SNYDER, S. H. "The Dopamine Hypothesis of Schizophrenia: Focus on the Dopamine Receptors," *American Journal of Psychiatry,* 133 (1976):197–202.

280. ———. "Dopamine Receptors, Neuroleptics and Schizophrenia," *American Journal of Psychiatry,* 138 (1981):960–964.

281. SNYDER, S. H., BANARJEE, S. P., and YAMAMURA H. I. "Drugs, Neurotransmitters and Schizophrenia," *Science,* 184 (1974):1243–1253.

282. SNYDER, S. H., CREESE, J., and BURT, D. R. "The Brain Dopaminergic Receptor: Labeling with (H^3) Dopamine and (H^3) Haloperidol," *Psychopharmacological Communication,* 1 (1975):663–673.

283. SOKOLOFF, B., et al. "The C-14 Deoxyglucose Method for the Measurement of Local Cerebral Glucose Utilization: Theory, Procedure, and Normal Values in the Conscious and Anesthetized Albino Rat," *Journal of Neurochemistry,* 28 (1977):897–916.

284. SOURKES, T. L. "On the Origin of Homovanillic Acid (HVA) in the Cerebrospinal Fluid," *Journal of Neural Transmission,* 34 (1973):153–157.

285. STAWARZ, R. J., et al. "On the Significance of the Increase in Homovanillic Acid (HVA) Caused by Antipsychotics in Corpus Striatum and Limbic Forebrain," *Federation Proceedings,* 32 (1976):246.

286. STEIN, L., and WISE, C. D. "Possible Etiology of Schizophrenia: Progressive Damage of the Noradrenergic Reward System by Hydroxydopamine," *Science,* 171 (1971):1032–1036.

287. STEIN, L., BELUZZI, J. D., and RITTERS, S. "Self Stimulation Reward Pathway: Norepinephrine versus Dopamine," *Journal of Psychiatric Research,* 11 (1974):115–124.

288. STERNBERG, D. E., VAN KAMMEN, D. P., and LAKE, C. R. "The Effect of Primozine on CSF Norepinephrine in Schizophrenia," *American Journal of Psychiatry,* 138 (1981):1045–1051.

289. STERNBERG, D. E., et al. "Schizophrenia: Dopamine Hydroxylase Activity and

Treatment Response," *Science*, 216 (1982):1423–1425.

290. STEVENS, J., WILSON, K., and FOOTE, W. "GABA Blockade, Dopamine and Schizophrenia: Experimental Studies in the Cat," *Psychopharmacologia*, 39 (1974): 105–119.

291. STEVENS, J. R. "Receptor Supersensitivity Relationship to Cerebral Anatomy and Histopathology of Schizophrenia," *Biological Psychiatry*, 16 (1981):1119–1122.

292. ———. "Neuropathology of Schizophrenia," *Archives of General Psychiatry*, 39 (1982):1131–1139.

293. STEVENS, J. R., et al. "Telemetered EEG-EOG During Psychotic Behavior of Schizophrenics," *Archives of General Psychiatry*, 36 (1979):251–262.

294. STEVENS, J. R., et al. "Viral Antigen in the Brain of Schizophrenic Patients?" in J. Mendlewicz and H. M. Van Praag, eds., *Advances in Biological Psychiatry*. Basal: Karger, 1983, pp. 76–95.

295. STJARN, L., and BRUNDIN, J. "Affinity of Noradrenaline and Dopamine for Neural Alpha Receptors Mediating Negative Feedback Control of Noradrenaline Secretion in Human Vasoconstrictor Nerves," *Acta Psychiatrica Scandinavica*, 95 (1975):89–94.

296. STORMS, L. J., CLANTON, J. M., and WRIGHT, T. C. "Effects of Gluten on Schizophrenics," *Archives of General Psychiatry*, 39 (1982):323–327.

297. SYNEK, V., and REUBEN, J. R. "The Ventricular Brain Ratio Using Planimetric Measurement of EMI Scans," *British Journal of Psychiatry*, 49 (1976):233–237.

298. TAMMINGA, C. A., and SCHAEFFER, M. H. "Gamma-Type Endorphins and Schizophrenia: In Reply," *Archives of General Psychiatry*, 38 (1981):1182–1183.

299. TAMMINGA, C. A., CRAYTON, G., and CHASE, T. "Muscimol: GABA Agonist Therapy in Schizophrenia," *American Journal of Psychiatry*, 135 (1978):746–747.

300. TAMMINGA, C. A., TIGHE, P. J., and CHASE, T. N. "Des-Tyrosine-Gamma-Endorphin Administration in Chronic Schizophrenics: A Preliminary Report," *Archives of General Psychiatry*, 38 (1981):167–168.

301. TERENIUS, L. "Characteristics of the Receptors for Narcotic Anagelsics in Synaptic Plasma Membrane Fraction from Rat Brain," *Acta Pharmacologia Toxicologia*, 33 (1973):377–384.

302. TINARI, P. "Schizophrenia in Finnish Male Twins," in M. H. Lader, ed., *Studies of Schizophrenia*. Ashford, England: Headley Brothers, 1975, pp. 29–35.

303. TOLLEFSON, G. D., and GARVEY, M. J. "Indomethacin and Prostaglandins: Their Behavioral Relationships in an Acute Toxic Psychosis," *Brief Reports*, 2 (1982):62–64.

304. TORREY, E. F., and PETERSON, M. R. "Slow and Latent Viruses in Schizophrenia," *Lancet*, 2 (1973):22–24.

305. ———. "Schizophrenia and the Limbic System," *Lancet*, 2 (1974):942–946.

306. ———. "The Viral Hypothesis in Schizophrenia," *Schizophrenia Bulletin*, 2 (1976):136–146.

307. TORREY, E. F., and TORREY, B. B. "A Shifting Seasonality of Schizophrenic Birth," *British Journal of Psychiatry*, 134 (1979):183–186.

308. TORREY, E. F., TORREY, B. D., and PETERSON, M. R. "Seasonality of Schizophrenia Birth in United States," *Archives of General Psychiatry*, 34 (1977):1065–1077.

309. TORREY, E. F., YOLLEN, R. H., and ALBRECHT, P. "Cytomegalovirus as a Possible Etiological Agent in Schizophrenia," in H. Mendlewicz and H. N. Van Praag, eds., *Advances in Biological Psychiatry*, vol. 12. Basel: Karger, 1983, pp. 150–159.

310. TORREY, E. F., YOLLEN, R. H., and WINFREY, C. J. "Cytomegalovirus Antibody in Cerebrospinal Fluid of Schizophrenic Patients Detected by Enzyme Immunoassay," *Science*, 216 (1982):892–894.

311. TUCKER, G. J., CAMPION, E. W., and SILBERFARB, P. M. "Sensorimotor Function and Cognitive Disturbance in Psychotic Patients," *American Journal of Psychiatry*, 132 (1975):17–21.

312. TUCKER, G. J., et al. "The Relationship of Subtle Neurologic Impairment to Disturbance Thinking," *Psychotherapy and Psychosomatics*, 24 (1974):165–169.

313. TURNER, P. "Schizophrenia as a Prosta-

glandin Deficiency Disease," *Lancet*, 1 (1977):1058.

314. UNGERSTEDT, U. "Stereotaxic Mapping of the Monoamine Pathways in the Rat Brain," *Acta Physiologica Scandinavica*, 367 (Supplement) (1971):1–48.

315. VAN KAMMEN, D. P., and BUNNEY, W. E., JR. "Heterogeneity in Schizophrenia: Effect of Placebo, Chronic Pimozide and Pimozide Withdrawal," in E. Usdin, J. Kopin, and J. D. Barchas, eds., *Catecholamines Basic and Clinical Frontiers*, vol. 2. New York: Pergamon Press, 1979, pp. 1896–1898.

316. VAN KAMMEN, D. P., DOCHERTY, J. P., and BUNNEY, W. E. "Prediction of Early Relapse After Pimozide Discontinuation by Response to d-Amphetamine During Pimozide Treatment," *Biological Psychiatry*, 17 (1982):233–242.

317. VAN KAMMEN, D. P., et al. "Antipsychotic Effect of Pimozide in Schizophrenia: Treatment Response Prediction with Acute Dextroamphetamine Response," *Archives of General Psychiatry*, 39 (1982):261–266.

318. VAN KAMMEN, D. P., et al. "Long-Term Pimozide Pretreatment Differentially Affects Behavioral Response to Dextroamphetamine in Schizophrenia: Further Exploration of the Dopamine Hypothesis in Schizophrenia," *Archives of General Psychiatry*, 39 (1982):275–281.

319. VAN KAMMEN, D. P., et al. "Dopamine-β-Hydroxylase Activity and Homovanillic Acid in Spinal Fluid of Schizophrenics with Brain Atrophy," *Science*, 220 (1983):974–977.

320. VAN KAMMEN, D. P., et al. "CSF Levels of Aminobutyric Acid in Schizophrenia," *Archives of General Psychiatry*, 39 (1982):91–97.

321. VAN PRAAG, H. M., and VERHOEVEN, W.M.A. "Endorphin Research in Schizophrenic Psychosis," *Comprehensive Psychiatry*, 22 (1981):135–144.

322. VERHOEVEN, W.M.A., VAN REE, J. M., and DEWIED, D. "Gamma-Type Endorphins and Schizophrenia," *Archives of General Psychiatry*, 38 (1981):1182.

323. VIGNERI, R., PAZZINO, V., and SQUATRIT, S. "Sleep-Associated Growth Hormone Release in Schizophrenia," *Neuroendocrinology*, 14 (1974):356–361.

324. VOLOVKE, J., MALLJA, A., and BAIG, S. "Naloxone in Chronic Schizophrenia," *Science*, 196 (1977):1227–1228.

325. WASCZAK, B., and WALTERS, J. "Effects of GABA Mimetics on Substantia Nigra Neurons," *Advances in Neurology*, 23 (1979):727–740.

326. WATSON, C. G., et al. "Schizophrenia Birth Seasonality in Relation to the Incidence of Infectious Diseases and Temperature Extremes," *Archives of General Psychiatry*, 41 (1984):85–90.

327. WATSON, S. J., BERGER, P. A., and AKIL, H. "Effect of Naloxone in Schizophrenia: Reduction in Hallucinations in a Subpopulation of Subjects," *Science*, 201 (1978):73–78.

328. WEINBERGER, D. R., and WYATT, R. J. "Cerebral Ventricular Size: A Biological Marker for Subtyping Chronic Schizophrenia," in E. Usdin and J. Hanin, eds., *Biological Markers in Psychiatry and Neurology*. New York: Pergamon Press, 1982, pp. 505–512.

329. WEINBERGER, D. R., WAGNER, R. L., and WYATT, R. J. "Neuropathological Studies of Schizophrenia: A Selective Review," *Schizophrenia Bulletin*, 9 (1983):193–212.

330. WEINBERGER, D. R., et al. "Lateral Cerebral Ventricular Enlargement in Chronic Schizophrenia," *Archives of General Psychiatry*, 36 (1979):735–739.

331. WEINBERGER, D. R., et al. "Cerebellar Pathology in Schizophrenia: A Controlled Postmortem Study," *American Journal of Psychiatry*, 137 (1980):359–361.

332. WEINBERGER, D. R. et al. "Cerebral Ventricular Enlargement in Chronic Schizophrenia: Association with Poor Response to Treatment," *Archives of General Psychiatry*, 37 (1980):11–14.

335. WEINBERGER, D. R., et al. "Familial Aspects of CT Abnormalities in Chronic Schizophrenic Patients," *Psychiatric Research*, 4 (1981):65–71.

334. WEINBERGER, D. R., et al. "CT Scan in Schizophreniform Disorders and Other Acute Psychiatric Patients," *Archives of General Psychiatry*, (1982):778–783.

335. WENDER, P. H., ROSENTHAL, D., and KETY, S. S. "A Psychiatric Assessment of the Adoptive Parents of Schizophrenics," in D. Rosenthal and S. S.

Kety, eds., *The Transmission of Schizophrenia.* Oxford: Pergamon Press, 1968, pp. 235–250.

336. WENDER, P. H., et al. "Crossfostering: A Research Strategy for Clarifying the Role of Genetics and Experiential Factors in the Etiology of Schizophrenia," *Archives of General Psychiatry,* 30 (1974):121–128.

337. WIDEN, L., et al. "PET Studies of Glucose Metabolism in Patients with Schizophrenia," *American Journal of Neurological Research,* 4 (1983):550–552.

338. WIESEL, F. A., and SEDVALL, G. "Effects of Antipsychotic Drugs on Homovanillic Acid Levels in Striatum and Olfactory Tubercule in Rat," *European Journal of Pharmacology,* 30 (1975): 364–367.

339. WILSON, R. D. "The Neural Associations of Nucleus Accumbens Septi in the Albino Rat." (Master thesis, Massachusetts Institute of Technology, 1972), unpublished.

340. WISE, C. D., BADEN, M. M., and STEIN, L. "Postmortem Measurements of Enzymes in Human Brain: Evidence of a Central Noradrenergic Deficit in Schizophrenia," *Journal of Psychiatric Research,* 11 (1974):185–189.

341. WISE, R. A. "Catecholamine Theories of Reward: A Critical Review," *Brain Research,* 152 (1978):215–247.

342. WOLF, L. E. "Elcosanoids: Prostaglandins, Tromboxanes, Leukotienes and Other Derivatives of Carbon 20 Unsaturated Fatty Acids," *Journal of Neurochemistry,* 38 (1982):1–14.

343. WOLF, P., et al. "GABAergic Inhibition of Neurons in the Ventral Tegmental Area," *Experientia,* 34 (1978):73–74.

344. WYATT, R. J., ERDELI, E., and WISE, C. D. "Dopamine Hydroxylase in Brain of Chronic Schizophrenic Patients," *Science,* 107 (1975):368–370.

345. WYATT, R. J., VAUGHAN, T., and GALANTE, R. "Behavioral Changes of Chronic Schizophrenic Patients Given L-5 Hydroxytrytophan," *Science,* 177 (1972):1124–1126.

346. WYATT, R. J., et al. "Dopamine Hydroxylase Activity in Brains of Chronic Schizophrenic Patients," *Science,* 187 (1975): 368–369.

347. WYATT, R. J., et al. "Difficulties in Comparing Catecholamine-Related Enzymes from Brains of Schizophrenics and Controls," *Biological Psychiatry,* 13 (1978):317–334.

348. YARYURA-TOBIAS, J. A., DIAMOND, B., and MERLIN, S. "The Action of L-DOPA on Schizophrenic Patients (A Preliminary Report)," *Current Therapeutic Research,* 12 (1970):528–531.

349. YOSHIDA, M., and PRECHT, W. "Monosynaptic Inhibition of Neurons of the Substantia Nigra by Caudal-Nigral Fibers," *Brain Research,* 32 (1981):225–228.

CHAPTER 18

BIOLOGICAL TREATMENT OF SCHIZOPHRENIC DISORDERS

John M. Davis and Marcelle A. Mostert

¶ Introduction

Chlorpromazine, the first modern anti-psychotic drug, was initially developed as an antihistamine by the French anesthesiologist-surgeon H. Laborit to reduce the autonomic response to surgical stress. The discovery that chlorpromazine had tranquilizing properties but did not alter level of consciousness led to Delay and Deniker's experimental trials of the drug with psychotic patients in 1952.[60] When it was found to produce a beneficial result unlike that of previous treatments, chlorpromazine's use spread throughout the world, and within a few years it had revolutionized the care of psychiatric patients. Reserpine, which had been used for many years as a medical herb in India, was introduced as an antipsychotic agent in the United States by Kline in 1952. Although reserpine was an effective antipsychotic, chlorpromazine was more effective and easier to use. Chlorpromazine became an antipsychotic of choice, and at present, reserpine is very rarely used.

¶ Controlled Clinical Trials

The discovery of chlorpromazine spurred scientific as well as therapeutic changes in psychiatry. The late 1950s saw a controversy regarding the true efficacy of the new class of drugs, a debate that could not be settled by the impressionistic and anecdotal nature of available clinical observations. Skeptics suggested that (1) the response was due to a placebo effect; (2) the effect was merely sedative, and there was no advantage over previously available sedatives; or (3) the net effect might, in fact, be detrimental to the patient's mental status. The result was the gradual development of the clinical trial using placebo in a double-blind, random design.[44,198] These methods could control for the expectations of both patient and observer, since neither knew who was receiving active medication and who was receiving placebo. Other variables could also be controlled, such as effects of the specific milieu in which the patient was being treated. In addition, the incidence of spontaneous improvement could be evaluated in the placebo group. The trials also necessitated the development of objective rating scales to provide more reliable measures by which to evaluate the study group.

¶ The General Effectiveness of Antipsychotic Drugs

Figure 18–1, from the National Institute of Mental Health (NIMH) Collaborative Study, portrays the typical result of an antipsychotic-placebo comparison.[45,46] Seventy percent

of the antipsychotic group improved significantly and only one-tenth deteriorated or were unimproved. By contrast, only one-quarter of the placebo group improved and almost half deteriorated, even while receiving psychosocial therapies. New psychotic symptoms frequently appeared in the placebo group, but not in the drug-treated group. Lehmann[166] coined the term psychostatic to describe the capacity of antipsychotics to both suppress existing psychotic symptoms and prevent the emergence of new ones. The efficacy of antipsychotic drugs has now been proven by hundreds of double-blind studies, which are summarized in table 18–1. In those studies that do not show antipsychotic to be superior to placebo, it can be demonstrated that the dose used is inadequate. The results of a number of placebo-controlled, double-blind studies are, in essence, the same as the results of the NIMH Collaborative Studies.[205] These include double-blind, placebo-controlled studies from different countries—Great Britain, Canada, the United States, Germany, Japan, and so forth—funded from several different sources and carried out in a variety of different facilities. The veterans' administration (VA) carried out several large collaborative studies,[24,25] as did Spring Grove State Hospital.[187] Thus there is a large data base of findings that essentially confirm the NIMH Double-Blind Collaborative Study No. 1,[46] which is a prototype for this type of study.

We have critically reviewed this literature previously and provided extensive analysis of the results.[44,52] New classes of drugs, such as indoles (molindone) and dibenzoxazepines (loxapine), have recently been introduced. They have received extensive investigation in random assignment, double-blind studies comparing each of the drugs with placebo and/or the standard antipsychotic, and both drugs have been proven superior to placebo and approximately equal in efficacy to the standard antipsychotic drugs (see tables 18–1 and 18–3).*

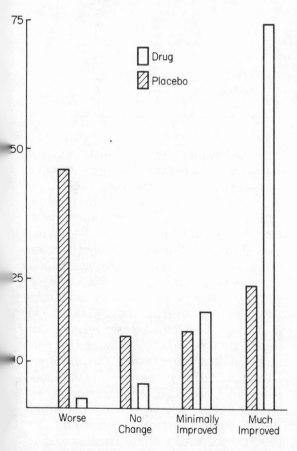

Figure 18–1. Doctors' global rating of improvement in patients after treatment with phenothiazines or placebo.

*See references 28, 37, 40, 41, 43, 68, 82, 85, 87, 88, 174, 191, 194, 198, 199, 213, 228, 236, 237, 238, 240, 242, 258, 268, and 271.

TABLE 18–1

Drug–Placebo Comparisons in Controlled Studies of Schizophrenia

Drug		No. of Studies in Which Drug Was	
Generic Name	Trade Name	More effective than placebo	Equal to placebo
Chlorpromazine	Thorazine	55	11
Reserpine	Serpasil, Sandril	20	9
Triflupromazine	Vesprin	9	1
Perphenazine	Trilafon	5	0
Prochlorperazine	Compazine	7	2
Trifluoperazine	Stelazine	16	2
Fluphenazine	Prolixin, Permitil	15	0
Butaperazine	Repoise	4	0
Thioridazine	Mellaril	7	0
Mesoridazine	Serentil	3	0
Mepazine	Pactal	2	3
Carphenazine	Proketazine	2	0
Pimoside	–	2	2
Promazine	Sparine	3	4
Chlorprothixene	Taractan	4	0
Thiothixene	Navane	2	0
Haloperidol	Haldol	9	0
Molindone	Moban, Lidone	1	0
Loxapine	Loxitane, Doxolin	5	1
Phenobarbital	Luminal, Solfoton	0	3

Cognitive-Behavioral Effects

Antipsychotics have a normalizing effect on both cognitive functioning and motor behavior, as demonstrated by ratings before and after treatment. Rating scales show a reduction in symptoms such as hallucinations, paranoid identification, hostility, belligerence, and negativism (see table 18–2). Hurt, Holzman, and Davis[139] followed the course of schizophrenic symptoms and thought disorder using the Brief Psychiatric Rating Scale (BPRS) and the Holzman-Johnston Thought Disorder Index (TDI)[132] in which schizophrenic patients respond to standardized stimuli (Rorschach cards and the Wechsler Adult Intelligence Scale). Raters, who were blind to treatment, found a parallel improvement in schizophrenic symptoms and thought disorder (see figure 18–2).

Psychologists attempting to characterize the cognitive abnormalities that may underlie schizophrenic symptomatology have discovered a peculiar difficulty in attending to and processing incoming perceptual stimuli, which has been crystalized in the attention deficit hypothesis of schizophrenia. In 1977 Spohn and his coworkers[255] demonstrated the effect of antipsychotics on these processes in chronic schizophrenic patients over the course of a six-week placebo washout period that was followed by random assignment to chlorpromazine or placebo. (Out of sixty-three patients, sixteen relapsed during the drug washout, yielding a relapse rate of 17 percent per month.) The remaining forty patients were tested on attentional, perceptual, and psychophysiological parameters at weeks 1, 4, and 8 on drug or placebo. Results showed that chlorpromazine (1) improved concentration and attention, (2) reduced overestimation and fixation time on a perceptual task, and (3) increased accuracy of perceptual judgment. Dysfunctions in at-

TABLE 18–2

Effect of Phenothiazines on Symptoms in Schizophrenia

	VA Study No. 1	VA Study No. 3	Spring-Grove Study	NIMH-PSC No. 1	VA Group Psychotherapy Study
Fundamental symptoms					
Thought disorder	++	++	++	++	++
Blunted affect-indifference				++	+
Withdrawal-retardation	++	++	o	++	++
Autistic behavior-mannerisms	++	++	o	++	+
Accessory symptoms					
Hallucinations	++	++	+	+	o
Paranoid ideation	o	++	o	+	+
Grandiosity	o	o	o	o	+
Hostility-belligerence	++	++	H.R.[a]	+	+
Resistiveness-uncooperativeness	++	++	H.R.	++	++
Nonschizophrenic symptoms					
Anxiety-tension, agitation	o	o	H.R.	+	o
Guilt depression	++	o	o	o	o
Disorientation				o	
Somatization					o

++, Symptom areas showing marked drug-control group differences; +, those showing significant but less striking differences; o, areas not showing differential drug superiority.

SOURCE: J. O. Cole, S. C. Goldberg, and J. M. Davis, "Drugs in the Treatment of Psychosis: Controlled Studies," in P. Solomon, ed. *Psychiatric Drugs* (New York: Grune & Stratton, 1966), pp. 153–181.

[a]H.R., heterogeneity of regression found on analysis of co-variance of the measures indicated. (This invalidates this particular statistical procedure but does not mean that there was no drug effect.)

tention, information processing, and autonomic responses were normalized on antipsychotics but not on placebo. The magnitude of the drug-placebo difference may well have been underestimated because of the large number of relapses during the washout period.

It should be evident from the preceding data that the term major tranquilizer is a misnomer for the class of drugs to which chlorpromazine belongs. Just as with cognitive functions, the effect on motor behavior is a normalizing one: Retarded schizophrenic patients are mobilized, and hyperactivity is slowed. Normal persons find the effect somewhat unpleasant. The effect is different from tranquilization because there is a cognitive restoration and a reduction in psychotic symptoms such as hallucinations and delusions as opposed to an across-the-board slowing of all symptoms in all patients (see table 18–2). The term tranquilizer is therefore

inappropriate. There is a clear-cut difference between the sedative and the antipsychotic properties of these agents. Furthermore, antipsychotics that are maximally "stimulating" are just as effective as those that are maximally sedating. It is therefore a mistake to think of these drugs as a special type of sedative. They are more appropriately referred to as "antipsychotics." It should be emphasized that antipsychotic activity is a general property, rather than the ability to specifically control an isolated symptom—for instance, psychotic agitation or hallucinations. The ability of antipsychotics to alleviate schizophrenic symptomatology results from a global cognitive restoration, as yet roughly characterized, that appears to be mediated by the drugs' effects on dopaminergic systems in the brain.

Although it is known that the antipsychotics alleviate psychosis by blocking dopamine (DA) receptors, we do not know the mech-

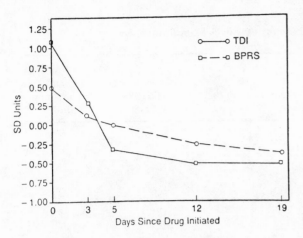

Figure 18–2. Antipsychotic drug effect on schizophrenic symptoms and thought disorder, measured by the Brief Psychiatric Rating Scale (BPRS) and the Holzman-Johnston Thought Disorder Index (TDI).

such paternalistic analogies can be misunderstood and are, in any case, imprecise. Until more is known about the connection of dopaminergic systems to the disease process, we will not know enough to specify a more appropriate analogy. What we know now are the empirical consequences of drug use: Psychotic patients become less psychotic. This change is manifested in all the symptoms of psychosis, including thought disorder and the disordered perceptual processes.

The antipsychotic drugs have a normalizing effect on schizophrenic patients, as shown in table 18–2. They lessen typical schizophrenic symptoms, such as hallucinations and delusions. However, to label the drugs as "antischizophrenic" is too restrictive, because they are also effective in psychotic depression, mania, and organic psychosis. Since the symptoms that are reduced by these drugs are not only typical of schizophrenia in particular but also of psychosis in general, the agents are best referred to as "antipsychotic" drugs. There is no evidence that certain specific symptoms are affected directly, uniquely, and specifically by antipsychotic drugs. These drugs lessen all

anisms by which the blocked DA receptors interrelate with whatever is causing the psychosis. Therefore, the analogy of "control" is imprecise. It is true that physicians sometimes speak of insulin as controlling diabetes, as if diabetes were a misbehaving child, but

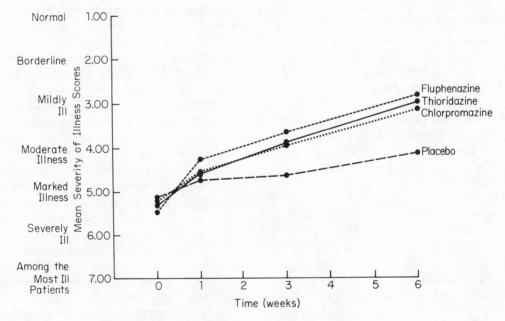

Figure 18–3. Time course of clinical improvement of patients taking phenothiazines.

TABLE 18–3

Effectiveness of the Antipsychotic Drugs Compared to Standard Antipsychotic (Chlorpromazine, Thioridazine, and Trifluoperazine)

Drug		No. of Studies in Which Drug Was		
Generic Name	Trade Name	More effective than standard	As effective as standard	Less effective than standard
Phenothiazines				
Acetophenazine	Tindal	0	2	0
Butaperazine	Repoise	0	5	0
Carphenazine	Proketazine	0	6	0
Chlorpromazine		–	–	–
Fluphenazine	Prolixin, Permitil	0	12	0
Mepazine	Pacatal	0	0	4
Mesoridazine	Serentil	0	10	0
Perphenazine	Trilafon	0	6	0
Piperacetazine	Quide	0	3	0
Prochlorperazine	Compazine	0	10	0
Promazine	Sparine	0	2	4
Thiopropazate	Dartal	0	1	0
Thioridazine	Mellaril	0	12	0
Trifluoperazine	Stelazine	0	11	0
Triflupromazine	Vesprin	0	10	0
Buterophenones				
Haloperidol	Haldol	0	11	0
Dibenzoxazepines				
Loxapine	Loxitane, Doxolin	0	14	1
Clozapine		–	–	–
Diphenylbutylpiperidines				
Pimozide		–	–	–
Indoles				
Molindone	Moban, Lidone	0	6	0
Thioxanthenes				
Chlorprothixene	Taractan	0	7	0
Thiothixene	Navane	0	4	0
Barbiturate (nonantipsychotic)				
Phenobarbital	Luminal, Solfoton	0	0	6

the symptoms of psychosis approximately equally. Just as insulin injections replace insulin absent from the body and hence restore a diabetic person to normal, antipsychotic drugs, through their property of blocking DA receptors, empirically lessen psychosis. Hence the correct term for their action is "antipsychotic."

Time Course of Improvement with Antipsychotic Drugs

The time course of the improvement produced by antipsychotics is shown in Figure 18–3.[45] About 40 percent of the improve-ment produced by six weeks is present at one week, but, nevertheless, the time course is rather gradual. The slow rate of improvement cannot be explained by slow rate of drug accumulation in brain, because steady state is achieved in the first week or so, and, in addition, use of a loading dose does not speed up the time to response. At present, there is no explanation of why it takes weeks for a schizophrenic patient to respond to an antipsychotic, but clinicians must appreciate the time course in making clinical decisions. Other studies show that patients continue to improve at least for twenty-five weeks or so, although at a slower rate. These improve-

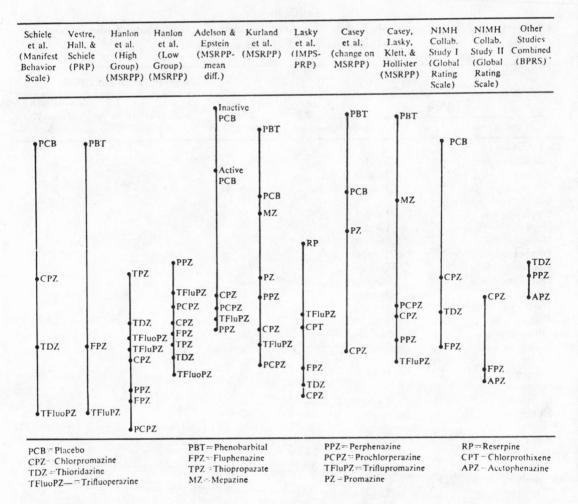

PCB = Placebo
CPZ = Chlorpromazine
TDZ = Thioridazine
TFluoPZ—= Trifluoperazine

PBT = Phenobarbital
FPZ = Fluphenazine
TPZ = Thiopropazate
MZ = Mepazine

PPZ = Perphenazine
PCPZ = Prochlorperazine
TFluPZ = Triflupromazine
PZ = Promazine

RP = Reserpine
CPT = Chlorprothixene
APZ = Acetophenazine

Figure 18–4. The rank-ordering of phenothiazine derivatives' efficacy in studies using rating scales as a measure of reduction in psychopathology.

ments are average data, and there is substantial variability between patients in the rate of improvement.

Comparative Effects of Antipsychotics

The search for effective antipsychotic action with fewer side effects has generated several structurally distinct new classes of antipsychotics in addition to the phenothiazines. These include (1) the butyrophenones (haloperidol); (2) the thioxanthenes (thiothixene), which are structural analogues of the phenothiazines; (3) the indoles (molindone); and (4) the dibenzoxazepines (loxapine). Members of these various classes are listed in table 18–3. Have any of these new agents been clearly demonstrated to be superior to chlorpromazine or to each other? The answer is no; the relevant studies are summarized in table 18–3. Eleven studies show trifluoperazine equivalent to chlorpromazine and twelve studies find thioridazine hydrochloride equal to chlorpromazine in efficacy. Most studies use chlorpromazine as the standard antipsychotic, but some use thioridazine or trifluoperazine. If a study used chlorpromazine, we considered it the standard and entered the results in table 18–3. If the study did not use chlorpromazine but did use thioridazine or trifluoperazine, we also entered it in the table, which gives the number of studies in which a given agent is inferior to standard antipsychotic, equal, or superior. All agents are equal in efficacy to chlorpromazine except phenobarbital, mepazine, or promazine hydrochloride,[25,138,158,159] of which only the last[158,159] is better than placebo. In order to assess whether or not there were nonsignificant trends for any one neuroleptic to be superior to the others, we inspected these drugs' evaluations on various continuous scales (see figure 18–4). Although the different studies used different scales, improvement on drugs can be placed on a quantitative scale, and the numbers generated can be expressed graphically.[44] We present a rank ordering of the improvement scores of different drugs in different studies in figure 18–4. Inspection of the figure does not show any drug to be consistently better than any other drug. Does a particular symptom or subtype of disease respond better to a particular agent? Again, the answer is no. The consistency in the pattern of response to antipsychotic agents is remarkable. This exceptional degree of similarity across a wide range of symptoms is consistent with their common and unique action on dopaminergic systems in the brain. Differences lie primarily with the particular balance of side effects produced by a given drug.

What should determine the choice of a particular agent for the individual patient? Even if the average effect of each agent is equivalent, it may be that an individual will respond best to a particular drug. For example, an individual may find sedation distressing and might do better on a nonsedating drug. Common psychiatric wisdom has it that a sedating drug, such as chlorpromazine or thioridazine, is best used for an agitated psychosis, such as mania, whereas a "stimulating" agent such as fluphenazine or trifluoperazine is better for withdrawn conditions. This premise has never been borne out by experiment and, in fact, some evidence— namely Goldberg and coworkers' 1967[100] and 1972[101] reports on the NIMH Collaborative Studies—has pointed in the opposite direction. Goldberg suggested that "apathetic and retarded" schizophrenics respond better

to chlorpromazine, although this finding was not duplicated in cross-validation. Results of any study must be cross-validated to lessen the likelihood of a chance relationship before the results can be accepted as fact.

Choice of an optimally effective antipsychotic drug for an individual patient is of necessity empirical. Although there are no clear indications for the use of a given agent for a given set of symptoms, clinicians occasionally observe that individuals respond best to one drug or class of drugs.[89] When a patient has been given an adequate trial on an appropriate dosage and still fails to respond optimally, another agent, of a maximally different class, may be substituted. For patients with acute symptoms, this may be done within days or weeks, whereas a more stable patient under chronic treatment could be switched after weeks or months, keeping in mind that the apparent acute response to the new agent may in fact be attributable to late response to the old agent. Any drug trial should ensure a reasonable time for an optimal dose of medication to exert its effect. It is inappropriate to change drugs every few days.

Do Antipsychotics Alter the Natural Course of Schizophrenia?

EFFECT OF ANTIPSYCHOTICS ON THE COURSE OF DISEASE

May[179] and coworkers studied first-break hospitalized schizophrenic patients over a period of six months. They compared the effect of phenothiazines and psychotherapy alone and in combination, including a treatment-free control group. Table 18–4 shows the results. All patients were switched to conventional therapy after the initial six-month (to one-year) study period. Ten years later they published a follow-up study of the same patients at intervals of three to five years after the index admission. Significant differences in outcome were evident when the total number of days spent in hospital since the study period and overall social functioning were assessed.[180,181,182,183]

TABLE 18–4

Assessment of Outcome in Schizophrenic Patients Treated
With and Without Antipsychotic Drugs and Psychotherapy

	No Drugs		Drug	
	No psychotherapy	Psychotherapy	No psychotherapy	Psychotherapy
Percent released	59	64	95	96
Nurses' rating MACC total	38	38	48	48
Menninger nurses' health-sickness rating	26	23	29	30
Nurses' idiosyncratic symptoms $(125\text{-}X)^a$	37	29	66	74
Therapists' rating on symptom rating sheet $(50\text{-}X)^a$	22	21	27	27
Analysis rating of insight	3.4	3.3	3.7	4.1

SOURCE: P.R.A. May, *Treatment of Schizophrenia: A Comparative Study of Five Treatment Methods.* New York: Science House, 1968).
[a] A higher number reflects greater improvement. In order to have the two scales fit with this convention, we subtracted scores from an arbitrary constant. See May[179] for definition of scales.

Figure 18–5 shows that the patients who received psychotherapy alone during the initial admission spent about twice as much time in the hospital subsequently as those who received pharmacotherapy and psychotherapy. Table 18–5 shows the carryover effect of initial treatment on work history in the follow-up period. Regarding the apparently detrimental effect of psychotherapy compared to control, it should be noted that psychotherapy was not uniformly provided by experienced therapists. It is also relevant to consider the "dose" of psychotherapy. Patients in the "no psychotherapy" groups (milieu only or drug only) actually did have some individual contact with therapists and during their hospital stay received approximately 10 and 8.5 hours, respectively, of, in effect, psychotherapy; whereas patients in the formal psychotherapy groups received 49 hours (no drug) and 33 hours (with drug) of formal psychotherapy. If we mean by "an intense psychotherapeutic involvement" three to five hours a week for two to five years (e.g., 4 hours a week for three years equals 600 hours of treatment), then dose of psychotherapy was rather small. We believe that what is particularly unique about this study is not the psychotherapy contrast but rather the drug-to-no-drug contrast. Most drug studies last three to six weeks. It is quite unusual to find a group of schizophrenic patients who have not received antipsychotic drugs for a substantial period of time. In this study, patients did not receive antipsychotic drugs for a period of roughly six months to one year, and data are provided on the subsequent three to five years. During this period of time, it is clear that the patients who received drugs during their initial episode did substantially better than those who did not receive drugs at the time. This is the closest evidence we have that drugs may alter the natural course of this illness: Therapy with antipsychotics during the initial episode resulted in a better outcome several years down the line. It has been suggested that a psychotic episode, particularly if untreated, will result in "psychic scarring." Anyone who has talked with a patient who has been unsuccessfully treated in the past can appreciate some of the reasons behind this, including damage to the person's sense of personal integrity and self-confidence resulting from the fear of a recurrent psychotic episode.

The Prophylactic Effects of Antipsychotics

RELAPSE RATES

Shortly after chlorpromazine came into wide use, it became clear that relapse of psy-

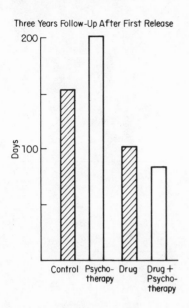

Three Years Follow-Up After First Release

Days

Control | Psycho-therapy | Drug | Drug + Psycho-therapy

Figure 18–5. Comparison of days spent in the hospital during a three-year period subsequent to treatment on initial hospitalization with psychotherapy, drugs, psychotherapy plus drugs, or none of these.

chosis frequently followed upon the heels of drug discontinuance. More precise investigational methods have made it possible to assess relapse rates over time, refuting the frequent assertion that only 50 percent of patients will relapse and therefore only that proportion requires maintenance medication. Relapses seem to occur at a constant rate over time. Even though many fewer patients will be unrelapsed at, for example, fifteen months, their relapse rate will be identical to what it was in the first month, when the overwhelming majority of the patients were still well. That is, a fixed proportion of the well patients remaining at any

point will relapse in the next month. The relapse rate is conceptually similar to radioactive decay, or plasma drug half-life ($t_{1/2}$), in that it fits an exponential curve. Let us review the evidence.

The suggestion that relapse rates might be constant was first investigated by Davis in 1975 and 1980 [53,58] by reassessing data from a number of earlier studies. It was found that the relapse rate was constant over time. A review of data from Caffey and associates' 1964 [20] study of VA inpatients disclosed a relapse rate of 15.7 percent per month. Hogarty and Goldberg's 1973 study [124] yielded a somewhat lower relapse rate for patients on placebo: 10.7 percent. The NIMH Collaborative Study [205] indicated a relapse rate of 8 percent per month (see figure 18–8). In each case, least-squares analysis demonstrated an excellent fit of the relapse rate to the exponential curve, with r^2 values of about 0.95, as shown in figures 18–6, 18–7, and 18–8.

Relapse rates prove more difficult to assess after longer time periods. The Hogarty and Goldberg [125,126,127] data showed a constant relapse rate only until eighteen months, at which time the number of survivors was extremely small. Survivors at this point may not be at risk for relapse, possibly because their disease is different in some way, generating a plateau of patients not subject to recurrent illness. In 1976 Hogarty and associates [128] sought to examine the outliers by calculating relapse rates of two-year survivors. There were so few in the drug-free group that meaningful analysis was impossible. The treated group, however, had a large pool of patients who were relapse-free at two years. Medication was discontinued for this group, generating the same constant relapse rate

TABLE 18–5
Mean Rating on Working for Pay at Two Years[a]

	Psychotherapy	No Psychotherapy	Psychotherapy Effect
Drug	1.8	2.3	−.5
No Drug	1.2	1.6	−.4
Drug Effect	0.6	0.7	

[a]See original studies for details on how the ratings were performed.[180, 181, 182, 183]

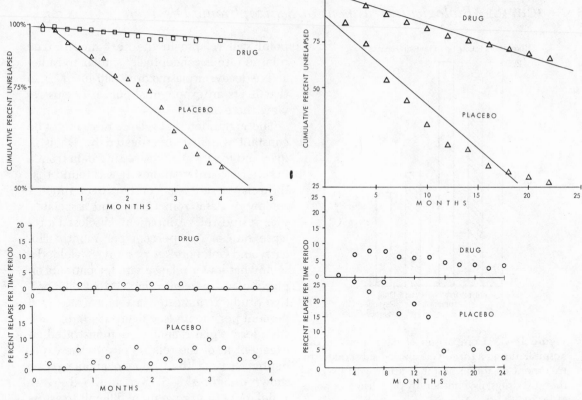

Figure 18–6. Relapse rates over time of outpatient treated with phenothiazines schizophrenics receiving placebo or antipsychotics.

Figure 18–7. Relapse rates over time of inpatient schizophrenics receiving placebo or antipsychotics.

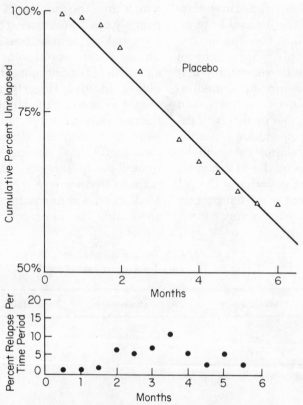

Figure 18–8. Relapse rates over time of schizophrenics receiving placebo.

found in the original study. Therefore, it does not appear that duration of drug use has any effect on relapse rate.

To prevent tardive dyskinesia (TD), it would be helpful to manage a long-term chronic hospital patient situation without medication. To do so, we need to select which patients would not relapse when antipsychotics are discontinued. Morgan and Cheadle[192] identified patients they felt could do well without drugs and selected 74 out of 475 patients as drug-free candidates. They believed the remaining 401 needed maintenance neuroleptics. Unfortunately, only 5 of these 74 patients remained relapse-free after several years off drug. The relapse of the other 69 patients occurred, on the average, about four and one-half months after drugs were discontinued. The study indicates that *most* chronic schizophrenic patients are at risk for relapse, including even those whom clinicians feel might be appropriate candidates for a drug-free trial.

Given the definite rate of relapse for drug-free schizophrenic patients, it is clear that many will need maintenance medication to ensure a sustaining remission. Double-blind studies have evaluated the effect of maintenance medication versus placebo prospectively in both inpatient and outpatient populations. Thirty-five controlled studies that documented patient number and ran for a minimum of six weeks for oral agents and two months for depot forms are summarized in table 18–6. This group of studies followed a total of 3,625 subjects for a period of from four to six months, and demonstrated an overall relapse rate of 53 percent on placebo versus 20 percent on drug. Combining the group according to the method of Mantel[84] generates a p value of less than 10^{-100}, which dramatically supports the value of antipsychotic therapy for maintenance purposes.

We will present some examples of these studies in more detail. Caffey and associates is a typical inpatient study, which followed 171 patients on placebo and 88 on either chlorpromazine or thioridazine.[20] Only 4 of the 88 patients on medication relapsed (5 percent), in contrast to fully 45 percent of the placebo group. Medication decreased the relapse rate from 15.7 percent to 1.5 percent per month. These figures are fairly certain because all medications were administered by nurses, rather than by the patients themselves. Because of the medication compliance problem, outpatient studies tend to generate a higher relapse rate for "medicated" patients. Hogarty and Goldberg[124] followed 374 recovered schizophrenic subjects after discharge from hospital. After an initial period of stabilization, half were randomized to placebo and half to maintenance chlorpromazine. Half of each group received individual psychotherapy and vocational counseling. After one year, 68 percent of placebo patients with psychotherapy had relapsed, compared to 73 percent without psychotherapy. In contrast, 26 percent of patients with drug and psychotherapy had relapsed, versus 33 percent with drug alone. Eliminating patients who discontinued medication without supervision produces a relapse rate of only 16 percent in the medicated group, indicating that half of relapses in medicated outpatients are due to drug discontinuance. Although the relapse rate of patients having the benefit of psychotherapy was lower in both groups, the difference was not statistically significant. Social functioning proved to be superior in the group with psychotherapy and drugs. Goldberg and associates[102] found that the individuals who tended to do best with psychotherapy tended to be those who were least symptomatic.

Virtually all the studies on maintenance treatment have used chronic schizophrenic patients who either are still symptomatic or would be predicted to relapse because they have relapsed in the past. Hence these studies can only be generalized to that type of schizophrenic patient. There are patients who have a single psychotic episode, or even occasionally two psychotic episodes, whose illness does not run a chronic remitting and /or deteriorating course.[259,260,266,267] These patients are sometimes called "reactive schizophrenics" or "schizophrenics of good prognosis," as opposed to "process schizo-

TABLE 18–6

Antipsychotic Prevention of Relapse

Study	Date	No. of patients	Relapse on placebo (%)	Relapse on drug (%)	Difference in relapse rate (placebo-drug) (%)
Caffey et al.[20]	1964	250	45	5	40
Prien and Cole[205]	1968	762	42	16	26
Prien, Cole, and Belkin[206]	1968	325	56	20	36
Schiele, Vestre, and Stein[228]	1961	80	60	3	57
Adelson and Epstein[2]	1962	281	90	49	41
Morton[193]	1968	40	70	25	45
Baro et al.[10]	1970	26	100	0	100
Hershon, Kennedy, and McGuire[115]	1972	62	28	7	21
Rassidakis et al.[214]	1970	84	58	34	24
Melynk, Worthington, and Laverty[185]	1966	40	50	0	50
Schawver et al.[226]	1959	80	18	5	13
Freeman and Alson[86]	1966	94	28	13	16
Whitaker and Hoy[274]	1963	39	65	8	57
Garfield et al.[91]	1966	27	31	11	20
Diamond and Marks[64]	1960	40	70	25	45
Blackburn and Allen[15]	1961	53	54	24	30
Gross and Reeves[109]	1961	109	58	14	44
Engelhardt et al.[71]	1967	294	30	15	15
Leff et al.[165]	1982	30	83	33	50
Hogarty et al.[124, 126]	1973,74	361	67	31	36
Troshinsky, Aaronson, and Stone[264]	1962	43	63	4	59
Hirsch et al.[121]	1973	74	66	8	58
Chien[30]	1975	31	87	12	94
Gross[108]	1975	61	65	34	31
Rifkin et al.[217]	1977	62	68	7	61
Clark et al.[42]	1975	35	78	27	51
Clark et al.[38]	1971	19	70	43	27
Kinross-Wright and Charalampous[154]	1965	40	70	5	65
Andrews, Hall, and Snaith[4]	1976	31	35	7	28
Wistedt[280]	1981	38	63	38	25
Cheung[29]	1981	28	62	13	48
Levine et al.[168, 169, 170] (PO)	1979,80	33	59	33	26
Levine et al.[168, 169, 170] (IM)	1979,80	34	30	18	12
Kane et al.[148, 149]	1983,83	16	88	13	75
Zissis (Johnson)[144]	1982	32	81	0	81

SOURCE: J. M. Davis, "Overview: Maintenance Therapy in Psychiatry: I. Schizophrenia," *American Journal of Psychiatry*, 132 (1975):1237–1245.
Summary statistics, p less than 10^{-100}.

phrenics." Indeed, it has been suggested that such patients may have a variant of affective disease and not true schizophrenia. Others suggest that such patients have a third "psychotic" disorder, which is neither an affective disorder variant or true "process" schizophrenia, in the European sense. Individuals in this category have a brief psychotic episode, which is often reactive in nature and remits quickly. These disorders have been termed brief reactive psychosis, atypical psychosis, and schizophreniform disorder in DSM-III terminology, as well as "psychogenic" or "hysterical" psychoses. This group has not been studied with respect to maintenance medication. It has been said that patients with good prognostic signs may not need medication at all. We would not necessarily recommend maintenance medication for all such patients.

Drug therapy should be tailored to the needs of the individual patient. Any acutely psychotic patient can benefit from an antipsychotic agent in a moderately high dose, which is titrated as needed. Once the patient is recovered, medication should be continued at a moderate but adequate dosage until it is certain that the improvement is sustained. This period can reasonably last from three months to a year. Patients who have a single psychotic episode do not need further maintenance, but as this is difficult to predict, they should be carefully followed after medication is gradually decreased and then discontinued. Patients who have relapsed in the past when medication has been discontinued, as well as those with continuing symptomatology, are candidates for long-term maintenance. Maintenance treatment meets the goals of prophylaxis, as well as supporting the patient at his or her maximum level of functioning. Psychosocial modalities are useful to all patients in facilitating adjustment to the community and further diminishing the likelihood of relapse.

In the interest of lessening long-term side effects, the author (J.M.D.) has suggested that it might be possible to discontinue medication in selected patients, who must then be followed closely for signs of relapse. At the first hint of recurrent symptomatology, an antipsychotic could then be reintroduced, hopefully aborting the episode. A pilot study by Herz and coworkers[116,120] on nineteen selected stable schizophrenic outpatients showed that fourteen could tolerate gradual tapering and discontinuance of medication. Ten of these were treated successfully for an average of eight months with an intermittent strategy—reinstituting drug treatment for two weeks at signs of recurrence and tapering again over two weeks; each time, prodromal but nonpsychotic symptoms recurred. The investigators do not recommend tapering or discontinuing medication for patients who remain symptomatic while on maintenance therapy, or for patients who are known to decompensate immediately upon drug discontinuance. They point out the usefulness of a relative or significant other in

monitoring symptom emergence, but found that both patient and family were frequently fearful of stopping drug treatment because of previous medical advice. Obviously the number of patients in this study is too small to allow generalization to the larger population, particularly since there was no control group. In a somewhat longer study, Carpenter and Heinrichs[21] followed forty-one schizophrenic outpatients over twenty-four months, with twenty-seven on continuous medication and fourteen treated with a "targeted" approach using four-week treatment periods upon signs of deterioration. Four targeted and two continuous-drug patients relapsed.

This "no drug but early intervention to abort relapse" strategy is an interesting idea. The research to prove that this idea actually works, however, has yet to be done. We must not wishfully accept the idea as correct and the pilot data as valid until blind study has verified the hypothesis. At this time, this idea is an unproven hypothesis.

Drug Holiday

There is very little information on drug holidays of weeks or months, but since patients relapse on placebo at a rate of about 10 percent per month, we can estimate the relapse in a drug holiday. Drug holidays of one or two days have little liability of relapse. We would favor decreasing the dose rather than using one- or two-day drug holidays as a means of reducing drug intake, because inconsistency in drug schedule can be confusing for patients, who are usually told that not taking medication will eventually cause relapse.

Long-acting Depot Agents

The problem of medication noncompliance has met a partial solution with the advent of long-acting intramuscular depot forms of antipsychotics.[8] Several studies have even suggested that certain patients do better on these agents than on oral forms of the same drug. The major factor is compliance. A minor factor may be that certain patients are rapid metabolizers who lose much of the orally administered drug in the first pass through the liver. Two studies found depot medication more effective.[48,61] Del Guidice, Clark, and Gocka's study, for example, showed that fluphenazine's 3 percent-per-month relapse rate dropped to 1 percent when patients were switched to the depot form.[61] Most studies, however, show oral and depot forms to be equally effective* in the sense of no statistically significant difference. Research with the subgroup of patients who do better on depot agents has been clouded by newer, more stringent criteria for acceptance of patients for research. Habitual noncompliers are unlikely to be willing to sign complicated consent forms, much less cooperate with the extensive evaluations required by most research protocols. On the other hand, those patients who do consent to be studied can be influenced by the Hawthorne effect, which skews results in favor of patients cooperating in taking their medication. This effect is brought about by the investment of investigators in their project. Their increased interest can translate into improved patient care, which can motivate patients to do better in remembering to take their medication. The distance between the noncompliant patient taking depot form and the more cooperative research subject taking oral forms may be widened by these effects; studies looking at these different individuals should be interpreted accordingly. Good compliance among patients taking oral medication may account for some of the observed therapeutic benefit of oral medication as compared with depot medication taken by noncompliant patients.

Since two of the smaller studies found the depot drug to produce fewer relapses and the two largest studies found a trend in the direction of the depot drug producing relapses, it is reasonable to consider combining all the five studies to see if the depot formulation does produce less relapse. When this is done, about 51 percent of patients relapse on oral phenothiazine and about 31 percent on depot fluphenazine ($p < 10^{-3}$). The most widely used depot forms in the United States are fluphenazine enanthate and fluphenazine decanoate. The latter is slightly more potent and therefore longer acting. It also has slightly fewer immediate neurological side effects.[66,147,269] Prolixin decanoate is probably marginally better than prolixin enanthate, but both drugs are highly effective. These drugs have been well studied in a variety of circumstances and clearly are an important addition to the psychiatrist's therapeutic tools.

Pipotiazine palmitate and several long-acting thioxanthines are available in Europe and have been shown to be as effective in maintenance management.[19] Haloperidol decanoate has likewise been shown to be as effective as oral haloperidol in several controlled studies. It is a promising new depot formulation.* Penfluridol is an unusual oral agent that has a duration of action of about one week.[212] It has been shown to be as effective as both oral and depot forms of fluphenazine. Pimozide is a well-studied, relatively specific DA blocker with demonstrated efficacy in maintenance treatment.[38,42,77]

Which patients are candidates for therapy with long-acting depot agents? Obviously, patients who are poorly compliant with daily oral medication are appropriate if they are able to come in every few weeks for an injection. Despite the increased incidence of immediate neurological side effects, it is even possible to use depot forms in the emergency room to circumvent the need for hospitalization, particularly for the patient who refuses admission but is not a candidate for involuntary hospitalization. Depot fluphenazine is effective in treating an acute episode. For those patients who remain on oral agents, one practical way of assessing compliance is to have them bring their medication containers to appointments, so the remaining pills can be counted and compared with expected amounts.

Although at the present time patients do

---

*See references 129, 217, 229, 230, and 231.

*See references 94, 135, 144, 220, 279, and 280.

not always do as well as one would like upon discharge to the community, before the advent of antipyschotic drugs in 1952, the prognosis for schizophrenia was dismal. A review of eight typical studies of the long-term prognosis of schizophrenic patients found that before the era of drug treatment, approximately two-thirds of these patients spent substantial parts of their lives in psychiatric hospitals.* It should be recognized from the outset that antipsychotic drugs are not "miracle" drugs and in no way represent a cure for schizophrenia. Although drugs often suppress symptoms, many patients continue to have residual symptoms in spite of drug treatment. There is no permanent cure, since maintenance drugs are often required to sustain improvement and they do not help all patients. However, they do help the majority of patients.

Clozapine: A Drug That Does Not Cause Extrapyramidal Side Effects

Clozapine is a relatively new antipsychotic that does not appear to cause extrapyramidal side effects (EPRs) and, presumably, does not cause TD.[32,95,96,239,241] Clozapine has been studied in one double-blind, placebo-controlled study and four controlled studies comparing it with standard antipsychotics, chlorpromazine, or haloperidol. A total of about 500 patients were studied in these random assignment, double-blind trials. Clinical improvement was assessed using BPRS total scores. In two studies, clozapine was clearly superior to standard drug ($p < 0.001$). The other two studies found a trend for clozapine to be effective ($p = 0.10$). When the results of these studies are combined, according to the method of Fleiss,[84] the larger sample size yields an even stronger finding for clozapine's superiority to standard drug ($p = 0.00001$). However, one must exercise caution in interpreting this finding since two studies found only a trend. Also, when a large sample of patients is studied, a relatively small effect can become quite statistically significant.

*See references 7, 11, 76, 114, 161, 162, 215, 223, and 256.

However, this evidence clearly establishes that clozapine is at least equal in efficacy to the standard antipsychotics, with the distinct possibility that it may even be slightly superior to them. Long-term studies of clozapine have demonstrated that improvement is maintained over time even with reduced doses, which indicates that patients do not develop tolerance to its antipsychotic properties. Clozapine is marketed and used in twenty-two countries; clinical experience and open trials also support its antipsychotic efficacy.

The major advantage of clozapine is that it does not produce EPRs. We would assume that since it does not produce acute EPRs, it would not produce TD when given on a long-term basis. This is only an assumption. We believe that it is possible but unlikely that a drug could produce EPRs but not produce TD or vice versa.

The disadvantage of clozapine is that it produces agranulocytosis. To measure incidence, the number of patients developing agranulocytosis and the number of patients included in the trial must be known. We estimate the incidence as about 1.5 in 1,000 patients, based on studies where the denominator and numerator are both known. This may be a falsely high incidence since it may be unduly influenced by the Finnish epidemic of agranulocytosis in patients taking clozapine. If the epidemic was not caused by clozapine per se but rather by "something" localized to those state hospitals where it occurred, then this estimate may be falsely high. We will elaborate on this and other side effects of antipsychotics in greater detail in a subsequent section.

Clozapine has been suggested to have a unique beneficial effect in some treatment-resistant schizophrenic patients. A design to test this particular point should use neuroleptic-treatment failures, randomly assigned to receive further drug treatment with a different "conventional DA-blocking" neuroleptic or with clozapine, to test if clozapine does produce a better result than a conventional neuroleptic.

There is no doubt that clozapine is an

effective antipsychotic drug that certainly should be considered for patients who either have TD or would be predicted to have TD based on provocative tests and so forth. Since most cases of agranulocytosis do not develop until after five weeks of treatment, clozapine can be given to treatment-resistant patients and, if they are significantly benefited, treatment can be continued into the period of the greatest risk for agranulocytosis (weeks 5 to 25). If no substantial benefit is observed, clozapine can be discontinued before that period.

In summary, clozapine is an interesting and theoretically important drug. There is some suggestion that it may possibly be superior to currently available antipsychotics in overall efficacy, and as such it may be useful in previously treatment-resistant patients. This would be truly interesting if it could be cross-validated. Because it does not appear to cause true EPRs, it may be postulated to have the additional benefit of not causing TD and therefore would be an appropriate treatment for psychotic patients already so afflicted. (If the term neuroleptic is considered to include both antipsychotic and extrapyramidal effects, then clozapine would not be considered a neuroleptic in the strict sense.) On the negative side, clozapine seems to carry an increased risk for precipitating agranulocytosis. Clozapine offers the hope that extrapyramidal and antipsychotic effects can be dissociated, so that the latter benefit may be obtained without the former risk.

¶ The Impact of Antipsychotics on the Treatment of Schizophrenia

Prior to the introduction of antipsychotics, two out of three schizophrenic patients spent most of their lives within the confines of state mental hospitals. Currently, 95 percent of schizophrenic patients are living in the community, although many do continue to have problems with relapses and residual symptoms. NIMH data show that the psychiatric inpatient population fell from a high in 1954 just before chlorpromazine was introduced

to the present much lower levels (see figure 18–9). These figures attest to the efficacy of antipsychotic drugs, although they also reflect the vigorous development of psychosocial therapies that were facilitated both by the effects of the drugs themselves and by the more optimistic atmosphere engendered by the reality of an efficacious psychiatric treatment. The focus of public mental health policy shifted from massive state institutions to community agencies for the many patients who were now able to function adequately in the community. Halfway houses and nursing homes were developed for those whose residual impairment did not permit independent functioning. The benefit to those who had to remain in the hospital was a more humane inpatient environment. This change in the health care system is a consequence of the antipsychotic efficacy of neuroleptics.

¶ Social Therapies

In this section we will consider "social therapy" to include psychological approaches involving the patient in a one-to-one interaction with a therapist, as well as family and group therapy. Critics of the use of antipsychotic drugs point to their potentially serious consequences and argue that schizophrenia can be cured by psychological means alone. They believe that antipsychotic treatment merely serves as a "chemical straitjacket" for violent or underclass in-

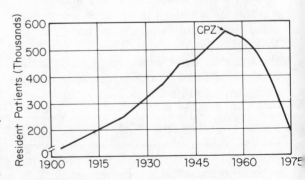

Figure 18–9. Psychiatric inpatient population before and after the advent of chlorpromazine in 1954.

dividuals who are denied access to more expensive but more effective psychosocial measures. Consonant with this belief, the legal profession is trying to outlaw antipsychotic use in certain classes of patients. In Massachusetts it is now illegal to administer medication to committed patients on an involuntary basis; treatment is permitted only when urgently needed. No one would deny that poor quality of mental health care exists in certain institutions, but does the use of psychotropic medication play any role in this? Perhaps mental health funding is the real issue here. But let us look at the premise underlying this aspect of mental health activism. Is the notion that schizophrenia responds to psychosocial treatments alone supported by the available evidence?

The group of studies on hospitalized subjects tends to be hampered by incomplete data collection and the confounding impact of variable drug use even in the "psychotherapy" groups. Medicated patients are often undermedicated, yielding results that are difficult to interpret. Karon and associates' study[150,151,152,265] fits in this category. Their control group, which received no treatment, was transferred to chronic care facilities that did not provide the same baseline treatment as that received by the study groups. Most important, many in the control group probably did receive medication throughout the two-year study. Furthermore, every subject received drugs acutely for the initial episode, and many received drugs on a more chronic basis. There was no separation of subjects in the psychotherapy group with and without chronic medication. Drugs are, therefore, an uncontrolled variable.

Paul and Lentz's study[201] provides another example of drug use as an uncontrolled variable. There is inadequate information on drug dosage and type of drug, hence the study is open to the criticism that most patients in the medicated group were on inadequate doses or inappropriate drugs. Paul's comparison of specific behavioral versus milieu treatment is more valid. He and his co-workers found that a behavioral "token economy" approach produced seemingly better results than a milieu approach. Food was used as a positive reward, tokens being required for food unless the body weight fell below 90 percent of ideal weight, at which time patients were fed what Paul calls a "medical meal," where the required food is combined in a tasteless blend served in a single container. Patients without tokens potentially could become very hungry before they lost enough weight to qualify for a "medical meal." As a negative reinforcer, Paul used up to seventy-two hours in a time-out (seclusion) room, which was made more aversive by the intermittent and unpredictable tooting of an aerosol air horn or spray of water mist through a high window, or an aversive high heat-humidity condition seclusion room was used. British "antipsychiatrist" R. D. Laing has reported encouraging but uncontrolled results from family-oriented therapy with schizophrenics, but his criteria for diagnosis are unclear, and, of particular relevance here, Esterson, Cooper, and Laing[75] note that 25 percent of their patients did not need tranquilizers, which implies that 75 percent did in fact receive drugs.

Well-controlled inpatient studies, such as that of May, Tuma, and Dixon[179,180,181,182] (outlined in tables 18–4 and 18–5 and figure 18–5), show that denial of drug treatment can in fact be detrimental. Even at long-term follow-up, those individuals who initially received no drugs, regardless of subsequent therapy, did not do as well. Drugs resulted in significantly more improvement than psychotherapy alone. Medicated patients who received psychotherapy did slightly, but not significantly, better than those who did not. The authors of this study point out that some patients may find psychotherapy too intrusive and deteriorate as a result. Despite its careful design, this study is open to the criticism that its therapists were inexperienced. Grinspoon, Ewalt, and Shader's study at the Massachusetts Mental Health Center[106,107,186] addresses this point: Senior psychoanalysts treated a small group of chronic schizophrenic patients who required continuing hospitalization. The patients deteriorated whenever placebo was substituted for thioridazine. Medication appeared to enhance the patients' ability to engage in psychotherapy, in contrast to suggestions that it will blunt emotional response. Drug improved involvement in therapy as well as awareness of events in the outside world.

Another study from the same institution, by Greenblatt and associates,[105] further demonstrates the complementarity of drugs and social approaches, looking at high versus low social therapy with and without drugs. A chronic-care state hospital was the setting for low social therapy. High social therapy included social work services, occupational therapy, psychodrama, "total push" therapy, and a variety of psychotherapies. Results, detailed in table 18–7, show the clear superiority of drug treatment across all categories. In medicated patients, there was a trend (nonsignificant) for more improvement from high (33 percent) versus low (23 percent) social therapy. Unmedicated patients did (nonsignificantly) better with low social therapy at the state hospital (10 percent) than with high social therapy at the Massachusetts Mental Health Center (0 percent). One possible explanation is that patients are more easily involved in aggressive social therapy when medicated. The results of several VA double-blind studies[104,134] of combinations of group therapy and phenothiazine treatment with both young and chronic elderly schizophrenic patients are similar. A number of other studies suggest synergism of drug and social approaches.

Rosen[221,222] used a "direct analytic" technique, with its roots in psychoanalysis, to bring about what he reported as permanent improvement in thirty-seven deteriorated schizophrenic patients. However, Horwitz and associates[137] provided follow-up that exposed Rosen's claim, showing that almost 40 percent of the group were not initially diagnosed as schizophrenic, with the bulk of these considered psychoneurotic. Of the remaining true schizophrenic patients, 75 percent had from two to five hospitalizations in the ten years subsequent to Rosen's treatment period; this can hardly be considered permanent improvement. Furthermore,

when Bookhammer and coworkers[16] attempted to replicate Rosen's work, they were unable to produce more favorable results in the experimental subjects than in the control group.

Comparisons of brief hospitalization with long-term inpatient hospitalization in four studies* have shown no difference in outcome. The data from Glick and Hargreaves' "Langley Porter Study"[99] is presented in table 18–8. Theirs is a disappointing result for inpatient psychotherapy.

Several studies compared day hospitals, hospital alternatives, or alternate facilities to regular hospitalization. Alternatives to hospital care or brief hospitalization are generally less expensive than full hospitalization, but sometimes the difference is not that large. The therapeutic efficacy of these settings is equal, an observation consistent with the fact that schizophrenic patients are treated with antipsychotics in all settings. The drugs seem effective in all settings. This body of data questions the cost effectiveness of long inpatient hospitalization.

Postdischarge outpatient psychotherapy appears much more promising than lengthy hospitalization. Hogarty, Goldberg, and associates[126,127] showed that whereas individual therapy alone could not prevent relapse, the addition of social approaches to drug treatment improved social function. Claghorn and associates[35] showed that for patients on maintenance medication, group therapy was able to improve patients' insight, although it made little impact on symptomatology. O'Brien and coworkers[197] demonstrated improvements in both insight and symptomatology from group over individual therapy, although there were no differences in readmission rates. Findings are similar with family therapy compared to individual therapy. Family therapy focuses on problem solving rather than on interpreting dynamics.

It has been suggested that families with high expressed emotions have a greater relapse rate than families with low expressed

*See references 99, 117, 118, 119, 157, and 202.

TABLE 18–7

Results of Four Treatments in Chronic Schizophrenia

	% Showing High Improvement at 6-month Evaluation		% Discharged After 6 to 9 Months		% Showing High Improvement After 36 Months	
	Drug Therapy	No Drug Therapy	Drug Therapy	No Drug Therapy	Drug Therapy	No Drug Therapy
High social therapy[a]	33	0	27	7[b]	35	26[b]
Low social therapy[c]	23	10	9	5[b]	19	6[b]

SOURCE: M. Greenblatt et al., eds., *Drug and Social Therapy in Chronic Schizophrenia* (Springfield, Ill.: Charles C Thomas, 1965).
[a]Patients transferred to Massachusetts Mental Health Center.
[b]No drug therapy for six months.
[c]Patients remained in state hospitals.

TABLE 18–8

Langley Porter Study: Outcome at Two Years After Covariate Adjustment for Prehospital Prognosis and Posthospital Treatment

	Hospitalization		Statistical Significance
	Short	Long	
Health Sickness Rating Scale[a]	38.0	40.7	NS
Psychiatric Evaluation Form[b] (Severity of Illness)	3.6	3.4	NS
Katz Adjustment Scale[b] (Relative Rating Social Performance)	31.0	30.9	NS
Historical Information Form[b] (Global Scale)	0.2	0.2	NS

[a]Higher number = good outcome.
[b]Lower number = good outcome.

emotions.[165] This suggests a vulnerability of schizophrenic patients to emotional confrontations. Several workers have randomly assigned patients to receive family therapy interventions to reduce expressed emotion or to improve the families' ability to interact and cope with the schizophrenic family member. In addition, families are educated about schizophrenic illness and the necessity for patients to take their maintenance medication. The model is to help the family cope with the disease. This is in marked contrast to the model in which schizophrenic mothers and fathers are considered the cause and pa-tients are hospitalized in order to separate them from the aversive family. All studies used patients treated with maintenance antipsychotics, and so all were testing whether education/family therapy has an additional effect over and above that produced by drugs. The results of these studies are presented in table 18–9. Any enthusiasm about the results is tempered by the fact that Leff and coworkers[163] had two suicides in their family therapy group.

Goldstein and associates' study[103] showed a significant positive effect of family therapy in the six weeks following a brief two-week

TABLE 18–9
Outcome of Social Skills and Family Therapy

	9 Months[a]		9 Months[b]		2 Years[c]	
	Well	Readmitted	Well	Relapsed	Well	Relapsed
Control	9	9	36	12	2	7
Family Therapy	16	2	17	0	6	4
Social Skills			12	5		
Family Therapy & Social Skills			19	1		

[a]Based on data from Falloon et al.[79]
[b]Based on data from Hogarty and Ulrich.[125]
[c]Based on data from Leff.[163]

Relapse According to Treatment Group (Goldstein et al.[103])

	Relapse At 6 Weeks		No Relapse	
	Mod. Dose	Low Dose	Mod. Dose	Low Dose
Family Therapy				
+	0	2	23	21
−	3	5	26	16

hospitalization. They suggested that such an approach further solidified the somewhat tentative reintegration present at the time of discharge by increasing patient and family insight and bolstering social supports. Combining the data of these four studies and considering the social skill subgroups as a separate study, the consistently better outcome for the family therapy/education intervention is statistically significant ($p < 4 \times 10^{-6}$).

We have critically reviewed this literature on social therapy at some length elsewhere, and our conclusion, drawn from available data, is that schizophrenia does *not* respond to social therapies used as the sole treatment modality.[56] Pharmacological intervention is essential for symptomatic improvement and has the further benefit of facilitating the patient's ability to respond to social measures. But drugs provide only the foundation for rehabilitation; social therapies are clearly necessary for improving social skills and facilitating readjustment to the community. Patients will require education as to the nature of their illness and a supportive environment in which to make sense of their experience. Both patient and family will respond better to an approach that presents the disease as essentially biological in nature but exacerbated by social stress. Combined pharmacological and social therapy therefore makes the best sense.

¶ Treatment with Antipsychotic Medication

Indications

Antipsychotic agents are properly used, as their name implies, for the treatment of psychosis, that is, loss of reality testing evidenced by such symptomatology as hallucinations and delusions. Double-blind studies have shown their efficacy in schizophrenia, schizophreniform disorders, late paraphrenia (onset of first paranoid symptoms after age fifty-five in clear sensorium without organicity), psychotic depression, mania, and organic psychosis. Antipsychotics are the drugs of choice in treating intoxication by amphetamine and similar drugs, and there is some evidence that antipsychotics with low anticholinergic potency are useful in PCP psychosis.[98] But given the existence of placebo response in many of these studies, one might ask whether drugs should be used in every case of psychosis. The NIMH Collaborative Study[259] showed that one in four cases of psychosis improves spontaneously. Even in selected good-prognosis patients, the overall improvement is greater for the drug group than the placebo group; medicated patients tend to do better.

Can one predict which patient will require antipsychotics and, conversely, which patient will tend not to respond to treatment? In 1973 Klein and Rosen[156] reported that asocial childhood schizophrenic patients do not do as well on chlorpromazine as nonsocial "good-prognosis" schizophrenic patients. This differential response points to what may be heterogeneity in the underlying etiology and neurochemistry of the disease. In 1960 Cole and an associate[45,46] looked at a group of 338 patients with schizophrenia, 74 of whom were on placebo, and attempted to find variables that correlated with spontaneous versus drug-induced remission. No single variable studied was found to be an excellent predictor of response in either category. In summary, antipsychotics are documented to live up to their name, and as a group, psychotic patients tend to do better when medicated. Unfortunately, there is no simple way of predicting whether an individual patient will improve spontaneously or whether medication will be required to induce a remission.

Dose-Response Relationships

There are differing perspectives on what dosage to employ when initiating therapy. Some clinicians opt for a high dose for rapid control of symptoms, to be tapered off according to response and tolerance of side effects. Others prefer, particularly with the pharmacologically naive subject, to start with a low dose and increase as necessary. Davis, Eriksen and Hurt[73,74] designed a double-blind study to test the usefulness of a loading dose, which is comparable to the use

of an initial high dose. Acutely decompensated schizophrenic patients were randomized into two groups, the first of which received 15 mg haloperidol orally daily. The second group received 60 mg haloperidol daily intramuscularly (which has greater bioavailability than the oral route) for five days before being switched to the same regimen as the first group. Response was measured on a global scale, the BPRS, and the Holzman-Johnston TDS. The two-part hypothesis under scrutiny held that, first, improvement would be more rapid in the loading-dose group and, second, that response would would be superior in this group at three weeks (see figure 18–10). Neither of these assertions was borne out by the study; normal dose and loading dose proved identical in both onset of action and extent of improvement at three weeks. The high-dose group predictably had a slightly higher incidence of side effects, particularly dystonias. Similar studies by other investigators have yielded similar results. In short, there is no inherent

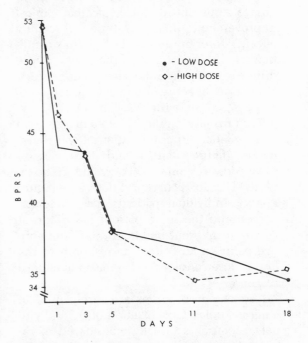

Figure 18–10. Comparison of clinical response, measured by the Brief Psychiatric Rating Scale (BPRS), of patients taking high versus low doses of haloperidol.

superiority of a high or loading dose over a lower, but adequate, dose.

The superiority of a higher dose may not be demonstrated for the group as a whole, but individual patients may require dosages that are considerably higher than average for an optimal response and will require careful titration of dose. In the initial phases of treatment, such titration will require administration of the drug several times daily. Because of the long half-life of all antipsychotics, the patient can be switched to a single daily dose after the first week or so of treatment. Many patients find a bedtime dose more convenient because it lessens the daytime experience of such side effects as sedation.

The use of high versus low dose can be best conceptualized in terms of the dose-response curve, as rendered in figure 18–11. The first part of the curve is flat, showing that low doses have no demonstrable effect. The second part is linear, indicating that gradual increases in dose are accompanied by increasing symptomatic improvement. The third part is a plateau in which a wide range in dosage results in identical maximal clinical improvement, demonstrating a "ceiling effect." Deterioration in the patient's condition sets in the last part of the curve, where drug toxicity obliterates therapeutic effect. Each side effect will have its own dose-response curve, with onset of clinically significant toxicity in different dose ranges, as in figure 18–11c. Superimposition of the therapeutic (figure 18–11b) and toxic (figure 18–11c) dose-response curves results in the inverted-U-shaped curve just described (figure 18–11d). Individual patients have different curves, and the same patient has different curves at different points in time. The optimal point on any curve corresponds to the lowest dose consistent with maximal clinical response.

Dose-response curves are rarely used in clinical studies. Optimization of the individual response is usually considered paramount, and the investigator consequently uses a flexible-dose design. This can only obscure the characteristics of the curve because it selects out only one of the parts, the pla-

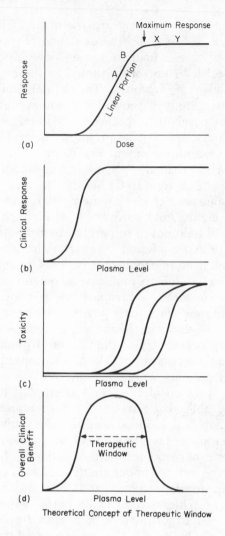

Figure 18–11. Dose/response (a), plasma-level/response (b, c), and theoretical concept of therapeutic window (d).

teau of optimal response. By excluding earlier points on the curve by design, these studies can teach us little about lowest optimal dose.

A small number of studies have randomly assigned subjects to different fixed doses, and these are summarized in table 18–10. These dose-response studies investigated newly admitted psychiatric patients with acute symptoms, using a fixed dose for several weeks. Another design that was studied investigated acutely ill patients in a psychotic break, using a fixed dose for a few hours or, at most, a day.

TABLE 18–10
Dose Versus Outcome in Dose-response Trials

Study	Higher Dose	Lower Dose	Drug	Result
Dose-response studies (acute patients)				
Quitkin et al.[212]	100,000	2,500	Fluphenazine[a]	H=S
Wijsenbeck, Steiner, and Goldberg[276]	21,000	2,100	Trifluoperazine[a]	H=S
Donlon, Hopkin, and Tupin[65]	6,200	1,700	Haloperidol[a]	H=S
Denber[62]	2,700	1,360	Thiothixene[a]	H=S
Modestin et al.[190]	3,600	1,250	Haloperidol[a]	H=S
Ericksen, Hurt, and Chang[73]	3,800	940	Haloperidol[a]	H=S
Donlon et al.[67]	6,250	625	Fluphenazine[a]	H=S
Donlon et al.[67]	2,700	625	Fluphenazine[a]	H=S
Neborsky et al.[196]	2,600	600	Haloperidol[a]	H=S
Fitzgerald[83]	1,600	300	Haloperidol[a]	H=S
Goldstein et al.[103]	293	73	Fluphenazine[a]	S better than L
1–2 Day Acute Studies (acute patients)				
Anderson, Kuenle, and Catanzano[3]	2,100	800	Haloperidol	H=S
Slotnick[246]	1,900	300	Haloperidol	H=S
Man and Chen[175]	2,200	300	Haloperidol	H=S
Reschke[216]	875	230	Haloperidol	H better than L
Gerstenzang and Krulisky[97]	313	50	Haloperidol	S better than L
Chronic-dose-response Studies				
Rimon et al.[218]	7,500	3,750	Haloperidol	H=S
Itil et al.[140]	67,000	2,500	Fluphenazine	H=S
DeBuck[59]	67,000	1,700	Fluphenazine	H=S
Bjorndal et al.[14]	10,800	800	Haloperidol	H=S
Itil et al.[141]	3,300	800	Fluphenazine	H=S
McCreadie and MacDonald[173]	6,250	600	Fluphenazine	H=S
Prien, Levine, and Cole[207]	2,900	540	Trifluoperazine	H=S
Carscallen, Rochman, and Lovegrove[23]	3,600	360	Trifluoperazine	H=L
Prien and Cole[205]	2,000	300	Chlorpromazine	H better than L
Clark et al.[36, 39]	600	300	Chlorpromazine	H better than L
McClelland et al.[172]	5,850	290	Fluphenazine	H=L
Dencker et al.[63]	5,300	270	Fluphenazine	H better than L
Gardose et al.[90]	910	230	Thiothixene	H=S
Lehmann et al.[167]	2,600	230	Fluphenazine	H better than L
Clark et al.[36, 39]	300	150	Chlorpromazine	H better than L
Simpson et al.[243]	440+	56	Butaperazine	S better than L
Kane et al.[147]	309	29–117	Fluphenazine	S better than L
Kane et al.[147]	309	15–59	Fluphenazine	S better than L

[a]High-dose drug.

Note: H= high dose; S = standard dose; L = low dose. H=S = high dose produces equal improvement to standard. H better than L = High dose produces better response than low dose. S better than L = Standard dose produces better response than low dose. Numbers represent chlorpromazine equivalents.

A third group of studies investigated continuously ill chronic schizophrenic patients or chronic schizophrenic patients in remission. We summarized the results for these three types of patients, indicating whether the higher dose of the drug produced a clearly statistically significant effect over the standard dose. We put the burden on the author to clearly show that the higher dose is better than the standard dose. In any study that compares patients in a wide variety of measures, there will be an occasional variable for which one dose will be superior to another dose. We required an evaluation of superiority, a statistically significant difference on the total score or Global Improvement Score, or on a substantial number of individual item scores.

We constructed a dose-response curve on the basis of data from these studies. The ability to draw a meaningful curve is, of course, qualified by the individuality of patient response. Very large samples are necessary to separate out small subgroups that may have different characteristics, for example, requirement for a comparatively high dose for optimal response. In other words, because these studies are all relatively small, they may miss a small group of patients who may "need" higher doses. There is clearly substantial variability in patient response to psychiatric drugs. For a study empirically to show a higher dose to be better than a lower dose, there must be sufficient nonresponding patients in the lower-dose group in comparison to patients in the higher-dose group in order to stand out from the background variabilities to produce a statistically reliable difference. These paired comparisons of fixed doses are used in defining the dose-response curve. Take, for example, theoretical points on the curve in figure 18–11a. If the dose at point A results in a response that is consistently inferior to that at point B, then it can be said with certainty that point A is on the linear part of the curve. Point B can be shown to be on the flat part of the curve only if a higher dose, corresponding to point C, results in equivalent response. Point D can be

shown to be on the declining part of the curve only in comparison to points B or C. The burden of proof, clinically, rests with those studies that demonstrate significant differences between doses, corresponding to points A and B on our theoretical curve.

Grouping the data from the studies summarized in table 18–11, it appears overall that the lowest dose of chlorpromazine, or equivalent, for adequate therapeutic response is about 300 mg. Doses ranging from 150 to 300 mg are on the linear part of the curve (that is, they do not produce an optimal response), and those above 800 mg appear to be on the declining part, with dosages in the range of 400 to 600 mg having identical and maximal response. The second group of studies in table 18–10 compares fixed doses of antipsychotic in the first one to two days of treatment. Even with this short time course, before plasma levels have reached a steady state, we find that the equivalent of 300 mg chlorpromazine produced as good a response as much higher doses. These data again speak against the need for a large loading dose of antipsychotic. In order to create a dose-response curve from the comparison of different doses shown in table 18–10, we have combined the data from these three sources and converted dosage amounts to chlorpromazine equivalents. The larger body of data on comparisons of fixed doses of chlorpromazine versus placebo gives the same result;

TABLE 18–11
Effectiveness of Different Dose Levels of Chlorpromazine

	Percentage of Studies in Which Chlorpromazine Was		
Dose (mg.)	More effective than placebo	Slightly more effective than placebo	Equal to placebo
300 or less	42	23	35
301–400	50	38	13
401–500	80	0	20
501–800	100	0	0
800 or more	100	0	0

whenever the lower dose was less than the equivalent of 400 mg chlorpromazine, the higher dose yielded better results.

As stated previously, it must be kept in mind that each patient may be thought of as having a unique dose-response curve, which can shift with time to the left, causing an increase in sensitivity to antipsychotic, or to the right, resulting in increased dose requirements. There is some suggestion from clinical observations that this shift is determined by disease activity, such that more disturbed patients have increased medication requirements, but insufficient data are available to state this with certainty. Most patients will respond adequately to between 400 and 700 mg chlorpromazine daily. Individual variation is reflected by differing plasma levels at steady-state between patients on the same dose.

Plasma-level Response Relationships

There are relatively few controlled investigations of plasma levels of antipsychotic drugs and clinical efficacy. Flexible-dose studies are methodologically flawed and are worthless in making conclusions about the relationship of plasma levels to efficacy. If flexible doses are used, the blood level will reflect dose, and the dose is determined by the clinician's reaction to the patient's clinical state. There are some patients who do not improve with neuroleptics because they are not floridly ill, their psychosis during hospitalization being about the same as before hospitalization. Their admission to a hospital was caused by deterioration in their social situation, not a true relapse. These patients are not appropriate for a blood-level study. Chronic, relatively stabilized long-term patients are similarly not suitable for correlational studies because drugs have produced all the effects of which they are capable. In a therapeutic blood-level trial, it is necessary to study patients who have florid illness and, therefore, have the capacity to show a substantial degree of therapeutic improvement. Valid plasma-level studies must exclude schizophrenic patients who have only residual symptoms and include only floridly ill pa-

tients. It is also important to distinguish rate of improvement from the maximal improvement possible. The former might be related to blood level, the latter to the underlying prognosis of the patient.

The greatest rate of drug-induced improvement is in the first week of treatment. After a few weeks of treatment, the rate of improvement decreases gradually as it approaches the maximal improvement that the drug is capable of producing. We believe that the best level of functioning that can be achieved with a drug is primarily a function of the disease process; and the rate of improvement in the first week or two is the best measure of improvement induced by the drug. For that reason, we suggest that the appropriate time to correlate plasma and red blood cell (RBC) level with drug-induced change of symptoms is the first week or so of treatment.

The first investigations were the studies by Curry, Marshall, Janowsky, Davis, and associates,[49,50,51] who noted that there were marked individual differences in plasma levels among patients on comparable doses, observing a wide twentyfold range (approximately 25 to 500 ng/ml) in plasma levels. A few patients with a very low level of chlorpromazine failed to show either side effects or clinical response. Other patients with a high chlorpromazine plasma level showed excessive sedation and failure to respond. When the dose was lowered, plasma levels fell, and these patients showed a clinical response. These findings suggest an inverted-U relationship between plasma level and clinical response. It is necessary that these exploratory open findings be verified by properly controlled studies.[57]

CONTROLLED STUDIES OF PLASMA-LEVEL RESPONSE RELATIONSHIPS

There have been very few methodologically sound investigations of the relationship between antipsychotic drug-plasma levels and clinical efficacy.[57] The first study by Curry, Lader, Sakalis,[160,224] and their co-workers treated a small number of schizophrenic and manic patients with 300 mg chlorpromazine daily. This original sample deliberately included nonfloridly ill patients (because investigators chose patients amenable to psychophysiological studies); but these subjects are too often inappropriate for the study of therapeutic effects. Lader extended the study to include floridly ill new patients. Since 300 milligrams is probably lower than the median effective dose of chlorpromazine (the average dose necessary to produce 50 percent of maximal improvement), it would be very unlikely that any patient would have plasma levels above the therapeutic window. The expected relationship between plasma level and clinical efficacy is a linear one at this dose. Hence patients with low plasma levels would be predicted to have poor clinical response, whereas patients with higher levels would be expected to have a good clinical response. In a report on the first thirty-two patients, these investigators found a correlation of -0.32 between clinical efficacy and plasma levels ($p = 0.04$ level, one-tailed).

Wode-Helgodt and coworkers[233,234,281] did a methodologically sound study on patients who were treated with randomly assigned fixed doses of 200, 400, or 600 mg chlorpromazine per day. A 200 mg or 400 mg fixed-dose schedule would be considered low, whereas 600 mg would be a moderate dose. In fifteen male schizophrenic patients, there was a positive correlation ($r = 0.82$, $p < 0.01$) between improvement and prolactin elevation at four weeks. There was a similar correlation between plasma levels and clinical response. This group recently reported a second fixed-low-dose chlorpromazine study and found similar results, with nonresponders having slightly low chlorpromazine plasma levels during the first week or so. Thus in the three chlorpromazine studies using low doses, there is a small and somewhat weak effect for nonresponders to have lower plasma levels.[113] Van Putten and coworkers[184] studied schizophrenic patients generally treated with chlorpromazine (6.6 mg/kg/day) for twenty-eight days. Plasma chlorpromazine levels did not differentiate between the patients who did or did not do well. This study did not report on data at one

or two weeks, where one would be most likely to see the correlation.

Chlorpromazine theoretically can be metabolized to 168 different metabolites, many of which may be active. If a chemical assay measures only the unchanged chlorpromazine, if the clinical effects are produced to a fair extent by metabolites, and if the amount of metabolite is not well correlated with the amount of unchanged drug, then the presence of active metabolites may obscure the correlation between plasma levels and therapeutic efficacy. If what are producing improvement in the brain are active metabolites, then stable plasma chlorpromazine levels would not be expected to correlate well with clinical efficacy.

HALOPERIDOL. Van Putten and associates, using one week's treatment data from a study performed at the Shanghai Psychiatric Institute;[270] Potkin and others;[204] Mavoroidis and Garver in Cincinnati;[176] Davis (unpublished data); and Smith and coworkers[251] have found an inverted-U-shaped relationship between haloperidol levels and clinical response. Brown and coworkers[18] found that for patients on maintenance antipsychotics, those who relapse tend to have low plasma levels. It is interesting that the results of all these studies were roughly consistent. They also show an inverted-U-shaped relationship, with roughly the same therapeutic window, with optimal response at about 5 to 20 ng haloperidol per cubic centimeter.

FLUPHENAZINE. Dysken and coworkers[69] and Mavoroidis and associates[178] have studied plasma fluphenazine levels and found an inverted-U-shaped relationship between fluphenazine and clinical response. Most nonresponders have either very low or very high fluphenazine levels.

BUTAPERAZINE. Most antipsychotic drugs exist bound to the plasma protein. Only about one-tenth is not bound to plasma proteins. The plasma concentration of "free" drug is in equilibrium with tissue-drug levels. It is technically impossible at this time to measure free drug level, yet this analysis is potentially quite important. In addition, drugs must cross the blood-brain barrier to reach central receptor sites. If the mechanisms involved in the drugs' distribution across the RBC membrane mimic those governing the passage of drug through the blood-brain barrier into brain, then RBC drug levels may give additional information beyond that given by total plasma levels. Probably the amount of free drug present in plasma determines RBC and also brain levels, but there may be other factors also present. Chang, Garver,[26,92,93] and their co-workers administered a constant dose of butaperazine to floridly ill schizophrenic patients, measuring plasma and RBC levels. Although both plasma and RBC levels versus response were best characterized by an inverted-U-shaped curve, the relationship using RBC levels was more striking (see figures 18–12 and 18–13).

OTHER NEUROLEPTICS. Some studies have found a therapeutic window for perphenazine and for thiothixene.

ANTIPSYCHOTIC THERAPEUTIC WINDOWS

Three chlorpromazine studies that used low doses found a hint of a lower limit to the inverted-U-shaped window. An inverted-U-shaped window has been found for haloperidol, butaperazine, thiothixene, and perphen-

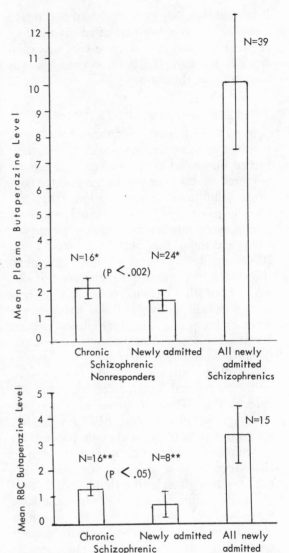

Figure 18–13. Mean plasma and red blood cell (RBC) butaperazine levels in chronic and newly admitted schizophrenics.

azine. All the data look similar in that the therapeutic window is not well defined and there is a substantial amount of scatter. Although these results achieve some degree of statistical significance, they are not highly significant. The relationship of plasma/RBC levels and clinical response is only an approximate one, with many values that do not fit. The results agree that there is only a modest effect of the inverted-U-relationship. We be-

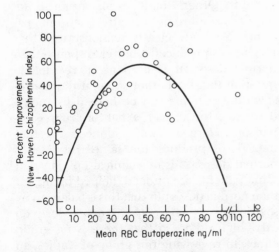

Figure 18–12. Illustration of therapeutic window with butaperazine red blood cell (RBC) levels.

lieve that there are two consistent findings in the data so far: (1) the hint of an inverted-U-relationship and (2) evidence that this relationship is weak. The latter conclusion is as important as the former.

TREATMENT-RESISTANT PATIENTS

Even though most schizophrenic patients respond to some degree to drugs and then return home, an occasional patient has no response whatsoever and needs to have continuous lifetime hospitalization. Our research group[249,250] studied such chronic, continuously hospitalized schizophrenic patients and found that both their plasma and RBC drug levels were substantially below those seen in the acute population. We also studied another group consisting of extremely unresponsive patients in an acute setting who were referred for clinical plasma levels after a test dose. Many of these patients had absolutely no clinical response to antipsychotic drugs; indeed, many were being considered for transfer to a chronic-care facility. These patients also had extremely low plasma and RBC levels that were similar to those of chronic patients. A fair number of these nonresponders did partially recover to a sufficient degree for discharge when given higher than normal doses of fluphenazine enanthate or decanoate. Since oral antipsychotics undergo first-pass metabolism, an intramuscular formulation can bypass this effect of gut metabolism so that an adequate plasma level can be achieved.

CEREBROSPINAL FLUID–PLASMA-LEVEL CORRELATION

Cerebrospinal fluid (CSF) level would be expected to closely parallel free plasma level. Several studies found that plasma-chlorpromazine levels are highly correlated to CSF chlorpromazine levels.[233,234,281]

Use of Megadoses

The data summarized in table 18–1 fail to demonstrate the overall superiority of mega-doses to conventional doses. Despite this, there are anecdotal reports of patients who do not respond to usual doses but are converted into responders on high doses of medication. An occasional "nonresponder" can be clinically shown to have a low plasma level on what is thought to be an adequate dose. Boosting the dose might therefore be expected to raise the plasma level and result in improvement. But the possibility exists that many patients who appear to be nonresponders may in fact be late responders. In these patients improvement may falsely be attributed to a megadose used as a last resort, while improvement might still have taken place if the patient had been left on the lower dose. Nevertheless, we do recommend a time-limited trial of a moderately high dose for the patient who does not respond to the standard dose in the event that this may be one of those uncommon individuals who has a higher requirement.

Included in the studies in table 18–10 are those that used substantially high doses. If we consider a so-called megadose greater than 2 g chlorpromazine equivalence and a standard dose of 0.5 to 1.0 g chlorpromazine equivalence, a substantial number of studies use megadoses in comparison to normal doses. Some of these studies (see table 18–10, dose-response studies) used relatively acute patients. Others (table 18–10, chronic-dose-response studies) used relatively chronic patients. No study clearly demonstrated that megadoses produced a better response than normal doses. It is certainly a reasonable question to ask whether some of the nonresponding patients can be helped by megadoses, and the answer is that for group comparisons, a large body of evidence shows that megadoses produce the same response as normal doses. It is our clinical opinion that some patients are, indeed, helped by higher than normal doses but that this is balanced by some patients who may do more poorly on extra-high doses, so that there is no group effect. In reviewing this group of studies, an occasional study finds a trend for megadose to be superior to standard dose. For example, certain studies, although they fail to find a clear-cut difference on global or summation scores, did find that the high-dose group did better on some individual items. This is balanced, however, by several other studies that found that the high-dose group actually did worse on several items. A substantial number of studies have found that the therapeutic results in the megadose group are almost the same as therapeutic results in the standard-dose group. One might argue occasionally about the significance of slight trends in one direction or the other, but our overall impression in reviewing these studies is that megadoses are equal to standard doses. We feel the clinician should be alert and perform a therapeutic trial of higher-than-normal doses for nonresponders on too-low doses. This is entirely empirical and is done by gradually raising the dose, even to quite high levels, to see if the patient will respond. The clinician should keep in mind that some patients respond relatively slowly and be aware that a clinical improvement occurs with the passage of time. The patient who responds to a gradual escalation of dose may actually be improved with the passage of time, not the extra-high dose.

The clinician should also try patients who are nonresponsive to high doses on a moderate dose, or even a low dose. In other words, the clinician should try a variety of doses to see which dose the patient responds to. In doing this, the clinician should keep in mind the rate of response to antipsychotic drugs as presented in figure 18–3. Certainly, the rate of response is relatively slow. About 40 percent of the responses that will be present by six weeks are already present by one week in the average patient. On the other hand, average patients still improved at twenty-five weeks above where they were at five weeks, although the increment in average improvement at twenty-five weeks over five weeks is relatively small. In the highly disturbed patient, it is certainly indicated to have dose adjustments every few days because of the emergency nature of the situation. However, for the average psychiatric patient, dose adjustments are made on a weekly or biweekly rather than a daily basis.

We know that, on an average, all drugs are equally effective, and we suspect that they all act through the same mechanism, namely the blockade of DA receptors. Nevertheless, experienced clinicians sometimes claim that a patient who had been relatively unresponsive to one neuroleptic may respond to another. Again, this may be an artifact of the passage of time. It may be that a given patient has a relatively slow time of response and responds to a second drug not because it is a different neuroleptic, but because of the passage of time or spontaneous "swings" in the underlying psychosis that would have taken place regardless of drug. A study by Gardose[89] hints that some patients may respond better to one neuroleptic than another, but this question has received little systematic investigation. For nonresponders, a trial of different neuroleptics as well as different doses is indicated.

Once the schizophrenic illness has remitted, hopefully completely or partially, the clinician should try to reduce the dose. It is important to use the minimal possible dose that is necessary for effective treatment on the theory that TD is dose-related and can be minimized when the drug dose is reduced as far as possible.

The Acute Psychotic Emergency

Loss of impulse control leading to unpredictability and violence constitutes a psychiatric emergency. Under these conditions, it is important to medicate the patient both rapidly and reliably. If the oral route is used, the peak action occurs in about ninety minutes. About 50 percent of the drug is lost in the first pass through the liver. If the patient is uncooperative, or if the clinician desires more rapid drug titration, the intramuscular route should be used. With intramuscular administration, the time to peak action is cut by two-thirds, to thirty minutes, and the delivered dose is greater than with the oral route because there is no first-pass effect. Intramuscular administration is the route of choice if the patient is dangerously disturbed. Patients frequently respond to rapid tranquilization—that is, repeated doses at intervals of thirty to ninety minutes—within hours, thereby averting serious harm to the patient and those around him or her. In these situations, it is wise to use moderately high rather than low or moderate doses. The dose-response curve is such that the increase in side effects is minimal, whereas the benefit is often the prevention of uncontrollable violence.

One may rightfully ask whether the use of such high doses is dangerous to the patient. The data summarized in table 18–10 show that patients can tolerate high doses—for example, 1,200 mg fluphenazine[217] or 700 mg trifluoperazine[276] (or loxapine, thiothixene, or haloperidol)[72,130,262]—for months without a significant excess of toxicity over standard doses. Rather than these massive doses, we recommend moderate or moderately high doses because the gain in effectiveness with a massive dose is negligible.

Dose and Cost of Medication

Equivalent doses and costs of the various antipsychotics, culled from comparative double-blind studies, are detailed in table 18–12.[54] Regardless of the particular agent chosen, from a practical standpoint it is important to know that cost is determined more by tablet number than by milligram content of the individual tablet. For example, a 100 mg tablet of chlorpromazine costs only slightly more than a 25 mg tablet. It therefore makes sense to prescribe the largest dose tablet appropriate in order to minimize cost to the patient.

It is sometimes useful for the physician or hospital pharmacist to be aware of the cost of medication. Sometimes when generic medication is available, there is a generic product from a reliable manufacturer that is less expensive than the original compound. Occasionally a nongeneric form may be less expensive than a generic. Although quality of product is important, some comparison shopping between equivalent products can result in cost savings, so the physician, purchasing agents, pharmacists, and pharmacy committee should consider cost along with other factors in arriving at sensible decisions. A single daily dose is sufficient, given the long half-life of these compounds. Delayed-release oral forms are superfluous. Once-daily dosage at bedtime can minimize waking experience of side effects and contribute to cost-saving, and it often facilitates compliance by simplifying medication use. It can also protect confidentiality by sparing patients the pressure to respond to the queries of acquaintances who may become aware of medication ingestion during the day.

Drug Combinations

A combination of more than one antipsychotic is generally unnecessary and only cumbersome to the patient. Whenever such combinations have been studied, the net effect is the same as that of the combined chlorpromazine equivalence of the agents given. It is best to prescribe the single agent to which the patient responds best, following the guidelines previously outlined.

Does combining antipsychotics with other classes of drugs contribute anything to the treatment of, for example, symptoms of anxiety or depression? The Spring Grove group[111,187] compared phenothiazine plus benzodiazepine to phenothiazine alone and found that antipsychotic alone was superior to the combination. Unfortunately, because of the flexible dose design, the combination group received a lower dose of antipsychotic (probably because clinicians were trying to minimize sedation, which would be more of a problem in that group).

But what about the combination of schizophrenia and depression? It is frequently difficult to differentiate apathetic, retarded, or catatonic schizophrenia from a severe or psychotic depression. Patients with a psychotic depression appear to respond better to a combination of antidepressant and antipsychotic than to either agent alone. Apathetic schizophrenic patients do not respond better to antipsychotic-antidepressant combinations than they do to anti-

TABLE 18-12

Comparative Costs of Antipsychotic Drugs

Generic Name	Trade Name	Average Dose (mg/day)[a]	Wholesale Cost a Month[b]
Molindone	Moban	44	6.46
Fluphenazine	Permitil	9	10.58
Haloperidol	Haldol	12	11.70
Fluphenazine HCl	Prolixin HCl	9	12.83
Chlorpromazine	Thorazine	734	14.56
Trifluoperazine	Stelazine	20	15.18
Carphenazine	Proketazine	183	16.71
Loxapine	Loxitane	64	17.28
Thiothixene	Navane	32	18.06
Chlorprothixene	Taractan	323	24.48
Prochlorperazine	Compazine	103	27.56
Acetophenazine	Tindal	169	31.59
Mesoridazine	Serentil	411	32.33
Fluphenazine decanoate	Prolixin Decanoate	5	32.64
Fluphenazine enanthate	Prolixin Enanthate	5	33.42
Piperacetazine	Quide	80	33.78
Perphenazine	Trilafon	66	36.99
Thioridazine	Mellaril	712	37.86
Triflupromazine	Vesprin	205	56.36

[a]Dosages represent empirically defined dose for acute treatment.[54] Most doses listed fall within dosage range listed in the *Physician's Desk Reference* (PDR); however, some do not. PDR doses for Thorazine, Trilafon, Vesprin, and Serentil are lower than empirically defined doses; PDR dose for Moban is higher than the empirically defined dose.
[b]Cost to retailer for one-month supply of drug for average acute treatment, based on wholesale prices of least expensive (largest) tablet or bottle purchased in largest quantity. Actual cost to the consumer is considerably greater because of physician's ordering of smaller-dose tablets, pharmacy ordering less than largest package of drug, and pharmacist markup.

psychotics alone.[244,272] A large collaborative VA study by Casey and associates[24] showed no benefit from adding a monoamine oxidase inhibitor to chlorpromazine in chronic schizophrenia. Addition of amphetamine produced some worsening of psychotic symptoms. Prusoff and coworkers[209,210] compared amitriptyline plus perphenazine to perphenazine alone in chronic schizophrenia. The combination resulted in somewhat less depression but somewhat more thought disorder. A relatively low dose of neuroleptic was used here, and it is quite possible that if a higher dose of neuroleptic was used, the combination would have shown a greater beneficial effect on depression without a worsening of thought disorder. Data from the Spring Grove group[187] indicate treatment results with the combination antipsychotic/tricyclic similar to treatment results with antipsychotic alone. This study did not find marginal improvement with the combination in certain subgroups. It is clear that schizophrenic apathy does not respond to antidepressants. These results suggest that the combination of an antidepressant and an antipsychotic will help only those patients who have a truly affective component, that is, atypical affective disorders, schizo-affective disorders, and bona fide affective disorders with a psychotic component, which may have been misdiagnosed as schizophrenia.

A study of chronic schizophrenic patients with secondary depression treated with neuroleptic plus either trazodone hydrochloride or placebo found the antidepressant produced significantly greater improvement in some depressive symptoms. Many schizophrenic patients will appear more depressed as they respond to antipsychotic therapy. Such a "postpsychotic" depression results from the patient's increasingly realistic appreciation of the severity of his or her illness as the thought disorder resolves and will not respond to antidepressant therapy any more than will normal grief; however, a major depression superimposed on schizophrenia will respond to antidepressants.

Siris and associates[245] did a retrospective study of twenty-five patients with schizophrenia or schizo-affective disorder who developed the clinical syndrome of depression after resolution of their schizophrenic episode. This secondary depression responded relatively well to the addition of a tricyclic (imipramine hydrochloride, amitriptyline hydrochloride) to neuroleptic. Only one patient experienced an exacerbation of psychosis.

There are occasional affective diseases that are misdiagnosed as schizophrenia. These may respond to lithium carbonate and/or antidepressants in a dramatic fashion. It is unfortunate that chronic apathetic schizophrenic patients do not have a variant of depression that responds to antidepressants; schizophrenic apathy is not helped by antidepressants. A body of empirical evidence shows that the addition of antidepressants to the treatment of schizophrenia is nonproductive. Some evidence indicates that schizophreniform disease responds well to lithium, and lithium should certainly be considered in any patient who has that disorder, which might be an affective variant.[122] By the same token, it is often useful to add carbamazepine (Tegretol), which is increasingly used in patients with affective disorders who cannot take lithium, to antipsychotics in treating patients with mixed affective and schizophrenic symptoms. Carbamazepine is also useful in patients who may have psychomotor epilepsy superimposed on schizophrenia. Antidepressants can occasionally be useful in a patient who has a depressed episode superimposed on the schizophrenic process. Electroconvulsive therapy (ECT) is occasionally useful in acute reactive psychosis, catatonic excitement, or retardation, as well as in variants of affective disorders.[225] ECT, lithium, propranolol hydrochloride, carbamazepine, and so forth are discussed elsewhere in the volume.

¶ Other Somatic Therapies

Before the advent of antipsychotics, somatic therapies such as insulin shock and ECT were the mainstay of inpatient treatment. Insulin shock has essentially fallen by the wayside, but it is worth mentioning that Ackner and Oldham in 1962[1] showed no beneficial effect in a controlled study of schizophrenic subjects. Insulin shock also was found inferior to antipsychotic medication in a recent Chinese study.[204]

In contrast, several studies show a beneficial effect of ECT on some schizophrenic patients. A 1967 study by Smith and coworkers[247] showed that a combination of ECT and antipsychotic resulted in more rapid improvement when compared with antipsychotic medication alone. ECT used alone is less effective than antipsychotics, but more effective[179,180,182,183] than psychotherapy alone. ECT may therefore be considered as an adjunct in the therapy of selected schizophrenic patients.

¶ Mode of Action of Antipsychotic Medications

Whereas the etiology of schizophrenia is as yet undetermined, the action of antipsychotic drugs is known to occur through their antidopaminergic effects. This appears to be the common denominator that ties together the diverse group of drugs that have antipsychotic properties, including phenothiazine derivatives, thioxanthene derivatives, butyrophenones, indoles, dibenzoxazepines, reserpine, and several experimental agents. In general, drugs that decrease DA activity have an antipsychotic effect.

The most clinically obvious evidence that DA is involved in the action of antipsychotics is the fact that the drugs induce parkinsonian side effects; Parkinson's disease is known to be a DA-deficiency disease. It can, therefore, be inferred that antipsychotics in some way decrease the effect of DA in the brain. It has been demonstrated *in vitro* that antipsychotics bind to DA receptors and that the affinity correlates exactly with the individual drug's antipsychotic potency.[235,254] Horn and Snyder[136] provided x-ray crystallographic evidence that chlorpromazine is structurally similar to DA. Furthermore, receptor affinity is known to be affected by specific molecular configuration; the isomer of flupenthixol that has the ability to bind to DA receptors *in vitro* is the only one that has clinically demonstrable antipsychotic properties.[146] All of the known antipsychotic drugs bind to, and thereby block, central nervous system DA receptors. The binding to and blocking of central DA receptors can be inferred to cause a compensatory increase in DA synthesis. The pharmacology of one antipsychotic, clozapine, suggests that there may be anatomically distinct (mesolimbic) subtypes of DA receptors that are more intimately involved in the schizophrenic defect. Sulperide, a specific blocker of D-2 DA receptors, has antipsychotic activity, and since all other neuroleptics also block the D-2 type of DA receptors, the antipsychotic properties of these drugs probably reside in D-2 receptor blockage.

Alpha-methyl-*p*-tyrosine inhibits DA synthesis. When it is co-administered with a neuroleptic drug such as chlorpromazine, it decreases the dosage of neuroleptic required to produce a clinically relevant therapeutic response. Interfering with dopaminergic function at points other than synthesis can also contribute to amelioration of psychosis. Agents that interfere with catecholamine storage, such as reserpine and tetrabenazine, have been shown to have antipsychotic properties. In preliminary studies apomorphine, a DA agonist, has been suggested to have antipsychotic activity when used in a dose range that stimulates presynaptic receptors to reduce DA synthesis and release.[47,248,261] This evidence comes from single-dose studies.

The psychomotor stimulants methylphenidate, amphetamine, and cocaine all increase release of DA and/or block its reuptake, thereby increasing DA availability in the synapse. A large oral, intramuscular, or intravenous (IV) dose of psychomotor stimulant can produce a paranoid psychosis. Indeed, a single large IV dose of amphetamine can rapidly induce a paranoid psychosis whose course parallels the duration of the drug in the body. We have found that small IV doses of methylphenidate, which have no effects either on normal subjects or on schizophrenic patients in remission, can markedly exacerbate symptoms in schizophrenic patients with active disease.[143] This again suggests an abnormality of dopaminergic function in schizophrenia. It should be noted that exacerbation of symptoms follows the pattern of the preexisting psychosis; there is no uniform production of a particular type of psychosis, as occurs when a large dose of psychomotor stimulant is given to nonpsychotic subjects. Methylphenidate is known to cause release of DA and norepinephrine from the reserpine-sensitive pool. It is more potent than d-amphetamine in this regard, which is in turn more potent than *L*-amphetamine. Evidence for the psychosis-exacerbating effects of increasing dopaminergic activity comes from the treatment of Parkinson's disease. The DA precursor DOPA is known to cause psychosis as a side effect, as are a variety of DA agonists in use in neurologic practice. Amantadine hydrochloride is another example of a dopaminergic drug that can trigger psychosis. Thus, while we do not know exactly how dopaminergic function is related to whatever causes schizophrenia specifically or psychosis in general, a substantial body of evidence indicates that the relevant mechanism of action of the antipsychotics is their blockade of D-2 DA receptors.

¶ Acknowledgment

We wish to gratefully acknowledge the support of the MacArthur Foundation.

¶ Bibliography

1. ACKNER, B., and OLDHAM, A. J. "Insulin Treatment of Schizophrenia," *Lancet*, 1 (1962):504.

2. ADELSON, D., and EPSTEIN, L. A. "A Study of Phenothiazines in Male and Female Chronically-Ill Schizophrenics," *Journal of Nervous and Mental Disease*, 134 (1962):543–554.

3. ANDERSON, W. H., KUENLE, J. C., and CATANZANO, D. M. "Rapid Treatment of Acute Psychosis," *American Journal of Psychiatry*, 133 (1976):1076–1078.

4. ANDREWS, P., HALL, J. N., and SNAITH, R. P. "A Controlled Trial of Phenothiazine Withdrawal in Chronic Schizophrenic Patients," *British Journal of Psychiatry*, 128 (1976):451–455.

5. APPLETON, W. S., and DAVIS, J. M. *Practical Clinical Psychopharmacology*, 4th ed. New York: Medcomb, 1980.

6. ARIK, M. Unpublished material made available by Lederle Laboratories, Pearl River, New York, 1974.

7. ASTRUP, C., FOSSUM, A., and HOLMBOE, R. *Prognosis in Functional Psychoses.* Springfield, Ill.: Charles C Thomas, 1962.

8. AYD, F. J., Jr. "The Depot Fluphenazines: A Reappraisal After Ten Years' Clinical Experience," *American Journal of Psychiatry*, 132 (1975):491–500.

9. BAKER, A. A., and THORPE, J. G. "Placebo Response," *Archives of Neurology and Psychiatry*, 78 (1957):57–60.

10. BARO, F., et al. "Maintenance Therapy of Chronic Psychotic Patients with a Weekly Oral Dose of R 16341," *Journal of Clinical Pharmacology*, 10 (1970): 330–341.

11. BECK, M. N. "Twenty-Five and Thirty-Five Year Follow-Up of First Admissions to Mental Hospitals," *Canadian Psychiatric Association Journal*, 13 (1968):219–229.

12. BENNETT, J. L., and KOOI, K. A. "Five Phenothiazine Derivatives," *Archives of General Psychiatry*, 4 (1961):413–418.

13. BISHOP, M. P., and GALLANT, D. M. "Loxapine: A Controlled Evaluation in Chronic Schizophrenic Patients," *Current Therapeutic Research*, 12 (1970): 594.

14. BJORNDAL, N., et al. "High Dosage Haloperidol Therapy in Chronic Schizophrenic Patients: A Double-Blind Study of Clinical Response, Side Effects, Serum Haloperidol, and Serum Prolactin," *Psychopharmacology*, 67 (1980):17–23.

15. BLACKBURN, H., and ALLEN, J. "Behavioral Effects of Interrupting and Resuming Tranquilizing Medication Among Schizophrenics," *Journal of Nervous and Mental Disease*, 133 (1961):303–307.

16. BOOKHAMMER, R. S., et al. "A Five Year Follow-Up Study of Schizophrenic Patients," *Current Therapeutic Research*, 12 (1966):594.

17. BRATFOS, O., and HAUG, J. O. "Comparison of Sulpiride and Chlorpromazine in Psychoses: A Double-Blind Multicentre Study," *Acta Psychiatrica Scandinavica*, 60 (1979):1–9.

18. BROWN, W. A., et al. "Low Serum Neuroleptic Levels Predict Relapse in Schizophrenic Patients," *Archives of General Psychiatry*, 39 (1982):998–1000.

19. BURCH, E. A., Jr., and AYD, F. J., Jr. "Depot Pipotiazine 1970–1982: A Review," *Journal of Clinical Psychiatry*, 44 (1983):242–247.

20. CAFFEY, E. M., et al. "Discontinuation or Reduction of Chemotherapy in Chronic Schizophrenics," *Journal of Chronic Disease*, 17 (1964):347–358.

21. CARPENTER, W. T., and HEINRICHS, D. W. "Early Intervention, Time-Limited, Targeted Pharmacotherapy of Schizophrenia," *Schizophrenia Bulletin*, 9 (1983):533–542.

22. CARRANZA, J., VARGAS, L., and GOMEZ, J. "A Double-Blind Evaluation of Sulpiride, a New Antipsychotic Compound," *Clinical Pharmacology and Therapeutics*, 14 (1973):132–133.

23. CARSCALLEN, H. B., ROCHMAN, H., and LOVEGROVE, T. D., "High Dosage Trifluoperazine in Schizophrenia," *Canadian Psychiatric Association Journal*, 13 (1968):459–461.

24. CASEY, J. F., et al. "Combined Drug Therapy of Chronic Schizophrenics. Controlled Evaluation of Placebo, Dextro-amphetamine, Imipramine, Isocarboxazid and Trifluoperazine Added to Maintenance Doses of Chlorpromazine," *American Journal of Psychiatry*, 117 (1961):997–1005.

25. CASEY, J. F., et al. "Drug Therapy in Schizophrenia: A Controlled Study of the Relative Effectiveness of Chlorpro-

mazine, Promazine, Phenobarbital and Placebo," *Archives of General Psychiatry,* 2 (1960):210–220.

26. CASPER, R. C., et al. "Phenothiazine Levels in Plasma and Red Blood Cells," *Archives of General Psychiatry,* 37 (1980): 301–307.

27. CASSANO, G. B., et al. "Sulpiride Versus Haloperidol in Schizophrenia: A Double-Blind Comparative Trial," *Current Therapeutic Research,* 17 (1975):189–201.

28. CHARALAMPOUS, K. D., et al. "Loxapine Succinate: A Controlled Double-Blind Study in Schizophrenia," *Current Therapeutic Research,* 16 (1974):829–837.

29. CHEUNG, H. K. "Schizophrenics Fully Remitted on Neuroleptics for 3–5 Years," *British Journal of Psychiatry,* 138 (1981):490–494.

30. CHIEN, C. P. "Drugs and Rehabilitation in Schizophrenia," in M. Greenblatt, ed., *Drugs in Combination with Other Therapies.* New York: Grune & Stratton, 1975, pp. 13–14.

31. CHIEN, C. P., and COLE, J. O. "Depot Phenothiazine Treatment in Acute Psychosis: A Sequential Comparative Clinical Study," *American Journal of Psychiatry,* 130 (1973):13–18.

32. CHOUINARD, G., and ANNABLE, L. "Clozapine in the Treatment of Newly Admitted Schizophrenic Patients: A Pilot Study," *Journal of Clinical Pharmacology,* 16 (1976):289–297.

33. CHOUINARD, G., et al. "Amitriptyline-Perphenazine Interaction in Ambulatory Schizophrenic Patients: A Controlled Study of Drug Interaction," *Archives of General Psychiatry,* 32 (1975):1295–1309.

34. CHOUINARD, G., et al. "A Double-Blind Controlled Clinical Trial of Haloperidol Decanoate and Fluphenazine Decanoate in the Maintenance Treatment of Schizophrenia," *Psychopharmacology Bulletin,* 20 (1984):108–110

35. CLAGHORN, J., et al. "Group Therapy and Maintenance Treatment of Schizophrenia," *Archives of General Psychiatry,* 31 (1974):361–385.

36. CLARK, M. L., et al. "Chlorpromazine in Chronic Schizophrenia: Behavioral Dose-Response Relationship," *Psychopharmacologia,* 18 (1970):260–270.

37. CLARK, M. L., et al. "Molindone in Chronic Schizophrenia," *Clinical Pharmacology and Therapeutics,* 11 (1970): 680.

38. CLARK, M. L., et al. "Pimozide (Oral): A Tolerance Study," *Clinical Trial Journal Supplement,* 2 (1971):25–32.

39. CLARK, M. L., et al. "Chlorpromazine in Chronic Schizophrenia. The Effect of Age and Hospitalization on Behavioral Dose-Response Relationships," *Archives of General Psychiatry,* 27 (1972): 479–483.

40. CLARK, M. L., et al. "Evaluation of Loxapine Succinate in Chronic Schizophrenia," *Diseases of the Nervous System,* 33 (1972):783–791

41. CLARK, M. L., et al. "Loxapine in Newly Admitted Chronic Schizophrenic Patients," *Journal of Clinical Pharmacology,* 15 (1975):286.

42. CLARK, M. L., et al. "Pimozide in Chronic Outpatients," *Diseases of the Nervous System,* 36 (1975):137–141.

43. CLARK, M. L., et al. "Evaluation of Two Dose Levels of Loxapine Succinate in Chronic Schizophrenia," *Diseases of the Nervous System,* 38 (1977):7–10.

44. COLE, J. O., and DAVIS, J. M. "Antipsychotic Drugs," in L. Bellak and L. Leob, eds., *The Schizophrenic Syndrome.* New York: Grune & Stratton, 1969, pp. 478–568.

45. COLE, J. O., GOLDBERG, S. C., and DAVIS, J. M. "Drugs in the Treatment of Psychosis: Controlled Studies," in P. Solomon, ed., *Psychiatric Drugs.* New York: Grune & Stratton, 1966, pp. 153–181.

46. COLE, J. O., GOLDBERG, S. C., and KLERMAN, G. L. "Phenothiazine Treatment in Acute Schizophrenia," *Archives of General Psychiatry,* 10 (1964):246–261.

47. CORSINI, G. U., et al. "A. Sedative, Hypnotic and Antipsychotic Effect of Low Doses of Apomorphine in Man," in E. Costa and G. L. Gessa, eds., *Symposium on Non-Striatal Dopaminergic Neurons.* New York: Raven Press, 1977, pp. 645–648.

48. CRAWFORD, R., and FORREST, A. "Controlled Trial of Depot Fluphenazine in Outpatient Schizophrenics," *British Journal of Psychiatry,* 124 (1974):385–391.

49. CURRY, S. H., et al. "Intrapatient Variation in Physiological Availability of Chlorpromazine as a Complicating Factor in Correlation Studies of Drug Metabolism and Clinical Effect," in A. Carletti and F.J. Bove, eds., *The Present Status of Psychotropic Drugs,* vol. 6. Amsterdam: Excerpta Medica Foundation, 1968, pp. 72–76.

50. CURRY, S. H., et al. "Chlorpromazine Plasma Levels and Effects," *Archives of General Psychiatry,* 22 (1970):289–296.

51. CURRY, S. H., et al. "Factors Affecting Chlorpromazine Plasma Levels in Psychiatric Patients," *Archives of General Psychiatry,* 22 (1970):209–215.

52. DAVIS, J. M. "Efficacy of Tranquilizing and Antidepressant Drugs," *Archives of General Psychiatry,* 13 (1965):552–566.

53. ———. "Overview: Maintenance Therapy in Psychiatry: I. Schizophrenia," *American Journal of Psychiatry,* 132 (1975):1237–1245.

54. ———. "Comparative Doses and Costs of Antipsychotic Medication," *Archives of General Psychiatry,* 33 (1976):858–861.

55. ———. "Recent Developments in the Drug Treatment of Schizophrenia," *American Journal of Psychiatry,* 133 (1976):208–214.

56. DAVIS, J. M., and CHANG, S. "Does Psychotherapy Alter the Course in Schizophrenia?" in J.P.B. Brady and H.K.H. Brodie, eds., *Controversy in Psychiatry.* Philadelphia: W. B. Saunders, 1978, pp. 595–620.

57. DAVIS, J. M., ERICKSEN, S., and DEKIRMENJIAN, H. "Plasma Levels of Antipsychotic Drugs and Clinical Response," in M. A. Lipton, A. DiMascio, and K. F. Killam, eds., *Psychopharmacology: A Generation of Progress.* New York: Raven Press, 1978, pp. 905–915.

58. DAVIS, J. M., et al. "Use of Survival Curves in Analysis of Antipsychotic Relapse Studies," in F. Cattabeni et al., eds., *Long-Term Effects of Neuroleptics, Advances in Biochemistry and Psychopharmacology,* vol. 24. New York: Raven Press, 1980, pp. 471–481.

59. DEBUCK, R. P. "Relative Safety and Efficacy of High and Low Dose Administration of Fluphenazine HCl to Psychotic Patients," in T. A. Ban et al., eds., *Pro-ceedings of the 8th International Congress of the C.I.N.P.* Amsterdam: North Holland Publishing Co., 1972, pp. 265–271.

60. DELAY, J., and DENIKER, P. "Le Traitement des Psychoses Par Une Methode Neurolytique Derivée de L'hibernotherapie," in J. Boudouresques and J. Bonnal, eds., *Congres des Medicins Alienistes et Neurologistes de France,* vol. 50. Paris: Masson & Cie Libraires de L'Academie de Medecine, 1952, p. 497.

61. DEL GUIDICE, J., CLARK, W. G., and GOCKA, E. F. "Prevention of Recidivism of Schizophrenics Treated with Fluphenazine Enanthate," *Psychosomatics,* 16 (1975):32–36.

62. DENBER, H.C.B. "High Dose Neuroleptic Therapy," Paper presented at the American Psychiatric Association 31st Institute on Hospital and Community Psychiatry, New Orleans, September 3–5, 1979.

63. DENCKER, S. J., et al. "High Doses of Fluphenazine Enanthate in Schizophrenia. A Controlled Study," *Acta Psychiatrica Scandinavica,* 57 (1978):405–414.

64. DIAMOND, L. S., and MARKS, J. B. "Discontinuance of Tranquilizers Among Chronic Schizophrenic Patients Receiving Maintenance Dosages," *Journal of Nervous and Mental Disease,* 131 (1960): 247–251.

65. DONLON, P. T., HOPKIN, J. T., and TUPIN, J. P. "Haloperidol for Acute Schizophrenic Patients: An Evaluation of Three Oral Regimens," *Archives of General Psychiatry,* 37 (1980):691–695.

66. DONLON, P. T., et al. "Comparison of Depot Fluphenazines: Duration of Action and Incidence of Side Effects," *Comprehensive Psychiatry,* 17 (1976): 369–376.

67. DONLON, P. T., et al. "High vs. Standard Dosage Fluphenazine HCl in Acute Schizophrenia," *Journal of Clinical Psychiatry,* 39 (1978):800–804.

68. DUBE, K. C., and KUMAR, N. "Loxapine Succinate: A Comparative Study with Chlorpromazine," *Current Therapeutic Research,* 19 (1976):653.

69. DYSKEN, M. W., et al. "Fluphenazine Pharmacokinetics and Therapeutic Re-

sponse," *Psychopharmacology,* 73 (1981):205–210.

70. EDWARDS, G. J., et al. "Controlled Trial of Sulpiride in Chronic Schizophrenic Patients," *British Journal of Psychiatry,* 137 (1980):522–529.

71. ENGELHARDT, D. M., et al. "Phenothiazines in the Prevention of Psychiatric Hospitalization," *Archives of General Psychiatry,* 16 (1967):98–99.

72. ERESHEFSKY, L., et al. "Management of Chronic, Refractory Schizophrenic Patients with High-dose Loxapine," *Psychopharmacology Bulletin,* 9 (1983): 600–603.

73. ERICKSEN, S. E., HURT, S. W., and CHANG, S. "Haloperidol Dose, Plasma Levels, and Clinical Response: A Double-blind Study," *Psychopharmacology Bulletin,* 14 (1978):15–16.

74. ERICKSEN, S. E., HURT, S. W., and DAVIS, J. M. "Dosage of Antipsychotic Drugs," *New England Journal of Medicine,* 294 (1976):1296.

75. ESTERSON, A., COOPER, D. G., and LAING, R. D. "Results of Family-oriented Therapy with Hospitalized Schizophrenics," *British Medical Journal,* 2 (1965):1462–1465.

76. FAERGEMAN, P. M. *Psychogenic Psychoses.* London: Butterworth & Co., 1963.

77. FALLOON, I., WATT, D. C., and SHEPHERD, M. "A Comparative Controlled Trial of Pimozide and Fluphenazine Decanoate in the Continuation Therapy of Schizophrenia," *Psychological Medicine,* 8 (1978):59–70.

78. FALLOON, I.R.H., et al. "Family Management in the Prevention of Exacerbations of Schizophrenia," *New England Journal of Medicine,* 306 (1982):1437–1440.

79. FALLOON, I.R.H., et al. "Family Management in the Prevention of Exacerbations of Schizophrenia: A Controlled Study," *New England Journal of Medicine,* 306 (1982):1437–1440.

80. FENTON, F. R., and STRUENING, E. L. "A Comparative Trial of Home and Hospital Psychiatric Care," *Archives of General Psychiatry,* 36 (1978):1074–1079.

81. FENTON, F. R., et al. "A Two-year Follow-up of a Comparative Trial of the Cost-effectiveness of Home and Hospital Psychiatric Treatment," *Canadian Journal of Psychiatry,* 29 (1984):205–211.

82. FILHO, V. V., CALDEIRA, M.V.N., and BUENO, J. R. "The Efficacy and Safety of Loxapine Succinate in the Treatment of Schizophrenia: A Comparative Study," *Current Therapeutic Research,* 18 (1975):476–490.

83. FITZGERALD, C. H. "A Double-blind Comparison of Haloperidol with Perphenazine in Acute Psychiatric Episodes," *Current Therapeutic Research,* 11 (1969):515–519.

84. FLEISS, J. L. *Statistical Methods for Rates and Proportions.* New York: John Wiley & Sons, 1981.

85. FREEMAN, H., and FREDERICK, A. N. "Comparison of Trifluoperazine and Molindone in Chronic Schizophrenic Patients," *Current Therapeutic Research,* 11 (1969):670–676.

86. FREEMAN, L. S., and ALSON, E. "Prolonged Withdrawal of Chlorpromazine in Chronic Patients," *Diseases of the Nervous System,* 23 (1966):321–325.

87. FRUENSGAARD, K., et al. "Loxapine Versus Haloperidol Parenterally in Acute Psychosis with Agitation: A Double-blind Study," *Acta Psychiatrica Scandinavica,* 56 (1977):256–264.

88. GALLANT, D. M., and BISHOP, M. P. "Molindone: Controlled Evaluation in Chronic Schizophrenic Patients," *Current Therapeutic Research,* 10:(1968): 441–447.

89. GARDOSE, G. "Are Antipsychotic Drugs Interchangeable"? *Journal of Nervous and Mental Disease,* 159 (1978):343.

90. GARDOSE, G., et al. "High and Low Dose Thiothixene Treatment in Chronic Schizophrenia," *Diseases of the Nervous System,* 35 (1974):53–58.

91. GARFIELD, S., et al. "Withdrawal of Ataractic Medication in Schizophrenic Patients," *Diseases of the Nervous System,* 27 (1966):321–325.

92. GARVER, D. L., et al. "Pharmacokinetics of Red Blood Cell Phenothiazine and Clinical Effects," *Archives of General Psychiatry,* 33 (1976):862–866.

93. GARVER, D. L., et al. "Neuroleptic Drug Levels and Therapeutic Response: Preliminary Observations with Red Blood

Cell Bound Butaperazine," *American Journal of Psychiatry*, 134 (1978):304–307.

94. GELDERS, Y. G., et al. "Twelve-Month Study of Haloperidol Decanoate in Chronic Schizophrenic Patients," *International Pharmacopsychiatry*, 17 (1982):247–254.

95. GELENBERG, A. J., and DOLLER, J. C. "Clozapine Versus Chlorpromazine for the Treatment of Schizophrenia: Preliminary Results From a Double-blind Study,"*Journal of Clinical Psychiatry*, 40 (1979):238–240.

96. GERLACH, J., et al. "Clozapine and Haloperidol in a Single-blind Crossover Trial: Therapeutic and Biochemical Aspects in the Treatment of Schizophrenia," *Acta Psychiatrica Scandinavica*, 50 (1974):410–424.

97. GERSTENZANG, M. L., and KRULISKY, T. V. "Parenteral Haloperidol in Psychiatric Emergencies: Double-blind Comparison with Chlorpromazine," *Diseases of the Nervous System*, 38 (1977):581–583.

98. GIANNINI, A. J., et al. "Comparison of Haloperidol and Chlorpromazine in the Treatment of Phencyclidine Psychosis," *Journal of Clinical Pharmacology*, 24 (1984):202–204.

99. GLICK, J. D., and HARGREAVES, W. A. *Psychiatric Hospital Treatment for the 1980's.* Lexington, Mass: Lexington Books, 1979.

100. GOLDBERG, S. C., et al. "Prediction of Improvement in Schizophrenia Under Four Phenothiazines," *Archives of General Psychiatry*, 16 (1967):107–117.

101. GOLDBERG, S. C., et al. "Prediction of Response to Phenothiazines in Schizophrenia: A Crossvalidation Study," *Archives of General Psychiatry*, 26 (1972):367–373.

102. GOLDBERG, S. C., et al. "Prediction of Relapse in Schizophrenic Outpatients Treated by Drug and Sociotherapy," *Archives of General Psychiatry*, 34 (1977):171–184.

103. GOLDSTEIN, M. J., et al. "Drug and Family in the Aftercare of Acute Schizophrenics," *Archives of General Psychiatry*, 35 (1978):1169–1177.

104. GORHAM, D. R., and POKORNY, A. D.

"Effects of Phenothiazine and/or Group Psychotherapy with Schizophrenics," *Diseases of the Nervous System*, 25 (1964):77.

105. GREENBLATT, M., et al., eds. *Drug and Social Therapy in Chronic Schizophrenia.* Springfield, Ill.: Charles C Thomas, 1965.

106. GRINSPOON, L., EWALT, J. R., and SHADER, R. "Psychotherapy and Pharmacotherapy in Chronic Schizophrenia," *American Journal of Psychotherapy*, 124 (1968):67–74.

107. ———. *Schizophrenia: Pharmacotherapy and Psychotherapy.* Baltimore: Williams & Wilkins, 1972.

108. GROSS, H. S. "A Double-blind Comparison of Once-a-day Pimozide, Trifluoperazine, and Placebo in the Maintenance Care of Chronic Schizophrenics," *Current Therapeutic Research*, 16 (1975): 696–705.

109. GROSS, M., and REEVES, W. P. "Relapse after Withdrawal of Ataractic Drugs in Mental Patients in Transition," in M. Greenblatt, ed., *Mental Patients in Transition.* Springfield, Ill.: Charles C Thomas, 1961, pp. 313–321.

110. GUIRGUIS, E., et al. "Clozapine (Leponex) vs. Chlorpromazine (Largactil) in Acute Schizophrenia (A Double-blind Controlled Study)," *Current Therapeutic Research*, 21 (1977):707–719.

111. HANLON, T. E., et al. "The Comparative Effectiveness of Amitriptyline, Perphenazine, and Their Combination in the Treatment of Chronic Psychotic Female Patients,"*Journal of New Drugs*, 4 (1964):52.

112. HANSEN, L. B., LARSEN, N. E., and GULMANN, N. "Dose-response Relationships of Perphenazine in the Treatment of Acute Psychoses," *Psychopharmacology*, 78 (1982):112–115.

113. HARNRYD, C., et al. "Clinical Evaluation of Sulpiride in Schizophrenic Patients— A Double-blind Comparison with Chlorpromazine," *Acta Psychiatrica Scandinavica*, 69 (Supplement) (1984): 7–30.

114. HASTINGS, D. W. "Follow-up Results in Psychiatric Illness," *American Journal of Psychiatry*, 114 (1958):1–11.

115. HERSHON, H. I., KENNEDY, P. F., and

McGUIRE, R. J. "Persistence of Extrapyramidal Disorders and Psychiatric Relapse After Withdrawal of Long-term Phenothiazine Therapy," *British Journal of Psychiatry*, 120 (1972):41–50.

116. HERZ, M. I., and MELVILLE, C. "Relapse in Schizophrenia," *American Journal of Psychiatry*, 137 (1980):801–805.

117. HERZ, M. I., ENDICOTT, J., and SPITZER, R. L. "Brief Hospitalization of Patients with Families: Initial Results," *American Journal of Psychiatry*, 132 (1975): 413–418.

118. ———. "Brief Versus Standard Hospitalization. The Families," *American Journal of Psychiatry*, 133 (1976):795–801.

119. ———. "Brief Hospitalization: A Two-year Follow-up," *American Journal of Psychiatry*, 134 (1977):502–507.

120. HERZ, M. I., SZYMANSKI, H. W., and SIMON, J. C. "Intermittent Medication for Stable Schizophrenic Outpatients: An Alternative to Maintenance Medication," *American Journal of Psychiatry*, 139 (1982):918–922.

121. HIRSCH, S. R., et al. "Outpatient Maintenance of Chronic Schizophrenic Patients with Long-acting Fluphenazine Double-blind Placebo Trial," *British Medical Journal*, 1 (1973):633–637.

122. HIRSCHOWITZ, J., et al. "Lithium Response in Good Prognosis Schizophrenia," *American Journal of Psychiatry*, 137 (1980):916–920.

123. HOGARTY, G. E. "Depot Neuroleptics: The Relevance of Psychosocial Factors —A United States Perspective," *Journal of Clinical Psychiatry*, 45 (1984):36–42.

124. HOGARTY, G. E., and GOLDBERG, S. C. "Drugs and Sociotherapy in the Aftercare of Schizophrenic Patients. One-year Relapse Rates," *Archives of General Psychiatry*, 28 (1973):54–64.

125. HOGARTY, G. E., and ULRICH, R. F. "Temporal Effects of Drug and Placebo in Delaying Relapse in Schizophrenic Outpatients," *Archives of General Psychiatry*, 34 (1977):297–301.

126. HOGARTY, G. E., GOLDBERG, S. C., and SCHOOLER, N. R. "Drugs and Sociotherapy in the Aftercare of Schizophrenic Patients: III. Adjustment of Nonrelapsed Patients," *Archives of General Psychiatry*, 31 (1974):609–618.

127. HOGARTY, G. E., et al. "Drugs and Sociotherapy in the Aftercare of Schizophrenic Patients," *Archives of General Psychiatry*, 31 (1974):603–608.

128. HOGARTY, G. E., et al. "Drug Discontinuation Among Long-term Successfully Maintained Schizophrenic Outpatients," *Diseases of the Nervous System*, 37 (1976):494–500.

129. HOGARTY, G. E., et al. "Fluphenazine and Social Therapy in the Aftercare of Schizophrenic Patients: Relapse Analyses of a Two-year Controlled Study of Fluphenazine Decanoate and Fluphenazine Hydrochloride," *Archives of General Psychiatry*, 36 (1979):1283–1294.

130. HOLLISTER, L. E., and KIM, D. Y. "Intensive Treatment with Haloperidol of Treatment-resistant Chronic Schizophrenic Patients," *American Journal of Psychiatry*, 139 (1982):1466–1468.

131. HOLLISTER, L. E., et al. "Perphenazine Combined with Amitriptyline in Newly Admitted Schizophrenics," *American Journal of Psychiatry*, 120 (1963):591–592.

132. HOLZMAN, P., and JOHNSTON, M. H. *Assessing Schizophrenic Thinking.* San Francisco: Jossey-Bass, 1980.

133. HOMMER, D. W., et al. "Prazosin, a Specific Alpha$_1$-noradrenergic Receptor Antagonist, Has No Effect on Symptoms but Increases Autonomic Arousal in Schizophrenic Patients," *Psychiatry Research*, 11 (1984):193–204.

134. HONIGFELD, G., et al. "Behavioral Improvement in the Older Schizophrenic Patient: Drugs and Social Therapies," *Journal of the American Geriatric Society*, 13 (1965):57–72.

135. HOPKIN, J. T., DONLON, P. T., and SCHAFFER, C. B. "Injectable Haloperidol in the Control of Acute Schizophrenics: Efficacy and Safety," *Current Therapeutic Research*, 27 (1980):620–625.

136. HORN, A. S., and SNYDER, S. H. "Chlorpromazine and Dopamine: Conformational Similarities that Correlate with the Antischizophrenic Activity of Phenothiazine Drugs," *Proceedings of the Academy of Science*, 65 (1971):2325.

137. HORWITZ, W. A., et al. "A Study of Cases

of Schizophrenia Treated by 'Direct Analysis,' " 114 (1958):780–783.

138. HURST, L. "Chlorpromazine and Perazine in Chronic Schizophrenia," *Journal of Mental Science*, 106 (1960):726–731.

139. HURT, S. W., HOLZMAN, P. S., and DAVIS, J. M. "Thought Disorder," *Archives of General Psychiatry*, 40 (1983):1281–1285.

140. ITIL, T., et al. "Treatment of Resistant Schizophrenics with Extremely High Dosage Fluphenazine Hydrochloride," *Psychosomatics*, 11 (1970):456–463.

141. ITIL, T., et al. "Clinical and Quantitative EEG Changes at Different Dosage Levels of Fluphenazine Treatment," *Acta Psychiatrica Scandinavica*, 47 (1971): 440–451.

142. ITIL, T. M., et al. "Comparison of the Clinical and Electroencephalographical Effects of Molindone and Trifluoperazine on Acute Schizophrenic Patients," *Behavioral Neuropsychiatry*, 3 (1971): 25–32.

143. JANOWSKY, D. S., et al. "Provocation of Schizophrenic Symptoms by Intravenous Administration of Methylphenidate," *Archives of General Psychiatry*, 28 (1973):185–191.

144. JOHNSON, D.A.W. *Haloperidol Decanoate and the Treatment of Chronic Schizophrenia*. New York: Adis Press, 1982.

145. JOHNSTON, M. H., and HOLZMAN, P. S. *Assessing Schizophrenic Thinking*. San Francisco: Jossey-Bass, 1979.

146. JOHNSTONE, E. C., et al. "Mechanism of the Antipsychotic Effect in the Treatment of Acute Schizophrenia," *Lancet*, 1 (1978):848.

147. KANE, J. M., et al. "Comparison of the Incidence and Severity of Extrapyramidal Side Effects with Fluphenazine Enanthate and Fluphenazine Decanoate," *American Journal of Psychiatry*, 135 (1978):539–542.

148. KANE, J. M., et al. "Low-dose Neuroleptic Treatment of Outpatient Schizophrenics: I. Preliminary Results for Relapse Rates," *Archives of General Psychiatry*, 40 (1983):893–896.

149. KANE, J. M., et al. "Minimum Dosage Requirements in Maintenance Treatment of Schizophrenia," Paper presented at the Collegium Internationale Neuro-psychopharmacologicum, 14th CINP Congress, Florence, Italy, 1984.

150. KARON, B., and O'GRADY, P. "Intellectual Test Changes in Schizophrenic Patients in the First Six Months of Treatment," *Psychotherapy: Theory, Research and Practice*, 6 (1969):88–96.

151. KARON, B. P., and VANDENBOS, G. R. "Experience, Medication and the Effectiveness of Psychotherapy with Schizophrenics," *British Journal of Psychiatry*, 116 (1970):427–428.

152. ———. "The Consequences of Psychotherapy to Schizophrenic Patients," *Psychotherapy: Theory, Research and Practice*, 9 (1972):111–119.

153. KILOH, L. G., WILLIAMS, S. E., and GRANT, D. A. "A Double-blind Comparative Trial of Loxapine and Trifluoperazine in Acute and Chronic Schizophrenia Patients," *Journal of International Medical Research*, 4 (1976):441–448.

154. KINROSS-WRIGHT, J., and CHARALAMPOUS, K. D. "A Controlled Study of a Very Long-acting Phenothiazine Preparation," *International Journal of Neuropsychiatry*, 1 (1965):66–70.

155. KLEIN, D. F., and DAVIS, J. M. *Diagnosis and Drug Treatment of Psychiatric Disorders*. Baltimore: Waverly Press, 1969.

156. KLEIN, D. F., and ROSEN, B. "Premorbid Asocial Adjustment and Response to Phenothiazine Treatment Among Schizophrenic Inpatients," *Archives of General Psychiatry*, 29 (1973):480–485.

157. KNIGHT, A., HIRSCH, S., and PLATT, S. D. "Clinical Change as a Function of Brief Admission to a Hospital in a Controlled Study Using the Present State Examination," *British Journal of Psychiatry*, 137 (1980):170–180.

158. KURLAND, A. A., and RICHARDSON, J. M. "A Comparative Study of Two Long-acting Phenothiazine Preparations, Fluphenazine Enanthate and Fluphenazine Decanoate," *Psychopharmacologia*, 4 (1966):320.

159. KURLAND, A. A., et al. "The Comparative Effectiveness of Six Phenothiazine Compounds, Phenobarbital and Inert Placebo in the Treatment of Acutely Ill Patients: Global Measures of Severity of

Illness," *Journal of Nervous and Mental Disease*, 133 (1961):1–18.

160. LADER, M. "Monitoring Plasma Concentrations of Neuroleptics," *Pharmacopsychiatry*, 9 (1976):170–177.

161. LANGFELD, G. "The Prognosis in Schizophrenia," *Acta Psychiatrica Neurologica Scandinavica*, 110 (Supplement) (1965):7–66.

162. ———. "Schizophrenia: Diagnosis and Prognosis," *Behavioral Science*, 14 (1969):173–182.

163. LEFF, J. "Psychosocial Relevance and Benefit of Neuroleptic Maintenance: Experience in the United Kingdom," *Journal of Clinical Psychiatry*, 45 (1984):43–49.

164. LEFF, J., and WING, J. K. "Trial of Maintenance Therapy in Schizophrenia," *British Medical Journal*, 3 (1971):599.

165. LEFF, J., et al. "A Controlled Trial of Social Intervention in the Families of Schizophrenic Patients," *British Journal of Psychiatry*, 141 (1982):121–134.

166. LEHMANN, H. E. "Drug Treatment of Schizophrenia," in N. S. Kline and H. E. Lehmann, eds., *International Psychiatry Clinics*, vol. 2, no. 4. Boston: Little, Brown, 1965, p. 717.

167. LEHMANN, H. E., et al. "Wirkungsdifferenzen bei Hoch-und Standarddosierung von Fluphenazin-Decanoat in Abhangigkeit von Patienten-Merkmalen," *Pharmakopsychiatrie*, 13 (1980):117–129.

168. LEVINE, J., SCHOOLER, N. R., and CASSANO, G. "The Role of Depot Neuroleptics in the Treatment of Schizophrenic Patients," *Psychological Medicine*, 9 (1979):383–386.

169. LEVINE, J., SCHOOLER, N. R., and SEVERE, J. "Discontinuation of Oral and Depot Fluphenazine in Schizophrenic Patients After One Year of Continuous Medication: A Controlled Study," *Advances in Biochemical Psychopharmacology*, 24 (1980):483–493.

170. LEVINE, J., et al. "Discontinuation of Oral and Depot Fluphenazine in Schizophrenic Patients After One Year of Continuous Medication," in E. Cattabeni, *Long-term Effects of Neuroleptics*. New York: Raven Press, 1980, pp. 483–484.

171. LINN, M. W., et al. "Hospital versus Community (Foster) Care for Psychiatric Patients: A Veterans Administration Cooperative Study," *Archives of General Psychiatry*, 34 (1977):78–83.

172. MCCLELLAND, H. A., et al. "Very High Dose Fluphenazine Decanoate: A Controlled Trial in Chronic Schizophrenia," *Archives of General Psychiatry*, 33 (1976):1435–1439.

173. MCCREADIE, R. G., and MACDONALD, I. M. "High Dosage Haloperidol in Chronic Schizophrenia," *British Journal of Psychiatry*, 131 (1977):310–316.

174. MALIK, S. C., and KUMAR, K. "Loxapine in Adolescent Schizophrenia," *Current Therapeutic Research*, 28 (1980):432–446.

175. MAN, P. L., and CHEN, C. H. "Rapid Tranquilization of Acutely Psychotic Patients with Intramuscular Haloperidol and Chlorpromazine," *Psychosomatics*, 13 (1973):59–63.

176. MAVOROIDIS, M. L., et al. "Therapeutic Blood Levels of Fluphenazine: Plasma or RBC Determinations?" *Psychopharmacology Bulletin*, 20 (1984):168–170.

177. MAVOROIDIS, M. L., et al. "Haloperidol Blood Levels and Response: Confounded Variables?" *Psychopharmacology Bulletin*, 21 (1985):62–65.

178. ———. "Fluphenazine Plasma Levels and Clinical Response," *Journal of Clinical Psychiatry*, in press.

179. MAY, P.R.A. *Treatment of Schizophrenia: A Comparative Study of Five Treatment Methods*. New York: Science House, 1968.

180. MAY, P.R.A., TUMA, A. H., and DIXON, W. J. "Schizophrenia: A Follow-up Study of Results of Treatments. I. Design and Other Problems," *Archives of General Psychiatry*, 33 (1976):474–480.

181. ———. "For Better or for Worse? Outcome Variance with Psychotherapy and Other Treatments for Schizophrenia," *Journal of Nervous and Mental Disease*, 165 (1977):231–239.

182. ———. "Schizophrenia: A Follow-up Study of the Results of Five Forms of Treatment," *Archives of General Psychiatry*, 38 (1981):776–784.

183. MAY, P.R.A., et al. "Schizophrenia: A Fol-

low-up Study of Results of Treatment. II. Hospital Stay Over Two to Five Years," *Archives of General Psychiatry*, 33 (1976):481.

184. MAY P.R.A., et al. "Chlorpromazine Blood and Saliva Levels and the Outcome of Treatment in Schizophrenic Patients," *Archives of General Psychiatry*, 38 (1981):202–207.

185. MELYNK, W. T., WORTHINGTON, A. G., and LAVERTY, S. G. "Abrupt Withdrawal of Chlorpromazine and Thioridazine From Schizophrenic Inpatients," *Canadian Psychiatric Association Journal*, 11 (1966):410–413.

186. MESSIER, M., et al. "A Follow-up Study of Intensively Treated Chronic Schizophrenic Patients," *American Journal of Psychiatry*, 125 (1969):1123–1127.

187. MICHAUX, M. H., KURLAND, A. A., and AGALLIANOS, D. "Chlorpromazine-Chlordiazepoxide and Chlorpromazine-Imipramine Treatment of Newly Hospitalized Acutely-ill Psychiatric Patients," *Current Therapeutic Research*, 8 (Supplement) (1968):117.

188. MICHAUX, M. H., et al. "Day and Full Psychiatric Treatment: A Controlled Comparison," *Current Therapeutic Research*, 14 (1972):279.

189. MICHAUX, M. H., et al. "Postrelease Adjustment of Day and Full-time Psychiatric Patients," *Archives of General Psychiatry*, 29 (1973):647–651.

190. MODESTIN, J., et al. "Haloperidol in Acute Schizophrenic Inpatients: A Double-blind Comparison of Two Dosage Regimens," *Pharmacopsychiatrie*, 16 (1983):121–126.

191. MOORE, D. F. "Treatment of Acute Schizophrenia with Loxapine Succinate (Loxitane) in a Controlled Study with Chlorpromazine," *Current Therapeutic Research*, 18 (1975):172.

192. MORGAN, R., and CHEADLE, J. "Maintenance Treatment of Chronic Schizophrenics with Neuroleptic Drugs," *Acta Psychiatrica Scandinavica*, 50 (1974):78–85.

193. MORTON, M. R. "A Study of Withdrawal of Chlorpromazine or Trifluoperazine in Chronic Schizophrenia," *American Journal of Psychiatry*, 124 (1968):1585–1588.

194. MOYANO, C. "A Double-blind Comparison of Loxitane (Loxapine Succinate) and Trifluoperazine Hydrochloride in Chronic Schizophrenic Patients," *Diseases of the Nervous System*, 36 (1975):301.

195. MUNK-ANDERSEN, E., et al. "Sulpiride versus Haloperidol, a Clinical Trial in Schizophrenia. A Preliminary Report," *Acta Psychiatrica Scandinavica*, 69 (Supplement) (1984):31–41.

196. NEBORSKY, R., et al. "Rapid Treatment of Acute Psychotic Symptoms with High- and Low-dose Haloperidol," *Archives of General Psychiatry*, 38 (1981):195–199.

197. O'BRIEN, C., et al. "Group vs. Individual Psychotherapy with Schizophrenics," *Archives of General Psychiatry*, 27 (1972):474–478.

198. PAPROCKI, J., and VERSIANI, M. "A Double-blind Comparison Between Loxapine and Haloperidol by Parenteral Route in Acute Schizophrenia," *Current Therapeutic Research*, 21 (1977): 80.

199. PAPROCKI, J., et al. "A Controlled Double-blind Comparison Between Loxapine and Haloperidol in Acute Newly Hospitalized Schizophrenic Patients," *Psychopharmacology Bulletin*, 12 (1976): 52–84.

200. PAREDES, A., et al. "Clinical Judgement in the Assessment of Psychopharmacological Effects," *Journal of Nervous and Mental Disease*, 142 (1966):153–160.

201. PAUL, G. L., and LENTZ, R. J. *Psychosocial Treatment of Chronic Mental Patients.* Cambridge, Mass.: Harvard University Press, 1977.

202. PLATT, S., HIRSCH, S. R., and KNIGHT, D. C. "Effects of Brief Hospitalization on Psychiatric Patients' Behavior and Social Functioning," *Acta Psychiatrica Scandinavica*, 63 (1981):117–128.

203. POTKIN, S. G., et al. "Failure of Insulin Coma and Presence of a Therapeutic Window for Haloperidol in Chinese Schizophrenics," Paper presented at the Collegium Internationale Neuropsychopharmacologicum, 14 CINP Congress, 1984, Florence, Italy.

204. ———. "Does a Therapeutic Window for Plasma Haloperidol Exist? Preliminary

Chinese Data," *Psychopharmacology Bulletin*, 21 (1985): 59–61.

205. PRIEN, R. F., and COLE, J. O. "High Dose Chlorpromazine Therapy in Chronic Schizophrenia: Report of National Institute of Mental Health Psychopharmacology Research Branch Collaborative Study Group," *Archives of General Psychiatry*, 18 (1968):482–495.

206. PRIEN, R. F., COLE, J. O., and BELKIN, N. F. "Relapse in Chronic Schizophrenics Following Abrupt Withdrawal of Tranquilizing Drugs," *British Journal of Psychiatry*, 115 (1969):679–686.

207. PRIEN, R. F., LEVINE, J., and COLE, J. O. "High Dose Trifluoperazine in Chronic Schizophrenia," *American Journal of Psychiatry*, 126 (1969):305–313.

208. PRIEN, R. F., LEVINE, J., and SWITALSKI, R. W. "Discontinuation of Chemotherapy for Chronic Schizophrenics," *Hospital and Community Psychiatry*, 22 (1971):4–7.

209. PRUSOFF, B. A., et al. "A Controlled Clinical Trial of Amitriptyline Added to Perphenazine in the Treatment of Depressed Schizophrenics," *Psychopharmacology Bulletin*, 15 (1978):80.

210. ———. "Treatment of Secondary Depression in Schizophrenia," *Archives of General Psychiatry*, 36 (1979):569.

211. QUITKIN, F., RIFKIN, A., and KLEIN, D. F. "Very High Dosage vs. Standard Dosage Fluphenazine in Schizophrenia," *Archives of General Psychiatry*, 32 (1975):1276–1281.

212. QUITKIN, F., et al. "Long Acting Oral Versus Injectable Antipsychotic Drugs in Schizophrenics," *Archives of General Psychiatry*, 35 (1978):889.

213. RAMSEY, R. A., et al. "A Comparative Study of Molindone and Trifluoperazine," *Current Therapeutic Research*, 12 (1970):438–440.

214. RASSIDAKIS, N. C., et al. "Withdrawal of Antipsychotic Drugs from Chronic Patients," *Bulletin of the Menninger Clinic*, 34 (1970):216–222.

215. RENNIE, T.A.C. "Follow-up Study of Five-hundred Patients with Schizophrenia Admitted to the Hospital from 1913 to 1923," *Archives of Neurological Psychiatry*, 42 (1939):877–891.

216. RESCHKE, R. W. "Parenteral Haloperidol for Rapid Control of Severe Common Disruptive Symptoms of Acute Schizophrenia," *Diseases of the Nervous System*, 35 (1974):112–115.

217. RIFKIN, A., et al. "Fluphenazine Decanoate, Oral Fluphenazine, and Placebo in the Treatment of Remitted Schizophrenics. I. Relapse Rates After One Year," *Archives of General Psychiatry*, 34 (1977):1215–1219.

218. RIMON, R., et al. "Serum and CSF Levels of Haloperidol by Radioimmunoassay and Radioreceptor Assay During High-dose Therapy of Resistant Schizophrenic Patients," *Psychopharmacology*, 73 (1981):197–199.

219. RITTER, R. M., DAVIDSON, D. E., and ROBINSON, T. A. "Comparison of Injectable Haloperidol and Chlorpromazine," *American Journal of Psychiatry*, 129 (1972):110–113.

220. ROOSE, K. "Haloperidol Decanoate as a Replacement for Maintenance Therapy with Intramuscular Fluphenazine Decanoate in Schizophrenia and Other Chronic Psychoses," *Acta Psychiatrica Belgica*, 2 (1982): 216–223.

221. ROSEN, J. N. "The Treatment of Schizophrenic Psychoses by Direct Analytic Therapy," *Psychiatric Quarterly*, 21 (1947):117–119.

222. ———. *Direct Analysis: Selected Papers*. New York: Grune & Stratton, 1953.

223. RUPP, C., and FLETCHER, E. "A Five- to Ten-year Follow-up Study of 641 Schizophrenic Cases," *American Journal of Psychiatry*, 96 (1939):877–888.

224. SAKALIS, G., et al. "Psychologic and Clinical Effects of Chlorpromazine and Their Relationship to Plasma Level," *Clinical Pharmacology and Therapeutics*, 13 (1972):931–946.

225. SALZMAN, C. "The Use of ECT in the Treatment of Schizophrenia," *American Journal of Psychiatry*, 137 (1980):9.

226. SCHAWVER, J., et al. "Comparison of Chlorpromazine and Reserpine in Maintenance Drug Therapy," *Diseases of the Nervous System*, 20 (1959):452–457.

227. SCHIELE, B. C. "Loxapine Succinate: A Controlled Double-blind Study in Chronic Schizophrenia," *Diseases of the Nervous System*, 18 (1975):361.

228. SCHIELE, B. C., VESTRE, N. D., and STEIN, K. E. "A Comparison of Thioridazine, Trifluoperazine, Chlorpromazine and Placebo: A Double-blind Controlled Study on the Treatment of Chronic, Hospitalized, Schizophrenic Patients," *Journal of Clinical and Experimental Psychopathology*, 21 (1961):151–162.

229. SCHOOLER, N. R., and LEVINE, J. "NIMH-PRB Collaborative Fluphenazine Study Group: The Initiation of Long-term Pharmacotherapy in Schizophrenia: Dosage and Side Effect Comparisons Between Oral and Depot Fluphenazine," *Pharmakopsychiatrie Neuro-psychopharmakologie*, 9 (1976):159–169.

230. ———. "Fluphenazine and Fluphenazine HCl in the Treatment of Schizophrenic Patients," in P. Deniker, C. Radouca-Thomas, and A. Villeneuve, eds., *Proceedings of the Meeting of the Collegium International Neuro-Psychopharmacologicum*. Oxford: Pergamon Press, 1978, p. 418.

231. SCHOOLER, N. R., LEVINE, J., and SEVERE, J. B. "Depot Fluphenazine in the Prevention of Relapse in Schizophrenia: Evaluation of a Treatment Regimen," *Psychopharmacology Bulletin*, 15 (1978):44.

232. SCHOOLER, N. R., et al. "Prevention of Relapse in Schizophrenia: An Evaluation of Fluphenazine Decanoate," *Archives of General Psychiatry*, 37 (1980):16–24.

233. SEDVALL, G. "Relationships Among Biochemical, Clinical, and Pharmacokinetic Variables in Neuroleptic-treated Schizophrenic Patients," in F. Cattabeni, ed., *Long Term Effects of Neuroleptics*. New York: Raven Press, 1980, pp. 521–528.

234. SEDVALL, G., and GRUMM, V. "Cerebrospinal Fluid and Plasma as Tools for Obtaining Biochemical and Pharmacologic Data in Neuroleptic Therapy," in G. O. Burrows, and T. Norman, eds., *Psychotropic Drugs: Plasma Concentration and Clinical Research*. New York: Dekker, 1981, pp. 331–356.

235. SEEMAN, P., et al. "Antipsychotic Drug Doses and Neuroleptic/dopamine Receptors," *Nature*, 261 (1976):717–719.

236. SELMAN, F. B., MCCLURE, R. F., and HELWIG, H. "Loxapine Succinate: a Double-blind Comparison with Haloperidol and Placebo in Acute Schizophrenics," *Current Therapeutic Research*, 19 (1976): 645.

237. SETH, S., MAHAL, A. S., and KUMAR, K. A. "A Double-blind Comparative Trial of Loxapine and Trifluoperazine in Chronic Schizophrenic Patients," *Current Therapeutic Research*, 25 (1979): 320–329.

238. SHOPSIN, B., et al. "A Controlled Double-blind Comparison Between Loxapine Succinate and Chlorpromazine in Acute Newly Hospitalized Schizophrenic Patients," *Current Therapeutic Research*, 14 (1972):739.

239. SHOPSIN, B., et al. "Clozapine Chlorpromazine and Placebo in Newly Hospitalized Acutely Schizophrenic Patients," *Archives of General Psychiatry*, 36 (1979):657–664.

240. SIMPSON, G. M., and CUCULIC, Z. "A Double-blind Comparison of Loxapine Succinate and Trifluoperazine in Newly Admitted Schizophrenic Patients," *Journal of Clinical Pharmacology*, 16 (1976):60–65.

241. SIMPSON, G. M., and VARGA, E. "Clozapine—A New Antipsychotic Agent," *Current Therapeutic Research*, 16 (1976):679–686.

242. SIMPSON, G. M., AMIN, M., and EDWARDS, J. G. "A Double-blind Comparison of Molindone and Trifluoperazine in the Treatment of Acute Schizophrenia," *Journal of Clinical Pharmacology*, 11 (1971):227–236.

243. SIMPSON, G. M., et al. "Problems in the Evaluation of the Optimal Dose of Phenothiazine (Butaperazine)," *Diseases of the Nervous System*, 29 (1968): 478–484.

244. SINGH, A. N., SAXENA, B., and NELSON, H. L. "A Controlled Study of Trazodone in Chronic Schizophrenic Patients with Pronounced Depressive Symptomatology," *Current Therapeutic Research*, 23 (1978):485–501.

245. SIRIS, S. G., RIFKIN, A. E., and REARDON, G.T. "Response of Postpsychotic Depression to Adjunctive Imipramine or Amitriptyline," *Journal of Clinical Psychiatry*, 43 (1982):485–486.

246. SLOTNICK, V. B. "Management of the

Acutely Agitated Psychiatric Patient with Parenteral Neuroleptics: The Comparative Symptom Effectiveness Profiles of Haloperidol and Chlorpromazine," in R. de la Fuente, and M. N. Weisman, eds., *Proceedings of the 5th World Congress of Psychiatry,* 1971, Amsterdam: Exerpta Medica, 1973, p. 531.

247. SMITH, K., et al. "ECT-Chlorpromazine and Chlorpromazine Compared in the Treatment of Schizophrenia," *Journal of Nervous and Mental Disease,* 144 (1967):284.

248. SMITH, R. C., TAMMINGA, C., and DAVIS, J. M. "Effects of Apomorphine on Chronic Schizophrenic Symptoms," *Journal of Neurological Transmitters,* 40 (1977): 171–176.

249. SMITH, R. C., et al. "Plasma Butaperazine Levels in Long-term Chronic Nonresponding Schizophrenics," *Communications in Psychopharmacology,* 1 (1977):319.

250. SMITH, R. C., et al. "Blood Levels of 6 Neuroleptic Drugs in Nonresponding Chronic Schizophrenic Patients," *Archives of General Psychiatry,* 36 (1979): 579–584.

251. SMITH, R. C., et al. "RBC and Plasma Levels of Haloperidol and Clinical Response in Schizophrenia," *American Journal of Psychiatry,* 139 (1982):1054–1056.

252. SMITH, R. C., et al. "Comparative Utility of Chemical and Radioreceptor Drug Level Assays for Evaluating the Relationship Between Neuroleptic Drug Levels and Clinical Response in Schizophrenia," Paper presented at the Collegium Internationale Neuropsychopharmacologicum, 14th CINP Congress, Florence, Italy, 1984.

253. SMITH, R. C., et al. "Red Cell and Plasma Haloperidol and Response in Acutely Ill Schizophrenics: Comparison of GLC and RRA," *Psychopharmacology Bulletin,* 21 (1985):57–59.

254. SNYDER, S. H., CREESE, I., and BURT, D. R. "The Brain's Dopamine Receptor: Labelling with ^{3}H-Dopamine and ^{3}H-Haloperidol," *Communications in Psychopharmacology,* 1 (1975):663–673.

255. SPOHN, H. E., et al. "Phenothiazine Effects on Psychological and Psychophysiological Dysfunction in Chronic Schizophrenics," *Archives of General Psychiatry,* 34 (1977):633.

256. STALKER, H. "Prognosis in Schizophrenia," *Journal of Mental Science,* 85 (1939):1224–1240.

257. STEIN, L., and TEST, M. "Alternative to Mental Hospital Treatment. I, II, and III," *Archives of General Psychiatry,* 37 (1980):392–411.

258. STEINBOOK, R. M., et al. "Loxapine: A Double-blind Comparison with Chlorpromazine in Acute Schizophrenic Patients," *Current Therapeutic Research,* 15 (1973):1–7.

259. STEPHENS, J. H. "Long-Term Course and Prognosis of Schizophrenia," *Seminars in Psychiatry,* 2 (1970):464–485.

260. STEPHENS, J. H., and ASTRUP, C. "Prognosis in 'Process' and 'Non-process' Schizophrenia," *American Journal of Psychiatry,* 119 (1963):945–953.

261. TAMMINGA, C. A., et al. "Schizophrenic Symptoms Improve with Apomorphine," *Science,* 200 (1978):567–568.

262. TEGELER, J. E., et al. "Expetrimenteller Vergleich Niedriger and hoher Haloperidol: Dosen in der Behandlung akut Schizophrener Patienten," *Arzneimittel-Forschung,* 32 (1982):887–888.

263. TORU, M., et al. "A Double-blind Comparison of Sulpiride with Chlorpromazine in Chronic Schizophrenia," *Journal of Clinical Pharmacology,* 12 (1972):221–229.

264. TROSHINSKY, C. H., AARONSON, H. G., and STONE, R. K. "Maintenance Phenothiazine in the Aftercare of Schizophrenic Patients," *Pennsylvania Psychiatric Quarterly,* 2 (1962):11–15.

265. TUMA, A. H., and MAY, P.R.A. "Psychotherapy, Drugs and Therapist Experience in the Treatment of Schizophrenia: A Critique of the Michigan State Project," *Psychotherapy: Theory, Research and Practice* 12 (1975):138–142.

266. VAILLANT, G. E. "The Prediction of Recovery in Schizophrenia," *Journal of Nervous and Mental Disease,* 133 (1962):534–543.

267. ———. "Prospective Prediction of Schizophrenic Remission," *Archives of General Psychiatry,* 11 (1964):509–518.

268. VAN DER VELDE, C. D., and KILTIE, H. "Effectiveness of Loxapine Succinate in Acute Schizophrenia: A Comparative Study with Thiothixene," *Current Therapeutic Research,* 17 (1975):1–2.

269. VAN PRAAG, H., and DOIS, L.C.W. "Fluphenazine Enanthate and Fluphenazine Decanoate: A Comparison of Their Duration of Action and Motor Side Effects," *American Journal of Psychiatry,* 130 (1973):801.

270. VAN PUTTEN, T., et al. "Is a Plasma Level of Haloperidol Clinically Useful?" *Psychopharmacology Bulletin,* 21 (1985):61–64.

271. VYAS, B. K., and KALLA, V. A. "Six Month Double-Blind Comparison of Loxapine Succinate and Chlorpromazine in Chronic Schizophrenic Patients," *Current Therapeutic Research,* 28 (1980):16–30.

272. WAEHRENS, J., and GERLACH, J. "Antidepressant Drugs in Anergic Schizophrenia: A Double-blind Crossover Study of Maprotiline and Placebo," *Acta Psychiatrica Scandinavica,* 61 (1980):438–444.

273. WASHBURN, S., et al. "A Controlled Comparison of Psychiatric Day Care and Inpatient Hospitalization," *Journal of Consulting and Clinical Psychology,* 44 (1976):665–675.

274. WHITAKER, C. B., and HOY, R. M. "Withdrawal of Perphenazine in Chronic Schizophrenia," *British Journal of Psychiatry,* 109 (1963):422–427.

275. WHITTIER, J. R., et al. "Mepazine (Pacatal): Clinical Trial with Placebo Control and Psychological Study," *Psychopharmacologia,* 1 (1960):280–287.

276. WIJSENBECK, H., STEINER, M., and GOLDBERG, S. C. "Trifluoperazine: A Comparison Between Regular and High Doses," *Psychopharmacologia* (Berlin), 36 (1974):147–150.

277. WILDER, J. F., LEVIN, G., and ZWELLING, J. "A Two-year Followup Evaluation of Acute Psychiatric Patients Treated in a Day Hospital," *American Journal of Psychiatry,* 122 (1966):1095–1106.

278. WING, J., and LEFF, J. "Trial of Maintenance Therapy in Schizophrenia," *British Medical Journal,* 3 (1971):599–604.

279. WISTEDT, B. "A Depot Neuroleptic Withdrawal Study," *Acta Psychiatrica Scandinavica,* 64 (1981):65–84.

280. ———. "Withdrawal of Long Acting Neuroleptics in Schizophrenic Outpatients," *Acta Universities Upsalienses,* 64 (1981):391–397.

281. WODE-HELGODT, et al. "Clinical Effects and Drug Concentrations in Plasma and Cerebrospinal Fluid in Psychotic Patients Treated with Fixed Doses of Chlorpromazine," *Acta Psychiatrica Scandinavica,* 58 (1978):149–173.

282. ZUARDI, A. W., et al. "Double-blind Comparison Between Two Forms of Haloperidol: An Oral Preparation and a New Depot Decanoate in the Maintenance of Schizophrenic Inpatients," *Current Therapeutic Research,* 34 (1983):253.

CHAPTER 19

ALTERNATIVE TREATMENTS FOR SCHIZOPHRENIC PSYCHOSES

Susan R. Donaldson, Alan J. Gelenberg, and Ross J. Baldessarini

¶ Introduction

Since the introduction of chlorpromazine in 1952, neuroleptic drugs have been the mainstay of treatment in schizophrenia. However, this class of agents has serious limitations: Some schizophrenic patients do not improve when given neuroleptic agents, while others suffer severe and sometimes irreversible adverse effects. The search therefore continues for other treatments that may prove more effective or less toxic than currently available neuroleptics. This chapter reviews recent research on some alternative treatments for schizophrenic psychoses, summarizing evidence for efficacy and safety.

"Schizophrenia" is a heterogeneous group of disorders, diverse in etiology, pathophysiology, and clinical description.* A particular

treatment may be effective for a certain subgroup of patients diagnosed as schizophrenic, but ineffective in others. The broad efficacy of the neuroleptics is clinically advantageous, but suggests that the drugs work on common features of various disorders that produce psychosis. Alternative agents that correct more specific defects would be welcome, yet might appear ineffective in clinical trials because they treat only one subgroup of patients. In this review, an attempt is made to define subgroups of patients for whom a particular treatment appears to be effective.

The difficulties of conducting and interpreting research in this area are considerable. The presumed heterogeneity of patient populations invites a particular Type II error, in which an effect pertaining to only a proportion of subjects is obscured in studies of a broader population, leading to a "false nega-

---

*At present, the term schizophrenia is often restricted to denote a chronic idiopathic psychotic disorder. However, many of the studies reviewed here have used broader definitions, based on a wide variety of diagnostic criteria. For clarity, we have highlighted such broader usages by the use of quotation marks in the text whenever the distinction seems especially significant.

tive" conclusion. Thus a particular agent might be successful in treating a subgroup comprising 5 percent of unselected "schizophrenics," but the proof of such effectiveness would require the independent identification of the subgroup and its separate evaluation.

A second factor that predisposes to Type II errors is the frequent selection of treatment-resistant patients as subjects. While concern for the patient's welfare may suggest that such patients should be offered alternative treatments, this practice hardly provides a fair trial for the treatment. Some of the agents reviewed here appear most effective in patients who had also responded to neuroleptic agents.

Other problems also plague this area of research. The complex nature of outcome measurements makes the evaluation of treatment effects uncertain. Studies using different outcome measures are difficult to compare. Spontaneous fluctuations in the course of the illness may also obscure treatment effects. Finally, the ubiquitous placebo effect makes the evaluation of uncontrolled studies hazardous, if not impossible, especially given unavoidable subjectivity in outcome ratings and the responsiveness of psychotic patients to environmental changes. Because of these uncertainties, the criteria for acceptance or rejection of a given treatment should be unusually rigorous. At the same time, the devastating nature of schizophrenic illnesses and the inadequacy of current treatments justify an openminded and adventurous spirit in approaching and evaluating innovative treatments.

The current discussion is limited to agents other than traditional neuroleptic drugs or their newer congeners. Other recent reviews cover the uses, limitations, actions, and future prospects of the pharmacological treatments for schizophrenia.[5,6,21]

¶ Lithium in Schizophrenia

There is a growing consensus that lithium carbonate may play a useful role in the treatment of some patients who meet current diagnostic criteria for "schizophrenia" or "schizophreniform psychosis." This idea contradicts the traditional view that lithium is effective only in affective disorders and at best may ameliorate affective symptoms in schizoaffective patients.[26,37] Indeed, some authors have suggested that lithium might be preferentially toxic to schizophrenic patients and is therefore contraindicated[64,73]—an idea not supported by other studies. In contrast, a recent review by Delva and Letemendia,[19] which provides detailed summaries of the major controlled and uncontrolled studies in this area, concludes that "between one-third and one-half of patients with schizophrenia will benefit from lithium" (p.391).

Obviously the question of *diagnosis* is crucial. Lithium is an effective treatment for mania, bipolar disorders, and perhaps other affective disorders,[6] and one might assume accordingly that all that responds to lithium must be affective illness. In fact, "schizophrenic" patients who respond to lithium have clinical features in common with affectively ill patients, and it has been suggested that these patients (DSM-III "schizophreniform," "schizoaffective," or "atypical psychosis") may be inseparable from affective patients.[27,63] However, several studies also suggest that some patients who meet DSM-III[20] criteria for a diagnosis of schizophrenic disorder may benefit from lithium.

The following sections examine, in the light of current literature, several hypotheses that have been advanced about patient characteristics that might predict a beneficial response to lithium.

Review of Studies

PREDICTIVE VALUE OF CURRENT SYMPTOMS

The Research Diagnostic Criteria (RDC) of Spitzer, Endicott, and Robins[80] provides a useful test of the value of affective symptoms alone in predicting lithium response. According to RDC, schizophrenic patients are distinguished from schizo-affective ones solely by the presence or absence of affective symptoms *at the time of evaluation.* Three studies allow the separate assessment of RDC schizophrenics versus schizo-affectives in their response to lithium, either alone or combined with an antipsychotic agent.[1,15,36] Summing individual patient outcomes in these studies, 35 percent (9/26) of the schizo-affective patients had a favorable response to lithium, compared to 31 percent (11/36) of the schizophrenic patients. Thus patients without affective symptoms responded approximately as often as patients who displayed such symptoms. A more recent study,[13] while not giving exact numbers of patients improved, also found that RDC diagnosis (as well as other *symptom-oriented* as opposed to *course-oriented* criteria) did not predict outcome, nor did it distinguish response to lithium from response to chlorpromazine. Thus it appears that affective symptoms alone do not predict a beneficial response to lithium treatment.

Other reviews have suggested that specific psychotic symptoms, including the first-rank symptoms of Schneider, also do not predict or preclude lithium responsiveness.[19,63]

PREDICTIVE VALUE OF PROGNOSTIC CATEGORY

A more useful division may be the distinction between "good-" and "poor-prognosis schizophrenia."[56] The former is characterized by good premorbid function, acute onset, a remitting course, and good recovery of function between psychotic episodes. Poor-prognosis schizophrenia has a more insidious onset, with a poor premorbid history and a deteriorating course in which prior functioning is not regained between exacerbations; this pattern accords with recent conceptualizations of schizophrenia as a chronic, idiopathic psychotic illness. DSM-III[20] has recognized this distinction in part by separating "schizophrenia" from "schizophreniform disorder," the latter being a psychosis of less than six months' duration without a full affective syndrome. Even the six months' criterion does not define chronicity, however, since

an untreated affective psychosis may persist for six to twelve months.

Table 19–1 summarizes ten recent studies of the use of lithium to treat schizophrenic patients. Where possible, patient descriptions have been included that allow some characterization of their illness and prognosis. Although conclusions are by no means clear, a number of impressions can be drawn from the table.

In poor-prognosis or chronic schizophrenia: *acute exacerbations* respond poorly to lithium alone; chlorpromazine may or may not produce a more favorable response. For *maintenance treatment,* lithium alone appears not to be of value. Surprisingly, however, several studies using specific contemporary diagnostic criteria found that the addition of lithium to an antipsychotic agent benefited about half of chronic, poor-prognosis patients.[11,15,79]

In good-prognosis schizophrenia: for *acute exacerbations,* lithium and chlorpromazine appear to be equally effective. *Maintenance* with lithium has not been studied in good-prognosis schizophrenic patients, but schizo-affective patients with a good prognosis appear to do better on lithium maintenance than on placebo.[2,63]

PREDICTIVE VALUE OF LEVEL OF ACTIVITY

A distinction not noted in table 19–1 separates highly active from less active psychotic patients. In two studies, highly active patients appeared to do better with chlorpromazine than with lithium during the acute phase of illness.[13,65] It is unclear to what extent this difference merely represents lithium's slower onset of action and the clinical difficulty of managing an "active" patient until lithium takes effect.

PREDICTIVE VALUE OF BIOLOGICAL MARKERS

Several recent studies have attempted to correlate lithium responsiveness with biochemical measurements to complement clinical observations. The following three

TABLE 19–1

Clinical Studies of Lithium in Schizophrenia

Study	Date	N	Diagnosis/Description	Study Design	Results	Comments
Johnson[41]	1970	11	"Schizo-affective" with insidious onset, residual personality impairment, poor function between psychotic episodes.	Lithium vs. chlorpromazine—double-blind.	6/11 worsened, apparently due to neurotoxicity.	"Manic" patients on same protocol improved. Lithium levels as high 2.55 mEq/liter.
Shopsin, Kimn, and Gershon[74]	1971	21	Newly hospitalized "acute schizophrenic" including chronic undifferentiated, paranoid, schizo-affective. 14/21 had affective symptoms.	Lithium vs. chlorpromazine—double-blind.	6/11 treated with lithium neurotoxic.	Lithium levels 0.65–1.2 mEq/liter.
Prien, Caffey, and Klett[65]	1972	83	Schizo-affective by DSM-II.	Lithium vs. chlorpromazine.	Lithium = chlorpromazine for "mildly active," chlorpromazine > lithium for "highly active."	2/83 became toxic; high dropout rate in high-activity/lithium group may account for findings: Lithium works more slowly.
Small et al.[79]	1975	22	"Very chronically ill" schizophrenic (14) or schizo-affective (8) by Feighner criteria: insidious onset, poor functioning.	Neuroleptic plus lithium or placebo.	10 patients improved and were continued on lithium after study. Cognitive symptoms improved as well as excitement.	1/22 toxic; no good predictors of improvement were found, including diagnostic subtype.
Biederman, Lerner, and Belmaker[11]	1979	36	Schizo-affective by RDC. Subdivided into "affective" (good interepisode function) and "schizophrenic" (chronic impairment).	Neuroleptic plus lithium or placebo.	Lithium benefited both groups. "Affective" group showed more improvement, but lithium accounted for more of improvement in "schizophrenic" group. Both cognitive and affective symptoms improved.	1/36 toxic.

Study	Date	N	Diagnosis/Description	Study Design	Results	Comments
Alexander, van Kammen, and Bunney[1]	1979	13	By DSM-II: 10 schizophrenic, 3 schizo-affective. By RDC: 8 schizophrenic, 5 schizo-affective. Also rated for prognosis.	Lithium vs. placebo.	7 "responders" of whom only 4 relapsed off lithium; 4 "nonresponders." Of 6 good-prognosis patients, 4 were responders.	Data given did not allow clear assessment of correlation of lithium response (including relapse status) with prognostic category. However, none of the diagnostic groupings used predicted lithium response vs. nonresponse.
Growe et al.[30]	1979	8	RDC: 6 schizophrenic, 2 schizo-affective. "Chronic, treatment-resistant."	Neuroleptic with lithium or placebo.	Of 8 scales used, only "psychotic excitement" showed significant decrease on lithium. No change in thought disorder. Trend for improvement on 2 other scales.	No toxicity seen. Small N makes lack of significance hard to assess.
Hirschowitz et al.[36]	1980	31	RDC schizophrenic or schizo-affective. By DSM-III: 9 schizophreniform, 15 schizophrenic, 7 others. Also rated for prognosis.	Uncontrolled; lithium alone.	Among schizophreniform patients: 7/9 improved, mean 50 percent improvement. Among DSM-III schizophrenics: 1 improved, mean 0.6 percent improvement. Among "other" patients: Prognosis predicted lithium response.	Schizophrenic vs. schizophreniform distinction also divided good from poor prognosis patients. No toxicity seen.
Carman, Bigelow, and Wyatt[15]	1981	18	RDC schizophrenic or schizo-affective. Chronic, poor pre- or intermorbid function, insidious onset.	Neuroleptic with lithium or placebo.	Approximately 50 percent benefited, mostly on "arousal" scale (of 3 scales). 3/4 relapsed on lithium alone.	Good premorbid history, episodic course, and affective symptoms were predictors of lithium response, but 3 patients with none of these showed clear improvement.
Braden et al.[3]	1982	78	New admissions with two or more symptoms of mania. By RDC: 12 schizophrenic, 30 affective, 31 schizo-affective, 5 "other." By DSM-III: 11 schizophrenic, 53 affective, 14 other.	Lithium vs. chlorpromazine.	No diagnostic system predicted differential drug response: In general, good-prognosis patients had better outcome than poor-prognosis ones. Patients with higher activity levels did better on chlorpromazine.	4 patients became "more confused" on lithium at therapeutic levels: 2 manic, 2 schizo-affective. No evidence that effect of lithium was confined to affective symptoms.

studies predicted lithium response at a statistically significant level using biological measures, although none has been replicated.

Hirschowitz, Zemlan, and Garver[35] studied thirty-one patients diagnosed by DSM-III criteria as schizophrenic (twenty-five) or schizophreniform (five). DSM-III diagnoses predicted lithium response for all but one patient in each diagnostic group (four of five schizophreniform patients improved, while twenty-four of twenty-five schizophrenic patients did not). However, response was similarly predicted by observations of the *in vitro* erythrocyte ratio of intra- to extracellular lithium combined with assessment of plasma growth hormone level increases in response to apomorphine.

Edelstein and associates[22] tested eleven patients with RDC diagnoses of schizophrenia or schizo-affective disorder, using intravenous physostigmine. Four of the eleven patients showed a transient reduction in psychotic thinking after physostigmine treatment and later improved on lithium treatment; the others responded to neither agent.

Alexander, van Kammen, and Bunney[1] studied thirteen patients with RDC diagnoses of schizophrenia or schizo-affective disorder. Six of their patients were classified as good-prognosis schizophrenics. They attempted to extend the findings of Carman, Bigelow, and Wyatt,[15] which suggested that a high pretreatment ratio of calcium to magnesium in serum predicted a good response to lithium in affectively ill patients. The findings of Alexander, van Kammen, and Bunney[1] were consistent with Carman, Bigelow, and Wyatt's hypothesis but did not reach statistical significance.

All of these studies used lithium alone as the treatment, and none included a placebo control. While it is not possible to construct a coherent biomedical theory incorporating all of these findings, it does appear that biochemical studies may usefully supplement clinical observations in predicting response to lithium. In view of many past difficulties in replicating biochemical studies in the idiopathic psychoses, however, replications of these results are needed.

SPECIFIC EFFECTS OF LITHIUM IN SCHIZOPHRENIC PATIENTS

Clinical lore has suggested that lithium can effectively treat affective symptoms in psychotic patients regardless of diagnosis but does not affect the presumed "core symptoms" of schizophrenia (withdrawal, illogical thought, mood-incongruent delusions).[26] As table 19–1 shows, some studies support this notion. However, three carefully documented studies found lithium to have a beneficial effect on symptoms of cognitive disorganization in schizophrenic patients.[11,13,79]

A small number of studies have suggested that lithium may be contraindicated in schizophrenic patients because of a supposedly increased risk of neurotoxicity at therapeutic blood levels.[64,73] While such cases have been reported, there is no controlled evidence that such toxicity occurs more frequently in schizophrenic patients than in manic-depressive patients. Furthermore, as can be seen in table 19–1, a majority of studies have found lithium to be well tolerated by schizophrenic patients.

Summary

In conclusion, it appears that lithium may benefit some patients diagnosed as schizophrenic, even by contemporary research criteria. Affective symptoms do not predict lithium response, nor do Schneiderian symptoms preclude it. Good-prognosis (or schizophreniform) patients may be treated acutely with lithium unless their activity level requires rapid control with an antipsychotic or sedative agent. Good-prognosis patients who are diagnosed "schizo-affective" may benefit from lithium prophylaxis between episodes. Chronically psychotic schizophrenic patients whose response to antipsychotic agents is incomplete may sometimes benefit from the addition of lithium to an antipsychotic agent, although this group is, almost by definition, less likely to respond than others. The fact that lithium is of value in these patients does not necessarily demand a rediagnosis, as treatment responses in psychiatry are not highly specific and may or may not serve as a useful part of the definition of a diagnostic category. However, it may well be that lithium-responsive schizophrenic patients constitute a biologically distinct subgroup that may prove to be more closely related to patients with affective disorder than to those with chronic poor-prognosis schizophrenia.

¶ Antidepressants in Schizophrenia

Schizophrenic patients are sometimes clinically depressed. Some clinicians consider depressive episodes to be a common component of chronic psychotic illness. In addition, some characteristic schizophrenic symptoms—anergy, anhedonia, flatness of affect—give the appearance of depression even in the absence of depressed mood and so, rightly or wrongly, may prompt treatment with an antidepressant. On such clinical grounds, over the past three decades, many schizophrenic patients have been treated with antidepressants. However, a review of the literature suggests that this practice may be on shaky ground, not only theoretically but empirically as well.

In 1978 Siris, van Kammen, and Docherty,[78] compiled a comprehensive review of controlled studies of antidepressants in schizophrenia. Their conclusions are worth reviewing in some detail, as they have remained largely unchallenged by more recent studies. Also worth reviewing, however, are the limitations of the individual studies they considered.

Review of Siris, van Kammen, and Docherty's Conclusions

Of the forty-two studies reviewed in 1978 by Siris, van Kammen, and Docherty, only eleven were published in the 1970s. This fact in itself bespeaks a waning enthusiasm for the use of antidepressants in schizophrenia. More important, it means that only a small number of studies used diagnostic criteria that can be translated accurately into current diagnostic practice. For example, one study assured the reader that subjects were drawn from "the hard core of long-stay schizophrenics"; no other description is given.[18] In addition, measures of clinical change are often idiosyncratic and difficult to evaluate: For example, an increase in the level of motor activity and speech was noted in several studies, but was interpreted as improvement in some, as worsening in others.

Despite these limitations, Siris, van Kammen, and Docherty[78] extracted the following impressions from their review.

ANTIDEPRESSANT AGENTS ALONE

There is little evidence that antidepressants given without an antipsychotic agent have beneficial effects in schizophrenic patients. This impression applies to both tricyclic antidepressants and monoamine oxidase inhibitors (MAOIs). An exception to this generalization was one study in which patients were specifically selected for depressive symptoms; these patients showed modest improvements in some affective symptoms, but apathy and withdrawal were not affected.

TRICYCLIC ANTIDEPRESSANTS WITH ANTIPSYCHOTIC AGENTS

Ten of twelve studies found an antipsychotic agent alone to be as effective in reducing schizophrenic symptoms as the combination of a tricyclic and an antipsychotic agent; the antidepressant agent conveyed no extra benefit. Again, exceptions were two studies in which patients with depressive symptoms were assessed separately; the depressed patients seemed to benefit more from the combination.

MAOIs WITH ANTIPSYCHOTIC AGENTS

Many of the studies of MAOIs with antipsychotic agents dealt with long-term hospitalized patients and sought to improve their characteristic apathy and anhedonia. There was no definite evidence of benefit, but several controlled studies showed trends for some withdrawn patients to improve when an MAOI was added. The improvement usually took the form of an increase in activity level or interest in the surroundings, rather than a reduction in psychotic symptoms. Uncontrolled studies also reported optimistic findings.[14]

Although a wide range of antidepressants is not represented in the studies reviewed by Siris, van Kammen, and Docherty[78] (which favored the combinations of amitriptyline hydrochloride–perphenazine and tranylcypromine sulfate–trifluoperazine hydrochloride), there was no indication that one member of a class was more effective than another.

Since 1978 interest has focused on the use of antidepressants combined with antipsychotics in schizophrenic patients with superimposed depression. Three studies have reported positive findings. One of these[77] is difficult to interpret because it lacks a control group. A second[66] reports that adding amitriptyline to perphenazine improved depressive symptoms at four months but, inconsistently, not at one, two, or six months. The third,[76] a well-controlled study using trazodone hydrochloride, found a small but significant improvement in depression with the drug, while psychotic symptoms were not exacerbated.

In contrast, three other studies found no advantage of antidepressants over placebo as adjunctives to an antipsychotic.[8,40,55] One of these studies found psychotic symptoms to worsen dramatically when nortriptyline hydrochloride was added to the treatment regimen.[55]

In summary, the evidence weighs against the usefulness of antidepressants in schizophrenic patients, even in the presence of superimposed depression. One exception to this finding may be the anxiolytic-sedative antidepressant trazodone, which deserves further trials in this setting.

Pharmacological Considerations

The pharmacology of antidepressant treatment in schizophrenia may also be revealing. Tricyclic antidepressants may, through competitive inhibition of hepatic enzymes, *increase* blood levels of simultaneously administered antipsychotic agents.[55] Any improvement during addition of an antidepressant agent may, therefore, reflect only a greater bioavailability of the antipsychotic agent. Alternatively, the anticholinergic action associated with many tricyclic antidepressant agents may counteract antipsychotic-induced extrapyramidal symptoms, some of which may mimic depression. This effect could produce a spurious impression of specific antidepressant effect. In general, however, antidepressants appear to have little use in schizophrenia, while their addition probably does increase the risk of toxic reactions.

¶ Propranolol in Schizophrenia

Review of Studies

A recent tantalizing entry into the field of putative antipsychotic medications has been propranolol hydrochloride, along with other beta-receptor blockers. In the early 1970s, several reports claimed dramatic improvements in both acute and chronic psychosis following treatment with high doses of propranolol.* Although early reports cited mixed groups of patients, including some with mania, organic psychosis, or puerperal psychosis, attention quickly focused on the startling remissions seen in some chronically ill "schizophrenic" patients who had been refractory to treatment with antipsychotic agents. In these early uncontrolled studies, very high doses of propranolol were typically used—up to 3 or 4 g per day in some series.[4,82,84,86] In some cases propranolol replaced an antipsychotic agent, while in others the two agents were combined; some successes were reported in both conditions. A review of representative reports on beta-blockers is provided in table 19–2.

Three points are worth noting in reviewing these reports. One is the ubiquitous lack

*See references 3, 4, 29, 72, 82, 84, and 86.

of clear diagnostic criteria, which is a problem for many later studies as well. A second point is the inconsistency in the time required for an apparent therapeutic effect. While some authors found improvement within a week of beginning treatment, others[73,85] maintained that several weeks or even months were needed to observe changes. Finally, the nature of the improvement varied: Some investigators documented a decrease in "positive" symptoms such as aggression and thought disorder, while others noted improvement in "negative" symptoms of withdrawal and apathy.

Since 1977, a series of controlled studies have given a more tempered verdict. Referring again to table 19–2 for details, the following two points should be noted.

First, one double-blind study[88] of *propranolol alone* found it to be only slightly less effective than chlorpromazine in treating acute exacerbations of psychosis; however, improvement was minimal in both the propranolol and chlorpromazine groups. Three other controlled studies of propranolol alone compared to chlorpromazine or to placebo failed to find any therapeutic effect or found it to be less effective than chlorpromazine.[12,46,62]

All of these studies used doses of propranolol comparable to those used in earlier studies reporting therapeutic success, and all allowed sufficient time to detect improvement (at least twelve weeks). One might argue that the populations used were particularly refractory to treatment, since chlorpromazine also failed to produce substantial effects in most cases. However, earlier studies had suggested that propranolol could treat such patients and in fact had proposed that the drug might be particularly effective in patients with psychosis that was resistant to vigorous neuroleptic treatment.

Second, four controlled studies of a *beta-blocker* versus placebo *in combination with a neuroleptic* found the beta-blocker to be a more effective adjunct than placebo.[43,51,67,72] Three of these studies used propranolol, while one[43] used oxprenolol hydrochloride. The report by Sheppard[72] was unconvinc-

ing, as patients improved early in the trial but then deteriorated. The other three studies showed modest but significant degrees of improvement attributable to the beta-blocker. These findings are particularly noteworthy in that the patients had not improved with vigorous neuroleptic treatment and, in two studies, were rigorously diagnosed chronic schizophrenics. These patients represent a group in which any improvement at all commands attention.

A fifth controlled study of propranolol added to a neuroleptic failed to find any advantage of propranolol over placebo.[57]

Adverse Effects

Although many psychotic patients have tolerated propranolol well, even at very high doses, unwanted effects have been reported. Dizziness, ataxia, hypotension, sleep disturbances, and delirium were not uncommon. Cardiovascular collapse has been reported.[62] Paradoxically, *hyper*tensive responses also have been described, with accompanying angina or encephalopathy.[3,4,23,86] Three patients were reported to have experienced grand mal seizures at high doses of propranolol (one during withdrawal); only one patient had a previous history of seizures.[46,81] Yorkston and associates[87] suggest that most of these serious adverse effects can be avoided by using a twice-daily dosage schedule, raising the dose not more than 40 to 80 mg per day, and monitoring patients carefully. Karniol and Portela[43] note that "practically no side effects" were observed with a slow-release preparation of oxprenolol, even at doses up to 640 mg per day. In fact, they record the tantalizing observation that symptoms of tardive dyskinesia decreased significantly in their patients on oxprenolol.

Two fatalities have been reported during high-dose propranolol treatment of psychosis. One patient bled to death from an unsuspected gastric ulcer while taking 2,880 mg propranolol.[29] A second unexplained and apparently sudden death occurred in a healthy eighteen-year-old outpatient who was taking 1,280 mg propranolol per day for treatment

TABLE 19–2

Clinical Studies of Propranolol in Schizophrenia

Author	Date	Type of Study	Number of Patients Completing Trial	Dosage of Propranolol mg/day	Concomitant Neuroleptic Medication	Results	Adverse Reactions
Atsmon et al.[4]	1972	Open.	12 (6 males; 6 females); 7 acute, 5 chronic.	400–4,280, av. 1,400.	N.A.	5 of 7 acute showed much improvement. 3 of 5 chronic showed some improvement.	Hypertension, ataxia.
Gardos et al.[29]	1973	Open.	8 (6 males; 2 females).	120–720. 1 patient up to 2,560; 1 patient up to 2,880.	None.	No antipsychotic effect.	Hypotensive episode, insomnia, fatigue, 1 fatal bleeding ulcer on 2,880 mg.
Yorkston et al.[84]	1974	Open.	14 (9 males; 5 females); not responding to phenothiazines.	500 to 3,000.	Phenothiazines.	6 complete remissions of symptoms; 5 improved; 2 minimal or transient improvement; 1 unchanged with severe toxic reaction.	Ataxia, confusional states, visual hallucinations.
Atsmon[3]	1976	Open.	44: 11 acute schizophrenics, 15 chronic schizophrenics, 8 postpartum psychosis, 5 manic psychosis, 5 psychosis due to organic brain syndrome (OBS).	Up to 2,600.	None.	18 markedly improved: 7/11 acute schizophrenics; 3/15 chronic schizophrenics; 5/8 postpartum psychosis; 3/5 manic psychosis; 0/5 psychosis due to OBS.	Acute hypertension, vomiting, and diarrhea; fatigue, vivid dreams, impaired coordination, slurred speech, 1 patient premature ventricular contractions, 1 mild congestive heart failure.

TABLE 19–2 (Continued)

Author	Date	Type of Study	Number of Patients Completing Trial	Dosage of Propranolol mg/day	Concomitant Neuroleptic Medication	Results	Adverse Reactions
Yorkston et al.[86]	1976	Open.	55.	160–3,000 (median 1,125).	Phenothiazine or butyrophenone.	28 complete remission of symptoms, 17 with propranolol alone and 11 with propranolol and a phenothiazine.	Ataxia, dysarthria, visual hallucinations, confusional state, congestive heart failure, hypertension, angina.
van Zerssen[82]	1976	Open.	17: 6 manic, 2 porphyria, 3 schizophrenics, 6 schizo-affective.	Up to 3,780. Oxprenolol: 1,480–4,720.	None.	2 organic psychoses —marked improvement; 6 manic, 2 improved 4 did not; 3 schizophrenics—no improvement; 6 schizo-affective psychosis—slight improvement.	Toxic psychoses, epileptic seizures (2 patients), gastrointestinal hemorrhage (latter on other medication as well).
Yorkston et al.[85]	1977	Propranolol vs. placebo.	14 (5 males; 9 females) not improved by major tranquilizers (chlorpromazine average 1,634 mg).	Av. 954.	Phenothiazines, butyrophenone.	"Both groups improved, but the propranolol group improved significantly more." 12-week trial: first change noted at 8 weeks.	No significant toxic effects.
Sheppard[72]	1979	Open.	8 male (Schneider's criteria), "acute;" partial response to antipsychotics.	Up to 2,400.	Phenothiazine, butyrophenone.	7 patients showed significant clinical evidence of psychiatric improvement (3-week trial), but 6/7 deteriorated later in trial.	Drowsiness, ataxia, hypotension.

TABLE 19-2 (*Continued*)

Author	Date	Type of Study	Number of Patients Completing Trial	Dosage of Propranolol mg/day	Concomitant Neuroleptic Medication	Results	Adverse Reactions
Bigelow, Zalcman, and Kleinman[12]	1978	Double-blind crossover, random assignment.	11	1,920.	None.	2/11 improved but not when repeated.	None reported.
Belmaker et al.[10]	1979	Open (to determine biological effect).	10	1,000.	None.	None did as well as on neuroleptics; had some effect on 3 (3 weeks).	None reported.
Elizur et al.[23]	1979	Single-blind.	10 (5 males; 5 females).	Up to 3,000	None.	3/10 marked improvement; 1/10 partial; 6/10 no improvement or deterioration.	Hypertensive encephalopathy.
Lindstrom and Persson[51]	1980	Double-blind, crossover.	12 (10 males; 2 females); incomplete response to antipsychotics.	1,280–1,920.	Fluphenthixol.	6 improved (2 weeks); 3 unchanged; 3 deteriorated.	Hypotension, ataxia.
Hanssen et al.[33]	1980	Open.	6 (2 males; 4 females) Schneiderian criteria: "refractory to phenothiazines."	1,440.	Antipsychotics (not added until after propranolol given 2–4 weeks) and benzodiazepines as needed.	3/6 improved (2–4 weeks).	Bradycardia, hypotension, sleep disturbance.
King et al.[46]	1980	Open, then double-blind.	8 patients, all male, results on 5; Feighner criteria.	1,000.	Trifluoperazine added in one section.	No statistically significant improvement. Some improvement when antipsychotic added (3 weeks).	1/5 seizures (history of seizures prior to study).

TABLE 19-2 *(Continued)*

Author	Date	Type of Study	Number of Patients Completing Trial	Dosage of Propranolol mg/day	Concomitant Neuroleptic Medication	Results	Adverse Reactions
Yorkston et al.[88]	1981	Double-blind, random assignment.	35 Schizophrenia Research Project criteria "acute."	670.	Rare p.r.n.	Propranolol equally effective as chlorpromazine, but neither very effective (3-month trial).	Ataxia, dizziness.
Peet et al.[62]	1981	Double-blind, randomized comparison of propranolol, chlorpromazine, placebo.	53 (19 on propranolol); Feighner criteria; long-term hospitalization.	640.	None.	Neither propranolol nor chlorpromazine different from placebo (3-month trial).	Cardiovascular collapse (1).
Myers et al.[57]	1981	Double-blind, random assignment.	20 (10 on propranolol); "treatment-resistant."	1,920.	Depot antipsychotics throughout.	No difference between propranolol and placebo.	Hallucinations, syncope (1), drowsiness, ataxia.
Karniol and Portela[43]	1982	Double-blind crossover.	8 ICD-9 chronic schizophrenic, hospitalized, symptomatic on neuroleptics.	Oxprenolol to 640.	Various.	Improvement over baseline with oxprenolol only.	"Practically no side effects"; tardive dyskinesia improved.
Pugh, Steinert, and Priest[67]	1983	Double-blind, propranolol versus placebo.	41 patients. Feighner criteria. Florid symptoms on neuroleptics.	Propranolol to 640.	Various.	Modest advantage of propranolol over placebo.	Similar to adverse effects on placebo.

SOURCE: P. E. Hayes and S. C. Schulz, "Review of the Efficacy of Beta-blocking Agents in Psychiatry: Anxiety Disorders and Schizophrenia," *Pharmacotherapy,* 3 (1983): 101–117.

of psychosis.[70] The patient was found dead at home, and autopsy revealed no physical abnormality or evidence of overdose.

Despite such sobering reports, propranolol has been well tolerated by the majority of schizophrenic patients when doses have been raised gradually. It may, however, carry the potential for unpredictable, severe, or even fatal reactions, and empirical trials should be limited to patients who fail to respond to vigorous application of more conventional treatments.

Theoretical Implications

Speculations as to why beta-adrenergic blockers might have antipsychotic activity have been offered by several investigators. Peet, Middlemiss, and Yates[61] demonstrated that adding propranolol to a constant dose of chlorpromazine markedly increased chlorpromazine blood levels. This is not an entirely satisfactory explanation, however, since at least two studies[43,72] note that patients who improved with beta-blockers had previously failed to improve at higher doses of neuroleptics than were given with the beta-blocker. Karniol and Portela[43] also point out that neuroleptic-induced parkinsonian symptoms did not increase in their patients when oxprenolol was added. This observation argues against increased neuroleptic activity. In addition, the assumption that "more is better" in antipsychotic therapy must be questioned.[17] Gruzelier and associates[31] found that propranolol corrected apparent abnormalities in habituation of alerting responses in schizophrenic patients and suggested that this response might be related to an antipsychotic effect.

With respect to the dramatic successes described with propranolol treatment in early trials, another observation is in order. At least some of the initial successes reported were not in schizophrenic patients, but rather in patients with mania or with organic mental syndromes such as acute intermittent porphyria.[3,82] In table 19–2, it is obvious that propranolol's apparent efficacy in schizo-phrenia wanes as diagnostic rigor increases. Included in the studies cited are three case histories of schizophrenic patients who responded well to treatment with propranolol.[33,84] Of the three cases, two are highly suggestive of temporal lobe epilepsy (one patient developed a chronic psychosis following a parietal skull fracture and had an abnormal electroencephalogram (EEG); the other complained of olfactory hallucinations and sudden attacks of agitation, both of which suggest temporal lobe dysfunction). It is possible, then, that propranolol has a specific antipsychotic effect in patients with coarse brain dysfunction, independent of any possible "antischizophrenic" effect. While not used as an anticonvulsant in humans, propranolol has anticonvulsant activity in animals,[84] and so might suppress temporal lobe dysrhythmias. Several recent reports also suggest that patients with brain damage who show violent or aggressive behavior may become calmer and more manageable after treatment with propranolol.[25,89] The mechanism of this action is not known. Another hypothesis concerning the apparent antipsychotic effect of propranolol rests on reports of its marked beneficial effect on the restless agitation (akathisia) routinely associated with neuroleptic treatment.[54] Such an effect might give the appearance of specific antipsychotic action when the two agents were combined.

Schizophrenia, as a heterogeneous clinical syndrome, undoubtedly includes patients with various kinds of brain dysfunction. In patients with rigorously diagnosed chronic schizophrenia, beta-blockers appear to produce modest improvement when given as adjuncts to neuroleptic treatment. This improvement may represent a specific antipsychotic action or may merely reflect a decrease in neuroleptic-induced akathisia. The beta-blockers may, however, also have a selective effect on patients whose "schizophrenic" symptoms are a manifestation of a cerebral dysrhythmia. Early reports of successful treatment of manic patients with beta-blockers also remain to be systematically investigated. The spectrum of efficacy of the beta-blockers in psychosis deserves further definition.

¶ Benzodiazepines in Schizophrenia

Benzodiazepines have been used in the treatment of schizophrenia and other psychotic disorders for several reasons. Many schizophrenic patients suffer from anxiety, and the use of anxiolytics seems clinically reasonable. This is particularly the case when the anxiety appears to be secondary to external stress or deficient coping skills rather than to the underlying psychosis.[69] Curiously, this use of benzodiazepines has not been adequately studied in its own right. However, studies cited in the next section provide enough data to suggest that even an antianxiety effect of benzodiazepines is not established in schizophrenic patients. Benzodiazepines are also used as hypnotics in psychotic patients, but again, efficacy remains to be established.[42] These drugs are given, with variable but often limited efficacy, to relieve the akathisia associated with antipsychotic medications. They also have an accepted place in the management of some hallucinogen-induced psychoses and in the management of acute psychotic agitation in mania.[5] But benzodiazepines also have themselves been used as primary antipsychotic agents and have been given in even heroic doses in hopes of ameliorating symptoms such as disordered thinking and hallucinations.

Review of Studies

The data emerging from studies of benzodiazepines in psychosis are mixed. In 1980 Nestoros[59] summarized the controlled studies then available. He argued that benzodiazepines had been wrongly maligned as ineffective antischizophrenic agents. He pointed to three studies in which a benzodiazepine was superior to placebo in treating psychosis and three others in which a benzodiazepine outperformed an antipsychotic. In the remaining eleven comparisons, however, benzodiazepines were at best as effective as placebo, and sometimes less effective. Nestoros cited doses used and pointed out that many studies in which benzodiazepines were ineffective used relatively low doses (e.g., 30 mg chlordiazepoxide). However, several of the favorable studies used similar doses. To add to the confusion, several of the comparison antipsychotic agents also were given in relatively low doses (e.g., 150 mg chlorpromazine; 2 to 8 mg trifluoperazine). In summary, little can be concluded from these studies.

The few additional studies since Nestoros's review have yielded equally mixed results (see table 19–3). No clear pattern is discernible correlating efficacy with dose or with the concomitant use of antipsychotic medication. Despite the lack of definitive data, however, some interesting points emerge. One is the repeated finding that, in a given group of patients, some prove to be completely unresponsive, while others improve markedly. Several investigators have remarked on this variability, but have been unable to find clinical predictors of response.[9,39] Three authors proposed that schizophrenic and schizoaffective patients may respond differentially,[9,39,48] but their hypotheses as to which diagnostic group will improve with benzodiazepines were mutually contradictory.

Despite the consistent anxiolytic effect of benzodiazepines in patients who are not psychotic, many "nonresponding" psychotic patients in these studies failed even to show decreased anxiety.[53,68] Conversely, schizophrenic patients who did respond to benzodiazepines not only became less anxious, but most also showed a decrease in psychotic symptoms. Hallucinations in particular appeared to be sensitive to benzodiazepines, while delusions and disordered thinking responded less.[9,45,52]

It is as yet unclear whether such antipsychotic effects represent a nonspecific response to decreased anxiety or whether the effect is specific. For example, one study

TABLE 19–3

Clinical Studies of Benzodiazepines in Schizophrenia

Study	Date	N	Patient Description	Study Design	Drug and Dose, mg/day	Concomitant Antipsychotic	Results
Kellner et al.[45]	1975	6	Anxious schizophrenic, selected for good response in open trial.	Double-blind.	Chlordiazepoxide, 300.	Yes.	2 patients improved "substantially," including hallucinations and thought disorder; a third showed moderate improvement; three showed no change.
Ruskin et al.[68]	1979	8	Unselected "chronic schizophrenic."	Open.	Diazepam, 40–80.	Not stated.	No clinical benefit, including measures of anxiety and tension.
Lingjaerde et al.[53]	1979	23	"Chronic schizophrenic or chronic psychotic reaction."	Double-blind.	Diazepam, 15.	Yes.	Small but statistically significant decrease in Brief Psychiatric Rating Scale score on diazepam, including symptoms of thought disorder, but not "anxiety."
Lingjaerde[52]	1982	58	Mostly "chronic schizophrenic" with auditory hallucinations, poorly responsive to antipsychotics.	Double-blind.	Estazolam, 6.	Yes.	Estazolam superior to placebo in reducing auditory and visual hallucinations and compulsive thoughts, also on global rating.
Karson et al.[44]	1982	13	RDC: chronic schizophrenic.	Double-blind.	Clonazepam, ? 1–5.	Yes.	No significant improvement for any symptom; trend toward decreased anxiety. 3 patients demonstrated unaccustomed violent behavior.
Beckmann and Haas[9]	1980	15	RDC: schizophrenic (9) and schizo-affective (6).	Open.	Diazepam, 400 maximum.	No.	All had decreased anxiety. 10 improved, 7 to "complete" remission; hallucinations remitted in all patients. 5 deteriorated and withdrew early: 3 showed loss of sexual and social inhibition. Nonresponders had only moderate response to antipsychotics.
Jimerson et al.[39]	1982	6	RDC: schizophrenic (5) and schizo-affective (1).	Double-blind, crossover.	Diazepam, 300 maximum.	No.	Only 3/6 patients tolerated high dose; others were ataxic, sedated. One (schizo-affective) improved substantially and relapsed when tapered; one other had mild improvement, the third was unchanged.
Nestoros et al.[60]	1982	12	RDC: schizophrenic; DSM-III: paranoid type.	Double-blind.	Diazepam, to 400.	No (p.r.n. only).	Substantial improvement in hours to days on diazepam, not on placebo. One patient developed a parkinsonian syndrome.

found intravenously administered diazepam to reduce acute psychotic symptoms at least as well as similar treatment with haloperidol over the first twenty-four hours of treatment.[50] The authors concluded that haloperidol's primary action during the first hours of treatment was probably sedation rather than a specific antipsychotic action. They acknowledged, however, the possibility that diazepam might have antipsychotic action—an interpretation supported by the dramatic decrease in measures of thought disorder. Conversely, a benzodiazepine-induced reduction in akathisia could give the impression of reducing psychotic agitation.

A recent development has been the treatment of schizophrenic patients with very high doses of diazepam (up to 400 mg/day). Two studies suggest considerable efficacy for this strategy: One open study[9] claimed "complete remission" in seven of fifteen patients, while a controlled study of newly admitted patients[60] showed high doses of diazepam to be more effective than placebo in reducing psychotic symptoms during the first days of treatment. A third study[39] found mixed results.

Adverse Effects

Few serious adverse effects have been reported with the use of benzodiazepines in schizophrenic patients. Sedation and ataxia could be controlled by lowering the dose. However, there are suggestions that even low or moderate doses of some benzodiazepines may "disinhibit" patients sufficiently to increase inappropriate sexual or aggressive activity.[44] This effect may reflect more than nonspecific intoxication and has sometimes been dramatic at high doses.[9,44] Significant withdrawal reactions were not reported in any of the studies cited. Addiction and drug-seeking behavior also were not reported in these studies, but certainly are not unknown to clinicians using benzodiazepines for other disorders.

Summary

Of the six recent double-blind studies cited, all but one have found benzodiazepines to outperform placebo in some, but not all, schizophrenic patients. It is noteworthy that psychotic symptoms as well as anxiety improved in those patients who responded favorably. Given the presumed heterogeneity of psychotic patients, an alternative treatment that consistently and safely benefits even a small proportion of them deserves further investigation. However, clinical use of benzodiazepines as antipsychotic agents requires further critical evaluation of efficacy and safety.

¶ Clonidine in Schizophrenia

Clonidine hydrochloride, currently approved as an antihypertensive agent, stimulates alpha-2 (presynaptic) and, to a lesser extent, alpha-1 (postsynaptic) adrenergic receptors. By stimulating inhibitory presynaptic sites, clonidine decreases norepinephrine release. Because the noradrenergic system may be implicated in psychosis, a few investigators have treated psychotic patients experimentally with clonidine. One presumptive advantage of this drug is that, like propranolol, it should be free of the adverse extrapyramidal neurologic effects associated with dopamine-blocking agents.

Review of Studies

At least six studies describe the treatment of schizophrenic patients with clonidine. Of these, only one was performed double-blind, and it involved only eight patients.[28] Only two studies found clonidine to have an apparent antipsychotic effect; one was the small double-blind study just mentioned. The other is an intriguing but uncontrolled study in which forty-one patients were assigned to either clonidine or the anticonvulsant, sedative benzodiazepine clonazepam on the basis of the response of distal colon motility to the same agents.[48] These treatments appeared to be remarkably successful. The authors note, without documenting the statement, that patients assigned to each treatment deteriorated when given the alternative treatment. If this finding was reproduced in a double-blind study, it would be of considerable interest.

Four other studies of clonidine in schizophrenic patients all report uniformly discouraging results, with two groups noting that patients became more hostile and aggressive when given the drug.[24,38,75,81] Some authors speculated that such deterioration might result from a postsynaptic alpha-adrenergic action of clonidine. Other adverse effects included hypotension, which limited dosage in many patients, and some sedation. Most investigators also noted a high incidence of psychotic exacerbations on withdrawal from the drug, often to a level described as worse than the original illness.

Patients who responded well to clonidine tended to have responded previously to neuroleptic agents. Both of the positive studies specifically chose patients with a history of good response to conventional antipsychotics.[28,48] Most other reports did not mention previous treatment response, but one negative report did note that both patients studied had previously been treated unsuccessfully with neuroleptics.[24] Two other investigators[75,81] appeared to have chosen their subjects from chronically hospitalized patients who presumably did not respond adequately to previous treatment.

Summary

The clinical usefulness of clonidine in psychosis is probably limited, especially in view of its adverse cardiovascular and sedative effects. It may be worth considering in some patients who develop unacceptable side effects on available antipsychotic agents. In this context, it is of interest that in two studies clonidine appeared to diminish the abnormal movements of tardive dyskinesia.*[28,48]

¶ Carbamazepine in Schizophrenia

Carbamazepine, currently used as an anticonvulsant and in the treatment of central pain syndromes, is finding increasing use in the treatment of affective disorders.[7] There are only rare reports on the use of carbamazepine in the treatment of schizophrenia. One is an uncontrolled pilot study of eight violent schizophrenic patients (no criteria were given for diagnosis, but patients were chronically hospitalized in a maximum-security hospital).[32] All eight had nonspecific EEG abnormalities, but none had a clinical diagnosis of epilepsy. After treatment with carbamazepine, "violent behavior disappeared almost completely in all eight patients" and six of the eight could be transferred to a less secure unit or discharged. A second, controlled trial compared carbamazepine and placebo in eleven diverse psychotic patients, all of whom had temporal lobe EEG abnormalities and were unresponsive to conventional antipsychotic agents.[58] Eight carried the diagnosis of "schizophrenia," but criteria were not stated. Carbamazepine was said to be significantly better than placebo, but specific details of improvement were not given.

It is possible that some of these patients were, in fact, suffering from temporal lobe dysfunction. However, all were diagnosed as schizophrenic, despite questionable EEG findings. One may conclude either that carbamazepine may be an effective treatment for "schizophrenic" patients with EEG abnormalities, or that some patients with temporal lobe disorders may be misdiagnosed as schizophrenic.

---

*As yet, the combination of clonidine and a neuroleptic as a treatment for psychosis has not been described in the literature. One could speculate that a combined dopaminergic and adrenergic blockade might be of value in some patients.

¶ General Conclusions

None of the alternative treatments reviewed has outperformed available neuroleptics in treating schizophrenic patients. In that sense, little has been learned that is clinically applicable, and findings have been predominantly negative (e.g., the failure of added antidepressants to better the performance of conventional antipsychotic treatment). For most of the treatments reviewed, the conflicting data make clinical recommendations premature, although further evaluation seems worthwhile.

Nonetheless, such studies may make a useful contribution to the definition of schizophrenic illnesses. Lehmann[49] suggested that "therapeutic responsiveness to particular psychotropic drugs may serve as external criteria for new diagnostic categories." In the past, psychotropic medications have been regarded as primarily symptom-specific rather than disease-specific. But currently, as in the studies reviewed here, patients whose symptoms are clinically similar seem to respond differently to medication. Borrowing a model from internal medicine, two patients with clinical evidence of pneumonia may have similar syndromes but respond to different antibiotic treatments because the bacterial etiology differs. While psychiatry lacks the equivalent of a bacteriology laboratory, it need not ignore clues that may arise out of differential treatment response; patients who respond to different treatments may have different illnesses.

¶ Acknowledgments

The authors are grateful to Drs. Peggy Hayes and Charles Schulz for permission to adapt their table on propranolol and schizophrenia. We also thank Ms. Ellen Poulos for her invaluable help in the preparation of this manuscript. This work was supported in part by NIMH Career Award MH-47370 and Program Award MH-31154.

This review is based in large part on a report requested by the NIMH and appearing in *Schizophrenia Bulletin,* 9 (1983):504–527.

¶ Bibliography

1. ALEXANDER, P. E., VAN KAMMEN, D. P., and BUNNEY W. E. "Antipsychotic Effects of Lithium in Schizophrenia," *American Journal of Psychiatry,* 136: (1979):283–287.

2. ANGST, J. et al. "Lithium Prophylaxis in Recurrent Affective Disorders," *British Journal of Psychiatry,* 116 (1970):604–614.

3. ATSMON, A. "Early Observations of the Effect of Propranolol on Psychotic Patients," *Advances in Clinical Pharmacology,* 12 (1976):86–90.

4. ATSMON, A., et al. "Further Studies with Propranolol in Psychotic Patients," *Psychopharmacology,* 27 (1972):249–254.

5. BALDESSARINI, R. J. "Antipsychotic Agents," in T. B. Karasu, ed., *The Psychiatric Therapies.* Washington D.C.: American Psychiatric Association, 1984, pp. 119–170.

6. ———. "Drugs Used in the Treatment of Psychiatric Disorders," in L. S. Goodman and A. Gilman, ed., *The Pharmacologic Basis of Therapeutics,* 7th ed. New York: Macmillan, forthcoming.

7. BALLENGER, J. C., and POST, R. M. "Carbamazepine in Manic-depressive Illness: A New Treatment," *American Journal of Psychiatry,* 137 (1980):782–790.

8. BECKER, R. E. "Implications of the Efficacy of Thiothixene and a Chlorpromazine-Imipramine Combination for Depression in Schizophrenia," *American Journal of Psychiatry,* 140 (1983):208–211.

9. BECKMANN, H., and HAAS, S. "High-dose Diazepam in Schizophrenia," *Psychopharmacology* (Berlin), 71 (1980):79–82.

10. BELMAKER, R. H., et al. "The Effect of Propranolol Treatment in Schizophrenia on CSF Amine Metabolites and Prolactin," *Psychopharmacology,* 63 (1979):293–296.

11. BIEDERMAN, J., LERNER, Y., and BEL-MAKER, R. H. "Combination of Lithium Carbonate in Schizoaffective Disorder," *Archives of General Psychiatry*, 36 (1979):327–333.

12. BIGELOW, L. G., ZALCMAN, S., and KLEIN-MAN, J. E. "Propranolol Treatment of Chronic Schizophrenia: Clinical Response, Catecholamine Metabolism and Lymphocyte Beta-receptors," *Fourth International Catecholamine Symposium*, 4 (1978):1851–1853.

13. BRADEN, W., et al. "Lithium and Chlorpromazine in Psychotic Inpatients," *Psychiatry Research*, 7 (1982):69–81.

14. BRENNER, R., and SHOPSIN, B. "The Use of MAOI's in Schizophrenia," *Biological Psychiatry*, 15 (1980):633–647.

15. CARMAN J. S., BIGELOW, L. B., and WYATT, R. J. "Lithium Combined with Neuroleptics in Chronic Schizophrenic and Schizo-affective Patients," *Journal of Clinical Psychiatry*, 42 (1981):124–128.

16. CARMAN, J. S., et al. "Divalent cations in Predicting Antidepressant Response to Lithium," *Lancet*, 2 (1974):1454.

17. COLE, J. O. "Antipsychotic Drugs: Is More Better?" *McLean Hospital Journal*, 7 (1982):61–87.

18. COLLINS, A. D., and DUNDAS, J. "A Double-blind Trial of Amitriptyline/Perphenazine, Perphenazine and Placebo in Chronic Withdrawn Inert Schizophrenics," *British Journal of Psychiatry*, 113 (1967):1425–1429.

19. DELVA, N. J., and LETEMENDIA, F.J.J. "Lithium Treatment in Schizophrenia and Schizo-affective Disorders," *British Journal of Psychiatry*, 141 (1982):387–400.

20. *Diagnostic and Statistical Manual of Mental Disorders*, 3rd ed. (DSM-III). Washington, D.C.: American Psychiatric Association, 1980.

21. DONALDSON, S. R., GELENBERG, A. J., and BALDESSARINI, R. J. "The Pharmacologic Treatment of Schizophrenia: A Progress Report," *Schizophrenia Bulletin*, 9 (1983):504–527.

22. EDELSTEIN, P. et al. "Physostigmine and Lithium Response in the Schizophrenias," *American Journal of Psychiatry*, 138 (1981):1078–1081.

23. ELIZUR, A., et al. "Antipsychotic Effect of Propranolol on Chronic Schizophrenics: Study of a Gradual Treatment Regimen," *Psychopharmacology*, 60 (1979):189–194.

24. ELIZUR, A., et al. "Preliminary Trial of Clonidine Treatment in Two Patients Suffering from Chronic Schizophrenia," *Communications in Psychopharmacology*, 4 (1980):507–517.

25. ELLIOTT, F. A. "Propranolol for the Control of Belligerent Behavior Following Acute Brain Damage," *Annals of Neurology*, 1 (1977):489–491.

26. FIEVE, R. R. "Lithium Therapy," in H. Kaplan, A. Freedman, and B. Sadock, eds., *Comprehensive Textbook of Psychiatry*, 3rd ed. Baltimore: Williams & Wilkins, 1980, pp. 2348–2352.

27. FOGELSON, D. L., COHEN B. M., and POPE, H. G. "A Study of DSM-III Schizophreniform Disorder, *American Journal of Psychiatry*, 139 (1982):1281–1285.

28. FREEDMAN, R., et al. "Clonidine Treatment of Schizophrenia: Double-blind Comparison to Placebo and Neuroleptic Drugs, *Acta Psychiatrica Scandinavica*, 65 (1982):35–45.

29. GARDOS, G., et al. "A Dose-response Study of Propranolol in Chronic Schizophrenics," *Current Therapeutic Research*, 15 (1973):314–323.

30. GROWE, G. A., et al. "Lithium in Chronic Schizophrenia," *American Journal of Psychiatry*, 136 (1979):454–455.

31. GRUZELIER, J. H., et al. "Influence of D- or DL-propranolol or Chlorpromazine on Habituation of Phasic Electrodermal Response in Schizophrenia," *Acta Psychiatrica Scandinavica*, 60 (1979):241–248.

32. HAKOLA, H. P. A., and LAULUMAA, V. A. "Carbamazepine in Treatment of Violent Schizophrenics," *Lancet*, 1 (1982):1358.

33. HANSSEN, T., et al. "Propranolol in Schizophrenia," *Archives of General Psychiatry*, 37 (1980):685–690.

34. HAYES, P. E., and SCHULZ, S. C. "The Use of Beta-adrenergic Blocking Agents in Anxiety Disorders and Schizophrenia," *Pharmacotherapy*, 3 (1983):101–117.

35. HIRSCHOWITZ, J., ZEMLAN, F. P., and GARVER, D. L. "Growth Hormone Lev-

els and Lithium Ratios as Predictors of Success of Lithium Therapy in Schizophrenia," *American Journal of Psychiatry,* 139 (1982):646–649.

36. HIRSCHOWITZ, J., et al. "Lithium Response in Good Prognosis Schizophrenia," *American Journal of Psychiatry,* 137 (1980):916–920.

37. JEFFERSON, J. W., and GREIST, J. H. *Primer of Lithium Therapy.* Baltimore: Williams & Wilkins, 1977.

38. JIMERSON, D. C., et al. "Preliminary Trial of the Noradrenergic Agonist Clonidine in Psychiatric Patients," *Biological Psychiatry,* 15 (1980):45–57.

39. JIMERSON, D. C., et al. "Diazepam in Schizophrenia: A Preliminary Double-blind Trial," *American Journal of Psychiatry,* 139 (1982):489–491.

40. JOHNSON, D.A.W. "Studies of Depressive Symptoms in Schizophrenia," *British Journal of Psychiatry,* 139 (1981):89–101.

41. JOHNSON, G. "Differential Response to Lithium Carbonate in Manic-depressive and Schizo-affective Disorder," *Diseases of the Nervous System,* 13 (1970):613–615.

42. JUS, K., et al. "The Utilization of Hypnotics in Chronic Schizophrenics: Some Critical Remarks," *Biological Psychiatry,* 14 (1979):955–960.

43. KARNIOL, I. G., and PORTELA, W. "Oxprenolol in Schizophrenic Patients with Tardive Dyskinesia: A Double-blind, Placebo-controlled, Crossover Study," *Brazilian Journal of Medical and Biological Research,* 15 (1982):389–394.

44. KARSON, C. N., et al. "Clonazepam Treatment of Chronic Schizophrenia: Negative Results in a Double-blind, Placebo-controlled Trial," *American Journal of Psychiatry,* 139 (1982):1627–1628.

45. KELLNER, R., et al. "Anxiety in Schizophrenia. The Responses to Chlordiazepoxide in an Intensive Design Study," *Archives of General Psychiatry,* 32 (1975):1246–1254.

46. KING, D. J., et al. "Some Clinical and Metabolic Aspects of Propranolol in Chronic Schizophrenia," *British Journal of Psychiatry,* 137 (1980):458–468.

47. KIRKPATRICK, B., and BURNETT, G. B. "Observations on Neuroleptic Use in Acutely Psychotic Patients," *Journal of*

Clinical Psychopharmacology, 2 (1982): 205–207.

48. LECHIN, F., and VAN DER DIJS, B. "Clonidine Therapy for Psychosis and Tardive Dyskinesia," (letter to ed.), *American Journal of Psychiatry,* 138 (1981):390.

49. LEHMANN, H. E. "The Impact of the Therapeutic Revolution on Nosology," in R. Carcro, ed., *The Schizophrenic Syndrome.* New York: Brunner/Mazel, 1971, pp. 136–153.

50. LERNER, Y., et al. "Acute High-dose Parenteral Haloperidol Treatment of Psychosis," *American Journal of Psychiatry,* 136 (1979):1061–1064.

51. LINDSTROM, L. H., and PERSSON, E. "Propranolol in Chronic Schizophrenia: A Controlled Study in Neuroleptic-treated Patients," *British Journal of Psychiatry,* 137 (1980):126–130.

52. LINGJAERDE, O. "Effect of the Benzodiazepine Derivative Estazolam in Patients with Auditory Hallucinations," *Acta Psychiatrica Scandinavica,* 65 (1982):339–354.

53. LINGJAERDE, O., et al. "Antipsychotic Effect of Diazepam When Given in Addition to Neuroleptics in Chronic Psychotic Patients: A Double-blind Clinical Trial," *Current Therapeutic Research,* 26 (1979):505–514.

54. LIPINSKI, J. F., et al. "Propranolol in the Treatment of Neuroleptic-induced Akathisia," *American Journal of Psychiatry,* 141 (1984):412–414.

55. LOGA, S., CURRY, S., and LADER, M. "Interaction of Chlorpromazine and Nortriptyline in Patients with Schizophrenia," *Clinical Pharmacokinetics,* 6 (1981):454.

56. MCCABE, M. S., et al. "Familial Differences in Schizophrenia with Good and Poor Prognosis," *Psychological Medicine,* 1 (1971):326–332.

57. MYERS, D. H., et al., "A Trial of Propranolol in Chronic Schizophrenia," *British Journal of Psychiatry,* 139 (1981):118–121.

58. NEPPE, V. M. "Carbamazepine in the Psychiatric Patient," *Lancet,* 2 (1982):334.

59. NESTOROS, J. N. "Benzodiazepines in Schizophrenia: A Need for Reassessment," *International Pharmacopsychiatry,* 15 (1980):171–179.

60. NESTOROS, J. N., et al. "Diazepam in High Doses Is Effective in Schizophrenia," *Progress in Neuropsychopharmacology and Biological Psychiatry*, 6 (1982):513–515.

61. PEET, M., MIDDLEMISS, D. N., and YATES, R. A. "Propranolol in Schizophrenia. II: Clinical and Biochemical Aspects of Combining Propranolol with Chlorpromazine," *British Journal of Psychiatry*, 139 (1981):112–117.

62. PEET, M., et al. "Propranolol in Schizophrenia. I: Comparison of Propranolol, Chlorpromazine and Placebo," *British Journal of Psychiatry*, 139 (1981):105–111.

63. POPE, H. C., and LIPINSKI, J. F. "Diagnosis in Schizophrenia and Manic Depressive Illness," *Archives of General Psychiatry*, 35 (1978):811–828.

64. PRAKASH, R., KELWALA, S., and BAN, T. A. "Neurotoxicity in Patients with Schizophrenia During Lithium Therapy," *Comprehensive Psychiatry*, 23 (1982):271–273.

65. PRIEN, R. F., CAFFEY, E. M., and KLETT, C. J. "A Comparison of Lithium Carbonate and Chlorpromazine in the Treatment of Excited Schizo-affectives," *Archives of General Psychiatry*, 27 (1972):182–189.

66. PRUSOFF, B. A., et al. "Treatment of Secondary Depression in Schizophrenia," *Archives of General Psychiatry*, 36 (1979):569–575.

67. PUGH, C. R., STEINERT, J., and PRIEST, R. G. "Propranolol in Schizophrenia: A Double-blind, Placebo-controlled Trial of Propranolol as an Adjunct to Neuroleptic Medication," *British Journal of Psychiatry*, 143 (1983):151–155.

68. RUSKIN, P., et al. "Benzodiazepines in Chronic Schizophrenia," *Biological Psychiatry*, 14 (1979):557–558.

69. SCHATZBERG, A. F., and COLE, J. O. "Benzodiazepines in the Treatment of Depressive Borderline Personality, and Schizophrenic Disorders," *British Journal of Clinical Pharmacology*, 11 (Supplement) (1981):17–22.

70. SCHULZ, S. C. Medical College of Virginia. Personal communication to Alan J. Gelenberg, M.D., 1982.

71. SETHI, B. B., and DUBE, S. "Propranolol in Schizophrenia," *Progress in Neuropsychopharmacology and Biological Psychiatry*, 7 (1983):89–99.

72. SHEPPARD, G. P. "High-dose Propranolol in Schizophrenia," *British Journal of Psychiatry*, 134 (1979):470–476.

73. SHOPSIN, G., JOHNSON, G., and GERSHON, S. "Neurotoxicity with Lithium: Differential Drug Responsiveness," *International Pharmacopsychiatry*, 5 (1970):170–182.

74. SHOPSIN, B., KIMN, S. S., and GERSHON, S. "A Controlled Study of Lithium vs. Chlorpromazine in Acute Schizophrenics," *British Journal of Psychiatry*, 199 (1971):435–440.

75. SIMPSON, G. M., KUNZ-BARTHOLINI, E., and WATTS, T.P.S. "A Preliminary Evaluation of the Sedative Effects of Catapres, a New Antihypertensive Agent, in Chronic Schizophrenic Patients," *Journal of Clinical Psychopharmacology*, 7 (1967):221–225.

76. SINGH A. N., SAXENA B., and NELSON, H. L. "A Controlled Clinical Study of Trazodone in Chronic Schizophrenic Patients with Pronounced Depressive Symptomatology," *Current Therapeutic Research*, 23 (1978):485–501.

77. SIRIS, S. G., RIFKIN, A. E., and REARDON, G. T. "Response of Postpsychotic Depression to Adjunctive Imipramine or Amitriptyline," *Psychopharmacology*, 43 (1982):485–486.

78. SIRIS, S. G., VAN KAMMEN, D. P., and DOCHERTY, J. P. "Use of Antidepressant Drugs in Schizophrenia," *Archives of General Psychiatry*, 35 (1978):1368–1377.

79. SMALL, J. G., et al. "A Placebo-controlled Study of Lithium Combined with Neuroleptics in Chronic Schizophrenic Patients," *American Journal of Psychiatry*, 132 (1975):1315–1317.

80. SPITZER, R. L., ENDICOTT J., and ROBINS, E. "Clinical Criteria for Psychiatric Diagnosis and DSM-III," *American Journal of Psychiatry*, 132 (1975):1187–1192.

81. SUGERMAN, A. A. "A Pilot Study of ST-155 (Catapres) in Chronic Schizophrenics," *Journal of Clinical Psychopharmacology*, 7 (1967):226–230.

82. VAN ZERSSEN, D. "Beta-adrenergic Block-

ing Agents in the Treatment of Psychoses," *Advances in Clinical Pharmacology,* 12 (1976):105–114.

83. YEOH, P. N., and WOLF, H. H. "The Effects of Some Adrenergic Agents in Low-frequency Electroshock Seizures," *Journal of Pharmaceutical Sciences,* 57 (1968):340–342.

84. YORKSTON, N. J., et al. "Propranolol in the Control of Schizophrenic Symptoms," *British Medical Journal,* 4 (1974):633–635.

85. YORKSTON, N. J., et al. "Propranolol as an Adjunct to the Treatment of Schizophrenia," *Lancet,* 2 (1977):575–578.

86. YORKSTON, N. J., et al. "Propranolol to Control Schizophrenic Symptoms: 55 Patients," *Advances in Clinical Pharmacology,* 12 (1976):91–104.

87. YORKSTON, N. J., et al. "Safeguards in the Treatment of Schizophrenia with Propranolol," *Postgraduate Medical Journal,* 52 (1976):175–180.

88. YORKSTON, N. J., et al. "DL-propranolol and Chlorpromazine Following Admission for Schizophrenia: A Controlled Comparison," *Acta Psychiatrica Scandinavica,* 63 (1981):13–27.

89. YUDOFSKY, S., WILLIAMS, D., and GORMAN, J. "Propranolol in the Treatment of Rage and Violent Behavior in Patients with Chronic Brain Syndrome," *American Journal of Psychiatry,* 138 (1981):218–220.

CHAPTER 20

THE BIOLOGY AND EXPERIMENTAL TREATMENT OF TARDIVE DYSKINESIA AND OTHER RELATED MOVEMENT DISORDERS

Dilip V. Jeste, Andrei C. Iager,
and Richard Jed Wyatt

¶ Introduction

History

Although neuroleptics* were introduced into psychiatry in 1952, the first
reports of neuroleptic-induced,
delayed-onset, persistent involuntary movement disorder appeared only in 1957, when
Schönecker [306] in Germany described orofacial dyskinesia following treatment with

*Neuroleptic (neuro—Old Greek, nerve; lepsis—Old
Greek, seizing): Substance that acts on the nervous system. (From *Stedman's Medical Dictionary*, 1980).

chlorpromazine. Sigwald and associates [315] in
France confirmed this finding, describing in
detail "facio-bucco-lingual-masticatory dyskinesia," which developed in four elderly
women after three to eight months of neuroleptic treatment and persisted for six to
twenty-seven months, despite discontinuation of the drug. They further subdivided
phenothiazine-induced dyskinesias into
three groups: acute, which had early onset
after beginning piperazine phenothiazines
and disappeared quickly; subacute, which
had a slower onset, were unrelated to the
type of neuroleptic treatment used, and remitted one to two weeks after the discon-

tinuation of the drug; and chronic, which persisted long after stopping the drug and were resistant to treatment.

Walter Kruse[234] was the first American to report persistent movement disorder after neuroleptic treatment. He noted muscular restlessness after phenothiazine treatment in three women, in whom the involuntary movements persisted long after neuroleptic withdrawal. While the lower extremities were most affected in these patients, there were involuntary movements of the lips and tongue in one patient and in the arms in another.

Uhrbrand and Faurbye[353] from Denmark published the first epidemiological study of twenty-nine patients with bucco-linguo-masticatory dyskinesias. Eleven of the seventeen patients in whom neuroleptics were discontinued had dyskinesias that persisted over four to twenty-two months. Uhrbrand and Faurbye[353] observed "the unmasking effect" of neuroleptic discontinuation in patients in whom dyskinesias increased or even appeared for the first time after withdrawal of neuroleptics. Faurbye and coworkers adopted the term tardive dyskinesia in their follow-up review article published in 1964.[143] They noted that tardive dyskinesia was seldom noticeable in the first six months of neuroleptic treatment but usually occurred after years of exposure to the drug. Further, they contended that the incidence of tardive dyskinesia was far greater than that of spontaneous orofacial dyskinesia occurring in nonmedicated patients.

With greater awareness of the syndrome, an increasing number of epidemiological, clinical, biochemical, neuropathological, and pharmacological studies of tardive dyskinesia have appeared in the last decade. In this chapter we will review some of these studies, focusing on the biological basis and possible treatment of this iatrogenic disorder.

Definition, Phenomenology, and Diagnosis

Tardive dyskinesia (TD) is a drug-induced syndrome characterized by abnormal, stereotyped involuntary movements, generally of choreoathetoid type and principally affecting the mouth, face, limbs, and trunk, which usually appear after at least three months of the drug treatment. This syndrome is reversible in slightly more than one-third of the patients treated with neuroleptics and virtually fully reversible in patients with dyskinesia due to nonneuroleptic drugs. The dyskinesia should be present for at least a month before a diagnosis of TD is made. One or more of the following three areas are affected in most cases: tongue, jaw, and extremities (see tables 20–1 and 20–2).

On examining a patient, certain guidelines may prove to be helpful in establishing the diagnosis of TD. The inspection of the tongue in the oral cavity may reveal fine vermicular contractions of intrinsic muscles of the tongue. Gross movements of the extrinsic muscles of the tongue inside the oral cavity producing the so-called bonbon sign may be present. Involuntary repetitive tongue protrusion outside the oral cavity resembling the "fly-catcher's tongue" may also occur.

Repetitive clenching of teeth, opening and closing of the mouth, or chewing movements may be observed in the jaw. Lower lip pouting, lip smacking, puckering, licking, and sucking are frequently seen. Other facial muscles may be involved: twitching or spasmodic contractions of orbicularis oculi, eyebrow lifting, retractions of the angle of the mouth, grimacing, puffing of cheeks, or frowning. Muscles of pharynx and larynx may also be involved: Grunting or similar sounds can sometimes be heard, and palatal dyskinesia can be observed.

Other manifestations can occur in the limbs: choreiform movements of the arm and forearm; athetoid movements of the forearm, hand, and fingers; and choreoathetoid movements or ballistic movements of arms may occur in varying degrees of intensity. In the lower limbs, spreading, retroflexion, or athetoid movements of the toes, stamping movements, inversion and eversion of the foot, shifting weight, and, rarely, ballistic movements may occur. Isolated involvement of the trunk and/or axial girdle is rare in TD.

TABLE 20–1
Topography of Tardive Dyskinesia

Authors	Date	N	Percentage of Patients with Dyskinesias			Comments
			Orofacial	Limb	Trunk	
Hunter, Earl, and Thornicroff[180]	1964	13	100	100	?	Elderly patients
Paulson[280]	1968	33	75.8	57.6	18.2	Elderly patients
Jones and Hunter[205]	1969	33	75.8	51.5	?	Patients over 40 years
Yagi[374]	1970	7	85.7	42.9	0	
Itoh et al.[183]	1971	10	60	70	30	
McAndrew, Case, and Treffert[247]	1972	10	60	100	?	Children, 4–16 years
Kinoshita, Inose, and Sakai[221]	1972	56	100	7.1	0	
Karasuyama, Fujii, and Takahashi[212]	1972	32	100	34.4	3.1	
Polizos et al.[289]	1973	34	2.9	100	100	Children (6–12 years) with withdrawal dyskinesia
Ogita, Yagi, and Itoh[274]	1975	24	100	29.2	25	French hospital
		22	100	31.8	27.5	Japanese hospital
Jeste and Wyatt[190]	1982	54	94.4	48.1	14.8	Patients over 50 years
		24	79.4	83.3	20.8	Patients under 50 years
Total		352	80.7	50.6	23.3	

TABLE 20–2
Prevalence of Tardive Dyskinesia in Orofacial Region and Limbs

Authors	Date	N	Tongue	Jaw	Lips	Face	Upper Extremities	Lower Extremities
Faurbye et al.[143]	1964	75	37.3	42.7	44	?	50.7	
Paulson[280]	1968	33[a]	33.3	66.7	–	?	48.5	21.2
Ogita, Yagi, and Itoh[274]	1975	46	95.7	100	–	?	4.3	26.1
Smith and Kiloh[329]	1979	88	47.7	18.2	26.1	4.5	27.3	28.4
Jeste and Wyatt[190, a]	1982	54[a]	66.7	64.8	71.4	29.6[b]	42.6	14.8
Jeste and Wyatt[190, c]	1982	24[c]	75	58.3	20.8	37.5[b]	79.2	37.5
Total		320	55.9	46.1	17.5	34.3	34.3	24.9

[a]Only patients over the age of 50.
[b]Usually of mild intensity.
[c]Only patients under the age of 50.

Variable portions of the trunk may rarely be involved in rocking, oscillatory, or twisting movements; respiratory irregularities and /or speech abnormalities; retching and vomiting. The neck muscles may produce nodding or rotatory movements and painless, repetitive torticollislike movements. The shoulder girdle muscles may engage in raising or shrugging of shoulders. The pelvic girdle muscles may also produce tortipelvislike movements. In addition, twisting or undulating movements may be seen upon lying down, standing, or walking.

The manifestations are generally bilateral; however, they may be unilateral or bilateral but asymmetrical in intensity. They are aggravated by emotional arousal and reduced by relaxation. They may be temporarily controlled by volitional effort, and they are absent during sleep. Tremors, acute dystonias, myoclonus, mannerisms, and compulsions are not a part of TD, even if they coexist. Increasing the neuroleptic dose often reduces the intensity of dyskinesia, while decreasing or withdrawing the neuroleptic tends to worsen or "unmask" the dyskinesia.

TABLE 20-3
Increasing Prevalence of Tardive Dyskinesia Among Chronically Ill
Psychiatric Inpatients Treated with Neuroleptics

Period	1960–1965	1966–1970	1971–1975	1976–1980
Number of studies	3	16	6	12
Number of patients	821	6800	2211	3048
Prevalence of TD (%)	5.5	14.6	20.2	25.6

Epidemiology and Etiology

According to Smith and Kane,[327] the prevalence of TD in studies where an involuntary movement rating scale was used was 24.4 percent compared with 13.9 percent in those in which a scale was not employed. Most recent studies have used the Abnormal Involuntary Movement Scale (AIMS) developed by the Psychopharmacology Research Branch of the National Institute of Mental Health. We use a global AIMS cut-off level of at least 2 (on a 0-to-4 scale) as one of the research criteria for TD.

Differences in methods and in the patient populations studied are largely responsible for differences in the findings of various epidemiologic surveys of spontaneous dyskinesia and TD. Eleven of the fourteen epidemiological studies we reviewed found the prevalence of TD significantly higher in neuroleptic-treated than in nonneuroleptic-treated patients. The three studies that did not find a significant difference were those of Demars,[114] Brandon, McClelland, and Protheroe,[32] and Owens, Johnstone, and Frith.[277] Demars's study did not match the two groups for age. The study by Brandon, McClelland, and Protheroe failed to match the severity of dyskinesia between the two groups and included patients with other neurological conditions known to produce "spontaneous dyskinesia," such as Huntington's chorea. The study of Owens, Johnstone, and Frith, besides failing to match the two groups for age, used highly selected samples of patients with severe institutionalized schizophrenia, in whom superimposed senile chorea and/or dementia could be responsible for clouding the results. Also, neurolep-tic-treated patients may differ from non-neuroleptic-treated patients on many variables (i.e., anxiety), which may at least in part influence the presence and/or severity of movement disorders.

Jeste and Wyatt[190] reviewed thirty-seven studies published between 1960 and 1980 that met certain selection criteria. After reanalyzing the data and excluding false positive cases of TD from a total of 12,930 patients, they found a mean prevalence of 17.6 percent. A careful look at these reports arranged in a chronological order shows that the reported prevalence of TD has risen progressively over the past two decades (see table 20–3 and figure 20–1), which may be at least partly explained by an increasing number of patients with a history of long-term neuroleptic treatment.

Risk Factors

Age

Based on the data available, we found the overall weighted mean prevalence of dyskinesia in patients over forty to be nearly three times that in younger patients (see table 20–4). Smith and Baldessarini[326] reported a strong correlation between age and severity of TD and a strong inverse correlation between age and rates of spontaneous remissions of TD.

TD occurs in 8 to 20 percent of children and adolescents treated with neuroleptics, although persistent dyskinesia is probably less common in these age groups as compared with adults.[190] The movement disorder in children predominantly involves

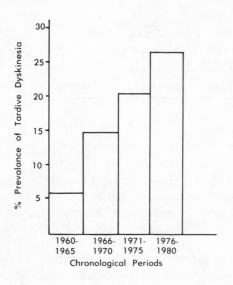

Figure 20–1. Weighted mean percentage prevalence of tardive dyskinesia among chronically ill psychiatric inpatients on neuroleptic treatment drawn from 37 studies published from 1960 through 1980.

the limbs, in contrast to the mainly orofacial involvement in adults.

GENDER

Of the twenty studies that gave prevalence by gender,[190] thirteen reported a higher prevalence in women, five found no difference, and two noted a higher prevalence in men. Combining data from all twenty studies, the overall weighted mean prevalence in women was 41 percent higher than that in men. There are, however, few studies reporting prevalence of dyskinesia in different age groups by gender. Smith and coworkers[328] noted a linear increase in the prevalence of dyskinesia with age in women, whereas Baldessarini and Tarsy[16] noted a decrease of prevalence after the age of seventy in men.

LENGTH OF DRUG EXPOSURE

Kane and Smith[210] reviewed eighteen studies exploring the relationship between cumulative neuroleptic use and prevalence of TD. Only four studies found a significant positive correlation. Of the twenty-one studies exploring length of drug exposure as a risk variable, only six found a positive relationship.

TYPE OF NEUROLEPTIC USED

All orally administered neuroleptics, when given in equivalent amounts and for a comparable length of time, probably have a similar propensity to produce TD—although data to prove this point are difficult to obtain, since few patients are treated with a single neuroleptic at a given dose over a period of years. Several recent studies seem to indicate that the use of depot fluphenazine or flupen-

TABLE 20–4

Distribution of Prevalence of Tardive Dyskinesia Among Chronic Psychiatric Inpatients, by Age

Authors	Date	N	Age Below 40 % with TD	N	Age Above 40 % with TD
Degkwitz and Wenzel[113]	1967	255	5.5	512	22.7
Crane and Paulson[85]	1967	46	4.3	136	16.2
Crane[76]	1968	116	20.7	263	30.8
Crane[77]	1970	49	24.5	78	28.2
Brandon, McClelland, and Protheroe[32]	1971	106	1.9[a]	806	26.2[a]
Fann, Davis, and Janowsky[137]	1972	29	17.2	175	38.9
Ogita, Yagi, and Itoh[274]	1975	44	0	87	27.6
		39	2.6	84	25
Perenyi and Arato[285]	1980	71	16.9	129	27.1
Jeste and Wyatt[190]	1982	28	14.3	67	38.8
Total		783	9.7	2337	26.8

[a]Total prevalence for TD and spontaneous dyskinesia.

thixol may be associated with an increase in prevalence of TD, although further studies are necessary. No controlled data suggest an association between neuroleptic polypharmacy and an increased risk for TD.

INTERRUPTIONS OF NEUROLEPTIC TREATMENT

The contribution of interruptions of medication to the prevention of TD is uncertain. Lengthy drug-free intervals may be associated with an apparent increase in the prevalence of TD.[29,112,195,376] One of the reasons for the relatively high prevalence of TD reported among affective disorder patients may be the intermittent use of neuroleptics in their treatment.[316] A note of caution in interpreting these results is due as a result of the intrinsic relationship between the number of drug-free intervals and the time elapsed since the first neuroleptic intake.

OTHER FACTORS

Although the published data show that anticholinergic drugs often aggravate preexisting dyskinesia,[220,224] there is no convincing evidence for the assertion that these drugs induce TD. Lengthy institutionalization, primary psychiatric illness (with the possible exception of affective disorders), and physical treatments such as electroconvulsive therapy, leukotomy, or insulin coma treatments do not alter significantly the prevalence of TD. Nonneuroleptic-induced dyskinesias will be discussed later.

Complications

There has been an increasing awareness of the deleterious effects of TD. Reports of physical complications and psychosocial sequelae affecting patients of all ages treated with neuroleptics have led to additions to the adverse reactions section of the package insert of all neuroleptic drugs.

Physical complications range from severe respiratory disturbances, characterized by irregularities in respiratory rate, depth, and rhythm accompanied by involuntary grunt-ing, snorting, and gasping noises; or severe gastrointestinal dyskinesia with persistent vomiting, aerophagia, retching, and paroxysmal contraction and distention of the abdominal wall; to less severe but more frequent and still disturbing swallowing disorders, hyperkinetic dysarthria, loosening of teeth, and traumatic ulcerations of the oral mucosa, which may become infected.

Psychosocial sequelae may range from embarrassment, anxiety, guilt, shame, and anger, to severe, full-blown reactive depression, decompensation of psychosis, and even suicide. Dyskinesia can result in a social and /or occupational handicap and stigmatization.

¶ Biology of Tardive Dyskinesia

Animal Models

An ideal animal model of an iatrogenic dyskinesia such as TD should reproduce a TD syndrome similar to that seen in humans. This would allow in-depth, longitudinal or cross-sectional studies and ongoing experimental procedures or neuropathological studies of brain tissue after controlled administration of a drug over varying lengths of time. Susceptibility of the animal model to the same risk factors as in humans is also important. Table 20–5 suggests a list of criteria against which animal models of TD may be evaluated.

Two major experimental models of TD have been used: neuroleptic-induced striatal postsynaptic dopamine (DA) receptor supersensitivity[226] and dyskinesias in primates following prolonged neuroleptic use.[172,281] The neuroleptic-induced striatal postsynaptic DA receptor supersensitivity model has been studied mainly in rodents. We believe that the neuroleptic-withdrawal-emergent-dyskinesia may be best explained with the help of this model. Dopaminergic supersensitivity may be a common response to chronic neuroleptic treatment[303] and hence is far from an ideal model. However, it is one

TABLE 20–5
Criteria for Evaluation of the Two Principal
Animal Models of Tardive Dyskinesia

| | Animal Model[a] | |
| | Postsynaptic Dopamine Receptor Supersensitivity | Dyskinesias in Monkeys |
Criterion		
Caused only by chronic, but not acute, neuroleptic administration	−	+
Higher incidence of greater effects in older animals	±	Not tested
Spontaneous appearance during or following neuroleptic administration	+	+
Persistence long after neuroleptic withdrawal	−	+
Suppression by acute neuroleptic administration	+	+
Nonresponse to, or aggravation by, anticholinergic administration	±	+

[a]+ indicates presence and − indicates absence of that requirement in the animal; ± indicates uncertain status.

model that can be pursued in lesser mammals. Although the primate dyskinesia model is more expensive, the chronic neuroleptic-induced dyskinesia in monkeys is a more satisfactory model of TD.

Biochemical Hypotheses

Neuroleptics are believed to exert their principal clinical effects by acting on the central neurotransmitter systems, especially the catecholaminergic ones. The most explored biochemical model of TD is that of postsynaptic DA receptor supersensitivity in the nigrostriatal system. According to some researchers, cholinergic and GABA (gamma-aminobutyric acid)-ergic mechanisms may also play an important role. We will briefly review the main biochemical theories of the pathogenesis of TD.

DOPAMINERGIC OVERACTIVITY

Indirect evidence of dopaminergic overactivity in TD is presented in table 20–6. There is as yet no consistent, direct clinical evidence to support this hypothesis. Dopaminergic overactivity can conceivably occur at postsynaptic or presynaptic levels.

Postsynaptic DA receptor supersensitivity represents a decrease in the threshold of postsynaptic receptors toward DA agonists or an increase in the number of these receptors. Thus smaller quantities of DA agonists are required to elicit a biological response and/or a stronger response is elicited using the standard amounts of agonists. Most neuroleptics are believed to block the effect of DA on postsynaptic receptors, thereby

TABLE 20–6
Indirect Evidence for Dopaminergic
Overactivity in Tardive Dyskinesia

Agents	DA Agonists	DA Antagonists
Administration:	Aggravate TD.	Temporarily suppress TD.
	Reduce parkinsonian symptoms.	Produce parkinsonian-like symptoms.
	Aggravate dyskinesias induced by levodopa in Parkinson's patients, as well as the abnormal movements in Huntington's and Tourette's patients.	Reduce dyskinesias in Huntington's chorea and Tourette's syndrome.
Withdrawal:	Improvement in dyskinesias in Parkinson's patients.	Initial worsening or unmasking TD.

NOTE: There are some clinical exceptions to the general statements in this table.

producing a functional denervation of those receptors. Ungerstedt[355] first demonstrated central catecholaminergic denervation supersensitivity by producing destruction of nigrostriatal dopaminergic neurons with 6-hydroxydopamine, and then showing heightened response to DA agonists. His work was confirmed by other investigators who also found a high positive correlation between supersensitivity and DA binding sites. According to Langer,[241] the relatively gradual evolution of supersensitivity to apomorphine, presumed to be a specific postsynaptic DA receptor agonist with little presynaptic stimulant action, suggests that such supersensitivity is postsynaptic. Chronic neuroleptic treatment results in supersensitivity to DA agonists in rodents;[303] sacrificed animals from this study exhibited an increase in the number of striatal DA receptors labeled with ^{3}H-spiperone, which confirms previous studies.[331] Rupniak, Jenner, and Marsden[303] demonstrated that withdrawal after chronic neuroleptic treatment in rodents was followed by persistent but not permanent supersensitivity to apomorphine. Over a one-year period, the gradual normalization of response to apomorphine was paralleled by a return of striatal DA receptor density to control values.

In human postmortem studies, evidence of increased D-2 DA binding was found in neuroleptic-treated schizophrenic patients, but not in untreated patients.[92,310] Although there is strong experimental evidence supporting postsynaptic DA receptor supersensitivity following chronic neuroleptic treatment, there is insufficient clinical evidence to prove that TD is a consequence of this phenomenon. Crow and associates[92] did not find significant differences in binding affinities and densities in brains obtained from neuroleptic-treated schizophrenic patients with or without a history of TD.

Crane[78] suggested that TD was more likely to develop in patients with neuroleptic-induced parkinsonism. Demars[114] noted that the two syndromes rarely occurred together, and Chouinard, De Montigny, and Annable[62] observed an inverse correlation

between the two. In contrast, five studies reviewed by Jeste and Wyatt[190] found no correlation, and Heinrich, Wagener, and Bender[176] and Wolf and coworkers[372] reported that pharmacogenic parkinsonism occurred frequently in patients with TD. Furthermore, TD does not always worsen following DA agonists such as bromocriptine[203,288,297] or apomorphine administration,[45,203,258,350] as one might expect to find in the case of postsynaptic receptor supersensitivity.

It is assumed that when DA is released into the synaptic cleft it binds to specific postsynaptic receptors, leading to a release (D-1 receptors) or inhibition (D-2 receptors) of cyclic3',5'-adenosine monophosphate (cAMP).[339] Also, DA is metabolized to homovanillic acid (HVA). Both cAMP and HVA are removed relatively quickly from the brain via interstitial pathways, first into the cerebrospinal fluid (CSF) and then into the bloodstream. Studies of CSF from TD patients analyzing cAMP and HVA levels do not seem to support consistently the supersensitivity hypothesis (see table 20–7). It is possible that only a proportion of dyskinetic patients with low CSF-HVA may have postsynaptic supersensitivity, although no consistent pattern is found in the literature. Kirch and associates,[222] for example, found a significant positive correlation between the level of plasma HVA and the severity of TD.

Finally, the receptor supersensitivity hypothesis cannot explain the increasing prevalence of TD with age. Makman and coworkers[251] demonstrated that functional DA receptors decrease in number in older animals, and Weiss, Greenberg, and Cantor[368] found a reduction in the capacity of aged tissues to increase the number of functional receptors in response to a lowering of neurotransmitter input.

Presynaptic overactivity usually indicates a breakdown in a self-inhibitory feedback system that is normally activated when the concentration of a neurotransmitter in the synapse exceeds a certain threshold. Increased synthesis or reduced reuptake of

TABLE 20–7
Studies of Monoamine Metabolites in Cerebrospinal Fluid

Authors	Date	N	Findings
Pind and Faurbye[287]	1970	8	HVA and 5-HIAA levels increased after probenecid similar to the controls. High levels in both groups? Controls were obtained from literature.[275]
Chase, Schnur, and Gordon[58]	1970	6	HVA and 5-HIAA levels lower in dyskinetic patients and in patients with drug-induced parkinsonism. Controls were 5 schizophrenic patients treated with neuroleptics.
Chase[56]	1973	8	HVA levels after probenecid lower than normal controls. Response to haloperidol also low in 6 dyskinetic patients. Lowest values in parkinsonian patients. Controls were patients with various neurological diseases.
Curzon[95]	1973		HVA and 5-HIAA similar to controls.
Gerlach, Thorsen, and Munkvad[161]	1975	7	Haloperidol reduced dyskinesia, increased HVA. Clozapine did not affect dyskinesia but reduced HVA and 5-HIAA. No controls.
Roccatagliata, Albano, and Besio[298]	1977	4	Trazadone reduced dyskinesia, increased HVA, reduced 5-HIAA. No controls.
Winsberg, Hurwic, and Perel[371]	1977	3 (children with withdrawal-emergent dyskinesia)	Lower HVA and 5-HIAA levels after probenecid in dyskinetic children; cAMP not different from controls (3 children without withdrawal-emergent dyskinesia).
Bowers, Moore, and Tarsy[28]	1979	11	HVA similar to controls; cAMP significantly lower compared to schizophrenic controls, but similar to depressed patients. Controls were 26 schizophrenic and 19 depressed patients.
Nagao et al.[266]	1979	12	HVA, MHPG, 5-HIAA, cAMP, and cGMP similar to controls. Sodium valproate or cyproheptadine reduced dyskinesia, reduced HVA, and increased cAMP and cGMP. Patients with drug-induced tremor (parkinsonism) had lowest HVA and 5-HIAA levels. Controls were 15 chronic schizophrenic patients (nondyskinetic).
Jeste, Doongaji, and Linnoila[191]	1984	13	NE levels significantly greater in TD patients. Controls were 15 schizophrenic patients (nondyskinetic).

NOTE: 5-HIAA = 5-hydroxyindoleacetic acid. MHPG = 3-methoxy-4-hydroxy-phenyl glycol; cGMP = cyclic guanosine monophosphate; NE = norepinephrine.

DA; reduced monoamine oxidase (MAO) activity and, thus, reduced presynaptic metabolism of DA; or subsensitivity of presynaptic inhibitory autoreceptors for DA can result in presynaptic overactivity.

Carlsson and Lindquist[43] first demonstrated an increase in DA turnover following neuroleptic administration in animals. Although this increase was found to be a short-lasting effect during the course of long-term

neuroleptic administration,[305] it could conceivably persist in some patients at risk for developing TD.

The high CSF-HVA levels and low CSF-cAMP concentrations reported in some patients with TD and the positive correlation of plasma HVA with the severity of dyskinesia[222] support the likelihood of presynaptic dopaminergic overactivity. Aggravation of TD by amphetamines and levodopa, which are believed to act presynaptically, may also support a presynaptic involvement.

NORADRENERGIC OVERACTIVITY

Hornykiewicz[178] suggested that norepinephrine (NE) sets up the sensitivity of those neural systems on which DA acts and thus controls locomotor activity. Most of the arguments supporting the hypothesis of dopaminergic overactivity in TD can also be applied to advancing a hypothesis of noradrenergic overactivity in some patients with this syndrome. Thus amphetamines and levodopa are also NE stimulants. Conversely, neuroleptics block noradrenergic receptors as well as DA receptors.

Jeste and collaborators, in a series of studies reviewed in 1982,[190] found that a proportion of patients with TD presented with low platelet and lymphocyte MAO activities, high plasma dopamine beta-hydroxylase (DBH) activity, and high plasma renin activity, indicating increased catecholaminergic activity at least in the periphery. Reports of encouraging results in the treatment of TD using noradrenergic antagonists such as fusaric acid;[363] the beta-blocker, propranolol hydrochloride[14,263]; and the presynaptic noradrenergic inhibitor, clonidine hydrochloride,[149] are consistent with this hypothesis. Among the thioridazine metabolites, sulforidazine has been shown to have maximum affinity for alpha-noradrenergic and dopaminergic receptors.[68] Jeste and Wyatt[190] found an association between TD and high serum levels of sulforidazine in a small group of patients.

CHOLINERGIC DEFICIT

The cholinergic deficit hypothesis of TD originated from two assumptions: first, that there is a reciprocal relationship between DA and acetylcholine (ACh) in basal ganglia, and second, that there is hypothesized nigrostriatal dopaminergic overactivity in TD. The striatal postsynaptic DA receptor lies, at least in part, on the cell body of cholinergic neurons, over which DA exerts an inhibitory control. Increasing striatal DA receptor activity by the administration of DA agonists was found to cause an increase in striatal ACh content, interpreted as being due to a decrease in cholinergic transmission.[311] Murugaiah and associates,[265] however, found that chronic neuroleptic treatment of rodents caused a significant increase in striatal ACh content, which was the opposite of what one might expect from the previous finding. Studies using cholinergic agents have not found consistent effects on TD. Also, there is too little evidence to date showing that anticholinergic drugs alone are capable of inducing TD.

GABAERGIC DEFICIT

The GABAergic deficit hypothesis was suggested as a result of the apparent antagonism between nigrostriatal dopamine and GABA in their effects on locomotion. Standefer and Dill[338] found that intrastriatal injections of GABA antagonists produced myoclonus in rats, whereas concomitant administration of GABA prevented these effects. Chlorpromazine and other neuroleptics are known to reduce GABA reuptake into the presynaptic neurons.[73] The CSF-GABA concentrations in four drug-free patients with TD were reported by Chase and Tamminga[57] to be significantly lower than those of twenty-one controls. A reduction in nigrostriatal GABA activity in TD is possible, but as yet unproven.

SEROTONERGIC DEFICIT

Serotonergic deficit in the basal ganglia was suggested to contribute to the pathogenesis of TD by Prange, Sisk, and Wilson.[290] Double-blind, controlled studies using L-tryptophan, a serotonin (5HT) precursor, yielded contradictory results.[208,291] Jeste and coworkers[200] found no significant differences in the plasma 5HT concentrations between patients with TD and matched controls. CSF 5-hydroxyindoleacetic acid (5-HIAA) studies have led to conflicting results.* These data do not support the hypothesis that the seroton-

*See references 58, 95, 266, 287, and 371.

ergic system is involved in the pathophysiology of TD.

ESTROGENS

Estrogens may have a neurolepticlike effect by both increasing the predisposition for development of TD and suppressing the presence of TD. This speculation is based on the higher prevalence of TD in women than in men and on some clinical observations. Bedard, Langelier, and Villeneuve[22] found increased prevalence of TD in postmenopausal as compared with premenopausal women. Raymond (unpublished, cited by Bedard, Langelier, and Villeneuve[22]) found that 17-estradiol reversed the effects of dopaminergic drugs on prolactin release, which may suggest that estrogens have antidopaminergic activity. Villeneuve, Langelier, and Bedard[361] observed improvement of levodopa-induced dyskinesia in one female patient and in neuroleptic-induced TD in another woman during periods of raised circulating estrogen activity. Gratton[169] noted that an apparent sensitization to neuroleptic-induced parkinsonism occurred in both genders following administration of estrogens. Villeneuve, Cazejust, and Cote[360] reported improvement of TD among male patients treated with conjugated estrogens in an open trial. On the other hand, Koller and coworkers[231] have reported estrogen-induced dyskinesia. Choreiform movements have been noted as a possible side effect of contraceptive pills containing estrogen. Nausieda and associates[270] found that supersensitivity to DA agonists was significantly reduced after oophorectomy in female guinea pigs. Subsequent chronic administration of estradiol increased the sensitivity to dopaminergic agents. Gordon, Borison, and Diamond[168] noted that long-term combined administration of estradiol and haloperidol increased DA receptor supersensitivity, whereas treatment with estradiol following haloperidol tended to reduce supersensitivity.

From these data it seems that estrogens may have a dyskinesia-suppressing action and that their prolonged use may aggravate TD. It is presumed that estrogens exert their effects by increasing the postsynaptic DA receptor density, although other mechanisms of action cannot be ruled out. Estrogens may explain only partially some of the variability encountered in the prevalence of TD in the two genders.

In summary, we believe that there are likely to be different subtypes of TD. These may be characterized by somewhat different, albeit overlapping, neurochemical disturbances. Mechanisms such as noradrenergic hyperactivity may be as crucial as postsynaptic DA receptor supersensitivity in a number of patients.

Neuropathology

THE NIGROSTRIATAL SYSTEM

The nigrostriatal system consists of the corpus striatum, substantia nigra, and their efferents and afferents. The basic anatomy and physiology of the nigrostriatal system is graphically represented in figures 20–2 and 20–3. The corpus striatum, the largest subcortical cell mass, consists of the caudate and lentiform nuclei, the latter being divided into the putamen and globus pallidus. The striatum is striped by the internal capsule white fibers. The caudate and putamen, which constitute the neostriatum, have embryologic, cytologic, and functional similarities.[44] The neostriatum receives afferent fibers from the cerebral cortex, intralaminar thalamic nuclei, and substantia nigra. The paleostriatum comprises the globus pallidus, which receives afferent fibers from the neostriatum and subthalamic nucleus of Luys. The major efferents from the striatum arise in the medial pallidal segment by way of the ansa lenticularis and fasciculus lenticularis and project to the ventral lateral and ventral anterior nuclei of the thalamus, which in turn project to the frontal motor cortex. A small pallidal output projects to the centromedian thalamic nucleus, which in turn may provide feedback to the striatum and to the midbrain (pedunculopontine nucleus).

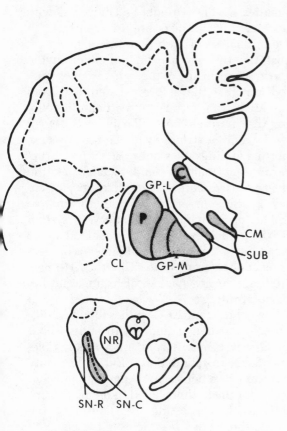

C = Caudate
CM = Centromedian Nucleus
(Thalmus)
CL = Claustrum
GP-m = Globus Pallidus-Medial Part
GP-L = Globus Pallidus-Lateral Part
P = Putamen
SUB = Subthalmic Nucleus
NR = Nucleus ruber
SN = Substantia nigra
SN-R = Pars reticulata
SN-C = Pars compacta

Figure 20–2. The anatomy of the striatum.

The lateral pallidal segment efferents terminate in the subthalamic nucleus of Luys.

The substantia nigra, which extends the length of the midbrain, consists of pars compacta and pars reticularis. Pars compacta sends nigrostriatal efferents, whereas pars reticularis sends nigrothalamic efferents. The substantia nigra receives its input from the striatum as part of a striato-nigro-striatal loop.

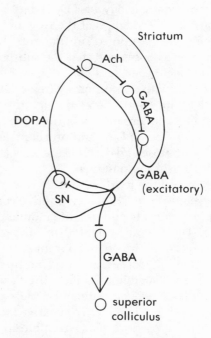

Figure 20–3. The putative functional connections of the striatum. Only one cholinergic neuron has been shown. Recent evidence indicates that there are two cholinergic interneurons in the striatum. SN = substantia nigra.

Nauta and Mehler[271] note that the striatum receives, in a topographic organization, afferents from all the major subdivisions of the neocortex, and its efferents to the thalamus terminate in the ventrolateral and ventroanterior nuclei, constituting the major gateway to the precentral cortex. Figure 20–3 shows the postulated interaction among dopaminergic, GABAergic, and cholinergic neurons in the nigrostriatal system. The principal functions of this system are concerned with postural adjustments, associated movements, and motoric integration. Lesions affecting parts of the system may result in disinhibition of involuntary activity.

The pathology of TD is poorly understood. According to Klawans and Rubovitz,[227] the areas of the caudate related to the complex fine movements of the face and hands may be particularly affected by long-term exposure to neuroleptics. There is no direct evidence, however, that the caudate is involved in the pathophysiology of TD. It has been demonstrated, though, that the caudate and putamen are atrophied in patients with Huntington's chorea and that the substantia nigra and locus coeruleus show degeneration in patients with Parkinson's disease. Also, hemiballismus and hemichorea are associated with lesions in the contralateral subthalamic nucleus of Luys and prerubral area, whereas athetosis and dystonia are associated with lesions in the putamen.

Only two of the fourteen studies reviewed by Jeste and Wyatt[190] found a positive correlation between TD and organic mental syndrome. The overall weighted mean prevalence of TD in schizophrenia, other "functional" psychoses, and organic mental syndrome did not differ significantly. Two recent studies, however, raise a possibility that patients with predominantly negative symptoms may be particularly susceptible to develop TD.[91,204] Chouinard and associates[63] reported that patients known to have brain damage tended to have more severe dyskinesias than other groups.

CLINICAL INVESTIGATIONS

Only a few investigators attempted to find associations between the presence of TD and a specific neurological abnormality. Six of the twelve studies we reviewed found a positive association.

Of the two pneumoencephalographic studies, Pandurangi and coworkers[278] found evidence of caudate atrophy in those three of the five patients who had persistent TD; an earlier study by Faurbye and associates[143] did not find any differences between seven elderly schizophrenic patients with TD and schizophrenic patients of the same age group without the movement disorder.

Interestingly, further conflicting findings were reported by researchers following computerized tomography (CT)-scan studies. Three out of four studies failed to detect a relevant relationship between TD and CT-scan findings.[155,199] Only one study, by Famuyiwa and coworkers,[136] found a significantly higher prevalence of CT-scan abnor-

malities in TD patients as compared with age-matched schizophrenic controls. A closer analysis of their data shows, however, that the two groups did not differ in the mean scores in any of the four variables studied, but that the difference stemmed from the use of an arbitrary cut-off point in defining the "normal ventricular index."

The lack of strong evidence for gross abnormal findings does not rule out fine structural abnormalities, undetectable at the degree of resolution that radiological technology can currently provide. Alternative modes of studying central nervous system (CNS) pathology in TD as reflected in its functions were attempted by means of electroencephalography (EEG), the H-reflex studies, neuropsychological testing, and behavioral ratings.

Two of the four EEG studies found no difference between patients with and without dyskinesia.[190,322] In contrast, Gardos, Cole, and Sokol[154] found that EEG abnormality discriminated between TD patients and controls, but the authors failed to define the criteria used in assessing the differences between the groups. Wegner and associates[365] observed a B-mitten EEG pattern in twenty of twenty-one dyskinesia patients and in only seven of twenty-one matched controls. The B-mitten EEG pattern consists of a sharp wave followed by a higher voltage slow wave —the whole complex resembles the thumb and hand of a mitten. It occurs bilaterally and synchronously over frontal and frontal-central areas during stages 3 and 4 of sleep, and may be found mostly in subjects between fifteen and fifty years of age. Wegner and coworkers[365] suggested that the presence of this pattern might indicate the susceptibility of younger patients to develop TD. This finding, however, remains to be confirmed.

The H-reflex studies assessed the excitability of the spinal alpha-motor neuron pool elicited by stimulation of sensory fibers, an electrically evoked spinal neurosynaptic reflex. The reflex-evoked muscle action potential was recorded with an electromyographic apparatus. Crayton and others[89] studied H-reflex curves in thirty-one schizophrenic patients with TD, schizophrenic patients without TD, and normal controls, and found an absence of H-reflex in nine patients with the movement disorder but in none of the other subjects. The absence of H-reflex was not related to the dyskinetic movements themselves. Surprisingly, the patients with severe dyskinesia had higher values for the peak of the H-reflex curve as compared to the patients with mild or no dyskinesia. There was no clinical evidence of peripheral neuropathy in any of the patients studied. The actual meaning of these findings is unclear.

Neuropsychological testing was employed by some investigators in an attempt to locate the substrate of the TD pathology. Pryce and Edwards[293] administered the Modified Word-Learning Test of Walton, White, and Black[364] to twenty-one elderly female patients with dyskinesia and twenty-one controls, matched for age, gender, primary psychiatric diagnosis, and length of current admission, and found no difference in the prevalence of pathology. Edwards[127] repeated this study, matching the controls for phenothiazine intake, and found significantly more impairment (73 percent) in dyskinetic patients as compared to controls (32 percent). Famuyiwa and coworkers[136] found that their dyskinesia patients performed significantly worse than controls on Inglis's Paired Associate Learning Test, but the two groups did not differ in the scores on the Withers-Hinton Clinical Test of the Sensorium. These findings may suggest a degree of cognitive impairment in the dyskinetic patients. Furthermore, Ivnik[185] administered the Halstead-Reitan battery to a fifty-eight-year-old man with dyskinesia, both before and after neuroleptic treatment, and noted that the patient improved both clinically and on the testing after withdrawal from neuroleptics. It appears that further study is warranted on the relationship of TD and neuroleptic treatment to the performance on neuropsychological testing.

Recently researchers found an association between TD in schizophrenic patients and negative symptoms such as affective blunting and paucity of thought content,[91,204] which may point toward a defect state responsible for both. These data will also need further confirmation and interpretation.

POSTMORTEM BRAIN STUDIES

Although neuropathological and neurochemical studies proved their usefulness in understanding other involuntary movement disorders such as Huntington's chorea and Parkinson's disease, few well-controlled postmortem studies have been completed on the brains of the patients who had a diagnosis of TD. In fact, only two of the eight studies we reviewed examined samples from more than three patients. The first, by Christensen, Moller, and Faurbye,[65] included twenty-eight patients and twenty-eight controls, although not well matched for gender and age. The dyskinetic patients had been selected from a group in which neuroleptic treatment was started unusually late (mean age sixty-nine years). Also, the degenerative changes found in the substantia nigra and the gliosis in the brain stem of the patients with TD were not significantly different from those found in patients with spontaneous dyskinesia.

The second study, published by Jellinger,[188] reported neuronal damage in the caudates of five of his nine patients with TD as compared to only one of the fourteen controls. The damage was not related to duration of neuroleptic treatment, nor was the clinical dyskinesia correlated to the degree of the neuropathological change.

Of the ten brains from dyskinetic patients examined in the remaining six studies, four had degenerative changes in the substantia nigra, three had atrophic lesions in the caudate, two in other areas of the striatum, and one in the olivary nucleus.[190]

In an extensive recent review on brain DA receptors, Seeman[310] advanced the hypothesis that TD may be a result of the long-term blockade of the DA receptors not linked to the DA-sensitive adenylate cyclase (also called D–2 receptors). According to this review, the D–2 receptors increase in number in the striata and limbic tissues of chronic neuroleptic-treated animals, and they are also found to be increased in postmortem striatum and nucleus accumbens of neuroleptic-treated schizophrenic patients. Crow and associates[92] also reported increased density of D-2 binding sites in the putamen of schizophrenic patients compared with age-matched controls. These researchers reported, however, that in postmortem studies of schizophrenic brains, neither the D-2 nor the D-1 binding was different between patients with and patients without movement disorders.[92] Also, D-2 receptors were found to mediate inhibition on striatal adenylate cyclase formation.[276,339]

These data are inconclusive, and further methodologically sophisticated postmortem studies of the brains of TD patients and well-matched controls are required in order to unveil the structural brain abnormalities specific to this disorder.

¶ Treatment Strategies Against Tardive Dyskinesia

Introduction

Before starting our review of treatment modalities, let us consider the potential pitfalls in assessing and interpreting the results of clinical trials in TD. First, the exact pathophysiology and neurochemistry of TD remain unknown. Moreover, current knowledge of the mechanisms of action of many drugs is far from complete. Hence it would be premature to speak of "rational pharmacotherapy" for TD (with the exception of neuroleptic withdrawal). Difficulties in measuring clinical response arise from the selection of patients for the studies and from the actual rating of change in the movement disorder. The patients' selection process should be clearly specified a priori, particularly with respect to issues such as clinical diagnosis, presence or absence of signs of brain damage, age-gender matching, concurrent use of

medications, medication history prior to the beginning of research, medication blood levels, and severity of movement disorder. In regard to the measurement of the degree of treatment response, the research design should provide for double-blind, placebo-controlled studies using valid, sensitive, and reliable rating scales. The movement disorder should preferably be rated in all subjects at approximately the same time of the day and in a similar environment. The length of treatment trials should be sufficiently long to differentiate among persistent, intermittent, and reversible dyskinesias.

For heuristic purposes, we may subdivide the treatment studies into three major groups: neuroleptic withdrawal studies, nondrug studies, and drug trials. Following the review of each of the three groups we will attempt to compare the efficacy of the various treatment modalities and to draw certain guidelines for the clinician.

Neuroleptic Withdrawal

In view of the chronic neuroleptic-treatment-induction of TD, it only seems logical that the first theoretical line of treatment considered for this syndrome should be neuroleptic withdrawal. In a recent review of the literature, Jeste and Wyatt[189] found twenty-three studies in which antipsychotics were withdrawn for periods varying from several weeks to three years, with an overall remission of dyskinetic symptoms in 36.5 percent of patients. It appeared that the longer the length of neuroleptic withdrawal, the greater the likelihood of the remission of dyskinesia. They also found that 33.5 percent of patients had a remission within the first three months of withdrawal, suggesting that the presence of dyskinesia beyond three months after withdrawal may be considered a valid research criterion for persistence of dyskinesia. Neuroleptic withdrawal usually leads to an initial aggravation of dyskinesia, which reaches a peak of intensity within one to two weeks; thereafter, the severity of dyskinesia subsides to complete dissolution in approximately one-third of patients, or persists at a more or less even level of severity in a majority of the remaining patients.

The persistent character of dyskinesia might be influenced by certain variables such as aging and brain damage. An inverse correlation between aging and spontaneous remission of TD was found by Smith and Baldessarini.[326] An association between organicity and persistent dyskinesia was reported by Uhrbrand and Faurbye[353] and Yagi and associates.[375] In recent years several researchers[29,112,195,376] found evidence for an association between interrupted neuroleptic treatment and persistent dyskinesia. Also, in animal studies[367] Weiss and Santelli found that monkeys became dyskinetic when treated intermittently with haloperidol. Simpson[316] pointed out that the reported high incidence of TD among certain affective disorder patients may be due in part to the intermittent pattern of their neuroleptic treatment. More systematic research needs to be directed at this aspect of the intermittent neuroleptic treatment in relation to persistent TD.

Nondrug Treatments

Nondrug treatments of TD have rarely been attempted and have consisted mostly of small numbers of patient case reports of open or poorly controlled studies. *Prosthodontia* has proven useful in some patients with ill-fitting dentures as a palliative treatment of orolingual dyskinesia. A *biofeedback* technique based on electromyographic feedback to the maseter muscles was used by Albanese and Gaarder[3] and Sherman[313] in dyskinetic patients, with some success. Betts, Johnston, and Pratt[24] used *transcutaneous nerve stimulation* for pain relief in a patient with severe TD and noted a decrease in the involuntary movement and alleviation of pain. *Electroconvulsive therapy* was used by Price and Levin[292] and Rosenbaum, O'Connor, and Duane[300] in depressed patients with TD. This reportedly resulted in notable improvement in both depression and dyski-

nesia. However, Asnis and Leopold[10] found no significant change in dyskinesia with this type of treatment in a single-blind, controlled study. Druckman, Seelinger, and Thulin[124] and Nashold[268] attempted *brain stereotaxic surgical procedures* in patients with TD, and Heath[175] obtained remission of dyskinesia in a young patient after cerebellar stimulation through an implanted pacemaker. The limited knowledge about the neuropathology of TD does not seem to warrant further surgical explorations of this kind at the present time.

Drug Treatments

In a review of all the studies on treatment of TD published over two decades, Jeste and Wyatt[189] noted a number of important specific obstacles in interpreting results of drug treatments: (1) With a sufficient number of patients in a study, even a 30 percent reduction in symptoms may yield statistically significant results. Hence statistically significant change may not necessarily represent clinically meaningful improvement. (2) There is a bias in the literature toward publishing positive rather than negative studies. (3) Whenever a new theory appears in conjunction with a new drug, the initial published reports tend to be encouraging, as happened in the case of deanol acetamidobenzoate. (4) The concurrent use of neuroleptics, although found more effective by several investigators, may make interpretation difficult because of complex drug interactions. In our review, we define "improvement" as at least 50 percent reduction in symptoms and "positive" studies as those in which at least 50 percent of the patients had improvement. For heuristic purposes, we classify the drug treatments according to the postulated neurochemical hypothesis.

DOPAMINE ANTAGONISTS

DA antagonists are believed to suppress TD by inhibiting the nigrostriatal dopaminergic activity. Among them are DA blockers and DA-depleting agents (see table 20–8).

Table 20–8
Dopamine Antagonists

Class	Generic Names	Most Used Representatives	Brand Name
DA blockers	Phenothiazines		
	• Aliphatic	Chlorpromazine	Thorazine
	• Piperidine	Thioridazine	Melarill
	• Piperazine	Trifluoperazine	Stelazine
		Fluphenazine	Prolixin
	Thioxanthenes		
	• Aliphatic	Chlorprothixene	Taractan
	• Piperazine	Thiothixene	Navane
	Butyrophenones	Haloperidol	Haldol
	Dibenzazepines	Loxapine	Loxitane
	Dibenzodiazepines	Clozapine	
	Dihidroindolones	Molindone	Moban
	Diphenylbutylpiperidines	Pimozide	Orap
	Benzamides	Sulpiride	
		Metoclopramide	
		Oxiperomide	
DA depleters	Rauwolfia alkaloids	Reserpine	Serpasil
	Benzoquinolizines	Tetrabenazine	
	Indol piperazines	Oxypertine	
	Methyrozine		
	Methyldopa		

Dopamine Blockers

DA blockers are represented by neuroleptic drugs. The use of neuroleptics as treating agents for tardive dyskinesia is paradoxical and controversial due to their virtually unmistakable contribution to the etiology of this disorder. Tables 20–9 and 20–10 show

Table 20–9
Review of Treatment Studies with Dopamine Blockers in Tardive Dyskinesia

Neuroleptic	No. of Studies	N	% Patients Improved[a]
Haloperidol	7	83	79
Thiopropazate	10	71	62
Clozapine[b]	8	75	51[c]
Others	16	164	84
Total[d]	41	393	72

[a]Improvement was defined as a reduction of dyskinesia by at least 50 percent.
[b]The precise mode of the antipsychotic action of clozapine is not yet known.
[c]The improvement with clozapine was significantly lower than that with haloperidol ($p < 0.002$ X^2 test)
[d]Totals include some repeats with different neuroleptics.

that in spite of the controversy surrounding the legitimacy of using neuroleptics in dyskinetic patients, these drugs are the most successful palliative treatment of TD.

Among the putative DA blockers, clozapine had a significantly lower effect on TD than did haloperidol ($p = 0.002$, X^2 test).[189] In fact, if we consider DA blocker studies, excluding the clozapine trials, approximately 85 percent of the patients had a reduction of at least 50 percent in the intensity of TD.

Table 20–10
Review of Treatment Studies with Antidopaminergic Drugs in Tardive Dyskinesia

Drug	No. of Studies	N	% Patients Improved[a]
Neuroleptics	41	393	72
Catecholamine depleters	23	278	62
Low-dose DA agonists	38	212	21

[a]Improvement was defined as a reduction of dyskinesia by at least 50 percent.

With regard to the specificity of this effect, Gerlach and Simmelsgaard[158] found that neuroleptics administered in doses that did not cause sedation produced a noticeable improvement in TD. Evidence that the antidyskinetic effect of neuroleptics is independent from sedation also comes from the observation that neuroleptics with variable sedative properties had comparable antidyskinetic effects. The fact that the severity of TD does not correlate with the severity of psychosis or parkinsonism suggests that the antidyskinetic properties may be independent of the antipsychotic and acute extrapyramidal effects of the DA blockers.

Long-term studies may help in weighing the risk/benefit ratio of the use of neuroleptics in treating TD. Jeste and Wyatt[189] compared results of short-term studies (patients treated for less than eight weeks) with those of longer term trials and found a trend for greater improvement with prolonged treatment. Except for two studies,[164,217] investigators did not confirm the development of tolerance to antidyskinetic effects of neuroleptics.

It is important to point out that the effect of the DA blockers on TD is only symptomatic and their discontinuation results in at least a temporary recurrence of the movement disorder. An exception to this rule occurred when Jus, Jus, and Fontaine[207] applied a "desensitization technique." These investigators postulated that a "desensitization" of those DA receptors implicated in the pathophysiology of this movement disorder might be achieved by a slow, progressive increase and then a gradual reduction of the neuroleptic dosages until their complete discontinuation. The researchers reported a 79 percent rate of improvement; 42 percent of all the patients had a remission. TD recurred in 29 percent of the patients, but when small regimens of haloperidol or reserpine were resumed, improvement was obtained again. Reversible dyskinesia was not ruled out in the remitted cases, and this study needs to be repeated before the value of its findings can be established.

As far as neuroleptic dosage is concerned, Jeste and Wyatt[189] calculated the overall mean daily dosage of neuroleptics used in the treatment of TD to be 304 mg chlorpromazine equivalents and did not find any significant correlation between the dosage of neuroleptic used and the percentage of patients who had improvement. It may be of interest to point out that similar dosages seem adequate for maintenance treatment of chronic schizophrenia.[15]

Increased D-2-binding in postmortem striatum and nucleus accumbens of neuroleptic-treated schizophrenic patients, and the correlation found between the average dose controlling schizophrenic symptoms and the D-2, but not the D-1, binding,[310] led researchers to specifically study the D-2 blockers (see table 20-11). These studies, particularly those using sulpiride and metoclopramide, need further confirmation.

Jeste, Olgiati, and Ghali[193] found that dividing the total daily dose of a neuroleptic into four equal doses was significantly more effective in suppressing dyskinesia than administering the once-a-day total dose at bedtime—a finding that was confirmed by our subsequent experience. One can speculate that this may be related to the maintenance of the neuroleptic blood (and maybe brain) levels above a certain antidyskinetic threshold.

To summarize, the DA blockers produce a significant symptomatic improvement in more than two-thirds of patients with TD and seem to possess potent antidyskinetic properties.

CATECHOLAMINE-DEPLETING AGENTS

Tables 20-10 and 20-12 summarize the treatment studies of TD with putative catecholamine-depleting agents. These drugs appear to have effects on TD approximately similar to the DA blockers. Of the patients in these sixteen studies, 63 percent improved, with a trend for tetrabenazine to be somewhat more effective (68 percent of the patients improved) and for oxypertine hydrochloride to be less effective (59 percent of the patients improved). Due to similarities in

TABLE 20–11

Review of Double-blind, Placebo-controlled Treatment Studies with D–2 Blockers in
Tardive Dyskinesia

| Drug | N | Investigators | Patients' Improvement | |
			Improved	%[a]
Sulpiride	11	Casey, Gerlach, and Simmelsgaard[53]	10	91
Metoclopramide	94	Bateman et al.[21] Karp et al.[213] Doongaji et al.[122]	79	84
Oxiperomide	10	Casey and Gerlach[51]	6	60
Total	115		95	83

[a]Improvement was defined as a reduction of dyskinesia by at least 50 percent.

both antipsychotic and antidyskinetic effects of DA depleters and blockers, most investigators tend to consider these agents as part of the neuroleptic family. Clinicians have to bear in mind, however, that certain potentially more severe adverse reactions may occur when using catecholamine depleters. Clinically severe major depressive disorder occurs in as many as 15 percent of all patients on long-term treatment with reserpine, many of whom require hospitalization and sustained antidepressant measures.[99]

DOPAMINE AGONISTS

Some DA agonists are postulated to have a prominent antagonistic effect on the presynaptic dopaminergic autoreceptor when administered in small doses, leading to a decrease in the presynaptic exocytosis of the

DA vesicles. A number of researchers have investigated the antidyskinetic effects of the DA agonists (see table 20–13). The overall improvement of TD as a result of treatments with these agents was disappointingly low (21 percent), ranging from zero percent when using d-amphetamine to 30 percent when apomorphine was used.

A novel strategy for treating TD was developed by Alpert and Friedhoff.[5] These researchers administered levodopa with the aim of producing a postulated "receptor sensitivity modification." Unfortunately, development of side effects, such as an aggravation of psychosis, limits the clinical use of levodopa in dyskinetic patients.

TABLE 20–12

Review of Treatment Studies with
Catecholamine Depleters in Tardive Dyskinesia

Drug	No. of Studies	N	% Patients Improved[a]
Tetrabenazine	5	38	68
Reserpine	7	96	64
Methyrosine	3	39	64
Oxypertine	4	68	59
Methyldopa	4	37	55
Total	23	278	62

[a]Improvement was defined as a reduction of dyskinesia by at least 50%.

TABLE 20–13

Review of Treatment Studies with
Miscellaneous Dopamine Agonists in Tardive
Dyskinesia

Drug	No. of Studies	N	% Patients Improved[a]
Apomorphine	8	31	30
Amantadine	9	65	22
Levodopa	12	51	22
Bromocriptine	3	26	20
Methylphenidate	1	17	18
Tiomergine	2	12	16
D-Amphetamine	3	10	0
Total	38	212	21

[a]Improvement was defined as a reduction of dyskinesia by at least 50 percent.

NORADRENERGIC DRUGS

The typical neuroleptic drugs tend to block nonspecifically both dopaminergic and noradrenergic receptors.[148] Therefore, it may be difficult to conclude whether their antidyskinetic effects are due to their activity on the dopaminergic receptor, the noradrenergic receptors, or on both. Furthermore, virtually the same arguments used in the support of dopaminergic overactivity as a primary cause of TD can be used in the support of the noradrenergic overactivity hypothesis of TD (see the section entitled "Biochemical Hypotheses"). Only a few investigators have tried more specific *antinoradrenergic drugs* for their antidyskinetic effects. Clonidine hydrochloride and propranolol hydrochloride are relatively pure antinoradrenergic drugs that have been tested as antipsychotic drugs.* Clonidine is an imidazoline derivative that is believed to inhibit central noradrenergic function when given in small doses, probably by stimulating alpha-2-noradrenergic autoreceptors. Freedman and coworkers[150] found that in eight dyskinetic patients with schizophrenia given daily doses of clonidine ranging from 0.2 to 0.9 mg, dyskinesia decreased by 63 percent compared with the drug-free ratings. These data should be interpreted with caution due to the short interval (three weeks) used for obtaining baseline drug-free ratings. In this study, clonidine was also found to have an antipsychotic effect. Interestingly, clonidine has been reported to be useful in the control of another movement disorder—Gilles de la Tourette's syndrome.[69]

Propranolol is a specific beta-adrenergic receptor blocker. Carroll, Curtis, and Kokmen[45] first tried 160 mg per day for eight days in one patient and obtained significant effects. Three subsequent studies found significant improvement either with low doses ranging from 20 to 40 mg propranolol per day[14,235] or high doses such as 800 mg per day.[263] Thus, eleven out of fifteen patients treated with propranolol had a significant decrease in TD, consistent with the suggestion of noradrenergic overactivity in some patients with TD. Propranolol, however, is known for its anxiolytic effects, which in turn might have contributed in part to the decrease in dyskinesia in these studies.

DBH inhibitors such as fusaric acid and disulfiram presumably reduce NE synthesis. Jeste and associates[194,200] reported elevated plasma DBH activity in a proportion of patients with TD. Although Viukari and Linnoila[363] reported some improvement of TD treated with fusaric acid, this effect needs further confirmation. Disulfiram was successfully tried in patients with levodopa-induced dyskinesia by Birket-Smith and Andersen.[25] Further well-designed studies using antinoradrenergic drugs in TD are needed.

CHOLINERGIC DRUGS

The striatal cholinergic deficit hypothesis of TD[159,162] encouraged investigators to try cholinergic drugs in this disorder. Two major types of cholinomimetic drugs have been used: ACh precursors and cholinesterase inhibitors.

Among the acetylcholine precursors, deanol, choline, and lecithin were used more extensively. Physostigmine is a centrally acting, reversible cholinesterase inhibitor that is usually administered parenterally, although an oral form is under investigation. The results obtained with these cholinomimetic drugs are reviewed in table 20–14. The available data do not seem to support routine use of these agents in the long-term treatment of TD. The overall improvement rate of dyskinesia in patients treated with cholinomimetics as calculated by Jeste and Wyatt[190] was 39 percent.

ANTICHOLINERGIC DRUGS

Anticholinergic drugs are thought by most investigators either to have no effect or to aggravate the dyskinesia. Jeste and Wyatt[190] reviewed fourteen systematic studies using anticholinergic drugs for the treatment of TD and found an overall rate of improvement of only 7 percent.

*See references 12, 149, 150, 152, 173, 283, and 378.

TABLE 20–14

Review of Treatment Studies with Cholinergic
Drugs in Tardive Dyskinesia

Drug	No. of Studies	N	% Patients Improved[a]
Physostigmine (IV)	15	69	52
Lecithin	7	25	48
Choline	7	36	44
Deanol	43	236	34
Total	72	406	36

[a]Improvement was defined as a reduction of dyskinesia by at least 50 percent.

GABAERGIC DRUGS

Putative GABAergic drugs were speculated to counterbalance the postulated reduction in nigrostriatal GABA activity in TD. In the nineteen studies we examined, 54 percent of the 204 patients treated with putative GABAergic drugs had a significant reduction in dyskinesia (see table 20–15). Only two of these studies,[52,324] however, involved drug administration for more than eight weeks, and both were open trials including relatively small numbers of patients. Also, no sustained effort was made in these studies to control for the sedative and muscle relaxant effects of these drugs, with the exception of

TABLE 20–15

Review of Treatment Studies with GABAergic
Drugs in Tardive Dyskinesia

Drug	No. of Studies	N	% Patients Improved[a]
Diazepam	4	26	65
Clorazepate	1	12	58
Clonazepam[b]	3	62	71
Sodium valproate	7	72	36
Gamma-acetylenic GABA	1	10	40
Total	16	182	54

[a]Improvement was defined as a reduction of dyskinesia by at least 50 percent.
[b]The results of the treatment studies with clonazepam are highly conflicting. In one study by O'Flanagan,[273] 100 percent of the patients treated with clonazepam improved. The other two studies found the results with this drug discouraging, but had small numbers of patients.

Singh and associates[325] who administered diazepam in doses that did not cause sedation but suppressed dyskinesia.

Combined treatment using a neuroleptic and valproate sodium has been reported to be more beneficial than either drug alone by Linnoila and Viukari.[243] Casey and coworkers[54] reported that gamma-acetylenic GABA (believed to increase brain GABA) was more useful in reducing dyskinesia when added to a DA blocker than either drug alone.

Korsgaard[232] used p-chlorophenyl-GABA (baclofen), a putative GABA analogue, in the treatment of TD, obtaining a high improvement rate. The mean overall improvement rate of dyskinesia in the seven studies using baclofen reviewed by Jeste and Wyatt[190] was 64 percent. While baclofen was originally thought to be a GABA agonist, subsequent work has shown that this may not be the case. Moore and Demarest[262] have reported a dose-related increase in brain DA concentrations with systemic administration of this drug.

Several authors have noted unpleasant side effects with GABAergic drugs. Sedman[308] found a high incidence of severe sedation and drowsiness. Tamminga, Crayton, and Chase[342] found that although a five-day trial of muscimol improved dyskinesia, it appeared to worsen the psychosis. Singh and associates[325] reported increased impulsiveness and belligerence in two of their patients treated with diazepam. Although it seems that the GABAergic drugs as a group are more effective than all the nonneuroleptic drugs in suppressing TD, there is no convincing evidence to suggest that their effect is specifically antidyskinetic. Nevertheless, the results obtained with these drugs are encouraging and deserve further replication and interpretation.

MISCELLANEOUS DRUGS

Estrogens may have an antidyskinetic effect. This speculation is based on a number of facts derived from prevalence and clinical studies (discussed earlier). Villeneuve, Cazejust, and Cote[360] conducted an open trial with conjugated estrogens in twenty male patients and observed a reduction of TD in 50 percent of the patients. Interestingly, Koller and associates[231] reported induction of choreiform movements in patients who received estrogens for prolonged periods. Further investigation in this area is warranted.

Dalen[98] and Prange and others[291] first reported successful use of *lithium carbonate* in dyskinetic patients. Although Bunney and associates[37] postulated that lithium blocks the development of DA receptor supersensitivity, subsequent trials have yielded generally disappointing results. Only 27 percent of the ninety patients who underwent treatment with lithium carbonate for TD in ten separate studies reviewed by Jeste and Wyatt[190] had a reduction of at least 50 percent of dyskinesia. Experimental work on animals reported by Klawans, Weiner, and Nausieda[228] and Pert and coworkers[286] found that concurrent administration of lithium carbonate and haloperidol prevented the development of DA receptor supersensitivity that would have occurred following long-term treatment with haloperidol alone. Tanimoto, Maeda, and Terada[345] also found evidence that short- or long-term lithium treatment may induce a reduction in neuroleptic binding site density (Bmax) tested with ^{3}H-spiperone in the limbic forebrain of rats, but not in the caudate and putamen. These findings are suggestive of a possible use of lithium as a "prophylactic" measure in the prevention of TD in long-term antipsychotic-treated patients. There is no clear clinical evidence, however, to support this suggestion.

Manganese chelation by phenothiazines prompted Kunin[238] to treat TD with a supplement of dietary manganese. He reported that fourteen out of fifteen patients were "cured" or much improved. Only five of his patients, however, appeared to have TD. Norris and Sams[272] replicated these findings in six patients with TD. Controlled trials with manganese in TD are lacking, and Weiner, Nausieda, and Klawans[366] reported that in guinea pigs, long-term chlorpromazine administration resulted in significant increases of manganese concentrations within the caudate nucleus. Moreover, in view of the reports of potentially irreversible neurological disorders, including movement disorders, caused by chronic manganese intoxication,[72] it is difficult to maintain a rationale for further experimental use of manganese in patients with TD.

Tryptophan combined with pyridoxine was first tried in TD by Prange and associates[291] after they noticed its effects of worsening parkinsonian symptoms. The investigators obtained improvement in all four patients, but when tryptophan was tried alone it did not appear to have any effect. Jus and coworkers[208] also reported negative results with D-L-tryptophan. The studies using *pyridoxine* alone reported negative results.[87,119,126]

Melanocyte-stimulating hormone release inhibiting factor-I, also called MIF-I (chemically, prolyl-leucyl-glycinamide), was reported to reduce levodopa-induced dyskinesia in parkinsonian patients. This led Ehrensing[128] to first use it in a depressed patient with TD. In spite of the first encouraging results, a subsequent trial on thirteen patients reported by Ehrensing and others[129] showed no significant effect, except for a temporary improvement in female patients at lower doses, suggesting a possible biphasic dose-related response. More recently, Davis and associates[108] found that MIF-I increased the stereotypy reaction to apomorphine in haloperidol-pretreated rats, suggesting that MIF-I, might, if anything, aggravate TD.

Bjorndal, Casey, and Gerlach[26] used a single-blind, single-injection design with three separate drugs: FK-33-824 (a synthetic *met-enkephalin* analogue), *morphine,* and *naloxone hydrochloride* in eight patients with TD. Only FK-33-824 appeared to reduce dyskinesia in two of the eight patients, who were also receiving high-dose neuroleptics. Korsgaard and others[233] gave five weeks of single-blind *lysine-8-vasopressin* to sixteen patients with negative schizophrenia and TD and found no change in dyskinesia.

Cyproheptadine hydrochloride (4-amine-3-p-chlorophenylbutyric acid), an antihistaminic, antiserotonergic compound, was tried in three separate trials for TD. Whereas Goldman[167] reported improvement in all three patients in his study, Gardos and Cole[152] and Nagao and associates[266] had negative results in their subjects.

Diphenylhydantoin sodium was tested by Jus and coworkers[208] in an acute intravenous infusion of 100 mg in fourteen patients with TD, based on reports of its usefulness in some cases of chorea minor. Eight of the fourteen patients had transient improvement, which was less dramatic than that following diazepam treatment.

Barbiturates were also tried in TD. Although Lipsius[245] reported improvement in dyskinesia in one patient treated with phenobarbital, most clinicians agree that barbiturates are of little use in this disorder.[24,124,133,333]

Fann, Davis, and Wilson[138] tried *caffeine, amphetamine,* and *methylphenidate hydrochloride* in a pilot study in dyskinetic patients. There was no response to the first two drugs, but mild improvement occurred with methylphenidate. A double-blind study with the latter, however, led to improvement in only three of the seventeen patients (18 percent). Crayton and associates[89] and Carroll, Curtis, and Kokmen[45] reported worsening of tardive dyskinesia with d-amphetamine. Roccatagliata, Albano, and Besio[298] studied the effects of *trazodone hydrochloride* on four patients with TD. This antidepressant of the triazolopyridine type is thought to have adrenolytic, dopaminergic, and serotonergic actions. All the four patients who participated in this study improved after a single intravenous dose of 50 mg trazodone.

Overview of the Comparative Values of Different Treatments

A comparative overview of the values of the different treatments previously outlined is summarized in table 20–16. The greatest number of dyskinetic patients reported in these studies were those who underwent withdrawal from neuroleptic drugs. It is worth noting that approximately one out of three patients with TD can attain complete remission of the movement disorder within three months of withdrawal. Most of these studies seem to agree that TD is more likely to remit in the younger and non-brain damaged patients.* Four studies, however, found a higher prevalence of persistent dyskinesia in patients given interrupted treatment.[29,112,195,376] Neuroleptics are the most effective suppressants of TD. This creates a critical clinical and ethical dilemma, for the drugs that appear to be the etiological agents of TD are also the best palliative agents for suppressing it. Furthermore, in many situations continued use of neuroleptics is required to help control recurrent psychotic episodes. Approximately three-fourths of the double-blind studies using neuroleptics in the treatment of TD report significant reductions in the movement disorder. Within this class of drugs, the D–2-blockers, and in particular metoclopramide and sulpiride, although very little studied, appear to provide the most potentially promising results. Among the other treatments, the ones that seem to merit our consideration are the noradrenergic blockers and the GABAergics.

The results of the treatment studies with noradrenergic blockers, propranolol and clonidine, have been impressive. These studies support the hypothesis of noradrenergic hyperactivity in a proportion of patients with TD. The number of patients treated has, however, been small.

The results obtained with the GABAergic drugs were promising in the open trials (65 percent of the patients improved), whereas the double-blind trials reported much lower improvement rates (43 percent). As with the treatment studies using noradrenergic blockers, well-designed studies with GABAergic drugs on large patient populations are needed for assessing the exact value of these agents in the treatment of TD.

---

*See references 112, 126, 127, 180, 279, 293, 352, 353, and 375.

TABLE 20–16
Overview of the Comparative Values of Various Treatment Modalities in Tardive Dyskinesia

Method of Treatment	No. of Studies	N	Open Studies	% Patients Improved[a] Double-Blind Studies	All Studies
DA blockers	41	393	68	74	72
Baclofen	7	55	67	63	64
Catecholamine depleters	23	278	67	53	62
GABAergic drugs	16	182	65	43	54
Cholinergic drugs	68	379	47	30	39
Lithium carbonate	10	84	38	20	26
DA agonists	38	212	27	15	21
Anticholinergic drugs	14	177	7	–	7
Estrogens	2	20	50	–	50
Neuroleptic withdrawal	23	1005	37	–	37
Nondrug studies	12	16	75	–	75
Noradrenergic blockers[b]	4	15	73	–	73

[a]Improvement was defined as a reduction of dyskinesia by at least 50 percent.
[b]Propranolol studies only.

There seems to be a general consensus that most of the other treatments listed in table 20–16 have either little value in the treatment of TD or have side effects that outweigh their beneficial effects.

In summary, there is no satisfactory treatment for the majority of patients with TD. Paradoxically, the neuroleptics appear to be the most effective dyskinesia-suppressing drugs. Several studies have shown that long-term administration of neuroleptic drugs for weeks to months does not result in a worsening of TD; however, more long-term studies are needed. Withdrawal of neuroleptics leads to complete remission of dyskinesia in about one-third of all patients.

Guidelines for Clinicians

The clinician may encounter one of the following three relevant situations: (1) patients presenting for the first time as candidates for neuroleptic treatment; (2) patients who are receiving neuroleptics and do not have TD; (3) patients who have developed TD. The first two situations call for a consideration of primary prevention against TD, whereas the latter requires secondary prevention, tertiary prevention, or both.

In the case of the patient who becomes a possible candidate for neuroleptic treatment, three major issues must be considered. First, the clinician needs to perform a thorough diagnostic workup before initiating long-term neuroleptic treatment. A neuroleptic should be used only when it is the drug of choice for a well-specified clinical condition. Baldessarini and Davis[15] have listed a number of primary clinical indications for this type of treatment. These include schizophrenia, paranoia, childhood psychosis, and certain neuropsychiatric disorders such as Gilles de la Tourette's syndrome and Huntington's chorea. Short-term use of neuroleptics is justifiable in most cases of acute psychosis, manic excitement, agitated depression, certain organic mental syndromes, and intractable nausea and vomiting.

Second, once the clinical decision for a long-term neuroleptic maintenance treatment is made, it becomes necessary to discuss in detail with the patient and his or her family the benefits and the risks associated with such a course of treatment. According to a recent survey,[15] most clinicians (approximately 80 percent) do not consider it necessary to obtain a written informed consent from their patients and/or patients' families before instituting neuroleptic treatment. There is an increasing trend, however, toward documenting that a discussion took place and providing justification for long-term treatment.

Third, as discussed earlier, there is little evidence to show that drug interruptions reduce the incidence of TD. Indeed, in some studies, lengthy drug holidays were associated with an increased prevalence of persistent dyskinesia. When neuroleptics are not indicated, they should not be used. Also, they should not be continued any longer than is necessary. At the same time, there is little justification for stopping neuroleptics repeatedly and for lengthy intervals with the hope of preventing TD in patients who need maintenance neuroleptic therapy. The role of neuroleptics in the maintenance therapy of schizophrenia is well established. On reviewing the literature on this subject, Davis[99] found that approximately half of the moderately ill schizophrenic patients relapsed within six months of discontinuation of their medication, whereas Hogarty and Goldberg[177] found that two-thirds of the schizophrenic patients discharged from the hospital decompensated on placebo within one year, as opposed to a 16 percent rate of relapse while on neuroleptic maintenance. Nevertheless, it is reasonable to decrease the neuroleptic dose to determine the lowest effective dose.

In the case of the patient who does not have TD, but receives maintenance neuroleptic treatment for clinically well-justified and documented reasons, the clinician needs to determine the *lowest effective dosage* that keeps the illness under control, while producing the least side effects. We did not find any evidence to prove that there is an antipsychotic drug of choice, or that a particular neuroleptic drug leads to less TD. Therefore, all treatment attempts should be highly *individualized* and in accordance with the clinical state of the patient, which may vary from time to time, and changes in treatment should be justified and well documented. Anticholinergic treatment should also be avoided when possible, and, when necessary for treating acute extrapyramidal reactions, the clinician should be aware that this need is usually only temporary, and that prolonged use of these drugs in psychiatric patients is not usually indicated.

In the case of the patient who already presents with dyskinesia, the risk of persistent TD has to be weighed against the risk of ravages elicited by the primary illness for which maintenance neuroleptic treatment has been prescribed. Development of TD warrants a *reassessment* of the need for continuing neuroleptics, and, whenever possible, an attempt should be made to taper off neuroleptics and to discontinue them. In many cases, neuroleptic withdrawal is fraught with the danger of a relapse of psychosis. If a neuroleptic was needed prior to the development of dyskinesia, it may still be needed afterward for the same primary illness. In such patients, the clinician may attempt a *dose reduction* and/or a *switch* to another class of neuroleptic drugs that the patient has never used before. It is advisable to document consent from a dyskinetic patient (and his family, when necessary) before continuing him or her on neuroleptics.

We estimate that in approximately one-third of these patients in whom neuroleptics are stopped, TD will disappear. The remaining two-thirds of these patients will have persistent TD. In patients with persistent dyskinesia who need to continue on neuroleptics, the clinician and the patient must decide whether some antidyskinetic treatment modality is worth considering. To date, there is no proven specific curative treatment for persistent TD. The clinician should explore options such as beta-adrenergic blockers and GABAergics, which have been found to be useful in suppressing TD in some patients, but which, like any other drugs, have their own drawbacks.

A periodic and systematic review of the patient's mental status and severity of dyskinesia must be recorded and used as the patient's treatment reference. Dental prosthetic work may be useful when indicated. Most other treatments are still considered experimental.

¶ Related Movement Disorders

Other Types of Neuroleptic-induced Dyskinesias

TD is not the only motor abnormality induced by neuroleptic drugs. Although insufficiently studied, the incidence of the other neuroleptic-induced, abnormal, involuntary movement disorders is probably much higher than commonly believed among clinicians. A useful classification of these involuntary movement disorders according to their time of onset in the course of neuroleptic treatment divides them into those that appear relatively early, from a few hours to a few weeks after starting the neuroleptic treatment, and those that manifest later. The early ones include acute dystonia, akathisia, and neuroleptic-induced parkinsonism. The late-onset group is represented by TD and by certain controversial entities such as tardive dystonia, tardive parkinsonism, tardive Tourette's syndrome, and other encephalopathies.

ACUTE DYSTONIAS

Acute dystonias are relatively fixed involuntary postures due to muscle spasms that usually involve midline structures of the facial muscles, tongue, and throat. Severe dystonia can cause patients unbearable discomfort, and require prompt action on the part of the treating clinician. In most cases this dystonia will be almost instantaneously relieved by intravenous injection of diphenhydramine hydrochloride (Benadryl, usual dose range 25 to 50 mg, which can be repeated if needed), an antihistamine with strong anticholinergic activity. After the acute episode, maintenance antidystonic treatment with an anticholinergic agent may be indicated for a few weeks. In recurrent dystonia, hypocalcemia should be ruled out as a possible cause, and alternative options such as reducing the dose of neuroleptic or switching to a lower-potency neuroleptic

should be considered. The acute dystonic reactions occur very rapidly (within minutes) after initiation or change in neuroleptic treatment. They seem to occur more frequently in younger than older patients and men are more susceptible than women.

AKATHISIA

Akathisia is a state of psychomotor restlessness that may be induced by neuroleptic treatment. The patients may complain of tension, being driven to move, pulling sensations in the legs, or an inability to tolerate inactivity. Many psychotic patients are not able, however, to complain, and the diagnosis is often missed or mistaken for psychotic phenomena. Akathisia is often dose-related. Van Putten[357] indicated that 40 percent of the patients receiving a 5 mg oral dose of haloperidol experienced akathisia and the incidence rose to 70 percent in those patients who took 10 mg haloperidol at night for four weeks. A similar incidence of akathisia was reported in patients treated with thiothixene.[357] These investigators called for a more sustained doctor-patient interaction aimed at improving diagnosis of akathisia and monitoring it as a potential side effect of neuroleptic treatment. The treatment of akathisia is not well established; the physician may need to try several modalities before selecting the most effective one. Among the drugs most commonly used are anticholinergic antiparkinsonian drugs, benzodiazepines, amantadine hydrochloride, and propranolol. The physician may also try lowering the neuroleptic dose and switching to a lower-potency neuroleptic.

NEUROLEPTIC-INDUCED PARKINSONISM

Neuroleptic-induced parkinsonism in its mild and subtle forms is frequently underestimated in the medical community. Some of its major features are akinesia, rigidity, and tremor, which may occur together or alone. Overemphasis on rigidity and cogwheeling as pathognomonic signs results in an underdiagnosis of neuroleptic-induced parkinsonism in patients who present with the reduced arm swing and mild reduction in facial expression that may be easily mistaken for negative symptoms of schizophrenia. The neuroleptic-induced parkinsonism is thought to be caused by inadequate dopamine neurotransmission with relative cholinergic over-

activity in the nigrostriatum, and it is accordingly treated with anticholinergic drugs, antihistamines acting by the anticholinergic route, or DA agonists such as amantadine. As with other movement disorders, the treatment of this condition should be strictly individualized. The physician should also be

TABLE 20–17

Dyskinesias Induced by Drugs Other than Neuroleptics and Levodopa

Authors	Date	Drug	N	Reversible Dyskinesia	Location of Dyskinesia
Cotzias et al.[75]	1970	Apomorphine	5	yes	Mouth
Pearce[282]	1970	Amantadine	1	yes	Lingual-facial
Ashcroft, Eccleston, and Waddell[9]	1965	Amphetamines[a]	?	yes	Oral-lingual-facial and limbs
Mattson and Calverley[255]	1968	Dextroamphetamine	4	?	Jaw (lateral movements)
Eveloff[134]	1968	Dextroamphetamine	1	?	Oral-facial and limbs and trunk
Mattson and Calverley[255]	1968	Methylphenidate	1	yes	
Golden[166]	1974	Methylphenidate	1	yes	
Denckla, Bemporad, and Mackay[116]	1976	Methylphenidate	20	yes	
Brandon[31]	1969	Fenfluramine	1	yes	Teeth (grinding) and facial
Stancer[337]	1979	MAOI and lithium	2	not on lithium alone	Jaw (chewing)
Sedivec, Valenova, and Paceltova[307]	1970	Tricyclics	5	yes?	Oral-facial
Fann, Sullivan, and Richman[139]	1976	Tricyclics	2	yes	Oral-facial (choreoathetosis)
Deckret et al.[111]	1977	Tricyclics	1	yes?	Oral
Woogen, Graham, and Angrist[373]	1981	Tricyclics	1	yes?	Oral
Thach, Chase, and Bosma[349]	1975	Antihistamines	2	50%	Oral-lingual-facial (blepharospasm), upper limbs
Davis[109]	1976	Antihistamines	1	yes	Left oral-facial (blepharospasm)
Kirschberg[223]	1975	Ethosuximide, phenobarbital, phenytoin	1	yes	
Joyce and Gunderson[206]	1980	Carbamazepine	1	yes	
Chadwick, Reynolds, and Marsden[55]	1976	Phenytoin	numerous	yes	
Kaplan and Murkofsky[211]	1978	Benzodiazepines		yes	Oral-buccal
Rosenbaum and De La Fuente[299]	1979	Benzodiazepines	5	yes	Oro-facial
Akindele and Odejide[2]	1976	4-aminoquinolines	4	yes	Lingual and neck
Umez-Eronini and Eronini[354]	1977	4-aminoquinolines	5	yes	Hands

[a] A large amount of the literature on dextroamphetamine-induced dyskinesias comes from Sweden, where these dyskinesias are considered a part of the "punding" syndrome.

aware of the potential for anticholinergic-induced delirium and other adverse effects of the combined anticholinergic activity of the antiparkinsonian and neuroleptic drugs.

Among the late-onset, neuroleptic-induced movement disorders other than TD, we have mentioned tardive dystonia, tardive parkinsonism, tardive Tourette's syndrome,[203,264] and other encephalopathies. There have been only a few case reports of these conditions, and their etiological relationship to neuroleptics is still controversial. As reported, disorders of these types tend to be disabling and do not show a tendency to improve with the passage of time, whether the neuroleptic treatment is continued or interrupted. They resemble the naturally occurring diseases of the CNS and tend to be underdiagnosed as neuroleptic-induced persistent side effects. It is very likely, however, that at least some movement disorders developing during or soon after discontinuation of neuroleptic treatment may have been caused by these drugs.

Nonneuroleptic Drug-induced Dyskinesias

The only nonneuroleptic drugs that have been commonly associated with TDs have been catecholaminergic agents such as levodopa, d-amphetamine, and methylphenidate hydrochloride (see table 20–17). Levodopa-induced dyskinesias usually occur after long-term and high-dosage treatment of patients with Parkinson's disease. Methylphenidate presumably induces movement disorders in some patients with minimal brain dysfunction, whereas dextroamphetamine is believed to induce it in some chronic amphetamine abusers.

In a recent paper, Karson and associates[214] compared regions of motor involvement as affected by levodopa-induced and neuroleptic-induced dyskinesias. The investigators reported that in neuroleptic-induced TD, there is a predominance of orofacial movement disorder, whereas in levodopa-induced dyskinesias the lower extremities were more commonly affected. These findings may suggest different pathophysiological mechanisms for these two different entities.

In most patients the movement disorders induced by nonneuroleptic drugs appear to be heterogenous in severity and quality,

TABLE 20–18
Other Movement Disorders

Disorders Primarily Affecting the Basal Ganglia

Huntington's chorea
Parkinson's disease
Striatonigral degeneration
Sydenham's chorea
Wilson's disease (hepatolenticular degeneration)
Fahr's syndrome
Hallervorden-Spatz disease

Disorders of the Cerebellum

Cerebellar ataxias, etc.

Miscellaneous Movement Disorders

Tourette's syndrome
Paroxysmal choreoathetosis
Creutzfeldt-Jakob disease (with myoclonus)
Progressive supranuclear palsy
Periodic dystonia
Dystonia musculorum deformans
Epilepsia partialis continua
Palatal myoclonus
Meige syndrome
Breughel syndrome
Spontaneous akathisia
Spontaneous movement disorders in psychiatric patients
Chorea gravidarum
Conversion disorders
Senile hyperkinesias

Movement Disorders Secondary to:

Multiple sclerosis
Hypoparathyroidism
Thyrotoxicosis
Systemic lupus erythematosus
Henoch-Schonlein's purpura
Encephalitis
Dementia
Post-anoxic syndromes
Cerebral trauma
Cerebrovascular accidents
Poisoning
Psychosis

TABLE 20-19

Summary of Movement Disorders Involving the Basal Ganglia

	Huntington's Chorea	Parkinson's Disease	Striatonigral Degeneration	Sydenham's Chorea	Wilson's Disease	Hallervorden-Spatz Disease
Average Age of Onset	30–50	50–60	50–65	5–15	20–30	10–15
Characteristic Abnormal Movements	Chorea	Bradykinesia, tremor (pill rolling)	Chorea, tremor	Chorea	Tremor (wing beating)	Dystonia, choreoathetosis
Common Neuropsychiatric Associations						
• Dementia	Yes	Yes	Yes	No	Yes	Yes
• Affective Disorders	Yes	Yes	Yes	Rare	Yes	?
• Psychoses	Yes	Uncommon (except drug-induced)	?	Schizophrenia?	Yes	?
Major Sites of Pathology in Basal Ganglia	Striatum	Substantia nigra	Striatum, Substantia nigra	Caudate ?, subthalamic nuclei ?	Globus pallidus, putamen	Substantia nigra, globus pallidus, red nucleus
Major Neurotransmitters Implicated	GABA, ? somatostatin	Dopamine, norepinephrine	Dopamine	?	?	?
Genetics	Autosomal dominant	a	a	a	Usually autosomal recessive	Autosomal recessive
Other Characteristics	Rigidity in Westphal variant (early onset)	Sometimes secondary to other etiologies	Nonresponsive to levodopa	Postgroup A streptococcal infection	Kayser-Fleisher rings in cornea; hepatic failure, low serum ceruloplasmin	Iron deposition in basal ganglia

SOURCE: D. V. Jeste, J. A. Grebb, and R. J. Wyatt, "Psychiatric Aspects of Movement Disorders and Demyelinating Diseases," in *Psychiatry Update*, vol. 4 (Washington, D.C.: American Psychiatric Press, 1985).

[a] No identified genetic basis; however, familial cases have been reported.

even within a patient group treated with an identical drug. The dyskinesias appear in many cases as an idiosyncratic reaction to the drug and tend to disappear within days to weeks after withdrawal of the responsible drugs.

Persistent "TDs" induced by non-neuroleptic drugs are rarely reported. There is no good evidence that nonneuroleptics have produced persistent TD in patients without firm evidence of structural brain damage.

Other Movement Disorders

In table 20–18 we have listed other movement disorders that may be encountered in neuropsychiatric practice. Many of these are discussed at length in other chapters in this volume.

Table 20–19 summarizes important clinical features of some of the spontaneously occurring movement disorders.

¶ Acknowledgment

The authors would like to express their appreciation to Dr. Craig N. Karson and Dr. Joel E. Kleinman for their suggestions in writing this chapter and to Ms. Denise Ondrish and Ms. Theresa Robbins for preparing the manuscript.

¶ Bibliography

1. AHMAD, S., et al. "Involuntary Movements Caused by Phenytoin Intoxication in Epileptic Patients," *Journal of Neurology, Neurosurgery and Psychiatry,* 38 (1975):225–231.
2. AKINDELE, M. O., and ODEJIDE, A. O. "Amodiaquine-induced Involuntary Movements," *British Medical Journal,* 2 (1976):214–215.
3. ALBANESE, H., and GAARDER, K. "Biofeedback Treatment of Tardive Dyskinesia: Two Case Reports," *American Journal of Psychiatry,* 134 (1977):1149–1150.
4. ALLEN, R. E., and STIMMEL, G. L. "Neuroleptic Dosage, Duration, and Tardive Dyskinesia," *Journal of Clinical Psychiatry,* 38 (1977):385–387.
5. ALPERT, M., and FRIEDHOFF, A. J. "Clinical Application of Receptor Modification," in W. E. Fann, et al., eds., *Tardive Dyskinesia: Research and Treatment.* New York: SP Medical & Scientific Books, 1980, pp. 471–473.
6. AMSTERDAM, J., and MENDELS, J. "Treatment-resistant Tardive Dyskinesia: A New Therapeutic Approach," *American Journal of Psychiatry,* 136 (1979): 1197–1198.
7. ———. "Baclofen and Tardive Dyskinesia," *American Journal of Psychiatry,* 137 (1980):634.
8. ANANTH, J. V., BAN, T. A., and LEHMANN, H. E. "An Uncontrolled Study with Thiopropazate in the Treatment of Persistent Dyskinesia," *Psychopharmacology Bulletin,* 13 (1977):9.
9. ASHCROFT, G. W., ECCLESTON, D., and WADDELL, J. L. "Recognition of Amphetamine Addicts," *British Medical Journal,* 1 (1965):57.
10. ASNIS, G. M., and LEOPOLD, M. A. "A Single-blind Study of ECT in Patients with Tardive Dyskinesia," *American Journal of Psychiatry,* 135 (1978):1235–1237.
11. ASNIS, G. M., et al. "A Survey of Tardive Dyskinesia in Psychiatric Outpatients," *American Journal of Psychiatry,* 134 (1977):1267–1370.
12. ATSMON, A., et al. "Further Studies with Propranolol in Psychotic Patients," *Psychopharmacologia,* 27 (1972):249–254.
13. AYD, F. J., JR. "Respiratory Dyskinesias in Patients with Neuroleptic-induced Extrapyramidal Reactions," *International Drug Therapy Newsletter,* 14 (1979):1–3.
14. BACHER, N. M., and LEWIS, H. A. "Low-dose Propranolol in Tardive Dyskinesia," *American Journal of Psychiatry,* 137 (1980):495–497.
15. BALDESSARINI, R. J., and DAVIS, J. M. "What Is the Best Maintenance Dose of Neuroleptics in Schizophrenia?" *Psychiatry Research,* 3 (1980):115–122.
16. BALDESSARINI, R. J., and TARSY, D. "Tardive Dyskinesia," in M. A. Lipton, A. DiMascio, and K. F. Killam, eds., *Psychopharmacology: A Generation of*

Progress. New York: Raven Press, 1978, pp. 993–1004.

17. ———. "Relationship of Actions of Neuroleptic Drugs to the Pathophysiology of Tardive Dyskinesia," *International Review of Neurobiology,* 21 (1979):1–45.

18. BARBEAU, A. "Lecithin in Neurologic Disorders," *New England Journal of Medicine,* 299 (1978):200–201.

19. BARTHOLINI, G., and PLETSCHER, A. "Atropine-induced Changes of Cerebral Dopamine Turnover," *Experientia,* 27 (1971):1302.

20. BARTHOLINI, G., and SANDLER, H. "Cholinergic and GABAergic Influence on the Dopamine Release in Extrapyramidal Centers," in O. Almgren, A. Carlsson, and J. Engel, eds., *Chemical Tools in Catecholamine Research,* vol. 2. Amsterdam: North-Holland, 1975, pp. 235–241.

21. BATEMAN, D. N., et al. "Metoclopramide and Haloperidol in Tardive Dyskinesia," *British Journal of Psychiatry,* 135 (1979):505–508.

22. BEDARD, P., LANGELIER, P., and VILLENEUVE, A. "Oestrogen and Extrapyramidal System," *Lancet,* 2 (1977): 1367–1368.

23. BEITMAN, B. D. "Tardive Dyskinesia Reinduced by Lithium Carbonate," *American Journal of Psychiatry,* 135 (1978):1229–1230.

24. BETTS, W. C., JOHNSTON, F. S., and PRATT, M. J. "An Effective Palliative Treatment for Phenothiazine-induced Tardive Dyskinesia," *North Carolina Medical Journal,* 40 (1979):286.

25. BIRKET-SMITH, E., and ANDERSEN, J. V. "Treatment of Side Effects of Levodopa," *Lancet,* 1 (1973):431.

26. BJORNDAL, N., CASEY, D. E., and GERLACH, J. "Enkephalin, Morphine, and Naloxone in Tardive Dyskinesia," *Psychopharmacology,* 69 (1980):133–136.

27. BOCKENHEIMER, S., and LUCIUS, G. "Zur Therapie mit Dimethylaminoethanol (Deanol) bei Neurolepikaninduzierten Extrapyramidalen Hyperkinesen," *Archiv für Psychiatrie und Nervenkrankheiten* (Berlin), 222 (1976):69–75.

28. BOWERS, M. B., JR., MOORE, D., and TARSY, D. "Tardive Dyskinesia: A Clinical Test of the Supersensitivity Hypoth-

esis," *Psychopharmacology,* 61 (1979): 137–141.

29. BRANCHEY, M., and BRANCHEY, L. "Patterns of Psychotropic Drug Use and Tardive Dyskinesia," *Journal of Clinical Psychopharmacology,* 4 (1984):41–45.

30. BRANCHEY, M. H., et al. "Lecithin in the Treatment of Tardive Dyskinesia," *Communications in Psychopharmacology,* 3 (1979):303–307.

31. BRANDON, S. "Unusual Effect of Fenfluramine." *British Medical Journal,* 4 (1969):557–558.

32. BRANDON, S., McCLELLAND, H. A., and PROTHEROE, C. "A Study of Facial Dyskinesia in a Mental Hospital Population," *British Journal of Psychiatry,* 118 (1971):171–184.

33. BRANDRUP, E. "Tetrabenazine Treatment in Persisting Dyskinesia Caused by Psychopharmacy," *American Journal of Psychiatry,* 118 (1961):551–552.

34. BUCCI, L. "The Dyskinesias: A New Therapeutic Approach," *Diseases of the Nervous System,* 32 (1971):324–327.

35. BULLOCK, R. J. "Efficacy of Thiopropazate Dihydrochloride (Dartalan) in Treating Persisting Phenothiazine-induced Choreoathetosis and Akathisia," *Medical Journal of Australia,* 2 (1972):314–316.

36. BUNNEY, B. S., and AGHAJANIAN, G. K. "Dopaminergic Influence in the Basal Ganglia: Evidence for Striatonigral Feedback Regulation," in M. D. Yahr, ed., *The Basal Ganglia.* New York: Raven Press, 1976, pp. 249–267.

37. BUNNEY, W. E., et al. "Mode of Action of Lithium," *Archives of General Psychiatry,* 36 (1979):898–901.

38. BURNETT, G. N., et al. "Adverse Effects of Anticholinergic Antiparkinsonian Drugs in Tardive Dyskinesia," *Neuropsychobiology,* 6 (1980):109–120.

39. CAINE, E. D., et al. "Gilles de la Tourette's Syndrome, Tardive Dyskinesia, and Psychosis in an Adolescent," *American Journal of Psychiatry,* 135 (1978):241–243.

40. CAINE, E. D., et al. "Trial Use of Clozapine for Abnormal Involuntary Movement Disorders," *American Journal of Psychiatry,* 136 (1979):317–320.

41. CALNE, D. B., et al. "Pimozide in Tardive

Dyskinesia," *Transactions of the American Neurological Association,* 99 (1974):166–170.

42. CARLSON, K. R. " 'Tardive Dyskinesia' Resulting from Chronic Narcotic Treatment," in W. E. Fann, et al., eds., *Tardive Dyskinesia: Research and Treatment.* New York: SP Medical & Scientific Books, 1980, pp. 27–33.

43. CARLSSON, A., and LINDQUIST, M. "Effect of Chlorpromazine on Formation of 3-methoxytyramine and Normetanephrine in Mouse Brain," *Acta Pharmacologica et Toxicologica,* 20 (1963):140–144.

44. CARPENTER, M. B. "Anatomical Organization of the Corpus Striatum and Related Nuclei," in M. D. Yahr, ed., *The Basal Ganglia.* New York: Raven Press, 1976, pp. 1–36.

45. CARROLL, B. J., CURTIS, G. C., and KOKMEN, E. "Paradoxical Response to Dopamine Agonists in Tardive Dyskinesia," *American Journal of Psychiatry,* 134, (1977):785–789.

46. CARRUTHERS, S. G. "Persistent Tardive Dyskinesia," *British Medical Journal,* 3 (1971):572.

47. CASEY, D. E. "Deanol in the Management of Involuntary Movement Disorders: A Review," *Diseases of the Nervous System,* 38 (Supplement), (1977):7–15.

48. ———. "Mood Alterations During Deanol Therapy," *Psychopharmacology,* 62 (1979):187–191.

49. CASEY, D. E., and DENNEY, D. "Dimethylaminoethanol in Tardive Dyskinesia," *New England Journal of Medicine,* 29 (1974):797.

50. ———. "Deanol in the Treatment of Tardive Dyskinesia," *American Journal of Psychiatry,* 132 (1975):864–867.

51. CASEY, D. E., and GERLACH, J. "Oxiperomide in Tardive Dyskinesia," *Journal of Neurology, Neurosurgery and Psychiatry,* 43 (1980):264–267.

52. CASEY, D. E., and HAMMERSTAD, J. P. "Sodium Valproate in Tardive Dyskinesia," *Journal of Clinical Psychiatry,* 40 (1979):483–485.

53. CASEY, D. E., GERLACH, J., and SIMMELSGAARD, H. "Sulpiride in Tardive Dyskinesia," *Psychopharmacology,* 66 (1979):73–77.

54. CASEY, D. E., et al. "Gamma-Acetylenic

GABA in Tardive Dyskinesia," *Archives of General Psychiatry,* 37 (1980):1376–1379.

55. CHADWICK, D., REYNOLDS, E. H., and MARSDEN, C. D. "Anticonvulsant-induced Dyskinesia: A Comparison with Dyskinesias Induced by Neuroleptics," *Journal of Neurology, Neurosurgery and Psychiatry,* 39 (1976):1210–1218.

56. CHASE, T. N. "Catecholamine Metabolism and Neurological Disease," in E. Usdin and S. H. Snyder, eds., *Frontiers in Catecholamine Research.* New York: Pergamon Press, 1973, pp. 1127–1132.

57. CHASE, T. N., and TAMMINGA, C. A. "GABA System Participation in Human Motor, Cognitive, and Endocrine Function," in P. Korsgaard-Larsen, J. Scheel-Kruger, and H. Kofod, eds., *GABA-Neurotransmitters.* New York: Academic Press, 1979.

58. CHASE, T. N., SCHNUR, J. A., and GORDON, E. K. "Cerebrospinal Fluid Monoamine Catabolites in Drug-induced Extrapyramidal Disorders," *Neuropharmacology,* 9 (1970):265–268.

59. CHEIN, C., DiMASCIO, A., and COLE, J. O. "Antiparkinsonian Agents and a Depot Phenothiazine," *American Journal of Psychiatry,* 131 (1974):86–90.

60. CHIEN, C., JUNG, K., and ROSS-TOWSEND, A. "Efficacies of Agents Related to GABA, Dopamine and Acetylcholine in the Treatment of Tardive Dyskinesia," *Psychopharmacology Bulletin,* 14 (1978):20–22.

61. CHOUINARD, G., and JONES, B. D. "Early Onset of Tardive Dyskinesia: Case Report," *American Journal of Psychiatry,* 136 (1979):1323–1324.

62. CHOUINARD, G., DE MONTIGNY, C., and ANNABLE, L. "Tardive Dyskinesia and Antiparkinsonian Medication," *American Journal of Psychiatry,* 136 (1979): 228–229.

63. CHOUINARD, G., et al. "Factors Related to Tardive Dyskinesia," *American Journal of Psychiatry,* 136 (1979):79–83.

64. CHRISTENSEN, A. V., and NIELSEN, I. M. "Dopaminergic Supersensitivity: Influence of Dopamine Agonists, Cholinergics, Anticholinergics, and Drugs Used for the Treatment of Tardive Dyskine-

sia," *Psychopharmacology*, 62 (1979): 111–116.

65. CHRISTENSEN, E., MOLLER, J. E., and FAURBYE, A. "Neurological Investigation of 28 Brains from Patients with Dyskinesia," *Acta Psychiatrica Scandinavica*, 46 (1970):14–23.

66. CLAVERIA, L. E., et al. "Tardive Dyskinesia Treated with Pimozide," *Journal of the Neurological Sciences*, 24 (1975): 393–401.

67. CLOW, A., et al. "Striatal Dopamine Receptors Become Supersensitive While Rats Are Given Trifluoperazine for Six Months." *Nature*, 278 (1979):59–61.

68. COHEN, B. M., HERSCHEL, M., and AOBA, A. "Neuroleptic, Antimuscarinic, and Antiadrenergic Activity of Chlorpromazine, Thioridazine, and Their Metabolites," *Psychiatry Research*, 1 (1979):199–208.

69. COHEN, D. J., et al. "Clonidine Ameliorates Gilles de la Tourette Syndrome," *Archives of General Psychiatry*, 37 (1980):1350–1357.

70. COLE, J. O., GARDOS, G., and GRANACHER, R. "Drug Evaluations in Tardive Dyskinesia." Paper presented at the annual meeting of the American Psychiatric Association, Miami Beach, Florida, May 1976.

71. COLE, J. O., et al. "Drug Trials in Persistent Dyskinesia," in W. E. Fann, et al., eds., *Tardive Dyskinesia: Research and Treatment*. New York: SP Medical & Scientific Books, 1980, pp. 419–427.

72. COOK, D. G., FAHN, S., and BRAIT, K. A. "Chronic Manganese Intoxication," *Archives of Neurology*, 30 (1974):59–65.

73. COOPER, J. R., BLOOM, F. E., and ROTH, R. H. *The Biochemical Basis of Neuropharmacology*, 3rd ed. New York: Oxford University Press, 1978.

74. COSTALL, B., and NAYLOR, R. J. "Neurolepetic Antagonism of Dyskinetic Phenomena," *European Journal of Pharmacology*, 33 (1975):301–312.

75. COTZIAS, G. C., et al. "Similarities Between Neurologic Effects of L-dopa and of Apomorphine," *New England Journal of Medicine*, 282 (1970):31–33.

76. CRANE, G. E. "Dyskinesia and Neurolep-

tics," *Archives of General Psychiatry*, 19 (1968):700–703.

77. ———. "High Doses of Trifluoperazine and Tardive Dyskinesia," *Archives of Neurology*, 22 (1970):176–180.

78. ———. "Prevention and Management of Tardive Dyskinesia," *American Journal of Psychiatry*, 129 (1972):126–127.

79. ———. "Pseudoparkinsonism and Tardive Dyskinesia," *Archives of Neurology*, 30 (1972):426–430.

80. ———. "Clinical Psychopharmacology in Its 20th Year," *Science*, 181 (1973):124–128.

81. ———. "Mediocre Effects of Reserpine on Tardive Dyskinesia," *New England Journal of Medicine*, 288 (1973):104–105.

82. ———. "Rapid Reversal of Tardive Dyskinesia," *American Journal of Psychiatry*, 130 (1973):1159.

83. ———. "Deanol for Tardive Dyskinesia," *New England Journal of Medicine*, 292 (1975):926.

84. ———. "The Prevention of Tardive Dyskinesia," *American Journal of Psychiatry*, 134 (1977):757–759.

85. CRANE, G. E., and PAULSON, G. W. "Involuntary Movements in a Sample of Chronic Mental Patients and Their Relation to the Treatment with Neuroleptics," *International Journal of Neuropsychiatry*, 3 (1967):286–291.

86. CRANE, G. E., and SMEETS, R. A. "Tardive Dyskinesia and Drug Therapy in Geriatric Patients," *Archives of General Psychiatry*, 30 (1974):341–343.

87. CRANE, G. E., TUREK, I. S., and KURLAND, A. A. "Failure of Pyridoxine to Reduce Drug-induced Dyskinesia," *Journal of Neurology, Neurosurgery and Psychiatry*, 33 (1970):511–512.

88. CRANE, G. E., et al. "Effects of Drug Withdrawal on Tardive Dyskinesia," *Journal of Neurology, Neurosurgery and Psychiatry*, 33 (1969):511–512.

89. CRAYTON, J. W., et al. "Electrophysiological (H-reflex) Studies of Patients with Tardive Dyskinesia," *American Journal of Psychiatry*, 134 (1977):775–781.

90. CREWS, E. L., and CARPENTER, A. E. "Lithium-induced Aggravation of Tardive Dyskinesia," *American Journal of Psychiatry*, 134 (1977):933.

91. CROW, T. J. Personal communication, 1983.

92. CROW, T. J., et al. "Tardive Dyskinesia: Disease Process on Drug Effect," in C. Perris, G. Strüwe, and B. Jansson, eds., *Proceedings of Third World Congress of Biological Psychiatry, Stockholm, 1981.* Amsterdam: Elsevier/North-Holland Publication, pp. 860–864.

93. CURRAN, D. J., NAGASWAMI, S., and MOHAN, K. J. "Treatment of Phenothiazine-induced Bulbar Persistent Dyskinesia with Deanol Acetamidobenzoate," *Diseases of the Nervous System,* 36 (1975):71–73.

94. CURRAN, J. P. "Management of Tardive Dyskinesia with Thiopropazate," *American Journal of Psychiatry,* 130 (1973):925–927.

95. CURZON, G. "Involuntary Movements Other than Parkinsonism: Biochemical Aspects," *Proceedings of the Royal Society of Medicine,* 66 (1973):873.

96. CUTLER, N. R., et al. "Depression-dependent Dyskinesias in Two Cases of Manic-depressive Illness," *New England Journal of Medicine,* 304 (1981):1088–1089.

97. DAHADELAH, M. P., SMALL, M., and THOMAS, D. J. "Dimethylaminoethanol in Blepharospasm and Hemifacial Spasm," *New England Journal of Medicine,* 293 (1975):98.

98. DALEN, P. "Lithium Therapy in Huntington's Chorea and Tardive Dyskinesia," *Lancet,* 1 (1973):107–108.

99. DAVIS, J. M. "Antipsychotic Drugs," in H. I. Kaplan, A. M. Freedman, and B. J. Sadock, eds., *Comprehensive Textbook of Psychiatry,* vol. 3, 3rd ed. Baltimore: Williams & Wilkins, 1980, pp. 2257–2289.

100. DAVIS, K. L., and BERGER, P. A. "Pharmacological Investigations of the Cholinergic Imbalance Hypothesis of Movement Disorders and Psychosis," *Biological Psychiatry,* 13 (1978):23–49.

101. DAVIS, K. L., BERGER, P. A., and HOLLISTER, L. E. "Choline for Tardive Dyskinesia," *New England Journal of Medicine,* 293 (1975):152.

102. ———. "Deanol in Tardive Dyskinesia," *American Journal of Psychiatry,* 134 (1977):807.

103. DAVIS, K. L., et al. "Choline Chloride in the Treatment of Huntington's Disease and Tardive Dyskinesia: A Preliminary Report," *Psychopharmacology Bulletin,* 13 (1977):37–38.

104. DAVIS, K. L., et al. "Choline in Tardive Dyskinesia and Huntington's Disease," *Life Sciences,* 19 (1976):1507–1516.

105. DAVIS, K. L., et al. "Choline Chloride in Animal Models of Tardive Dyskinesia," *Life Sciences,* 22 (1978):1699–1708.

106. DAVIS, K. L., et al. "Dimethylaminoethanol (Deanol): Effect on Apomorphine-induced Sterotypy and an Animal Model of Tardive Dyskinesia," *Psychopharmacology,* 63 (1979):143–146.

107. DAVIS, K. L., et al. "Cholinergic Aspects of Tardive Dyskinesia: Human and Animal Studies," in W. E. Fann, et al., eds., *Tardive Dyskinesia: Research and Treatment.* New York: SP Medical & Scientific Books, 1980, pp. 395–403.

108. DAVIS, K. L., et al. "MSH and MIF-I in Animal Models of Tardive Dyskinesia," *Pharmacology, Biochemistry and Behavior,* 13 (1980):37–40.

109. DAVIS, W. A. "Dyskinesia Associated with Chronic Antihistamine Use," *New England Journal of Medicine,* 294 (1976):113.

110. DECKER, B. L., et al. "Amantadine Hydrochloride Treatment of Tardive Dyskinesia," *New England Journal of Medicine,* 285 (1971):860.

111. DECKRET, J. J., et al. "A Case of Oral Dyskinesia Associated with Imipramine Treatment," *American Journal of Psychiatry,* 134 (1977):1297–1298.

112. DEGKWITZ, R. "Extrapyramidal Motor Disorders Following Long-term Treatment with Neuroleptic Drugs," in G. E. Crane and J. R. Gardner, Jr., eds., *Psychotropic Drugs and Dysfunctions of the Basal Ganglia* (U.S. Public Health Service Publication No. 1938). Washington, D.C.: U.S. Government Printing Office, 1969, pp. 22–33.

113. DEGKWITZ, R., and WENZEL, W. "Persistent Extrapyramidal Side Effects After Long-term Application of Neuroleptics," in H. Bril, ed., *Neuro-Psycho-Pharmacology* (International Congress Series No. 129). New York: Excerpta Medica Foundation, 1967, pp. 608–615.

114. DEMARS, J. C. A. "Neuromuscular Effects of Long-term Phenothiazine Medication, Electroconvulsive Therapy and Leucotomy," *Journal of Nervous and Mental Disorders*, 143 (1966):73–79.

115. DE MONTIGNY, C., CHOUINARD, G., and ANNABLE, L. "Ineffectiveness of Deanol in Tardive Dyskinesia: A Placebo Controlled Study," *Psychopharmacology*, 65 (1979):219–222.

116. DENCKLA, M. B., BEMPORAD, J. R., and MACKAY, M. C. "Tics Following Methylphenidate Administration," *Journal of the American Medical Association*, 235 (1976):1349–1351.

117. DESILVA, L., and HUANG, C. Y. "Deanol in Tardive Dyskinesia," *British Medical Journal*, 3 (1975):466.

118. DEVEAUGH-GEISS, J. "Aggravation of Tardive Dyskinesia by Phenytoin," *New England Journal of Medicine*, 298 (1978):457–458.

119. DEVEAUGH-GEISS, J., and MANION, L. "High-dose Pyridoxine in Tardive Dyskinesia," *Journal of Clinical Psychiatry*, 39 (1978):573–575.

120. DIAMOND, B. I., and BORISON, R. L. "The Role of Enkephalins in Tardive Dyskinesia," *Neurology*, 29 (1979):605–606.

121. DOONGAJI, D. R. "The Treatment of Tardive Dyskinesia with Penfluperidol: A Case Report," *Neurology India*, 25 (1977):244–246.

122. DOONGAJI, D. R., et al. "Effects of Intravenous Metoclopramide in 81 Patients with Tardive Dyskinesia," *Journal of Clinical Psychopharmacology*, 2 (1983):376–379.

123. DRAVET, C., et al. "Dyskinesies paroxystiques au cours des traitements par la diphenylhydantoine," *Revue Neurologique*, 136 (1980):1–14.

124. DRUCKMAN, R., SEELINGER, D., and THULIN, B. "Chronic Involuntary Movements Induced by Phenothiazines," *Journal of Nervous and Mental Diseases*, 135 (1962):69–76.

125. DUVOISIN, R. C. "Reserpine for Tardive Dyskinesia," *New England journal of Medicine*, 286 (1972):611.

126. DYNES, J. B. "Oral Dyskinesias—Occurrence and Treatment," *Diseases of the Nervous System*, 31 (1970):854–859.

127. EDWARDS, H. "Significance of Brain Damage in Persistent Oral Dyskinesia," *British Journal of Psychiatry*, 116 (1970):271–275.

128. EHRENSING, R. H. "Lithium and M.R.I.H. in Tardive Dyskinesia," *Lancet*, 2 (1974):1459–1460.

129. EHRENSING, R. H., et al. "Melanocyte-stimulating Hormone Release-inhibiting Factor-1 and Tardive Dyskinesia," *Diseases of the Nervous System*, 38 (1977):303–306.

130. ENGELHARDT, D. M., POLIZOS, P., and WAIZER, J. "CNS Consequences of Psychotropic Drug Withdrawal in Autistic Children: A Follow-up Report," *Psychopharmacology Bulletin*, 11 (1975):6–7.

131. ERESHEFSKY, L., RUBIN, T. N., and FRIEDMAN, S. "Treatment of Tardive Dyskinesia and Mania with RBC Lithium Determinations," *American Journal of Psychiatry*, 136 (1979):570–573.

132. ESCOBAR, J. I., and KEMP, K. F. "Dimethylaminoethanol for Tardive Dyskinesia," *New England Journal of Medicine*, 292 (1975):317–318.

133. EVANS, J. H. "Persistent Oral Dyskinesia in Treatment with Phenothiazine Derivatives," *Lancet*, 1 (1965):458–460.

134. EVELOFF, H. H. "A Case of Amphetamine-induced Dyskinesia," *Journal of the American Medical Association*, 204 (1968):933.

135. FAHN, S. "Treatment of Tardive Dyskinesia with Combined Reserpine and Alpha-methyl-tyrosine," *Transactions of the American Neurological Association*, 103 (1978):100–103.

136. FAMUYIWA, O. O., et al. "Tardive Dyskinesia and Dementia," *British Journal of Psychiatry*, 135 (1979):590–594.

137. FANN, W. E., DAVIS, J. M., and JANOWSKY, D. S. "The Prevalence of Tardive Dyskinesia in Mental Hospital Patients," *Diseases of the Nervous System*, 33 (1972): 590–594.

138. FANN, W. E., DAVIS, J. M., and WILSON, I. C. "Methylphenidate in Tardive Dyskinesia," *American Journal of Psychiatry*, 130 (1973):922–924.

139. FANN, W. E., SULLIVAN, J. L., and RICHMAN, B. W. "Tardive Dyskinesia Associated with Tricyclic Antidepressants," *British Journal of Psychiatry*, 128 (1976):490–493.

140. FANN, W. E., et al. "Cholinergic Suppression of Tardive Dyskinesia," *Psychopharmacologia* (Berlin), 37 (1974):101–107.

141. FANN, W. E., et al. "Deanol in Tardive Dyskinesia: A Preliminary Report" *Psychopharmacologia* (Berlin), 42 (1975): 135–137.

142. FAURBYE, A. "The Structural and Biochemical Basis of Movement Disorders in Treatment with Neuroleptic Drugs and in Extrapyramidal Diseases," *Comprehensive Psychiatry*, 11 (1970):205–225.

143. FAURBYE, A., et al. "Neurological Symptoms in Pharmacotherapy of Psychoses," *Acta Psychiatrica Scandinavica*, 40 (1964):10–27.

144. FEDER, R., and MOORE, D. C. "Baclofen and Tardive Dyskinesia," *American Journal of Psychiatry*, 137 (1980):633–634.

145. FRANGOS, E., and CHRISTODOULIDES, H. "Clinical Observations on the Treatment of Tardive Dyskinesia with Haloperidol," *Acta Psychiatrica Belgica*, 75 (1975):19–32.

146. FRATTOLA, L., et al. "Treatment of Dyskinetic and Dystonic Disorders with CF 25-397: Clinical and Pharmacological Aspects," in M. Goldstein, et al., eds., *Ergot Compounds and Brain Function*. New York: Raven Press, 1980, pp. 381–386.

147. FREEDMAN, H., and SONI, S. D. "Oxypertine for Tardive Dyskinesia," *British Journal of Psychiatry*, 137 (1980):522–523.

148. FREEDMAN, R. "Interactions of Antipsychotic Drugs with Norepinephrine and Cerebellar Neuronal Circuitry: Implications for the Psychobiology of Psychosis," *Biological Psychiatry*, 12 (1977):181–197.

149. FREEDMAN R., BELL, J., and KIRCH, D. "Clonidine Therapy for Coexisting Psychosis and Tardive Dyskinesia," *American Journal of Psychiatry*, 137 (1980): 629–630.

150. FREEDMAN, R., et al. "Clonidine Treatment of Schizophrenia. Double-blind Comparison to Placebo and Neuroleptic Drugs," *Acta Psychiatrica Scandinavica*, 65 (1982):25–45.

151. GARDOS, G., and COLE, J. O. "Papverine for Tardive Dyskinesia?" *New England Journal of Medicine*, 292 (1975):1355.

152. ———. "Pilot Study of Cyproheptadine (Periactin) in Tardive Dyskinesia." *Psychopharmacology Bulletin*, 14 (1978): 18–20.

153. GARDOS, G., COLE, J. O., and SNIFFIN, C. "An Evaluation of Papaverine in Tardive Dyskinesia," *Journal of Clinical Pharmacology*, 16 (1976):304–310.

154. GARDOS, G., COLE, J. O., and SOKOL, M. "Pitfalls in the Assessment of Tardive Dyskinesia." Paper presented at the Sixth World Congress of Psychiatry, Honolulu, August 28-September 3, 1977.

155. GELENBERG, A. J. "Computerized Tomography in Patients with Tardive Dyskinesia," *American Journal of Psychiatry*, 133 (1976):578–579.

156. GELENBERG, A. J., DOLLER-WOJCIK, J. C., and GROWDON, J. H. "Choline and Lecithin in the Treatment of Tardive Dyskinesia: Preliminary Results from a Pilot Study, *American Journal of Psychiatry*, 136 (1979):772–776.

157. GERBINO, L., SHOPSIN, B., and COLLORA, M. "Clozapine in the Treatment of Tardive Dyskinesia: An Interim Report," in W. E. Fann, et al., eds., *Tardive Dyskinesia: Research and Treatment*. New York: SP Medical & Scientific Books, 1980, pp. 475–489.

158. GERLACH, J., and SIMMELSGAARD, H. "Tardive Dyskinesia During and Following Treatment with Haloperidol, Haloperidol + Biperiden, Thioridazine, and Clozapine," *Psychopharmacology*, 59 (1978):105–112.

159. GERLACH, J., REISBY, N., and RANDRUP, A. "Dopaminergic Hypersensitivity and Cholinergic Hypofunction in the Pathophysiology of Tardive Dyskinesia," *Psychopharmacologia* (Berlin), 34 (1974): 21–35.

160. GERLACH, J., RYE, T., and KRISTJANSEN, P. "Effect of Baclofen on Tardive Dyskinesia," *Psychopharmacology*, 56 (1978):145–151.

161. GERLACH, H., THORSEN, K., and MUNKVAD, I. "Effect of Lithium on Neuroleptic-induced Tardive Dyskinesia Compared with Placebo in a Double-blind

Cross-over Trial," *Phamrakopsychiatrie*, 8 (1975):51–56.

162. GIANUTSOS, G., and LAL, H. "Alteration in the Action of Cholinergic and Anticholinergic Drugs After Chronic Haloperidol: Indirect Evidence for Cholinergic Hyposensitivity," *Life Sciences*, 18 (1976):515–520.

163. GIBSON, A. C. "Depot Injections and Tardive Dyskinesia," *British Journal of Psychiatry*, 132 (1978):361–365.

164. ———. "Sodium Valproate and Tardive Dyskinesia," *British Journal of Psychiatry*, 133 (1978):82.

165. GODWIN-AUSTEN, R. B., and CLARK, T. "Persistent Phenothiazine Dyskinesia Treated with Tetrabenazine," *British Medical Journal*, 4 (1971):25–26.

166. GOLDEN, G. S. "Gilles de la Tourette's Syndrome Following Methylphenidate Administration," *Developmental and Medical Child Neurology*, 16 (1974):76–78.

167. GOLDMAN, D. "Treatment of Phenothiazine-induced Dyskinesia," *Psychopharmacology*, 47 (1976):271–272.

168. GORDON, J. H., BORISON, R. L., and DIAMOND, B. I. "Estrogen in Experimental Tardive Dyskinesia," *Neurology*, 30 (1980):551–554.

169. GRATTON, L. "Neuroleptiques, parkinsonisme et schizophrenie," *Union Medicale du Canada*, 89 (1960):679–694.

170. GROWDON, J. H., et al. "Oral Choline Administration to Patients with Tardive Dyskinesia," *New England Journal of Medicine*, 297 (1977):524–527.

171. GROWDON, J. H., et al. "Lecithin Can Suppress Tardive Dyskinesia," *New England Journal of Medicine*, 298 (1978):1029–1030.

172. GUNNE, L. M., and BARANY, S. "Haloperidol-induced Tardive Dyskinesia in Monkeys," *Psychopharmacology*, 50 (1976):237–240.

173. HANSSEN, T., et al. "Propranolol in Schizophrenia," *Archives of General Psychiatry*, 37 (1980):685–690.

174. HARGREAVES, W. A., and GAYNOR, J. "Risk of Tardive Dyskinesia: Preliminary Hypotheses," *Psychopharmacology Bulletin*, 16 (1980):48–50.

175. HEATH, R. G. "Modulation of Emotion with a Brain Pacemaker," *Journal of Nervous and Mental Disease*, 165 (1977):300–317.

176. HEINRICH, K., WAGENER, I., and BENDER, H.-J. "Spate Extrapyramidal Hyperkinesen Bei Neuroleptischer Langzeittherapie," *Pharmakopsychiatrie, Neuro-Psychopharmakologie*, 1 (1968):169–195.

177. HOGARTY, G. E., and GOLDBERG, S. E. "Drugs and Sociotherapy in the Aftercare of Schizophrenic Patients," *Archives of General Psychiatry*, 28 (1973):54–59.

178. HORNYKIEWICZ, O. "Neurohumoral Interactions and Basal Ganglia Function and Dysfunction," in M. D. Yahr, ed., *The Basal Ganglia*. New York: Raven Press, 1976, pp. 269–280.

179. HUANG, C. C., et al. "Evaluation of Reserpine and Alphamethyldopa in the Treatment of Tardive Dyskinesia," *Psychopharmacology Bulletin*, 16 (1980):41–43.

180. HUNTER, R., EARL, C. J., and THORNICROFF, S. "An Apparently Irreversible Syndrome of Abnormal Movements Following Phenothiazine Medication," *Proceedings of the Royal Society of Medicine*, 57 (1964):758–762.

181. ITIL, T., UNVERDI, C., and MEHTA, D. "Clorazepate Dipotassium in Tardive Dyskinesia," *American Journal of Psychiatry*, 131 (1974):1291.

182. ITOH, H., and YAGI, G. "Reversibility of Tardive Dyskinesia," *Folia Psychiatrica et Neurologica Japonica*, 33 (1979):43–54.

183. ITOH, H., et al. "Irreversible Dyskinesia Associated with Long-term Usage of Psychotropic Drugs," *Annual Reports of the Pharmacopsychiatry Research Foundation*, 3 (1971):190–195.

184. ITOH, H., et al. "Serum Level of Haloperidol and Its Clinical Significance," *Progress in Neuro-psychopharmacology*, 4 (1980):171–183.

185. IVNIK, R. J. "Pseudodementia in Tardive Dyskinesia," *Psychiatric Annals*, 9 (1979):211–216.

186. JACKSON, I. V., et al. "Treatment of Tardive Dyskinesia with Lecithin," *American Journal of Psychiatry*, 136 (1979):1458–1460.

187. JANOWSKY, D. S., et al. "Effects of Amantadine on Tardive Dyskinesia and Pseudoparkinsonism," *New England Journal of Medicine*, 286 (1972):785.

188. JELLINGER, K. "Neuropathologic Findings After Neuroleptic Long-term Therapy," in L. Roizin, H. Shiraki, and N. Grcevic, eds., *Neurotoxicology*. New York: Raven Press, 1977, pp. 25–42.

189. JESTE, D. V., and WYATT, R. J. "Therapeutic Strategies Against Dyskinesia," *Archives of General Psychiatry*, 39 (1982): 803–816.

190. ———. *Understanding and Treating Tardive Dyskinesia*. New York: Guilford Press, 1982.

191. JESTE, D. V., DOONGAJI, D. R., and LINNOILA, M. "Elevated Cerebrospinal Fluid Norepinephrine in Tardive Dyskinesia," *British Journal of Psychiatry*, 144 (1984):177–180.

192. JESTE, D. V., GREBB, J. A., and WYATT, R. J. "Psychiatric Aspects of Movement Disorders and Demyelinating Diseases," in *Psychiatry Update*, vol. 4. Washington, D. C.: American Psychiatric Press, 1985.

193. JESTE, D. V., OLGIATI, S. G., and GHALI, A. Y. "Masking of Tardive Dyskinesia with Four-times-a-day Administration of Chlorpromazine," *Diseases of the Nervous System*, 38 (1977):755–758.

194. JESTE, D. V., et al. "Platelet monoamine oxidase and Plasma Dopamine-β-hydroxylase in Tardive Dyskinesia," *Lancet*, 2 (1979):850–851.

195. JESTE, D. V., et al. "Tardive Dyskinesia: Reversible and Persistent," *Archives of General Psychiatry*, 36 (1979):585–590.

196. JESTE, D. V., et al. "High Serum Neuroleptic Levels in Tardive Dyskinesia?" *New England Journal of Medicine*, 301 (1979):1184.

197. JESTE, D. V., et al. "Amphetamine Sensitivity and Dyskinesia—An Animal Model," *Indian American Journal of Psychiatry*, 21 (1979):362–369.

198. JESTE, D. V., et al. "Evaluation of CT Scans in Tardive Dyskinesia," *American Journal of Psychiatry*, 137 (1980):247–248.

199. JESTE, D. V., et al. "Computed Tomography in Tardive Dyskinesia," *British Journal of Psychiatry*, 136 (1980):606–607.

200. JESTE, D. V., et al. "A Biochemical Study of Tardive Dyskinesia in Young Male Patients," *Psychiatry Research*, 4 (1981):327–331.

201. JESTE, D. V., et al. "Lymphocyte Monoamine Oxidase and Plasma Prolactin and Growth Hormone in Tardive Dyskinesia," *Journal of Clinical Psychiatry*, 42 (1981):75–77.

202. JESTE, D. V., et al. "Ex Uno Multi: Subtyping the Schizophrenic Syndrome," *Biological Psychiatry*, 17 (1982):199–222.

203. JESTE, D. V., et al. "Low-dose Apomorphine and Bromocriptine in Neuroleptic-induced Movement Disorders," *Biological Psychiatry*, 8 (1983):1085–1091.

204. JESTE, D. V., et al. "Association of Abnormal Movement and Negative Symptoms," *Psychopharmacology Bulletin*, 20 (1984): 380–381.

205. JONES, M., and HUNTER, R. "Abnormal Movements in Patients with Chronic Psychiatric Illness," in G. E. Crane and R. Gardner, Jr., eds., *Psychotropic Drugs and Dysfunctions of the Basal Ganglia* (U.S. Public Health Service Publication No. 1938). Washington, D.C.: U.S. Government Printing Office, 1969, pp. 53–65.

206. JOYCE, R. P., and GUNDERSON, C. H. "Carbamazepine-induced Orofacial Dyskinesia," *Neurology*, 30 (1980):1333–1334.

207. JUS, A., JUS, K., and FONTAINE, P. "Long-term Treatment of Tardive Dyskinesia," *Journal of Clinical Psychiatry*, 40 (1979):72–77.

208. JUS, A., et al. "Studies on the Action of Certain Pharmacological Agents on Tardive Dyskinesia and on the Rabbit Syndrome," *International Journal of Clinical Pharmacology*, 9 (1974):138–145.

209. JUS, A., et al. "Deanol, Lithium and Placebo in the Treatment of Tardive Dyskinesia," *Neuropsychobiology*, 4 (1978): 140–149.

210. KANE, J., and SMITH, M. D. "Tardive Dyskinesia. Prevalence and Risk Factors, 1959 to 1979," *Archives of General Psychiatry*, 39 (1982):473–486.

211. KAPLAN, S. R., and MURKOFSKY, C. "Oral-buccal Dyskinesia Symptoms As-

sociated with Low-dose Benzodiazepine Treatment," *American Journal of Psychiatry,* 135 (1978):1558–1559.

212. KARASUYAMA, N., FUJII, K., and TAKAHASHI, R. "Tardive Dyskinesia," *Clinical Neurology,* 12 (1972):687.

213. KARP, J. M., et al. "Metoclopramide Treatment of Tardive Dyskinesia," *Journal of the American Medical Association,* 246 (1981):1934–1935.

214. KARSON, C. N., et al. "A Comparison of Two Iatrogenic Dyskinesias," *American Journal of Psychiatry,* 140 (1983):1504–1506.

215. KAZAMATSURI, H. "Treatment of Tardive Dyskinesia with Oxypertine: Preliminary Clinical Experience and a Brief Review of the Literature," *Comprehensive Psychiatry,* 21 (1980):352–357.

216. KAZAMATSURI, H., CHIEN, C., and COLE, J. O. "Treatment of Tardive Dyskinesia. I. Clinical Efficacy of a Dopamine-depleting Agent, Tetrabenazine," *Archives of General Psychiatry,* 27 (1972):95–99.

217. ———. "Treatment of Tardive Dyskinesia: II. Short-term Efficacy of Dopamine-blocking Agents, Haloperidol and Thiopropazate," *Archives of General Psychiatry,* 27 (1972):100–103.

218. ———. "Treatment of Tardive Dyskinesia: III. Clinical Efficacy of a Dopamine Competing Agent, Methyl-dopa," *Archives of General Psychiatry,* 27 (1972): 842–827.

219. ———. "Long-term Treatment of Tardive Dyskinesia with Haloperidol and Tetrabenazine," *American Journal of Psychiatry,* 130 (1973):479–483.

220. KILOH, L. G., SMITH, J. S., and WILLIAMS, S. E. "Antiparkinson Drugs as Causal Agents in Tardive Dyskinesia," *Medical Journal of Australia,* 2 (1973):591–593.

221. KINOSHITA, J., INOSE, T., and SAKAI, H. "Tardive Dyskinesia—Studies on Its Clinical Survey and Postmortem Examination of a Case," *Annual Reports of the Pharmacopsychiatry Research Foundation,* 4 (1972):221–228.

222. KIRCH, D. G., et al. "Plasma Homovanillic Acid and Tardive Dyskinesia During Neuroleptic Maintenance and Withdrawal," *Psychiatry Research,* 9 (1983): 217–223.

223. KIRSCHBERG, G. J., "Dyskinesia—An Unusual Reaction to Ethosuximide," *Archives of Neurology,* 32 (1975):137–138.

224. KLAWANS, H. L., JR. "The Pharmacology of Tardive Dyskinesia," *American Journal of Psychiatry,* 130 (1973):82–86.

225. ———. "Therapeutic Approaches to Neuroleptic-induced Tardive Dyskinesia," in M. D. Yahr, ed., *The Basal Ganglia.* New York: Raven Press, 1976, pp. 447–457.

226. KLAWANS, H. L., and RUBOVITZ, R. "An Experimental Model of Tardive Dyskinesia," *Journal of Neural Transmission,* 33 (1972):235–246.

227. ———. "Effect of Cholinergic and Anticholinergic Agents on Tardive Dyskinesia," *Journal of Neurology, Neurosurgery and Psychiatry,* 27 (1974):941–947.

228. KLAWANS, H. L., WEINER, W. J., and NAUSIEDA, P. A. "The Effect of Lithium on an Animal Model of Tardive Dyskinesia," *Progress in Neuro-psychopharmacology,* 1 (1977):53–60.

229. KLAWANS, H. L., et al. "Animal Models of Dyskinesia," in I. Hanin and E. Usdin, eds., *Animal Models in Psychiatry and Neurology.* New York: Pergamon Press, 1977, pp. 351–364.

230. KLAWANS, H. L., et al. "Gilles de la Tourette Syndrome After Long-term Chlorpromazine Therapy," *Neurology,* 28 (1978):1064–1066.

231. KOLLER, W. C., et al. "Oral Contraceptive-induced Chorea: Clinical and Experimental Observations," *Neurology,* 29 (1979):604.

232. KORSGAARD, S. "Baclofen (Lioresal) in the Treatment of Neuroleptic-induced Tardive Dyskinesia," *Acta Psychiatrica Scandinavica,* 54 (1976):17–24.

233. KORSGAARD, S., et al. "Vasopressin in Anergic Schizophrenia. A Cross-over Study with Lysine-8-vasopressin and Placebo," *Psychopharmacology,* 74 (1981):379–382.

234. KRUSE, W. "Persistent Muscular Restlessness After Phenothiazine Treatment: Report of 3 Cases," *American Journal of Psychiatry,* 117 (1960):152–153.

235. KULIK, F. A., and WILBUR, R. "Propranolol for Tardive Dyskinesia and Extrapyramidal Side Effects (Pseudoparkinsonism) from Neuroleptics," *Psy-*

chopharmacology Bulletin, 16 (1980):18–19.

236. KUMAR, B. B. "Treatment of Tardive Dyskinesia with Deanol," *American Journal of Psychiatry*, 133 (1976):978.

237. KUNIN, R. A. "Manganese in Dyskinesias," *American Journal of Psychiatry*, 133 (1976):105.

238. ———. "Manganese and Niacin in the Treatment of Drug-induced Dyskinesias," *Orthomolecular Psychiatry*, 5 (1976):4–27.

239. LAL, S., and ETTIGI, P. "Comparison of Thiopropazate and Trifluoperazine in Oral Dyskinesia: A Double-blind Study," *Current Therapeutic Research*, 16 (1974):990–997.

240. LAMBERT, P. O., et al. "Le Dimethylaminoethanol dans le Traitement des Dyskinesies Tardives Induites par les Neuroleptiques," *Annales Medico-Psycologiques*, 136 (1978):625–629.

241. LANGER, S. Z. "Denervation Supersensitivity," in L. L. Iversen, S. D. Iversen, and S. H. Snyder, eds., *Handbook of Psychopharmacology*, vol. 2. New York: Plenum Press, 1975, pp. 245–280.

242. LATERRE, E. C., and FORTEMPS, E. "Deanol in Spontaneous and Induced Dyskinesias," *Lancet*, 1 (1975):301.

243. LINNOILA, M., and VIUKARI, M. "Sodium Valproate and Tardive Dyskinesia," *British Journal of Psychiatry*, 134 (1979):223.

244. LINNOILA, M., VIUKARI, M., and HIETALA, O. "Effect of Sodium Valproate on Tardive Dyskinesia," *British Journal of Psychiatry*, 129 (1976):114–119.

245. LIPSIUS, L. H. "Barbiturates and Tardive Dyskinesia," *American Journal of Psychiatry*, 134 (1977):1162–1163.

246. LONOWSKI, D. J., STERLING, F. E., and KING, H. A. "Electromyographic Assessment of Dimethylaminoethanol (Deanol) in Treatment of Tardive Dyskinesia," *Psychological Reports*, 45 (1979):415–419.

247. McANDREW, J. B., CASE, Q., and TREFFERT, D. A. "Effects of Prolonged Phenothiazine Intake on Psychotic and Other Hospitalized Children," *Journal of Autism and Childhood Schizophrenia*, 2 (1972):75–91.

248. MacCALLUM, W. A. G. "Tetrabenazine for Extrapyramidal Movement Disorders," *British Medical Journal*, 1 (1970):-760.

249. MACKAY, A. V. P., and SHEPPARD, G. P. "Pharmacotherapeutic Trials in Tardive Dyskinesia," *British Journal of Psychiatry*, 135 (1979):489–499.

250. MAJUMDAR, S. K. "Mechanism of Chloroquine-induced Involuntary Movements," *British Medical Journal*, 1 (1977):1350.

251. MAKMAN, M. H., et al. "Aging and Monoamine Receptors in the Brain," *Federation Proceedings*, 38 (1979):1922–1926.

252. MALLYA, A., et al. "Antiparkinsonics, Neuroleptics and Tardive Dyskinesia," *Biological Psychiatry*, 14 (1979):645–649.

253. MARTENSSON, E., and ROOS, B. E. "Serum Levels of Thioridazine in Psychiatric Patients and Healthy Volunteers," *European Journal of Clinical Pharmacology*, 6 (1973):181–186.

254. MARTZ, E., et al. "Clozapine: A Potential Antipsychotic Drug Without Extrapyramidal Manifestations," *Current Therapeutic Research*, 16 (1974):687–695.

255. MATTSON, R. H., and CALVERLEY, J. R. "Dextroamphetamine-sulfate-induced Dyskinesia," *Journal of the American Medical Association*, 204 (1968):108–110.

256. MEHTA, D., MEHTA, S., and MATHEW, P. "Failure of Deanol in Treating Tardive Dyskinesia," *American Journal of Psychiatry*, 135 (1978):371–372.

257. MELTZER, H. Y. "Biochemical Studies in Schizophrenia," in L. Bellak, ed., *Disorders of the Schizophrenia Syndrome.* New York: Basic Books, 1979, pp. 45–135.

258. MELTZER, H. Y., et al. "Dopamine and Schizophrenia," *Lancet*, 2 (1976):1142.

259. MERREN, M. D. "Amantadine in Tardive Dyskinesia," *New England Journal of Medicine*, 286 (1972):268.

260. MILLER, E. M. "Dimethylaminoethanol in the Treatment of Blepharospasm," *New England Journal of Medicine*, 289 (1973):697.

261. ———. "Deanol: A Solution for Tardive Dyskinesia?" *New England Journal of Medicine*, 291 (1974):796–797.

262. MOORE, K. E., and DEMAREST, K. T. "Effects of Baclofen on Different

Dopaminergic Neuronal Systems," *Brain Research Bulletin,* 5 (Supplement 2), (1980), 531–535.

263. MOREIRA, M. J. C., and KARNIO, I. G. "Improvement of Tardive Dyskinesia with High Doses of Propranolol: A Case Report," *Revista Paulista de Medicina,* 93 (1979):76–78.

264. MULLER, J., and AMINOFF, M. J. "Tourette-like Syndrome After Long-term Neuroleptic Drug Treatment," *British Journal of Psychiatry,* 141 (1982):191–193.

265. MURUGAIAH, K., et al. "Alterations in Cerebral Dopamine Function Caused by Administration of Cis- or Trans-flupenthixol for Up to 18 Months," *Neuroscience,* 10 (1983):811–819.

266. NAGAO, T., et al. "Cerebrospinal Fluid Monoamine Metabolites and Cyclic Nucleotides in Chronic Schizophrenic Patients with Tardive Dyskinesia or Drug-induced Tremor," *Biological Psychiatry,* 14 (1979):509–523.

267. NAIR, N. P. V., et al. "Baclofen in the Treatment of Tardive Dyskinesia," *American Journal of Psychiatry,* 135 (1978):1562–1563.

268. NASHOLD, B. S. "The Effects of Central Tegmental Lesions on Tardive Dyskinesia," in G. E. Crane and J. R. Gardner, Jr. eds., *Psychotropic Drugs and Dysfunctions of the Basal Ganglia* (U.S. Public Health Service Publication No. 1938). Washington, D.C.: U.S. Government Printing Office, 1969, pp. 111–119.

269. NASRALLAH, H. A., PAPPAS, N. J., and CROWE, R. R. "Oculogyric Dystonia in Tardive Dyskinesia," *American Journal of Psychiatry,* 137 (1980):850–851.

270. NAUSIEDA, P. A., et al. "Modification of Postsynaptic Dopaminergic Sensitivity by Female Sex Hormones," *Life Sciences,* 25 (1979):521–526.

271. NAUTA, W. J. H., and MEHLER, W. R. "Fiber Connections of the Basal Ganglia," in G. E. Crane and J. R. Gardner, Jr. eds., *Psychotropic Drugs and Dysfunctions of the Basal Ganglia* (U.S. Public Health Service Publication No. 1938). Washington, D.C.: U.S. Government Printing Office, 1969, pp. 68–74.

272. NORRIS, J. P., and SAMS, R. E. "More on the Use of Manganese in Dyskinesia," *American Journal of Psychiatry,* 134 (1977):1488.

273. O'FLANAGAN, P. M. "Clonazepam in the Treatment of Drug-induced Dyskinesia," *British Medical Journal,* 1 (1975): 269–270.

274. OGITA, K., YAGI, G., and ITOH, H. "Comparative Analysis of Persistent Dyskinesia of Long-term Usage with Neuroleptics in France and Japan," *Folia Psychiatrica et Neurologica Japonica,* 29 (1975):315–320.

275. OLSSON, R., and ROOS, B.E. "Concentration of 5-hydroxyindoleacetic Acid and Homovanillic Acid in the Cerebrospinal Fluid After Treatment with Probenecid in Patients with Parkinson's Disease," *Nature,* 219 (1968):502–503.

276. ONALI, P., OLIANAS, M. C., and GESSA, G. L. "Selective Blockade of Dopamine D_1 Receptors by SCH23390 Discloses Striatal Dopamine D_2 Receptors Mediating the Inhibition of Adenylate Cyclase in Rats," *European Journal of Pharmacology,* 99 (1984):127–128.

277. OWENS, D. G. C., JOHNSTONE, E. C., and FRITH, C. D. "Spontaneous Involuntary disorders of Movement," *Archives of General Psychiatry,* 39 (1982):452–461.

278. PANDURANGI, A. K., DEVI., V., and CHANNABASAVANNA, S. M. "Caudate Atrophy in Tardive Dyskinesia (A Pneumoencephalographic Study)," *Journal of Clinical Psychiatry,* 41 (1980):229–231.

279. PAULSON, G. W. "An Evaluation of the Permanence of 'Tardive Dyskinesia,'" *Diseases of the Nervous System,* 29 (1968):692–694.

280. ———. "'Permanent' or Complex Dyskinesias in the Aged," *Geriatrics,* 23 (1968):105–110.

281. ———. "Dyskinesia in Monkeys," *Advances in Neurology,* 1 (1973):647–650.

282. PEARCE, J. "Mechanism of Action of Amantadine," *British Medical Journal,* 3 (1970):529.

283. PEET, M., MIDDLEMISS, D. N., and YATES, R. A. "Propranolol in Schizophrenia: II. Clinical and Biochemical Aspects of Combining Propranolol with Chlorpromazine," *British Journal of Psychiatry,* 138 (1981):112–117.

284. PENOVICH, P., et al. "Double-blind Evaluation of Deanol in Tardive Dys-

kinesias," *Journal of the American Medical Association*, 239 (1978):1997–1998.

285. PERENYI, A., and ARATO, M. "Tardive Dyskinesia on Hungarian Psychiatric Wards," *Psychosomatics*, 21 (1980):904–909.

286. PERT, A., et al. "Long-term Treatment with Lithium Prevents the Development of Dopamine Receptor Supersensitivity," *Science*, 201 (1978):171–173.

287. PIND, K., and FAURBYE, A. "Concentration of Homovanillic Acid and 5-hydroxyindoleacetic Acid in the Cerebrospinal Fluid After Treatment with Probenecid in Patients with Drug-induced Tardive Dyskinesia," *Acta Psychiatrica Scandinavica*, 46 (1970):323–326.

288. POLDINGER, W. "Therapy of Extrapyramidal Side Effects, with Particular Reference to Persistent Dyskinesia and Lithium Tremor," *International Pharmacopsychiatry*, 13 (1978):230–233.

289. POLIZOS, P., et al. "Neurological Consequences of Psychotropic Drug Withdrawal in Schizophrenic Children," *Journal of Autism and Childhood Schizophrenia*, 3 (1973):247–253.

290. PRANGE, A. J., SISK, J. L., and WILSON, I. C. "Balance, Permission and Discrimination Among Amines: A Theoretical Consideration of the Actions of I-tryptophan in Disorders of Movement and Affect," in J. D. Barchas and E. Usdin, eds., *Serotonin and Behavior*. New York: Academic Press, 1973, pp. 539–548.

291. PRANGE, A. J., et al. "Preliminary Experience with Tryptophan and Lithium in the Treatment of Tardive Dyskinesia," *Psychopharmacology Bulletin*, 9 (1973):36–37.

292. PRICE, T. R. P., and LEVIN, R. "The Effects of Electroconvulsive Therapy on Tardive Dyskinesia," *American Journal of Psychiatry*, 135 (1978):991–993.

293. PRYCE, I. G., and EDWARDS, H. "Persistent Oral Dyskinesia in Female Mental Hospital Patients," *British Journal of Psychiatry*, 112 (1966):983–987.

294. RAY, I. "Tardive Dyskinesia Treated with Deanol Acetamidobenzoate," *Canadian Medical Association Journal*, 117 (1977):129.

295. RE, O. N. "Deanol in L-dopa and Tardive Dyskinesia: A Review," *Current Therapeutic Research*, 18 (1975):872–875.

296. REDA, F. A., ESCOBAR, J. I., and SCANLAN, J. M. "Lithium Carbonate in the Treatment of Tardive Dyskinesia," *American Journal of Psychiatry*, 132 (1975):560–562.

297. RINGWALD, E. "Behandlung von Neuroeptischen Spathyperkinesien mit Antiparinsonika," *Pharmacopsychiatrica*, 11 (1978):294–298.

298. ROCCATAGLIATA, G., ALBANO, C., and BESIO, G. "Discinesie Croniche Tardive da Neurolettici—Data Farmacologici e Liquorali," *Rivista di Patologia Nervosa e Mentale*, 98 (1977):228–232.

299. ROSENBAUM, A. H., and De La FUENTE, J. R. "Benzodiazepines and Tardive Dyskinesia," *Lancet*, 2 (1979):900.

300. ROSENBAUM, A. H., O'CONNOR, M. K., and DUANE, D. D. "Treatment of Tardive Dyskinesia in an Agitated, Depressed Patient," *Psychosomatics*, 21 (1980):765–766.

301. ROSENBAUM, A. H., et al. "Tardive Dyskinesia in Depressed Patients: Successful Therapy with Antidepressants and Lithium," *Psychosomatics*, 21 (1980):715–719.

302. ROXBURGH, P. A. "Treatment of Persistent Phenothiazine-induced Oral Dyskinesia," *British Journal of Psychiatry*, 116 (1970):277–280.

303. RUPNIAK, N. M. J., JENNER, P., and MARSDEN, C. D. "The Effect of Chronic Neuroleptic Administration on Cerebral Dopamine Receptor Function," *Life Sciences*, 32 (1983):2289–2341.

304. SATO, S., DALY, R., and PETERS, H. "Reserpine of Phenothiazine-induced Dyskinesia," *Diseases of the Nervous System*, 32 (1971):680–685.

305. SCATTON, B., GARRET, C., and JULOU, L. "Acute and Subacute Effects of Neuroleptics on Dopamine Synthesis and Release in the Rat Striatum," *Archives of Pharmacology*, 289 (1975):419.

306. SCHÖNECKER, M. "Ein Eigentumliches Syndrom im Oralen Bereich bei Megaphen Applikation," *Nervenarzt*, 28 (1957):35.

307. SEDIVEC, V., VALENOVA, Z., and PACELTOVA, L. "Persistent Extrapyramidal Oral Dyskinesia Following Treatment

with Thymoleptics," *Activitas Nervosa Superior*, 12 (1970):67–68.

308. SEDMAN, G. "Clonazepam in the Treatment of Tardive Oral Dyskinesia," *British Medical Journal*, 2 (1976):583.

309. SEEMAN, M. V., PATEL, J., and PYKE, J. "Tardive Dyskinesia with Tourette-like Syndrome," *Journal of Clinical Psychiatry*, 42 (1981):357–358.

310. SEEMAN, P. "Brain Dopamine Receptors," *Pharmacological Reviews*, 32 (1980): 229, 313.

311. SETHY, V. H., and VAN WOERT, M. H. "Modification of Striatal Acetylcholine Concentration by Dopamine Receptor Agonists and Antagonists," *Research Communications in Chemistry, Pathology, and Pharmacology*, 8 (1974):13–28.

312. SHAPIRO, A. K., et al. *Gilles de la Tourette's Syndrome*. New York: Raven Press, 1978.

313. SHERMAN, R. A. "Successful Treatment of One Case of Tardive Dyskinesia with Electromyographic Feedback from the Masseter Muscle," *Biofeedback and Self-Regulation*, 4 (1979):367–370.

314. SHOULSON, I., and CHASE, T. N. "Fenfluramine and Dyskinesia," *New England Journal of Medicine*, 291 (1974): 850–851.

315. SIGWALD, J., et al. "Quatre Cas de Dyskinesie Facio-bucco-linguo-masticatrice à Evolution Prolongée Secondaire à un Traitment par les Neuroleptiques," *Revue Neurologique*, 100 (1959):751–755.

316. SIMPSON, G. M. "The Current Status of Tardive Dyskinesia," *International Drug Therapy Newsletter*, 15 (1980):22–24.

317. SIMPSON, G. M., and KLINE, N. S. "Tardive Dyskinesia: Manifestations, Incidence, Etiology and Treatment," in M. D. Yahr, ed., *The Basal Ganglia*. New York: Raven Press, 1976, pp. 427–432.

318. SIMPSON, G. M., and SHRIVASTAVA, R. K. "Abnormal Gaits in Tardive Dyskinesia," *American Journal of Psychiatry*, 135 (1978):865.

319. SIMPSON, G. M., LEE, J. H., and SHRIVASTAVA, R. K. "Clozapine in Tardive Dyskinesia," *Psychopharmacology*, 56 (1978):75–80.

320. SIMPSON, G. M., et al. "Lithium in Tardive

Dyskinesia," *Pharmacopsychiatrie*, 9 (1976):76–80.

321. SIMPSON, G. M., et al. "Deanol in the Treatment of Tardive Dyskinesia," *Psychopharmacology*, 52 (1977):257–261.

322. SIMPSON, G. M., et al. "Baclofen in the Treatment of Tardive Dyskinesia and Schizophrenia," *Psychopharmacology Bulletin*, 14 (1978):16–18.

323. SINGER, K., and CHENG, N. M. "Thiopropazate Hydrochloride in Persistent Dyskinesia," *British Medical Journal*, 4 (1971):22–25.

324. SINGH, M. M. "Diazepam in the Treatment of Tardive Dyskinesia," *International Pharmacopsychiatry*, 11 (1976): 232–234.

325. SINGH, M. M., et al. "Treatment of Tardive Dyskinesia with Diazepam: Indirect Evidence for the Involvement of Limbic, Possibly GABAergic Mechanisms," *Brain Research Bulletin*, 5 (Supplement 2), (1980):673–680.

326. SMITH, J. M., and BALDESSARINI, R. J. "Changes in Prevalence, Severity and Recovery in Tardive Dyskinesia with Age," *Archives of General Psychiatry*, 37 (1980):1368–1373.

327. SMITH, J. M., and KANE, J. "Epidemiology of Tardive Dyskinesia," in J. DeVeaugh-Geiss, ed., *Tardive Dyskinesia and Related Involuntary Movement Disorders*. Boston: PSG Inc., 1982, pp. 41–50.

328. SMITH, J. M., et al. "Tardive Dyskinesia: Age and Sex Differences in Hospitalized Schizophrenics," *Psychopharmacology*, 58 (1978):918–922.

329. SMITH, J. S., and KILOH, L. G. "Six Month Evaluation of Thiopropazate Hydrochloride in Tardive Dyskinesia," *Journal of Neurology, Neurosurgery and Psychiatry*, 42 (1979):576–579.

330. SMITH, R. C., TAMMINGA, C., and DAVIS, J. M. "Behavioral Effects of Apomorphine and Amphetamine in Tardive Dyskinesia Patients," in W. E. Fann, et al., eds., *Tardive Dyskinesia: Research and Treatment*. New York: SP Medical & Scientific Books, 1980, pp. 333–344.

331. SNYDER, S. H. "The Dopamine Hypothesis of Schizophrenia: Focus on the Dopamine Receptor," *American Journal of Psychiatry*, 133 (1976):197–202.

332. SOVNER, R., and DiMASCIO, A. "The

Effect of Benzotropine Mesylate in the Rabbit Syndrome and Tardive Dyskinesia," *American Journal of Psychiatry*, 134 (1977):1301–1302.

333. SOVNER, R., and LOADMAN, A. "More on Barbiturates and Tardive Dyskinesia," *American Journal of Psychiatry*, 135 (1978):382.

334. STADLER, H., et al. "Enhanced Striatal Acetylcholine Release by Chlorpromazine and Its Reversal by Apomorphine," *Brain Research*, 55 (1973):476–480.

335. STAFFORD, J. R., and FANN, W. E. "Deanol Acetamidobenzoate (Deaner) in Tardive Dyskinesia," *Disorders of the Nervous System*, 38 (Supplement), (1977): 3–6.

336. STAHL, S. M. "Tardive Tourette Syndrome in an Autistic Patient After Long-term Neuroleptic Administration," *American Journal of Psychiatry*, 137 (1980):1267–1269.

337. STANCER, H. C. "Tardive Dyskinesia Not Associated with Neuroleptics," *American Journal of Psychiatry*, 136 (1979): 727.

338. STANDEFER, J. J., and DILL, R. E. "The Role of GABA in Dyskinesias Induced by Chemical Stimulation of the Striatum," *Life Sciences*, 21 (1977):1515–1520.

339. STOFF, J. C., and KEBABIAN, J. W. "Opposing Roles for D_1 and D_2 Dopamine Receptors in Efflux of Cyclic AMP from Rats' Striatum," *Nature*, 294 (1981):366–368.

340. SUTCHER, H. D., et al. "Orofacial Dyskinesia: A Dental Dimension," *Journal of the American Medical Association*, 216 (1971):1459–1463.

341. TAMMINGA, C. A., and CHASE, T. N. "Bromocriptine and CF 25-397 in the Treatment of Tardive Dyskinesia," *Archives of Neurology*, 37 (1980):204–205.

342. TAMMINGA, C. A., CRAYTON, J. W., and CHASE, T. N. "Improvement in Tardive Dyskinesia After Muscimol Therapy," *Archives of General Psychiatry*, 36 (1979):595–598.

343. TAMMINGA, C. A., SMITH, R. C., and DAVIS, J. M. "The Effects of Cholinergic Drugs on the Involuntary Movements of Tardive Dyskinesia," in W. E. Fann, et al., eds., *Tardive Dyskinesia: Re-search and Treatment*. New York: SP Medical & Scientific Books, 1980, pp. 411–418.

344. TAMMINGA, C. A., et al. "Cholinergic Influences in Tardive Dyskinesia," *American Journal of Psychiatry*, 134 (1977): 769–774.

345. TANIMOTO, K., MAEDA, K., and TERADA, T. "Inhibitory Effect of Lithium on Neuroleptic and Serotonin Receptors in Rat Brain," *Brain Research*, 265 (1983): 148–151.

346. TARSY, D., and BRALOWER, M. "Deanol Acetamidobenzoate Treatment in Choreiform Movement Disorders," *Archives of Neurology*, 34 (1977):756–758.

347. TARSY, D., LEOPOLD, N., and SAX, D. "Physostigmine in Choreiform Movement Disorders," *Neurology* (Minneapolis), 23 (1973):392.

348. ———. "Physostigmine in Choreiform Movement Disorders," *Neurology* (Minneapolis), 24 (1974):28–33.

349. THACH, B. T., CHASE, T. N., and BOSMA, J. F. "Oral Facial Dyskinesia Associated with Prolonged Use of Antihistaminic Decongestants," *New England Journal of Medicine*, 293 (1975):486–487.

350. TOLOSA, E. S. "Modification of Tardive Dyskinesia and Spasmodic Torticollis by Apomorphine," *Archives of Neurology*, 35 (1978):459–462.

351. ———. "Clinical Features of Meige's Disease (Idiopathic Orofacial Dystonia)—A Case Report of 17 Cases," *Archives of Neurology*, 38 (1981):147–151.

352. TURUNEN, S., and ACHTE, K. A. "Buccolingual Masticatory Syndrome as a Side Effect of Neuroleptic Therapy," *Psychiatric Quarterly*, 41 (1967):268–279.

353. UHRBRAND, L., and FAURBYE, A. "Reversible and Irreversible Dyskinesia After Treatment with Perphenazine, Chlorpromazine, Reserpine, and Electroconvulsive Therapy," *Psychopharmacologia*, 1 (1960):408–418.

354. UMEZ-ERONINI, E. M., and ERONINI, E. A. "Chloroquine-induced Involuntary movements," *British Medical Journal*, 1 (1977):945–946.

355. UNGERSTEDT, U. "Postsynaptic Supersensitivity After 6-hydroxydopamine-

induced Degeneration of the Nigro-striatal Dopamine System," *Acta Physiologica Scandinavica*, 367 (Supplement), (1971):69–93.

356. VALE, S., and ESPEJEL, J. A. "Amantadine for Dyskinesia Tarda," *New England Journal of Medicine*, 284 (1971):673.

357. VAN PUTTEN, T. "Vulnerability to Extrapyramidal Side Effects," *Clinical Neuropharmacology*, 6 (Supplement 1), (1983):27–34.

358. VAN WOERT, M. H., et al. "Gilles de la Tourette's Syndrome: Biochemical Approaches," in M. D. Yahr, ed., *The Basal Ganglia*. New York: Raven Press, 1976, pp. 459–465.

359. VILLENEUVE, A., and BOSZORMENYI, Z. "Treatment of Drug-induced Dyskinesias," *Lancet*, 1 (1980):353–354.

360. VILLENEUVE, A., CAZEJUST, T., and COTE, M. "Estrogens in Tardive Dyskinesias in Male Psychiatric Patients," *Neuropsychobiology*, 6 (1980):145–151.

361. VILLENEUVE, A., LANGELIER, P., and BEDARD, P. "Estrogens, Dopamine and Dyskinesias," *Canadian Psychiatric Association Journal*, 23 (1978):68–70.

362. VIUKARI, M., and LINNOILA, M. "Effect of Methyldopa on Tardive Dyskinesia in Psychogeriatric Patients," *Current Therapeutic Research*, 18 (1975):417–424.

363. ———. "Effect of Fusaric Acid on Tardive Dyskinesia and Mental State in Psychogeriatric Patients," *Acta Psychiatrica Scandinavica*, 56 (1977):57–61.

364. WALTON, D., WHITE, J. G., and BLACK, D. A. "A Modified Word-learning Test: A Cross-Validation Study," *British Journal of Medical Psychology*, 32 (1959): 213–220.

365. WEGNER, J. T., et al. "Relationship Between the B-mitten EEG Pattern and Tardive Dyskinesia," *Archives of General Psychiatry*, 36 (1979):599–603.

366. WEINER, W. J., NAUSIEDA, P. A., and KLAWANS, H. L. "Regional Brain Manganese Levels in an Animal Model of Tardive Dyskinesia," in W. E. Fann, et al., eds., *Tardive Dyskinesia: Research and Treatment*. New York: SP Medical & Scientific Books, 1980, pp. 159–163.

367. WEISS, B., and SANTELLI, S. "Dyskinesia Evoked in Monkeys by Weekly Administration of Haloperidol," *Science*, 200 (1978):799–801.

368. WEISS, B., GREENBERG, L., and CANTOR, E. "Age-related Alterations in the Development of Adrenergic Denervation Supersensitivity," *Federation Proceedings*, 38 (1979):1915–1921.

369. WEISS, K. J., CIRAULO, D. A., and SHADER, R. I. "Physostigmine Test in Rabbit Syndrome and Tardive Dyskinesia," *American Journal of Psychiatry*, 137 (1980):-627–628.

370. WIDROWE, J. J., and HEISLER, S. "Treatment of Tardive Dyskinesia," *Diseases of the Nervous System*, 37 (1976):162–164.

371. WINSBERG, B. G., HURWIC, M. J., and PEREL, J. "Neurochemistry of Withdrawal-emergent Symptoms in Children," *Psychopharmacology Bulletin*, 13 (1977):38–40.

372. WOLF, M., et al. "The Clinical Association of Tardive Dyskinesia and Drug-induced Parkinsonism," *Biological Psychiatry*, 18 (1983):1181–1188.

373. WOOGEN, S., GRAHAM, J., and ANGRIST, B. "A Tardive Dyskinesia-like Syndrome After Amitriptyline Treatment," *Journal of Clinical Psychopharmacology*, 1 (1981):34–36.

374. YAGI, G. "Irreversible Extrapyramidal Disturbance Induced by Psychotropic Drugs," Paper presented at the meeting of the Kanagowaken Seishin Igakukai, Tokyo, 1970.

375. YAGI, G., et al. "Persistent Dyskinesia After Long-term Treatment with Neuroleptics in Japan," *Keio Journal of Medicine*, 25 (1976):27–35.

376. YASSA, R., GHADIRIAN, A. M., and SCHWARTZ, G. "Tardive Dyskinesia Developmental Factors," Paper presented at the 32nd annual meeting of the Canadian Psychiatric Association, Montreal, Quebec, 1982.

377. YESAVAGE, J. A., et al. "Serum Level Monitoring of Thiothixene in Schizophrenia: Acute Single-dose Levels at Fixed Doses," *American Journal of Psychiatry*, 139 (1982):174–178.

378. YORKSTON, N. J., et al. "DL-propranolol and Chlorpromazine Following Admission for Schizophrenia," *Acta Psychiatrica Scandinavica*, 63 (1981):13–27.

CHAPTER 21

THE NEUROBIOLOGY OF ANXIETY: THE ROLE OF THE GABA/BENZODIAZEPINE RECEPTOR COMPLEX

Steven M. Paul, Jacqueline N. Crawley, and Phil Skolnick

¶ **Introduction**

Anxiety is a subjective emotional state that has become popularized of late because it is a primary presenting symptom of such common clinical disorders as generalized anxiety, panic/agoraphobia, and obsessive-compulsive disorder.[1,29,30] It has been estimated that anywhere from 2 to 8 percent of the general population suffers from anxiety of sufficient severity to warrant medical intervention, and within the subpopulation of psychiatric patients, the incidence of severe anxiety may be as high as 27 percent.[60,72] In addition, certain neuropsychiatric conditions, such as chronic alcoholism, appear to have an unusually high rate of associated anxiety[10] such that anxiety has been proposed as being of etiological significance in this disorder. It is also widely believed (although as yet unproven) that excessive anxiety may contribute to a variety of medical conditions, since the physiological manifestations of anxiety affect a variety of homeostatic systems (e.g., cardiovascular, endocrine, immune, and gastrointestinal).

Before considering the neurobiological substrates of anxiety, however, it is important to emphasize that anxiety per se is neither a disease nor solely a symptom of one, but is a normal and fundamental component of human emotion. From an evolutionary standpoint, anxiety, like fear, is clearly an adaptive emotional state that is frequently evoked and probably has survival value for virtually all species.[15] Although anxiety cannot be directly measured in animals, its presence can be inferred by studying the effects of antianxiety drugs on a variety of anxiety-related behaviors.[13,20,21,36] Thus the neurobiological systems governing the development of anxiety (and/or its attenuation) are likely to be operative independent of a clinically apparent anxiety disorder.

For conceptual purposes, it is reasonable to think of anxiety as a derivative of fear, except that the latter is more often associated with situations of actual rather than perceived danger. In some respects, anxiety can also be viewed as the cognitive and emotional component of the behavioral "alarm" (so-called fight or flight) reaction serving to mobilize and alert the organism to impending danger. In man, with the development of the cerebral cortex and an increased capacity for associative processes, as well as memory consolidation and retrieval, anxiety can be triggered by much more complex developmental and environmental stimuli. Freud, in fact, pointed out that the source of the perceived threat or danger may be imaginary or subconscious, and thus, in his view, anxiety represented a "signal" for anticipating potential danger.[19] Such signals have a multiplicity of origins, and it is not surprising, therefore, that anxiety as a symptom is perhaps the most common of all psychiatric complaints.

On the basis of epidemiological and pharmacological data, it appears that the anxiety disorders themselves may represent a group of distinct (but perhaps overlapping) clinical disorders; and each may, therefore, have its own unique neurochemical basis.[30,40,72] In this review, we will not discuss the current classification schemes or the biological hypotheses concerning the various anxiety disorders but will focus on an area of research that has attempted to define the neurobiological substrata of anxiety itself.* These studies have been facilitated by the availability of relatively specific and potent antianxiety drugs, the development of a variety of

animal models of anxiety that are sensitive to these agents, and the relatively recent discovery of the neurochemical mechanisms by which these drugs reduce anxiety. Taken together, these findings have allowed for the formulation of a neurobiological hypothesis that highlights the role of the major central inhibitory neurotransmitter system (the gamma-aminobutyric acid [GABA]–ergic neuron) in both the physiology and pathophysiology of anxiety.* Current work on whether or not this system (which serves as the primary target for antianxiety drugs) is involved in the pathogenesis of human anxiety is in progress and will be reviewed briefly.

The Neuropharmacological Bridge: Benzodiazepines as Selective Anxiolytics

The basic premise of much of the work to be presented is that the neurochemical events underlying anxiety can be derived from an understanding of the precise mechanisms of action of antianxiety drugs. This approach is not new to psychiatry; many of the biological theories concerning the etiology of neuropsychiatric disorders have evolved from extrapolating neurochemical data on the mode of action of psychotropic drugs. The "dopamine hypothesis of schizophrenia" and the "catecholamine theory of depression," for example, are based primarily on the accumulated preclinical and clinical data concerning the mechanism(s) of action of drugs that either mimic or antagonize the symptoms of depression and schizophrenia respectively[6,63] (see also Chapters 12 and 17).

The utility of this approach obviously depends on the specificity of antianxiety drugs for reducing the symptoms of anxiety. In the case of the anxiety disorders, a wide variety of psychopharmacological agents have been employed as effective therapeutic agents (e.g., barbiturates, propanediol carbamates, benzodiazepines, beta-adrenergic blockers,

---

*See the DSM-III[1] and Klein et al.[30] for comprehensive reviews on the nosology of pathological anxiety states.

*See references 28, 36, 40, 42, 61, and 74.

antidepressants, etc.).[10] However, these drugs vary in their specificity and potency and some (e.g., the tricyclic antidepressants) are complex pharmacological agents with many diverse neurochemical actions.[43] Benzodiazepines, on the other hand, are potent anxiolytics and at therapeutic doses (generally *low* μg/kg doses) are devoid of the anticholinergic, antihistaminic, and alpha- and beta-adrenolytic actions of most psychotropic agents.[22,23] Benzodiazepines are also generally regarded as being relatively ineffective antidepressant and antipsychotic agents, and antidepressants and antipsychotic agents are not particularly effective for treating generalized anxiety disorders. Thus, in so far as benzodiazepines are specific as anxiolytics, they may be useful as probes in delineating the neurobiology of anxiety.

Recent work has shown that, in general, certain anxiolytics are far more effective in reducing some forms of anxiety (e.g., tricyclic antidepressants and monoamine oxidase inhibitors in agoraphobia/panic disorder and benzodiazepines in generalized anxiety) than in others (e.g., benzodiazepines in agoraphobia/panic disorder).[29,30] The specificity of a given anxiolytic agent will therefore depend on the type of anxiety being studied. There is now substantial clinical evidence that benzodiazepines are effective anxiolytics, both in healthy individuals and in patients with so-called generalized anxiety disorder.[10,22,23,46] Again, these findings support the view that the "anxiety" that is sensitive to benzodiazepines will not be unique or confined to a specific anxiety disorder but will be present, to a certain extent, in all of us. In this context, pathological anxiety can be viewed as an inappropriate or exaggerated response rather than a qualitatively unique state.

Before proceeding with a discussion of the benzodiazepines, it is worth mentioning the other antianxiety drugs of the same general class. Barbiturates (e.g., pentobarbital and phenobarbital) and subsequently the propanediol carbamates (e.g., meprobamate) were both widely prescribed as anxiolytics but because of their side effects and toxicity,

their use has decreased dramatically since the introduction of benzodiazepines in the early 1960s.[31] Nevertheless, all three compounds, despite having chemically different structures, are pharmacologically quite similar and show cross-tolerance and dependence with each other when chronically administered to either laboratory animals or man.[10,60] Moreover, man's oldest and most widely used anxiolytic, ethanol, shares many pharmacological properties with the benzodiazepines and barbiturates; and all three agents can be substituted for each other in instances of tolerance and withdrawal.[10] This suggests that barbiturates, propanediol carbamates, alcohols, and benzodiazepines may share a common neurochemical mechanism of action and that this mechanism may be involved in the antianxiety effects of all four agents. If a common mechanism of action for such chemically disparate drugs is identified, it will be an important clue for understanding the pathophysiology of anxiety.

In addition to reducing anxiety, benzodiazepines have anticonvulsant, muscle relaxant, and sedative properties.[22,23] Although it has been suggested that the anxiolytic actions of benzodiazepines may result from a combination of their muscle relaxant and sedative properties, it now appears that neither is required to achieve a clinically apparent anxiolytic action. Sedation is generally considered to be the major side effect of the benzodiazepines, and, in clinical studies, the sedative effects of these drugs are sometimes difficult to separate from their antianxiety action. Nevertheless, it is clear that sedation per se is not required for the antianxiety action of benzodiazepines, since tolerance to the former, but not the latter, develops rather quickly. In animals it has been much easier to show that the sedation produced by benzodiazepines is quite distinct from their "antianxiety" actions. As already mentioned, the notion that animals experience anxiety requires a "leap of faith" that can only be approached indirectly. Nevertheless, the effects of anxiolytics on various animal behaviors support the specificity of these agents, and a closer look at "anxiolytic-sensitive" behaviors in animals reveals many parallels to their effects on human behavior.

In laboratory animals, benzodiazepines (as well as the other anxiolytics just mentioned) selectively attenuate the behavioral effects of three classes of environmental stimuli.[20,21] These include behaviors associated with punishment or conflict, nonreward, and novelty. Gray[21] has proposed that these three types of environmental stimuli activate a "behavioral inhibition system" in brain whose output results in the inhibition of ongoing behavior with corresponding increases in arousal and attention. According to his hypothesis, the behavioral inhibition system consists of several anatomically associated brain structures, including the septo-hippocampal pathway and the ascending serotonergic and noradrenergic afferents to this region. Benzodiazepines and other antianxiety drugs impair activity in the behavioral inhibition system and thus "release" behaviors suppressed by these stimuli. By contrast, benzodiazepines fail to alter behavior that is associated with simple punishment or the aversive effects of noxious environmental stimuli.

In addition to reducing the behavioral effects of punishment, nonreward, and novelty, benzodiazepines attenuate the autonomic and endocrine changes that accompany these behaviors; for the most part, these are the same physiological changes that are characteristic of human anxiety states as well.[30,72] The behaviors that are sensitive to benzodiazepines in animals can thus be anthropomorphized to threats of punishment, frustration, and uncertainty. Most clinicians would agree that the latter represent the primary components of human anxiety, strengthening the hypothesis that similar forms of anxiety may exist in animals.

Perhaps the most widely studied behavioral action of the benzodiazepines in animals relates to their ability to reduce the behavioral inhibition produced by punishment.[20] In one such paradigm, animals are simultaneously presented with rewarding (e.g., food or water) and aversive

(e.g., foot or tail shock) stimuli. The animals are thus in a "state of conflict"; when they approach their reward, they receive an aversive shock. Under such conditions, animals will dramatically reduce their response rate for the rewarding stimulus. Benzodiazepines inhibit or attenuate the reduction in behavior produced by this "conflict" situation, as do all clinically effective anxiolytics. The anticonflict action of benzodiazepines occurs at doses well below those that produce sedation and, in fact, the latter will nonspecifically reduce motor behavior and thus counteract the anticonflict or "anxiolytic" effects of benzodiazepines in this paradigm. Furthermore, at similar doses, benzodiazepines fail to alter a variety of other naturally occurring and conditioned behaviors that have been shown to be sensitive to other classes of psychotropic drugs. Perhaps most important is the observation that the relative potencies of a large series of benzodiazepines in producing an anticonflict action in animals is highly correlated with their potencies as antianxiety agents in man (reviewed in Skolnick and Paul[60] and Tallman et al.[70]). This suggests that the mechanisms responsible for the anticonflict effect of benzodiazepines in laboratory animals may be similar, if not identical, to those responsible for their antianxiety effects in man. As we shall see, the anticonflict action of benzodiazepines has proven to be a useful model for exploring the neurobiology of anxiety.

¶ The Benzodiazepine/GABA Receptor Complex: Central Targets for Anxiolytic Drugs

Although the benzodiazepines are among the most widely prescribed of all drugs,* very little was known about how benzodiaze-

*In 1982 over 70 million prescriptions were written for benzodiazepines in the United States alone! More impressive, however, is the prevalence rate for the use of antianxiety drugs, which is approximately 11 percent. This means that 11 percent of the adult population (ages 18 to 74 years old) would have taken an antianxiety drug at least once in the preceding twelve months and over 80 percent of these are benzodiazepines.[31]

pines produce their antianxiety effects until the middle to late 1970s. It is noteworthy that even as late as the second volume in this series,[10] no tentative biochemical theory on the mechanism(s) of action of these drugs was offered. Early workers had reported a variety of neurochemical changes in brain following the administration of benzodiazepines to laboratory animals. Alterations, for example, in the "turnover" of a number of neurotransmitters including acetylcholine, norepinephrine, and serotonin were reported,[70] but these changes were subtle and not universally observed. Some studies even suggested that the antianxiety and muscle-relaxant effects of benzodiazepines were mediated by peripheral rather than central mechanisms.

In 1977 two groups of investigators reported the presence of saturable, high-affinity, and stereospecific recognition sites for benzodiazepines in rat brain.[34,35,65] Moreover, in studying the relative affinities of a large series of benzodiazepines for these binding sites, both groups observed striking correlations between their binding affinities *in vitro* and their clinical potencies as anxiolytic agents. Similar correlations were observed between relative binding affinity and the behavioral potencies of benzodiazepines as anticonflict agents in animals. These data were exciting because, like previous studies on the opiate receptor and their naturally occurring peptide ligands, they provided strong evidence for the presence of a pharmacological receptor for benzodiazepines in brain and, in essence, reoriented thinking on the possible neurobiological substrates of human anxiety.

Since the initial discovery of benzodiazepine receptors, literally thousands of reports have been published further validating and extending the role of the benzodiazepine receptor in the mechanism(s) of action of these agents. It is now known that all of the major pharmacological actions of benzodiazepines (muscle-relaxant, anticonvulsant, and hypnotic effects) are mediated through benzodiazepine receptors (see Mendelson et al.[32,33] and Skolnick and Paul[60]). Benzodiazepine receptors have also been

demonstrated in a variety of species, including man,[35] and to date, no major species differences in the biochemical or pharmacological characteristics of these receptors have been demonstrated. Benzodiazepine receptors are, however, rather recent phylogenetic additions, since they are not found in invertebrates and are enriched in the more highly evolved brain regions.

Using autoradiographic techniques,[75] the anatomical distribution of benzodiazepine receptors has been carefully mapped in both rat and human brain. Relatively high densities of benzodiazepine receptors have been found in the cerebral cortices, hippocampus, and amygdala, while lower concentrations are found in the thalamus and brain stem. We and others have previously speculated that the broad spectrum of pharmacological effects of benzodiazepines may result from this widespread distribution of benzodiazepine receptors in brain.[60,74] In this regard, recent work suggests that the anticonflict, anticonvulsant, and hypnotic properties of benzodiazepines may be mediated by discretely localized populations of receptors, such as those in the amygdala/hippocampus, cerebral cortex, and brain stem, respectively.[8,33,57]

Benzodiazepine receptors can also be demonstrated and visualized using *in vivo* or *ex vivo* techniques.[9,73] Under these more "physiological" conditions, almost identical correlations between receptor binding affinity and clinical potency have been observed.[9,73] More recently, a suitable technique for visualizing benzodiazepine receptors in the living human brain using positron emission tomography (PET) has been reported,[11] and as will be discussed later, this method should prove useful in delineating a possible physiological role for the receptor in man. At this point, however, it is important to emphasize the almost exclusive localization of benzodiazepine receptors to the central nervous system. Peripheral recognition sites for benzodiazepines have been amply demonstrated,[70] and it appears that these may also represent "receptors" for heretofore unrecognized pharmacological effects of the benzodiazepines.[52] Nevertheless, the peripheral benzodiazepine "receptor" does not as yet appear to be related to the important behavioral and pharmacological actions of benzodiazepines described earlier.

Benzodiazepines and GABA

Even prior to the discovery of benzodiazepine receptors, it had been observed that benzodiazepines could potentiate the inhibitory actions of GABA as measured by electrophysiological and pharmacological techniques.[12,25] GABA is one of the most ubiquitous and important inhibitory neurotransmitters in brain and has been estimated to be present in as many as 30 percent of all synapses.[18,47] Surprisingly, the initial reports describing the presence of benzodiazepine receptors in brain failed to observe any significant interaction between a number of naturally occurring neurotransmitters, including GABA, and the binding of radioligands to the benzodiazepine receptor.

The definitive link between the benzodiazepine receptor and GABA came when Tallman and coworkers[69,70] found that GABA increased the affinity of benzodiazepines for their receptor when added to well-washed brain membranes. The effects of GABA in "allosterically" enhancing benzodiazepine receptor affinity *in vivo* were mimicked by GABA receptor agonists, like muscimol, and blocked by the GABA receptor antagonist, bicuculline. Shortly thereafter, it was shown that permeable anions such as chloride and bromide also enhanced the binding of benzodiazepines to their receptor,[70] suggesting the involvement of an ion channel (perhaps a chloride channel) in the action of benzodiazepines. Significantly, previous electrophysiological studies had shown that GABA inhibits neuronal excitability by selectively activating membrane chloride conductance. Together, these findings indirectly suggested that the benzodiazepine and GABA receptors were intimately associated with one another and that GABAergic transmission was, indeed, directly involved in the mechanisms of action of benzodiazepines.

More recent studies on the solubilization and purification of the benzodiazepine receptor have confirmed its close association with the GABA receptor, and, in fact, it now appears that the binding sites for benzodiazepines and GABA exist on the same protein subunit.[54] Thus the benzodiazepine receptor may simply be a phylogenetically recent subclass of GABA receptors.[54] It is now generally accepted that the benzodiazepine receptor is structurally associated with the GABA receptor and, along with a chloride channel, forms a "supramolecular receptor complex" whose ultimate function is to regulate the transport of chloride ions across neuronal membranes.[44]

Thus, when GABA is released into the synaptic cleft, it activates a specific postsynaptic receptor (the so-called $GABA_A$ receptor),* resulting in an opening of the chloride channel. The movement of chloride from the extracellular space to the inside of the neuron results in an increase in the negative potential across the membrane, making the neuron less likely to be depolarized. This state of "hyperpolarization" induced by GABA reduces neuronal excitability, yielding significant behavioral effects depending on the brain region in question. Benzodiazepines produce little or no effect on membrane chloride conductance alone, but in the presence of GABA, they markedly potentiate GABA-mediated increases in chloride permeability. On a molecular level, the effect of benzodiazepines on GABA receptor-mediated chloride transport appears to be due to an increase in the frequency of chloride channel openings rather than an enhanced conductance of chloride by each channel.[67]

---

*GABA, like most neurotransmitters, interacts with more than one membrane receptor. To date, two GABA receptors have been delineated: $GABA_A$ receptors are associated with benzodiazepine receptors and chloride channels, while $GABA_B$ receptors are associated with adenylate cyclase and do not appear to be modulated by benzodiazepines.[18]

The Benzodiazepine/GABA Receptor as a Final Common Pathway for Anxiolytic Drug Action

We cited evidence earlier that a variety of chemically dissimilar antianxiety drugs (e.g., benzodiazepines, barbiturates, propanediol carbamates, and ethanol) shared a number of pharmacological properties including their ability to reduce anxiety-related behaviors in both laboratory animals and man.[10,21] We also suggested that if these agents shared a common underlying neurochemical mechanism, this mechanism may very likely represent an important neurobiological clue to understanding the pathophysiology of anxiety. In the initial reports describing the presence of benzodiazepine receptors in brain,[65] it was also reported that most nonbenzodiazepine anxiolytics, including the barbiturates, failed to compete with [^{3}H]-diazepam for binding to the receptor. In other words, the barbiturates, propanediol carbamates, and ethanol did not directly interact with the benzodiazepine binding site (as do the benzodiazepines), and it was therefore concluded that these drugs had different mechanisms of action.

The striking electrophysiological and pharmacological similarities between barbiturates and benzodiazepines, as well as the reported effects of GABA and chloride in enhancing benzodiazepine receptor binding, prompted a more extensive examination of the possible interaction of barbiturates with benzodiazepine receptors.[37,44,62] In these experiments, pentobarbital was used as a prototype barbiturate and was shown to enhance the binding of benzodiazepines to the benzodiazepine receptor *in vitro*. At low sedative-hypnotic concentrations, pentobarbital potentiated the ability of submaximal concentrations of GABA to enhance benzodiazepine receptor binding, while at higher (i.e., anesthetic) concentrations, barbiturates directly stimulated the binding of benzodiazepines to their receptor. The enhancement of benzodiazepine binding is due to an increase in the apparent affinity of radioligand for the receptor and, like the effects of GABA, is dependent on the presence of chloride ions.[62]

The dual actions of barbiturates on the benzodiazepine receptor are similar to the reported electrophysiological actions of these compounds[65] and provide further evidence that the barbiturates do interact, albeit indirectly, with the binding site for benzodiazepines to potentiate GABAergic transmission. In addition to barbiturates, a number of other anxiolytic and anticonvulsant drugs have been reported to interact in a similar fashion with the benzodiazepine receptor (see Skolnick and Paul[61] for review).

More recently, it has been possible to directly measure the effects of barbiturates on GABA receptor function *in vitro*.[55,56] Schwartz and coworkers[55] have developed a sensitive method for studying radioactive chloride transport in a subcellular brain preparation. Using this method, both barbiturates and GABA have been shown to stimulate chloride uptake into resealed neuronal membranes; these effects are blocked by specific GABA receptor antagonists such as picrotoxin and bicuculline, confirming that they are mediated by a functional GABA$_A$ receptor. The potencies of a series of barbiturates in stimulating chloride uptake and in enhancing benzodiazepine receptor binding are also highly correlated,[55] and thus it appears that the GABA receptor being measured is, in fact, coupled to the benzodiazepine receptor. With the development of this method, it has been possible to examine the effects of other anxiolytic drugs believed to work via the receptor complex. Significantly, ethanol, at concentrations that occur in blood during acute intoxication, increases chloride uptake in a manner quite similar to that of the barbiturates and GABA.[68] These experiments suggest that ethanol stimulates the benzodiazepine/GABA receptor complex like pentobarbital and GABA, and at concentrations that may explain ethanol's antianxiety properties.[10]

Although these studies substantiate the hypothesis that all of the previously-mentioned antianxiety drugs enhance GABAergic neurotransmission by interacting with the benzodiazepine/GABA receptor complex, it should be emphasized that there are important differences in their precise molecular mechanisms of action. For example, benzodiazepines produce little or no effect on chloride conductance in the absence of GABA, while the barbiturates and ethanol can directly activate chloride conductance, resulting in membrane hyperpolarization. These differences may account for the greater toxicity and side-effect profile of barbiturates and ethanol compared with the benzodiazepines. In addition, barbiturates increase the actual time of chloride channel opening rather than the frequency of openings, and this may also contribute to pharmacological differences between the barbiturates and benzodiazepines.[67] Nonetheless, from the abundant biochemical and pharmacological data, it appears that the benzodiazepine/GABA receptor actually represents an oligomeric protein complex consisting of several subunits and containing multiple but interacting binding sites for a variety of antianxiety and sedative agents. In this regard, the benzodiazepine/GABA receptor complex resembles other neurotransmitter-gated ion channels such as the nicotinic-cholinergic receptor. The ultimate function of this complex is to modulate GABAergic neurotransmission by directly regulating GABA receptor-mediated chloride conductance. The fact that virtually all antianxiety drugs of the same class potentiate GABAergic neurotransmission makes this an extremely intriguing locus for exploring the neurobiology of anxiety.

Anxiety and the Benzodiazepine/GABA Receptor Complex

The discovery of a specific receptor for benzodiazepines and the demonstration that this receptor complex mediates the anxiolytic actions of many antianxiety drugs raises the possibility that the benzodiazepine receptor may also mediate the physiological responses underlying "fear" or "anxiety."

However, simply knowing the mechanisms of action of a drug does not necessarily equate with understanding the mechanism(s) responsible for the pathological processes that are responsive to that drug. Cardiac glycosides, for example, are effective in the treatment of congestive heart failure, but their action in inhibiting adenosine triphosphatase has not proven particularly useful in understanding the pathogenesis of this disorder. Nonetheless, why has a drug recognition site for benzodiazepines evolved in brain, and why is it associated with a naturally-occurring neurotransmitter such as GABA?[40,70] One possibility, of course, is that the benzodiazepine receptor is itself subserved by a neuromodulator substance. In other words, the benzodiazepine receptor (like the opiate receptor) may have its own endogenous ligand(s). If such a compound exists, it could theoretically mimic the benzodiazepines and reduce anxiety, or it could antagonize their effects and produce an anxiety-provoking or anxiogenic action.

In searching for an endogenous ligand for the benzodiazepine receptor, Braestrup and colleagues[3,4] isolated a beta-carboline derivative (beta-carboline 3-carboxylate ethyl ester, or beta-CCE) from human urine. Although now known not to be a naturally occurring compound, beta-CCE possesses an extremely high affinity for the benzodiazepine receptor compared with the other isolated putative endogeneous ligands,[60] and surprisingly, when administered to rodents, beta-CCE effectively antagonized the anticonvulsant and sedative effects of the benzodiazepines.[71]

At first it was thought that beta-CCE simply blocked the effects of benzodiazepines, but later it was shown that this compound had intrinsic pharmacological activity that was essentially opposite that of the benzodiazepines.[4] In rodents, such intrinsic actions are difficult to observe, but in primates, Ninan and coworkers[28,36] reported marked behavioral agitation (e.g., struggling in the restraint chair, piloerection, distress vocalizations, etc.) following intravenous administration of beta-CCE. Significantly, the behavioral effects of beta-CCE in the rhesus monkey were also accompanied by increases in heart rate, blood pressure, and the stress hormones adrenocorticotrophic hormone/cortisol, epinephrine, and norepinephrine. Moreover, all of the behavioral and physiological changes produced by beta-CCE were blocked by pretreatment with diazepam or the selective benzodiazepine receptor antagonist Ro 15-1788.[14,27,28,36] These data clearly implicate the benzodiazepine receptor in mediating the "anxiogenic" effects of beta-CCE and argue against a nonspecific action of beta-CCE in producing arousal.

Although the behavioral, physiological, and endocrine effects of beta-CCE in subhuman primates are reminiscent of those seen in extremely anxious patients,[51,53] it is still not certain how similar the beta-CCE–induced syndrome is to naturally occurring "fear" or "anxiety." In this regard, Insel and coworkers[28] and Crawley and associates[13] observed that lower doses of beta-CCE produced highly individualistic behavioral and physiological responses in rhesus monkeys that were also correlated with the animals' subsequent response to threatening environmental stimuli.[28] Thus the behavioral responses to beta-CCE, while varying from animal to animal, were highly characteristic of that animal and were similar to those observed under a variety of stressful or anxiety-provoking situations. If, for example, an animal became highly aroused and agitated when approached by a stranger, its response to beta-CCE administration would also be robust. Similarly, animals with low overt behavioral and physiological responses to beta-CCE would also be low responders to environmental "stress."[13,28] The fact that low pharmacologically relevant doses of benzodiazepines reversed or blocked the anxiety-related behaviors produced by beta-CCE supports the hypothesis that this syndrome may represent a reliable pharmacological model of human anxiety. Furthermore, other nonbenzodiazepine anxiolytic compounds including the alpha-adrenoceptor agonist clonidine hydrochloride also attenuated the beta-CCE–induced syndrome.[13]

Despite the rather impressive similarities between the beta-CCE–induced behavioral syndrome in animals and many of the signs and symptoms of human anxiety, it is, as already mentioned, impossible to conclusively demonstrate the presence or absence of anxiety in any animal other than man. Recently, Dorow and associates[16] administered a closely related beta-carboline derivative (FG 7142) to several human volunteers. The administration of FG 7142 resulted in symptoms of muscle tension, autonomic hyperactivity, and extreme apprehension. These effects were interpreted subjectively as being quite similar to anxiety and were characterized by feelings of "inner tension, excitation, and sensations of physical disturbance." The subjective effects of beta-CCE were accompanied by significant elevations in heart rate, blood pressure, and plasma cortisol. In one volunteer, these symptoms were so severe that intravenous lormetazepam was administered; the symptoms subsided within only a few minutes.

For obvious reasons, clinical studies on the anxiogenic actions of beta-carboline esters have been rather limited, but other anxiogenic compounds that work via the GABA receptor complex have also been shown to produce anxiety in man. Pentylenetetrazol, for example, is a convulsant that binds to the benzodiazepine/GABA receptor complex[66] and has been shown to produce "anxiety" in man when administered at subconvulsant doses.[50]

Do the behavioral effects of functional GABA receptor antagonists like beta-CCE, FG 7142, and pentylenetetrazol resemble human anxiety? In assessing the signs and symptoms of "anxiety" from large populations of anxious patients, several classification schemes have emerged (see Klein et al.[30]). In the most commonly used classification,[1] the syndrome of generalized anxiety can be divided into four symptom subgroups that include motor (i.e., muscle) tension, autonomic hyperactivity, apprehensive-expectation, and vigilance and scanning (e.g., insomnia). In comparing the pharmacological spectrum of action of both benzodiazepine receptor agonists (i.e., the anxiolytic benzodiazepines) and inverse agonists (e.g., beta-CCE, FG 7142),[28,74] it is apparent that the syndrome of generalized anxiety consists of symptoms that are selectively attenuated by agonists and mimicked by inverse agonists (see table 21–1). We have concluded that if the benzodiazepine/GABA receptor model of anxiety is involved in pathological anxiety in man, it might be most relevant to the group of patients suffering from generalized anxiety disorder.

Since both the beta-carboline esters and pentylenetetrazol effectively antagonize GABA-mediated chloride conductance,[47,67] it appears that a decrease in GABAergic activity is associated with these drug-induced anxiety states. Could a decrease in GABAergic neuronal activity in certain brain regions underlie the development of anxiety? If so, how could this disinhibition occur?

Recently Costa and his colleagues[24] have isolated, purified, and a sequenced a family of peptides that compete with benzodiazepines and beta-carbolines for binding to the receptor and that they have proposed as being endogenous ligands for the benzodiazepine receptor. One of these peptides (diazepam binding inhibitor, or DBI) has been shown to have proconflict actions in animals[24] and to selectively inhibit the effects of GABA in electrophysiological experiments. It appears,

TABLE 21–1

Effects of Benzodiazepine Receptor Agonists and Inverse Agonists on the Symptoms of Anxiety

DSM-III Criteria for Generalized Anxiety Disorder	Benzodiazepine Agonist Effects[a]	Benzodiazepine Inverse Agonist Effects[b]
Motor Tension		
Shakiness, jitteriness, trembling	↓	↑
Muscle aches, tension	↓	↑
Fatiguability	—	—
Fidgeting, restlessness	↓	↑
Autonomic Hyperactivity		
Heart pounding, racing	↓	↑
Dizziness	—	—
Lightheadedness	↓	—
High respiratory rate	?	—
Paresthesias	?	—
Upset stomach	?	↑
Frequent urination	?	↑
Sweaty, cold, clammy hands	—	—
Flushing	—	↑
Apprehension/Expectation		
Anxiety	↓	↑
Fear, worry	↓	↑
Anticipation of misfortune	↓	↑
Vigilance and Scanning		
Insomnia	↓	↑

[a]From D. J. Greenblatt and R. I. Shader, *Benzodiazepines in Clinical Practice* (New York: Raven Press, 1974).
[b]From R. Dorow et al., "Severe Anxiety Induced by FG 7142, a β-carboline Ligand for Benzodiazepine Receptors," *Lancet*, 2 (1983): 98–99; W. Mendelson et al., "Do Benzodiazepine Receptors Play a Role in Sleep Regulation: Studies with the Benzodiazepine Antagonist, 3-hydroxymethylcarboline (3-HMC)," in E. Usdin, ed., *Beta-Carbolines and Tetraisoquinolines* (New York: Alan R. Liss, 1982), pp. 253–261; and W. Mendelson et al., "A Benzodiazepine Receptor Antagonist Decreases Sleep and Reverses the Hypnotic Actions of Flurazepam," *Science*, 219 (1983): 414–416.

therefore, that this peptide (or a related fragment) may function as an endogenous "anxiogenic" substance serving to attenuate GABAergic activity. The release of DBI or a related peptide during "stress" may serve to attenuate the inhibitory effects of GABA, resulting in the behavioral and physiological manifestations of anxiety. The availability of these peptides from commercial sources, as well as the development of specific antibodies directed against them, should help to clarify their exact physiological role, including their possible involvement in states of pathological anxiety.

Other evidence that the benzodiazepine/GABA receptor complex may be involved in the physiological expression of anxiety derives from recent studies on the effects of environmental "stress" on the benzodiazepine/GABA receptor complex in laboratory animals. Biggio[2] and coworkers were among the first to demonstrate that the receptor can be rapidly altered following exposure to various "stressors." In these experiments, rather rapid decreases in $[^3H]$-GABA binding to brain membranes were observed in animals subjected to inescapable foot shock, and the opposite was found in animals that were habituated to stress. The authors suggest that the release of an endogenous beta-carboline-like substance could result in a decrease in GABA receptor binding, since the latter was mimicked by beta-CCE and blocked by either diazepam or the selective receptor antagonist Ro 15-1788. It is tempting to speculate that the stress-induced changes in $[^3H]$-GABA binding to the GABA receptor (a presumed measure of decreased GABA receptor activity) reported by Biggio[2] are due to the release of a beta-carboline-like peptide such as DBI.[24]

More recently, Havoundjian and associates in unpublished work have demonstrated that "swim" stress rapidly alters the conformation of the benzodiazepine/GABA receptor complex at the chloride/barbiturate recognition site, an effect that is manifested by an enhanced sensitivity of benzodiazepine receptor binding to permeable anions. Functionally, these changes equate to stress-induced enhancement of GABAergic receptor sensitivity, a conclusion that has been recently confirmed both biochemically and electrophysiologically in our laboratory (unpublished observations).

Thus, immediately following "stress," a compensatory enhancement of GABA receptor sensitivity occurs directly at the postsynaptic benzodiazepine/GABA receptor complex. Interestingly, previous behavioral studies have already demonstrated increases in seizure threshold for GABA receptor antagonists like picrotoxin and pentylenetetrazol following similar "stressors" in rodents.[21,64] It appears that such alterations in "inhibitory tone" may serve to attenuate the physiological and perhaps cognitive components of "stress." We have proposed that this enhanced GABAergic sensitivity might represent a homeostatic feedback mechanism for coping with fear or anxiety-provoking stimuli.

Previous work by Robertson and colleagues has demonstrated decreased numbers of benzodiazepine receptors in genetically inbred strains of rats (Maudsley reactive) and mice that have been bred for hyperactivity to stress.[48,49] It is therefore possible that these hyperemotional and "anxious" animals have decreased benzodiazepine/GABA receptor activity, which results in their hypersensitivity to environmental stress. Conversely, the ability of the GABA receptor to alter its conformation may also be impaired in these animals. Recent developments in assessing benzodiazepine receptor sensitivity *in vivo* using such noninvasive techniques as PET[11] and a recently developed protocol for measuring benzodiazepine receptor-mediated slowing of saccadic eye velocity[26] should prove useful in determining whether the benzodiazepine/GABA receptor complex may be altered in anxious patients.

Anxiety, Depression, and the Benzodiazepine/GABA Receptor

Numerous studies in the psychiatric literature have suggested that anxiety may not simply be a symptom of depression but may, in fact, be essential to the development of at least some subtypes of depression. The issue as to whether "anxiety" and "depression" are causally related has been recently reviewed by Gray[21] and is beyond the scope of this chapter. Nevertheless, certain animal models of depression have been developed that involve the administration of inescapable aversive or "anxiety-provoking" environmental stimuli,[17,21] resulting in the development of what has been called "learned helplessness." In rodents, the "lack of control" over aversive experiences such as inescapable shock results in a behavioral syndrome characterized by failure to learn an escape task twenty-four hours later; reduction in aggression and social dominance; opioid-mediated, stress-induced analgesia; depressed lymphocyte proliferation, with increased growth of implanted tumors; decreased food intake; and ulcer formation.[17,21] Many of the components of this syndrome have been shown to be responsive to antidepressant drugs, and as such, it has been proposed as a model of depression.

Since the "stressors" that induce learned helplessness are similar, if not identical, to those used in the conflict test of anxiety, we wondered whether pharmacologically induced "anxiety" might be related to the development of this "learned helplessness" syndrome. Consequently, we administered the anxiogenic beta-carboline FG 7142 to rats and tested them for deficits in learning on a subsequent shuttlebox escape task. When administered to rats, FG 7142, like inescapable shock, resulted in a syndrome of learned helplessness that was blocked by pretreatment with benzodiazepines or the selective antagonist Ro 15-1788.[17] Interestingly, pretreatment with benzodiazepines also blocked the development of learned helplessness when induced by inescapable shock, but was ineffective in reversing the syndrome once it had already developed. These data suggest that certain animal models of anxiety may be biochemically related to the learned helplessness model of depression. Whether such information is related to the vulnerability factors that determine the progression of anxiety to depression in man is unknown but is actively being investigated.

¶ Summary

The data reviewed in this chapter strongly support a pivotal role for the GABAergic neurotransmitter system in mediating the anxiolytic actions of many, if not all, of the commonly used minor tranquilizers. The specific site of action of these agents is the postsynaptic benzodiazepine/GABA receptor complex, which serves to regulate the excitability of neurons by increasing chloride permeability and hyperpolarizing the nerve membrane. In addition to anxiolytic drugs that potentiate GABAergic inhibition, a series of compounds have been discovered that inhibit GABA-mediated chloride conductance, resulting in an increase in neuronal excitability and a behavioral action(s) that is essentially opposite that of the benzodiazepines. This "anxiogenic" action has been observed in laboratory animals as well as in man and is selectively blocked by antianxiety drugs such as the benzodiazepines. More recent data on the isolation of an endogenous anxiogenic peptide ligand and the demonstration of "stress"-induced conformational changes in the receptor complex suggest that the benzodiazepine/GABA receptor complex may be involved in the neurochemical events underlying "anxiety" and "fear." Much more work will obviously be required before we will know whether the benzodiazepine/GABA receptor is directly involved in human anxiety, including the anxiety disorders. However, at the very least we now have a comprehensive and testable hypothesis concerning the neurobiology of what is probably the most common of all human emotions.

¶ Bibliography

1. AMERICAN PSYCHIATRIC ASSOCIATION. *Diagnostic and Statistical Manual of Mental Disorders*, 3rd ed. Washington,

D.C.: American Psychiatric Association, 1980.

2. BIGGIO, G. "The Action of Stress, β-carbolines, Diazepam and Ro 15–1788 on GABA Receptors in the Rat Brain," in: G. Biggio and E. Costa, eds., *Advances in Biochemical Psychopharmacology*, vol. 38, New York: Raven Press, 1983, pp. 105–119.

3. BRAESTRUP, C., NIELSEN, M., and OLSEN, C. F. "Urinary and Brain β-carboline-3-carboxylates as Potent Inhibitors of Brain Benzodiazepine Receptors," *Proceedings of the National Academy of Science* (USA), 77 (1980): 2288–2292.

4. BRAESTRUP, C., et al. "β-Carboline-3-carboxylates and Benzodiazepine Receptors," in E. Costa, G. DiChiara, and G. Gessa, eds., *GABA and Benzodiazepine Receptors*. New York: Raven Press, 1981.

5. BREZNITZ, S. "Denial Versus Hope: Concluding Remarks," in S. Breznitz, ed., *The Denial of Stress*. New York: International Universities Press, 1983.

6. BUNNEY, W. E., JR., and DAVIS, J. M. "Norepinephrine in Depressive Reactions: A Review," *Archives of General Psychiatry*, 13 (1965): 483–494.

7. BUTLER, P. W., BESSER, G. M., and STEINBERG, H. "Changes in Plasma Cortisol induced by Dexamphetamine and Chlordiazepoxide Given Alone and in Combination in Man," *Journal of Endocrinology*, 40 (1968): 391–392.

8. CANANZI, A., COSTA, E., and GUIDOTTI, A. "Potentiation by Intraventricular Muscimol of the Anticonflict Effect of Benzodiazepines," *Brain Research*, 196 (1980): 447–453.

9. CHANG, R.S.L., and SNYDER, S. H. "Benzodiazepine Receptors: Labelling in Intact Animals with [³H] Flunitrazepam," *European Journal of Pharmacology*, 48 (1978): 213–218.

10. COLE, J. O., and DAVIS, J. M. "Antianxiety Drugs," in D. X. Freedman and J. E. Dyrud, eds., *American Handbook of Psychiatry*, 2nd ed. New York: Basic Books, 1975, pp. 427–440.

11. COMAR, D., et al. "Positron Emission Tomography in Psychopharmacological Research," *Progress in Neuro-Psychopharmacology* (abstract), 132 (Supplement) (1980): 111.

12. COSTA, E., et al. "New Concepts on the Mechanism of Action of Benzodiazepines," *Life Sciences*, 17 (1975): 167–186.

13. CRAWLEY, J. N., et al. "Neuropharmacological Antagonism of the β-carboline-induced "Anxiety" Response in Rhesus Monkeys,' *Journal of Neuroscience*, 5 (1985): 477–485.

14. DARRAGH, A., et al. "Investigation in Man of the Efficacy of a Benzodiazepine Antagonist, Ro 15–1788," *Lancet*, 2 (1981): 8–10.

15. DARWIN, C. *The Expression of the Emotions in Man and Animals*. Chicago: University of Chicago Press, 1965.

16. DOROW, R., et al. "Severe Anxiety Induced by FG 7142, a β-carboline Ligand for Benzodiazepine Receptors," *Lancet*, 2 (1983): 98–99.

17. DRUGAN, R. C., et al. "An Anxiogenic Benzodiazepine Receptor Ligand Induces Learned Helplessness," *European Journal of Pharmacology*, 113 (1985): 453–457.

18. ENNA, S. J., and GALLAGHER, J. P. "Biochemical and Electrophysiological Characteristics of Mammalian GABA Receptors," *International Review of Neurobiology*, 24 (1983): 181–212.

19. FREUD, S. *The Problem of Anxiety*, trans. H. A. Bunker. New York: The Psychoanalytic Quarterly Press and W. W. Norton, 1936.

20. GELLER, I., and SEIFTER, J. "The Effects of Meprobamate, Barbiturates, D-amphetamine and Promazine on Experimentally-induced Conflict in the Rat," *Psychopharmacologia*, 1 (1960): 482–492.

21. GRAY, J. A. *The Neuropsychology of Anxiety: An Enquiry into the Functions of the Septo-Hippocampal System*. New York: Oxford University Press, 1982.

22. GREENBLATT, D. J., and SHADER, R. I. *Benzodiazepines in Clinical Practice*. New York: Raven Press, 1974.

23. GREENBLATT, D. J., SHADER, R. I., and ABERNETHY, D. R. "Current Status of Benzodiazepines," *New England Journal of Medicine*, 309 (1983): 354–358, 410–416.

24. GUIDOTTI, A., et al. "Isolation, Characterization, and Purification to Homogeneity of an Endogenous Polypeptide

with Agonistic Action on Benzodiazepine Receptors," *Proceedings of the National Academy of Science* (USA), 80
(1983):3531–3535.

25. HAEFELY, W., et al. "Possible Involvement of GABA in the Central Actions
of Benzodiazepines," *Advances in
Biochemical Psychopharmacology*, 14
(1975):131–151.

26. HOMMER, D. W., et al. "Benzodiazepine
Receptor Sensitivity in Humans," *Archives of General Psychiatry*, in press.

27. HUNKELER, W., et al. "Selective Antagonists of Benzodiazepines," *Nature*, 290
(1981):514–516.

28. INSEL T. R., et al. "A Benzodiazepine
Receptor-mediated Model of Anxiety:
Studies in Non-human Primates and
Clinical Implications," *Archives of Gen-
eral Psychiatry*, 41 (1984):741–750.

29. KLEIN, D. F. "Delineation of Two Drug-
responsive Anxiety Syndromes," *Psychopharmacologia*, 5 (1964):397–408.

30. KLEIN, D. F., et al. *Diagnosis and Drug
Treatment of Psychiatric Disorders:
Adults and Children*, 2nd ed. Balti-
more: Williams & Wilkins, 1980.

31. MELLINGER, G. D., and BALTER, M. B.
"Psychotherapeutic Drugs: A Current
Assessment of Prevalence and Patterns
of Use," in J. P. Morgan and D. V.
Kagan, eds., *Society and Medication:
Conflicting Signals for Prescribers and
Patients*. Lexington, Mass.: D. C. Heath
Co., 1983, pp. 137–154.

32. MENDELSON, W., et al. "Do Benzodiazepine Receptors Play a Role in Sleep
Regulation: Studies with the Benzodiazepine Antagonist, 3-hydroxyme-
thylcarboline (3-HMC)," in E. Usdin,
ed., *Beta-Carbolines and Tetraisoquinolines*. New York: Alan R. Liss, 1982.

33. MENDELSON, W., et al. "A Benzodiazepine Receptor Antagonist Decreases
Sleep and Reverses the Hypnotic Actions of Flurazepam," *Science*, 219
(1983):414–416.

34. MOHLER, H., and OKADA, T. "Benzodiazepine Receptor: Demonstration
in the Central Nervous System," *Science*, 198 (1977):849–851.

35. ———"Biochemical Identification of the
Site of Action of Benzodiazepines in
Human Brain by ^{3}H-diazepam Binding," *Life Sciences*, 22 (1978):985–
996.

36. NINAN P. T., et al. "Benzodiazepine
Receptor-mediated Experimental 'Anxiety' in Primates," *Science*, 218 (1982):
1332–1334.

37. OLSEN, R. W. "GABA-benzodiazepine-
barbiturate Receptor Interactions,"
Journal of Neurochemistry, 37 (1981):
1–37.

38. PATEL, J. B., and MALICK, J. B. "Neuropharmacological Profile of an Anxiolytic," in J. B. Malick, S. J. Enna, and H.
Yamamura, eds., *Anxiolytics: Neurochemical, Behavioral and Clinical Perspectives*. New York: Raven Press, 1983,
pp. 173–192.

39. PAUL, S. M., and SKOLNICK, P. "Rapid
Changes in Brain Benzodiazepine
Receptors After Experimental Sei-
zures," *Science*, 202 (1978):892–894.

40. ———."Benzodiazepine Receptors and
Psychopathological States: Towards a
Neurobiology of Anxiety," in D. F.
Klein and J. Rabkin, eds., *Anxiety: New
Research and Changing Concepts*. New
York: Raven Press, 1981, pp. 215–230.

41. ———."Comparative   Neuropharmacology of Antianxiety Drugs," *Pharmacology, Biochemistry and Behavior*, 17
(supplement 1) (1982):37–41.

42. ———."The Biochemistry of Anxiety:
From Pharmacotherapy to Pathophysiology," in D. Klein, ed., *Psychiatry Update: The APA Annual Review*, vol. 13.
Washington, D.C.: American Psychiatric Association, 1984, pp. 482–490.

43. PAUL, S. M., JANOWSKY, A., and SKOL-
NICK, P. "Monoaminergic Neurotransmitters and Antidepressant Drugs," in
R. E. Hales, and A. J. Frances, eds., *Psychiatry Update: The APA Annual Review*, vol. 4. Washington, D.C.: American Psychiatric Associaton, 1985, pp.
37–48.

44. PAUL, S. M., MARANGOS, P. J., and SKOL-
NICK, P. "The Benzodiazepine-GABA-
chloride Ionophore Receptor Complex:
Common Site of Minor Tranquilizer Action," *Biological Psychiatry*, 16 (1981):
213–229.

45. POLC, P., ROPERT, N., and WRIGHT, D. M.
"Ethyl-β-carboline-3-carboxylate   Antagonizes the Action of GABA and Ben-

zodiazepine in the Hippocampus," *Brain Research,* 217 (1981):216–220.

46. RICKELS, K. "Use of Anti-anxiety Agents in Anxious Outpatients," *Psychopharmacology,* 58 (1978):1–17.

47. ROBERTS, E., CHASE, T. W., and TOWER, D. B. *GABA in Nervous System Function.* New York: Raven Press, 1976.

48. ROBERTSON, H. "Benzodiazepine Receptors in 'Emotional' and 'Nonemotional' Mice: Comparison of Four Strains," *European Journal of Pharmacology,* 56 (1979):163–167.

49. ROBERTSON, H. A., MARTIN, I. L., and CANDY, J. M. "Differences in Benzodiazepine Receptor Binding in Maudsley Reactive and Maudsley Nonreactive Rats," *European Journal of Pharmacology,* 50 (1978):455–457.

50. RODIN, E. "Metrazol Tolerance in a 'Normal' and Volunteer Population," *EEG Clinical Neurophysiology,* 10 (1958): 433–446.

51. ROSE, R. M., and SACHAR, E. "Psychoendocrinology," in R. H. Williams, ed., *Textbook of Endocrinology,* 6th ed. Philadelphia: W. B. Saunders, 1981, pp. 654–657.

52. RUFF, M. R., et al. "Benzodiazepine Receptor-mediated Chemotaxis of Human Monocytes," *Science,* 229 (1985):1281–1283.

53. SACHAR, E. J. "Psychological Factors Relating to Activation and Inhibition of the Adrenocortical Stress Response in Man: A Review," *Progress in Brain Research,* 32 (1970):316.

54. SCHWARTZ, R. D., et al. "Radiation Inactivation Studies of the Benzodiazepine/GABA/chloride Ionophore Receptor Complex," *Journal of Neurochemistry,* 45 (1985):108–115.

55. SCHWARTZ, R. D., et al. "Characterization of Barbiturate-stimulated Chloride Efflux from Rat Brain Synaptoneurosomes," *Journal of Neuroscience,* 5 (1985):2963–2970.

56. SCHWARTZ, R. D., et al. "Demonstration of GABA/barbiturate-receptor Mediated Chloride Transport in Rat Brain Synaptoneurosomes: A Functional Assay of GABA Receptor-effector Coupling," in G. Biggio and E. Costa, *Advances in Biochemical Pharmacology,* New York: Raven Press, forthcoming.

57. SCHEEL-KRUGER, J., and PETERSEN, F. "Anticonflict Effects of the Benzodiazepines Mediated by a GABAergic Mechanism in the Amygdala," *European Journal of Pharmacology,* 82 (1982): 115.

58. SELIGMAN, M.E.P. *Helplessness. On Depression, Development and Death.* San Francisco: W. H. Freeman, 1975.

59. SHEEHAN, D. V. "Current Concepts in Psychiatry: Panic Attacks and Phobias," *New England Journal of Medicine,* 307 (1982):156–158.

60. SKOLNICK, P., and PAUL, S. M. "Benzodiazepine Receptors in the Central Nervous System," *International Review of Neurobiology,* 23 (1982):103–140.

61. ———."New Concepts in the Neurobiology of Anxiety," *Journal of Clinical Psychiatry,* 44 (1983):12–19.

62. SKOLNICK, P., et al. "Pentobarbital Has Dual Actions to Increase Brain Benzodiazepine Receptor Affinity," *Science,* 211 (1981):1448–1450.

63. SNYDER, S. H., et al. "Drugs, Neurotransmitters and Schizophrenia," *Science,* 184 (1974):1243–1253.

64. SOUBRIE, P., et al. "Decreased Convulsant Potency of Picrotoxin and Pentetrazol and Enhanced [^{3}H]flunitrazepam Cortical Binding Following Stressful Manipulations in Rats," *Brain Research* 189 (1980):505–517.

65. SQUIRES, R. F., and BRAESTRUP, C. "Benzodiazepine Receptors in Rat Brain," *Nature,* 266 (1977):732–734.

66. SQUIRES, R. F., et al. "Convulsant Potencies of Tetrazoles Are Highly Correlated with Actions on GABA/benzodiazepine Picrotoxin Receptor Complexes in Brain," *Life Sciences* 35 (1984):1439–1444.

67. STUDY, R. E., and BARKER, J. L. "Cellular Mechanisms of Benzodiazepine Actions," *Journal of the American Medical Association,* 247 (1982):2147–2151.

68. SUZDAK, P., et al. "Ethanol Stimulates ^{36}Cl Uptake into Synaptoneurosomes via the GABA Receptor Complex" Unpublished.

69. TALLMAN, J. D., THOMAS, J., and GALLAGER, D. "GABAergic Modulation of

Benzodiazepine Site Sensitivity," *Nature*, 274 (1978):383–395.

70. TALLMAN, J. F., et al. "Receptors for the Age of Anxiety: Pharmacology of the Benzodiazepines," *Science*, 207 (1980): 274–281.

71. TENEN, S. S., and HIRSCH, J. D. "β-Carboline-3-carboxylic Acid Ethyl Ester Antagonizes Diazepam Activity," *Nature*, 288 (1980):609–610.

72. UHLENHUTH, E. H., et al. "Symptom Checklist Syndromes in the General Population: Correlations with Psychotherapeutic Drug Use," *Archives of General Psychiatry*, 40 (1983):1167–1173.

73. WILLIAMSON, M. J., PAUL, S. M., and SKOLNICK, P. "Labelling of Benzodiazepine Receptors *in vivo*," *Nature*, 275 (1978):551–553.

74. WOLKOWITZ, O. W., and PAUL, S. M. "Neural and Molecular Mechanisms in Anxiety," in G. C. Curtis, B. A. Thyer, and J. M. Rainey, eds., *Psychiatric Clinics of North America*, vol. 8. Philadelphia: W. B. Saunders, 1985, pp. 145–158.

75. YOUNG, W. S., and KUHAR, M. J. "Autoradiographic Localization of Benzodiazepine Receptor in the Brains of Humans and Animals," *Nature*, 280 (1979):393–395.

CHAPTER 22

SOME PRACTICAL APPROACHES TO THE UNDERSTANDING AND TREATMENT OF THE SYMPTOMS OF ANXIETY AND STRESS

Richard I. Shader and David J. Greenblatt

¶ Introduction

Despite the vast amount of effort and research that has gone into clarifying the concepts of fear, stress, and anxiety, much semantic confusion persists; the relationships among fear, stress, and anxiety remain obscure. With the introduction of meprobamate in the 1950s and the benzodiazepines in the 1950s and 1960s, a new era of progress was ushered in. These and other agents serve not only as treatments but also as pharmacological tools to modify and study the experience of anxiety. Even with the use of these probes, the etiology and un-

derlying pathophysiology of anxiety, fear, and stress are unknown. The development of the new classification system in the third edition of the *Diagnostic and Statistical Manual* (DSM-III) of the American Psychiatric Association[4] also has helped to promote more specificity in diagnostic and semantic thinking, but it has not accomplished enough of the task; promised revisions to DSM-III, one hopes, will take us a step closer.

In order to treat patients with anxiety disorders and stress, it is important to have at

Portions of this chapter are based on R. I. Shader and D. J. Greenblatt, "Some Current Treatment Options for the Symptoms of Anxiety," *Journal of Clinical Psychiatry,* 44 (1983): 21–29.

least some working or practical perspectives about these concepts. Let us start with the concept of fear. A clinically useful perspective is to consider fear as a normal and appropriate reaction to threats to survival or to danger. It is an emotional response to signals from our perceptual organs. Fear alerts us both to external threats and to internally perceived changes in our functioning that suggest danger. For example, the experience of impending suffocation that is associated with hypoxia produces a threat to survival, and fear can ensue. Fear, then, is an affective experience that provides the basis for cautious adaptations to our external and internal experiences during which we weigh these factors in our environment and prepare for action. A patient may find a lump somewhere in the body and fear it is cancerous. In turn, there may be a fear that the illness will cause death, disability, or loss of income, either through the actual high cost of medical care or from loss of work. These are understandable fears, but some individuals may be inappropriately fearful (anxious) and then not seek help. In the latter circumstances, denial, displacement, rationalization, acting out, and conversion symptoms are not unusual. Clinicians need to recognize that fear may underly such presentations. These patients need to share their concerns and get as much time, reassurance, and education as is appropriate. Although it is normal to feel fear about a threat to one's integrity or survival, fear should dissipate as soon as the circumstances change and the conditions move from threat to safety. Usually the memory of the threatening experience is integrated; this allows the individual to mobilize coping skills and behaviors that will either permit avoidance of similar experiences in the future or will promote the capacity for the mastery of such situations.

Anxiety involves similar emotional and physiological experiences to those that are felt in fear. However, in anxiety the threat to survival is either not apparent or the response to the perceived threat is clearly disproportionate to the intensity of the threatening stimulus. Anxiety is at times a conditioned response in which the linkages to the original fear-producing stimulus or situation are now forgotten or repressed.

Anxiety can be a fear of fear or stem from unrecognized emotional conflict. Anxiety is an experience of unwanted and uncontrolled autonomic nervous system arousal. Anxiety may be persistent, leading to a sense of being constantly "uptight" or nervous, or it can have an attacklike course. Only when patients' symptoms appear to have no cause, or when responses to fear-provoking situations seem irrational, excessive, unremitting, or unwarranted, is it considered appropriate to label patient's complaints as anxiety disorder. In these instances, patients who seek help almost always show or relate a history of autonomic nervous system overactivity, manifesting some combination of apprehension (worry, premonition), excessive arousal or dysautonomia (tachycardia, sweating), muscle tension (soreness, trembling, jumpiness), and hyperattentiveness (vigilance). In acute situations of both anxiety and fear, laboratory studies may reveal elevations in catecholamines, free fatty acids, and cortisol, although wide individual differences are found in these responses. At the present time, there is no reliable or consistent laboratory test that differentiates between anxiety and fear.

Repeated fear-linked exposures can lead to a sense of vulnerability, helplessness, powerlessness, or impotent rage. Here it is useful to introduce the concept of stress. Stress is a direct consequence of feeling too helpless to cope. It may occur from having to deal with change, ambiguity, novel stimuli, or uncertainty. Stress may occur from a wide variety of other life experiences ranging from social isolation or physical immobility and confinement—the extreme being sensory deprivation—to overstimulation or excessive responsibility such as in decision-making stress. How one behaves in stressful situations may influence the degree of stress; some individuals show good judgment in terms of when to get out of stress-provoking situations, and others seem to remain too long and become the captive of the stressful situation. Stress is both a cause and result of "dysease" and disease. In anxiety states or with fear or stress, individuals will vary in their seeking of assistance; in their abilities to develop action strategies, plan for contingencies, or cope psychologically through the use of denial, displacement, and rationalization; or in their use of others for support in surmounting the danger or stress.

T. S. Eliot's observation that "humankind cannot bear very much reality" (*Murder in the Cathedral*, 1935) underlies man's susceptibility to stress. Humankind is bombarded by the complexities and vulnerabilities of modern life, lack of control or mastery, and conflict with significant persons. Humankind is also particularly sensitive to unwanted separations, the unexpected loss of love, and the involuntary disruption of attachment bonds. The ability to bear such stress may be even more compromised today when there is a general weakening in the strength of family and religious ties and when supporting and trusting relationships with neighbors are becoming more rare. The strain of such situations can be acute but is usually chronic and recurrent. It can produce significant impairment of functioning, especially through headache, muscle tension and fatigue, mental tension, and distress, which is another form of stress. Yet not all individuals exposed to comparably troubling experiences will reveal evidence of stress. What makes some "deniers," others "minimizers," and still others "exaggerators" in their encounters with problematic or disruptive situations remains a mystery.

¶ Simple Approaches to Stress Management

General steps and approaches to stress reduction include recognition of the sources and of the causes, reassurance, support, removal of or from the "stressors" when possible, strategies to promote feelings of being able to cope or manage, and techniques for relaxation. The aim is to try to relax the "taut rubber band" feeling that such patients often describe. When stress is work-related, certain techniques can be recommended and applied that may directly promote a reduction in stress. In addition to the steps and approaches just noted, it may be helpful to: (1) review short- and long-range goals and eliminate those that are not attainable; (2) create a hierarchy of tasks or assignments that establishes appropriate priorities and estimates reasonable and realistic time allotments; (3) divide undone work into manageable units or parts; (4) start with initial tasks that are "do-able"— starting with complicated or difficult work often leads to procrastination; (5) be assertive when appropriate and necessary— learning to say no and doing no more than can be handled; (6) create needed time for sharing and discussions with others as well as time out for relaxation and rest; and (7) modify periods of feeling stressed, anxious, or blocked by utilizing specific relaxation strategies such as taking six to ten deep breaths, trying to fill the chest, while sitting in a relaxed way and with adequate support for the arms, shoulders, and neck, or closing the eyes for a few moments picturing a favorite vacation spot and trying to capture the sights, sounds, smells, and textures of the experience. Be sure that nonwork hours are a change of pace with adequate sharing, distraction, exercise, nutrition, and sleep.

To further minimize and treat the symptoms of stress, simple exercises can be carried out while sitting in a classroom, an office chair, or any other appropriate location. These will help to relax taut muscles. The aim is to further stretch and then relax any tense muscle groups. Since the muscles in the back of the head and in the neck and shoulders are the ones most often affected, starting with these is often best and, in many instances, actually may be sufficient:

1. Lower the head forward toward the chest, stretching the muscles in the back of the neck (if a tie is being worn, it should be loosened; collars should be unbuttoned).
2. Alternately lower the head toward each shoulder, keeping the face forward, and, without raising the shoulders, stretch the side muscles of the neck.

3. Let the head fall back, arching the muscles of the back, stretching the muscles under the chin.
4. Folding the forearms over each other, right over left, alternately move the right shoulder toward the left and the left toward the right, stretching the outer muscles of each shoulder and the lateral shoulder blades.
5. Shrug the shoulders, tensing and then relaxing the lateral muscles of the neck and the upper shoulders.
6. Alternately push the shoulders back and then forward, stretching the muscles of the back—with the backward movement, arch the lower back and keep the neck straight.

Working out some variation of this plan for your patients that takes into account individual differences in posture and sitting habits can reduce tension and related aspects of work strain. Taking five to ten minutes twice a day from the typical coffee break to accomplish such exercises will probably be beneficial by itself—any reduction in caffeine and sugar intake will probably be a secondary benefit. Other muscles can be involved as is necessary (e.g., hand tension can be relieved by squeezing a tennis ball). With these and other personally created techniques, some of the consequences of stress can be reduced and thereby endured.

¶ Approaches to the Treatment of Anxiety

While the goals of the treatment of anxiety are clear—namely, reducing symptomatology—choosing the best approach for the individual patient can be a complicated process, depending on the diagnosis as well as the patient's age, medical status, drug history, personality, and social context. Fortunately, refinements in diagnosis and treatment resulting from extensive research are enhancing our ability to manage anxiety effectively.

Clinicians need to become comfortable enough in their clinical interactions to use phrases or questions that will elicit underlying fears and anxiety. Examples include: (1)

You seem worried. (2) Were you worried when you felt the . . . (or noticed the . . .)? (3) What did you worry would happen to you in the hospital? (4) Are there things (or people) that will be neglected while you are in the hospital? (5) Have you been anxious recently? (6) What brings on such feelings? or (7) What do you fear most?

It is also important to elicit and examine for the typical signs and symptoms of anxiety (e.g., tremulousness, avoidance behaviors, trouble falling asleep, fatigue) to establish the degree, patterning, and pervasiveness of the anxiety and any associated impairment of functioning. With experience, clinicians can learn to obtain relevant material without worrying their patients and without becoming entangled in the contagion of patients' anxieties.

When the patient has been appropriately identified as suffering from an anxiety disorder, further classification is necessary. The symptoms may be chronic or sporadic, free-floating or focused. They may occur alone or with other symptoms, such as depression, anger, or depersonalization; somatic complaints commonly accompany anxiety. Anxiety may be the primary problem, as in a phobic disorder or primary anxiety state, or a secondary yet intrinsic aspect of a documented or medical problem, such as hyperthyroidism, multiple small pulmonary emboli, Addison's disease, hypocalcemia or pheochromocytoma; drug intoxication or withdrawal from hypnotics, stimulants, anxiolytics, over-the-counter preparations, alcohol, or caffeine (see chapters 29 and 30); or an affective disorder or schizophrenia (see chapters 13 and 18). Whether the diagnosis is anxiety disorder per se or whether the symptoms are secondary to some other condition is crucial, since appropriate treatment options may differ considerably.

Even if a primary anxiety disorder is strongly suspected, a careful history and a thorough physical examination, including laboratory tests, must be performed. This assessment may in itself be therapeutic, as it conveys concern, support, and involvement with the patient and his or her problems.

When appropriate, the patient can be taught during the assessment that there is therapeutic value to identifying the experience as anxiety, putting it into words, and remembering that these attacks pass. These and similar expressed phrases can help with coping with anxiety: I'm feeling anxious. I'm not falling apart. These feelings will pass; they are familiar. I know I can be treated and I will feel better.

Once other etiologies for the anxiety symptoms have been ruled out, the diagnosis and classification of a primary anxiety disorder can be made. The two major categories of anxiety, according to DSM-III, are Phobic Disorders, such as agoraphobia, social phobia, and simple phobia, and Anxiety States, such as panic disorder, obsessive-compulsive disorder, and generalized anxiety disorder. While not frequently diagnosed, another important category is post-traumatic stress disorder. Unfortunately, this subtype has become linked too exclusively to Viet Nam war veterans. As a result, other traumatic experiences, such as pathological family experiences, are not understood in this way. However, the symptoms and response to treatment of the disorders that follow traumatic events are similar to those of the classic post-traumatic stress disorder described for Viet Nam veterans.

Therapeutic options are numerous. Whether a single or combination treatment is chosen, it must be individualized not only to the specific diagnosis but also to the patient. For example, if a candidate for pharmacotherapy is an alcoholic or elderly patient or is prone to drug abuse, drug choice or dosage may need to be changed.

The approach to treatment should be conservative initially, beginning with the safest option and adding or substituting another therapy if necessary. In general, nonpharmacological interventions have the lowest potential for adverse effects unless they produce unnecessary dependency or cause financial distress. When properly selected and administered, however, pharmacotherapy can be both rational and safe and can be prescribed with confidence.

Therapeutic communication aimed at clarification and understanding remains the foundation of treatment for anxiety. Supportive and behavioral therapies are widely used and have been found effective in some patients with anxiety states. Among the currently marketed psychopharmacological interventions, benzodiazepines remain the drugs of choice; when prescribed and administered correctly, they are relatively effective and safe. However, these drugs are not devoid of hazards and side effects, and new antianxiety agents, with comparable or improved efficacy and less potential for unwanted effects, must be and are being sought.

Some of the difficulty in determining the best treatment for anxiety can be minimized by remembering that what patients call anxiety is actually a clustering of symptoms, not a diagnosis; effective therapy is aimed at treating underlying causes and associated problems rather than merely responding to symptoms. Understanding the underlying causes of each patient's anxiety and therefore arriving at the correct diagnosis is of paramount importance in treatment planning, because a therapeutic approach that works well for one anxiety disorder may not work well for another.

¶ Nonpharmacological Options for the Treatment of Anxiety

Theoretical, philosophical, and ethical issues of traditional psychotherapeutic approaches versus behavioral methods have been debated for many years. The psychotherapist typically views behavior and symptoms essentially as manifestations of underlying processes, postulating that only by recognition and modification of such unconscious factors can troublesome behavior be changed. The behaviorist, on the other hand, maintains that actions are in themselves dynamically significant and that changing unwanted responses can also effect more profound changes.

The fundamental impact of both views

may in fact be the same. It is reasonable to postulate a synergistic effect when such approaches are used in combination. Behavioral therapy may complement psychotherapy by removing uncomfortable symptoms, and psychotherapy may enhance behavioral therapy by assuring that these changes are permanent and not replaced by other maladaptive behaviors. The "working through" done in typical psychodynamically oriented psychotherapies can easily be understood as a form of desensitization.

Psychodynamically Oriented Psychotherapy

Every patient being treated for anxiety should receive some form of therapeutic communication. For the stressed or situationally anxious patient, understanding, reassurance, support, and education are often sufficient. However, primary anxiety disorders may require more intense approaches.

The element of interpretation, or insight, that classically distinguishes psychodynamically oriented psychotherapy from behavioral therapy can lead to profound alterations in both attitude and behavior, but relief or change from insight alone is not a common experience. When a patient's symptoms appear to arise from conflict, psychodynamically oriented psychotherapy is probably the most effective approach in the long run, but this requires a strong commitment by the patient and may be a very slow process.

The psychodynamically oriented psychotherapist seeks to identify unresolved or unexpressed anger, sexual concerns, grief, or troubles with the patient's spouse, children, or significant others. Underlying principles include the following sequential linkages: anxiety becomes linked to specific situations, displacement may occur, avoidance develops, avoidance spreads or generalizes as anxiety mounts, and withdrawal occurs. Another important sequence is that young people look to their parents as protectors, that loss of the sense of being protected causes anxiety, that loss of a protecting figure can become linked to loss of love, and that loss of love can

produce anxiety. In general, a key underlying concept is that exposure and resolution of repressed or unexpressed conflict will diminish anxiety. It is also important to recognize that different issues may be the sources of conflict at different ages.

Group formats can also be useful. They can be helpful with educational objectives about anxiety, provide a "buddy system" that encourages counterphobic behaviors, diminish isolation for those who feel alone, allow members to see that their symptoms are not unique, reinforce a focus on the here and now, encourage coping rather than retreat, provide support to those who need to look at anger or loss, or promote an effort to float through an anxiety experience rather than resorting to fight or flight.

Behavioral Therapy

Whereas insight is the central characteristic of psychotherapy, desensitization has been defined by Eysenck and Rachman[35] as the essential element in behavioral therapy. According to Wolpe and others,[116,140,153] desensitization gradually weakens the anxiety response habit in patients sensitized to particular situations or dissociates the anxiety response from its usual stimuli. However, it does not, as a rule, influence nonspecific, nonfocused responses.[14,116,140,153] Thus behavioral interventions would appear to be best suited for phobia, panic symptoms, and obsessive-compulsive disorders. For many behavioral therapists, some form of traditional psychotherapy is usually an essential element in the treatment plan.[45] Since anxious patients are often socially withdrawn and may feel inadequate, cognitive therapies, social skills enhancement, and assertiveness training may be employed.

The interventions that have been attempted range from general relaxation techniques, such as transcendental meditation (TM), muscle relaxation, and biofeedback, to more specific desensitization processes, including Wolpe's systematic desensitization, forced immersion, thought stopping, and aversion relief.

Relaxation Techniques

Deep relaxation is felt to be essential to the success of many behavioral techniques. However, specific relaxation techniques have also been employed with varying degrees of efficacy for generalized anxiety, panic symptoms, and situational anxiety. Migraine and tension headaches, some forms of insomnia, chronic pain, and essential hypertension may also be improved through relaxation training.

Meditation, a technique that is widely practiced today, most often consists of sitting comfortably, with eyes closed, for twenty minutes twice a day, while maintaining a constant awareness of a mantra or sound. Physiological changes that occur during meditation are opposite to those that occur during anxiety states. Studies[147,148] of what typically is called transcendental meditation suggest that TM lowers physiological arousal, stabilizes autonomic functioning,[94] increases electroencephalographic alpha density,[147,148] and decreases blood lactate concentrations.[147,148] Benson, in his classic study, termed these effects the "relaxation response."[16]

Clinical trials by Orme-Johnson,[95] Farwell,[39] and Hjelle[68] conclude that TM is effective in reducing anxiety. Criticism that the beneficial effects found are due solely to the act of sitting quietly has been somewhat silenced by a study comparing TM with passive relaxation.[33] However, long-term exposure is necessary for good results; studies have shown that the efficacy of short-term meditation is no greater than that of placebo.[19,46,134] Unfortunately, many patients discontinue treatment before positive effects can be perceived. Many patients are too distressed or distracted to sit still or concentrate long enough to use this approach. This limitation is often evident in the more severe cases of generalized anxiety disorder and in patients with panic disorder.

Another common relaxation technique involves deep-muscle relaxation and is based on the premise that anxiety and relaxation cannot coexist.[120,150,154] The fact that muscle relaxation apparently induces a "trophotropic" physiological state[45] and may reduce sympathetic adrenal medullary activity[67] seems to support this view. Muscle relaxation therapy is suggested to be superior to nonspecific treatments in reducing anxiety[101,102,114,141] and is intended to give patients a sense of being able to exert some control over their own symptoms.

Muscle relaxation techniques, although said to have been first described in 1938 by Jacobsen,[72] were actually described much earlier by Schultz.[119] Jacobsen's "progressive relaxation" method is still used today and depends on systematically tensing and relaxing some ten to twenty muscle groups. The tensing and relaxing of different muscle groups promotes a contrasting experience for patients and thus develops a sense of discrimination. Since this method requires prolonged training (five to ten sessions at a minimum), a variation was developed by Schultz and Luthe that emphasizes the patient's ability to relax quickly and at will.[120] The systematic contraction and release can produce a residual relaxation over baseline, which is maintained with regular practice. Advantages of progressive relaxation are as follows: There are no equipment costs, the technique can be easily taught and used indefinitely, and it can be carried out in any place that is quiet (a dimly lit room equipped with a reclining chair that supports the head is preferable). It can be coupled to the stress-relieving exercises described earlier.

In a recent study involving patients and controls, the effects of "anxiety management training" were compared with those of "applied relaxation training," relaxation only, and placebo.[71] Anxiety management training, which included detailed instructions on the use of relaxation in everyday life, proved superior to the other techniques, suggesting that for some patients, muscle relaxation is most effective when incorporated into daily situations. The success of muscle relaxation will depend on the type and severity of a patient's anxiety.

The use of electromyographic biofeedback may provide the patient with a mechanism for profoundly altering the rates of certain biological functions and levels of relaxation. Relaxation of the frontalis muscle is now used in a wide range of clinical situations, including anxiety. Despite claims of its usefulness,[15,133] however, a consistent correlation has not been demonstrated between profound reduction in frontalis muscle potentials and subjectively experienced relaxation.[27,109]. Thus any observed effect may be due to general relaxation rather than to the biofeedback techniques per se. Raskin and coworkers,[107,108] in two separate studies of biofeedback alone or in combination with TM, found that neither approach was more effective than muscle relaxation alone in alleviating chronic anxiety, and although there was improvement for the patients taken as a group, the majority were not substantially helped by these techniques.

Systematic Desensitization

Systematic desensitization was first used by Wolpe[153] as a means of weakening the bond between anxiety-provoking stimuli and the anxiety response, through the phenomenon of reciprocal inhibition. The technique involves the initiation of deep relaxation, using Jacobsen's method of progressive muscle relaxation, hypnosis, antianxiety agents, or intravenous methohexital sodium, which has been found to be extremely safe as well as practical for outpatient use.[106] After careful assessment of the patient, a system of anxiety hierarchies is constructed that includes all sources of anxiety. These are then presented for the patient's imagination, beginning with the least and progressing to the most threatening stimulus. The patient learns to relax in the face of each of the threatening images.

Systematic desensitization is reported to be effective in clinical trials* for the treatment of some phobic disorders. However, it is not considered the behavioral treatment of choice for agoraphobia.[43] Two variants of

*See references 42, 43, 79, 81, and 100.

systematic desensitization are successive approachment, in which the patient is rewarded for approaching the feared object,[85] and self-observation, in which the patient gradually approaches the anxiety stimulus with instructions to stop when anxiety becomes too great.[29]

Forced Immersion

Forced immersion requires that the patient be presented with highly anxiety-producing stimuli at the outset of therapy, either through imagination, as in implosion therapy, or by confrontation with the feared object, a technique termed flooding.

Some investigators have found flooding superior to systematic desensitization in the treatment of agoraphobia.[86,139] Stern and Marks recommend individual or group sessions of approximately two hours, held weekly or biweekly for several months.[139] Concomitant antianxiety medication is discouraged,[87] and antidepressants have been given[157] (see section entitled "Pharmacological Options"), but combined approaches have not been sufficiently studied to merit support or avoidance.

Thought Stopping

This technique is applied primarily to obsessive-compulsive behavior and, like systematic desensitization, employs hierarchies. The patient is asked to evoke an obsessional thought, whereupon the therapist makes a noise, such as tapping on a table, and the patient shouts, "Stop!" In time, the patient learns to eradicate the thought by merely thinking the word "Stop."[138]

Response prevention is similar to thought stopping. Using muscle relaxation and/or antianxiety medication, the patient attempts to keep the obsessive response within limits. Results of a recent study[137] indicate that response prevention is successful when combined with prolonged flooding as well as imagined exposure (implosion).

Other Behavioral Approaches

Other behavioral approaches include assertiveness training,[103] modeling,[11] and aversion relief,[136] all of which appear effective for some phobic disorders. Choosing from among the available interventions is largely a matter of clinical judgment and personal preference. Most likely, as with many therapeutic strategies, the choice is a function of where and by whom the practitioner was trained. However, there is some evidence that for focal phobias, flooding may be superior to therapies in which the anxiety-provoking stimulus is merely imagined.[82]

¶ Pharmacological Options for the Treatment of Anxiety

When anxiety is severe and for some specific anxiety disorders, nonpharmacological intervention alone is usually insufficient. Especially for patients whose anxiety seriously hinders normal functioning, the value of pharmacotherapy as a short-term and/or intermittent adjunct to nondrug approaches cannot be overstated.

The pharmacological options are numerous and diverse; diagnosis seems the best guideline to choosing an appropriate agent. The following section concentrates on the specific applications of currently marketed pharmacological agents. Discussion of agents that are rarely used or no longer recommended, such as barbiturates, meprobamate, glutethimide, and chloral hydrate derivatives, can be found elsewhere.[9,49,50,127]

Phobic Disorders and Panic Attacks

The most frequently treated phobic disorder is considered to be agoraphobia; it is said to affect at least six out of every thousand Americans. The term was first coined by Carl Westphal in 1872 to describe three male patients who were too scared to enter and cross the town square unless they were fortified with alcohol. Today agoraphobia is not seen merely as a fear of open spaces. Rather it is an avoidance of any of a variety of anxiety-provoking places in order to prevent panic attacks from occurring when easy or quick access to reassuring persons or places is not available. In essence then, agoraphobia is an attempt to avoid anxiety about anxiety. At the height of panic attacks, patients so affected typically worry about choking, dying, "going crazy," losing control, being embarrassed, or some other overwhelming or catastrophic outcome. Panic attacks usually have their onset in the teenage years or early twenties; later, once agoraphobia has set in, the patient may never or only rarely leave home until effectively treated with medication or unless accompanied by a reassuring and significant companion.

Klein has hypothesized and described a model in which the patient first experiences spontaneous panic attacks and subsequently develops anticipatory anxiety (worry that panic will recur) and avoidance behaviors.[76] Others propose a broader view.[130] DSM-III criteria require a minimum of three panic attacks in a three-week period to establish clearly the diagnosis of panic disorder. Panic attacks with secondary agoraphobia are often effectively managed with monoamine oxidase inhibitors (MAOIs), currently available heterocyclic antidepressants, or alprazolam. These treatments appear to block the panic attacks,[58,59] thereby lessening the anticipatory anxiety and breaking the cycle. The blocking effect of these approaches has been supported by studies employing sodium lactate infusion, which frequently precipitates panic in patients with this disorder but typically does not so affect control subjects.[105]

Present clinical data are insufficient to give preference to MAOIs, other antidepressants, or alprazolam in panic and agoraphobic disorders.[146] Bupropion is the only antidepressant to date that has not been shown to be effective.[132] Klein and Fink[77] first reported the antipanic effects of imipramine hydrochloride in 1962. Subsequent placebo-controlled trials have shown imipramine hydrochloride to be more effective than placebo in agoraphobic patients undergoing current psychotherapy or behavioral therapy. The required dose of imipramine is highly variable. The average effective dosage appears to be approximately 150 mg per day; higher dosages are rarely required. However, about 25 percent of patients are sensitive to rather small dosages, and a positive response can occur with as little as 10 mg per day. Major clinical effects may not be apparent until three weeks after initiation of treatment, which should be continued for at least six to twelve weeks. Since symptoms tend to recur when the medication is withdrawn, imipramine therapy may be best viewed as an integral part of a comprehensive treatment program that includes psychotherapy and behavioral modification.

MAOIs have also been found to be effective in the treatment of panic disorder [145] and agoraphobia. [74,83,131] Placebo-controlled studies have shown that phenelzine sulfate, in dosages of at least 45 mg per day or higher, is effective in reducing panic attacks, phobias, and associated symptoms. [131,143] However, higher dosages (60–90 mg/day) are sometimes given for six to eight weeks for maximum effects. [143,145] Just as with imipramine, however, some patients will respond to very low dosages of phenelzine, such as 15 mg per day.

Adverse reactions can occur with the MAOIs. Also, their interactions with various drugs affecting the sympathetic nervous system, as well as with foods containing tyramine, must be considered. (See chapter 13 for a discussion of the clinical use and side effects of MAOIs and other antidepressants.) At this time, phenelzine may be the most consistently and broadly effective medication, but, even so, symptoms rarely disappear totally and tend to recur with discontinuation of the medication.

When an MAOI or a heterocyclic antidepressant blocks the panic attacks but the anticipatory anxiety remains, a benzodiazepine may be a useful addition. Beta-blockers have been studied in some patients with panic disorder [47] and simple phobias. [17] Al-though they decrease autonomically mediated symptoms such as tachycardia, they have negligible behavioral or subjective effects. This may be a problem in design, since dosage regimens in these studies were not usually individually tailored to assure a meaningful degree of beta-blockade in each patient.

Although alprazolam's use in panic disorders has been relatively extensive on an informal or nonblind basis for the last few years, controlled trials, though completed, have not yet been published. The mean daily effective dose for blocking panic attacks seems to be about 6 mg; however, individual variation is high, with some patients requiring lower doses (1.0–2.0 mg) and others requiring higher doses (e.g., up to 12 mg). In rare cases even higher doses have been employed and found to be beneficial. Unfortunately, data are not yet available to understand fully the safety of these dosage regimens or be able to assess addiction potential adequately.

Obsessive-compulsive Disorder

Obsessive-compulsive disorder is notoriously difficult to treat by any method; fortunately, as a disorder rather than as a symptom, it is also relatively rare. Tricyclic antidepressants, especially chlorimipramine hydrochloride, have been found effective for some obsessive-compulsive patients in both uncontrolled [5] and comparative studies. [6,23,149,156]

Thoren and coworkers found 150 mg per day chlorimipramine significantly superior to placebo and somewhat more effective than 150 mg per day nortriptyline hydrochloride in decreasing obsessive-compulsive and depressive symptoms. [6] However, social function and self-report measures of improvement did not differ among the three groups. During a higher-dose, open phase of the study, the response rate to chlorimipramine was about 50 percent. High spinal fluid levels of 5-hydroxyindoleacetic acid, a metabolite of serotonin, appeared to correlate with clinical benefit. Other agents that affect serotonin may also prove useful in the management of obsessive-compulsive disorders.

Generalized Anxiety Disorder

Situational anxiety related to specific stressful experiences usually subsides gradually over a course of two to three weeks and should be treated by nonpharmacological means if at all possible. Generalized anxiety that persists for at least one month and is accompanied by symptoms of motor tension, autonomic hyperactivity, apprehensive expectation, vigilance, or scanning may require drug intervention. For these patients, benzodiazepines are currently the drugs of choice. Adverse publicity notwithstanding, their relatively consistent clinical efficacy has been established,[126] and proper administration minimizes the potential risks.

¶ The Use of Benzodiazepines in Treatment of Generalized Anxiety Disorder*

The benzodiazepines are the safest and most effective pharmacological treatment for anxiety. This safety and efficacy has been demonstrated in numerous controlled clinical trials.[51,55,110] Pharmacological and receptor investigations of the twelve benzodiazepines that are currently available in the United States (see table 22–1) have clearly established large quantitative differences in the potency of these compounds. However, the qualitative differences among these compounds that are frequently emphasized in advertisements are at best subtle differences. All of the currently available benzodiazepines are anxiolytic (i.e., useful in the treatment of anxiety), sedative-hypnotic (i.e., useful in the treatment of insomnia), and anticonvulsant and have muscle-relaxing activity. It is also difficult to find consistent scientific evidence to support the differences

*Portions of this section are based on D. J. Greenblatt, R. I. Shader, and D. R. Abernethy, "Current Status of Benzodiazepines, Parts I and II," *New England Journal of Medicine,* 309 (1983): 354–358 and 410–416.

among drugs in approved clinical indications. Thus, while some benzodiazepines are approved for the treatment of anxiety and others for the treatment of insomnia, there is little scientific evidence to support the division of currently marketed benzodiazepines on the basis of predominant anxiolytic versus predominant hypnotic activity.

This lack of evidence greatly complicates the practicing physician's task of choosing a benzodiazepine. The physician is faced with an increasing number of marketed benzodiazepines, each promoted as having unique clinical properties and specific clinical indications based on inadequate or selectively obtained scientific evidence. One oversimplified view suggests that all benzodiazepine needs can be adequately met by only one or two such drugs. Some cost-conscious hospital formulary committees list only chlordiazepoxide, since it can be inexpensively obtained as a generic compound. Such oversimplification has been resisted by many physicians, who state that important differences in clinical action do exist among the benzodiazepines despite their neuropharmacological similarities.[13] Sophisticated studies of the pharmacokinetics of benzodiazepines have partly corroborated these clinical observations in terms of rapidity of onset and duration of drug effects, safety in certain populations (the aged, liver disease patients, smokers, alcoholic patients, etc.), and drug interactions.[22,63,65,78]

The Pharmacokinetics of Benzodiazepines

The speed of onset of action and the intensity and duration of clinical activity after single doses of benzodiazepines are of great importance to physicians in the treatment of anxiety. An important factor in these temporal characteristics of the clinical activity of the benzodiazepines is their lipid solubility. All benzodiazepines are highly lipophilic compounds that rapidly cross the blood-brain barrier[7]; nevertheless, benzodiazepines do differ in relative lipid solubility. The onset of clinical anxiolytic activity of all ben-

TABLE 22–1

Characteristics of Benzodiazepines Used in the United States

Administered Drug (Year Introduced)	Approved Indications	Rate of Appearance after Oral Dose	Active Substances in Blood[a]	Overall Rate of Elimination
Chlordiazepoxide (1960)	Anxiety Alcohol withdrawal Preoperative sedation	Intermediate	Chlordiazepoxide Desmethylchlordiaze-poxide Demoxepam Desmethyldiazepam	Slow
Diazepam (1961)	Anxiety Alcohol withdrawal Muscle spasm Preoperative sedation Status epilepticus	Rapid	Diazepam Desmethyldiazepam	Slow
Oxazepam (1963)	Anxiety Anxiety-depression Alcohol withdrawal	Intermediate to slow	Oxazepam	Intermediate to rapid
Flurazepam (1970)	Insomnia	Rapid to intermediate	Hydroxyethyl flurazepam [Flurazepam aldehyde] Desalkylflurazepam	Slow
Clorazepate (1972)	Anxiety Seizure disorders Alcohol withdrawal	Rapid	Desmethyldiazepam	Slow
Clonazepam (1974)	Seizure disorders	Intermediate	Clonazepam	Intermediate
Lorazepam (1977)	Anxiety Anxiety-depression Preoperative sedation	Intermediate	Lorazepam	Intermediate
Prazepam (1977)	Anxiety	Slow	Desmethyldiazepam	Slow
Temazepam (1981)	Insomnia	Intermediate to slow	Temazepam	Intermediate
Alprazolam (1981)	Anxiety Anxiety-depression	Intermediate	Alprazolam	Intermediate
Halazepam (1981)	Anxiety	Intermediate to slow	[Halazepam] Desmethyldiazepam	Slow
Triazolam (1983)	Insomnia	Intermediate	Triazolam	Rapid

[a]Brackets indicate compounds of minor quantitative importance.
NOTE: Reprinted, by permission of the publisher, from D. J. Greenblatt, R. I. Shader, and D. R. Abernethy, "Drug Therapy: Current Status of Benzodiazepines, Part I," *New England Journal of Medicine*, 309 (1983):355.

zodiazepines injected intravenously is rapid, and there are few consistent differences based on relative lipid solubility. However, the duration of anxiolytic action differs considerably among the benzodiazepines. The more lipophilic ones have a shorter duration of clinical anxiolytic activity after a single intravenous dose, because increasing lipophilicity increases the extent of the drug's distribution into peripheral sites, mainly adipose tissue. This in turn causes the rapid egress of the drug from the blood and the brain into these inactive storage sites, diminishing the drug's effects in the brain.

Thus benzodiazepines that are relatively less lipophilic may have a longer duration of action because of reduced peripheral drug distribution. This dependence of duration of anxiolytic action on drug distribution rather than on rate of elimination explains the apparent paradox that benzodiazepines with a long half-life of elimination, such as diazepam, may have a shorter duration of anxiolytic action than benzodiazepines with a short half-life, such as lorazepam, when given in single doses.

After a single oral dose of benzodiazepines, the onset of action is based on the absorption from the gastrointestinal tract into the blood rather than on the more rapid transfer from blood to brain.[18,60,128] Diazepam and clorazepate dipotassium are the two benzodiazepines most rapidly absorbed from the gastrointestinal tract and therefore have a rapid onset to anxiolytic action. At the other extreme, prazepam is slowly transformed into its active metabolite desmethyldiazepam, which then slowly appears in the blood. Other benzodiazepines fall between these extremes (see table 22–1). The clinical anxiolytic effects of diazepam and clorazepate are therefore rapid in onset after a single oral dose. This may be appreciated by patients who welcome the rapid onset of anxiolytic action but less desirable for other patients who experience the rapid onset as an uncomfortable level of sedation.

The clinical anxiolytic effects of the benzodiazepines during and after repeated doses are related to the rate and extent of drug accumulation, which is a function of the elimination half-life and metabolic clearance. When the half-life is long, accumulation is slow and extensive; at the other extreme, when the drug has a short half-life, the steady state is achieved rapidly and accumulation is minimal. The elimination half-lives of the benzodiazepines are listed in table 22–1.

While these pharmacokinetic predictions of accumulation based on half-life have been repeatedly confirmed with the benzodiazepines,[22,63,65,78] speculation about the clinical risks and benefits of greater versus lesser accumulation have only been incompletely confirmed. While some investigations show that excessive drug accumulation can cause drowsiness, mental confusion, and motor incoordination,* most studies of sedation and performance show no consistent differences between benzodiazepines with long half-lives and those with short half-lives.[73] However, the possible increase in sedation produced by benzodiazepines with long half-lives should be kept in mind by physicians when prescribing these drugs.

When sedative effects do occur, they frequently develop early in the course of treatment and then either increase no further or decrease despite continued drug use and accumulation.[44,92,98] This phenomenon is operationally described as "tolerance" and explains why chronic users of benzodiazepines with long half-lives are not severely handicapped by sedation.

Benzodiazepines do not cure anxiety, and thus symptom recurrence can be expected when the drugs are discontinued. This recrudescence of symptoms is a function of a benzodiazepine's elimination half-life. Thus the return of anxiety will be more rapid when a short-acting benzodiazepine is terminated. The time course of the disappearance of drug side effects has a similar profile; sedation will persist longer after the discontinuation of a benzodiazepine with a long half-life.[117]

Liver metabolism is responsible for benzodiazepine elimination in humans. The two

*See references 24, 25, 93, 97, and 135.

major pathways involve hepatic microsomal oxidation or glucuronide conjugation. Oxidation can be impaired by age and disease states and by the coadministration of certain drugs such as cimetidine, estrogens, disulfiram, or isoniazid.[48,57] Conjugation is not affected by these factors.[48,57] Thus it would be logical to suppose that conjugated benzodiazepines would be safer for the elderly, patients with liver disease, or individuals receiving other drugs that impair oxidation. Interestingly, these speculations have been only incompletely confirmed in clinical studies. The explanation for this is probably the high therapeutic index of benzodiazepines and the fact that increase in plasma concentration may be partly or completely offset by tolerance.[92] Nevertheless, the physician should keep these metabolic considerations in mind when prescribing benzodiazepines.

The Practical Aspects of the Benzodiazepine Treatment of Anxiety

The efficacy studies evaluating benzodiazepines as anxiolytics are commonly of four weeks' duration, and in these studies, efficacy has been consistently and repeatedly demonstrated.[51,55,110] However, as a practical matter, many anxious patients are prescribed benzodiazepines for periods of months or years. Concern about the continued efficacy and possible dangers of long-term benzodiazepine use has led the Food and Drug Administration (FDA) to mandate caution against anxiolytic treatment lasting more than four months. Methodological and logistical problems make long-term investigations of the efficacy and hazards of the benzodiazepines difficult. This means that there is little evidence based on controlled investigations to either support or refute the FDA's position and that a controversy remains on the long-term efficacy of the benzodiazepines.

On one hand, recent investigations are reassuring in that they demonstrate continued anxiolytic benefit for periods up to six months, with a recrudescence of symptoms to pretreatment baseline levels when medication is discontinued.[38] In one investigation, long-term users of benzodiazepines had symptom recurrence with placebo substitution compared to a control group taking their usual dose who had no recurrence of symptoms.[20] On the other hand, there are a few controlled studies suggesting that the benzodiazepines may become ineffective during continuous, long-term treatment over months or years.[52,53,56] Two reports by Bowden and Fischer[20,21] further complicate interpretation of chronic dosage regimens, because they suggest that optimal or at least minimally adequate plasma concentrations are not always achieved in chronic benzodiazepine users due to problems with compliance.

While further controlled studies of these critical issues are needed, an individualized, commonsense approach to the treatment of anxiety can decrease the risks of benzodiazepine treatment.[115,121] In general, situational anxiety that is not out of proportion to the situation may improve performance and is probably best left untreated. Pathological anxiety lasting more than one month without panic attacks and avoidance behavior with and without obsessive-compulsive thinking and ritualistic behavior should probably be classified as generalized anxiety disorder and treated appropriately.[4]

As this chapter has emphasized, anxiolytic benzodiazepines are only one option available to patients with maladaptive generalized anxiety. Decisions about which patients are candidates for benzodiazepines are matters for individually tailored clinical judgment. When benzodiazepine treatment is begun, it is not always possible to predict how long it will be needed. The physician should closely monitor patients, particularly early in the course of treatment. Regular attempts to discontinue the drug can help establish whether treatment continues to be needed. Most clinicians have had experience with patients who required and benefited from chronic treatment with benzodiazepines. For these patients with chronic anxiety, long-term benzodiazepine anxiolytic treatment could be argued to be necessary and appropriate in much the same way as are diuretics for patients with hypertension, salicylates for patients with rheumatoid arthritis, or insulin for diabetics. Chronically anxious individuals are seldom physiologically addicted to benzodiazepines and should not be considered drug abusers. While it is obvious that the benzodiazepines do not cure anxiety, they can make life not only bearable but also productive for individuals who otherwise would be incapacitated by anxiety.

Benzodiazepines are effective in alleviating anxiety associated with such medical problems as gastrointestinal disorders or cardiovascular disorders such as hypertension or arteriosclerotic heart disease.[3] Benzodiazepines, however, have no effect on the underlying disease process. Anxiety associated with medical disease is clearly different from the anxiety-like symptoms associated with such medical conditions as thyroid disease, hypoxia, pheochromocytoma, or hypoglycemia, where treatment of the medical cause of such conditions is needed to alleviate the anxiety.

The use of benzodiazepines in the treatment of depression has become an unnecessarily complicated subject because the terms depression and anxiety refer to heterogeneous syndromes, and individuals frequently present mixed syndromes of both depression and anxiety.[118] True major affective disorders occurring cyclically and alternating with periods of normal mood, as in unipolar depression, or with mania, as in bipolar depression, respond best to treatment with heterocyclic antidepressants, MAOIs, lithium carbonate, and electroconvulsive therapy (see chapters 13 and 33). Many depressed patients who also have anxiety may have some of these symptoms alleviated by benzodiazepines, but the drugs are of little benefit for the underlying depressive disorder. Many patients who are primarily anxious but who also have some symptoms of depression will benefit from benzodiazepines, probably in proportion to the extent to which anxiety contributes to their overall disability. However, preliminary investigations with the new benzodiazepine alprazolam suggest that this compound may have some specific efficacy in the treatment of major depressive disorder that has not been previously reported with other benzodiazepines (see chapter 13; see also Fabre and McLendon[37] and Rickels et al.[113]).

Adverse Reactions, Side Effects, and Hazards of Benzodiazepine Treatment

The most common side effect associated with benzodiazepine use is related to excessive depression of the central nervous system. This can lead to drowsiness, sleepiness, impaired intellectual function, reduced motor coordination, and impairment of memory and recall.* The potential dangers of these effects should be jointly evaluated by the physician and patient as they assess the risks and benefits of benzodiazepine treatment.

Terrifying and sensationalistic descriptions of benzodiazepine abuse and addiction have become a popular subject for the lay media. These reports often suggest the existence of a national epidemic of benzodiazepine addiction caused by a pharmaceutical industry interested only in profit and a medical profession that overprescribes tranquilizers instead of taking the time to talk with a patient.[12] When these alleged problems with benzodiazepines are evaluated in scientific studies, results do not confirm such journalistic conclusions.[26,111] These studies find that prescriptions for and clinical use of benzodiazepines are for patients who do have symptoms that respond to benzodiazepines and that the majority of patients taking the drugs derive clinical benefit from them even over long periods. Evidence of benzodiazepine abuse or excessive increase in dosage is generally lacking, and there is no consistent evidence that the benzodiazepine treatment of anxiety impairs a patient's desire to seek more definitive solutions.[10,70] When benzodiazepines are discontinued, most individuals have a recurrence of symptoms consistent with their original condition.[20,38,80,112]

*See references 24,31,84,99,124, and 152.

Nonetheless, physiological addiction to benzodiazepines does occur.[54,89] Such physiological addiction is most common with high dosages but has also been documented with usual therapeutic doses.[90,104,151] Such addiction is more likely to occur with longer drug exposure, and therefore drug exposure should be limited to the minimum amount consistent with the chronicity of the patient's anxiety syndrome. Patients should be counseled to expect the occurrence of symptoms after long-term benzodiazepine use, but this does not always suggest addiction. Recurring symptoms of the original anxiety disorder will resemble those of the pretreatment emotional state and may gradually reappear over a period of weeks after benzodiazepine discontinuation. Benzodiazepine withdrawal symptoms, on the other hand, appear more rapidly, reach a peak intensity, and then decrease over time.

Such withdrawal symptoms[66,75,90] include tremulousness, sweating, increased sensitivity to light and sound, insomnia, gastrointestinal distress, and systolic hypertension. Seizures and psychosis, which certainly can occur, are fortunately rare.[32,41] Physicians should taper the dose to minimize the impact of drug discontinuation. This gradual discontinuation is particularly important for the benzodiazepines with short half-lives. Unpleasant autonomic symptoms can be treated with a beta-adrenergic blocking drug such as propranolol hydrochloride.[1,144]

Despite the more than one hundred scientific manuscripts on the subject, there are no consistent conclusions on the pharmacokinetic and clinical consequences of benzodiazepine administration with ethanol.[122] Coadministration of single doses of benzodiazepines with single doses of alcohol causes a small pharmacokinetic interaction, if any at all,[123] but causes greater central nervous system depression than either agent given alone.[122] In addition, just as with alcohol, benzodiazepines occasionally produce a paradoxical increase in aggression, which may represent a disinhibition or release of "anxiety-bound" hostility. Fortunately, there is no evidence for the supra-additive "knockout drop" effect of the combination of alcohol and benzodiazepines.

When taken alone, massive quantities of benzodiazepines rarely, if ever, have a fatal outcome.* The replacement of barbiturates by benzodiazepines as the primary treatments for anxiety and insomnia has greatly reduced the morbidity and mortality associated with sedative hypnotic overdose. However, many drug overdoses involve combinations of benzodiazepines and drugs of other classes. These syndromes can be extremely dangerous depending on the coingested drugs. One hopes that the specific benzodiazepine antagonists that are described in the literature will soon be clinically available and used in the diagnosis and treatment of benzodiazepine intoxication.[30,91]

Benzodiazepines do not produce clinically significant microsomal enzyme induction at therapeutic doses and can, therefore, be safely coadministered with oral anticoagulants and with other drugs metabolized by hepatic microsomal enzymes.

¶ Summary

Anxiety and stress are ubiquitous, and current approaches to their management and treatment are numerous. Formulating appropriate, effective treatment programs involves accurate diagnosis as well as consideration of the patient's age, medical status, and personality.

Psychotherapy is generally considered the foundation of treatment for anxiety, although behavioral therapies are often highly successful in ameliorating or eliminating certain anxiety disorders. Stress is best managed by prevention; it can be reduced by various tension-relieving techniques. Pharmacological interventions are varied, and attention should be paid to selecting the right agent(s) for each patient's particular presentation and needs.

*See references 2,34,40,61, and 62

¶ Bibliography

1. ABERNETHY, D. R., GREENBLATT, D. J., and SHADER, R. I. "Treatment of Diazepam Withdrawal Syndrome with Propranolol," *Annals of Internal Medicine*, 94 (1981):354–355.

2. ALLEN, M. D., et al. "Pharmacokinetic Study of Lorazepam Overdosage," *American Journal of Psychiatry*, 137 (1980):1414–1415.

3. AMEER, B., and GREENBLATT, D. J. "Lorazepam: A Review of Its Clinical Pharmacological Properties and Therapeutic Uses," *Drugs*, 21 (1981):161–200.

4. AMERICAN PSYCHIATRIC ASSOCIATION. *Diagnostic and Statistical Manual of Mental Disorders*, 3rd ed. Washington, D.C.: American Psychiatric Association, 1980.

5. ANANTH, J. "Treatment of Obsessive-compulsive Neurosis with Clomipramine (Anafranil). *Journal of International Medical Research*, 5 (1977):38–41.

6. ANANTH, J., et al. "Chlorimipramine Therapy for Obsessive-compulsive Neurosis," *American Journal of Psychiatry*, 136 (1979):700–701.

7. ARENDT, R. M., et al. "In vitro Correlates of Benzodiazepine CSF Uptake, Pharmacodynamic Action, and Peripheral Distribution," *Journal of Pharmacology and Experimental Therapeutics*, 227 (1983):98–106.

8. AYD, F. J. "Social Issues: Misuse and Abuse," *Psychosomatics*, 21 (1980):21–25.

9. BALDESSARINI, R. J. "Drugs and the Treatment of Psychiatric Disorders," in A. G. Gilman, L.S. Goodman, and A. Gilman, eds., *The Pharmacologic Basis of Therapeutics*. New York: Macmillan, 1980, pp. 391–447.

10. BALMER, R., BATTEGAY, R., and VON MARSCHALL, R. "Long-term Treatment with Diazepam: Investigation of Consumption Habits and the Interaction Between Psychotherapy and Psychopharmacology: A Prospective Study," *International Pharmacopsychiatry*, 16 (1981):221–234.

11. BANDURA, A. "Modeling Approaches to the Modification of Phobic Disorders," *International Psychiatry Clinics*, 6 (1969):201–223.

12. BARGMANN, E., et al. *Stopping Valium.* Washington, D.C.: Public Citizen's Health Research Group, 1982.

13. BASKIN, I., and ESDALE, A. "Is Chlordiazepoxide the Rational Choice Among Benzodiazepines?" *Pharmacotherapy*, 2 (1982):110–119.

14. BEDELL, J. R., ARCHER, R. P., and ROSMANN, M. "Relaxation Therapy, Desensitization and the Treatment of Anxiety-based Disorders," *Journal of Clinical Psychology*, 35 (1979):840–843.

15. BELAR, C. D. "A Comment on Silver and Blanchard's (1978) Review of the Treatment of Tension Headaches via EMG Feedback and Relaxation Training," *Journal of Behavioral Medicine*, 2 (1979):215–220.

16. BENSON, H., BEARY, J. R., and CAROL, M. P., "The Relaxation Response," *Psychiatry*, 37 (1974):37–46.

17. BERNARDT, M. V., SILVERSTONE, T., and SINGLETON, W. "Behavioral and Subjective Effects of Beta-adrenergic Blockage in Phobic Subjects," *British Journal of Psychiatry*, 137 (1980):452–457.

18. BLIDING, A. "Effects of Different Rates of Absorption of Two Benzodiazepines on Subjective and Objective Parameters," *European Journal of Clinical Pharmacology*, 7 (1974):201–211.

19. BOSWELL, P. C., and MURRAY, E. J. "Effects of Meditation on Psychological and Physiological Measures of Anxiety," *Journal of Consulting and Clinical Psychology*, 47 (1979):606–607.

20. BOWDEN, C. L., and FISCHER, J. G. "Safety and Efficacy of Long-term Diazepam Therapy," *Southern Medical Journal*, 73 (1980):1581–1584.

21. ———. "Relationship of Diazepam Serum Level to Antianxiety Effects," *Journal of Clinical Psychopharmacology*, 2 (1982):110–114.

22. BREIMER, D. D., JOCHEMSEN, R., and VON ALBERT, H. H. "Pharmacokinetics of Benzodiazepines: Short-acting Versus Long-acting," *Arzneimittelforsch*, 30 (1980):875–881.

23. CAPSTICK, N. "Chlorimipramine in

Obsessional States," *Psychosomatics*, 12 (1971):322–335.

24. CARSKADON, M. A., et al. "Daytime Carryover of Triazolam and Flurazepam in Elderly Insomniacs," *Sleep*, 5 (1982): 361–371.

25. CHURCH, M. W., and JOHNSON, L. C. "Mood and Performance of Poor Sleepers During Repeated Use of Flurazepam," *Psychopharmacology*, 61 (1979): 309–316.

26. COLE, J. O., HASKELL, D. S., and ORZACK, M. H. "Problems with the Benzodiazepines: An Assessment of the Available Evidence," *Mclean Hospital Journal*, 6 (1981):46–74.

27. COURSEY, R. D. "Electromyograph Feedback as a Relaxation Technique," *Journal of Consulting and Clinical Psychology*, 43 (1975):825–834.

28. COVI, L., et al. "Length of Treatment with Anxiolytic Sedatives and Response to Their Sudden Withdrawal," *Acta Psychiatrica Scandinavica*, 49 (1973):51–64.

29. CROINE, M. J., et al. "Time limited Desensitization, Implosion and Shaping for Phobic Patients: A Crossover Study," *Behaviour Research and Therapy*, 10 (1972):319–328.

30. DARRAGH, A., et al. "Investigation in Man of the Efficacy of a Benzodiazepine Antagonist, Ro 15-1788," *Lancet*, 2 (1981): 8–10.

31. DE GIER'T HART, B. J., NELEMANS, F. A., and BERGMAN, H. "Psychomotor Performance and Real Driving Performance of Outpatients Receiving Diazepam," *Psychopharmacology*, 73 (1981):340–344.

32. DE LA FUENTE, J. R., et al. "Lorazepam-related Withdrawal Seizures," *Mayo Clinic Proceedings*, 55 (1980):190–192.

33. DILLBECK, M. C. "The Effect of the Transcendental Meditation Technique on Anxiety Level," *Journal of Clinical Psychology*, 33 (1977):1076–1078.

34. DIVOLL, M., et al. "Benzodiazepine Overdosage: Plasma Concentrations and Clinical Outcome," *Psychopharmacology*, 73 (1981):381–383.

35. EYSENCK, H. J., and RACHMAN, S. *The Causes and Cures of Neurosis*. San Diego: Knapp Press, 1958.

36. FABRE, L. F., and HARRIS, R. T. "An Analysis of Clinical Factors in the Abuse Potential of New Anti-anxiety and Antidepressant Drugs," in F. Kagan et al., ed., *Hypnotics: Methods of Development and Evaluation*. New York: SP Publications, 1975, pp. 283–291.

37. FABRE, L. F., and MCLENDON, D. M. "A Double-blind Study Comparing the Efficacy and Safety of Alprazolam with Imipramine and Placebo in Primary Depression," *Current Therapeutic Research*, 27 (1980):474–482.

38. FABRE, L. F., MCLENDON, D. M., and STEPHENS, A. G. "Comparison of the Therapeutic Effect, Tolerance and Safety of Ketazolam and Diazepam Administered for Six Months to Out-patients with Chronic Anxiety Neurosis," *Journal of International Medical Research*, 9 (1981):191–198.

39. FARWELL, L. "Effect of Transcendental Meditation on Levels of Anxiety," in D. W. Orme-Johnson, L. Domask, and J. Farrow, eds., *Scientific Research on Transcendental Meditation: Collected Papers*. Los Angeles: Maharishi International University Press, 1974.

40. FINKLE, B. S., MCCLOSKEY, K. L., and GOODMAN, L. S. "Diazepam and Drug-associated Deaths," *Journal of the American Medical Association*, 242 (1979):429–433.

41. FRUENSGAARD, K. "Withdrawal Psychosis: A Study of 30 Consecutive Cases," *Acta Psychiatrica Scandinavica*, 53 (1976):105–118.

42. GELDER, M. J., and MARKS, I. M. "Desensitization and Phobia: A Cross-over Study," *British Journal of Psychiatry*, 114 (1968):320–328.

43. GELDER, M. G., MARKS, I. M., and WOLFF, H. "Densensitization and Psychotherapy in the Treatment of Phobic States. A Controlled Inquiry," *British Journal of Psychiatry* 113 (1967):53–57.

44. GHONEIM, M. M., et al. "Memory and Performance Effects of Single and 3-week Administration of Diazepam," *Psychopharmacology*, 73 (1981):147–151.

45. GOLDBERG, R. J. "Anxiety Reduction by Self-regulation: Theory, Practice and Evaluation," *Annals of Internal Medicine*, 96 (1982):483–487.

46. GOLDMAN, B. L., DOMITOR, P. J., and

MURRAY, E. J. "Effects of Zen Meditation on Anxiety Reduction and Perceptual Function," *Journal of Consulting and Clinical Psychology,* 47 (1979):551–556.

47. GRANVILLE-GROSSMAN, K. L., and TURNER, P. "The Effects of Propranolol on Anxiety," *Lancet,* 1 (1966):788–790.

48. GREENBLATT, D. J. "Clinical Pharmacokinetics of Oxazepam and Lorazepam," *Clinical Pharmacokinetics,* 6 (1981):89–105.

49. GREENBLATT, D. J., and SHADER, R. I. "Meprobamate: A Study of Irrational Drug Use," *American Journal of Psychiatry,* 127 (1971):1297–1303.

50. ———. "The Clinical Choice of Sedative-hypnotics," *Annals of Internal Medicine,* 77 (1972):91–100.

51. ———. *Benzodiazepines in Clinical Practice.* New York: Raven Press, 1974.

52. ———. "Drug Therapy: Benzodiazepines, Part I," *New England Journal of Medicine,* 291 (1974):1011–1015.

53. ———. "Drug Therapy: Benzodiazepines, Part II," *New England Journal of Medicine,* 291 (1974):1239–1243.

54. ———. "Dependence, Tolerance, and Addiction to Benzodiazepines: Clinical and Pharmacokinetic Considerations," *Drug Metabolism Reviews,* 8 (1978):13–28.

55. ———. "Pharmacotherapy of Anxiety with Benzodiazepines and β-adrenergic Blockers," in M. A. Lipton, A. DiMascio, and K. F. Killam, eds., *Psychopharmacology: A Generation of Progress.* New York: Raven Press, 1978, pp. 1381–1390.

56. ———. "Clinical Use of Benzodiazepines," *Rational Drug Therapy,* 15 (1981):3–6.

57. GREENBLATT, D. J., SELLERS, E. M., and SHADER, R. I. "Drug Disposition in Old Age," *New England Journal of Medicine,* 306 (1982):1081–1088.

58. GREENBLATT, D. J., SHADER, R. I., and ABERNETHY, D. R. "Drug Therapy: Current Status of Benzodiazepines, Part I," *New England Journal of Medicine,* 309 (1983):354–358.

59. ———. "Drug Therapy: Current Status of Benzodiazepines, Part II," *New En-gland Journal of Medicine,* 309 (1983):410–416.

60. GREENBLATT, D. J., et al. "Absorption Rate, Blood Concentrations, and Early Response to Oral Chlordiazepoxide," *American Journal of Psychiatry,* 134 (1977):559–562.

61. GREENBLATT, D. J., et al. "Acute Overdosage with Benzodiazepine Derivatives," *Clinical Pharmacology & Therapeutics,* 21 (1977):497–514.

62. GREENBLATT, D. J., et al. "Rapid Recovery from Massive Diazepam Overdose," *Journal of the American Medical Association,* 240 (1978):1872–1874.

63. GREENBLATT, D. J., et al. "Benzodiazepines: A Summary of Pharmacokinetic Properties," *British Journal of Clinical Pharmacology,* 11 (Supplement) (1981): 115–165.

64. GREENBLATT, D. J., et al. "Benzodiazepine Hypnotics: Kinetic and Therapeutic Options," *Sleep,* 5 (1982):18S–27S.

65. GREENBLATT, D. J., et al. "Benzodiazepine Kinetics: Implications for Therapeutics and Pharmacogeriatrics," *Drug Metabolism Reviews,* 14 (1983):251–292.

66. HALLSTROM, C., and LADER, M. "Benzodiazepine Withdrawal Phenomena," *International Pharmacopsychiatry,* 16 (1981):235–244.

67. HENRY, J. P., and STEPHENS, P. M. *Stress, Health, and the Social Environment. A Sociobiologic Approach to Medicine.* New York: Springer-Verlag, 1977

68. HJELLE, L. A. "Transcendental Meditation and Psychologic Health," *Perceptual and Motor Skills,* 39 (1974):623–628.

69. HOLLISTER, L. E., MOTZEBECKER, F. P., and SEGAN, R. O. "Withdrawal Reactions from Chlordiazepoxide (Librium)," *Psychopharmacologia,* 2 (1961): 63–68.

70. HOLLISTER, L. E., et al. "Long-term Use of Diazepam," *Journal of the American Medical Association,* 246 (1981):1568–1570.

71. HUTCHINGS, D. F., et al. "Anxiety Management and Applied Relaxation in Reducing General Anxiety," *Behaviour Research and Therapy,* 18 (1980):181–190.

72. JACOBSEN, E. *Progressive Relaxation,* 2nd

ed. Chicago: University of Chicago Press, 1938.

73. JOHNSON, L. C., and CHERNIK, D. A. "Sedative-hypnotics and Human Performance," *Psychopharmacology*, 76 (1982):101–113.

74. KELLY, D., et al. "Treatment of Phobic States with Antidepressants," *British Journal of Psychiatry*, 116 (1970):387–398.

75. KHAN, A., JOYCE, P., and JONES, A. V. "Benzodiazepine Withdrawal Syndromes," *New Zealand Medical Journal*, 92 (1980):94–96.

76. KLEIN, D. F. "Importance of Psychiatric Diagnosis in Prediction of Clinical Drug Effects," *Archives of General Psychiatry*, 16 (1967):118–126.

77. KLEIN, D. F., and FINK, M. "Psychiatric Reaction Patterns to Imipramine," *American Journal of Psychiatry*, 119 (1962):432–438.

78. KLOTZ, U., KANGAS, L., and KANTO, J. "Clinical Pharmacokinetics of Benzodiazepines," *Progress in Pharmacology*, 3 (1980):1–72.

79. LANG, P. J., LAZOVICK, A. D., and REYNOLDS, D. J. "Desensitization, Suggestibility, and Pseudotherapy," *Journal of Abnormal Psychology*, 70 (1965):395–402.

80. LAPIERRE, Y. D., et al. "A Therapeutic and Discontinuation Study of Clobazam and Diazepam in Anxiety Neurosis," *Journal of Clinical Psychiatry*, 43 (1982):372–374.

81. LAZARUS, A. A. "The Treatment of Chronic Frigidity by Systematic Desensitization," *Journal of Nervous and Mental Disease*, 136 (1963):272–278.

82. LINDEN, W. "Exposure Treatments for Focal Phobias," *Archives of General Psychiatry*, 38 (1981):769–775.

83. LIPSEDGE, M. S., et al. "The Management of Severe Agoraphobia: A Comparison of Iproniazid and Systematic Desensitization," *Psychopharmacologia*, 32 (1973):67–80.

84. McNAIR, D. M. "Antianxiety Drugs and Human Performance," *Archives of General Psychiatry*, 29 (1973):611–617.

85. MARKS, I. M. "Behavioral Treatments of Phobic and Obsessive-compulsive Disorders: A Critical Appraisal," in M.

Hersen, R. Eisler, and P. Miller, eds., *Progress in Behavior Modification*, vol 1. New York: Academic Press, 1975, pp. 65–168.

86. MARKS, I. M., BOULOUGOURIS, J., and MARSET, P. "Flooding Versus Desensitization in the Treatment of Phobic Patients: A Crossover Study," *British Journal of Psychiatry*, 119 (1971):353–357.

87. MARKS, I. M., et al. "Enhanced Relief of Phobias by Flooding During Waning Diazepam Effect," *British Journal of Psychiatry*, 121 (1972):493–505.

88. MARKS, J. "The Benzodiazepines: Use, Overuse, Misuse, Abuse," *Lancet*, 1 (1973):1101–1102.

89. ———. *The Benzodiazepines: Use, Overuse, Misuse, Abuse*. Baltimore: University Park Press, 1978.

90. MELLOR, C. S., and JAIN, V. K. "Diazepam Withdrawal Syndrome: Its Prolonged and Changing Nature," *Canadian Medical Association Journal*, 127 (1982): 1093–1096.

91. MENDELSON, W. B., et al. "A Benzodiazepine Receptor Antagonist Decreases Sleep and Reverses the Hypnotic Actions of Flurazepam," *Science*, 219 (1983):414–416.

92. OCHS, H. R., et al. "Repeated Diazepam Dosing in Cirrhotic Patients; Cumulation and Sedation," *Clinical Pharmacology and Therapeutics*, 33 (1983): 471–476.

93. OGURA, C., et al. "Residual Effects of Hypnotics Triazolam, Flurazepam, and Nitrazepam," *Psychopharmacology*, 68 (1980):61–65.

94. ORME-JOHNSON, D. W. "Autonomic Stability and Transcendental Meditation," *Psychosomatic Medicine*, 35 (1973):341–349.

95. ———. "Transcendental Meditation for Drug Abuse Counselors," in D. W. Orme-Johnson, L. Domask, and J. Farrow, eds., *Scientific Research on Transcendental Meditation: Collected Papers*. Los Angeles: Maharishi International University Press, 1974.

96. OSWALD, I. "The Why and How of Hypnotic Drugs," *British Medical Journal*, 1 (1979):1167–1168.

97. OSWALD, I., et al. "The Effects of Two

Hypnotics on Sleep, Subjective Feelings and Skilled Performance," in P. Passouant and I. Oswald, eds., *Pharmacology of the States of Alertness.* Oxford: Pergamon Press, 1979, pp. 51–63.

98. PALVA, E. S., et al. "Acute and Subacute Effects of Diazepam on Psychomotor Skills; Interaction with Alcohol," *Acta Pharmacologica et Toxicologica* (Copenhagen), 45 (1979):257–264.

99. PALVA, E. S., et al. "Actions and Interactions of Diazepam and Alcohol on Psychomotor Skills in Young and Middle-aged Subjects," *Acta Pharmacologica et Toxicologica* (Copenhagen), 50 (1982): 363–369.

100. PAUL, G. L. *Insight vs. Desensitization in Psychotherapy.* Stanford, Calif.: Stanford University Press, 1965.

101. ———. "Outcome of Systematic Desensitization II: Controlled Investigations of Individual Treatment, Technique Variations and Current Status," in C. M. Franks, ed., *Behavior Therapy: Appraisal and Status.* New York: McGraw-Hill, 1969, pp. 105–159.

102. PAUL, G. L., and TRUMBLE, R. W. "Recorded vs. 'Live' Relaxation Training and Hypnotic Suggestion: Comparative Effectiveness for Reducing Physiological Arousal and Inhibiting Stress Response," *Behavior Therapy,* 1 (1970): 285–302.

103. PERCELL, L. P., BERWICK, P. T., and BEIGEL, A. "The Effects of Assertive Training on Self-concept and Anxiety," *Archives of General Psychiatry,* 31 (1974):502–504.

104. PEVNICK, J. S., JASINSKI, D. R., and HAERTZEN, C. A. "Abrupt Withdrawal from Therapeutically Administered Diazepam; Report of a Case," *Archives of General Psychiatry,* 35 (1978):995–998.

105. PITTS, F. N., and McCLURE, J. N., JR. "Lactate Metabolism in Anxiety Neuroses," *New England Journal of Medicine,* 277 (1967):1328–1336.

106. RANZONI, J. "Treatment of Phobias by Systematic Desensitization," *Archives of General Psychiatry,* 30 (1974):291–293.

107. RASKIN, M., BALI, L. R., and PEEKE, H. V. "Muscle Biofeedback and Transcendental Meditation," *Archives of General Psychiatry,* 37 (1980):93–97.

108. RASKIN, M., JOHNSON, G., and RONDESTVEDT, J. W. "Chronic Anxiety Treated by Feedback-induced Muscle Relaxation," *Archives of General Psychiatry,* 28 (1973):263–267.

109. REINKING, R. H. J., and KOHL, M. L. "Effects of Various Forms of Relaxation Training on Physiologic and Self-report Measures of Relaxation," *Journal of Consulting and Clinical Psychology,* 43 (1975):595–600.

110. RICKELS, K. "Use of Antianxiety Agents in Anxious Outpatients," *Psychopharmacology,* 58 (1978):1–17.

111. ———. "Are Benzodiazepines Overused and Abused?" *British Journal of Clinical Pharmacology,* 11 (Supplement) (1981):71–83.

112. RICKELS, K., CASE, W. G., and DIAMOND, L. "Relapse After Short-term Drug Therapy in Neurotic Outpatients," *International Pharmacopsychiatry,* 15 (1980):186–192.

113. RICKELS, K., et al. "Alprazolam and Imipramine in Depressed Outpatients: A Controlled Study," *Current Therapeutic Research,* 32 (1982):157–164.

114. RIDDICK, C., and MEYER, R. G. "The Efficacy of Automated Relaxation Training with Response Contingent Feedback," *Behavior Therapy* 4 (1973):331–337.

115. ROSENBAUM, J. F. "The Drug Treatment of Anxiety," *New England Journal of Medicine,* 306 (1982):401–404.

116. SALTER, A. *Conditioned Reflex Therapy.* New York: Creative Age Press, 1950.

117. SALZMAN, C., et al. "Long v. Short Half-life Benzodiazepines in the Elderly: Kinetics and Clinical Effects of Diazepam and Oxazepam," *Archives of General Psychiatry,* 40 (1983):293–297.

118. SCHATZBERG, A. F., and COLE, J. O. "Benzodiazepines in Depressive Disorders," *Archives of General Psychiatry,* 35 (1978):1359–1365.

119. SCHULTZ, J. H. *Autogenic Training: A Psychophysiologic Approach in Psychotherapy.* New York: Grune & Stratton, 1969.

120. SCHULTZ, J. H., and LUTHE, W. *Autogenic Training. A Psychophysiological Ap-*

proach to Psychotherapy. New York: Grune & Stratton, 1959.

121. SELLERS, E. M. "Clinical Pharmacology and Therapeutics of Benzodiazepines," *Canadian Medical Association Journal*, 118 (1978):1533–1538.

122. SELLERS, E. M., and BUSTO, U. "Benzodiazepines and Ethanol: Assessment of the Effects and Consequences of Psychotropic Drug Interactions," *Journal of Clinical Pharmacology* 1982; 22:249–262.

123. SELLERS, E. M., and HOLLOWAY, M. R. "Drug Kinetics and Alcohol Ingestion," *Clinical Pharmacokinetics*, 3 (1978): 440–452.

124. SEPPALA, T., LINNOILA, M., and MATTILA, M. J. "Drugs, Alcohol and Driving," *Drugs*, 17 (1979):389–408.

125. SHADER, R. I., and GREENBLATT, D. J. "Clinical Implications of Benzodiazepine Pharmacokinetics," *American Journal of Psychiatry*, 134 (1977):652–656.

126. ———. "Management of Anxiety in the Elderly: The Balance Between Therapeutic and Adverse Effects," *Journal of Clinical Psychiatry*, 43 (1982):8–18.

127. SHADER, R. I., WEINBERGER, D. R., and GREENBLATT, D. J. "Psychopharmacologic Approaches to the Medically Ill Patient," in T. B. Karasu and R. I. Steinmuller, eds., *Psychotherapeutics in Medicine*. New York: Grune & Stratton, 1978, pp. 117–156.

128. SHADER, R. I., et al. "Impaired Absorption of Desmethyldiazepam from Clorazepate by Magnesium Aluminum Hydroxide," *Clinical Pharmacology and Therapeutics*, 24 (1978):308–315.

129. SHADER, R. I., et al. *Emergency Study of Sedative-Hypnotic Overdosage: A Study of the Issues*. USDHHS Publication (ADM) 82–118. Washington, D.C.: U.S. Government Printing Office, 1982.

130. SHEEHAN, D. V. "Current Concepts in Anxiety: Panic Attacks and Phobias," *New England Journal of Medicine*, 307 (1982):156–158.

131. SHEEHAN, D. V., BALLENGER, J., and JACOBSEN, G. "Treatment of Endogenous Anxiety with Phobic, Hysterical, and Hypochondriacal Symptoms," *Ar-*

chives of General Psychiatry, 37 (1980): 51–59.

132. SHEEHAN, D. V., et al. "Lack of Efficacy of a New Antidepressant (Bupropion) in the Treatment of Panic Disorder with Phobias," *Journal of Clinical Psychopharmacology*, 3 (1983):28–31.

133. SILVER, B. V., and BLANCHARD, E. B. "Biofeedback and Relaxation Training in the Treatment of Psychophysiological Disorders: Or Are the Machines Really Necessary," *Journal of Behavioral Medicine*, 1 (1978):217–239.

134. SMITH, J. C. "Psychotherapeutic Effects of Transcendental Meditation with Controls for Expectation of Relief and Daily Setting," *Journal of Consulting and Clinical Psychology*, 44 (1976):630–637.

135. SOLOMON, F., et al. "Sleeping Pills, Insomnia and Medical Practice," *New England Journal of Medicine*, 300 (1979): 803–808.

136. SOLYOM, L., et al. "Behavior Therapy Versus Drug Therapy in the Treatment of Phobic Neurosis," *Canadian Psychiatric Association Journal*, 18 (1973):25–32.

137. STEKETEE, G., FOA, E. B., and GRAYSON, J. B. "Recent Advances in the Behavioral Treatment of Obsessive Compulsives," *Archives of General Psychiatry*, 39 (1982):1365–1371.

138. STERN, R. "Treatment of a Case of Obsessional Neurosis Using Thought-stopping Technique," *British Journal of Psychiatry*, 117 (1970):441–442.

139. STERN, R. S., and MARKS, I. M. "Brief and Prolonged Flooding: A Comparison in Agoraphobic Patients," *Archives of General Psychiatry*, 28 (1973):270–276.

140. STEVENSON, I. "Direct Instigation of Behavioral Changes in Psychotherapy," *Archives of General Psychiatry*, 1 (1959):99–107.

141. TAYLOR, C. B., et al. "Relaxation Therapy and High Blood Pressure," *Archives of General Psychiatry*, 34 (1977):339–342.

142. THOREN, P., et al. "Clomipramine Treatment of Obsessive-compulsive Disorders," *Archives of General Psychiatry*, 37 (1980):1281–1295.

143. TYRER, P., CANDY, J., and KELLY, D. "A Study of the Clinical Effects of Phenelzine and Placebo in the Treatment of

Phobic Anxiety," *Psychopharmacologia*, 32 (1973):237–254.

144. TYRER, P., RUTHERFORD, D., and HUGGETT, T. "Benzodiazepine Withdrawal Symptoms and Propranolol," *Lancet*, 1 (1981):520–522.

145. TYRER, P., et al. "Clinical and Pharmacokinetic Factors Affecting Response to Phenelzine," *British Journal of Psychiatry*, 136 (1980):359–365.

146. UHLENHUTH, E. H. "Specific Anxiety Syndromes: Current Therapeutic Options," *Journal of Clinical Psychiatry*, 42 (1981):27–33.

147. WALLACE, R. K., and BENSON, H. "The Physiology of Medication," *Scientific American*, 226 (1972):84–96.

148. WALLACE, R. K., BENSON, H., and WILSON, A. F. "A Wakeful Hypometabolic Physiologic State," *American Journal of Physiology*, 221 (1971):795–799.

149. WAXMAN, D. "An Investigation into the Use of Anafranil in Phobic and Obsessional Disorders," *Scottish Medical Journal* (Glasgow), 20 (1975):61–66.

150. WHATMORE, G. B., and KOHLI, D. R. *The Physiopathology and Treatment of Functional Disorders.* New York: Grune & Stratton, 1974.

151. WINOKUR, A., et al. "Withdrawal Reaction from Long-term, Low-dosage Administration of Diazepam: A Double-blind, Placebo-controlled Case Study," *Archives of General Psychiatry*, 37 (1980): 101–105.

152. WITTENBORN, J. R. "Effects of Benzodiazepines on Psychomotor Performance," *British Journal of Clinical Pharmacology*, 7 (Supplement) (1979): 61–67.

153. WOLPE, J. "The Systematic Desensitization Treatment of Neurosis," *Journal of Nervous and Mental Disease*, 132 (1961): 189–203.

154. ———. *The Practice of Behavior Therapy.* New York: Pergamon Press, 1973.

155. WOODY, G. E., O'BRIEN, C. P., and GREENSTEIN, R. "Misuse and Abuse of Diazepam: An Increasingly Common Medical Problem." *International Journal of Addictions*, 10 (1975):843–848.

156. YARYURA-TOBIAS, J. A., and BHAGAVAN, H. N. "L-tryptophan in Obsessive-compulsive Disorders," *American Journal of Psychiatry*, 134 (1977):1298–1299.

157. ZITRIN, C. M., KLEIN, D. F., and WOERNER, M. G. "Treatment of Agoraphobia with Group Exposure in Vivo and Imipramine," *Archives of General Psychiatry*, 37 (1980):63–72.

CHAPTER 23

BIOLOGICAL ASPECTS OF AND DRUG TREATMENTS FOR SELECTED CHILDHOOD MENTAL DISORDERS

Glen R. Elliott and Roland D. Ciaranello

¶ Introduction

In 1984 the Institute of Medicine, National Academy of Sciences, published a report entitled *Research on Mental Illness and Addictive Disorders: Progress and Prospects.* [19] The section on mental disorders of childhood and adolescence begins with the following observation: "In a field with a series of overwhelming needs, childhood mental disorders remain noteworthy" (p. 31). The report notes that an estimated 2 million children in the United States have serious mental disorders needing immediate attention and that another 8 to 10 million children could benefit from care for less incapacitating but still severe developmental difficulties; yet the mental health care system in this country currently offers help of any kind to only 500,000 children. Increasingly, evidence suggests that many of the most severe and disabling childhood mental disorders have a major biological component and are likely to require pharmacological interventions.

This chapter describes the results of work over the past several decades that has moved the field of child psychiatry from an almost exclusive focus on psychological and environmental influences toward an increasing awareness of the importance of also understanding the effects of dysfunctions in biological substrates of development and brain organization. Also, we discuss the use of psychopharmacological agents in treating mental disorders of childhood and adolescence. As with most adult mental disorders, the ability of selected drugs to ameliorate or reverse symptoms of some childhood mental disorders is one type of evidence implicating the importance of biological factors.

Nothing in this chapter is meant to imply that the suffering and problems caused by severe mental disorders of childhood and adolescence are exclusively biological. Children develop within a complex context of genetic potential and physical, psychological, and social environment. Few childhood disorders are apt to remit strictly to a drug intervention, because a child's entire family and social structure also are affected; yet failure to treat the core problem vigorously with drugs, when appropriate, may doom a child needlessly to lifelong disability. Assessment of the full range of problems and construction of a complete treatment plan to address them constitutes the art and science of child psychiatry.

¶ Classification of Childhood Psychopathology

Difficulties in identifying and classifying childhood mental disorders continue to hinder researchers and therapists alike. Although still unresolved even for adult mental disorders, the problem is worse with childhood disorders, because developmental processes and varying rearing habits often cloud distinctions between normal and pathological behavior. A child's behavior changes constantly as new cognitive and physical abilities emerge, affecting his or her interests and skills. At the same time, the child has little or no control over the external environment imposed by adult caregivers. As a result, a particular behavior may be well within the acceptable range for some children in some environments yet be pathological for others in a different context.

Childhood psychosis is an excellent example of problems that can arise in diagnosing childhood mental disorders. In adults, the diagnosis depends on eliciting from the afflicted individual evidence of such symptoms as a thought disorder, delusions, or hallucinations. For children or adolescents whose cognitive growth is relatively complete, this approach still obtains; however, a child who has been psychotic since two or three years of age is likely to present an entirely different clinical picture that can be understood only within the context of a departure from normal development. In such children, abnormal play behavior or an absence of expected social interactions may be the predominant symptom.

The nosology of childhood disorders has changed substantially over the past twenty years, but authorities in child psychiatry still lack a universally acceptable classification system. The American Psychiatric Association's *Diagnostic and Statistical Manual,* second edition (DSM-II),[2] which was widely used in the mental health field until the late 1970s, had been constructed for use with adults and was unsuitable for diagnosing many childhood disorders.

The Committee on Child Psychiatry of the Group for the Advancement of Psychiatry[93] proposed a classification scheme more suited to the developing child. Its ten major diagnostic categories were: healthy responses, reactive disorders, developmental deviations, psychoneurotic disorders, personality disorders, psychotic disorders, psychophysiological disorders, brain syndromes, mental disorders, and other disorders. In addition, the scheme provided an elective symptom list with which the clinician could describe more precisely the behavioral, cognitive, and emotional disturbances in a particular child.

Unlike its predecessor, the third edition of the American Psychiatric Association's *Diagnostic and Statistical Manual* (DSM-III)[3] has specific diagnostic categories for children and adolescents. It now is the most widely used system in the United States for classifying mental disorders. DSM-III provides specific criteria for each diagnosis, based on observable or reportable signs and symptoms; it also uses a multiaxial scheme. Table 23–1 lists childhood-specific Axis I diagnoses; but children who meet the criteria also may receive an adult diagnosis, including schizophrenia, affective disorder, or substance abuse. Axis II is used to indicate either a specific type of personality disorder or a specific develop-

TABLE 23–1

DSM-III Axis I Diagnoses of Mental Disorders of Childhood and Adolescence

Pervasive Developmental Disorders (PDDs)
    Infantile autism
    Childhood onset pervasive developmental disorder
    Atypical childhood onset pervasive developmental
      disorder
Attention Deficit Disorders (ADDs)
    With or without hyperactivity
    Residual type
Anxiety Disorders of Childhood or Adolescence
    Separation anxiety disorder
    Avoidant disorder of childhood or adolescence
    Overanxious disorder
Conduct Disorders
    Undersocialized, aggressive
      or nonaggressive
    Socialized, aggressive
      or nonaggressive
    Atypical
Stereotyped Movement Disorders
    Transient or chronic motor tic disorder
    Tourette's disorder
    Atypical tic disorder
    Atypical stereotyped movement disorder
Eating disorders
    Anorexia nervosa
    Bulimia
    Pica
    Rumination disorder of infancy
    Atypical eating disorder
Mental Retardation
    Mild, moderate, severe, or profound
Other disorders of infancy, childhood, or adolescence
    Reactive attachment disorder of infancy
    Schizoid disorder of childhood or adolescence
    Elective mutism
    Oppositional disorder
    Identity disorder
Other Disorders with Physical Manifestations
    Stuttering
    Functional enuresis or encopresis
    Sleepwalking disorder
    Sleep terror disorder

SOURCE: American Psychiatric Association, *Diagnostic and Statistical Manual of Mental Disorders*, vol. 3 (Washington, D.C.: American Psychiatric Association, 1980), p. 15.

mental disorder, for example, in reading, arithmetic, or language. Axis III is used for concurrent medical conditions or symptoms that may arise from, contribute to, or complicate the mental disorder. Axes IV and V indicate the severity of accompanying psychoso-

cial stressors and the highest level of functioning during the preceding year, respectively.

Overall, DSM-III has had a beneficial effect for child psychiatry. It has generated considerable controversy about the clinical validity of those categories of childhood disorders that were included, which has, in turn, led to some rigorous studies of their clinical utility. Again, examples of such research are described later for some specific disorders. However, few child psychiatrists view DSM-III as the final word in diagnosing and classifying mental disorders of childhood and adolescence, and much work remains to be done in this area.

¶ Epidemiology of Childhood Mental Disorders

Continuing controversies about how best to categorize mental disorders in childhood have hampered efforts to define the magnitude of the problem. Even so, there is a distressing absence of reliable estimates of the prevalence and types of mental illnesses to which children and adolescents are prone. Too often these age groups are treated as an "other" category. For example, the American Psychiatric Association's 1983 *Economic Fact Book for Psychiatry*[4] reports data on admissions to mental health facilities for the following age groups, in years: over sixty-five, forty-five to sixty-four, twenty-five to forty-four, eighteen to twenty-four, and under eighteen. The youngest age group accounted for 18 percent of the total admissions; yet there was no information about which ages within that age range are involved most heavily. The superb effort that the National Institute of Mental Health recently sponsored to obtain a large-scale population survey of mental disorders looks only at individuals eighteen years of age or older.[175]

The incomplete information available about mental disorders in childhood and adolescence serves at least to document the general magnitude of the problem. Gould,

Wunsch-Hitzig, and Dohrenwend[85] reviewed a heterogeneous group of twenty-five studies of childhood psychopathology in the United States done between 1928 and 1975. Because of the diverse methods of data collection and diagnostic criteria used in these studies, the authors could only document the prevalence of a broad indicator of difficulty, which they called clinical maladjustment. Based on the available studies, they concluded that the overall prevalence of clinical maladjustment among children and adolescents was at least 12 percent, with actual prevalence rates varying with age, ethnic group, social class, and geographical region.

From a different perspective, Goldberg and associates[82] studied the prevalence of mental health problems among children seeing pediatricians. In this ambulatory population, 5 percent were identified as having some type of mental health difficulty at first visit, based on physician report. Among children with problems, the most common diagnoses were: adaptation reactions, 32 percent; speech and language disorder, 18 percent; other specific learning disorder, 17 percent; hyperkinetic disorder, 17 percent; and conduct disorder, 15 percent. Factors that affected the reported prevalence rates included type of pediatric practice, gender of the child, and age of the child. Two-thirds of the children had been afflicted with the diagnosed problem for more than two years, and over half of them were at least moderately impaired.

As mentioned earlier, a major hurdle to studying the epidemiology of mental disorders in children and adolescents has been and continues to be the absence of a widely accepted nosology or of a reliable, easy-to-use method of making a diagnosis. Fortunately, as criteria for specific types of childhood mental disorders such as autism and childhood depression are being defined and applied to various research populations, a clearer picture is emerging at least about the prevalence of these syndromes. Examples of such results are given later in discussions of those disorders.

¶ General Principles of Psychopharmacology of Childhood Mental Disorders

The overall principles for using psychoactive drugs to treat children are analogous to those for using drugs to treat adults:

1. The patient should have clearly identifiable signs or symptoms that are interfering with personal or social functioning.
2. There should be a reasonable chance that the drug selected will alleviate these signs or symptoms.
3. Parents and, to whatever extent possible, the child patient should know why the drug is being given, what side effects it may produce, and what precautions are needed in taking it.
4. If control of some specific constellation of symptoms is the goal rather than a complete remission of the disorder, the limited scope of the drug treatment and the relative merits and disadvantages of such treatment should be stated and discussed thoroughly in advance of treatment.
5. The drug should be given in the appropriate dosage range, neither too high nor too low.
6. Physician, parents, and patient should agree explicitly on the goals of treatment, how long treatment will continue if the goals are not attained, and how long treatment will last if these goals are achieved.

Having a child for a patient does complicate drug treatment in several ways. First, psychoactive drugs have not been studied nearly as well in children as in adults. The large-scale studies that established the efficacy of such drug classes as antidepressants and antipsychotics were all done on adult patient populations; they may not apply even to those children who have an "adult" form of a disorder. With few exceptions, basic information about which childhood mental disorders in what age groups respond best to a specific drug is accumulating at a distressingly slow pace. Often, drug treatments with children aim more at alleviating target symptoms than at treating an underlying disorder.[223] Second, little is known about the short- and long-term effects, good or bad, of psychoactive drugs on a developing organism, but abundant evidence confirms that side effects in children may differ markedly from those in adults. For example, central nervous system (CNS) stimulants retard growth in preadolescent children; much research has gone into determining the long-term consequences of this effect on children who benefit from such drugs and may need to take them for years.[88] Third, psychological meanings of medication to children and to their families can, at times, overwhelm any potential pharmacological action.[5] Depending on a child's cognitive capacity, pills may be viewed as magical, punitive, or restorative. Either the child or the family may view the child as defective, feel guilty about or ashamed of relying on medication, or conclude that pills are the answer to every problem. Such concerns further underscore the need for considered use of psychoactive agents within the context of an overall treatment plan.

Table 23–2 lists some representative drugs often prescribed to children and indicates the disorders or symptoms for which they are used most commonly. Unknowns about drug use in children and a continued emphasis in many parts of the United States on psychodynamic aspects of childhood disorders combine to affect actual prescription patterns in a variety of ways. Thus Pfefferbaum and Overall[158] surveyed twenty-five child psychiatrists from across the nation, asking them how they might make use of various psychoactive drugs in each of nine case vignettes. The respondents differed markedly in how often they were likely to use drugs for any given kind of patient. For example, one vignette described a six-year-old boy with attention deficit disorder (ADD) with hyperactivity. On average, the respondents indicated that they would use drugs to treat about 69 percent of patients with such symptoms; but the range of responses by individual child psychiatrists was from a low of 2 percent to a high of 100 percent. That report and others[1,223] indicate that thioridazine hydrochloride and other antipsychotics are among the most frequently used medicines in child psychiatry, generally used to control symptoms such as explosive behavior or excessive activity, rather than as a specific treatment for a disorder. Such results once again emphasize the need for more precise methods for diagnosing childhood mental disorders and better information about appropriate drug uses for each disorder.

¶ Specific Childhood Mental Disorders

Over the past few decades, researchers and clinicians in child psychiatry have begun to amass the information needed to identify and study the biological substrates of and define optimal drug treatments for some specific disorders. This section presents five examples of this vital type of endeavor.

Pervasive Developmental Disorders

The severe disorders of development especially highlight some of the difficulties unique to child psychiatry. For example, as noted earlier, defining psychosis becomes problematic for children in the early stages of cognitive development. Child psychiatrists continue to disagree about the best criteria for defining childhood psychosis. In addition, many hesitate to place such a diagnostic label on a child, fearing the social and psychological consequences of doing so; their decision is made more difficult by the paucity of knowledge about expected outcomes for psychotic children and about how maturation, environment, and various types of treatment affect outcome. Few researchers are prepared to tackle the complex task of studying how psychosis evolves during the continuous changes of development—or how psychosis itself alters that process.

CLINICAL PRESENTATION
The most widely known pervasive developmental disorder (PDD) is infantile autism, first defined by Kanner[107,108] in the mid-

TABLE 23-2
Representative Drugs Commonly Used in Treating Childhood Disturbances

Drug Generic (Brand)	Oral Dosage mg/day (doses/day)	Indications	Common Side Effects
Antipsychotics			
Chlorpromazine (Thorazine)	10–200 (2–4)	Psychosis, severe agitation, severe anxiety, uncontrollable assaultiveness	Anticholinergic effects, dystonic reactions, Parkinsonian symptoms, akathisia, seizures, blood dyscrasias, postural hypotension, cardiac dysrhythmias, tardive dyskinesia
Trifluorperazine (Stelazine)[a]	1–20 (1–2)		
Thioridazine HCl (Mellaril)[b]	10–200 (1–2)		
Thiothixene HCl (Navane)[c]	1–30 (1–2)		
Haloperidol (Haldol)[c]	2–16 (1–2)	Above, plus Tourette syndrome	
Pimozide	1–10 (1)		
Tricyclic Antidepressants		Depressive states, enuresis, school phobia	Anticholinergic effects, seizures, cardiac dysrhythmias
Imipramine HCl (Tofranil)[b]	50–250 (1–3)		
Amitriptyline HCl (Elavil)[c]	50–250 (1–3)		
Nortriptyline HCl (Aventyl HCl)	10–75 (1–3)		
Central Stimulants	Sulfate		
Dextroamphetamine (Dexedrine)	5–40 (2–3)	Attention deficit disorder, narcolepsy	Anorexia, GI complaints, weight loss, decreased growth rate, insomnia, irritability
Methylphenidate HCl (Ritalin HCl)[b]	10–60 (2–3)		
Pemoline (Cylert)[b]	37.5–150 (1)		
Fenfluramine (Pondimin)[c]	10–100 (2–3)	Autism[d]	
Sedative Hypnotics			
Diphenhydramine HCl (Benadryl)	25–100 (1–4)	Acute insomnia, transient anxiety, acute dystonias, sleepwalking, sleep talking, night terrors	Anticholinergic effects, daytime drowsiness
Chlordiazepoxide HCl (Librium)[c]	25–100 (1)		
Diazepam (Valium)	2.5–10 (1)		
Less Commonly Used Drugs			
Lithium carbonate	300–1800 (2–4)	Bipolar affective disorder, hyperaggression	Leucocytosis, hyperthyroidism, nephrotoxicity, polydipsia, weight gain, GI complaints
Clonidine HCl (Catapres)	0.1–0.8 (1–2)	Tourette syndrome[d]	Anticholinergic effects, GI complaints
Propranolol HCl (Inderal)	50–1000 (3–4)	Uncontrolled rage outbursts[d]	Somnolence, lethargy, hypotension, bradycardia, depression

[a] Food and Drug Administration (FDA) approval only for children over two years of age.
[b] FDA approval only for children over six years of age.
[c] FDA approval only for children over twelve years of age.
[d] Not approved by the FDA for this use and not established as effective.

1940s. He noted a small group of young children whose development was markedly abnormal before they were two and one-half years of age. For some children, symptoms were present from birth; for others, symptoms were progressive. Such children displayed symptoms of withdrawal, isolation, aloofness, delayed language, ritualisms, and strong resistance to change. These continue to be the basic criteria for infantile autism, as defined in DSM-III (see table 23–3).[3]

Often children with autism first come to medical attention because the parents are concerned about a failure to acquire language skills. Some never learn to speak; others start normally but then fail to progress; and still others develop some language, which they later lose.[107,233] Autistic children who can speak typically do so much later than usual and almost always have peculiarities in speech rhythm, structure, and word choice. Interestingly, nonverbal aspects of language also are impaired, so that autistic children often have trouble learning even to gesture for things they want.

Parents seek medical assistance for children who eventually are diagnosed as autistic for other reasons as well. As infants, these children may be exceptionally "good" babies who will lie quietly in their cribs for hours, playing with their fingers or just staring blankly; however, others may launch without warning into hours of unremitting crying or screaming.[53,148] Often parents will report that their baby never liked to be held or cuddled and never developed a social smile.[108,229] As they grow older, many of these children are thought to be deaf, because they seem not to notice or fail to respond to noises.[146] Yet seemingly trivial changes in daily routine, even minor rearrangements of familiar objects in a room, can set off prolonged tantrums.[83,117] For some children with autism, the most disconcerting

TABLE 23–3
DSM-III Criteria for Pervasive Developmental Disorders

Infantile Autism

- Onset before 30 months of age
- Pervasive lack of responsiveness to other people (autism)
- Gross deficits in language development
- If speech is present, peculiar speech patterns
- Bizarre responses to various aspects of the environment
- Absence of delusions, hallucinations, loosening of associations, or incoherence as in schizophrenia

---

Childhood-onset Pervasive Developmental Disorder

- Marked, chronic deficits in relationships with others
- Peculiarities evinced by at least three of the following:
    a) sudden excessive anxiety
    b) constricted or inappropriate affect
    c) resistance to change in the environment
    d) oddities in motor movement
    e) abnormalities of speech
    f) hyper- or hyposensitivity to sensory stimuli
    g) self-mutilation
- Onset of full syndrome after 30 months of age and before 12 years of age
- Absence of delusions, hallucinations, loosening of associations, or incoherence as in schizophrenia

---

NOTE: Reprinted by permission of the American Psychiatric Association, from *Diagnostic and Statistical Manual of Mental Disorders*, vol. 3 (Washington, D.C.: American Psychiatric Association, 1980), pp. 89–91.

early symptoms are extensive ritualistic activities such as twirling, head-banging, toe-walking, and flapping of hands or arms.[139,204]

Because of the diversity of potential symptoms, many of which may occur at least transiently during normal development, autism often is difficult to diagnose, especially in the first few years of life. No single symptom or set of symptoms is pathognomonic; rather, autism is characterized by a marked but individually variable disruption in the order and extent to which the child achieves developmental milestones.[12,28] Typically, the diagnosis becomes clear by age three years, when the marked delay in the acquisition of language and communication skills becomes apparent. Although there may be islands of normal or even exceptional ability, most children with autism have some degree of mental retardation.[148]

DSM-III distinguishes infantile autism from other childhood-onset PDDs (see table 23-3). However, in many instances the choice of a diagnosis rests on an assessment of whether problems began before or after thirty months of age. Many who work with such children find this distinction less than compelling. It seems likely that careful analyses of various symptom clusters within the PDDs will suggest subtypes that are more relevant to treatment and outcome.[199]

There are no distinct criteria in DSM-III for childhood schizophrenia. As noted in table 23-3, signs and symptoms of schizophrenia are explicit exclusion criteria for either infantile autism or childhood-onset PDD. Children with overt evidence of adult-like psychosis, including hallucinations, thought disorder, and delusions, receive an adult diagnosis—brief reaction psychosis, schizophreniform disorder, schizophrenia, or atypical psychosis, depending on the type and duration of symptoms.[3] Such diagnoses almost never are made in children under three years of age but are not uncommon in early and midadolescence. Schizophrenic children reportedly are somewhat less likely than adults with schizophrenia to have delusions, but thought disorders and hallucinations are common.[87]

EPIDEMIOLOGY

Estimates of the prevalence of infantile autism in the United States range from 1 to 5 per 10,000, depending on the definition used.[3,19,132,215] The prevalence of schizophrenia and related psychotic illnesses in childhood is in a similar range.[95] Infantile autism occurs about three to four times as often in boys as in girls.[53,212,215] Although adolescent boys also are at greater risk than girls for schizophrenia, that differential appears to be closer to two to one.[95,116] Overall, in the United States, at least 1 million children have these forms of severe developmental disorders.[19]

BIOCHEMICAL AND NEUROPHYSIOLOGICAL CORRELATES

Causes of the PDDs and childhood psychoses still are unknown. In fact, it has been difficult even to define the number of distinct disorders and how they interrelate. For example, some investigators believe that infantile autism is an early manifestation of schizophrenia,[10] but others argue that they are distinct syndromes.[185,229] Overall, the latter school of thought appears to be more in accord with available research evidence. Thus studies have shown that siblings of autistic children are at somewhat greater risk than are children in the general population for autism; but schizophrenia does not occur with unexpected frequency in families of autistic children.[95,147]

Among the childhood mental disorders, infantile autism probably has raised some of the most intense controversies about etiology. In the initial observations of these children, Kanner[107] concluded that the cause was most likely an inborn disturbance. However, studies of the markedly abnormal social behavior of these children led to the hypothesis that such disturbances were central to the syndrome and resulted from poor mothering.[16,69] This hypothesis attracted considerable attention. It also led to additional research such as efforts to define more precisely the range of normal interactions of mothers with their children and studies not only of how mothers interacted with their autistic child but also how they interacted with their nonautistic children. That research has failed to demonstrate any consistent differences between mothers or fathers of autistic and normal children.[116]

The weight of available evidence suggests that autism results from some abnormality of brain function and probably is the end stage of a heterogeneous assortment of insults to the CNS.[212] Several lines of research support this statement. The evidence for familial transmission was mentioned earlier. In addition, the risk of autism among children exposed to the rubella virus during gestation is one in ten,[66] and autism rates among children exposed to other viral infections *in utero* also are elevated.[148] Furthermore, about one-fourth of autistic children will develop a seizure disorder by adolescence.[187]

Although as a group, autistic children have an increased prevalence of biochemical and neurological peculiarities, no abnormalities have been found that are specific to this syndrome or present even most of the time. A direct neuropathological study of four children with autisticlike symptoms—one of whom had phenylketonuria—was unrevealing.[228] Computed x-ray tomography (CT) studies of autistic children have revealed a few instances of clear tissue damage, but the majority have no observable abnormalities or only nonspecific minor ones.[171,183,216] Electroencephalography (EEG) studies also have been inconclusive and contradictory,[60,102] as have electrophysiological studies of auditory, vestibular, and cardiovascular regulatory systems.[117,208]

The only consistent biochemical finding in autism has been that of hyperserotonemia, which occurs in about one-third of all autistic children.[84,190,234] Despite many efforts to clarify the meaning of this finding, little progress has been made. It is not even clear that peripheral serotonin (5HT) in any way reflects brain serotonergic activity. For example, Gillberg, Svennerholm, and Hamilton-Hellberg[79] found no differences in cerebrospinal fluid (CSF) concentrations of 5-hydroxyindoleacetic acid (5-HIAA), the major 5HT metabolite, when comparing autistic children with age-matched neurological controls. Hyperserotonemia also occurs in about 40 percent of children with mental retardation,[234] but this association with retardation does not account for the finding in autism. It seems likely that interest in 5HT will increase again with the recent report of several autistic children who had both peripheral and central antibodies to 5HT receptors.[212] It remains to be determined whether this finding, if confirmed, will lead to evidence of a specific role for 5HT in autism.

Most of the work just described does not distinguish reliably among such diagnostic subgroups as infantile autism, childhood-onset PDD, and childhood psychoses. As mentioned earlier, failure to differentiate between the first two categories may make little practical difference; but the available evidence suggests that childhood psychoses more closely resemble adult schizophrenia than autism.

Given the many unresolved questions about biological causes of adult schizophrenia, it is perhaps not surprising that few researchers have attempted to extend the research to psychotic children. In a small study, Gillberg, Svennerholm, and Hamilton-Hellberg[79] reported that 5-HIAA was increased in the CSF of psychotic but not autistic children, compared with sex- and age-matched neurological controls without psychiatric disorders; homovanillic acid (HVA), the major dopamine (DA) metabolite, was elevated in both experimental groups compared with controls. This study has many limitations but does suggest the value of broadening inquiries about biochemical aspects of these disorders beyond 5HT.

DRUG TREATMENT

Childhood psychoses are treated with the same drugs used to treat adult psychoses (see table 23-2).[29,53] Antipsychotics are the best available treatment for such target symptoms as hallucinations and thought disorder and can also help control violent outbursts and excessive excitation. However, there is a general perception that they are less effective in children than in adults and that children may be more susceptible to the full range of side effects, including tardive dyskinesia. Therefore, for each child, the physician and parents must weigh carefully the severity of the symptoms and degree of remission achieved with a drug against its potential short- and long-term risks. Parents must know in advance about the very real risk of tardive dyskinesia with prolonged use and be given a chance to help decide when a drug trial should be initiated and under what circumstances it would be stopped.

Antipsychotics differ in their relative potency and in the frequency with which they produce various side effects. Some—for example, chlorpromazine (Thorazine) and thioridazine hydrochloride (Mellaril)—are quite sedating; others, including haloperidol (Haldol) and fluphenazine hydrochloride (Prolixin), are less sedating but more likely to produce extrapyramidal reactions that may be extremely frightening for a child. With few practical guidelines, practitioners often adopt a few antipsychotics with which they have become most familiar and comfortable. Those who write reviews on this topic typically recommend a medium-potency antipsychotic such as trifluoperazine hydrochloride (Stelazine) or thiothixene hydrochloride (Navane).[29,53,212] Yet in studies of actual practice, thioridazine is the most popular and widely used antipsychotic for children.[1,158]

Antipsychotics are also the drugs used most often with infantile autism and childhood-onset PDD. For these children, the drugs typically are used for nonspecific benefits in decreasing hyperactivity and reducing the risk of violent, explosive behavior. The choice of the drug and the dosage must be tailored individually to achieve optimal response with minimal side effects. Dosage must be monitored carefully and may need to be adjusted over time, as the symptom picture changes and the child matures.

Lithium carbonate has been tried to a limited extent in infantile autism. A study of ten children, three to six years old, showed no positive effects for either chlorpromazine or lithium compared with placebo; however, one child with severe symptoms of violent temper and self-mutilation did have many fewer maladaptive behaviors while on lithium.[33] Another study of nine children with "infantile psychosis" concluded that lithium decreased disturbed activity, abnormal mood, and aggressiveness.[86]

Recently, Ritvo and his colleagues described the use of fenfluramine hydrochloride (Pondimin) to treat a small group of autistic children.[78,178,179] They reported that fenfluramine improved both the behavior and the IQ scores of some of the subjects. In addition to its obvious therapeutic implications, the result is of interest to researchers because, among other actions, fenfluramine depletes brain 5HT. These reports generated the first multicenter drug trial on autism in the United States, the results of which should be published in 1985. Unfortunately, although not all of the centers have completed their studies, our experience with fenfluramine at Stanford suggests that its benefits are much more limited than initially hoped.[200] At present, use of fenfluramine to treat autism is strictly experimental, and it should not be considered for routine use.[52]

Attention Deficit Disorder

Attention deficit disorder (ADD) is the DSM-III diagnostic label for a syndrome that has had many names, including minimal brain dysfunction, brain damage syndrome, hyperactive child syndrome, and hyperkinetic syndrome. Heinrich Hoffmann[100] first described this general cluster of symptoms in 1845. Although these terms all refer largely to the same cluster of problems, none completely overlaps with any other. The interchangeable use of such terms is only one source of the confusion and controversy that has plagued this area of child psychiatry.[94] Yet the syndrome remains one of the few in child psychiatry about which there is widespread agreement that specific drug treatment often is appropriate and can be markedly beneficial.

CLINICAL PRESENTATION

DSM-III defines ADD as a triad of symptoms: inattention, impulsivity, and hyperactivity.[3] Inattention is defined with such behaviors as failure to finish work or play activities, poor listening, easy distractibility, and inability to carry out tasks requiring sustained attention. Evidence of impulsivity includes a tendency to act without thinking, frequent shifts from activity to activity, a need for close supervision, poor organizational skills, and trouble waiting for a turn in school and play. Hyperactivity refers to excessive levels of motor activity, with constant fidgeting and generally purposeless movement, often even during sleep. If this last symptom is absent, the diagnosis is ADD without hyperactivity. Typically, symptoms are present at least by age three years, but the diagnosis usually is made after children start school, where the symptoms interfere markedly with performance.

Children with ADD can be extremely trying for parents, teachers, and peers. Often they first come to medical attention because parents or schools can no longer tolerate the constant activity. Under such circumstances, the pressure for the physician to "do something"—for example, prescribe a CNS stimulant—is usually intense. Few of the behaviors are likely to occur in a brief, structured office visit, so physicians typically must rely on parent and school reports. However, such information must be sifted carefully for evidence of specific developmental disorders in reading, arithmetic, or language; of external causes of inattention and hyperactivity, such as poor nutrition, understimulation, or excessive anxiety; or of some other primary diagnosis, including mental retardation, narcolepsy, or psychosis.[5,36]

The DSM-III focus on attention and impulsivity as the primary symptoms of ADD diverges substantially from an earlier tendency to view hyperactivity as the key feature of the syndrome.[5] This change of emphasis seems appropriate; although hyperactivity typically subsides as children enter adolescence, problems with attention often remain.[97,130] However, some research suggests that ADD without hyperactivity differs sufficiently from ADD with hyperactivity to be viewed as a different disorder. ADD children with hyperactivity are apt to have an aggressive conduct disorder, be quite unpopular, behave in bizarre ways, and lack any guilt for misbehavior, but those without hyperactivity typically are more anxious and shy, socially withdrawn, poor in sports, and less intensely unpopular.[112,124] Undoubtedly, formulations of relevant subgroupings of this syndrome will continue to evolve as more information about symptom clusters and long-term outcome emerges.

A detailed developmental history of children with ADD usually uncovers problems even during the toddler period.[6] Among common early symptoms are fussy eating habits, an irritable disposition, and marked delays in sleeping through the night. Also, these children are likely to have had difficulties adhering to limits, to have been excessively aggressive with siblings or playmates, and to have repeatedly gotten into things they were supposed to leave alone.

EPIDEMIOLOGY

ADD is one of the most common of the childhood mental disorders, with a prevalence of 3 percent among prepubertal children.[3] The ratio of boys to girls is in the order of ten to one. The ratio of ADD children with hyperactivity to those without hyperactivity is unknown.[124] Surveys looking for any of the symptoms of ADD report prevalence rates as high as 10 to 16 percent for prepubertal children.[38,189]

Several studies suggest a genetic, or at least familial, component to ADD.[35] For example, a total of seven pairs of monozygotic twins reported in two independent studies had a 100 percent concordance rate for ADD, compared with only two of six dizygotic twin pairs.[98,131] Family studies suggest that parents of children with ADD have an unexpectedly high prevalence of alcoholism, sociopathy, and hysteria and are more likely to report having had symptoms of ADD themselves as children.[34,143] All these studies have serious design flaws that prevent any firm conclusions about the genetics of ADD. For example, the diagnosis of a parent as having had the syndrome must be retrospective. Also, the twin studies involve very small sample sizes and cannot control for effects of prematurity, low birth weight, and prenatal compromise, all of which are themselves risk factors for ADD.[18,202]

BIOCHEMICAL AND NEUROPHYSIOLOGICAL CORRELATES

"Soft" neurological signs and minor physical anomalies such as large, low-set ears, poor fine-motor coordination, and impaired spatial orientation have been described in many children with ADD, but their prevalence and meaning remain unclear.[141,225] Such findings, along with the evidence of familial transmission, have encouraged a search for evidence of a developmental lag or of frank defects in brain function, for example, in the reticular activating system.[222]

CT studies have been relatively noncontributory.[171] Although investigators have found abnormalities in from 5 to 35 percent of patients, most changes were minor, and none seemed to be specific for the syndrome.[15,43,209] EEG studies[26,104,203] similarly have yielded inconclusive or negative results. In general, studies of physiological arousal indicate that many children with ADD have relatively low levels of CNS arousal,[188] which does not fit well with the clinical picture.

Several groups have obtained CSF from children with ADD and analyzed monoamine metabolites. Attention has focused especially on the DA metabolite HVA, because DA has long been thought to be involved in the etiology of the syndrome.[197,198] Shetty and Chase[198] reported that steady-state levels of HVA were the same in controls and children with ADD. However, Shaywitz, Cohen, and Bowers[197] measured HVA concentrations following a dose of probenecid, which inhibits the transport mechanisms that rapidly remove monoamine metabolites from the CSF. They reported that CSF HVA in children with ADD was 60 percent of the value for neurological controls. As with so many biological studies in child psychiatry, the meaning of this result hinges on the "normality" of the controls, which is unknown. Artifacts introduced by the use of probenecid also are impossible to assess.[71]

DRUG TREATMENT

The use of CNS stimulants to treat ADD and its diagnostic precursors was the first and remains the best-known success story in child psychopharmacology. Bradley first discovered the ability of dextroamphetamine (Benzedrine) to control the symptoms of hyperactivity in 1934.[21] Amphetamine was again used for that purpose in 1957,[125] and methylphenidate hydrochloride (Ritalin) was introduced the next year.[115] Amphetamine, methylphenidate, and more recently pemoline (Cylert) remain the drugs of choice for treating ADD.

An ideal drug for treating ADD would treat the full spectrum of essential and associated features of the syndrome, reducing impulsivity and hyperaggressiveness, increasing frustration tolerance and attention span, enhancing fine-motor coordination and visual and auditory perception, and controlling hyperactivity. Naturally, the drug would do all those things without producing any side effects. Although the CNS stimulants fall short of that ideal in several major ways, they are remarkably useful and relatively safe.

After over twenty-five years, methylphenidate remains the drug most often used in treating ADD.[5,39,59] In a typical treatment schedule, methylphenidate is given in an initial dosage of 0.25 mg/per kg daily in two doses—breakfast and lunch. Appetite suppression is a nearly universal acute side effect of all the CNS stimulants, and the drug can be given before or after meals, depending on the child's weight. The dose then is doubled each week as tolerated until symptoms have resolved, up to an average optimal dosage of 1 mg/per kg/per day.[223] Target symptoms should be identified clearly in advance, so that parents and schoolteachers can monitor changes. Analogous regimens can be used for amphetamine or for pemoline (see table 23–2). Pemoline is the longest-acting of the three drugs and can be given as a single morning dose.[59,67]

About 70 percent of children with ADD improve with medication, but 10 percent deteriorate. Tolerance of the side effects of each of the drugs varies among individuals. Because of concern about side effects and about the development of tolerance to the beneficial drugs, drug schedules typically include "holidays" over weekends and during the summer, if the family can cope with the behavior in other ways.

All of the CNS stimulants have side effects. One of the most worrisome is a direct suppression of growth in developing children.[67,88,89,138] The primary effect is a reduction of the rate at which weight is gained, although the rate of height gain also is slowed for some individuals. Some reports have not confirmed growth retardation[92,135,145]; however the bulk of the literature suggests that it does occur, at least at high, chronic doses in susceptible children. The cause of growth retardation remains unclear. It does not seem to be secondary to the anorexic side effects of CNS stimulants, because tolerance to that effect typically develops after a few weeks. The effects of methylphenidate appear to be mainly on weight, but amphetamine and pemoline decrease the rate of both weight and height gain.

Less serious but still bothersome side effects of the CNS stimulants include irritability and argumentativeness, gastrointestinal complaints such as stomachaches and nausea, and headaches. Typically, these are transient and resolve with time or with a slightly lower drug dosage. Another interesting side effect is sleep disturbance. Although the majority of children or their parents note restless sleep as a side effect, sleep EEG studies show only minor changes in actual sleep patterns.[90] The CNS stimulants are given early in the day to try to avoid adverse effects on sleep. However, Chatoor and associates[51] have suggested that some children actually sleep better when they also receive a dose at night; a nighttime dose of amphetamine produced subjective reports of more satisfactory sleep and EEG recordings showed a marked increase in sleep stages 1 and 2, with a corresponding decrease in rapid-eye-movement (REM) sleep and sleep stages 3 and 4. Based on these findings, Chatoor and coworkers[53] have suggested that, for some children, restless sleep may be a part of the syndrome and actually may improve with treatment.

The mode of action of the CNS stimulants on ADD is unknown. Initially investigators thought that the calming effects of these drugs was "paradoxical" and specific for children with this syndrome. Subsequent research has not supported either of those conclusions. Studies have shown that normal children[173] and enuretic children without ADD[224] respond to CNS stimulants in much the same way as children with ADD. Many children with conduct disorders, especially those who are aggressive, also respond well to stimulants.[30,36]

Although they are the most widely used, CNS stimulants are not the only drugs effective for ADD. Sporadic reports suggest that, at least in selected cases, other appropriate drug treatments include antipsychotics[114]; a combination of antipsychotic plus CNS stimulant[221]; lithium and a stimulant[23]; and antidepressants.[77,172] Where aggression and rage outbursts are a prominent feature, propranolol hydrochloride also might be considered.[227] Much remains to be learned about the appropriate use of these additional drugs, alone or in combination.

Functional Enuresis

Bedwetting, or enuresis, can be enormously discomfiting for both the afflicted persons and their families. Often patients and families are hesitant to seek help for enuresis, and many physicians are equally reluctant to offer it. Enuresis is only a symptom, with a number of both common and rare causes in the differential diagnosis. Although much remains unclear about enuresis, there has been progress in defining its major subtypes and defining a reasonable overall strategy for approaching the problem.[56,75]

CLINICAL PRESENTATION

Enuresis is a symptom, not a disorder or a syndrome, and there is no single typical presentation. Physicians need to obtain a detailed history of the problem. Information about the symptom itself should include whether wetting occurs during the day, the night, or both; whether the child has ever had a period of months when he or she was dry; and when during the night wetting occurs. A full physical evaluation of the genitourinary tract is vital, including observation of urination and a urinalysis, to rule out organic causes of incontinence. Often careful questioning may reveal that enuresis is related to acute or chronic stresses for the patient such as, for example, struggles for control between the child and parent or an acute traumatic loss. In such cases a full exploration of the problem may be helpful in itself and is invaluable for formulating a treatment plan.

Enuresis can be categorized in several ways (see table 23–4).[6] One important distinction is between primary and secondary enuresis: Primary enuretics have never had a period of reliable dryness; secondary enuretics were dry for at least six months, but then enuresis recurred. Most primary enureses are likely to result from anatomical abnormalities or developmental immaturity, whereas secondary enureses more typically reflect psychosocial factors. Enuresis also can be subdivided according to etiology as either organic or functional. Organic enureses include those caused by anatomic or metabolic problems and those related to certain stages of sleep. Among functional enureses are those associated with traumatic regression and adolescent adjustment problems.

EPIDEMIOLOGY

Enuresis is a relatively common disorder, affecting about 7 to 12 percent of the preadolescent population.[6,105] Prevalence decreases with age, from as high as 25 percent among four-year-olds to about 2 percent among fourteen-year-olds.[75,105] More than twice as many boys are affected as girls.[3,201] There is good evidence of heritability for primary enuresis: If both parents were enuretic, a child has a 77 percent chance of being enuretic, compared with a 44 percent chance if only one parent was enuretic.[9]

BIOCHEMICAL AND NEUROPHYSIOLOGICAL CORRELATES

Aside from anatomical and metabolic causes of enuresis, little is known about mechanisms underlying familial primary enuresis. There is no evidence of characteristic neurological anomalies.[140,226] Still, the steady decline in rates of enuresis up to early adolescence is consistent with the idea of late maturation of some key system. For several years there was intense interest in the possible role of sleep-stage transitions.[6] In sleep

TABLE 23–4
Major Subtypes of Enuresis

	Organic	Functional
Primary	Anatomic/metabolic	Sociocultural
	With NREM dyssomnia	Separation-individuation
	With mental retardation	
Secondary	Anatomic/metabolic	Regressive
	With hypersomnia	Adolescent
	With mental retardation	With depression

SOURCE: T. F. Anders and R. D. Ciaranello, "Psychopharmacology of Childhood Disorders," in J. D. Barchas et al., eds., *Psychopharmacology: From Theory to Practice* (New York: Oxford University Press, 1977), p. 419.

EEG studies on enuretic children, Broughton[22] found that enuresis often seemed to occur during the early hours of sleep, at the transition into the first REM period of sleep. However, subsequent sleep studies on large populations have failed to confirm this attractive hypothesis.[140,174]

DRUG TREATMENT

Enuresis became important in child psychopharmacology because of the discovery that imipramine hydrochloride and other tricyclic antidepressants, often at surprisingly low doses, were effective in preventing certain types of primary enuresis. Initially imipramine was used because of its peripheral anticholinergic actions, but these proved to be irrelevant to its effects on enuresis.[152,174] Typically, imipramine is administered as a single nighttime dose of 40 mg to a maximum of 150 mg per day. It is effective in 20 to 40 percent of children. When it works, it should be maintained for several months. Unfortunately, relapse rates when imipramine is discontinued may be as high as 60 percent.

Tourette Syndrome

First described by Georges Gilles de la Tourette[80] in 1885, this syndrome attracted little attention until the late 1960s. The discovery that Tourette syndrome (TS) responds dramatically to the antipsychotic haloperidol led to a renewed interest in its etiology that has continued to expand. The March 1984 issue of the *Journal of the American Academy of Child Psychiatry* examines progress being made in understanding this interesting and distressing disorder.

CLINICAL PRESENTATION

The key feature of TS is recurrent muscular and vocal tics; usually the disorder appears after two years of age and almost invariably by early adolescence.[3] The syndrome can be extremely embarrassing and socially disruptive. Diagnosis often is delayed for years, especially in milder forms, because even when children or parents finally seek medical attention, many physicians dismiss the symptoms as idiosyncracies of childhood.[24]

Among features commonly associated with TS are the irresistible urge to utter offensive words (coprolalia) and a tendency to mirror the movements of others (echokinesis) or to repeat one's own words or phrases (palilalia). Some patients also have obsessions or compulsions of varying intensity, which can range from prolonged repetitions of harmless and seemingly meaningless tasks to severe self-mutilation. The disorder has an uneven course, with unpredictable exacerbations and remissions. The frequency of spontaneous remissions for a year or longer may be over 15 percent, but no precise information exists about the frequency of permanent remissions.[194]

EPIDEMIOLOGY

With increasing awareness of TS and other tic disorders, and especially as clinicians have learned to recognize milder forms of the syndrome, its estimated prevalence has risen to a current level of 1 to 5 in 10,000.[3] TS is three times more common in boys than in girls. Families of patients with TS have a 40 percent prevalence of tics, suggesting a genetic contribution.[149] However, the syndrome can also develop secondary to some types of brain trauma such as encephalitis[24] and following administration of some psychoactive drugs, especially those that increase the activity of the brain dopaminergic systems.[73,205]

BIOCHEMICAL AND NEUROPHYSIOLOGICAL CORRELATES

Individuals with TS have a high incidence of minor EEG abnormalities of unknown significance.[196,218] Caparulo and associates[43] obtained CT scans on sixteen children with TS and found minor but nonspecific abnormalities in 37 percent.

Because DA antagonists markedly ameliorate the symptoms of TS, investigators have been interested in the possible role of brain dopaminergic systems in its etiology. This connection is strengthened by the observation that agents which increase DA activity can precipitate a transient "toxic" TS, which abates when the stimulation stops.[73,205] Some investigators have suggested that TS results from a relative excess of DA and deficiency of acetylcholine activity.[206] However, a study of CSF monoamine metabolites in children with TS was more consistent with decreased, rather than increased, DA activity.[27] In addition, noradrenergic systems may be involved, especially with respect to obsessive-compulsive behavioral symptoms.[55,128] These complex findings have yet to be synthesized into a convincing hypothesis about the underlying etiology of this debilitating disorder.

Drug Treatment

TS has been another relative success story for child psychopharmacology. The discovery over twenty years ago that haloperidol could produce a complete, long-lasting suppression of symptoms[50] led to a series of careful clinical trials that have helped to refine its use.[24,144] Usually patients are started on 0.25 to 0.5 mg haloperidol per day, with a slow increase of no more than 0.5 mg per week until maximum benefit is achieved with minimum side effects.[24] The dose often must be adjusted periodically to compensate for changes in the severity of the disorder. Haloperidol is effective for about 80 percent of patients with TS. About one-fourth of the treatment failures are a result of the patient's inability to tolerate the adverse side effects of the appropriate drug dosage.[195]

Although haloperidol remains the first drug of choice in treating TS, two drugs are emerging as alternatives in selected cases. The United States Food and Drug Administration (FDA) recently has approved the use of pimozide, a second-generation antipsychotic, for this purpose.[195] The dosage typically begins at 1 mg per day at bedtime, increasing by 1 mg every two to three days until maximum benefit is attained; the total daily dose should not exceed 20 mg in adults or 10 mg in children. Pimozide appears to produce cardiotoxicity in some people, so it must be used cautiously and with careful attention to cardiac status. No large-scale studies are yet available to assess pimozide's cardiovascular effects in children or to provide good dose-response curves.

Clonidine hydrochloride (Catapres), although still experimental, also shows promise of being useful for some patients[20,128] with TS. This alpha-adrenergic agonist is best known as an antihypertensive agent. Studies suggest that clonidine can work well alone or in combination with haloperidol. Recommended dosages begin at 0.05 mg once or twice a day, with gradual increases of 0.05 mg every one to two weeks as tolerated to a maximum daily dose of 0.8 mg.[24] Reported side effects include irritability, insomnia, emotional lability, and nightmares. Clonidine's efficacy raises a series of interesting questions about possible interactions between brain dopaminergic and noradrenergic systems and their relevance to the etiology of TS.

Affective Disorders

A marked change in child psychiatry since the early 1970s has been the growing recognition of affective disorders as a mental disorder[42,111] of childhood and early adolescence. At least in the United States, the prevailing opinion in the 1950s and 1960s was that children did not have affective disorders. Psychoanalysts argued that depression could not occur until the process of internalizing a superego and incorporating a well-formed ego ideal was complete in midadolescence.[177,182] Others granted that depressive symptoms might exist in some children but dismissed such symptoms as a normal, transient aspect of development.[129]

However, in the late 1960s and early 1970s reports began to appear about children with incontrovertible presentations of severe depression.[61,136,137,159] As the possibility of childhood depression came to be appreciated, clinicians also began to explore the possibility that children might have unique ways of presenting with depression, including masked depression.[58,62,81,176] Efforts are continuing to create useful classification schemes for childhood depression[41,61] and instruments for diagnosing it.[17,118,162,211] Although many areas of controversy remain, affective disorders in childhood do appear to be firmly established as an important area of inquiry within child psychiatry (see Cantwell and Carlson[42] for an excellent survey of this area).

CLINICAL PRESENTATION

Caveats about the imprecision of the term depression have long been emphasized in consideration of adult depression,[13] and they pertain equally to depression in children and adolescents.[37] Thus clinicians may use the term to describe a mood, a specific clinical syndrome, or a disorder. These distinctions involve more than the intensity or duration of the dysphoric mood. In both depressive syndrome and depressive disorder, mood is only one aspect of a cluster of symptoms, which may include changes in appetite, motor activity, cognitive function, and functional capacity. Depressive disorder implies a more self-contained process, with a characteristic course, clinical picture, and associated features, such as family history and biological abnormalities. The challenge in child psychiatry has been to define the depressive syndrome and depressive disorder for children and adolescents.

As mentioned earlier, there now is general agreement that some children have a depressive syndrome that fulfills strict criteria for adult major depressive disorder, as defined by DSM-III.[3] If questioned with sufficient care, some children, like adults, will report such symptoms as feelings of sadness or depression, excessive or inappropriate guilt, lack of usual interest in activities, changes in sleep patterns, suicidal ideation or attempts, changes in appetite and weight, poor concentration, and excessive tiredness.[162,166,211]

What is less clear and must be settled with additional research is the status of other diagnostic groups that some investigators have suggested may contain subsets of children for

whom the primary diagnosis is depression, including school phobia or refusal,[62,210] conduct disorder,[40,165] anorexia nervosa,[99,230] fire-setting behavior,[121] and childhood borderline disorder.[154] The importance of identifying such individuals, of course, lies in the hope that they might respond best to treatment of the underlying depression, a hypothesis that also largely remains to be tested.

One of the most dramatic potential consequences of depression is suicide. Of course, not every suicide in adults or children is the result of a depressive disorder; impulsive acts engendered by dysphoria or rage can also result in death. One of the most disturbing health trends in the United States is an unexplained increase in suicide rates among teenagers. Suicide rates for youths in the fifteen- to twenty-four-year-old range have risen from 5 in 100,000 in 1961 to 13 in 100,000 in 1983, making it the third highest cause of death in this age group.[19,45] Suicide below the age of fifteen is a much rarer event, less than one in 100,000; but even for this age group, death from suicide now equals the combined death rates for influenza and pneumonia.[45]

Suicide attempts are, of course, much more frequent than successful suicides.[156] One recent study of normal, nine- to ten-year-old schoolchildren reported that 9 percent had suicidal ideas, 2 percent had made threats, and 1 percent had made a mild attempt; this contrasts with a group of inpatients of similar age, of whom 26 percent had suicidal ideas, 26 percent had made threats, 20 percent had made a mild attempt, and 6 percent had made a serious attempt.[157] Evidence suggests that, as is true for adults, more young males successfully kill themselves by violent means and more young women make suicide attempts of lower lethality.[45]

Causes of suicides and suicide attempts in children and adolescents are not firmly established, but they often appear to occur in the context of a mental disorder, especially depression.[46] No systematic psychological assessment of individuals in this age group who successfully committed suicide has yet been published. Anecdotal reports of suicide attempts by young children suggest that they almost invariably come from highly disturbed settings and have long histories of psychosocial trauma.[57,150,214] To date, the youngest reported case of suicide behavior was two and one-half years old.[184] Such reports often emphasize that current statistics on suicide attempts may substantially underreport actual rates in this age group because of a strong tendency by many coroners and physicians to attribute deaths and injuries to accidents.

Whether mania and bipolar disorder manifest themselves in prepubertal children also remains controversial. As with depression, some clinicians argue that such cases do exist, but others insist that the observed symptoms are overinterpretations of normal fluctuations in mood.[8,44] Adult criteria for mania, such as excessive talking and movement, poor judgment and impulse control, irritability and argumentativeness, and high distractibility, are not transposed readily to children, because many of these symptoms are normal aspects of development and because similar symptoms occur in other mental disorders of childhood, for example, ADD with hyperactivity.[44,161]

Weinberg and Brumback[219] have suggested modified criteria for mania in childhood: presence of either euphoria or some combination of irritability and agitation, along with at least three symptoms from the following: hyperactivity, flight of ideas, grandiosity, pressured speech, sleep disturbance, and distractibility. Using these and other less strict criteria, investigators have reported relatively rare examples of manic behavior in children as young as four years old.[65,161,219] One way in which mania in children, especially in young ones, may differ from mania in adults is an absence of clear episodes in the former.[65] Elation and euphoria seem to be especially unusual symptoms in young children, but again they have been reported.[44,65]

The evidence for the presentation of bipolar affective disorder in adolescence is stronger.[48,96] Most sources of confusion about such cases have arisen from two sources. Often initial episodes during adolescence are quite mild and, therefore, may be either completely overlooked or diagnosed as some other disorder, such as adjustment reactions or behavior disorders; alternatively, physicians have often diagnosed severe episodes with psychotic features as schizophrenia.[47] It is reasonable to speculate that the early onset of bipolar affective disorder in childhood or adolescence has a worse prognosis than late-onset bipolar affective disorder, either because the disease is worse or because it interferes with acquisition of vital social and educational skills during that critical time in the life course; however, evidence to date has not supported that hypothesis.[44]

Epidemiology

Given the controversies over diagnosis, it should not be surprising that prevalence estimates of depression and bipolar affective disorder in childhood and adolescence are imprecise. In a survey of junior and senior high school students, using the Beck Depression Inventory, Kaplan, Hong, and Weinhold[109] reported a prevalence of depression of 8.6 percent in their sample. Depending on the populations studied and criteria used, estimated prevalence rates for children and early adolescents range from a high of 59 percent among psychiatric patients to about 1 to 2 percent in the general population, with much higher rates of persistent sadness.[37,111] Children of parents with bipolar affective disorder also seem to be at higher risk for depression.[64] No conclusive evidence exists about the relative risk of boys versus girls.

Even less information is available about the prevalence of bipolar affective disorder in younger age groups.[42] Some studies suggest that 30 to 40 percent of adults with bipolar affective disorder first became ill as adolescents.[151,230]

Biochemical and Neurophysiological Correlates

Relatively few investigators have looked explicitly at biological and neurophysiological aspects of depression in children. Part of the problem has been the confusion over diagnosis; also, it is substantially harder to justify any invasive diagnostic procedures in studies of children. As diagnostic reliability improves and safer and more sensitive probes of biological function become available, such research on children is increasingly more feasible.

The extensive literature on biochemical and neurophysiological correlates of affective disorders in adults is reviewed in chapters 4, 8, and 12 (cf. also Berger and Barchas,[14] Lowe and Cohen,[133] and Puig-Antich[166]). In brief summary, over the past several decades many researchers have searched diligently for evidence of an abnormality in brain noradrenergic or serotonergic activity, with inconclusive results. On the other hand, studies of neuroendocrine function have shown repeatedly that about 50 to 60 percent of depressed adult patients have an abnormally active pituitary-adrenal axis, most commonly demonstrated with the dexamethasone suppression test (DST)[49]; about 40 to 50 percent reportedly secrete less than normal amounts of growth hormone in response to insulin-induced hypoglycemia[91]; and a comparable number have a blunted thyroid-stimulating hormone secretion in response to an intravenous injection of thyrotropin-releasing hormone.[163]

Most of the endocrine studies in children have entailed assessments of DST responses in major depression.[101,113,160,181] The general conclusion from these studies is that, at least in adolescents, the DST appears to have a sensitivity (correctly identifying depressed children) of 40 to 60 percent and a specificity (correctly identifying nondepressed children) of 85 to 95 percent, which is comparable to the results in adults. However, Leckman[126] has cautioned appropriately that much work remains to be done, including a careful assessment of the effects of diet and acute weight change on the DST response and a careful analysis of age-dependent changes in DST. The few studies on growth hormone also have generally supported the

impression that adolescent depression resembles the adult form.[133,166,170]

One of the most robust findings in research on adult depression is the observation of specific changes in the sleep EEG architecture, including decreased total sleep time, shortened REM latency, decreased delta sleep, decreased sleep efficiency, intermittent awakenings, increased sleep latency, and early-morning awakenings.[122,166] However, studies of sleep EEG architecture in children with major depression have produced largely negative or contradictory[106,123,169,235] results. These findings have led to suggestions that maturational factors may affect sleep EEG architecture in ways that alter the expected findings in depressed prepubertal children.[166] To increase the feasibility of doing the studies needed to gain additional data about normal and abnormal sleep patterns in children, investigators are exploring the use of automated EEG systems that can be used in the child's home.

DRUG TREATMENT

Trials of antidepressants and lithium in child populations have been slow in coming.[42,111] Most still use small sample size and have design flaws such as unclear diagnostic criteria, lack of a placebo control, lack of a double-blind design, inadequate drug dosage, or inadequate follow-up, which make interpretation of these trials difficult. Even among studies that are reasonably well controlled, the results are contradictory. Researchers find that imipramine[155,168] and also amitriptyline[110,134] are superior to placebo for some children with depression, but not all.[120] Much more information is needed about possible age-related differences in the way antidepressants are metabolized that might affect their blood concentrations.[168] No systematic studies have yet been done on monoamine oxidase inhibitors or on the newer generation of antidepressants such as trazodone hydrochloride.

As an example of antidepressant use, amitriptyline or imipramine is usually started at

50 to 100 mg per day in two to four divided doses.[120,153] The dosage can be increased by 25 mg each time every day or two, as tolerated, to a maximum FDA recommended dosage of 5 mg per kg per day. Likely side effects include dry mouth, constipation, blurred vision, and postural hypotension. Patients and parents should know about such side effects in advance and can be assured that such symptoms typically become less bothersome over time. If side effects become severe, a slight, temporary reduction in dosage often is helpful. The tricyclic antidepressants can have cardiovascular side effects, including first-degree block and T-wave changes.[232] A careful history of any cardiovascular problems is mandatory, and electrocardiogram monitoring is highly recommended for any child on a dosage close to the recommended maximum. As is true for treating adult depression, the antidepressants typically take two to four weeks at adequate doses to work. No criteria have yet been established for children with respect to how long those who respond to the medication should remain on it.

Considering its widespread use in adults, lithium is a remarkably minor drug in child psychiatry.[158] This may be due, in part, to the complexities for the physician of monitoring the drug. Whatever the cause, few clinical trials of lithium for childhood disorders are available.[31,32,236] In reviewing the scant available evidence, Youngerman and Canino concluded that individuals who present with symptoms resembling adult bipolar affective disorder are apt to respond to lithium, whatever their age, and that in cases where the parents have bipolar affective disorder and the child has some sort of mood disturbance, lithium may be useful.

No specific guidelines for when to start a child or adolescent on lithium have been formulated. Ultimately, the decision has to rest with the treating physician, patient, and family, based on the severity of symptoms and likelihood of impending harm. Before starting lithium, the physician should order screening tests for thyroid and kidney func-

tion because of potential side effects.[103] Many young people seem to tolerate and to require higher doses of lithium than do adults, to blood levels of 0.8 to 1.4 mEq per liter, possibly as a result of more efficient renal clearance.[192] Again, there presently are no guidelines about how long a patient should stay on lithium if it is effective. Few patients want to hear that they may be on the drug for life, but this possibility does need to be broached when appropriate.

¶ Conclusion

Child psychiatry is emerging into an exciting and demanding time with respect to biological and pharmacological aspects of mental disorders. For the past several decades, progress has been relatively slow, as issues over diagnostic approaches were debated and as investigators of adult mental disorders accumulated the analytic tools needed to probe biological function. Although substantial amounts of work on both these fronts remain to be done, the innovative and well-done new studies cited throughout this chapter give hope that the pace of research progress is quickening.

Those interested in studying biological aspects of mental disorders in children and adolescents have been hampered severely by the lack of techniques that were sufficiently safe to be used in this population. The work on automated studies of sleep EEG architecture[54] is but one example of promising new techniques on the horizon. Computerized topographic mapping techniques for EEG and evoked-potential research should provide a valuable tool for assessing electrophysiological parameters of childhood mental disorders.[68,142] CT scans are now used to analyze brain structure in astonishing detail[220]; yet developments in nuclear magnetic resonance (NMR) imaging already promise to far outperform x-rays, especially for brain imaging.[74] (See chapter 11.) More distant but even more exciting for child psychiatry is the use of NMR as a spectrometer, which eventually should enable investigators to assay important brain substances *in vivo* in intact, living human beings.[70,164] (See chapter 11.)

Over the past several decades, the general perception of the relative importance of biological factors in severe childhood mental disorders has increased substantially, especially for the affective disorders and infantile autism. This chapter has focused on some of the products of the continuing efforts to learn more about the developing nervous system and what can go wrong with it. It seems reasonable to hope that new, more effective treatments may emerge from such knowledge. However, such directions of research are best pursued with the clear recognition that the mental disorders of childhood and adolescence reflect a closely interwoven pattern of biological predisposition, developmental stage, and psychosocial influences.

¶ Bibliography

1. AHSANUDDIN, K. M., et al. "Psychotropic Medication Prescription Patterns in 100 Hospitalized Children and Adolescents," *Journal of the American Academy of Child Psychiatry*, 22 (1983):361–364.
2. AMERICAN PSYCHIATRIC ASSOCIATION. *Diagnostic and Statistical Manual of Mental Disorders, vol 2*. Washington, D.C.: American Psychiatric Association, 1965.
3. ———. *Diagnostic and Statistical Manual of Mental Disorders, vol. 3*. Washington, D.C.: American Psychiatric Association, 1980.
4. ———. *Economic Fact Book for Psychiatry*. Washington, D.C.: American Psychiatric Press, 1983.
5. ANDERS, T. F., and CIARANELLO, R. D. "Pharmacological Treatment of the Minimal Brain Dysfunction Syndrome," in J. D. Barchas et al., eds., *Psychopharmacology: From Theory to Practice*. New York: Oxford University Press, 1977, pp. 425–435.
6. ———. "Psychopharmacology of Childhood Disorders," in J. D. Barchas et al., eds., *Psychopharmacology: From The-*

7. ory to Practice. New York: Oxford University Press, 1977, pp. 407–424.
7. ANDERSON, G. M., et al. "Developmental and Pharmacological Aspects of Attention Deficit Disorder (ADD)," *Progress in Clinical and Biological Research*, 135 (1983):207–223.
8. ANTHONY, J., and SCOTT, P. "Manic Depressive Psychosis in Childhood," *Journal of Child Psychology and Psychiatry*, 1 (1960):52–72.
9. BAKWIN, H. "The Genetics of Enuresis," in I. Kolvin, S. MacKeith, and R. Meadow, eds., *Bladder Control and Enuresis*. London: Lavenhan Press, 1973, pp. 73–77.
10. BENDER, L. "Alpha and Omega of Childhood Schizophrenia," *Journal of Autism and Childhood Schizophrenia*, 1 (1971):115–118.
11. ———. "Schizophrenic Spectrum Disorders in the Families of Schizophrenic Children," in R. R. Fieve, D. Rosenthal, and H. Brill, eds., *Genetic Research in Psychiatry*. Baltimore: Johns Hopkins University Press, 1975, pp. 125–134.
12. BENDER, L., and FREEDMAN, A. M. "A Study of the First Three Years in the Maturation of Schizophrenic Children," *Quarterly Journal of Child Behavior*, 4 (1952):245–272.
13. BERGER, P. A. "Antidepressant Medications and the Treatment of Depression," in J. D. Barchas, et al., eds., *Psychopharmacology: From Theory to Practice*. New York: Oxford University Press, 1977, pp. 174–207.
14. BERGER, P. A., and BARCHAS, J. D. "Biochemical Hypotheses of Affective Disorders," in J. D. Barchas, et al., eds., *Psychopharmacology: From Theory to Practice*. New York: Oxford University Press, 1977, pp. 151–173.
15. BERGSTROM, K., and BILLE, B. "Computed Tomography of the Brain in Children with Minimal Brain Damage: A Preliminary Study of 46 Children," *Neuropediatrie*, 9 (1978):378–384.
16. BETTLEHEIM, B. *The Empty Fortress—Infantile Autism and the Birth of the Self*. New York: Free Press, 1967.
17. BIRLESON, P. "The Validity of Depressive Disorder in Childhood and the Development of a Self-Rating Scale: A

Research Report," *Journal of Child Psychology and Psychiatry*, 22 (1981): 73–88.

18. BJERRE, I. "Neurological Investigation of Five-Year-Old Children with Low Birth Weight," *Acta Paediatrica Scandinavica*, 64 (1975):859–864.

19. BOARD ON MENTAL HEALTH AND BEHAVIORAL MEDICINE, INSTITUTE OF MEDICINE. *Research on Mental Illness and Addictive Disorders: Progress and Prospects.* Publication Number IOM-84-07. Washington, D.C.: Institute of Medicine, 1984. (Also appears as supplement to *American Journal of Psychiatry*, 142 (1985).

20. BORISON, R. L., et al. "New Pharmacological Approaches in the Treatment of Tourette Syndrome," *Advances in Neurology*, 35 (1982):377–382.

21. BRADLEY, C. "The Behavior of Children Receiving Benzadrine," *American Journal of Psychiatry*, 94 (1973):577–585.

22. BROUGHTON, R. J. "Sleep Disorders: Disorders of Arousal?" *Science*, 159 (1968): 1070–1078.

23. BROWN, R. P., INGBER, P. S., and TROSS, S. "Pemoline and Lithium in a Patient with Attention Deficit Disorder," *Journal of Clinical Psychiatry*, 44 (1983): 146–148.

24. BRUUN, R. D. "Gilles de la Tourette's Syndrome. An Overview of Clinical Experience," *Journal of the American Academy of Child Psychiatry*, 23 (1984):126–133.

25. BRUUN, R. D., et al. "A Follow-Up of 78 Patients with Gilles de la Tourette's Syndrome," *American Journal of Psychiatry*, 133 (1976):944–947.

26. BUSBY, K., FIRESTONE, P., and PIVIK, T. "Sleep Patterns in Hyperkinetic and Normal Children," *Sleep*, 4 (1981):366–383.

27. BUTLER, I. J., et al. "Neurotransmitters in Neurological Disorders of Childhood," in E. Usdin, I. J. Kopin, and J. Barchas, eds., *Catecholamines: Basic and Clinical Frontiers, vol. 2.* New York: Pergamon Press, 1979, pp. 1578–1580.

28. CAIN, A. C. "Special 'Isolated' Abilities in Severely Psychotic Young Children," *Psychiatry*, 32 (1969):137–149.

29. CAMPBELL, M. "Pharmacotherapy in Early Infantile Autism," *Biological Psychiatry*, 10 (1975):339–423.

30. CAMPBELL, M., COHEN, I. L., and SMALL, A. M. "Drugs in Aggressive Behavior," *Journal of the American Academy of Child Psychiatry*, 21 (1982):107–117.

31. CAMPBELL, M., PERRY, R., and GREEN, W. H. "Use of Lithium in Children and Adolescents," *Psychosomatics*, 25 (1984):95–105.

32. CAMPBELL, M., SCHULMAN, D., and RAPAPORT, J. "The Current Status of Lithium Therapy in Child and Adolescent Psychiatry," *Journal of the American Academy of Child Psychiatry*, 17 (1978):717–729.

33. CAMPBELL, M., et al. "A Controlled Crossover Study of Hyperactive Severely Disturbed Young Children," *Journal of Autism and Child Schizophrenia*, 2 (1972):234–263.

34. CANTWELL, D. P. "Psychiatric Illness in the Families of Hyperactive Children," *Archives of General Psychiatry*, 27 (1972):414–417.

35. ———. "Genetics of Hyperactivity," *Journal of Child Psychology and Psychiatry*, 16 (1975):261–264.

36. ———. "Hyperactivity and Antisocial Behavior Revisited: A Critical Review of the Literature," in D. O. Lewis, ed., *Vulnerabilities to Delinquency.* New York: Spectrum Publications, 1981, pp. 21–38.

37. ———. "Depression in Childhood," in D. P. Cantwell and G. A. Carlson, eds., *Affective Disorders in Childhood and Adolescence. An Update.* New York: SP Medical and Scientific Books, 1983, pp. 3–18.

38. CANTWELL, D. P., ed. *The Hyperactive Child: Diagnosis, Management, Current Research.* New York: Spectrum Publications, 1975.

39. CANTWELL, D. P., and CARLSON, G. A. "Stimulants," in J. S. Werry, ed., *Pediatric Psychopharmacology: The Use of Behavior Modifying Drugs in Children.* New York: Brunner/Mazel, 1978, pp. 171–207.

40. ———. "Unmasking Masked Depression," *American Journal of Psychiatry*, 137 (1980):445–449.

41. ———. "Issues in Classification," in D. P.

Cantwell and G. A. Carlson, eds., *Affective Disorders in Childhood and Adolescence. An Update.* New York: SP Medical and Scientific Books, 1983, pp. 19–38.

42. ———., eds. *Affective Disorders in Childhood and Adolescence. An Update.* New York: SP Medical and Scientific Books, 1983.

43. CAPARULO, B., et al. "Computed Tomographic Brain Scanning in Children with Developmental Neuropsychiatric Disorders," *Journal of the American Academy of Child Psychiatry,* 20 (1981): 338–357.

44. CARLSON, G. A. "Bipolar Affective Disorders in Childhood and Adolescence," in D. P. Cantwell and G. A. Carlson, eds., *Affective Disorders in Childhood and Adolescence. An Update.* New York: SP Medical and Scientific Books, 1983, pp. 61–83.

45. ———. "Depression and Suicidal Behavior in Children and Adolescents," in D. P. Cantwell and G. A. Carlson, eds., *Affective Disorders in Childhood and Adolescence. An Update.* New York: SP Medical and Scientific Books, 1983, pp. 335–352.

46. CARLSON, G. A., and CANTWELL, D. P. "Suicidal Behavior and Depression in Children and Adolescents," *Journal of the American Academy of Child Psychiatry,* 21 (1982):361–368.

47. CARLSON, G. A., and STROBER, M. "Affective Disorder in Adolescence: Issues in Misdiagnosis," *Journal of Clinical Psychiatry,* 39 (1978):63–66.

48. ———. "Manic Depressive Illness in Early Adolescence: A Study of Clinical and Diagnostic Characteristics in Six Cases," *Journal of the American Academy of Child Psychiatry,* 17 (1978):138–153.

49. CARROLL, B. J. "Use of the Dexamethasone Suppression Test in Depression," *Journal of Clinical Psychiatry,* 43 (1982):44–48.

50. CHALLAS, G., and BRAUER, W. "Tourette's Disease: Relief of Symptoms with R1625," *American Journal of Psychiatry,* 120 (1963):283–284.

51. CHATOOR, I., et al. "The Effects of Nocturnally Administered Stimulant Medication on EEG Sleep and Behavior in Hy-

peractive Children," *Journal of the American Academy of Child Psychiatry,* 22 (1983):337–342.

52. CIARANELLO, R. D. "Hyperserotonemia and Early Infantile Autism. Editorial," *New England Journal of Medicine,* 307 (1982):181–183.

53. CIARANELLO, R. D., and ANDERS, T. F. "Drug Treatment of Childhood Psychotic Disorders," in J. D. Barchas et al., eds., *Psychopharmacology: From Theory to Practice.* New York: Oxford University Press, 1977, pp. 436–447.

54. COBLE, P. A., et al. "EEG Sleep 'Abnormalities' in Preadolescent Boys with a Diagnosis of Conduct Disorder," *Journal of the American Academy of Child Psychiatry,* 23 (1984):438–447.

55. COHEN, D. J., et al. "Clonidine Ameliorates Gilles de la Tourette Syndrome," *Archives of General Psychiatry,* 37 (1979):1350–1357.

56. COHEN, M. W. "Enuresis," *Pediatric Clinics of North America,* 22 (1975):545–560.

57. COHEN-SANDLER, R., BERMAN, A. L., and KING, R. A. "Life Stress and Symptomatology: Determinants of Suicidal Behavior in Children," *Journal of the American Academy of Child Psychiatry,* 21 (1982):178–186.

58. CONNELL, H. M. "Depression in Childhood," *Child Psychiatry and Human Development,* 4 (1973):71–85.

59. CONNERS, C. K., and WERRY, J. S. "Pharmacotherapy," in H. C. Quary and J. S. Werry, eds., *Psychopathological Disorders of Childhood,* 2nd ed. New York: John Wiley & Sons, 1979, pp. 336–386.

60. CREAK, M., and PAMPIGLINE, G. "Clinical and EEG Studies on a Group of 35 Psychotic Children," *Developmental Medicine and Child Neurology,* 11 (1969):218–227.

61. CYTRYN, L., and MCKNEW, D. H. "Proposed Classification of Childhood Depression," *American Journal of Psychiatry,* 129 (1972):149–155.

62. ———. "Factors Influencing the Changing Clinical Expression of the Depressive Process in Children," *American Journal of Psychiatry,* 131 (1974):879–881.

63. CYTRYN, L., MCKNEW, D. H., and BUNNEY, W. E., JR. "Diagnosis of Depres-

sion in Children: A Reassessment," *American Journal of Psychiatry*, 137 (1980):22–25.

64. CYTRYN, L., et al. "Offspring of Patients with Affective Disorders: II," *Journal of the American Academy of Child Psychiatry*, 21 (1982):389–391.

65. DEJONG, C. R. "Lithium Carbonate Treatment of Select Behavior Disorder in Children Suggesting Manic-Depressive Illness," *Journal of Pediatrics*, 93 (1978):389–394.

66. DESMOND, M. M., et al. "Congenital Rubella Encephalitis," *American Journal of Diseases of Children*, 118 (1969):30–31.

67. DICKINSON, L. C., LEE, J., and RINGDAHL, I. L. "Impaired Growth in Hyperkinetic Children Receiving Pemoline," *Journal of Pediatrics*, 94 (1979):538–541.

68. DUFFY, F. H. "Topographic Display of Evoked Potentials: Clinical Applications of Brain Electrical Activity Mapping (BEAM)," *Annals of the New York Academy of Sciences*, 388 (1982):183–196.

69. EISENBERG, L., and KANNER, L. "Early Infantile Autism, 1943–1955," *American Journal of Orthopsychiatry*, 26 (1956): 556–566.

70. ELLIOTT, G. R. "Applications of Magnetic Resonance (MR) for Studying Structural and Metabolic Aspects of Brain in Living Human Beings," in J. D. Barchas, and W. E. Bunney, eds., *Perspectives in Neuropsychopharmacology*. New York: Alan R. Liss, forthcoming.

71. FAULL, K. F., et al. "Clinical Application of the Probenecid Test for Measurement of Monoamine Turnover in the CNS," *Biological Psychiatry*, 16 (1981): 879–899.

72. FEINSTEIN, S. C., and WOLPERT, E. "Juvenile Manic Depressive Illness: Clinical and Therapeutic Considerations," *Journal of the American Academy of Child Psychiatry*, 12 (1973):123–135.

73. FOG, R., and PAKKENBERG, H. "Theoretical and Clinical Aspects of the Tourette Syndrome (Chronic Multiple Tics)," *Journal of Neural Transmission*, 6 (Supplement) (1980):211–215.

74. FOSTER, M. A. *Magnetic Resonance in Medicine and Biology*. Oxford: Pergamon Press, 1984.

75. FRITZ, G. K., and ANDERS, T. F. "Enuresis: the Clinical Application of an Etiologically Based Classification System," *Child Psychiatry and Human Development*, 10 (1979):103–113.

76. FRITZ, G. K., and ARMBRUST, J. "Enuresis and Encopresis," *Psychiatric Clinics of North America*, 5 (1982):283–296.

77. GARFINKEL, B. D., et al. "Tricyclic Antidepressant and Methylphenidate Treatment of Attention Deficit Disorder in Children," *Journal of the American Academy of Child Psychiatry*, 22 (1983):343–348.

78. GELLER, E., et al. "Preliminary Observations on the Effect of Fenfluramine on Blood Serotonin and Symptoms in Three Autistic Boys," *New England Journal of Medicine*, 307 (1982):165–169.

79. GILLBERG, C., SVENNERHOLM, L., and HAMILTON-HELLBERG, C. "Childhood Psychosis and Monoamine Metabolites in Spinal Fluid," *Journal of Autism and Developmental Disorders*, 13 (1983): 383–396.

80. GILLES DE LA TOURETTE, G. "Etude sur une Affection Nerveuse, Characterisée par de l'Incoordination Motrice Accompagnée d'Echolalie et de Coprolalie," *Archives of Neurology*, 9 (1885):158–200.

81. GLASER, K. "Masked Depression in Children and Adolescents," *American Journal of Psychotherapy*, 21 (1967):565–574.

82. GOLDBERG, I. D., et al. "Mental Health Problems Among Children Seen in Pediatric Practice: Prevalence and Management," *Pediatrics*, 73 (1984):278–293.

83. GOLDFARB, W. "Self-awareness in Schizophrenic Children," *Archives of General Psychiatry*, 8 (1963):45–60.

84. GOLDSTEIN, M., et al. "Dopamine-beta-Hydroxylase and Endogenous Total 5-Hydroxyindole Levels in Autistic Patients and Controls," in M. Coleman, ed., *The Autistic Syndromes*. New York: American Elsevier, 1976.

85. GOULD, M. S., WUNSCH-HITZIG, R., and DOHRENWEND, B. "Estimating the Prevalence of Childhood Psychopathology: A Critical Review," *Journal of the American Academy of Child Psychiatry*, 20 (1981):462–476.

86. GRAM, L., and RAFAELSEN, O. J. "Lithium Treatment of Psychotic Children," in A. L. Annell, ed., *Depressive States in Childhood and Adolescence*. Stockholm: Almquist and Wiksell, 1972, pp. 286–290.

87. GREEN, W. H., et al. "A Comparison of Schizophrenic and Autistic Children," *Journal of the American Academy of Child Psychiatry*, 23 (1984):399–409.

88. GREENHILL, L. L. "Stimulant-Related Growth Inhibition in Children: A Review," in M. Gittelman, ed., *Strategic Interventions for Hyperactive Children*. Armonk, N.Y.: M. E. Sharpe, 1981, pp. 39–63.

89. GREENHILL, L. L., et al. "Growth Hormone, Prolactin, and Growth Responses in Hyperkinetic Males Treated With d-Amphetamine," *Journal of the American Academy of Child Psychiatry*, 20 (1981):71–84.

90. GREENHILL, L. L., et al. "Sleep Architecture and REM Sleep Measures in Prepubertal Children with Attention Deficit Disorder with Hyperactivity," *Sleep*, 6 (1983):91–101.

91. GREGOIRE, F., et al. "Hormone Release in Depressed Patients Before and After Recovery," *Psychoneuroendocrinology*, 32 (1977):303–312.

92. GROSS, M. D. "Growth of Hyperkinetic Children Taking Ritalin, Dexedrine, or Imipramine/Desipramine," *Pediatrics*, 58 (1976):423–431.

93. GROUP FOR THE ADVANCEMENT OF PSYCHIATRY. *Psychopathological Disorders in Childhood: Theoretical Considerations and a Proposed Classification*. New York: Group for the Advancement of Psychiatry, 1966.

94. GUALTIERI, C. T., HICKS, R. E., and MAYO, J. P. "Hyperactivity and Homeostasis—Editorial," *Journal of the American Academy of Child Psychiatry*, 22 (1983):382–384.

95. HANSON, D. R., and GOTESMAN, I. I. "The Genetics of Childhood Psychoses, in L. Wing, and J. K. Wing, eds., *Handbook of Psychiatry*, vol. 3. Cambridge: Cambridge University Press, 1983, pp. 222–232.

96. HASSANYEH, F., and DAVISON, K. "Bipolar Affective Psychosis with Onset Before Age 16: Report of Ten Cases," *British Journal of Psychiatry*, 137 (1980):530–539.

97. HECHTMAN, L., et al. "Hyperactivities as Young Adults: Initial Predictors of Adult Outcome," *Journal of the American Academy of Child Psychiatry*, 23 (1984):250–260.

98. HEFFRON, W. A., MARTIN, C. A., and WELSH, R. J. "Attention Deficit Disorder in Three Pairs of Monozygotic Twins: A Case Report," *Journal of the American Academy of Child Psychiatry*, 23 (1984):299–301.

99. HENDREN, R. L. "Depression in Anorexia Nervosa," *Journal of the American Academy of Child Psychiatry*, 22 (1983):59–62.

100. HOFFMANN, H. *Der Struwwelpeter: Oder Lustige Geschichtern und Drollige Bilder*. Leipsiz: Insel Verlag, 1845.

101. HSU, L.K.G., et al. "The Dexamethasone Suppression Test in Adolescent Depression," *Journal of the American Academy of Child Psychiatry*, 22 (1983):470–473.

102. HUTT, C., et al. "A Behavioral and Electroencephalographic Study of Autistic Children," *Journal of Psychiatric Research*, 3 (1965):181–197.

103. JEFFERSON, J. W., and GREIST, J. H. *Primer of Lithium Therapy*. Baltimore: Williams & Wilkins, 1977.

104. KAHN, A. U. "Sleep REM Latency in Hyperkinetic Boys," *American Journal of Psychiatry*, 139 (1982):1358–1369.

105. KALES, A., and KALES, J. "Sleep Disorders; Recent Findings in the Diagnosis and Treatment of Disturbed Sleep," *New England Journal of Medicine*, 200 (1974):487–499.

106. KANE, J., et al. "EEG Sleep in a Child With Severe Depression," *American Journal of Psychiatry*, 134 (1977):813–814.

107. KANNER, L. "Autistic Disturbances of Affective Contact," *Nervous Child*, 2 (1943):217–250.

108. ———. "Early Infantile Autism," *Journal of Pediatrics*, 25 (1944):211–217.

109. KAPLAN, S. L., HONG, G. K., and WEINHOLD, C. "Epidemiology of Depressive Symptomatology in Adolescents," *Journal of the American Academy of Child Psychiatry*, 23 (1984):91–98.

110. KASHANI, J. H., SHEKIM, W. O., and REID, J. C. "Amitriptyline in Children with Major Depressive Disorder: A Double-Blind Crossover Pilot Study," *Journal of the American Academy of Child Psychiatry*, 23 (1984):348–351.

111. KASHANI, J. H., et al. "Current Perspectives on Childhood Depression: An Overview," *American Journal of Psychiatry*, 138 (1981):143–153.

112. KING, C., and YOUNG, R. D. "Attentional Deficits With and Without Hyperactivity: Teacher and Peer Perceptions," *Journal of Abnormal Child Psychology*, 10 (1982):483–495.

113. KLEE, S. H., and GARFINKEL, B. D. "Identification of Depression in Children and Adolescents: The Role of the Dexamethasone Suppression Test," *Journal of the American Academy of Child Psychiatry*, 23 (1984):410–415.

114. KLEIN, D. F., et al. *Diagnosis and Drug Treatment of Psychiatric Disorders: Adults and Children.* Baltimore: Williams & Wilkins, 1980.

115. KNOBEL, M. "Psychopharmacology for the Hyperkinetic Child—Dynamic Considerations," *Archives of General Psychiatry*, 6 (1962):198–202.

116. KOLVIN, I., et al. "Six Studies in the Childhood Psychoses," *British Journal of Psychiatry*, 118 (1971):381–419.

117. KOOTZ, J. P., MARINELLI, B., and COHEN, D. J. "Modulation of Response to Environmental Stimuli in Autistic Children," *Journal of Autism and Developmental Disorders*, 12 (1982):185–193.

118. KOVACS, M. "Rating Scales to Assess Depression in School-Aged Children," *Acta Paedopsychiatrica*, 46 (1981):305–315.

119. KOVACS, M., et al. "Depressive Disorders in Childhood. I. A Longitudinal Prospective Study of Characteristics and Recovery," *Archives of General Psychiatry*, 41 (1984):229–237.

120. KRAMER, A. D., and FEIGUINE, R. J. "Clinical Effects of Amitriptyline in Adolescent Depression," *Journal of the American Academy of Child Psychiatry*, 20 (1981):636–644.

121. KUHNLEY, E. J., HENDREN, R. L., and QUINLAN, D. M. "Fire-setting in Children," *Journal of the American Academy of Child Psychiatry*, 21 (1982):560–563.

122. KUPFER, D. "REM Latency: A Psychobiological Marker for Primary Depressive Disease," *Biological Psychiatry*, 11 (1976):159–174.

123. KUPFER, D., et al. "Imipramine and EEG Sleep in Children with Depressive Symptoms," *Psychopharmacology*, 60 (1979):117–123.

124. LAHEY, B. B., et al. "Are Attention Deficit Disorders With and Without Hyperactivity Similar or Dissimilar Disorders?" *Journal of the American Academy of Child Psychiatry*, 23 (1984):302–309.

125. LAUFER, M., and DENHOOF, E. "Hyperkinetic Behavior Syndrome in Children," *Journal of Pediatrics*, 50 (1957):463–474.

126. LECKMAN, J. F. "The Dexamethasone Suppression Test—Editorial," *Journal of the American Academy of Child Psychiatry*, 22 (1983):477–479.

127. LECKMAN, J. F., et al. "Acute and Chronic Clonidine Treatment in Tourette's Syndrome: A Preliminary Report on Clinical Response and Effect on Plasma and Urinary Catecholamine Metabolites, Growth Hormone, and Blood Pressure," *Journal of the American Academy of Child Psychiatry*, 22 (1983):433–440.

128. LECKMAN, J. F., et al. "Growth Hormone Response to Clonidine in Children Ages 4–17: Tourette's Syndrome vs. Children with Short Stature," *Journal of the American Academy of Child Psychiatry*, 23 (1984):174–181.

129. LEFKOWITZ, M. M., and BURTON, N. "Childhood Depression: A Critique of the Concept," *Psychological Bulletin*, 85 (1978):716–726.

130. LONEY, J., KRAMER, J., and MILICH, R. "The Hyperactive Child Grows Up: Predictors of Symptoms, Delinquency, and Achievement at Follow-Up," in K. Gadow, and J. Loney, eds., *Psychosocial Aspects of Drug Treatment for Hyperactivity* (AAAS Selected Symposium Serial Number 44). Boulder, Co.: Westview Press, 1981, pp. 381–415.

131. LOPEZ, R. C. "Hyperactivity in Twins," *Canadian Psychiatric Association Journal*, 10 (1965):421–426.

132. LOTTER, V. "Epidemiology of Autistic Conditions in Young Children. I. Prevalence," *Social Psychiatry*, 1 (1966):124–137.

133. LOWE, T. L., and COHEN, D. J. "Biological Research on Depression in Childhood," in D. P. Cantwell and G. A. Carlson, eds., *Affective Disorders in Childhood and Adolescence. An Update.* New York: SP Medical and Scientific Books, 1983, pp. 229–248.

134. LUCAS, A. R., LOCKETT, H. J., and GRIMM, F. "Amitriptyline in Childhood Depression," *Diseases of the Nervous System*, 26 (1965):105–110.

135. MCNUTT, B. A., BALLARD, J. E., and BOILEAU, R. "The Effects of Long-Term Stimulant Medication on the Growth and Body Composition of Hyperactive Children; II. Report on Two Years," *Psychopharmacology Bulletin*, 13 (1977):36–38.

136. MALMQUIST, C. P. "Depressions in Childhood and Adolescence: I," *New England Journal of Medicine*, 284 (1971):887–893.

137. ———. "Depressions in Childhood and Adolescence: II," *New England Journal of Medicine*, 284 (1971):955–961.

138. MATTES, J., and GITTELMAN, R. "Growth of Hyperactive Children on Maintenance Methylphenidate," *Archives of General Psychiatry*, 40 (1983):317–321.

139. MAURER, R. G., and DAMASIO, A. R. "Childhood Autism from the Point of View of Behavioral Neurology," *Journal of Autism and Developmental Disorders*, 12 (1982):195–205.

140. MIKKELSEN, E. J., et al. "Childhood Enuresis. I. Sleep Patterns and Psychopathology," *Archives of General Psychiatry*, 37 (1980):1139–1144.

141. MIKKELSEN, E. J., et al. "Neurologic Status in Hyperactive, Enuretic, Encopretic, and Normal Boys," *Journal of the American Academy of Child Psychiatry*, 21 (1982):75–81.

142. MORIHISA, J. M. *Brain Imaging in Psychiatry*. Washington, D.C.: American Psychiatric Press, forthcoming.

143. MORRISON, J. R., and STEWARD, M. A. "The Psychiatric Status of the Legal Families of Adopted Hyperactive Children," *Archives of General Psychiatry*, 28 (1973):888–891.

144. NEE, L. E., et al. "Gilles de la Tourette Syndrome: Clinical and Family Study in 50 Cases," *Annals of Neurology*, 7 (1980):41–49.

145. OETTINGER, L., GANCH, R. R., and MAJORSKY, L. V. "Maturity and Growth in Children with MBD," *Learning Disabilities and Related Disorders*, 16 (1977):141–149.

146. ORNITZ, E. M. "Disorders of Perception Common to Early Infantile Autism and Schizophrenia," *Comprehensive Psychiatry*, 10 (1969):259–274.

147. ———. "Childhood Autism: A Review of Clinical and Experimental Literature," *California Medicine*, 118 (1973):21–47.

148. ORNITZ, E. M., and RITVO, E. R. "The Syndrome of Autism: A Critical Review," *American Journal of Psychiatry*, 133 (1976):609–621.

149. PAULS, D. L., et al. "Familial Pattern and Transmission of Gilles de la Tourette Syndrome and Multiple Tics," *Archives of General Psychiatry*, 38 (1981):1091–1093.

150. PAULSON, M. J., STONE, D., and SPOSTO, R. "Suicide Potential and Behavior in Children Ages 4 to 12," *Suicide and Life Threatening Behavior*, 8 (1978):225–269.

151. PERRIS, C. "A Study of Bipolar (Manic-depressive) and Unipolar Recurrent Depressive Psychoses," *Acta Psychiatrica Scandinavica*, 194 (Supplement) (1966):9–189.

152. PETERSEN, I., ANDERSON, O., and HANSEN, T. "Mode of Action of Imipramine and Relative Value of Similar Drugs in the Treatment of Nocturnal Enuresis," *European Journal of Clinical Pharmacology*, 7 (1974):187–194.

153. PETTI, T. A. "Imipramine in the Treatment of Depressed Children," in D. P. Cantwell and G. A. Carlson, eds., *Affective Disorders in Childhood and Adolescence. An Update.* New York: SP Medical and Scientific Books, 1983, pp. 375–415.

154. PETTI, T. A., and LAW, W., III. "Borderline Psychotic Behavior in Hospitalized Children: Approaches to Assessment and Treatment," *Journal of the Ameri-*

can Academy of Child Psychiatry, 21 (1982):197–202.

155. ——. "Imipramine Treatment of Depressed Children: A Double-Blind Pilot Study," *Journal of Clinical Psychopharmacology,* 2 (1982):107–110.

156. PFEFFER, C. R., et al. "Suicidal Behavior in Latency-Age Children: An Outpatient Population," *Journal of the American Academy of Child Psychiatry,* 19 (1980):703–710.

157. PFEFFER, C. R., et al. "Suicidal Behavior in Normal School Children: A Comparison with Child Psychiatric Inpatients," *Journal of the American Academy of Child Psychiatry,* 23 (1984):416–423.

158. PFEFFERBAUM, B., and OVERALL, J. E. "Decisions About Drug Treatment in Children," *Journal of the American Academy of Child Psychiatry,* 23 (1984):209–214.

159. POZNANSKI, E., and ZRULL, J. P. "Childhood Depression: Clinical Characteristics of Overtly Depressed Children," *Archives of General Psychiatry,* 23 (1970):8–15.

160. POZNANSKI, E., et al. "The Dexamethasone Suppression Test in Prepubertal Depressed Children," *American Journal of Psychiatry,* 139 (1982):321–324.

161. POZNANSKI, E., et al. "Hypomania in a Four-Year-Old," *Journal of the American Academy of Child Psychiatry,* 23 (1984):105–110.

162. POZNANSKI, E., et al. "Preliminary Studies of the Reliability and Validity of the Children's Depression Rating Scale," *Journal of the American Academy of Child Psychiatry,* 23 (1984):191–197.

163. PRANGE, A. J. "Patterns of Pituitary Responses to TRH in Depressed Patients," in W. Fann et al., eds., *Phenomenology and Treatment of Depression.* New York: Spectrum Publications, 1977, pp. 1–16.

164. PRICHARD, J. W. "Cerebral Metabolic Studies In Vivo by 31P NMR," *Proceedings of the National Academy of Sciences, USA,* 80 (1983):2748–2751.

165. PUIG-ANTICH, J. "Major Depression and Conduct Disorder in Prepuberty," *Journal of the American Academy of Child Psychiatry,* 21 (1982):118–128.

166. ——. "Neuroendocrine and Sleep Correlates of Prepubertal Major Depressive Disorder: Current Status of the Evidence," in D. P. Cantwell and G. A. Carlson, eds., *Affective Disorders in Childhood and Adolescence. An Update.* New York: SP Medical & Scientific Books, 1983, pp. 211–227.

167. PUIG-ANTICH, J., CHAMBERS, W. J., and TABRIZI, M. A. "The Clinical Assessment of Current Depressive Episodes in Children and Adolescents: Interviews with Parents and Children," in D. P. Cantwell and G. A. Carlson, eds., *Affective Disorders in Childhood and Adolescence. An Update.* New York: SP Medical & Scientific Books, 1983, pp. 157–179.

168. PUIG-ANTICH, J., et al. "Plasma Level of Imipramine and Desmethylimipramine and Clinical Response in Prepubertal Major Depressive Disorder," *Journal of the American Academy of Child Psychiatry,* 18 (1979):616–627.

169. PUIG-ANTICH, J., et al. "Sleep Architecture and REM Sleep Measures in Prepubertal Major Depressives: Studies During Recovery from the Depressive Episode in a Drug-Free State," *Archives of General Psychiatry,* 40 (1983):187–192.

170. PUIG-ANTICH, J., et al. "Cortisol and Prolactin Responses to Insulin-Induced Hypoglycemia in Prepubertal Major Depressives During Episode and After Recovery," *Journal of the American Academy of Child Psychiatry,* 23 (1984):49–57.

171. RAPOPORT, J. L. and ISMOND, D. R. "Biological Research in Child Psychiatry," *Journal of the American Academy of Child Psychiatry,* 21 (1982):543–548.

172. RAPOPORT, J. L., et al. "Imipramine and Methylphenidate Treatments of Hyperactive Boys," *Archives of General Psychiatry,* 30 (1974):789–793.

173. RAPOPORT, J. L., et al., "Dextroamphetamine: Cognitive and Behavioral Effects in Normal Prepubertal Boys," *Science,* 199 (1978):560–563.

174. RAPOPORT, J. L., et al. "Childhood Enuresis: II. Psychopathology, Tricyclic Concentration in Plasma, and Antienuretic Effect," *Archives of General Psychiatry,* 37 (1980):1146–1152.

175. REGIER, D. A., et al. "The NIMH Epidemiologic Catchment Area Program," *Archives of General Psychiatry*, 41 (1984):934–941.

176. RENSHAW, D. C. "Suicide and Depression in Children," *Journal of School Health*, 44 (1974):487–489.

177. RIE, H. E. "Depression in Childhood: A Survey of Some Pertinent Contributions," *Journal of the American Academy of Child Psychiatry*, 5 (1966):653–685.

178. RITVO, E. R., et al. "Correlation of Psychiatric Diagnoses and EEG Findings: A Double-Blind Study of 184 Hospitalized Children," *American Journal of Psychiatry*, 126 (1970):988–996.

179. RITVO, E. R., et al. "Effects of Fenfluramine on 14 Outpatients with the Syndrome of Autism," *Journal of the American Academy of Child Psychiatry*, 22 (1983):549–558.

180. RITVO, E. R., et al. "Study of Fenfluramine in Outpatients with the Syndrome of Autism," *Journal of Pediatrics*, 105 (1984):823–828.

181. ROBBINS, D. R., et al. "The Dexamethasone Suppression Test in Psychiatrically Hospitalized Adolescents," *Journal of the American Academy of Child Psychiatry*, 22 (1983):467–469.

182. ROCHLIN, G. "The Loss Complex," *Journal of the American Psychoanalytic Association*, 7 (1959):229–316.

183. ROSENBLOOM, S., et al. "High Resolution CT Scanning in Infantile Autism: A Quantitative Approach," *Journal of the American Academy of Child Psychiatry*, 23 (1984):72–77.

184. ROSENTHAL, P. A. "Sudden Disappearance of One Parent with Separation and Divorce: The Grief and Treatment of Preschool Children," *Journal of Divorce*, 3 (1979).

185. RUTTER, M. "Childhood Schizophrenia Reconsidered," *Journal of Autism and Child Schizophrenia*, 2 (1972):315–337.

186. RUTTER, M., and BARTAK, L. "Causes of Infantile Autism: Some Considerations from Recent Research," *Journal of Autism and Child Schizophrenia*, 1 (1971):20–32.

187. RUTTER, M., et al. "A Five to Fifteen Year Follow-Up Study of Infantile Psychosis. II. Social and Behavioral Outcome," *British Journal of Psychiatry*, 113 (1967):1183–1200.

188. SATTERFIELD, J. "Neurophysiologic Studies with Hyperactive Children," in D. Cantwell, ed., *The Hyperactive Child: Diagnosis, Management, Current Research*. New York: Spectrum Publications, 1975, pp. 67–82.

189. SCHACHAR, R., RUTTER, M., and SMITH, A. "The Characteristics of Situationally and Pervasively Hyperactive Children: Implications for Syndrome Definition," *Journal of Child Psychology and Psychiatry*, 22 (1981):375–392.

190. SCHAIN, R. J., and FREEDMAN, D. X. "Studies on 5-Hydroxyindole Metabolism in Autistic and Other Mentally Retarded Children," *Journal of Pediatrics*, 58 (1961):315–329.

191. SCHOPLER, E., and MESIBOV, G. B., eds. *Autism in Adolescents and Adults*. New York: Plenum Press, 1983.

192. SCHOU, M. "Lithium in Psychiatric Therapy and Prophylaxis. A Review with Special Regard to Its Use in Children," in A. L. Annell, ed., *Depressive States in Childhood and Adolescence*. Stockholm: Almquist and Wiksell, 1971, pp. 479–487.

193. SHAPIRO, A. K., and SHAPIRO, E. "Clinical Efficacy of Haloperidol, Pimozide, Penfluridol, and Clonidine in the Treatment of Tourette Syndrome," *Advances in Neurology*, 35 (1982):383–386.

194. ———. "An Update on Tourette Syndrome," *American Journal of Psychotherapy*, 36 (1982):379–389.

195. ———. "Controlled Study of Pimozide vs. Placebo in Tourette's Syndrome," *Journal of the American Academy of Child Psychiatry*, 23 (1984):373–384.

196. SHAPIRO, A. K., et al. "Organic Features in Gilles de la Tourette Syndrome," *British Journal of Psychiatry*, 122 (1973):639–644.

197. SHAYWITZ, B. A., COHEN, D. J., and BOWERS, M. B., JR. "CSF Monoamine Metabolites in Children with Minimal Brain Dysfunction: Evidence for Alteration of Brain Dopamine," *Journal of Pediatrics*, 90 (1977):67–71.

198. SHETTY, T., and CHASE, T N. "Central Monoamines and Hyperkinesis of

Childhood," *Neurology*, 26 (1976):1000–1002.

199. SIEGEL, B., et al. "Empirically Derived Subclassification of the Autistic Syndrome," *Journal of Autism*, in press.

200. SIEGEL, B., et al. "A Double-Blind Clinical Trial of Fenfluramine on Children With Autism. I. Behavioral Characteristics and Treatment Response," in preparation.

201. SIMONDS, J. F., and ASTON, L. "Preterm Birth, Low Birth Weight, and Hyperkinetic Behavior in Children," *Southern Medical Journal*, 73 (1980):1237–1238.

202. SIMONDS, J. F., and PARRAGA, H. "Prevalence of Sleep Disorders and Sleep Behaviors in Children and Adolescents," *Journal of the American Academy of Child Psychiatry*, 21 (1982):383–388.

203. SMALL, A., SATOCHI, H., and FEINBERG, I. "Effects of Dextroamphetamine Sulfate on EEG Sleep Patterns of Hyperactive Children," *Archives of General Psychiatry*, 25 (1971):369–380.

204. SOROSKY, A. D., et al. "Systematic Observations of Autistic Behavior," *Archives of General Psychiatry*, 18 (1968):439–449.

205. STAHL, S. M. "Tardive Tourette Syndrome in an Autistic Patient After Long-Term Neuroleptic Administration,"*American Journal of Psychiatry*, 137 (1980):1267–1269.

206. STAHL, S. M., and BERGER, P. A. "Cholinergic and Dopaminergic Mechanisms in Tourette Syndrome," *Advances in Neurology*, 35 (1982):141–150.

207. TANGUAY, P. E. "Toward a New Classification of Serious Psychopathology in Children," *Journal of the American Academy of Child Psychiatry*, 23 (1984):373–384.

208. TANGUAY, P. E., and EDWARDS, R. M. "Electrophysiological Studies of Autism: The Whisper of the Bang," *Journal of Autism and Developmental Disorders*, 12 (1982):117–184.

209. THOMPSON, J., ROSS, R., and HORWITZ, S. "The Role of Computed Axial Tomography in the Study of the Child with Minimal Brain Dysfunction," *Archives of General Psychiatry*, 38 (1981):562–568.

210. TISHER, M. "School Refusal: A Depressive Equivalent?" in D. P. Cantwell and G. A. Carlson, eds., *Affective Disorders in Childhood and Adolescence. An Update*. New York: SP Medical & Scientific Books, 1983, pp. 129–144.

211. TISHER, M., and LANG, M. "The Children's Depression Scale: Review and Further Developments," in D. P. Cantwell and G. A. Carlson, eds., *Affective Disorders in Childhood and Adolescence. An Update*. New York: SP Medical & Scientific Books, 1983, pp. 181–203.

212. TODD, R. D., and CIARANELLO, R. D. "Infantile Autism and the Childhood Psychoses," in *Handbook of Clinical Neurology*, forthcoming.

213. ———. "Demonstration of Inter- and Intraspecies Differences in Serotonin Binding Sites by Antibodies from an Autistic Child," *Proceedings of the National Academy of Sciences, USA*, 82 (1985):612–616.

214. TOOLAN, J. M. "Suicide in Children and Adolescents," *American Journal of Psychotherapy*, 29 (1975):339–344.

215. TREFFERT, D. A. "Epidemiology of Infantile Autism," *Archives of General Psychiatry*, 22 (1970):431–438.

216. TSAI, L., et al. "Unfavorable Left-Right Asymmetries of the Brain and Autism: A Question of Methodology," *British Journal of Psychiatry*, 140 (1982):312–319.

217. VARLEY, C. K. "Diet and the Behavior of Children with Attention Deficit Disorder," *Journal of the American Academy of Child Psychiatry*, 23 (1984):182–185.

218. VOLKMAR, F. R., et al. "EEG Abnormalities in Tourette's Syndrome," *Journal of the American Academy of Child Psychiatry*, 23 (1984):352–353.

219. WEINBERG, W., and BRUMBACK, R. "Mania in Childhood: Case Studies and Literature Review," *American Journal of Diseases of Children*, 130 (1976):380–385.

220. WEINBERGER, D. R., et al. "Computed Tomography in Schizophreniform Disorder and Other Psychiatric Disorders," *Archives of General Psychiatry*, 39 (1982):778–783.

221. WEIZMAN, A., et al. "Combination of Neuroleptic and Stimulant Treatment

in Attention Deficit Disorder with Hyperactivity," *Journal of the American Academy of Child Psychiatry*, 23 (1984):295–298.

222. WENDER, P. *Minimal Brain Dysfunction in Children.* New York: Wiley-Interscience, 1971.

223. WERRY, J. S. "An Overview of Pediatric Psychopharmacology," *Journal of the American Academy of Child Psychiatry*, 21 (1982):3–9.

224. WERRY, J. S., and AMAN, M. G. "Methylphenidate in Hyperactive and Enuretic Children," in L. Greenhill and B. Shopson, eds., *The Psychobiology of Childhood: Profile of Current Issues.* New York: Spectrum Publications, 1984.

225. WERRY, J. S., et al. "Studies on the Hyperactive Child. VII. Neurological States Compared with Neurotic and Normal Children," *American Journal of Orthopsychiatry*, 127 (1972):824–825.

226. WERRY, J. S., et al. "Imipramine in Enuresis," *Journal of Child Psychology and Psychiatry*, 16 (1975):289–299.

227. WILLIAMS, D. T., et al. "The Effect of Propranolol on Uncontrolled Rage Outbursts in Children and Adolescents with Organic Brain Dysfunction," *Journal of the American Academy of Child Psychiatry*, 21 (1982):129–135.

228. WILLIAMS, R. S., et al. "Autism and Mental Retardation: Neuropathologic Studies Performed in Four Retarded Persons with Autistic Behavior," *Archives of Neurology*, 37 (1980):749–753.

229. WING, J. K. "Diagnosis, Epidemiology, Etiology," in J. K. Wing, ed., *Early Childhood Autism.* London: Pergamon Press, 1966, pp. 3–49.

230. WINOKUR, A., MARCH, V., and MENDELS, J. "Primary Affective Disorder in Relatives of Patients with Anorexia Nervosa," *American Journal of Psychiatry*, 137 (1980):695–698.

231. WINOKUR, A., CLAYTON, P. J., and REICH, T. *Manic Depressive Illness.* St. Louis: C. V. Mosby, 1969.

232. WINSBERG, B. G., et al. "Imipramine and Electrocardiographic Abnormalities in Hyperactive Children," *American Journal of Psychiatry*, 128 (1972): 1425–1431.

233. WOLFF, S., and CHESS, S. "An Analysis of the Language of Fourteen Schizophrenic Children," *Journal of Child Psychology and Psychiatry*, 6 (1965):29–41.

234. YOUNG, J. G., et al. "Clinical Neurochemistry of Autism and Associated Disorders," *Journal of Autism and Developmental Disorders*, 12 (1982):147–165.

235. YOUNG, W., et al. "The Sleep of Childhood Depressives: Comparison with Age-Matched Controls," *Biological Psychiatry*, 17 (1982):1163–1168.

236. YOUNGERMAN, J., and CANINO, I. "Lithium Carbonate Use in Children and Adolescents: A Survey of the Literature," *Archives of General Psychiatry*, 35 (1978):216–224.

CHAPTER 24

THE BIOLOGY AND SOMATIC EXPERIMENTAL TREATMENT OF AGGRESSIVE DISORDERS

Burr Eichelman

¶ Introduction

Clinicians in the behavioral sciences must deal with aggressive and violent behavior. Within our society, statistics of interpersonal violence remain at alarming levels. Death by homicide is more common than death by bronchitis, emphysema, and asthma combined (10.3 per 100,000 in 1981).[227] Battery is the single major cause of injury to women, more significant than automobile accidents, rape, or mugging.[160] In 1981, 413,000 reports of child abuse were tabulated by the American Humane Association for the United States.[133] Victimization by violence, particularly of women and children as a class, is a phenomenon of epidemic proportion in our society. A clinical response to violence is therefore imperative, just as it has been for suicide and alcoholism.

As with most human behavior, factors that induce, direct, and maintain human violent behavior are many. While this complicates our understanding and prediction[147] of human violence, it also offers the clinician multiple avenues of intervention, including biological intervention, behavioral modification, and social change aimed at reducing social acceptance of violence or access to the means to violence (e.g., firearms), as well as reducing stressors, including poverty and crowding.

This chapter reviews biological elements that may be relevant to the understanding of human personal violence and biological interventions that are available to the clinician. The clinical field is complicated by the fact that while violent behavior is a symptom in many disorders in the *Diagnostic and Statistical Manual of Mental Disorders* (DSM-III), it may also characterize a patient who does not meet any DSM-III mental disorder criteria. Biological interventions to reduce violence in humans have frequently been reported in uncontrolled studies. In general, tightly controlled, double-blind treatment studies are the exception in this area.

Given these considerations, some working definitions are necessary. Aggression can be defined as "behavior that leads to, or appears to an observer to lead to the damage or destruction of a goal entity."[154] This restrictive definition of aggression does not include assertive or intrusive behaviors. Clinically, violence can be defined as destructive aggression that inflicts physical damage on persons or property.[45] Both research and treatment of human violent behavior have been hampered by a highly variable and poorly developed nosology. According to DSM-III mental disorder criteria, violent behavior in the adolescent might generate a conduct disorder diagnosis (Conduct Disorder, Undersocialized, Aggressive; or Conduct Disorder, Socialized, Aggressive).[4] In the adult such behavior might be categorized as either an Isolated or Intermittent Explosive Disorder, or such behavior might not be classified as a mental disorder at all. For example, in certain cases of child abuse, the behavior might be categorized as a DSM-III "V Code" of Parent-Child Problem. Violent behavior might also be considered a symptom of other psychiatric disorders including dementia, schizophrenia, alcohol or other drug intoxication, depression, mania, antisocial personality disorder, mental retardation, or attention-deficit disorder.

¶ Theories of Aggressive Behavior

Several theories have attempted to explain human aggressive behavior. These reflect in part the persistent nature-nurture conflicts that permeate psychology. Freud[72] hypothesized a drive state—*thanatos*—that was directed toward death and destruction. The drive theory of aggression was popularized by Konrad Lorenz's book *On Aggression,*[130] in which Lorenz described a drive state in humans that builds up aggressive urges which eventually "spill over" and are released. Intervention in such a theoretical system requires a rechanneling of the release of these urges in less destructive ways.

The frustration-aggression theory proposed by Dollard and associates[50] in the 1930s also conceptualized a type of reservoir of aggressive energy seeking an outlet. According to this theory, the interruption of goal-directed behavior by the external environment increases the probability of aggressive behavior. If the interrupted behavior is highly motivated, the probability of aggression is greater than in low-motivation situations. If the goal-directed behavior is repeatedly blocked, the probability of aggression increases proportionally with the "frustration."

In contrast to the drive theories of aggression are the social learning theories.[11] Within this theoretical system, organisms learn violent behavior through modeling or random activity. Violence is sustained by positive reinforcement contingencies. Moreover, the cognitive paradigms of the learning theory can be utilized to "disinhibit" aggressive behavior by overcoming either innate or early-learned inhibitions toward violence through the use of such techniques as desensitization or dehumanization of the victim.

The biological treatment of human aggressive disorders fits most easily into the conceptualization of aggression as a drive state seeking expression. Interventions can affect the development of the drive; for example, by decreasing "frustration" or the organism's perception of frustration. They can also block the discharge of the drive or render the discharge less impulsive. Upon this biological matrix, learning theory can also be applied. Clinical intervention most often utilizes both approaches.

¶ Biological Elements of Aggressive Behavior

Study of various animal models of aggressive behavior has generated many hypotheses regarding the etiology and maintenance of human violent behavior. In some cases, it has underscored our dearth of human data, pointing the way toward new areas of clinical research that encompass genetics, sensory processing of stimuli to incite aggression, neurophysiological mechanisms, hormonal regulation, neurochemistry, and psychopharmacology.

Mammalian research has been based predominantly on various animal models of aggressive behavior because of the necessity to rapidly assess the effects of drugs and other experimental manipulations. Animal populations have two advantages; they rapidly reproduce and can be sacrificed at the end of experiments to assess central biochemical changes. While expedient for research purposes, these models often appear far removed from the ethologically observed agonistic behavior of free-living mammals. Consequently, findings from studies of such models cannot be projected to either the wild state of the test animal or to other mammalian systems (e.g., humans), albeit such extrapolation may offer the best current hypotheses concerning neural mechanisms of human aggressive behavior.

Many categories of aggressive behavior exist. Moyer[154] classified aggressive behavior as predatory, intermale, fear-induced, irritable, territorial, maternal, and instrumental. These behaviors may be regrouped into two broad categories[174]: predatory and affective aggression. Predatory aggression characteristically leads to destruction of prey, usually for food. The attack involves minimal autonomic arousal and vocalization and no elaborate behavioral displays. Models of predatory aggression include mouse killing by rats,[10] rat killing by cats,[228] and cricket killing by mice.[31]

Affective aggression is displayed as "irritable," "intermale," "territorial," or "maternal" aggression. Threatening stimuli initiate an intense and patterned activation of the autonomic nervous system, coupled with threatening and defensive postures and threatening vocalization. The form of attack in this type of aggression varies with species but is generally characteristic for any given species. It may have both offensive and defensive sterotypic postures.[15] The affective display may often be an end in itself, serving to signal the intent of attack. Most models of affective aggression entail a lowering of the threshold for aggressive behavior, in some way producing an "irritable" animal. Models of affective aggression include sham rage in cats induced by electrical brain stimulation or decortication[173] and shock-induced fighting (SIF)[219] in which rats paired and subjected to inescapable foot-shock attack each other. Isolation-induced fighting[220] has been the most commonly utilized model. Male mice are isolated for approximately one month and then paired, and the ensuing fighting is quantified in terms of latency and quantity. In the intruder model,[159] a strange rat or mouse is placed into an established group of rodents. When the intruder is attacked, behavioral parameters of latency and attack duration can be measured.

Genetics

Animal research literature presents a compelling argument to support a hereditary role in animal disposition or predisposition to engage in aggressive behavior. Mouse[203] and rat[56] strains show marked variations in laboratory paradigms of intermale or pain-induced fighting. In the mouse, selective breeding can generate two lines of mice that differ in intermale aggression.[119] Genetic crosses and back crosses in the mouse have implicated autosomal, X, and Y chromosomal contributions. This work has been well reviewed by Maxson.[141] The role of genetics in the disposition toward aggression is commonly noted in domestic dog strains.[189] The biological mechanisms that produce these behavioral differences are poorly understood. For example, these mechanisms have been linked to catecholamine metabolism,[37] cerebral cyclic nucleotide concentrations,[161] and hormone surges during puberty.[190]

Genetic contributions to human aggressive behavior have been difficult to document, perhaps due to the major role acculturation plays in human behavior. Genetic research has been reviewed by several investigators.[60,143] Abnormal sex chromosomes, particularly the XYY genotype, were proposed to be associated with increased aggressive behavior.[105] Additional studies seem to confirm an increase in socially deviant behavior in people with abnormal sex chromosomal number, but the behavior is not necessarily an increase in aggression.[237]

From a sociological approach, Hutchings and Mednick[97] observed that the rate of criminal behavior among the biological fathers of Danish criminal adoptees was higher than among their adoptive fathers; that is, when the biological fathers were not criminals, the rate of criminal behavior of adoptees was lower than when the biological fathers were criminals. However, the highest rates of criminality occurred when both biological and adoptive fathers were criminals, supporting both genetic and environmental influences. Once again, the distinction between criminal and aggressive behavior must be clarified, since these behaviors are not synonymous.

Processing of Sensory Input

Sensory stimuli are crucial in the modulation of mammalian aggressive behavior. Olfactory bulb ablation abolishes intermale aggression in mice.[179] Removal of the vibrissae from rats severely suppresses shock-induced fighting.[28] Conversely, olfactory bulb ablation in rats increases predatory aggression (mouse killing).[110] Tactile stimulation in cats induces a grasping response that initiates the prey-catching behavior necessary for cats to kill rats. The "trigger zone" on the cat's forepaw can be enlarged by appropriate ipsilateral hypothalamic stimulation.[35] We know

little about whether sensory stimuli are processed differently in aggressive versus nonaggressive individuals.

Personal space, territory, or "body buffer zones"[114] also play a role in mammalian aggression. Wild animal trainers utilize the aversive effect of intrusion into their animals' personal space. Humans vary in their personal space. Although this is in part culturally determined, Kinzel[114] showed that American prisoners convicted of violent crimes had larger "body buffer zones" than those convicted of nonviolent crimes. We do not yet know whether violent individuals find various kinds of sensory input more aversive than do nonviolent people, nor do we know whether behavioral or biological treatment affects the sensory processing of aversive stimuli.

Brain Lesions

Brain pathology has been linked to aggressive behavior in animals and humans. For instance, septal lesions in rats[21] and lesions of the ventromedial nucleus of the hypothalamus in the cat[232] induce irritability. Conversely, lesions of the amygdala can produce a taming effect.[188]

In humans, specific case histories report aggressive behavior in patients with a third ventricle lesion,[3] a ventral medial hypothalamic tumor,[172] a cyst impinging on the septum pellucidum,[124] or a temporal lobe tumor.[210] However, there is not a one-to-one correlation of violence with brain pathology. For instance, in a review of eighteen cases of patients with limbic tumors, Malamud[134] found that in none of these cases was aggressive behavior the primary symptom.

Epilepsy

Electrical disturbances in the brain have been implicated as a cause of episodic human violent behavior.[138] Distinction must be made among aggressive behavior that occurs during a seizure, during the postictal period of confusion, and during relatively seizure-free periods. Rodin[178] recorded psychomotor seizures in 150 patients and observed no aggressive behavior. In contrast, Mark, Sweet, and Ervin[139] reported an association of temporal lobe spiking after limbic electrical stimulation and destruction of property. Extensive recent review of the behavior of patients during complex (temporal lobe) seizures demonstrated only exceedingly rare outbursts of violent behavior during the seizure.[47] However, some clinicians describe personality characteristics of temporal lobe epileptics that they believe lead to increased aggressive behavior.[16]

A number of studies report an increased incidence of violent behavior in patients with seizure disorders or abnormal electroencephalograms (EEGs). For example, Gunn[89] reported an increased incidence of epilepsy in a British prison population compared to national figures. Sixty-five percent of habitually aggressive prisoners in a study by Williams[234] showed abnormal EEGs compared with 12 percent of a normal population. Monroe[150] reported an association between activated EEGs (induced provocatively with alpha chloralose) and histories of episodic aggressive behavior.

Hormones

Aggressive behavior between the sexes shows a marked dichotomy. In most mammalian species, the male is more aggressive. This has prompted a study of the role of hormones in aggressive behavior. Many studies have attempted to measure circulating levels of sex hormones, particularly androgens, and to correlate them with the frequency of violent behavior. Such research has stemmed from animal husbandry observations that castrated farm animals, such as geldings and oxen, are less aggressive and more easy to domesticate. A few clinical studies reported positive correlations between circulating testosterone and aggressive behavior.[52,162] However, larger studies failed to find such a correlation.[116,144,152]

However, hormones can alternatively be regarded as organizers and sensitizers of the brain for future behavioral modulation. In the rat, Conner and associates[40] demonstrated that the presence of testosterone during the perinatal period was necessary to sensitize the brain to testosterone in adult life in a way that enhanced aggressive behavior. Male rat pups were castrated at birth (while the brain was still developing) or at weaning (when brain development was essentially complete). Both castrated male groups fought less than normal males. The group castrated at weaning was testosterone-sensitive and, with exogenous testosterone treatment, developed aggressive behavior comparable to normal male rats. The group castrated at birth was testosterone-insensitive and failed to increase aggressive behavior even when administered exogenous testosterone. Thus hormone levels present during brain development *in utero* may be a more relevant determinant of adult human aggression than absolute values of circulating hormone measurable at maturity. Accordingly, more knowledge concerning sex hormones and human aggression might be gleaned from "natural experiments" of *in utero* exposure to altered levels of sex hormones than from a search for correlations in the adult. Examples of such studies include Money and Ehrhardt's research[149] on the development of children with the adrenogenital syndrome and Yalom, Green, and Fisk's study[239] of male children exposed to increased estrogen and progesterone during pregnancy. Extensive reviews of hormonal studies and aggression have been published by Conner[39] and Brain.[22,23,24]

Neurotransmitters and Animal Aggression

Animal research focusing on the neurochemistry of behavior has demonstrated several principles of aggressive behavior:

1. No single neurotransmitter system appears responsible for the modulation of mammalian aggressive behavior.
2. Mammalian aggression is not a single behavior. There are several classes of aggressive behavior. Modulation of a given neurotransmitter system may decrease the

frequency of one type of aggression and in-crease the frequency of another. For exam-ple, tricyclic antidepressants suppress pred-atory aggression in the rat[96] but enhance SIF.[57]

3. Neurotransmitter systems are linked to neuroanatomic loci and neurophysiological mechanisms. For example, electrolytic le-sions of the septal nuclei in the rat alter biogenic amine concentrations in other re-gions (e.g., decreasing serotonin [5HT] in the hippocampus).[107]

4. External interventions can alter brain chemistry and behavior. While one can readily see this effect with administration of biologically active agents such as drugs, this principle is often overlooked in relation to environmental manipulations. Environ-mental stress can alter brain chemistry and behavior.[121]

ACETYLCHOLINE

Acetylcholine (ACh) apparently functions as a neurotransmitter that facilitates aggres-sive behavior. The cholinomimetic agent carbachol induced aggressive behavior in the cat when injected into the amygdala.[88] Phy-sostigmine injected into the amygdala of rats increased SIF,[177] while SIF was suppressed with cholinergic blockage.[165] Cholinergic stimulation also enhances predatory aggres-sion. Mouse killing in rats can be induced with lateral hypothalamic injections of carba-chol[200] and blocked with centrally applied methylatropine.[200] Cholinergic mechanisms also enhanced predatory behavior in the cat.[13,111]

GABA

The gamma aminobutyric acid (GABA) system in the brain appears to act in an inhib-itory way. GABA levels in the olfactory bulbs of mouse-killing rats are lower than in non-killers.[132] GABA injections into mouse-kill-ing rats transiently inhibited mouse killing.[137] A similar effect is obtained by treating rats with N-dipropylacetate,[137] a competitive in-hibitor of GABA transaminase (effectively raising brain GABA levels). GABAergic mechanisms seemed to decrease isolation-

induced fighting in mice[166] as well as SIF in mice.[167]

SEROTONIN

The 5HT system, like the GABA system, appears to inhibit aggressive behavior. Low-ering brain concentrations of 5HT by re-stricting dietary tryptophan,[79] inhibiting the synthesizing enzyme tryptophan hydroxy-lase,[48] or lesioning the 5HT cell bodies of the raphe nucleus[83] all induce predatory aggres-sion in the rat. Conversely, administration of 5-hydroxytryptophan (5-HTP) can block mouse killing.[118]

Similar changes occur with affective ag-gression. Tryptophan restriction in diet,[109] tryptophan hydroxylase inhibition with para-chlorophenylalanine (PCPA),[65] lesions of the raphe nuclei,[104] or treatment of rats with the 5HT neurotoxin 5,7-dihydroxytryptamine[108] all increase aggressive behavior while lower-ing brain 5HT. Elevated levels of brain 5HT in rats do not necessarily suppress aggressive behavior.[109] Yet in certain situations of brain injury (i.e., septal lesions or neurotoxin treat-ment) where shock-induced aggressive be-havior is increased, dietary tryptophan sup-plementation raises brain 5HT levels toward normal levels and blocks the increase in ag-gression observed in the pathological state.[107] Lithium's antiaggression effect may also operate by enhancement of central sero-tonergic systems.[185]

DOPAMINE

Dopaminergic stimulation appears to en-hance fighting. Levodopa treatment induces aggressive behavior in mice[66] and rats.[120] The dopaminergic agonist apomorphine in-duces "spontaneous fighting" in rats.[191] This behavior is potentiated with either levodopa or apomorphine in rats pretreated with 6-hydroxydopamine, suggesting an en-hanced effect on aggression in rats showing denervation supersensitivity to catechola-mines.[212] Dopamine (DA) infusions into rat cerebroventricles enhance SIF.[76] DA an-tagonists tend to suppress fighting.[93,241]

NOREPINEPHRINE

The experimental literature connecting noradrenergic systems to aggressive behavior implicates an enhancing effect of norepinephrine (NE). For example, there is a positive correlation between the frequency of sham rage attacks in the cat and the disappearance of brain-stem NE.[175] A comparable correlation in NE metabolism and fighting was observed in rat SIF.[207] Rats with supersensitive beta-adrenergic receptors (increased receptor number as indicated by ligand binding) showed increased SIF while supersensitivity lasted.[92] Rats treated with clonidine, which decreases locus coeruleus firing and NE function, showed decreased fighting, while the converse was seen with piperoxane treatment.[196] Drugs that decrease beta-adrenergic receptor number through increased adrenergic activity, such as tricyclic antidepressants or monoamine oxidase inhibitors (MAOIs), increased fighting in rodents.[57] Rubidium treatment increased NE turnover in the rat brain[206] and enhanced fighting and irritability.[61,205] Pedestal stress in the rat increased brain stem tyrosine hydroxylase (TH) activity and induced a down-regulation of cortical beta-adrenergic receptors.[58] This treatment also increased irritability and fighting behavior.[59]

However, in support of an inhibitory role for NE is the observation that the neurotoxin 6-hydroxydopa—which depletes brain NE—enhances SIF.[213] While this has been explained as a result of supersensitivity to remaining endogenous NE, there is also a report that intracerebroventricular injections of NE suppress aggressive behavior.[76]

Catecholaminergic agonists generally inhibit predatory aggression.[112] However, it must be recognized that the examples just presented are merely illustrative. Additional in-depth literature reviews are available.[55,60,146]

Neurotransmitters and Human Aggression

The neurochemistry of human aggression is but an embryonic field of research. However, certain consistencies with the animal literature are sufficient to generate excitement. Brown and associates[27] found a positive correlation between a history of aggressive behavior in a population of military personnel and their cerebrospinal fluid (CSF) levels of 3-methoxy-4-hydroxy-phenylglycol (MHPG), a NE metabolite, suggesting enhanced central NE turnover in the more aggressive individuals. Sandler and others[184] reported increased levels of the monoamine phenylethylamine in aggressive prisoners, raising the possibility of its function as an endogenous amphetaminelike compound.

Several human studies related to aggressive behavior have implicated 5HT; lower 5HT levels or activity have been correlated with increased aggressive behavior. Brown and coworkers[27] observed an inverse relationship between CSF levels of the 5HT metabolite 5-hydroxyindoleacetic acid (5-HIAA) and rating scores of lifelong patterns of aggressive behavior. Linnoila and associates[126] also reported a correlation between low 5-HIAA levels and impulsive aggressive behavior. Yaryura-Tobias and Neziroglu[240] reported lower 5HT levels in the whole blood of aggressive patients compared to nonaggressive patients. Aggressive behavior in hyperactive children has been linked to lowered blood concentrations of 5HT and 5-HIAA.[85]

Differences in body chemistry associated with aggression are not related solely to the central nervous system. Aggressive behavior has been linked to hypoglycemia[224,225] and hypercholesterolemia.[226]

Environmental and Social Influences

The frustration-aggression hypothesis of aggression asserts that an organism does not behave in a vacuum; the environment impinges upon the subject and can alter its behavior. Environmental manipulations clearly induce biological changes in organisms, some of which may be correlated with alterations in aggressive behavior. Animal models serve to illustrate this point.

Male mice isolated for a period of several

weeks develop a number of biological changes. These animals have reduced brain 5HT turnover compared with group-housed mice,[77] as well as central changes in the turnover of catecholamines.[230] Behaviorally, they are more aggressive than group-housed mice.[241]

Chronic immobilization stress in rats induces hypertension, peripheral catecholamine release, and increased activity of the enzyme TH in the hypothalamus—suggestive of increased noradrenergic turnover. Coupled with these changes is an increase in fighting.[121] If the stress is removed for one month, the rats again become normotensive. However, the change in brain TH activity and increased aggression persist for at least a month beyond the removal of the stress. Such a finding raises the possibility that stress in humans, especially during development, might alter brain chemistry for a prolonged period in ways that could render the person more susceptible to aggression. Such a model might apply to child abuse. We do know that abusing parents were often abused themselves as children.

Sleep deprivation can induce rapid biochemical changes in the brain that are associated with increased aggressive behavior. Rats placed on small pedestals surrounded by water cannot experience rapid-eye-movement sleep without losing muscle tone and falling into the surrounding water. By the end of five days, these rats are exceedingly irritable and SIF is markedly increased.[59] Neurochemical indicators of central noradrenergic metabolism are increased. TH activity in the brain stem is enhanced, and the number of cortical beta-adrenergic receptors is reduced.[58] Many forms of mental illness or simple stress responses in the human are coupled with a sleep disturbance. This could be linked to observed increases in aggressive behavior.

The social hierarchy of animal groups is associated with biogenic amine metabolism and drug effects. For example, dominant male vervet monkeys have whole-blood 5HT levels twice those of subordinate males. This elevation disappears if the dominant male is isolated from the social group.[169] Alcohol has been reported to affect the aggressive behavior of both rodents[117] and primates[236] differentially, depending on the position of the animal in the social hierarchy.

¶ Clinical Pharmacological Interventions in Human Aggression

Theories, animal models, and even basic neurochemical studies in humans are fascinating and instructional. Yet the clinician is often left with a patient who requests immediate "treatment" for episodic violent behavior. In what direction does the literature point the clinician?

First, the reported violence, the mental state of the patient, and characteristics of the victim must be carefully assessed. Lion[127] has outlined such an assessment. What are the patterns of violent behavior? What are the risk factors, such as available weapons? Is there a coexisting mental disorder, such as schizophrenia? Is the behavior exclusively linked to drugs, such as alcohol? What role does the victim exercise in precipitating or inhibiting the violence?

Second, any treatment plan must take into account and utilize behavioral as well as biological interventions. These might include uncovering or cognitive psychotherapy for a depressed patient, supportive therapy for a schizophrenic patient, or rigorously structured behavioral modification techniques for a mentally retarded patient. New patterns of behavior can also be taught that are often described under assertiveness training.[1] Techniques aimed at changing behavior may be broader, including instruction to change the cognitive sets associated with the initiation of anger as well as the response to a provocative situation.[80]

Third, in the course of treating an assaultive patient, usually a male, adequate support and protection must be afforded to potential victims, frequently women and children. This might involve temporary placement of children in foster homes or of battered women in shelters. It also entails obtaining supportive therapy for women and children to assist them in dealing with their victimization. Such intervention might also require legal interventions or the encouragement of the victim to seek such action.

Finally, one can consider biological interventions. In North America, these have been predominantly pharmacological interventions.

Acute Chemical Restraint

Psychiatrists in the field of emergency psychiatry have suggested the use of antipsychotic medication, barbiturates, or benzodiazepines in managing aggressive behavior in a medical setting—drugs that act as a "chemical restraint." Tupin proposes the use of sodium amobarbital orally or intramuscularly (IM) in a dose range of 200 to 500 mg. When given intravenously (IV), he suggests administration of a 2.5 to 5 percent solution given at a rate of 1 ml per min.[216]

Antipsychotic regimens such as haloperidol in doses of 5 mg IM or 10 mg *per os* (PO), repeated as frequently as every hour or half hour, have been proposed.[54,216] High-dose, low-potency antipsychotic medications such as chlorpromazine are given less preference due to an increased risk of postural hypotension.

The unreliable intramuscular absorption of benzodiazepines initially led to their use in emergency conditions only when given IV. Diazepam has been suggested, administered at a rate and dose of 5 mg per min for a total dose of 10 to 30 mg.[54,216] The development of more reliably absorbed intramuscular preparations has now encouraged their use. Lorazepam in doses of 1 mg given IM every thirty minutes has been used in emergency situations[182] and may become a standard intervention for the chemical restraint of aggressive behavior.

Chronic Pharmacological Treatment

The general clinical rule for the pharmacological treatment of aggressive behavior is to treat the underlying disorder if known or suspected.[54] Thus violence associated with delirium tremens requires the use of benzodiazepines. Violence associated with acute schizophrenia or manic states can be treated acutely with antipsychotic medications. Aggressive behavior in a child with an attention-deficit disorder may respond to direct treatment of the attention disorder with stimulants. Irritability associated with medical conditions such as hyperthyroidism or sepsis needs medical intervention targeted at the primary illness.

However, even after direct pharmacological intervention, a large number of patients remain for whom the primary intervention only partially succeeds or totally fails. There is also a population of patients who do not have major diagnoses like schizophrenia. These populations have been the subjects of various drug trials in an attempt to decrease their aggressive behavior. Representative studies of various classes of drugs are reviewed in the following sections.

NEUROLEPTIC AGENTS

Antipsychotic drugs, all of which are DA antagonists, have a long history in the treatment of aggressive behavior. They have been used to treat the primary illness associated with the violence (e.g., mania or schizophrenia) and also empirically to reduce aggression in demented, retarded, or personality-disordered individuals. Leventhal and Brodie,[125] Itil and Seaman,[100] and Itil and Wadud[101] have extensively reviewed this literature.

The literature is replete with clinical reports of the use of antipsychotic drugs spanning most chemical classes. While various antipsychotic drugs have been touted from time to time as having specific antiaggressive properties, no persistently replicated finding allows for the selection of one drug over another except on the basis of its potency, side effects, and ease of administration.

Phenothiazines were early reported to decrease aggressive behavior associated with schizophrenia.[73] Chlorpromazine has been reported effective in reducing aggressive behavior in both psychotic[35] and nonpsychotic patients.[38,43] Thioridazine,[168] mesoridazine,[74] and pericyazine,[181] a piperidylalkyl phenothiazine not available in the United States, have all been reported to decrease schizophrenic aggressive behavior. Pericyazine, as reviewed by Itil and Mukhopadhyay,[99] has been recommended for aggressive behavior associated with personality-disordered patients. Piperazine phenothiazines have also been reported as effective.[73] Doses of all phenothiazines used are in the standard clinical range.

Other classes of neuroleptic agents have comparable efficacy in reducing aggressive behavior. The butyrophenone haloperidol, which reduces aggressive symptoms associated with psychosis,[67,81] has been used to decrease violence in demented patients,[209] to treat conduct-disordered[33] and retarded children,[30] and to reduce aggressive behavior in a criminal population.[46]

Thioxanthenes such as thiothixene are effective in partially decreasing agitation and aggression in schizophrenia.[95] A similar efficacy has been noted with the indolic neuroleptic agent molindone hydrochloride[103] and the potent DA antagonist pimozide.[18]

Review of this extensive literature in regard to the partial efficacy of neuroleptic drugs should caution the clinician about their use in nonpsychotic patients. While these drugs may decrease aggressive behavior in nonpsychotic individuals, chronic use raises the risk of tardive dyskinesia. Therefore, whenever possible, it is prudent to try to suppress aggressive behavior in nonpsychotic patients with drugs whose chronic use has minimal risk (i.e., less long-term risk than that associated with antipsychotic medication). Failure to succeed with other drugs could then provide a partial justification for a trial of a neuroleptic agent.

MINOR TRANQUILIZERS

Valzelli notes that "the pharmacology of the benzodiazepines is dominated by the taming and antiaggressive properties of these compounds which, at first glance, look more potent and specific than any other substances such as barbiturates, phenothiazines, butyrophenones or meprobamates" (p. 149).[222] These taming effects have been reported with various benzodiazepines in various animal models.[36,171,221] However, animal studies are not uniform. There have been reports of increased aggressive behavior in group-housed mice fed benzodiazepines[70,71] and mixed reports[96,122,201] about the effects of benzodiazepines on predatory aggression. Azcarate[7] and DiMascio[49] have provided extensive clinical reviews of the use of minor tranquilizers in treating aggressive behavior.

As with neuroleptic drugs, benzodiazepines are claimed to decrease aggressive behavior in patients of many diagnostic classes. Boyle and Tobin[19] reported symptomatic improvement in "psychotic" patients treated with chlordiazepoxide hydrochloride. Over half of this population also had organic pathology. Kalina[106] reported a decrease in aggressive outbursts in prisoners reported as having schizophrenia or schizoidal personality disorders who were treated with diazepam. Monroe[150,151] suggests that chlordiazepoxide be used in patients with an episodic dyscontrol syndrome. Drug efficacy was linked to patients who had an abnormal activation of their EEGs with alphachloralose stimulation. Monroe suggests that the chlordiazepoxide can be increased to a ceiling of 200 mg per day. Neurotic patients have also been reported as responsive to chlordiazepoxide.[164] Oxazepam, in doses of 120 or 240 mg per day, was more effective than placebo and chlordiazepoxide (100 or 200 mg/day) in decreasing reported symptoms of anxiety and hostility in outpatients with a history of hostile outbursts associated with anxiety.[128]

The widespread use of benzodiazepines has been limited by reports of paradoxical rage reactions in certain patients treated with these drugs. Tobin, Bird, and Boyle[214] reported a 3.6 percent incidence of rage reactions in a patient group treated with chlordiazepoxide. Enhanced aggressive behavior in patients has also been noted for diazepam and clorazepate.[82,86,129] Chlordiazepoxide increased verbal hostility in an experimental group paradigm.[115] Future study and clinical observation are required to discern whether there is a differential effect on the induction of aggressive or hostile behavior from different benzodiazepines. In the study of Gardos and associates,[75] oxazepam did not increase verbal hostility. In Lion's study of fourteen oxazepam-treated and sixteen chlordiazepoxide-treated patients, no paradoxical rage responses were noted.[128]

Certain patient characteristics, environmental factors, or drug specificity could play a role in the development of violent paradoxical responses. At this time, the Boston research on group verbal hostility and Lion's report suggest a preference for the use of oxazepam. This has been substantiated in an open clinical trial of oxazepam versus diazepam in a prison population.[26]

LITHIUM

After the efficacy of lithium carbonate in the treatment of mania was noted, this alkali metal cation was tested in animal models of aggression, presumably because increased aggressive behavior can be manifested in manic episodes. Weischer[229] demonstrated a taming effect of lithium in fish and rodents. This was followed by other corroborative reports.[61,193] Both the animal and human literature has been reviewed by Sheard.[195]

In an attempted double-blind study, Sheard and coworkers[197] demonstrated a significant decrease in aggressive infractions in a prison population treated with lithium at serum levels ranging between 0.6 and 0.9 mEq per l. Sheard had previously reported similar findings in a single-blind study.[194] Tupin and others[217] corroborated Sheard's observations. Gram and Rafaelsen[84] reported lithium's efficacy in reducing aggressive behavior in a double-blind study of psychotic children. A more recent double-blind study by Campbell and associates[33] demonstrated that both lithium and

haloperidol reduced aggressive behavior in children with a diagnosis of Conduct Disorder, Aggressive Type.

Lithium trials have been given to many different patient populations, including criminal populations,[197] psychotic children,[84] personality-disordered aggressive patients,[69,192] paranoid schizophrenic patients,[140] self-mutilating patients,[44] and other unipolar depressed psychiatric patients.[238] Reports of lithium's efficacy in treating children have been mixed. Dostal and Zvolsky[51] reported an effect of decreased aggression with severely retarded adolescents, and Annell[6] reported a positive effect with aggressive children of mixed psychiatric diagnoses. However, Whitehead and Clark[233] failed to find a difference between the effects of lithium and placebo on hyperactive children. A recent case report suggests that lithium might exacerbate the interictal aggressive behavior observed in some patients with temporal lobe epilepsy.

ANTICONVULSANT DRUGS

There is substantial literature suggesting that abnormal brain electrical dysfunction can be associated with human aggression, a position popularized by Mark and Ervin.[138] Other literature reviews are less conclusive. In an extensive collaborative videotape review, Delgado-Escueta and coworkers[47] recently demonstrated the occurrence of violent epileptic automatisms. However, the frequency of such behavior is very, very rare.

In addition to the question of whether epileptic seizures produce violent behavior, many populations of violent or criminal individuals appear to have a higher incidence of abnormal EEGs than would be expected in a random sampling.[89,234] Monroe reported abnormal brain-wave patterns induced by alpha-chloralose anesthesia in patients with episodic dyscontrol syndromes.[150,151] Such observations have encouraged the trial of anticonvulsants in the treatment of aggressive disorders.

Open trials of phenytoin have been reported to decrease violence in episodic dyscontrol patients.[8,135] Phenytoin attenuated rage reactions.[218] It also reduced hostility and aggressiveness in prisoners and juvenile delinquents.[176] Stephens and Shaffer[204] reported decreased anger, irritability, and anxiety in "neurotic" outpatients. By contrast, Rosenblatt, Schaeffer, and Rosenthal[180] reported that phenytoin did not change aggressive or hostile attitudes of child-abusing parents.

Controlled studies have reported contradictory findings. Maletzky and Klotter[136] reported a positive effect of phenytoin on dyscontrol patients in a double-blind study. Gottschalk, Covi, and Uliana[83] and Lefkowitz[123] failed to find positive effects. Conners and associates[42] failed to find phenytoin effective in aggressive delinquents. Discrepant reports of efficacy also occur regarding the use of phenytoin in schizophrenic patients.[91,199]

Monroe[151] has suggested that primidone, either alone or in combination with chlordiazepoxide, is effective in treating the dyscontrol syndrome. Carbamazepine, a drug with anticonvulsant and psychotropic properties, has been reported in an open study to decrease violent behavior in patients with a dyscontrol syndrome.[215] Hakola and Laulamaa[90] reported a decrease in aggressive behavior in eight violent schizophrenic females. Neppe[157] reported improvement in aggressive behavior in eight of eleven psychiatric inpatients also treated with neuroleptic agents. Luchins[131] noted a similar effect of carbamazepine when added to ongoing neuroleptic treatment.

STIMULANT AND ANTIDEPRESSANT DRUGS

Examples of studies from the animal literature suggest that when given chronically, tricyclic antidepressants or MAOIs can enhance various types of intraspecies aggressive behavior.[55] Clinical lore suggests that treatment with antidepressants improves the symptoms of patients manifesting irritability who also have signs of major depression. Paradoxical rage with antidepressant treatment in humans is rare, but reported.[170]

The animal literature regarding psychostimulants such as amphetamine is divided. Experiments report increases, decreases, and "no change" with the use of amphetamines in various paradigms and at different doses.[145] The clinical literature has not changed substantially since a review by Allen, Safer, and Covi in 1975.[2] Cases of violence associated with amphetamine use appear linked to paranoid, delusional, or frightening ideation rather than to a generally enhanced aggressiveness.[63] Numerous papers have reported that stimulants such as amphetamine or methylphenidate might be appropriate in treating symptoms of aggressive behavior in patients diagnosed as having attention-deficit disorder (a hyperactive or minimal brain dysfunction diagnosis). Representative reports of clinical efficacy include studies by Conners,[41] Eisenberg and others,[62] Fish,[68] and Wender.[231] In patients with a conduct disorder, however, stimulants are reported as generally ineffective.[32] Stringer and Josef[208] published case reports of adult antisocial–personality-disordered patients with a clinical history of attention-deficit disorder who responded to treatment with methylphenidate.

PROPRANOLOL

An increased number of recent reports suggest that the beta-adrenergic antagonist propranolol hydrochloride is effective in reducing episodic violent behavior, particularly in organically impaired patients. These reports are especially interesting in light of biogenic amine hypotheses relating to aggressive behavior that have been generated by animal research. Elliott[64] initially reported the clinical observation that propranolol could attenuate intermittent aggressive behavior. This observation has been extended to other centers that treat patients with organic brain syndromes[87,163,243]; to treatment of Korsakoff's psychosis[244]; and to treatment of organically impaired children with rage outbursts.[235] Propranolol may also have an aggression-attenuating effect when used in combination with neuroleptic agents in schizophrenic patients.[198,242]

Patients are started on twice-daily dose schedules, with dose increases in healthy adults of 20 mg per day to daily levels usually in the range of 300 mg, although certain patients receive 600 or more mg per day. Pulse rate below 50 or 55 or hypotension can limit dosage in some patients.

SEROTONIN PRECURSORS

Neurochemical data already reviewed suggest that 5HT might be a neurotransmitter that plays an active role in inhibiting aggressive behavior. Violent patients have been reported to have low levels of CSF 5-HIAA, 5HT's metabolite.[27] Rats, ordinarily more aggressive as a consequence of electrolytic or neurotoxin lesions, can have this increased aggression blocked by the administration of dietary tryptophan, the precursor of 5HT.[107]

Such observations have suggested trials of 5HT precursors in humans. Soulairac, Lambinet, and Aymard[202] reported a decrease in aggressive behavior in a patient treated with the 5HT precursor, 5-HTP. A comparable finding was reported in the treatment of XYY aggressive males.[14] In schizophrenic patients with high Buss-Durkee scores and a high lifetime frequency of aggressive behavior, Morand, Young, and Ervin[153] reported a decrease in aggression with doses of 4 or 8 g of tryptophan per day.

HORMONAL TREATMENT

Based on the hypothesis that androgens organize the neural control systems that mediate adult aggressive behavior and act on these control systems to enhance aggression,[25] trials of "antiandrogens" have been given to violent patients. Two agents, medroxyprogesterone acetate (MPA) and cyproterone acetate (CPA), have been used clinically to treat the sexually dangerous patient,[113] as well as patients whose aggressive behavior is not necessarily associated with sexual violence. O'Connor and Baker[158] reported a decrease in violence in two schizophrenic patients treated with MPA. Blumer and Migeon[17] reported successful decreases in aggressive outbursts in temporal lobe epileptics and XYY patients whose behavior was predominantly characterized by episodic irritability and rage reactions. Doses of MPA in this uncontrolled study ranged from 100 to 300 mg every seven to ten days. Lower doses were reported as therapeutic in patients not requiring suppression of sexual arousal.

Suppression of sexually aggressive or deviant behavior has been reported in non-blinded studies described by Money[148] and Barry and Ciccone.[12] Doses in Money's study were 300 to 400 mg CPA every ten days and in Barry and Ciccone's study, 300 mg MPA every ten days.

¶ Clinical Surgical Interventions for Aggression

Based on animal studies, several centers have attempted to decrease human aggressive behavior by producing selective limbic lesions. The patients reported in these studies often carry a diagnosis of epilepsy. Groups that have reported success with establishing amygdala lesions include neurosurgical programs in Japan,[156] Great Britain,[94] and the United States.[139] However, not all programs have found a decrease in aggressive behavior with amygdala lesions.[155] In Japan, Sano and others[186] reported a series of patients in whom posterior hypothalamic lesions were produced to decrease violent behavior. Of the forty-four patients treated, twelve were reported to have had "excellent" results, while two were assessed as unchanged and two died. In the United States, Andy[5] also reported the use of thalamic lesions to decrease aggressive behavior.

¶ Clinical Applications of Treatments for Aggression

This chapter has reviewed aspects of the biology of aggression and biological therapies for aggressive behaviors. Such a cataloging of therapies can leave the primary treating physician with many references but no clear treatment plan. At this time, there is no uniformly accepted biological treatment protocol for aggressive patients. However, given the material discussed, it is possible to propose a paradigm for chronic biological treatment.

A first principle in constructing such a paradigm must be to *treat the primary illness*. Thus violence associated with delirium tremens requires benzodiazepine management for alcohol withdrawal as the primary intervention. Treatment of violent behavior associated with command hallucinations or delusional beliefs in a patient with paranoid schizophrenia requires the use of antipsychotic medication.

A second principle for developing a treatment paradigm is to *use the most benign interventions initially when embarking on empirical treatment*. Thus, in dealing with a patient who has explosive outbursts but no clearly diagnosable major mental illness, the clinician—if choosing a pharmacological treatment trial—would begin with benzodiazepines, drugs with relatively minor risks when judiciously used, rather than carbamazepine, which offers the slight but serious risk of inducing bone marrow suppression.

A third principle for treatment is to *have some quantifiable means of assessing efficacy*, which both the clinician and the patient can agree upon in advance, that determine whether to continue or discontinue a medication trial. These might be rule infractions for violence in a penal system, or threatening or violent behavior on a psychiatric ward, or the frequency and intensity of verbal or physical threats or behaviors toward a spouse in an outpatient setting.

A fourth principle is to *institute drug trials systematically*; that is, to introduce drugs as a single variable in treatment whenever possible. This also means that drugs should be introduced for a preplanned treatment period that has a clear beginning and a predetermined ending when efficacy can be assessed. It further means that drug levels should be monitored whenever possible during treatment to confirm therapeutic levels (especially with routinely assayable drugs such as lithium or carbamazepine).

Empirical treatment also appears to be biased at this time toward the early use of certain drugs in various clinical situations. An early trial of benzodiazepines—for example, oxazepam—is suggested for patients whose history and mental state manifests anxiety associated with agitation. If the individual can describe prodromal anticipatory feelings of anxiety or rage, short-acting benzodiazepines could also be used intermittently as a pharmacological adjunct to other behavioral coping strategies to abort a violent outburst. In contrast, the emotionally labile, impulsive patient has great difficulty predicting outbursts and requires regular medication. Since the symptoms of these patients appear similar to those of manic patients, a trial of lithium may be warranted. Initial trials of propranolol suggested its usefulness in patients with documented organic brain injury (e.g., a ruptured cerebral aneurysm or dementia). This drug may therefore merit early trial in such patients.

For patients who do not clearly fit primary treatment patterns or for whom traditional primary treatment has failed to attenuate violent behavior, an empirically ordered treatment can be proposed: for example, (a) benzodiazepine; (b) lithium or propranolol; and (c) an antipsychotic or anticonvulsant.

A clinical vignette can illustrate such an empirical treatment approach. John W. is a thirty-four-year-old, married white male who works in a lumber yard. His first marriage ended in divorce due to serious assaultive behavior. He has been remarried for two years, but once again his marriage is jeopardized by his episodic, unpredictable violent outbursts, both verbal and physical, associated with property destruction and physical abuse of his wife. In response to his wife's threats to leave, he has sought treatment. He has entered traditional behavioral therapy (a group program for abusive husbands), but is also seeking pharmacological treatment. Psychiatric evaluation does not confirm psychosis or a major depression. The most likely DSM-III diagnosis would be an Axis I diagnosis of Intermittent Explosive Disorder and an Axis II diagnosis of a Mixed

Personality Disorder, with no diagnosis of alcohol abuse.

An initial medication trial could be the administration of oxazepam four times a day for a daily dose of 120 mg, limiting the dosage if sedation develops. This trial could continue for one month, during which time both patient and spouse would separately log the intensity and frequency of violent behavior for the clinician. If the violence did not subside after one month, a trial of lithium (with a serum level of at least 0.7 mEq/l for six weeks) or propranolol (maintaining a dosage of perhaps 240–320 mg for several months) could be tried as second or third alternatives. Of course, this protocol would require appropriate pretreatment medical evaluation of the patient, and certain drugs would not be used if complicated by medical illnesses such as renal compromise with lithium or asthma with propranolol. If neither lithium nor propranolol proved successful, fourth- and fifth-line trials of an antipsychotic medication (e.g., haloperidol, 5–10 mg/day) or an anticonvulsant (e.g., carbamazepine at blood levels of anticonvulsant efficacy) could be attempted.

Severely disturbed inpatients undergoing a comparable treatment protocol could be administered higher doses of propranolol if monitored closely for bradycardia and hypotension. Failure of all such medication interventions probably exhausts "innovative treatment" options for such patients unless there is reason to suspect a secondary diagnosis, such as an attention-deficit disorder, that might prompt a trial of a stimulant.

Other biological interventions such as tryptophan, drug combinations (e.g., tryptophan and lithium), antiandrogens, or psychosurgery seem to this author to be experimental in nature, requiring protocol description and explicit patient consent. They are "last resorts," to be implemented only with severely violent patients at selected national centers, with close scrutiny of consent and outcome issues. A summary of this manner of considering the pharmacological treatment of human aggressive behavior is provided in table 24–1.

¶ New Directions for Clinical Research on Aggression

A chapter such as this highlights several areas of potential human research necessary to strengthen our understanding of the biological elements influencing human aggressive behavior. Basic research is needed to explore further the genetic or environmental influences of violent behavior on unaltered and cross-fostered siblings. Ethological study of human aggressive behavior is needed to identify those unconsciously perceived cues of threat, counterthreat, and submission that are exchanged between the violent perpetrator and victim or intervener. The work could be further extended to study the effects of various drugs on these cues and other trigger stimuli associated with the induction or inhibition of human violent behavior. A more comprehensive nosology of human aggressive behavior that might include biochemical parameters (e.g., CSF–5-HIAA levels) and distinguish between impulsive, controlled, drug-induced, or delusional violence might lead to more predictive pharmacological treatment.

Drug studies require the research community to standardize and accept evaluation scales for in- and outpatient treatment trials that can be shared from center to center for replication of initial findings of drug efficacy. Increased support for blinded, more tightly controlled studies is needed to limit the current expansion of "innovative treatment" that fails to generate a literature of solid and reproducible results. Since many of these drug treatments cannot be fully blinded due to biological indicators, such as a lithium-induced tremor or a propranolol-induced bradycardia, incompletely blinded studies may need to be legitimized. Small research populations may require well-monitored $N = 1$ protocols of *ABAB* design rather than those comprised of large population samples. Certainly the magnitude of the clinical problem of violent behavior requires a greater clinical research investment than has heretofore occurred.

TABLE 24–1

Pharmacologic Interventions for Violent Behavior
Associated with Various Psychiatric Disorders

Disorder	Suggested Medications
Schizophrenia	Antipsychotics
	Propranolol (?)
Mania	Antipsychotics
	Lithium
Major Depression	Antidepressants
Organic Brain Disorders	Antipsychotics
	Propranolol (?)
Mental Retardation	Antipsychotics (?)
	Propranolol (?)
	Lithium (?)
Attention-deficit Disorders	Stimulants
Conduct Disorders	Antipsychotics
	Lithium
Personality Disorders	Anticonvulsants (?)
Intermittent Explosive Disorders	Antipsychotics
	Benzodiazepines (?)
	Lithium
	Propranolol (?)
Seizure Disorders	Anticonvulsants
Alcohol Abuse	Disulfiram (?)
Sexual Disorders	Antiandrogens (?)

While currently available drugs merit more extensive testing, there is also the potential to develop new agents. In the early 1970s, Itil, Stock, and Duffy[102] reported positive findings with an experimental benzodiazepine, SCH-12679. More recently, Bradford and associates[20] have been studying a new class of compounds that they have labeled "serenics," which are reported to have relatively specific antiaggressive effects in animal models.

¶ Ethical Issues in Treating Aggression

Both research and innovative clinical applications related to the pharmacological treatment of human aggressive behavior raise difficult ethical issues.[53] Pharmacological research with aggressive individuals raises the issues of informed consent, confidentiality, responsibility, and retribution for harm during the research, as well as the withholding of potentially efficacious agents due to political and social moral standards.

Obtaining informed consent is complicated in research protocols designed to reduce aggressive behavior. First, many violent individuals are unable to give truly informed consent. These subjects include severely demented or retarded individuals as well as severely regressed psychotic patients. However, aggressive patients within these groups might benefit substantially in terms of enhanced care and socialization if their assaultive behaviors were decreased. Conduct-disordered or antisocial personality-disordered individuals are often angry and uncooperative with those who attempt to alter their aggressive behavior. Often, consent to participate in "experiments" is most difficult to obtain, tending to exclude a large research population from study.

Once consent is obtained and research treatment is begun, there are special issues related to confidentiality. Unlike the suicidal patient, the violent, often homicidal patient poses a risk to others. Rating scales and structured interviews, if honestly reported, might disclose threats of violence to others. Detailed history of such individuals tends to uncover episodes of other violence, often to children and frequently of a felonious nature. Breaking confidentiality can lead to the subject's withdrawal from the research, while the silence of the researcher can further endanger potential victims or allow a felon to go unpunished. Protocols with violent patients generally must include a caution that patient confidentiality can be breached when the researcher fears imminent, substantial harm to others.

Medical research has traditionally recognized the need to address potential injury to the research subject during an experiment. The pharmacological risks to these violent patients remain similar to those of other psychiatric populations, but there is a new risk factor—the risk to potential victims. Who is both morally and legally responsible for injury to a victim, perhaps a spouse or child, when violence occurs during a treatment period? What responsibility does the investigator have if, for example, a violent protocol patient in a benzodiazepine study has a paradoxical rage reaction and assaults his wife? Informed consent is not usually obtained from potential victims, yet they can be affected by the research.

Finally, research faces social restraints. Animal research suggests that opioids[78] and marijuana[34] can decrease aggressive behavior. Many users of marijuana allege that it reduces their anger and threshold for violent behavior. This has been supported in a research format.[183,211] However, approval to use potentially addictive or illegal drugs under present research regulations has been difficult and sometimes impossible to obtain, regardless of the potential benefits that might accrue to both the individual and society.

Ethical issues in treatment are also substantial. The use of pharmacological agents as controllers of violent behavior for social or political reasons is conceivable. Complaints regarding the use of pharmacological intervention for political purposes have been lodged against Soviet psychiatrists[142] and could be alleged in the United States if a broader use of "antiaggressive agents" were condoned. This North American culture has also failed to support coercive "rehabilitation" in the prison system in the manner of *A Clockwork Orange.*[29] Attempts at restrictive environments or aversive pharmacological treatment have been forbidden by the courts.[98] Whether such restrictions are more humane than incarceration in environments that are often marred with both physical and sexual violence remains open to debate.

¶ **Summary**

In conclusion, this chapter has illustrated how biological elements can influence aggressive behavior through genetics, the processing of sensory information, or the induction of neurochemical change by environmental stress; and the possible role of various neurotransmitters in aggressive behavior has been reviewed. Multiple neurotransmitter systems appear to interact in concert to modulate an organism's propensity for various types of aggressive behavior. The prediction of various drug interventions is complicated not only by dose effects, but also by the animal's place in the social hierarchy, its preexisting brain integrity, the type of aggressive behavior that might be elicited, the genetic substrate of a given organism, and its previous experience.

Such complexity leaves the clinician with poorly defined treatment options. Well-controlled and blinded studies are rare in this area of clinical pharmacology. Nevertheless, currently available drugs have been reported to reduce violent behavior in various clinical populations. Systematic trial of these agents with a careful monitoring for adverse effects is feasible and offers some potential relief for the patient seeking clinical assistance in diminishing the frequency and intensity of dystonic violent behaviors.

¶ **Acknowledgments**

This manuscript is supported by the Veterans Administration. Editorial assistance was provided by the VA Research Service staff.

¶ **Bibliography**

1. ALBERTI, R. E., and EMMONS, M. L. *Your Perfect Right: A Guide to Assertive Living*, 4th ed.. San Luis Obispo: California Impact Publishers, 1982.

2. ALLEN, R. P., SAFER, D., and COVI, L. "Effects of Psychostimulants on Aggression," *Journal of Nervous and Mental Disease*, 160 (1975):138–145.

3. ALPERS, B. J. "Relation of the Hypothalamus to Disorders of Personality," *Archives of Neurology*, 38 (1937):291–303.

4. AMERICAN PSYCHIATRIC ASSOCIATION. *Diagnostic and Statistical Manual of Mental Disorders*, 3rd ed. (DSM-III). Washington, D.C.: American Psychiatric Association, 1980.

5. ANDY, O. J. "Thalamotomy in Hyperactive and Aggressive Behavior," *Confinia Neurologica*, 32 (1970):322–325.

6. ANNELL, A. L. "Lithium in the Treatment of Children and Adolescents," *Acta Psychiatrica Scandinavica*, 207 (Supplement) (1969):19–33.

7. AZCARATE, C. L. "Minor Tranquilizers in the Treatment of Aggression," *Journal of Nervous and Mental Disease*, 160 (1975):100–107.

8. BACH-Y-RITA, G., et al. "Episodic Dyscontrol: A Study of 130 Violent Patients," *American Journal of Psychiatry*, 127 (1971):1473–1478.

9. BANDLER, R. J., JR., and FLYNN, J. P. "Control of Somatosensory Fields for Striking During Hypothalamically Elicited Attack," *Brain Research*, 38 (1972): 197–201.

10. BANDLER, R. J., JR., and MOYER, K. E. "Animals Spontaneously Attacked by Rats," *Communications in Behavioral Biology*, 5 (1970):177–182.

11. BANDURA, A. "Social Learning Theory of Aggression," in J. F. Knutson, ed., *Control of Aggression: Implications from Basic Research*. Chicago: Aldine, 1971, pp. 201–250.

12. BARRY, D. J., and CICCONE, J. R. "Use of Depo-Provera in the Treatment of Aggressive Sexual Offenders: Preliminary Report of Three Cases," *Bulletin of the American Academy of Psychiatry and the Law*, (1975):179–184.

13. BERNSTON, G. G., and LEIBOWITZ, S. F. "Biting Attack in Cats: Evidence for Central Muscarinic Mediation," *Brain Research*, 51 (1973):366–370.

14. BIOULAC, B., et al. "Serotonergic Dysfunction in the 47 XYY Syndrome," *Biological Psychiatry*, 15 (1980):917–923.

15. BLANCHARD, R. J., et al. "Attack and Defensive Behaviour in the Albino Rat," *Animal Behaviour*, 25 (1977):622–634.

16. BLUMER, D. "Temporal Lobe Epilepsy and its Psychiatric Significance," in D. F. Benson and D. Blumer, eds., *Psychiatric Aspects of Neurological Disease*. New York: Grune & Stratton, 1975, pp. 171–198.

17. BLUMER, D., and MIGEON, C. "Hormone and Hormonal Agents in the Treatment of Aggression," *Journal of Nervous and Mental Disease*, 160 (1975):127–137.

18. BOBON, D., et al. "Clinical Toxicology and Efficacy of Pimozide," *International Pharmacopsychiatry*, 4 (1970):194–203.

19. BOYLE, D., and TOBIN, J. M. "Pharmaceutical Management of Behavior Disorders; Chlordiazepoxide in Covert and Overt Expressions of Aggression," *Journal of the Medical Society of New Jersey*, 58 (1961):427–429.

20. BRADFORD, L. L., et al. "Serenics: The Pharmacology of Fluprazine and DU 28412," in K. A. Miczek, M. R. Kruk, and B. Olivier, eds., *Ethopharmacological Aggression Research*. New York: Alan R. Liss, 1984, pp. 191–207.

21. BRADY, J. V. and NAUTA, W.J.H. "Subcortical Mechanisms in Emotional Behavior: Affective Changes Following Septal Forebrain Lesions in the Albino Rat," *Journal of Comparative and Physiological Psychology*, 46 (1953):339–346.

22. BRAIN, P. F. *Hormones and Aggression*, vol. 1. Montreal: Eden Press, 1977.

23. ————. *Hormones and Aggression*, vol. 2. Montreal: Eden Press, 1979.

24. ———. *Hormones, Drugs, and Aggression,* vol. 3. Montreal: Eden Press, 1979.

25. BRONSON, F. H., and DESJARDIN, C. "Aggressive Behavior and Seminal Vesicle Function in Mice: Differential Sensitivity to Androgen Given Neonatally," *Endocrinology,* 85 (1969):971–974.

26. BROWN, C. R. "The Use and Misuse of Anxiolytics in the Violent, Aggressive Individual," in S. Fielding and R. C. Effland, eds., *New Frontiers in Psychotropic Drug Research.* New York: Futura, 1979, pp. 241–258.

27. BROWN, G. L., et al. "Human Aggression and Its Relationship to Cerebrospinal Fluid 5-Hydroxyindole Acetic Acid, 3-Methoxy-4-Hydroxyphenylglycol and Homovanillic Acid," in M. Sandler, ed., *Psychopharmacology of Aggression.* New York: Raven Press, 1979, pp. 131–148.

28. BUGBEE, N. M., and EICHELMAN, B. "Sensory Alterations and Aggressive Behavior in the Rat," *Physiology and Behavior,* 8 (1972):981–985.

29. BURGESS, A. *A Clockwork Orange.* New York: Norton, 1963.

30. BURK, H. W., and MENOLASCINO, F. "Haloperidol in Emotionally Disturbed Retarded Individuals," *American Journal of Psychiatry,* 124 (1968):1589–1591.

31. BUTLER, K. "Predatory Behavior in Laboratory Mice: Sex and Strain Comparisons," *Journal of Comparative and Physiological Psychology,* 85 (1973): 243–249.

32. CAMPBELL, M., COHEN, I. L., and SMALL, A. M. "Drugs in Aggressive Behavior," *Journal of the American Academy of Child Psychiatry,* 21 (1982):107–117.

33. CAMPBELL, M., et al. "Behavioral Efficacy of Haloperidol and Lithium Carbonate," *Archives of General Psychiatry,* 41 (1984):650–656.

34. CARLINI, E. A. "Effects of Cannabinoid Compounds on Aggressive Behavior," *Modern Problems of Pharmacopsychiatry,* 13 (1978):82–102.

35. CASEY, J. F., et al. "Treatment of Schizophrenic Reactions with Phenothiazine Derivatives," *American Journal of Psychiatry,* 117 (1960):97–105.

36. CHRISTMAS, A. J., and MAXWELL, D. R. "A Comparison of the Effects of Some Benzodiazepines and Other Drugs on Aggressive and Exploratory Behaviour in Mice and Rats," *Neuropharmacology,* 9 (1970):17–29.

37. CIARANELLO, R. D., LIPSKY, A., and AXELROD, J. "Association Between Fighting Behavior and Catecholamine Biosynthetic Enzyme Activity in Two Inbred Mouse Strains," *Proceedings of the National Academy of Science,* 71 (1974):3006–3008.

38. COHEN, M., et al. "Family Interaction Patterns, Drug Treatment, and Change in Social Aggression," *Archives of General Psychiatry,* 19 (1968):50–56.

39. CONNER, R. L. "Hormones, Biogenic Amines, and Aggression," in S. Levine, ed., *Hormones and Behavior.* New York: Academic Press, 1972, pp. 209–233.

40. CONNER, R. L., et al. "Hormonal Determinants of Aggressive Behavior," *Annals of the New York Academy of Sciences,* 159 (1969):760–776.

41. CONNERS, C. K. "Psychological Effects of Stimulant Drugs in Children with Minimal Brain Dysfunction," *Pediatrics,* 49 (1972):702–708.

42. CONNERS, C. K., et al. "Treatment of Young Delinquent Boys with Diphenylhydantoin Sodium and Methylphenidate. A Controlled Comparison," *Archives of General Psychiatry,* 24 (1971):156–160.

43. COOK, L., and KELLEHER, R. T. "Effects of Drugs on Behavior," *Annual Review of Pharmacology,* 3 (1963):205–222.

44. COOPER, A.F., and FOWLIE, H. D. "Control of Gross Self-Mutilation with Lithium Carbonate," *British Journal of Psychiatry,* 122 (1973):370–371.

45. DANIELS, D. N., GILULA, M. F., and OCHBERG, F. M., eds. *Violence and the Struggle for Existence.* Boston: Little, Brown, 1970.

46. DARLING, H. F. "Haloperidol in Sixty Criminal Psychotics," *Diseases of the Nervous System,* 32 (1971):31–34.

47. DELGADO-ESCUETA, A. V., et al. "The Nature of Aggression During Epileptic Seizures," *New England Journal of Medicine,* 305 (1981):711–716.

48. DiCHIARA, G., CAMBA, R., and SPANO, P. F. "Evidence for Inhibition by Brain

Serotonin of Mouse Killing Behaviour in Rats," *Nature*, 233 (1971):272–273.

49. DIMASCIO, A. "The Effects of Benzodiazepines on Aggression," in S. Garattini, W. Mussini, and L. O. Randall, eds., *The Benzodiazepines*. New York: Raven Press, 1973, pp. 433–440.

50. DOLLARD, J., et al. *Frustration and Aggression*. New Haven: Yale University Press, 1939.

51. DOSTAL, T., and ZVOLSKY, P. "Antiaggressive Effect of Lithium Salts in Several Mentally Retarded Adolescents," *International Pharmacopsychiatry*, 5 (1970):203–207.

52. EHRENKRANTZ, J., BLISS, E., and SHEARD, M. H. "Plasma Testosterone: Correlation with Aggressive Behavior and Social Dominance in Man," *Psychosomatic Medicine*, 36 (1974):469–475.

53. EICHELMAN, B. "Toward Maintaining Ethical Research on Violent Behavior," *Clinical Research*, 24 (1976):322–328.

54. ———. "Pharmacological Treatment of Aggressive Disturbances," in J. Barchas et al., eds., *Psychopharmacology: From Theory to Practice*, New York: Oxford University Press, 1977, pp. 260–269.

55. ———. "Role of Biogenic Amines in Aggressive Behavior," in M. Sandler, ed., *Psychopharmacology of Aggression*. New York: Raven Press, 1979, pp. 61–93.

56. ———. "Variability in Rat Irritable and Predatory Aggression," *Behavioral and Neural Biology*, 29 (1980):498–505.

57. EICHELMAN, B., and BARCHAS, J. "Facilitated Shock-Induced Aggression Following Antidepressive Medication in the Rat," *Pharmacology Biochemistry and Behavior*, 3 (1975):601–604.

58. EICHELMAN, B., and HEGSTRAND, L. "Stress-induced Alterations in Aggression and Brain Biochemistry," Paper presented at the 13th Collegium Internationale Neuro-Psychopharmacologicum, Jerusalem, Israel, June 1982.

59. EICHELMAN, B., and THOA, N. B. "The Aggressive Monoamines," *Biological Psychiatry*, 6 (1973):143–164.

60. EICHELMAN, B., ELLIOTT, G. R., and BARCHAS, J. D. "Biochemical, Pharmacological, and Genetic Aspects of Aggression," in D. Hamburg and M. B. Trudeau, eds., *Biobehavioral Aspects of Aggression*. New York: Alan R. Liss, 1981, pp. 51–84.

61. EICHELMAN, B., THOA, N. B., and PEREZ-CRUET, J. "Alkali Metal Cations: Effects on Aggression and Adrenal Enzymes," *Pharmacology, Biochemistry and Behavior*, 1 (1973):121–123.

62. EISENBERG, L., et al. "A Psychopharmacologic Experiment in a Training School of Delinquent Boys. Methods, Problems, and Findings," *American Journal of Orthopsychiatry*, 33 (1963):434–437.

63. ELLINWOOD, E. "Assault and Homicide Associated with Amphetamine Abuse," *American Journal of Psychiatry*, 127 (1971):1170–1175.

64. ELLIOTT, F. A. "Propranolol for the Control of Belligerent Behavior Following Acute Brain Damage," *Annals of Neurology*, 1 (1977):489–491.

65. ELLISON, G. D., and BRESLER, D. E. "Tests of Emotional Behavior in Rats Following Depletion of Norepinephrine, of Serotonin, or of Both," *Psychopharmacologia*, 34 (1974):275–288.

66. EVERETT, G. M., and WIEGAND, R. G. "Central Amines and Behavioral States: A Critique and New Data," in W.D.M. Paton, ed., *First International Pharmacological Meeting (Stockholm)*. London: Pergamon Press, 1963, pp. 85–92.

67. FELDMAN, P., et al. "Parenteral Haloperidol in Controlling Patient Behavior During Acute Psychotic Episodes," *Current Therapeutic Research*, 11 (1969):362–366.

68. FISH, B. "The 'One-Child One-Drug' Myth of Stimulants in Hyperkinesis," *Archives of General Psychiatry*, 25 (1971):193–203.

69. FORSSMAN, M., and WALINDER, J. "Lithium Treatment on Atypical Indication," *Acta Psychiatrica Scandinavica*, 207 (Supplement) (1969):34–40.

70. FOX, K. A., and SNYDER, R. L. "Effect of Sustained Low Doses of Diazepam on Aggression and Mortality in Grouped Male Mice," *Journal of Comparative and Physiological Psychology*, 69 (1969):663–666.

71. FOX, K. A., TUCKOSH, J. R., and WILCOX, A. H. "Increased Aggression Among Grouped Male Mice Fed Chlor-

diazepoxide," *European Journal of Pharmacology,* 11 (1970):119–121.

72. FREUD, S. "Civilization and Its Discontents," in J. Strachey, ed., *The Standard Edition of the Complete Psychological Works of Sigmund Freud.* London: Hogarth Press, 1958, vol. 21.

73. FREYHAN, F. A. "Therapeutic Implications of Differential Effects of New Phenothiazine Compounds," *American Journal of Psychiatry,* 115 (1959):577–585.

74. GALLANT, D. M., BISHOP, M. P., and SPREHE, D. "TPS-23; A New Thioridazine Derivative," *Current Therapeutic Research,* 7 (1965):102–104.

75. GARDOS, G., et al. "Differential Actions of Chlordiazepoxide and Oxazepam on Hostility," *Archives of General Psychiatry,* 18 (1968):757–760.

76. GEYER, M. A., and SEGAL, D. S. "Shock-Induced Aggression: Opposite Effects of Intraventricularly Infused Dopamine and Norepinephrine," *Behavioral Biology,* 10 (1974):99–104.

77. GIACALONE, E., et al. "Brain Serotonin Metabolism in Isolated Aggressive Mice," *Biochemical Pharmacology,* 17 (1968):1315–1327.

78. GIANUTSTOS, G., and LAL, H. "Narcotic Analgesics and Aggression," in L. Valzelli, ed., *Modern Problems of Pharmacopsychiatry,* vol. 13. Basel: Karger, 1978, pp. 114–138.

79. GIBBONS, J. L., et al. "Manipulations of Dietary Tryptophan: Effects on Mouse Killing and Brain Serotonin in the Rat," *Brain Research,* 169 (1979):139–153.

80. GOLDSTEIN, A. P., et al. *In Response to Aggression: Methods of Control and Prosocial Alternatives.* Elmsford, N.Y.: Pergamon Press, 1981.

81. GOLDSTEIN, B., CLYDE, D., and CALDWELL, J. "Clinical Efficacy of the Butyrophenones as Antipsychotic Drugs," in D. Efron, ed., *Psychopharmacology: A Review of Progress.* Washington, D.C.: U.S. Printing Office, USPHS no. 1836, 1968, pp. 1085–1091.

82. GORDON, E. B. "Tranquilizers Causing Aggression," *British Medical Journal,* 2 (1975):36–37.

83. GOTTSCHALK, L., et al. "Effects of Diphenylhydantoin on Anxiety and Hostility in Institutionalized Prisoners," *Comprehensive Psychiatry,* 14 (1973): 503–511.

84. GRAM, L. F., and RAFAELSEN, O. J. "Lithium Treatment of Psychotic Children and Adolescents: A Controlled Clinical Trial," *Acta Psychiatrica Scandinavica,* 48 (1972):253–260.

85. GREENBERG, A. S., and COLEMAN, M. "Depressed 5-Hydroxyindole Levels Associated with Hyperactive and Aggressive Behavior," *Archives of General Psychiatry,* 33 (1976):331–336.

86. GREENBLATT, D. J., SHADER, R. I., and KOCH-WESER, J. L. "Flurazepam Hydrochloride," *Clinical Pharmacology and Therapeutics,* 17 (1975):1–14.

87. GREENDYKE, R. M., SCHUSTER, D. B., and WOOTON, J. A. "Propranolol in the Treatment of Assaultive Patients with Organic Brain Disease," *Journal of Clinical Psychopharmacology,* 4 (1984):282–285.

88. GROSSMAN, S. P. "Chemically Induced Epileptiform Seizures in the Cat," *Science,* 142 (1963):409–411.

89. GUNN, J. C. "The Prevalence of Epilepsy Among Prisoners," *Proceedings of the Royal Society of Medicine,* 62 (1969): 60–63.

90. HAKOLA, H. P., and LAULAMAA, V. A. "Carbamazepine in Treatment of Violent Schizophrenics (Letter)," *Lancet,* 1 (1982):1358.

91. HAWARD, L.R.C. "Differential Modifications of Verbal Aggression by Psychotropic Drugs," in S. Garattini and E.B. Sigg, eds., *Aggressive Behaviour.* Amsterdam: Excerpta Medica Foundation, 1969, pp. 317–321.

92. HEGSTRAND, L., and EICHELMAN, B. "Increased Shock-Induced Fighting with Supersensitive β-Adrenergic Receptors," *Pharmacology, Biochemistry and Behavior,* 19 (1983):313–320.

93. HEIMSTRA, N. W. "Effects of Chlorpromazine on Dominance and Fighting Behaviour in Rats," *Behaviour,* 18 (1961):313–321.

94. HITCHCOCK, E. "Amygdalotomy for Aggression," in M. Sandler, ed., *Psychopharmacology of Aggression.* New York: Raven Press, 1979, pp. 205–215.

95. HOLDEN, J., et al. "The Clinical Effects of

Intramuscular Thiothixene and Trifluoperazine in Chronic Schizophrenia: A Comparative Study," *Current Therapeutic Research*, 13 (1971):298–310.

96. HOROVITZ, Z. P., et al. "Effects of Drugs on the Mouse-Killing (Muricide) Test and Its Relationship to Amygdaloid Function," *International Journal of Neuropharmacology*, 5 (1966):405–411.

97. HUTCHINGS, B., and MEDNICK, S. A. "Registered Criminality in the Adoptive and Biological Parents of Registered Male Criminal Adoptees," in R. R. Fieve and B. Rosenthal, eds., *Genetic Research in Psychiatry*. Baltimore: Johns Hopkins University Press, 1975, pp. 105–116.

98. *Individual Rights and the Federal Role in Behavioral Modification*. Washington D.C.: U.S. Government Printing Office, 1974.

99. ITIL, T. M., and MUKHOPADHYAY, S. "Pharmacological Management of Human Violence," in L. Valzelli, ed., *Modern Problems of Pharmacophsychiatry: Psychopharmacology of Aggression*, vol. 13. Basel: Karger, 1978, pp. 139–158.

100. ITIL, T. M., and SEAMAN, P. "Drug Treatment of Human Aggression," *Progress in Neuropsychopharmacology*, 2 (1979):659–669.

101. ITIL, T. M., and WADUD, A. "Treatment of Human Aggression with Major Tranquilizers, Antidepressants, and Newer Psychotropic Drugs," *Journal of Nervous and Mental Disease*, 160 (1975):83–99.

102. ITIL, T. M., et al. "Therapeutic Trials and EEG Investigations with SCH-12679 in Behaviorally Disturbed Adolescents," *Current Therapeutic Research*, 14 (1972):136–150.

103. ITIL, T. M., et al. "Comparison of the Clinical and Electroencephalographical Effects of Molindone and Trifluoperazine in Acute Schizophrenic Patients," *Behavioral Neuropsychiatry*, 3 (1971):6–13.

104. JACOBS, B. L., and COHEN, A. "Differential Behavioral Effects of Lesions of the Median or Dorsal Raphe Nuclei in Rats: Open Field and Pain-Elicited Aggres-

sion," *Journal of Comparative and Physiological Psychology*, 90 (1976): 102–108.

105. JACOBS, P. A., et al. "Aggressive Behaviour, Mental Sub-normality, and the XYY Male," *Nature*, 208 (1965):1351–1352.

106. KALINA, R. K. "Diazepam: Its Role in a Prison Setting," *Diseases of the Nervous System*, 25 (1964):101–107.

107. KANTAK, K. M., HEGSTRAND, L. R., and EICHELMAN, B. "Dietary Tryptophan Reversal of Septal Lesion and 5,7-DHT Lesion Elicited Shock-Induced Fighting," *Pharmacology Biochemistry and Behavior*, 15 (1981):343–350.

108. ———. "Facilitation of Shock-induced Fighting Following Intraventricular 5,7-Dihydroxytryptamine and 6-Hydroxydopa," *Psychopharmacology*, 74 (1981):157–160.

109. KANTAK, K. M., et al. "Effects of Dietary Supplements and a Tryptophan-Free Diet on Aggressive Behavior in Rats," *Pharmacology Biochemistry and Behavior*, 12 (1980):173–179.

110. KARLI, P., VERGNES, M., and DIDIER-GEORGES, F. "Rat-Mouse Interspecific Aggressive Behaviour and Its Manipulation by Brain Ablation and by Brain Stimulation," in S. Garattini and E. B. Sigg, eds., *Aggressive Behaviour*. Amsterdam: Excerpta Medica Foundation, 1969, pp. 47–55.

111. KATZ, R. J. "Effects of the Cholinomimetic Drug Arecoline upon Aggression: Intra vs. Inter-Specific Allocation of Attack," *Aggressive Behavior*, 2 (1976): 205–212.

112. ———. "Catecholamines in Predatory Behavior: A Review and Critique," *Aggressive Behavior*, 4 (1978):153–172.

113. KELLY, J. R., and CAVANAUGH, J. L. "Treatment of the Sexually Dangerous Patient," in J. Masserman, ed., *Current Psychiatric Therapies*, vol. 21. New York: Grune & Stratton, 1982, pp. 101–113.

114. KINZEL, A. F. "Body-Buffer Zone in Violent Prisoners," *American Journal of Psychiatry*, 127 (1970):59–64.

115. KOCHANSKY, G. E., et al. "Effects of Chlordiazepoxide and Oxazepam Administration on Verbal Hostility," *Ar-

chives of General Psychiatry, 34 (1977): 1457–1459.

116. KREUZ, L. E., and ROSE, R. M. "Assessment of Aggressive Behavior and Plasma Testosterone in a Young Criminal Population," *Psychosomatic Medicine,* 34 (1972):321–332.

117. KRSIAK, M. "Effect of Ethanol on Aggression and Timidity in Mice," *Psychopharmacology,* 51 (1976):75–80.

118. KULKARNI, A. S. "Muricidal Block by 5-Hydroxytryptophan and Various Drugs," *Life Sciences,* 7 (1968):125–128.

119. LAGERSPETZ, K.Y.H., TIRRI, R., and LAGERSPETZ, K.M.J. "Neurochemical and Endocrinological Studies of Mice Selectively Bred for Aggressiveness," *Scandinavian Journal of Psychology,* 9 (1968): 157–160.

120. LAMMERS, A.J.J.C., and VAN ROSSUM, J. M. "Bizarre Social Behaviour in Rats Induced by a Combination of a Peripheral Decarboxylase Inhibitor and DOPA," *European Journal of Pharmacology,* 5 (1968):103–106.

121. LAMPRECHT, F., et al. "Rat Fighting Behavior: Serum Dopamine-Beta-Hydroxylase and Hypothalamic Tyrosine Hydroxylase," *Science,* 177 (1972):- 1214–1215.

122. LEAF, R. C., et al. "Chlordiazepoxide and Diazepam Induced Mouse-Killing by Rats," *Psychopharmacologia,* 44 (1975): 23–28.

123. LEFKOWITZ, M. "Effects of Diphenylhydantoin in Disruptive Behavior: Study of Male Delinquents," *Archives of General Psychiatry,* 20 (1969):643–651.

124. LESLIE, W. "Cysts of the *Cavum Vergae,*" *Canadian Medical Association Journal,* 43 (1940):433–435.

125. LEVENTHAL, B. L., and BRODIE, H.K.H. "The Pharmacology of Violence," in D. A. Hamburg and M. B. Trudeau, eds., *Biobehavioral Aspects of Aggression.* New York: Alan R. Liss, 1981, pp. 85–106.

126. LINNOILA, M., et al. "Low Cerebrospinal Fluid 5-Hydroxyindoleacetic Acid Concentration Differentiates Impulsive from Nonimpulsive Violent Behavior," *Life Sciences,* 33 (1983):2609–2614.

127. LION, J. R. *Evaluation and Management of the Violent Patient.* Springfield, Ill.: Charles C Thomas, 1972.

128. ———. "Benzodiazepines in the Treatment of Aggressive Patients," *Journal of Clinical Psychiatry,* 40 (1979):70–71.

129. LION, J. R., AZCARATE, C. L., and KOEPKE, H. H. "Paradoxical Rage Reactions During Psychotropic Medication," *Diseases of the Nervous System,* 36 (1975):557–558.

130. LORENZ, K. *On Aggression.* New York: Harcourt, Brace & World, 1966.

131. LUCHINS, D. J. "Carbamazepine for the Violent Psychiatric Patient," *Lancet,* 2 (1983):766.

132. MACK, G., SIMLER, S., and MANDEL, P. "Système Inhibiteur GABA-nergique Dans L'Agressivité Interspécifique Rat-Souris," *Journal de Physiologie* (Paris), 71 (1975):162A.

133. MAGNUSON, E. "Child Abuse: The Ultimate Betrayal," *Time,* 5 September 1983, pp. 20–22.

134. MALAMUD, N. "Psychiatric Disorder with Intracranial Tumors of Limbic System," *Archives of Neurology,* 17 (1967):113–123.

135. MALETZKY, B. M. "The Episodic Dyscontrol Syndrome," *Diseases of the Nervous System,* 34 (1973):178–185.

136. MALETZKY, B. M., and KLOTTER, J. "Episodic Dyscontrol: A Controlled Replication," *Diseases of the Nervous System,* 35 (1974):175–179.

137. MANDEL, P., et al. "Molecular Aspects of a Model of Aggressive Behavior: Neurotransmitter Interactions," in S. Garattini, J. F. Pujol, and R. Samanin, eds., *Interactions Between Putative Neurotransmitters in the Brain.* New York: Raven Press, 1968, pp. 285–303.

138. MARK, V. H., and ERVIN, F. R. *Violence and the Brain.* New York: Harper & Row, 1970.

139. MARK, V. H., SWEET, W., and ERVIN, F. R. "Deep Temporal Lobe Stimulation and Destructive Lesions in Episodically Violent Temporal Lobe Epileptics," in W. S. Fields and W. H. Sweet, eds., *Neural Bases of Violence and Aggression.* St. Louis: Warren H. Green, 1975, pp. 379–391.

140. MARTORANO, J. T. "Target Symptoms in Lithium Carbonate Therapy," *Comprehensive Psychiatry,* 13 (1972):533–537.

141. MAXSON, S. C. "The Genetics of Aggression in Vertebrates," in P. F. Brain and

D. Benton, eds., *The Biology of Aggression.* Alphen aan den Rijn, The Netherlands: Sijthoff and Noordhoff, 1981, pp. 69–104.

142. MEDVEDEV, Z. A., and MEDVEDEV, R. A. *A Question of Madness.* New York: Knopf, 1971.

143. MEYER-BAHLBURG, H. F. L. "Sex Chromosomes and Aggression in Humans," in P. F. Brain and D. Benton, eds., *The Biology of Aggression.* Alphen aan den Rijn, The Netherlands: Sijthoff and Noordhoff, 1981, pp. 109–123.

144. MEYER-BAHLBURG, H.F.L., et al. "Aggressiveness and Testosterone Measures in Man," *Psychosomatic Medicine,* 36 (1974):269–274.

145. MICZEK, K. A., and BARRY, H. "Pharmacology of Sex and Aggression," in S. D. Glick, and J. Goldfarb, eds., *Behavioral Pharmacology.* St. Louis: Mosby, 1976, pp. 176–257.

146. MICZEK, K. A., and KRISIAK, M. "Pharmacological Analysis of Attack and Flight," in P. F. Brain and D. Benton, eds., *Multidisciplinary Approaches to Aggression Research.* Amsterdam: Elsevier, 1981, pp. 341–354.

147. MONAHAN, J. *The Clinical Prediction of Violent Behavior.* DHHS Pub. No. (ADM) 81–921, Washington D.C.: U.S. Government Printing Office, 1980.

148. MONEY, J. "Use of an Androgen-Depleting Hormone in the Treatment of Male Sex Offenders," *Journal of Sex Research,* 6 (1970):165–172.

149. MONEY, J., and EHRHARDT, A. "Gender Dimorphic Behavior and Fetal Sex Hormones," *Recent Progress in Hormone Research,* 28 (1972):735–754.

150. MONROE, R. *Episodic Behavioral Disorders.* Cambridge, Mass.: Harvard University Press, 1970.

151. ———. "Anticonvulsants in the Treatment of Aggression," *Journal of Nervous and Mental Disease,* 160 (1975):119–126.

152. MONTI, P. M., BROWN, W. A., and CORRIVEAU, D. P. "Testosterone and Components of Aggressive and Sexual Behavior in Man," *American Journal of Psychiatry,* 134 (1977):692–694.

153. MORAND, C., YOUNG, S. N., and ERVIN, F. R. "Clinical Response of Aggressive Schizophrenics to Oral Tryptophan," *Biological Psychiatry,* 18 (1983):575–578.

154. MOYER, K. E. "Kinds of Aggression and Their Physiological Basis," *Communications in Behavioral Biology* (Part A), 2 (1968):65–87.

155. NADORNICK, P., POGADY, J., and SRAMKA, M. "The Results of Stereotaxic Treatment of the Aggressive Syndrome," in L. Laitinen and K. E. Livingston, eds., *Surgical Approaches in Psychiatry.* Baltimore: University Park Press, 1973, pp. 125–128.

156. NARABAYASKI, H., et al. "Stereotaxic Amygdalotomy for Behavior Disorders," *Archives of Neurology,* 9 (1963): 1–16.

157. NEPPE, V. M. "Carbamazepine in the Psychiatric Patient," *Lancet,* 2 (1982):334.

158. O'CONNOR, M., and BAKER, H.W.G. "Depo-Medroxy Progesterone Acetate as an Adjunctive Treatment in Three Aggressive Schizophrenic Patients," *Acta Psychiatrica Scandinavica,* 67 (1983):399–403.

159. OLIVIER, B., et al. "Behavioral Effects of Psychoactive Drugs on Agonistic Behavior of Male Territorial Rats (Resident-Intruder Model)," in K. A. Miczek, M. R. Kruk, and B. Olivier, eds., *Ethopharmacological Aggression Research.* New York: Alan R. Liss, 1984, pp. 137–156.

160. O'REILLY, J. "Wife Beating: The Silent Crime," *Time,* 5 September 1983, pp. 23–26.

161. ORENBERG, E. K., et al. "Genetic Determination of Aggressive Behavior and Brain Cyclic AMP," *Psychopharmacology Communications,* 1 (1975):99–107.

162. PERSKY, H., SMITH, K. D., and BASU, G. K. "Relation of Psychologic Measures of Aggression and Hostility to Testosterone Production in Man," *Psychosomatic Medicine,* 33 (1971):265–267.

163. PETRIE, W. M., and BAN, T. A. "Propranolol in Organic Agitation," *Lancet,* 1 (1981):324.

164. PODOBNIKAR, I. G. "Implementation of Psychotherapy by Librium in a Pioneering Rural-Industrial Psychiatric Practice," *Psychosomatics,* 12 (1971):205–209.

165. POWELL, D. A., MILLIGAN, W. L., and

WALTERS, K. "The Effects of Muscarinic Cholinergic Blockade Upon Shock-Elicited Aggression," *Pharmacology Biochemistry and Behavior*, 1 (1973):389–394.

166. PUGLISI-ALLEGRA, S., and MANDEL, P. "Effects of Sodium N-Diprophlacetate, Muscimol Hydrobromide and (R.S.) Nipecotic Acid Amide on Isolation-Induced Aggressive Behavior in Mice," *Psychopharmacology*, 70 (1980):287–290.

167. PUGLISI-ALLEGRA, S., et al. "Involvement of the GABAergic System on Shock-Induced Aggressive Behavior in Two Strains of Mice," *Pharmacology Biochemistry and Behavior*, 14 (Supplement 1) (1981):13–18.

168. RADA, R. T., and DONLON, P. T. "Piperacetazine vs. Thioridazine for the Control of Schizophrenia in Outpatients," *Psychosomatics*, 13 (1972):373–376.

169. RALEIGH, M. J., et al. "Social and Environmental Influences on Blood Serotonin Concentrations in Monkeys," *Archives of General Psychiatry*, 41 (1984):405–410.

170. RAMPLING, D. "Aggression: A Paradoxical Response to Tricyclic Antidepressants," *American Journal of Psychiatry*, 135 (1978):117–118.

171. RANDALL, L. O., et al. "The Psychosedative Properties of Methaminodiazepoxide," *Journal of Pharmacology and Experimental Therapeutics*, 129 (1960): 163–171.

172. REEVES, A. G., and PLUM, F. "Hyperphagia, Rage, and Dementia Accompanying a Ventromedial Hypothalamic Neoplasm," *Archives of Neurology*, 20 (1969):616–624.

173. REIS, D. J. "The Relationship Between Brain Norepinephrine and Aggressive Behavior," *Research Publications of the Association for Research in Nervous and Mental Disease*, 50 (1972):266–297.

174. ———. "Central Neurotransmitters in Aggression," *Research Publications of the Association for Research in Nervous and Mental Disease*, 52 (1974):119–148.

175. REIS, D. J., and FUXE, K. "Brain Norepinephrine: Evidence that Neuronal Release Is Essential for Sham Rage Behavior Following Brainstem Transection in Cat," *Proceedings of the National Academy of Sciences USA*, 64 (1969):108–112.

176. RESNICK, O. "The Psychoactive Properties of Diphenylhydantoin: Experiences with Prisoners and Juvenile Delinquents," *International Journal of Neuropsychiatry*, 3 (1967):530–547.

177. RODGERS, R. J., and BROWN, K. "Amygdaloid Function in the Central Cholinergic Mediation of Shock-Induced Aggression in the Rat," *Aggressive Behavior*, 2 (1976):131–152.

178. RODIN, E. "Psychomotor Epilepsy and Aggressive Behavior," *Archives of General Psychiatry*, 28 (1973):210–213.

179. ROPARTZ, P. "The Relation Between Olfactory Stimulation and Aggressive Behaviour in Mice," *Animal Behaviour*, 16 (1968):97–100.

180. ROSENBLATT, S., SCHAEFFER, D., and ROSENTHAL, J. S. "Effects of Diphenylhydantoin on Child-Abusing Parents: A Preliminary Report," *Current Therapeutic Research*, 19 (1976):332–336.

181. ST. JEAN, A., et al. "Clinical Studies with Propericiazine (R.P. 8909)," *Diseases of the Nervous System*, 28 (1967):526–531.

182. SALZMAN, C. Personal communication, 1984.

183. SALZMAN, C., VANDERKOLK, B. A., and SHADER, R. I. "Marijuana and Hostility in a Small Group Setting," *American Journal of Psychiatry*, 133 (1976):1029–1033.

184. SANDLER, M., et al. "Phenylethylamine in Human Aggressive Behavior," in M. Sandler, ed., *Psychopharmacology of Aggression*. New York: Raven Press, 1979, pp. 149–158.

185. SANGDEE, C., and FRANZ, D. N. "Lithium Enhancement of Central 5-HT Transmission Induced by 5-HT Precursors," *Biological Psychiatry*, 15 (1980):59–75.

186. SANO, K., et al. "Results of Stimulation and Destruction of the Posterior Hypothalamus in Man," *Journal of Neurosurgery*, 33 (1970):689–707.

187. SCHIFF, H. B., et al. "Lithium in Aggressive Behavior," *American Journal of Psychiatry*, 139 (1982):1346–1348.

188. SCHREINER, L., and KLING, A. "Behavioral Changes Following Rhinence-

phalic Injury in the Cat," *Journal of Neurophysiology*, 16 (1953):643–659.

189. SCOTT, J. P., and FULLER, J. L. *The Genetics and Social Behavior of the Dog*. Chicago: University of Chicago Press, 1965.

190. SELMANOFF, M. K., et al. "Correlated Effects of the Y-Chromosome of Mice on Developmental Changes in Testosterone Levels of Intermale Aggression," *Life Sciences*, 20 (1977):359–365.

191. SENAULT, B. "Comportement D'Agressivite Intraspecific Induit Par L'Apomorphine Chez le Rat," *Psychopharmacologia*, 18 (1970):271–287.

192. SHADER, R. I., JACKSON, A. H., and DODES, L. M. "The Antiaggressive Effects of Lithium in Man," *Psychopharmacologia*, 40 (1974):17–24.

193. SHEARD, M. H. "Effect of Lithium on Footshock Aggression in Rats," *Nature*, 228 (1970):284–285.

194. ———. "Effect of Lithium on Human Aggression," *Nature*, 230 (1971):113–114.

195. ———. "Lithium in the Treatment of Aggression," *Journal of Nervous and Mental Disease*, 160 (1975):108–118.

196. ———. "The Role of Drugs Affecting Catecholamines on Shock-Elicited Fighting in Rats," in E. Usdin, ed., *Catecholamines: Basic and Clinical Frontiers*. New York: Pergamon Press, 1979, pp. 1690–1692.

197. SHEARD, M. H., et al. "The Effect of Lithium on Impulsive Aggressive Behavior in Man," *American Journal of Psychiatry*, 133 (1976):1409–1413.

198. SHEPPARD, G. P. "High Dose Propranolol in Schizophrenia," *British Journal of Psychiatry*, 134 (1979):470–476.

199. SIMOPOULIS, A. M., et al. "Diphenylhydantoin Effectiveness in Treatment of Chronic Schizophrenics," *Archives of General Psychiatry*, 30 (1974):106–111.

200. SMITH, D. E., KING, M. B., and HOEBEL, B. G. "Lateral Hypothalamic Control of Killing: Evidence for a Cholinoceptive Mechanism," *Science*, 167 (1970):900–901.

201. SOFIA, R. D. "Effects of Centrally Active Drugs on Four Models of Experimentally-Induced Aggression in Rodents," *Life Sciences*, 8 (1969):705–716.

202. SOULAIRAC, A., LAMBINET, H., and AYMARD, N. "Action du Précurseur de la Sérotonine, le 5-Hydroxy-Tryptophane sur la Symptomatologie Agressive," *Annales Médico Psychologiques*, 2 (1976):459–463.

203. SOUTHWICK, C. H., and CLARK, L. H. "Interstrain Differences in Aggressive Behavior and Exploratory Activity of Inbred Mice," *Communications in Behavioral Biology*, 1 (1968):49–59.

204. STEPHENS, J. H., and SHAFFER, J. W. "A Controlled Study of the Effects of Diphenylhydantoin on Anxiety, Irritability and Anger in Neurotic Outpatients," *Pharmacologia*, 17 (1970):169–181.

205. STOLK, J., CONNER, R., and BARCHAS, J. "Rubidium-Induced Increase in Shock-Elicited Aggression in Rats," *Psychopharmacologia*, 22 (1971):250–260.

206. STOLK, J. M., et al. "Brain Norepinephrine: Enhanced Turnover After Rubidium Treatment," *Science*, 168 (1970):501–503.

207. STOLK, J. M., et al. "Brain Norepinephrine Metabolism and Shock-Induced Fighting Behavior in Rats: Differential Effects of Shock and Fighting on the Neurochemical Response to a Common Footshock Stimulus," *Journal of Pharmacology and Experimental Therapeutics*, 190 (1974):193–209.

208. STRINGER, A. Y., and JOSEF, N. C. "Methylphenidate in the Treatment of Aggression in Two Patients with Antisocial Personality Disorder," *American Journal of Psychiatry*, 140 (1983):1365–1366.

209. SUGARMAN, A. A., WILLIAMS, B. H., and ADLERSTEIN, A. M. "Haloperidol in the Psychiatric Disorders of Old Age," *American Journal of Psychiatry*, 120 (1964):1190–1192.

210. SWEET, W. H., ERVIN, F. R., and MARK, V. H. "The Relationship of Violent Behaviour to Focal Cerebral Disease," in S. Garattini and E. B. Sigg, eds., *Aggressive Behaviour*. Amsterdam: Excerpta Medica, 1969, pp. 336–352.

211. TAYLOR, S. P., et al., "The Effects of Alcohol and Δ^9- Tetrahydrocannabinol on Human Physical Aggression," *Aggressive Behavior*, 2 (1976):153–161.

212. THOA, N. B., EICHELMAN, B., and NG, K. Y. "Shock-induced Aggression: Effects of 6-Hydroxydopamine and Other

Pharmacologic Agents," *Brain Research,* 43 (1972):467–475.

213. THOA, N. B., et al. "6-Hydroxydopa Depletion of Brain Norepinephrine and the Facilitation of Aggressive Behavior," *Science,* 178 (1972):75–77.

214. TOBIN, J. M., BIRD, I. F., and BOYLE, D. F. "Preliminary Evaluation of Librium (Ro50690) in the Treatment of Anxiety Reactions," *Diseases of the Nervous System,* 21 (1960):11–19.

215. TUNKS, E. R., and DERMER, S. W. "Carbamazepine in the Dyscontrol Syndrome Associated with Limbic Dysfunction," *Journal of Nervous and Mental Disease,* 164 (1977):56–63.

216. TUPIN, J. P. "Management of Violent Patients," in R. I. Shader, ed., *Manual of Psychiatric Therapeutics.* Boston: Little, Brown, 1975, pp. 125–136.

217. TUPIN, J. P., et al. "The Long-term Use of Lithium in Aggressive Prisoners," *Comprehensive Psychiatry,* 14 (1973):311–317.

218. TURNER, W. J. "The Usefulness of Diphenylhydantoin in Treatment of Nonepileptic Emotional Disorders," *International Journal of Neuropsychiatry,* 3 (Supplement 2) (1967):8–20.

219. ULRICH, R. E., and AZRIN, N. H. "Reflexive Fighting in Response to Aversive Stimulation," *Journal of the Experimental Analysis of Behavior,* 5 (1962):511–520.

220. VALZELLI, L. "Aggressive Behaviour Induced by Isolation," in S. Garattini and E. B. Sigg, eds., *Aggressive Behaviour.* Amsterdam: Excerpta Medica, 1969, pp. 70–76.

221. ———. "Activity of Benzodiazepines on Aggressive Behavior in Rats and Mice," in S. Garattini, E. Mussini, and L. O. Randall, eds., *The Benzodiazepines.* New York: Raven Press, 1973, pp. 405–417.

222. ———. "Effects of Sedatives and Anxiolytics on Aggressivity," in L. Valzelli, ed., *Modern Problems of Pharmacopsychiatry,* vol. 14. Basel: Karger, 1979, pp. 143–156.

223. VERGNES, M., MACK, G., and KEMPF, E. "Lésions du Raphé et Réaction D'Agression Interspécifique Rat-Souris. Effets Comportementaux et Bio-

chimiques," *Brain Research,* 57 (1973): 67–74.

224. VIRKKUNEN, M. "Reactive Hypoglycemia Tendency Among Habitually Violent Offenders: A Further Study by Means of the Glucose Tolerance Test," *Neuropsychobiology,* 8 (1982):35–40.

225. ———. "Insulin Secretion During the Glucose Tolerance Test in Antisocial Personality," *British Journal of Psychiatry,* 142 (1983):598–604.

226. VIRKKUNEN, M., and PENTTINEN, H. "Serum Cholesterol in Aggressive Conduct Disorder: A Preliminary Study," *Biological Psychiatry,* 19 (1984):435–439.

227. *Vital Statistics Report (Final Data),* vol. 33, suppl. 22 June 1984, p. 27, table 8.

228. WASMAN, M., and FLYNN, J. P. "Directed Attack Elicited from Hypothalamus," *Archives of Neurology,* 6 (1962):220–227.

229. WEISCHER, M. L. "Über die Antiaggressive Wirkung von Lithium," *Psychopharmacologia,* 15 (1969):245–254.

230. WELCH, B. L., and WELCH, A. S. "Greater Lowering of Brain and Adrenal Catecholamines in Group-Housed than in Individually Housed Mice Administered DL Alpha-Methyl-Tyrosine," *Journal of Pharmacy and Pharmacology,* 20 (1968):244–246.

231. WENDER, P. "The Minimal Brain Dysfunction Syndrome in Children," *Journal of Nervous and Mental Disease,* 155 (1972):55–71.

232. WHEATLEY, M. D. "The Hypothalamus and Affective Behavior in Cats: A Study of the Effects of Experimental Lesions with Anatomic Correlations," *Archives of Neurology and Psychiatry,* 52 (1944): 296–316.

233. WHITEHEAD, P. L., and CLARK, L. D. "Effect of Lithium Carbonate, Placebo, and Thioridazine on Hyperactive Children," *American Journal of Psychiatry,* 127 (1970):824–825.

234. WILLIAMS, D. "Neural Factors Related to Habitual Aggression," *Brain,* 92 (1969): 503–520.

235. WILLIAMS, D. T., et al. "The Effect of Propranolol on Uncontrolled Rage Outbursts in Children and Adolescents with Organic Brain Dysfunction," *Journal of*

the American Academy of Child Psychiatry, 21 (1982):129–135.

236. WINSLOW, J. T., and MICZEK, K. A. "Social Status as Determinant of Alcohol Effects on Aggressive Behavior in Squirrel Monkeys (Saimiri sciureus)," *Psychopharmacology*, in press.

237. WITKIN, H. A., et al. "Criminality in XYY and XXY Men," *Science*, 193 (1976):547–555.

238. WORRALL, E. P., MOODY, J. P., and NAYLOR, G. J. "Lithium in Non-Manic Depressives: Antiaggressive Effect and Red Blood Cell Lithium Values," *British Journal of Psychiatry*, 126 (1975): 464–468.

239. YALOM, I. D., GREEN, R., and FISK, N. "Prenatal Exposure to Female Hormones," *Archives of General Psychiatry*, 28 (1973):554–561.

240. YARYURA-TOBIAS, J. A., and NEZIROGLU, F. A. "Aggressive Behavior, Clinical Interfaces," in L. Valzelli and L. Morgese, eds., *Aggression and Violence: A Psychobiological and Clinical Approach*. St. Vincent, Italy: Centro Culturale, 1981, pp. 195–210.

241. YEN, C. Y., STANGER, R. L., and MILLMAN, N. "Ataractic Suppression of Isolation-Induced Aggressive Behavior," *Archives Internationales de Pharmacodynamie*, 123 (1959):179–185.

242. YORKSTON, N. J., et al. "Propranolol as an Adjunct to the Treatment of Schizophrenia," *Lancet*, 2 (1977):575–578.

243. YUDOFSKY, S., WILLIAMS, D., and GORMAN, J. "Propranolol in the Treatment of Rage and Violent Behavior in Patients with Chronic Brain Syndromes," *American Journal of Psychiatry*, 138 (1981):218–220.

244. YUDOFSKY, S., et al. "Propranolol in the Treatment of Rage and Violent Behavior Associated with Korsakoff's Psychosis," *American Journal of Psychiatry*, 141 (1984):114–115.

CHAPTER 25

THE BIOLOGY AND EXPERIMENTAL TREATMENT OF ALZHEIMER'S DISEASE

Celeste A. Johns and Kenneth L. Davis

¶ Introduction

Senile dementia affects approximately 4.4 percent of the 25 million Americans over the age of 65.[147,192] By far the most common form is senile dementia of the Alzheimer's type; as many as 70 to 80 percent of autopsied brains from demented patients beyond age sixty-five have characteristic histopathological changes of Alzheimer's disease, although 20 percent may also have changes consistent with vascular dementias.[57,157,248] As the proportion of the population in the United States sixty-five years and older is increasing, this major mental health problem will reach epidemic proportions. At present, the disease cannot be arrested or reversed, nor can it be definitively diagnosed prior to death. However, current studies to elucidate the histological and biochemical abnormalities that are the pathological hallmarks of Alzheimer's disease suggest rational approaches for research

attempting to facilitate diagnosis and treatment.

Alzheimer's disease has traditionally been defined as a progressive dementing illness with a presenile onset. Patients with a similar process whose illness begins to manifest itself clinically after age sixty-four have been diagnosed as senile dementia of the Alzheimer type. Since the work of many neuropathologists in the 1950s and 1960s[247,248] found that neuropathological changes in patients dying with dementia that started after age sixty-four are indistinguishable from those in cases of classical presenile Alzheimer's disease, most investigators have decided to treat Alzheimer's disease (AD) and senile dementia of the Alzheimer type as a single entity.

However, recent work suggests that there may be subtypes of AD that are biologically and behaviorally distinct. One line of evidence is the genetic work of Heston and colleagues[132,133] demonstrating that autopsy-confirmed cases with an apparent familial linkage are much more likely to have presenile onset than nonfamilial cases. Neurochemical work also suggests that early-onset cases may be distinct, since such cases are more likely to have a loss of noradrenergic cells of the locus coeruleus along with the more universal finding of a loss of cholinergic cells.[24,62,274] Cognitive studies also suggest possible subtypes. For example, agraphia was found to identify patients most likely to have a family history of AD[99,100] from among a large number of AD patients. Similarly, patients with presenile onset, determined by history, seem more likely to have agraphia and severe language disturbance than patients who meet similar diagnostic criteria but who by clinical history have a later onset.[222] Finally, it is worth noting that at least one large series found differential distribution and concentrations of senile plaques and tangles in patients with presenile versus senile onset.[114]

AD is characterized clinically by an insidious onset of memory impairment that begins in middle or late life and progresses relentlessly, usually over a five- to seven-year period, to a state of profound dementia. The early memory deficit is specifically a difficulty in recording and retrieving recent facts and experiences, while long-term memory and very short-term recall remain intact. Patients may appear to have a deterioration in the ability to reason, infer, and think abstractly. This is followed by progressive aphasia, apraxia, and agnosia. Afflicted individuals will simultaneously manifest deterioration of self-care, uncharacteristic emotional lability or blunting, and impairment of social adjustment. Paranoid ideation, agitation, sleep disturbance, and depressive symptoms may occur. Neurological signs, such as sucking and snout reflexes and gegenhalten, palmomental, grasp, and corneomandibular reflexes, have been frequently reported in the later stages of AD, but none is pathognomonic for the disease. Ultimately, motor disturbances and incontinence develop, and a terminal vegetative state precedes a premature death.[55,214,224]

On macroscopic examination, AD brains show nonspecific ventricular dilation and cortical atrophy with widening of the sulci. Microscopic examination reveals characteristic lesions on which the diagnosis of AD is based: neurofibrillary tangles, neuritic plaques, and granulovacuolar degeneration of neurons. These pathological hallmarks of AD are concentrated in the hippocampus and cortex[141] and correlate quantitatively with severity of dementia.[22,264] Neurofibrillary tangles are twisted helical protein filaments and are indicative of disrupted distal axonal transport. Plaques appear to be the condensation of degenerated distal neuronal elements surrounded by microglia, astrocytes, and perivascular amyloid. Histological studies of evolving plaques have revealed that immature plaques contain acetylcholinesterase (AChE)-rich dystrophic axons, which disappear as the plaques condense with age,[236] suggesting that some plaques are the end products of degenerated cholinergic nerve axons. While neither plaques nor tangles are found exclusively in AD brains, a large concentration of both changes in the brain of a demented individual is diagnostic of AD.

The etiology of the dramatic intra- and extracellular neuronal pathology that characterizes AD is currently being sought on a molecular level. *In vitro* studies suggesting that messenger ribonucleic acid (RNA)–directed protein synthesis declines in AD brains[221] are consistent with positron emission tomography (PET) studies that showed decreased incorporation of methionine into brain protein of AD patients.[38,39] Quantification of cortical RNA levels and associated ribonuclease activity has been conducted, and a decrease of total cellular RNA and polyadenylated messenger RNA has been demonstrated in conjunction with increased ribonuclease activity.[220] This provocative finding suggests that the neurotransmitter and cellular abnormalities that characterize AD are associated with decreased inhibition of cortical ribonuclease activity and resultant increases of RNA degradation and decreased protein synthesis, although it is not yet clear whether this observation is an etiological factor in AD or another manifestation of an as-yet unknown disease process.

The Neurochemistry of Alzheimer's Disease

In numerous investigations of neurotransmitters, multiple central nervous system (CNS) dysfunctions have been identified in AD, including changes in the concentration of norepinephrine (NE), serotonin (5HT), dopamine (DA), gamma-aminobutyric acid (GABA), and various neuropeptides. However, data on these systems are somewhat contradictory and, with some exceptions, inconclusive. The most consistent finding in AD is a major disruption of the cholinergic system, which has led to the development of a cholinergic hypothesis of AD. Practical developments of this hypothesis have been the exploration of peripheral markers of central cholinergic activity to establish clinical diagnostic tests for AD and treatment trials of agents that may selectively enhance cholinergic transmission.

A review of the biochemical evidence that led to the development of the cholinergic hypothesis necessitates the clarification of a reasoning process whereby the etiological significance of observed neurotransmitter deficiencies can be evaluated. Thus the following criteria for etiological significance provide a framework for a critical review of the currently available neurochemical data[120]:

1. At least one of the histopathological changes characteristic of AD should correlate positively with the degree of neurotransmitter deficit.
2. The neurotransmitter abnormality should lie in a brain substrate that primarily subserves learning and memory functions.
3. The extent of neurotransmitter deficit should correlate with performance on psychological tests by persons with AD.
4. Pharmacologically induced reduction in activity of the neurotransmitter should produce some of the symptoms of AD.
5. The pharmacologically induced enhancement of the neurotransmitter's activity should improve some aspects of memory functioning in normal persons or patients with AD.

The significance of the major neurotransmitter postmortem findings in AD brains are evaluated in the light of these criteria in the following sections.

Serotonin

Assessments of serotonergic neurotransmission in several autopsy series* have reported some diminution of serotonergic activity in AD brains, with deficiencies most pronounced in the temporal lobe. This reduction, however, has not been shown to relate closely to cognitive impairment as measured by the Blessed test of memory and information.[63] Furthermore, evidence from other studies that would satisfy the aforementioned criteria is lacking. Drugs that diminish serotonergic activity, such as cyproheptadine, methysergide, and cinanserin, are not reported to produce symptoms characteristic of AD. Similarly, neither precursors, reuptake blockers of 5HT, nor monoamine oxidase inhibitors appear to enhance learning and memory. Nevertheless, since many of these drugs have complex effects on brain activity, studies of the cognitive and behavioral effects of selective manipulation of serotonergic neurotransmission are required in order to clarify the role of this neurotransmitter deficiency in AD.

Gamma-aminobutyric Acid

Various components of GABA neurotransmission have been investigated in patients with AD. These include measurements of the activity of the synthesizing enzyme glutamic acid decarboxylase (GAD),† free hippocampal[241] and cortical[184,206,212] GABA, and GABA receptor binding.[29,200] While GAD activity was decreased in most studies of the midbrain, hippocampus, and cortex, the significance of this finding is confounded by the demonstration that GAD activity is dependent on the agonal state of the patient.[261] GABA receptor binding studies have been

*See references 30, 45, 63, 118, and 119.
†See references 27, 28, 67, 68, 180, and 233.

equivocal. Cortical GABA concentration declines significantly with age,[210,234] but whether a further decrement occurs in AD remains controversial.

One explanation for these contradictory results was found when autopsied AD brains were divided into two groups based on age of death; brains from AD patients who died before age seventy-nine had significantly lower concentrations of GABA in the frontal and temporal cortices than did controls, while cortices from older AD patients did not differ from non-AD autopsied specimens in this respect.[212] Thus any pathophysiological role for diminished GABA neurotransmission in AD requires further clarification, with careful attention paid to the age of patients at the time of autopsy.

Dopamine

Measurements of DA, of DA receptor binding, and of the DA metabolite homovanillic acid (HVA) have been assessed in AD brains with contradictory results.* While some areas of the brain have been reported to have decrements in at least one marker of the DA neurotransmitter system, the majority of careful histopathologically diagnosed studies suggest that the DA system is spared in AD. Pharmacological studies likewise offer little support for an involvement of DA in AD. Studies of the effect of levodopa on AD patients found no improvement of symptoms[86,151,252] and bromocriptyline, a post-synaptic DA agonist, similarly failed to improve cognition in AD patients.[191] Cognitive processes are not demonstrably enhanced by drugs that increase dopaminergic activity, and neuroleptics, which are potent dopaminergic receptor blocking agents, do not induce symptoms that resemble AD.

Norepinephrine

Numerous studies indicate that there is an abnormality of noradrenergic activity in the brain areas involved in learning and memory in at least a subgroup of patients with AD. The most consistent finding in this avenue of investigation is a loss of neurons in the locus coeruleus,* a finding of particular importance because this region has been implicated in the function of memory.[193,276] While this cell loss was not quantitatively related to scores on mental status examination in one investigation,[249] another study that compared older AD patients to younger patients with significantly greater cognitive impairment found increased cell loss in the younger patients.[24]

The preponderance of neurochemical studies of the noradrenergic system in AD brains have demonstrated decreased NE content in the hypothalamus, caudate nucleus, and cerebral cortex[2,158] and decreased dopamine-beta-hydroxylase activity in cerebral cortex.[62] This has been contradicted, however, by an investigation in which AD patients were stratified based on the severity of dementia. Plasma and cerebrospinal fluid (CSF) NE and 3-methoxy-4-hydroxyphenylglycol (MHPG) were found to be significantly higher in the group of patients with severe dementia than in either the group of normal controls or subjects with moderately advanced AD, while these two measures did not differentiate moderately severe AD patients from normal controls.[198] Elevated brain MHPG content had been reported by an earlier study that did not, however, find associated increases of NE,[267] and other CSF analyses have confirmed that MHPG levels do not differ significantly between moderately demented AD subjects and normal controls.[160,269] Furthermore, no correlation between noradrenergic activity and clinical severity of dementia as measured by the Blessed scale has been found.[183] It is conceivable that noradrenergic abnormalities are more closely linked to noncognitive symptoms of AD, such as pacing, agitation, or depression. The role of the observed locus coeruleus deficit is difficult to incorporate into

*See references 2, 46, 63, 119, 159, 200, and 273.

*See references 24, 102, 103, 159, and 249.

this model of AD; the neurohistological and neurochemical findings may in fact be independent variables operating in different subgroups of AD patients.

Pharmacological evidence for a relationship between the noradrenergic abnormalities and clinical symptomatology in AD is not convincing at this time. Clinical trials of drugs that augment noradrenergic activity in normals and AD patients have not shown enhancement of learning or memory. Methamphetamine does affect learning and memory, but this has been attributed to a generalized facilitation of attention and arousal rather than to a direct effect on encoding or retrieval from memory stores.[163] Methylphenidate had no effect on cognitive functions in a mixed group of cognitively impaired elderly.[61]

There have been few controlled studies designed to evaluate whether cognitive deficits are produced by drugs that diminish central noradrenergic activity, although this class of compound is widely used in the treatment of hypertension. Animal studies have indicated that learning and memory may be impaired by these drugs,* but with the exception of anecdotal accounts,[1,93,112] only one such investigation has been reported in humans.[231] Both the noradrenergic blocker methyldopa and the specific beta-NE-blocking agent propranolol hydrochloride were found to significantly impair both immediate and delayed verbal memory, as well as verbal recall, in both hypertensive and normotensive adults, while visual memory remained intact. This finding suggested that demonstrated abnormalities of the noradrenergic system in AD may have a role in producing cognitive symptoms; however, further biological analyses and investigations of specific cognitive task responses to noradrenergic blockade, as well as investigation of possible interactions between the noradrenergic and cholinergic systems, are required to elucidate the extent and contribution of noradrenergic system disruption in AD.

Neuropeptides

Neuropeptides coexist with and serve to potentiate the action of neurotransmitters in some neurons[135] and may themselves act as neurotransmitters in some brain areas. The significance of their action as neuromodulators is underscored by one study,[154] done in cat submandibular glands, in which vasoactive intestinal polypeptide (VIP) released with acetylcholine (ACh) increased ACh-induced salivary secretion. The mechanism for this action was a VIP-induced 10^5-fold enhancement of muscarinic receptor affinity for ACh.[154]

The concentrations of a number of neuropeptides, including somatostatin, VIP, cholecystokinin, arginine vasopressin, and substance P, have been measured in autopsied brains of AD patients and, with the exception of somatostatin, have not been found to differ from normal levels.* Somatostatin levels, however, are significantly reduced in the hippocampus and cortex of AD patients, and the degree of reduction appears to parallel decreases in cholinergic markers in these brain areas.[17,69,208,212] A recent finding has added considerable strength to the hypothesis that somatostatin may be closely involved with cholinergic neurons. AChE and somatostatin immunoreactivity in cortical neurons of the rat were found to coexist.[80]

Despite the close correlation of decreased somatostatin levels and cholinergic markers in AD and the coexistence of somatostatin and AchE in the rat cerebrum, there is substantial evidence from animal studies that lesions of the nucleus basalis of Meynert (nbM) and medial septum lead to the depletion of cholinergic markers without affecting cortical and hippocampal somatostatin levels.[156] One possible interpretation of these seemingly conflicting results is that somatostatin may be only intimately involved with cholinergic cells that are intrinsic to the cortex and hippocampus. Although the central and behavioral effects of

*See references 25, 82, 98, 127, 195, 196, and 202.

*See references 182, 185, 207, 208, 209, and 275.

somatostatin are not well understood, it is clear that its involvement in AD and its possible role and interaction with central cholinergic function and behavior need to be studied in detail.

One reason for the paucity of experimental data on the role of somatostatin in behavior has been the absence of specific pharmacological tools for manipulating central somatostatin levels. Recently a number of reports have shown that the systemic administration of cysteamine results in the relatively specific partial depletion of somatostatin from central pools.[176,219] The mechanism of action of cysteamine is not understood; however, it has been shown that cysteamine, when administered systemically, results in 40 to 60 percent depletion of somatostatin in a variety of central sites, including the cerebral cortex, hypothalamus, striatum, and pons, within two to four hours of administration.[219] The central effect of cysteamine is not permanent, as somatostatin levels return to normal within one to seven days depending on the region sampled. These effects may be relatively selective, affecting somatostatin levels but not the levels of a variety of other neuropeptides such as luteinizing hormone–releasing hormone (LHRH), vasopressin, enkephalin, VIP, and cholecystokinin[176]; however, the effects of cysteamine on neurotransmitters such as ACh, the catecholamines, and the indoleamines have not yet been established. Thus cysteamine may be a useful tool for the investigation of the role of somatostatin in the CNS. Haroutunian has reported in preliminary unpublished results in rats treated with cysteamine that somatostatin may play a role in memory processes, as cysteamine-induced somatostatin depletion led to a marked and significant deficit in the retention of a passive avoidance task.

Further investigations of neuropeptide deficits and of the complex interactions of this class of compounds with classical neurotransmitter systems will be essential to the understanding of the pathophysiological basis of AD.

Acetylcholine

The most consistent and persuasive evidence of a significant neurotransmitter deficit in AD is found in studies of the cholinergic system. Choline acetyl transferase (CAT), the enzyme that mediates the synthesis of ACh from its precursors, is localized in cholinergic neurons and serves as a marker for these neurons in histological studies. The activity of this enzyme is consistently and markedly reduced in the hippocampus and cortex of AD brains.* As these brain areas have been linked to learning and memory, a functional significance for this deficit in AD is suggested. Furthermore, the CAT deficit is quantitatively correlated to both plaque number and severity of dementia,[181,182,265] although the CAT abnormality may in fact precede the development of plaques and may be more closely related to cognitive impairment than plaque number.[182]

This decrease of CAT activity is likely to be due, in part, to selective degeneration of cholinergic neurons that originate in the nbM. Large AChE-rich neuronal bodies in the nbM project widely to the cerebral cortex, and similar neurons in the adjacent diagonal band of Broca and medial septum project to the hippocampus,[94,144,162,258] providing the major source of extrinsic cholinergic input to these areas. A decrease of up to 80 percent of these neurons has been demonstrated in the nbM of AD patients,[58,186,262] and cells in the medial septum and diagonal band are also subject to degeneration in AD.[58,186] This neuronal loss, however, may not be as extensive in senile-onset AD patients as it is in patients with a presenile onset, despite severe reductions of cortical CAT activity in both groups.[186,240]

These data have led to the suggestion that the cortex may be the site of the primary degenerative process in AD, with secondary axonal damage, retrograde neuronal degeneration, and dropout of cell bodies in subcortical nuclei. Regardless of the pathological mechanism, the histological and neuro-

---

*See references 7, 30, 68, 178, 184, 200, 211, and 261.

chemical data strongly suggest that a selective loss of cholinergic neurons in the nbM is a major, specific pathological feature of AD.

Detailed histological study of the hippocampus in AD brains is further characterizing specific neuronal losses in AD.[138] Input and output of the hippocampus is formed by axons that arise from discrete cell populations, namely layers II, III, and IV of the entorhinal cortex and the subiculum plus the adjacent CA1 pyramids. Marked cell loss has been identified in the subiculum and CA1 pyramids, as well as in layers II and IV of the entorhinal cortex in AD brains, and significant numbers of neurofibrillary tangles have been shown to be present in these layers, while layers III, V, and VI appear to be spared both pathological findings. As layer II receives cortical input and gives rise to the major cortical afferent source for the hippocampus, disruption of this layer effectively disconnects the cerebral cortex from the hippocampus with regard to its cortical input. Likewise, the subiculum and CA1 zone are the major source of hippocampal output to the thalamus, hypothalamus, basal forebrain, amygdala, and cerebral cortex, so the described AD pathology deprives these structures of hippocampal output. The subiculum also projects to layer IV of the entorhinal cortex, which in turn projects to the basal forebrain, the anatomical site of the nbM.

These findings, coupled with current knowledge of the cholinergic deficiency and diminished cell density in the nbM, begin to more clearly define the structural abnormalities in AD brains and indicate that specific focal abnormalities can result in widespread functional pathology, such as the effective isolation of the hippocampus and resultant devastating clinical symptomatology.

In contrast to this selective decrement of presynaptic cholinergic neurons, AD brains do not differ from age-matched controls in their ability to bind muscarinic antagonists in the cortex,* which suggests that postsynaptic muscarinic cholinergic receptors are not affected in AD. Nondemented elderly brains have been found to have small but significant decreases in cortical postsynaptic muscarinic receptor binding,[177,261] and this indicates that decrements of muscarinic receptor density are no greater in AD than in normal aged brains.

The role of ACh in learning and memory has been bolstered by the results of clinical pharmacological studies. Memory enhancement in young normal subjects follows administration both of the AChE inhibitor physostigmine and arecoline, a muscarinic agonist. The component of memory that is specifically enhanced by these agents is encoding of new information beyond immediate memory (i.e., long-term memory [LTM]).[75,225] This is one aspect of cognitive function that is typically diminished in AD.[250] Physostigmine and arecoline have no effect on short-term memory (STM) or on retrieval of information from LTM.[75,225] Conversely, administration of the centrally acting anticholinergic drug scopolamine to normal young adults results in transient cognitive impairments that appear to be phenomenologically similar to those seen in elderly people showing age-related memory loss.[84] These effects are reversed by physostigmine, but not by amphetamines,[83] a fact that specifically implicates the anticholinergic action of scopolamine in impairing cognition rather than its more general sedating effects, which impair attention and alertness. Similar results have been demonstrated in nonhuman primate studies,[11,14] while pharmacological agents that block neurotransmitters other than ACh did not reproduce naturally occurring memory deficits.[13]

The effectiveness of scopolamine in reliably and safely producing a cholinergic deficit encourages its use in diverse study populations for further investigation of anticholinergic "amnesia" and its similarity to AD. This approach could help elucidate the contribution of the cholinergic deficit to the symptoms of AD. Given that ACh deficit is only one of a series of neurotransmitter abnormalities that can be present in an AD patient, the extent that a pure, pharmacologically in-

*See references 3, 26, 70, 174, 177, 179, 180, 181, 200, and 261.

duced, cholinergic deficit does or does not mimic the core symptoms of AD takes on additional significance.

There is a considerable literature on "scopolamine dementia." The amnestic properties of scopolamine in normal subjects have been tested in seventeen studies to date.* Word list learning, a subtest of verbal memory, has been the most extensively used measure in these studies and has been shown to be impaired in twenty-eight of thirty-six (78 percent) tests.[33] Word fluency, another test of verbal memory, has been employed to a lesser extent and found to be impaired slightly by relatively high doses of scopolamine.[84] However, nonverbal memory tests have been given rarely; in these few studies, performance has not been impaired by scopolamine except for the paired associate tasks[64,175] and maze-type tasks.[74,199] Thus the extent to which scopolamine dementia can serve as a model for AD has not been fully explored. Specifically, although it is clear that the drug can impair the ability of new information to enter permanent memory, anticholinergic agents' effect on language and praxis, two common symptoms in AD, has not been systematically tested.

These studies have prompted a more detailed exploration of the nature of cognitive deficits produced in young normal subjects by scopolamine.[169] Once again, scopolamine markedly impaired performance in free recall tasks; however, no effect was seen on either verbal fluency or constructional praxis ability. These results raise the possibility that substantial language and praxis impairments cannot be produced by disruption of the cholinergic system alone and that disruption of other neurotransmitter or neuromodulatory systems is necessary for these symptoms to appear. At the very least, language and praxis functions appear to be less susceptible to disruption by anticholinergics than are aspects of memory.

In summary, a large body of preclinical, animal, and human data supports the hypothesis that a cholinergic deficit is a central etiological factor in AD. The cholinergic system is the only neurotransmitter system that has been demonstrated to meet all of the previously outlined criteria for etiological significance:

1. There is a significant reduction in CAT activity in the brains of persons with histological diagnoses of AD.
2. Reduced CAT activity is found in the brain regions subserving language and memory functions.
3. The CAT reduction correlates significantly with increased severity of mental dysfunction.
4. A pharmacologically induced diminution in central cholinergic activity consistently produces a learning deficit that is similar to the learning deficit that exists in AD.
5. Cholinomimetic agents enhance learning in young normal subjects and patients with AD.

It must be stressed that the empirical support for the centrality of the cholinergic deficit in AD does not imply that this deficit is the exclusive pathological factor in the disease, nor does it address the question of whether a cholinergic deficit is specific to AD or is more generally an etiological factor in dementias seen in different syndromes. Parkinson's disease, for example, is frequently associated with dementia. Reduced cortical cholinergic activity has been demonstrated in some Parkinson's disease brains and has been shown to be associated with clinical evidence of cognitive impairment.[187,216] The most likely neuropathological basis of this cholinergic deficit in a subgroup of Parkinson's patients is an extensive loss of neurons in the nbM,[44,263] the subcortical nucleus also implicated in AD. Parkinson's brains with reduced cholinergic activity, however, have usually not been found to have the classic histopathological hallmarks of AD,[187] indicating that a cholinergic deficit may be a final common pathway to dementia in both Parkinson's disease and AD, although the underlying basis for the deficit may be distinct in each disease. Further exploration of these and other de-

*See references 41, 64, 74, 75, 84, 85, 110, 111, 163, 165, 175, 189, 190, 199, 218, 225, and 256.

mentias to establish similarities and differences, both of pathophysiology and of clinical presentation, will ultimately increase our understanding of the contribution of the cholinergic deficit to the clinical syndrome seen in AD and may clarify the extent to which other neurotransmitter deficits are involved in this dementing illness.

¶ Clinical Diagnosis of and Assessment Instruments for Alzheimer's Disease

AD cannot be diagnosed with complete accuracy on clinical grounds, as definitive diagnosis requires autopsy or biopsy demonstration of the classical histopathology of the condition. Initial clinical diagnoses of AD given to patients when they first come to medical attention may not agree with the final diagnosis determined after complete medical, neurological, and psychiatric examinations and long-term follow-up in as many as 35 percent of cases.[161,204] Diagnosis is particularly likely to be incorrect in younger patients and those with less severe dementias. However, the development of stringent diagnostic inclusion and exclusion criteria has led to an increase in the proportion of correctly diagnosed patients to over 90 percent.[21,88,108,243] These criteria (see table 25–1) exclude patients with significant risk factors for multi-infarct, depressive, and other toxic-metabolic dementias and employ several autopsy-verified scales as part of the diagnostic evaluation.

The Memory and Information Test (MIT)[148,215] and the Blessed scale,[22] which rate LTM and cognition, and the Dementia Rating Scale (DRS),[22,148] which quantifies aspects of behavior, are clinically developed AD severity rating scales that have been shown to correlate significantly with the amount of CAT deficiency and the extent of histopathological changes seen on autopsy.[22,181] Long-term follow-up studies have confirmed that these scales have validity as diagnostic instruments when used in conjunction with standard medical dementia workups; patients with an MIT of less than ten or a DRS greater than 4 have a high probability of having autopsy-verifiable AD, while patients with scores that do not meet these criteria are statistically more likely to have non-AD dementias of various etiologies.[148]

The Hachinski Ischemic Scale[124] is another clinically developed scale that later received autopsy validation.[205] This scale aids in the differential diagnosis of AD and multi-infarct dementia. Features classically associated with cerebral ischemic damage are assessed by history and physical examinations and weighted scores are assigned; total scores less than five are likely to distinguish AD patients from multi-infarct dementia patients, who score in the seven to fourteen range. While such summary scores have been shown to be successful in differentiating autopsy-verified AD patients from multi-infarct dementia patients, certain individual characteristics, such as fluctuating course, atherosclerosis, and history of hypertension, were found in both groups and thus should not be considered to be absolute contraindications to the diagnosis of AD.

These restrictive criteria for the diagnosis of AD probably create false negatives by underdiagnosing early AD cases and eliminating patients with two or more concurrent potentially dementing processes. They do, however, greatly decrease false-positive diagnoses and are thus of great value when assessing patients for research and clinical treatment trials.

¶ Antemortem Biological Markers for Alzheimer's Disease

Antemortem markers of AD are actively being sought, since at present the definitive diagnosis of AD depends on the availability of brain specimens usually obtained at autopsy. The first phase of these investigations is the characterization of a number of neurochemical measures in AD patients and normal nondemented elderly subjects in order that potentially distinguishing neurochemical parameters can be identified. After this

TABLE 25–1
General Diagnostic Criteria for Alzheimer's Disease

Subjects must:

1. Have a Memory and Information Test score less than 10.
2. Have a Dementia Rating Scale score above 4.
3. Not meet DSM-III criteria for affective or schizophrenic disorder; have no past history of psychosis.
4. Not have a severe loss of hearing or sight.
5. Have insidious, not acute, onset of memory loss, with a continuous and not a steplike course of deterioration over at least one year.
6. Have no focal localizing neurological signs.
7. Have no history of strokes.
8. Have an unmedicated resting blood pressure of less than 150/95.
9. Have a score on the Hachinski Ischemia Scale of 4 or less.
10. Have normal electrolytes, renal, liver, and endocrine function by laboratory tests.
11. Have no laboratory signs of neurosyphilis.
12. Have normal serum folate and B_{12} levels.
13. Have normal skull x-ray and chest x-ray.
14. Have computed tomography scan ruling out a focal lesion. Subjects often display cortical atrophy.
15. Have no electroencephalogram abnormalities except for diffuse slowing.
16. Have normal cerebrospinal fluid protein, cell count, and glucose.
17. Not meet DSM-III criteria for alcoholism or drug abuse now or in the past.
18. Have no history of head trauma with loss of consciousness.
19. Have no evidence of Huntington's disease, Parkinson's disease, or Wilson's disease.

preliminary work has been accomplished, the determination of an actual, specific antemortem marker requires histopathologically confirmed evidence that the marker discriminates AD patients from both normal elderly and patients with other forms of dementia.

Although other neurotransmitters or neuromodulators, particularly NE and somatostatin, are deficient in some but not all patients with AD and these may interact with the cholinergic deficit of AD to affect the symptom profile, no neurotransmitter has been implicated so extensively in the symptoms of AD as ACh. The pervasiveness of the cholinergic deficit in AD leads logically to the hypothesis that a clinical test useful in the diagnosis of AD might be established if an *in vivo* marker that accurately reflects central cholinergic activity could be identified. Plasma cortisol, plasma and red blood cell (RBC) choline concentrations, CSF ACh concentration, and auditory evoked potentials can all be related to central cholinergic activity, and these are currently being investigated in AD patients and nondemented age-matched controls.

Cortisol Secretion Studies

The regulation of cortisol secretion has been linked to a number of neurotransmitters that are diminished in the brains of patients with AD. For example, NE and ACh can affect cortisol concentrations.* Cholinergic input has been shown to elevate plasma cortisol concentrations.† Thus a cholinergic deficit that extended to the hypothalamus could produce diminished cortisol secretion in AD. Noradrenergic input can be inhibitory on the hypothalamic-pituitary-adrenal (HPA) axis,‡ and the loss of noradrenergic cells in younger AD patients could be invoked to hypothesize mild hypercortisolemia in AD patients. Thus there is abundant reason to study the HPA axis in AD.

Nocturnal secretion of cortisol and single 9:00 A.M. cortisol samples were measured in AD patients and normal elderly controls in one recent study,[78] and group differences as well as relationships between cortisol secre-

*See references 59, 60, 71, 94, 109, 120, 134, 150, 153, 217, and 235.
†See references 59, 60, 71, 94, 109, 120, 134, and 150.
‡See references 109, 134, 153, 217, and 235.

tion and other clinical parameters, including CSF neurotransmitter metabolite levels and degree of dementia as measured by the MIT,[148,215] have been explored. Nocturnal cortisol levels during the period of maximal cortisol secretion, between 2:00 A.M. and 8:00 A.M., were significantly higher in AD patients than in controls, and were highest in the most severely demented patients, with a robust relationship demonstrable between MIT score and mean nocturnal cortisol. When CSF neurotransmitter values were correlated with mean nocturnal cortisol, CSF MHPG and cortisol demonstrated a significant inverse relationship, while significant correlations were not found for either CSF HVA or 5-hydroxyindoleacetic acid (5-HIAA). AD patients and normal controls were also found to be significantly differentiated by single 9:00 A.M. plasma cortisol measurements, with higher cortisol values seen in AD patients, which, like mean nocturnal cortisol, correlated with dementia severity.

Thus two measures of basal cortisol concentrations, mean nocturnal cortisol from 2:00 A.M. to 8:00 A.M. and a single 9:00 A.M. plasma cortisol, were elevated in AD patients compared to controls. The more definitive demonstration of higher cortisol concentrations in AD patients derived from the 9:00 A.M. sample, although both studies provided rather persuasive evidence that plasma cortisol concentrations are lower in normal nondemented elderly than patients with AD.

Indirect information was derived regarding the neurotransmitter basis of these elevated cortisol concentrations. Although the loss of ACh-containing cells is so extensive in AD patients that it extends to the hypothalamus,[242] this deficit cannot explain current findings.* The elevated concentrations of cortisol are more compatible with the noradrenergic deficiency† and pronounced degeneration in the locus coeruleus.[24,183,249] In fact, CSF MHPG and nocturnal cortisol were significantly correlated in the predicted direction. Cell loss in the locus coeruleus occurs in a large spectrum of AD patients, but is particularly prominent in younger patients[24] and patients with a presenile onset.[103]

These data suggest that AD patients have a mild hypercortisolemia. However, they provide little information regarding the dynamic processes of the HPA axis (i.e., suppressibility). One means of evaluating that aspect of cortisol regulation would be to perform a dexamethasone suppression test (DST) in AD patients.

Several studies of the DST have been conducted in elderly demented populations.* The majority of these studies report a 50 percent or greater incidence of dexamethasone nonsuppression in demented patients, without significant differences in depression scale scores between suppressors and nonsuppressors.[8,197,232] Nevertheless, the question has been raised as to whether those patients displaying dexamethasone nonsuppression are patients who have pseudodementia of depression, or at least both depression and dementia.

To further elucidate whether the DST could be useful in identifying depression in demented patients, a population of AD patients who did not meet the DSM-III criteria for depression was studied.[77,121] This inquiry was directed at whether DST nonsuppression would exist in such patients, and if so, whether any clinical characteristics might distinguish suppressors from nonsuppressors. Additionally, the study design afforded the opportunity to investigate both the relationship between severity of dementia, symptoms of depression, and HPA suppressibility. Fifty percent of AD patients studied were dexamethasone nonsuppressors. Nonsuppressors were older than suppressors, including all patients with a senile onset of dementia who were nonsuppressors. When depressive symptoms were analyzed, it was found that nonsuppressors and suppressors did not differ in total number of depressive symptoms, although those patients who spe-

---

*See references 59, 60, 71, 94, and 150.
†See references 109, 134, 153, 217, and 235.

*See references 8, 47, 48, 49, 197, and 232.

cifically did not suppress at 8:00 A.M., unlike nonsuppressors at 4:00 P.M. and 11:00 P.M., did have more total depressive symptoms than the remaining sample, and symptom number correlated with this one cortisol measurement. No relationship was revealed between results of the DST and any measure of dementia severity. These results cast doubt on the utility of the standard DST for distinguishing patients with depression and dementia from those with dementia alone.

Cerebrospinal Fluid Studies

CSF concentrations of ACh would appear to be a straightforward potential marker of a central cholinergic deficiency in AD patients. While CSF ACh originates in both the brain and the spinal cord, the CAT deficit in AD has been shown to extend to the spinal cord,[275] thus furthering the possibility that CSF ACh might be a valid and useful marker. However, the activity of AChE in CSF is quite high,[271] and as remaining ACh concentrations might approach the lower limits of sensitivity of the ACh gas chromatography/mass spectrometry (GC/MS) assay, the practicality of this approach is unclear. Nevertheless, neurotransmitter metabolites including ACh and choline have been measured in a pilot study of a small group of AD patients.

Fifteen AD patients (eleven male and four female, mean age sixty-five, standard error of mean [SEM] = 2.25 years) in whom degree of dementia had been rated using the MIT, had 9:00 A.M. lumbar punctures. CSF was analyzed for ACh and choline, HVA, 5-HIAA, and MHPG by GC/MS. The ACh assay had a minimum sensitivity of between 0.015 and 0.025 nmol per ml; the interassay variability is 16 percent for ACh and 6.8 percent for choline; the intraassay variability is 16 percent for ACh and 8.5 percent for choline. Patients with the greatest memory impairment were found to have the lowest CSF ACh (Pearson correlation coefficient of MIT with ACh was 0.70, $p = 0.004$), and there was a nonsignificant trend for these patients to have higher choline levels. No other neuro-

transmitter metabolite measured correlated with severity of dementia.[76,143]

AChE activity in CSF is another marker that might reflect central cholinergic cell loss in AD, and it too has been investigated as a possible diagnostic tool in AD. Measurements of total AChE activity include two major types of AChE: true AChE, which is found mainly in brain and erythrocyte, and pseudo- or butyrylcholinesterase (BChE), which is found mainly in plasma. AChE activity in CSF, therefore, reflects both true AChE, which has originated in the CNS, and BChE, which is believed to diffuse into the CSF from the plasma.[72] Degeneration of central cholinergic neurons in AD might be expected to result in decreased levels of true AChE in CSF, while BChE levels should not be similarly affected and have, in fact, been shown to increase in AD.[228] Investigations of total AChE activity in the CSF of AD patients have not provided consistent findings. Reports of decreased total AChE activity in AD patients[4,229,251] have been contradicted by other investigations that do not replicate this decrement.[81,269] The ratio of AChE to BChE activity in CSF might be a more appropriate diagnostic index for AD, as this ratio would be sensitive to variations in brain-derived true AChE and would factor out the contribution of plasma-derived BChE. This calculated ratio did in fact completely differentiate a small group of AD patients from age-matched controls, while either value examined independently overlapped to some degree between the two groups.[5]

Thus the marked cholinergic deficits observed in postmortem studies may be reflected in the CSF of AD patients. As the mean level of ACh reported for normal subjects approaches the CSF ACh concentrations of the least demented AD patients,[76,257] it is conceivable that CSF ACh might be a useful discriminant between AD patients and normal controls. Likewise, the ratio of AChE to BChE activity may be useful in confirming the diagnosis of AD in moderately demented patients. A far more critical determination would be whether either measure successfully differentiated between AD and other forms of dementia, especially multi-infarct dementia, which should have far less impairment of CAT activity than AD. Further investigation should show whether CSF ACh levels or AChE activity might reflect these differences in CAT activity and facilitate diagnosis.

Red Blood Cell Choline Studies

RBC and plasma choline concentrations have been measured in a number of conditions in which there is evidence of a cholinergic involvement, including affective illness, tardive dyskinesia, Huntington's disease, Gilles de la Tourette syndrome, and Friedreich's ataxia.[130] Unusual RBC choline concentrations or RBC/plasma choline ratios have been reported in some of these disorders.[128,129,130] If anything, the evidence that there is involvement of cholinergic mechanisms in AD is stronger than in those conditions in which RBC or RBC/plasma choline ratios differed significantly from normals. In fact, the mean ratio of RBC to plasma choline was higher in fourteen nondepressed demented patients than in four simultaneous controls or in twenty-three historical controls evaluated by similar techniques.[9] Parameters of choline uptake into RBCs have yielded[113,145] conflicting data. It has also been suggested that RBC choline may predict the response to the combination of piracetam and lecithin.[107] Taken together, these studies provide an adequate rationale for investigating the utility of RBC choline as an antemortem marker of AD.

One study has been conducted to date comparing RBC and plasma choline concentrations as well as the kinetics of choline transport across the RBC in AD and normal controls.[122] In seventeen AD patients (ten male and seven female, mean age 63.9, SEM = 1.8) and fifteen healthy elderly controls (nine male and six female, mean age 65.9, SEM = 2.0), blood was drawn at 9:00 A.M. after a ten-hour fast and was processed for RBC and plasma choline concentration by GC/MS and for RBC choline uptake kinetics.

RBC choline levels ranged from 14.3 to 198 nmol per ml, with a mean of 48.1 ± 11.4 in AD patients, and from 9.3 to 120 nmol per ml, with a mean of 43.7 ± 9.5 in normal elderly controls. Plasma choline levels ranged from 5.1 to 24.5 nmol per ml, with a mean of 11.2 $\pm$ 1.1 in the AD group, and from 7.8 to 29.0 nmol per ml, with a mean of 12.8 ± 1.3 in the normal elderly population. RBC/plasma choline ratios in AD patients ranged from 1.2 to 14.0, with a mean of 4.6 ± 1.0, and 1.0 to 8.5, with a mean of 3.4 ± 1.0, in normal controls. None of these mean values were significantly different in age- and sex-matched AD and nondemented subjects.

Other factors that might affect choline parameters were examined in the same investigation. When analyzed separately, the age of the normal population but not of the AD sample correlated significantly with RBC choline and RBC/plasma ratio. The correlation between increasing age and RBC choline remained significant when the entire group was considered. In contrast to earlier studies, none of the choline parameters were significantly related to severity of dementia.

Like RBC and plasma choline and their ratios, neither the dissociation constant (K_d) nor the maximum velocity (V_{max}) of choline uptake distinguished AD patients and controls. When theoretical choline uptake was calculated, it did not discriminate between AD patients and controls, although it was robustly related to severity of dementia.[146]

Thus neither measurement of RBC nor plasma choline appears likely to aid in the differentiation of AD patients from other elderly populations. However, the relationship between severity of dementia and theoretical choline uptake requires replication and extension to other demented populations to determine if the relationship may in fact be limited to AD patients alone or to all demented patients who have a significant CAT deficiency.

Auditory Evoked Potential Studies

The AEP is an electrophysiological measure recorded from the scalp depicting a series of positive and negative deflections occurring from 40 msec to 600 msec following the presentation of an auditory stimulus. Of greatest interest has been the positive deflection at 300 msec or the P300. There is evidence that the generation of the P300 may reside in the hippocampus.[123,126,194] Furthermore, the latency of the P300 seems to be related to cholinergic activity.[42] Thus it is not surprising that a heterogeneous population of "demented" patients had a significantly greater P300 latency than historical controls.[117] The measurement of P300 latency in a more carefully diagnosed population of AD confirmed this difference between AD and normals.[239] Hence there is both a preclinical and clinical rationale for investigating midlatency AEP changes as potential antemortem markers of AD.

Twenty-eight subjects (twelve AD patients and sixteen normal healthy elderly controls) participated in a study of AEP.[136] As is common in AEP paradigms, subjects heard two different stimuli: frequent "hoops" at 500 Hz and rare "beeps" at 2,000 Hz, with an 85 to 15 ratio. They were instructed to press the button to the beeps only, and to count them. Stimuli were delivered at a rate of seven stimuli per ten seconds.

Amplitude and latency of P1, N1, and P2 did not distinguish AD patients and controls. However, following the rare tones there was a distinct prolongation of the N2 and P3 components in AD patients. Furthermore, the amplitude of the N2 was increased in AD, while the amplitude of the P3 was decreased. The AEP variables were examined for predictive power through the construction of a stepwise discriminant function. Four coefficients that did not correlate with each other, N2 and P3 latency and N2 and P5 amplitude, when taken together in a discriminant function were able to clarify twelve of twelve cases as AD, and correctly identify fifteen of sixteen patients as normals by the statistical technique of "jackknifing." As with other biological markers described in this section, expansion of AEP work will reveal if this test is capable of discriminating AD patients from patients with dementias of other etiologies.

Brain Imaging Studies

Computed tomography (CT) scanning, PET scanning, and nuclear magnetic resonance (NMR) are imaging techniques capable of yielding information about brain morphology and physiology. All three techniques have been applied to AD, but their utility as diagnostic indicators remains controversial. While CT scans are considered to be an integral part of the diagnostic workup of demented patients in order to rule out mass lesions or areas of infarction, there are no CT scan findings that are diagnostic of AD. The degree of cerebral cortical atrophy and calculation of ventricular brain ratios using CT have been investigated as measures that might differentiate AD patients from the normal elderly, but this has proven to be inconclusive.[87,101,137,203] Both cerebral atrophy and ventricular brain ratio increase with age.* Patients with dementia do, as a group, demonstrate a greater degree of cerebral atrophy than age-matched nondemented elderly, but considerable overlap exists between the two groups.[140,248] Ventricular dilation by CT has been reported to be a more useful diagnostic index,[230] but again this measure cannot predict clinical status in all cases due to overlap of the two groups.[65] Likewise, although CT measurement of density of specific brain regions has been reported to be significantly different in the medial temporal lobe, anterior frontal lobe, and head of the caudate in AD patients,[23] another investigation found no differences in density between AD patients and age-matched controls.[266] Thus single CT scans in individual patients have not been shown to be useful in establishing that patient's diagnosis with any degree of certainty.

Serial CT scans, however, may provide more conclusive diagnostic information. One preliminary study found that the increase of ventricular size as measured by CT scans taken thirteen to thirty-five months apart was significantly greater in a small cohort of demented patients than would have been

*See references 10, 35, 101, 116, and 139.

predicted from published normative data,[34] while another two-year follow-up study reported that ventricular brain ratio increased in those patients whose cognitive function had deteriorated over the two-year period while no significant increase occurred in patients whose level of dementia remained stable.[172]

PET scanning allows the quantification of cerebral glucose metabolism via the measurement of uptake of radiolabeled fluorine-18-fluorodexoyglucose. The utilization of this technique is at an early stage and no conclusions can be drawn concerning its role in the diagnostic workup of dementia. Research studies have, however, been consistent in their demonstration of overall cortical hypometabolism in demented patients, with the amount of metabolic abnormality being proportional to the degree of cognitive impairment.*

In addition, specific sites of cortical hypometabolism have been identified in AD, although these findings must be regarded as preliminary data until larger patient cohorts are studied. The site of major cortical metabolic abnormality has been suggested to be the parietal lobes,[52,106,152] although in individual patients, the major focus of hypometabolism varies in a manner that correlates with the individual's predominant cognitive deficits.[52] These data indicate that PET scanning is a promising technique that may increase our understanding of localized abnormalities in AD whether or not it ultimately proves to be a clinically useful diagnostic tool.

NMR imaging is the newest *in vivo* technique for the visualization of local physiological alterations in abnormal brain tissue. Due to the instrument's limited availability, there has been little data published thus far on the significance of this imaging technique in AD. The clinical and research potential of this noninvasive technique, however, appears to be enormous. Early work comparing AD patients, multi-infarct dementia patients, and controls reported that the three groups could

be distinguished from each other, although there was some overlap between dementia groups: spin-lattice relaxation time (T_1) significantly differentiated normals from demented patients, and proton density value of all white matter areas was significantly greater in AD than in multi-infarct dementia.[19] These changes in proton density were seen in the absence of observed lesions on visual inspection of the images. Thus proton NMR may prove useful in the differential diagnosis of dementia by virtue of its capacity to pick up subtle variations of tissue abnormality. As the number of operational NMR instruments increases, larger patient series will be studied and the clinical applications of the technique to dementia will be elucidated.

¶ Cholinergic Treatment Strategies in Alzheimer's Disease

Evidence that the cholinergic deficit is a major factor in all AD patients suggests that a rational treatment approach would be to attempt the pharmacological enhancement of cholinergic activity. Agents that produce such enhancement can be grouped into three categories: presynaptic agents that might increase ACh synthesis and release, synaptic agents that increase ACh availability by limiting its breakdown, and postsynaptic agents that directly stimulate ACh receptors.

Presynaptic agents such as choline and lecithin have been attractive as potential therapeutic agents due to both their safety and their ease of administration and to preclinical studies that suggest that under some conditions large amounts of these agents can induce increases in ACh concentration.[56,131] However, the extent to which peripherally administered precursors can increase central cholinergic activity *in vivo* is controversial. Increasing available amounts of precursor has not been shown to alter spontaneous release of ACh,[20] as ACh synthesis in presynaptic terminals appears to be linked to choline uptake via a sodium-dependent, high-affinity

*See references 50, 51, 92, 96, and 104.

transport system that is almost completely saturated under normal conditions.[125,272] Fifteen trials of precursor administration in AD patients* and three in normal elderly[95,167,168] have confirmed these negative assessments of the utility of precursor therapy; in all but one trial, no significant cognitive improvement was seen, regardless of dose or length of treatment.

An alternative presynaptic treatment approach is to combine choline or lecithin with agents that enhance the firing rate of presynaptic neurons. The normal depletion of ACh that is the result of increased firing of presynaptic neurons, whether induced indirectly by atropine[255] or by direct electrical stimulation,[164] can be reversed by pretreatment with choline. The proposed mechanism for the pretreatment effect, which is not consistent with the observation of a high-affinity uptake system that is completely saturated and therefore rate-limiting under normal circumstances, is that under conditions of increased neuronal demand, a low-affinity uptake system transports the extra choline needed for ACh synthesis.[115] Therefore, the combination of precursor with an agent that would increase the firing activity of central presynaptic cholinergic neurons might, in fact, provide clinically meaningful enhancement of the cholinergic system.

While no pharmacological agent readily available for human use has convincingly demonstrated such an effect on firing rate, piracetam and its analogue pramiracetam are being studied as potential enhancers of neuronal metabolic activity. These agents have been shown to improve CNS functioning in hypoxic conditions[173] and to reduce hippocampal ACh levels, possibly secondary to accelerated ACh release,[270] although their precise mechanism of action has not been delineated. Administration of piracetam plus lecithin to aged rats improved retention of a passive avoidance task,[16] which encouraged extension of clinical trials to human subjects. Cognitive test scores in three of ten AD pa-

*See references 31, 36, 37, 53, 89, 90, 91, 105, 188, 201, 223, 227, 245, 254, and 260.

tients improved significantly after one week of combined piracetam/lecithin treatment in the first of such studies,[107] and four of ten AD patients improved on the same combination, while four other patients had their best performance on piracetam alone in a second study.[142] Pramiracetam given to AD patients had no demonstrable effect on objective cognitive test scores, but subjective ratings indicated that behavior, including depression, anxiety, hostility, and goal-directed activity was perceived by patients' relatives to be improved during the drug trial.[32]

These pilot studies suggest that piracetam or its analogue, given alone or in combination with ACh precursors, may have some beneficial effect in a subgroup of AD patients. If such a subgroup does exist, it would be expected to consist of those patients in whom the degenerative process had spared some quantity of functionally intact cholinergic neurons. RBC and plasma choline levels were studied in both piracetam trials as potential in vivo markers of cholinergic activity that might identify treatment responders. In the first report,[107] AD patients who responded to piracetam plus choline differed significantly from nonresponders, in that the responders exhibited higher baseline RBC choline, accumulated RBC choline at a greater rate during treatment, and had a higher RBC to plasma choline ratio both prior to and during drug administration. While the second study of lecithin plus piracetam in AD did not replicate the finding of correlations between baseline RBC choline levels and treatment response, this patient cohort did demonstrate a similar trend toward higher baseline RBC to plasma choline ratios in treatment responders, with three of the four responders to combination therapy evidencing the highest ratios in the cohort.[142]

Another type of drug that might enhance utilization of exogenously administered precursors is that group of agents which facilitate transmembrane calcium influx, such as guanidine and 4-aminopyridine. By altering calcium influx, these agents result in increased amounts of ACh as well as other transmitters released per nerve impulse and may directly stimulate neurotransmitter synthesis.[155,253] Both agents have been used to enhance peripheral cholinergic activity in Eaton-Lambert syndrome and both can be administered safely and effectively, although only 4-aminopyridine crosses the blood-brain barrier. This, however, does not eliminate the potential utility of guanidine in the treatment of AD, since in this disease the blood-brain barrier may not be intact.[268] Thus there exists a theoretical rationale for the testing of both agents alone and in combination with choline or lecithin in patients with AD, although only one such study has been published to date.[259]

When given to fourteen AD patients over six weeks, 4-aminopyridine was effective in improving memory.[259] As only one dose was given to all patients and 4-aminopyridine was not given in conjunction with precursor, these results encourage future studies in which individual optimal doses of 4-aminopyridine are selected and then combined with choline or lecithin.

Precursor therapies can be of benefit in AD only if intact cholinergic neurons remain that are capable of utilizing exogenous choline and increasing ACh synthesis to compensate for the loss of surrounding neurons. This may not be possible under normal physiological conditions of the cholinergic neurons. One means of circumventing this problem might be to administer agents that would increase available ACh by blocking its degradation at the synapse, such as physostigmine or tetrahydroaminoacridine (THA).

THA, a centrally acting reversible AChE inhibitor, has not yet been extensively tested in AD patients; only one parenteral[238] and one oral[149] trial have been reported. Both studies suggest that THA might be therapeutically useful in a subgroup of demented patients; intravenous THA administration resulted in improvement in orientation and global ratings in moderately demented, but not severely demented, patients, and oral THA, when administered with lecithin, was likewise beneficial in moderately impaired patients but was without effect in severely demented patients. In the latter study no improvement could be measured when either agent was tested singly.

Physostigmine, which produces chronic enhancement of the cholinergic system by competitively inhibiting AChE, has a shorter half-life than THA and has been more widely studied in AD patients, with some promising results. However, clinical studies of all cholinesterase (ChE) inhibitor therapies are not straightforward, and a review of appropriate study design and patient selection is necessary in order that previous results of clinical trials with cholinergic drugs can be critically examined.

Patient selection can be a major variable in treatment trials. Despite the use of clinical criteria to eliminate patients with dementias of non-AD etiologies, as discussed earlier, definitive diagnosis of AD patients cannot be made on clinical grounds but can only be made at autopsy by demonstration of the condition's classical histopathology. The use of autopsy-validated rating scales such as the MIT,[148,215] the DRS,[22,148] and the Blessed scale,[22] as well as the Hachinski Ischemic Scale,[124,205] can, in conjunction with strict inclusion and exclusion criteria (table 25–1), improve diagnostic accuracy. Patients who do not meet criteria or whose scores do not conform with those that have been autopsy-verified to be associated with a high probability of an AD diagnosis are more likely to have dementias of various etiologies misclassified as AD.[148] These non-AD patients would not be expected to respond to cholinomimetics and could, in fact, worsen when cholinergic agents, which theoretically may exacerbate depression, are administered. These issues become especially crucial when small patient cohorts are being tested, as is the case in most AD treatment studies.

The methodology of experimental trials with cholinergic agents is likewise not straightforward. Animal and human studies with intravenously administered physostigmine, an AChE inhibitor, have demonstrated that this drug has an extremely narrow therapeutic window, and while this phenomenon has not been widely studied in other cholinergic drugs, the possibility that it may exist mandates the use of unique study designs in cholinergic treatment trials. In aged monkeys, reliable and replicable facilitation of memory occurs during intravenous physostigmine administration, but the optimal dose varies dramatically—from 0.005 mg per kg to 0.05 mg per kg—between animals.[12] Doses that exceed the therapeutic window may, in fact, worsen performance on cognitive tests, as was demonstrated in healthy young human volunteers who received intravenous physostigmine in doses exceeding 1.5 to 2.0 mg.[74] Therefore, an adequate test of physostigmine's efficacy and, by extrapolation, of the efficacy of many cholinergic drugs, requires that multiple doses be administered to each patient to establish individual "best doses."[73] The drug dose associated with the subject's best performance can then be tested against a placebo dose in order to replicate the dose-finding phase response.

In summary, valid trials of physostigmine in AD require a specialized study design in which individualized optimal physostigmine doses are chosen and tested in a large population of stringently diagnosed AD patients. Testing devices must be chosen that are suitable for each patient's capabilities and should measure alterations of function in several areas. Those studies that have most closely approximated these conditions have demonstrated that low doses of parenteral physostigmine significantly improve learning and memory.

Five* of seven studies[6,188] have demonstrated that parenteral physostigmine produces mild to moderate transient improvements in AD patients. Four of the seven studies administered multiple different doses to each AD patient, and three of these[54,73,237] found that significant improvement resulted at some but not all doses. The fourth[188] reported improvement in one of only three patients tested. The narrowness of the dose-response window is underlined by the fact that in two of these studies,[54,237] improvement was seen on doses lower than 0.5 mg

*See references 54, 73, 171, 226, and 237.

administered intravenously but was not maintained on higher doses. It should be noted that despite the use of various doses of physostigmine, these two studies did not test each patient at his own unique "best dose," but rather grouped and analyzed data by dose. The two-phase protocol outlined previously, designed to test each patient at his or her own best dose, was employed only in one investigation,[73] in which best-dose physostigmine tested against placebo significantly enhanced cognitive performance.

Positive results are less likely to be seen when only one dose of physostigmine is tested, as was done in three investigations. One[6] failed to show any cognitive improvement. The other two, each of which tested only one patient, could not demonstrate learning and memory improvement, although one reported significant improvement of constructional skills,[171] and the other found that incorrect answers, or "intrusion errors," were significantly reduced by physostigmine.

Outcome measures used to assess physostigmine's effect varied from study to study. In general, studies that included recognition tasks in their cognitive batteries (tests in which AD patients are shown words or pictures and are then asked to identify them in a series of familiar and unfamiliar items)[166] established that significant improvement on these tasks[54,73,237] occurred with physostigmine. When recall tasks were utilized, improvement was not seen,[6,171,188] perhaps because such tasks are more difficult and often incomprehensible to patients and therefore without utility in assessing change in AD patients. Thus all three studies that utilized an appropriate recognition task and employed a multiple-dose study design confirmed that low-dose parenteral physostigmine improves learning and memory in AD patients.

Improvements produced by intravenous physostigmine are of theoretical importance, but whether this can be translated into practical pharmacological intervention in AD requires trials of safe, long-acting oral cholinomimetic drugs. Physostigmine given orally has a short half-life, but in multiple small doses it produces chronic enhancement of cholinergic activity. Clinical trials of oral physostigmine are made difficult by the lack of information equating parenteral and oral doses of physostigmine; this, combined with the demonstrated variability in individual response to different parenteral doses of physostigmine, makes a variable dosage procedure, similar to the one described for intravenous physostigmine, imperative. This strategy has been utilized in several studies and has yielded modest improvements, both in specific cognitive areas and overall functioning, in a majority of AD patients tested. * One additional investigation, in which physostigmine was administered at a fixed dose, reported variable response to physostigmine with four of eight patients showing behavioral improvement. [43]

The observation that many, but not all, AD patients improve during oral physostigmine treatment trials led to the exploration of biochemical measures that might correlate with treatment responses and differentiate responders from patients who derived no benefit from physostigmine treatment. Plasma cortisol is one such potential marker, as it is a readily obtainable peripheral neuroendocrine measure that can provide an indirect reflection of central cholinergic activity. Average nocturnal cortisol levels were obtained during sleep studies performed while AD patients were receiving oral physostigmine and again during placebo administration, and a strong correlation between symptom improvement and increases in mean cortisol secretion during physostigmine treatment was demonstrated. [170] Since central cholinergic input increases cortisol,† this correlation between treatment response and increased nocturnal cortisol suggests that physostigmine can be effective in AD patients only to the extent that it can induce increases in central cholinergic activity. Thus individualized CNS responses to physostigmine appear to mediate treatment response and may be based on the degree of deterioration of the

cholinergic system as well as penetrance of physostigmine into the CNS.

A second study of biochemical correlates of physostigmine treatment response substantiates the conclusions drawn from the measurement of nocturnal cortisol. CSF ChE activity was measured during oral physostigmine treatment, and increasing inhibition of ChE activity was found to correlate with memory improvement. [246] This suggests that variable treatment response may reflect individualized activity or penetrance of physostigmine in the CNS. A similar conclusion can be drawn from correlations of cortisol levels and memory improvement during oral physostigmine treatment.

Physostigmine's efficacy requires some functional cholinergic neurons to provide a substrate for the drug's activity. This requirement may not be satisfied in patients with profound cholinergic cell loss. To circumvent these problems, an alternative strategy would be to administer cholinergic agonists that act directly at postsynaptic sites, since the number of postsynaptic muscarinic receptor binding sites is not affected by AD. Three such agents are arecoline, pilocarpine, and oxotremorine. Arecoline has been shown to enhance learning in normal young humans [225] and in aged nonhuman primates [15] and has yielded statistically significant cognitive improvement when infused intravenously in a small group of AD patients. [54] This agent, however, is clinically impractical, since it has an extremely short half-life. Oral pilocarpine has not been shown to be useful either given alone or with lecithin, although this negative report results from only one study using a very small, mixed-diagnosis patient cohort. [40] Oxotremorine, a longer-acting muscarinic agent, may be a more useful compound, although an unpublished preliminary attempt by us to administer this drug orally to AD patients suggested that significantly distressing cholinergic side effects may preclude its clinical utility.

All postsynaptic muscarinic agonist drugs share a fundamental limitation in that their action may not be physiologically equivalent to ACh release from an intact presynaptic

---

*See references 18, 79, 170, 224, and 246.
†See references 59, 60, 71, 94, 109, 37, and 150.

neuron. Rather than selectively stimulating neurons, such agents might flood receptors, resulting in unusual temporal patterns of receptor activation. Additionally, these agents are toxic at high doses and at lower doses can cause discomfort due to their peripheral cholinergic activity. Within a narrow therapeutic range, however, these agents could be promising, and less toxic cholinergic receptor agonists are being sought for clinical trials.

¶ Conclusion

Alzheimer's disease is a multisymptom disease that may ultimately prove to be mediated by multiple neurochemical abnormalities. Alterations of many neurotransmitter systems, neuropeptides, and receptor sites may contribute to clinical impairment but have yet to be completely elucidated. In particular, the contribution of the noradrenergic system to the evolution of symptoms of AD patients is only beginning to be clarified, and its relevance to potential treatment regimens has yet to be explored. Despite these qualifications, compelling evidence supports the hypothesis that any ultimate pharmacological treatment of AD will have to address the problem of diminished cholinergic activity. A profound cholinergic deficit exists in the cortex and hippocampus of AD patients, areas of the brain associated with learning and memory, and the amount of deficit correlates both with the extent of · classical histological hallmarks of AD and with severity of dementia. Cognitive deficits typical of AD can be reliably produced in normal subjects by pharmacologically induced reduction of cholinergic activity. This collective evidence has led to treatment trials of cholinergic drugs and concurrent attempts to define biological markers that correlate with cholinergic deficit. However, the success of cholinomimetic treatment strategies thus far has been modest. Perhaps the development of valid antemortem markers combined with careful clinical diagnosis and attention to the unique pharmacological properties of cholinergic drugs may ultimately identify a group of AD patients who can derive meaningful benefit from ChE inhibitors or cholinergic agonists. Definitive treatment of AD undoubtedly awaits clarification of complex neurochemical variables, delineation of parameters that can predict response, and development of appropriate pharmacological probes and treatment agents.

¶ Bibliography

1. ADLER, S. "Methyldopa-induced Decrease in Mental Activity," *Journal of the American Medical Association*, 230 (1974):1428–1429.
2. ADOLFSSON, R., et al. "Changes in the Brain Catecholamines in Patients with Dementia of the Alzheimer Type," *British Journal of Psychiatry*, 135 (1979):216–223.
3. ANTUONO, P., et al. "A Discrete Sampling Technique in Senile Dementia of the Alzheimer Type and Alcoholic Dementia: Study of the Cholinergic System," in L. Amaducci, A. N. Davison, and P. Antuono, eds., *Aging of the Brain and Dementia*, vol. 13 of *Aging* series. New York: Raven Press, 1980, pp. 151–158.
4. APPLEYARD, M. E., et al. "Decreased CSF Acetylcholinesterase Activity in Alzheimer's Disease," *Lancet*, 2 (1983):452.
5. ARENDT, T., et al. "Decreased Ratio of CSF Acetylcholinesterase to Butyrylcholinesterase Activity in Alzheimer's Disease," *Lancet*, 1 (1984):173.
6. ASHFORD, J. W., et al. "Physostigmine and Its Effect on Six Patients with Dementia," *American Journal of Psychiatry*, 138 (1981):829–830.
7. BALL, M. J., et al. "Hippocampal Morphometry," in R. Katzman, ed., *Biological Aspects of Alzheimer's Disease*. New York: Cold Spring Harbor Laboratory, 1983, pp. 45–64.
8. BALLDIN, J., et al. "Dexamethasone Suppression Test and Serum Prolactin in Dementia Disorders," *British Journal of Psychiatry*, 143 (1983):277–281.
9. BARCLAY, L. L., et al. "Red-Cell/Plasma Choline Ratio in Dementia," *New En-*

gland *Journal of Medicine*, 307 (1982): 501.

10. BARRON, S. A., JACOBS, L., and KINKEL, W. R. "Changes in Size of Normal Lateral Ventricles During Aging Determined by Computerized Tomography," *Neurology*, 26(1976):1011–1013.

11. BARTUS, R. T. "Evidence for a Direct Cholinergic Involvement in the Scopolamine-Induced Amnesia in Monkeys: Effects of Concurrent Administration of Physostigmine and Methylphenidate with Scopolamine," *Pharmacology, Biochemistry and Behavior*, 9 (1978):833–836.

12. ———. "Physostigmine and Recent Memory Effects in Young and Aged Nonhuman Primates," *Science*, 206 (1979): 1087–1089.

13. ———. "Cholinergic Drug Effects on Memory and Cognition in Animals," in L. W. Poon, ed., *Aging in the 1980's: Psychological Issues*. Washington, D.C.: American Psychological Association, 1980, pp. 163–180.

14. BARTUS, R. T., and JOHNSON, H. R. "Short-Term Memory in the Rhesus Monkey: Disruption from the Anticholinergic Scopolamine," *Pharmacology, Biochemistry and Behavior*, 5 (1976):39–46.

15. BARTUS, R. T., DEAN, R. L., and BEER, B. "Memory Deficits in Aged Cebus Monkeys and Facilitation with Central Cholinomimetics," *Neurobiology of Aging*, 1 (1980):145–152.

16. BARTUS, R. T., et al. "Profound Effects of Combining Choline and Piracetam on Memory Enhancement and Cholinergic Function in Aged Rats," *Neurobiology of Aging*, 2 (1981):105–111.

17. BEAL, M. F., and MARTIN, J. B. "Somatostatin: Normal and Abnormal Observations in the Central Nervous System," in S. Corkin, J. Growdon, and R. J. Wurtman, eds., *Alzheimer's Disease: Advances in Basic Research and Therapies*. Massachusetts: Center for Brain Sciences and Metabolism, 1984, pp. 229–258.

18. BELLER, S. A., et al. "Oral Physostigmine in Senile Dementia of the Alzheimer Type: A Two-Phase Study" (Abstract). Paper presented at the American Psychiatric Association Annual Meeting, Los Angeles, 1984.

19. BESSON, J.A.O., et al. "Differentiating Senile Dementia of the Alzheimer Type and Multi-infarct Dementia by Proton NMR Imaging," *Lancet*, 2 (1983):789.

20. BIERKAMPER, G. G., and GOLDBERG, A. M. "The Effect of Choline on the Release of Acetylcholine from the Neuromuscular Junction," in A. Barbeau, J. H. Growden, and R. J. Wurtman, eds., *Nutrition and the Brain*, vol. 5. New York: Raven Press, 1979, pp. 243–251.

21. BIRD, T. D., et al. "Alzheimer's Disease: Choline Acetyltransferase Activity in Brain Tissue from Clinical and Pathological Subgroups," *Annals of Neurology*, 14 (1983):284–293.

22. BLESSED, G., TOMLINSON, B. E., and ROTH, M. "The Association Between Quantitative Measures of Dementia and of Senile Change in the Cerebral Gray Matter of Elderly Subjects," *British Journal of Psychiatry*, 114 (1968): 797–811.

23. BONDAREFF, W., BALDY, R., and LEVY, R. "Quantitative Computed Tomography in Senile Dementia," *Archives of General Psychiatry*, 38 (1981):1365–1368.

24. BONDAREFF, W., MOUNTJOY, C. G., and ROTH, M. "Loss of Neurons of Origin of the Adrenergic Projections to Cerebral Cortex (Nucleus Locus Coeruleus) in Senile Dementia," *Neurology*, 32 (1982):164–168.

25. BOTWINICK, C. Y., and QUARTERMAIN, D. "Recovery From Amnesia Induced by Pre-Test Injection of Monoamine Oxidase Inhibitors," *Pharmacology, Biochemistry and Behavior*, 2 (1974):375–379.

26. BOWEN, D. M., and DAVISON, A. N. "Biochemical Changes in the Cholinergic System of the Aging Brain and in Senile Dementia," *Psychological Medicine*, 10 (1980):315–319.

27. BOWEN, D. M., et al. "Brain Decarboxylase Activities as Indices of Pathological Change in Dementia," *Lancet*, 1 (1974): 1247–1249.

28. BOWEN, D. M., et al. "Neurotransmitter-Related Enzymes and Indices of Hypoxia in Senile Dementia and Other

Abiotrophies," *Brain*, 99 (1976):459–495.

29. BOWEN, D. M., et al. "Accelerated Aging or Selective Neuronal Loss as an Important Cause of Dementia," *Lancet*, 1 (1979):11–14.

30. BOWEN, D. M., et al. "Behavioral Assessment of Serotonergic and Cholinergic Dysfunction and Cerebral Atrophy in Alzheimer's Disease," *Journal of Neurochemistry*, 41 (1983):266–272.

31. BOYD, W. D., et al. "Clinical Effects of Choline in Alzheimer's Senile Dementia," *Lancet*, 2 (1977):711.

32. BRANCONNIER, R. J., et al. "The Therapeutic Efficacy of Piracetam in Alzheimer's Disease: Preliminary Observations" (Abstract). Paper presented at the American College of Neuropsychopharmacology Meeting, San Juan, P.R., 1982.

33. BRINKMAN, S. D., and GERSHON, S. "Measurement of Cholinergic Drug Effects on Memory in Alzheimer's Disease," *Neurobiology of Aging*, 4 (1983):139–145.

34. BRINKMAN, S. D., and LARGEN, J. W. "Changes in Brain Ventricular Size with Repeated CAT Scans in Suspected Alzheimer's Disease," *American Journal of Psychiatry*, 141 (1984):81–83.

35. BRINKMAN, S. D., et al. "Quantitative Indexes of Computed Tomography in Dementia and Normal Aging," *Radiology*, 138 (1981):89–92.

36. BRINKMAN, S. D., et al. "A Dose-Ranging Study of Lecithin in the Treatment of Primary Degenerative Dementia (Alzheimer's Disease)," *Journal of Clinical Psychopharmacology*, 2 (1982):281–285.

37. BRINKMAN, S. D., et al. "Lecithin and Memory Training in Suspected Alzheimer's Disease," *Journal of Gerontology*, 37 (1982):4–9.

38. BUSTANY, P., et al. "Regional Human Brain Uptake and Protein Incorporation of C-L-Methionine Studied *in vivo* with PET," *Journal of Cerebral Blood Flow and Metabolism*, 1 (Supplement 1) (1981):17–18.

39. BUSTANY, P., et al. "Brain Protein Synthesis in Normal and Demented Patients—A Study by Positron Emission Tomography with "C-L-Methionine," in P. E.

Magistretti, ed., *Functional Radionuclide Imaging of the Brain*. New York: Raven Press, 1983, pp. 319–326.

40. CAINE, E. D. "Cholinomimetic Treatment Fails to Improve Memory Disorders," *New England Journal of Medicine*, 303 (1980):585–586.

41. CAINE, E. D., et al. "Qualitative Analysis of Scopolamine-Induced Amnesia," *Psychopharmacology (Berlin)*, 74 (1981):74–80.

42. CALLAWAY, E. "Human Information Processing: Some Effects of Methylphenidate, Age and Scopolamine," *Biological Psychiatry*, in press.

43. CALTAGIRONE, C., GAINOTTI, G., and MASULLO, C. "Oral Administration of Chronic Physostigmine Does Not Improve Cognitive or Amnesic Performances in Alzheimer's Presenile Dementia," *International Journal of Neuroscience*, 16 (1982):247–249.

44. CANDY, J. M., et al. "Pathological Changes in the Nucleus Basalis of Meynert in Alzheimer's and Parkinson's Disease," *Journal of the Neurological Sciences*, 54 (1983):277–289.

45. CARLSSON, A. "Changes in Neurotransmitter System in the Aging Brain and in Alzheimer's Disease," in B. Reisberg, ed., *Alzheimer's Disease, The Standard Reference*. New York: Free Press, 1983, pp. 100–106.

46. CARLSSON, A., ADOLFSSON, R., and AQUILONIUS, S. M. "Biogenic Amines in Brain in Normal Aging, Senile Dementia and Chronic Alcoholism," *Advances in Biochemical Psychopharmacology*, 23 (1980):295–304.

47. CARNES, M., et al. "Effects of Chronic Medical Illness and Dementia on the Dexamethasone Suppression Test," *Journal of the American Geriatrics Society*, 31 (1983):267–271.

48. CARNES, M., et al. "The Dexamethasone Suppression Test in Demented Outpatients With and Without Depression," *Psychiatry Research*, 9 (1983):337–344.

49. CASTRO, P., et al. "Depression, Dementia and the Dexamethasone Suppression Test (Letter to Editor)," *American Journal of Psychiatry*, 140 (1983):1386.

50. CHASE, T. N., FOSTER, N. L., and MANSI,

L. "Alzheimer's Disease and the Parietal Lobe," *Lancet*, 2 (1983):225.

51. CHASE, T. N., et al. "Alzheimer's Disease: Local Cerebral Metabolism Studies Using the ^{18}F-Fluorodeoxyglucose Positron Emission Tomography Technique," in D. Samuel et al., eds., *Aging of the Brain*. New York: Raven Press, 1983, pp. 143–154.

52. CHASE, T. N., et al. "Regional Cortical Dysfunction in Alzheimer's Disease as Determined by Positron Emission Tomography," *Annals of Neurology* 15 (Supplement) (1984):170–174.

53. CHRISTIE, J. E., et al. "Effects of Choline and Lecithin on CSF Choline Levels and in Cognitive Function in Patients with Presenile Dementia of the Alzheimer Type," in A. Barbeau, J. Growden, and R. J. Wurtman, eds., *Nutrition and the Brain*, vol. 5. New York: Raven Press, 1979, pp. 377–389.

54. CHRISTIE, J. E., et al. "Physostigmine and Arecoline: Effects of Intravenous Infusions in Alzheimer Presenile Dementia," *British Journal of Psychiatry*, 138 (1981):46–50.

55. COBLENTZ, J. M., et al. "Presenile Dementia: Clinical Aspects and Evaluation of Cerebrospinal Fluid Dynamics," *Archives of Neurology*, 29 (1973):299–308.

56. COHEN, E. L., and WURTMAN, R. J. "Brain Acetylcholine: Increase After Systemic Choline Administration," *Life Science*, 16 (1975):1095–1099.

57. CORSELLIS, J. A. N. *Mental Illness and the Aging Brain*. London: Oxford University Press, 1962.

58. COYLE, J. T., PRICE, D. L., and DeLONG, M. R. "Alzheimer's Disease: A Disorder of Cortical Cholinergic Innervation," *Science*, 219 (1983):1184–1190.

59. COZANITIS, D. A. "Galanthamine Hydrobromide Versus Neostigmine," *Anaesthesia*, 29 (1974):163–168.

60. COZANITIS, D. A., DESSYPRIS, A., and NUUTTILA, K. "The Effect of Galanthamine Hydrobromide on Plasma ACTH in Patients Undergoing Anaesthesia and Surgery," *Acta Anaethesiologica Scandinavica*, 24 (1980):166–168.

61. CROOK, T., et al. "The Effect of Methylphenidate on Test Performance in the Cognitive Impaired Aged," *Psychopharmacology*, 52 (1977):251–255.

62. CROSS, A. J., et al. "Reduced Dopamine-Beta Hydroxylase Activity in Alzheimer's Disease," *British Medical Journal*, 282 (1981):93–94.

63. CROSS, A. J., et al. "Monoamine Metabolism in Senile Dementia of Alzheimer Type," *Journal of the Neurological Sciences*, 60 (1983):383–392.

64. CROW, T. J., and GROVE-WHITE, I. G. "Differential Effect of Atropine and Hyoscine on Human Learning Capacity," *British Journal of Pharmacology*, 43 (1971):464.

65. DAMASCIO, H., et al. "Quantitative Computed Tomographic Analysis in the Diagnosis of Dementia," *Archives of Neurology*, 40 (1983):715–719.

66. DAVIES, P. "Studies on the Neurochemistry of Central Cholinergic Systems in Alzheimer's Disease," in R. Katzman, R. D. Terry, and D. L. Bick, eds., *Alzheimer's Disease, Senile Dementia and Related Disorders*, vol. 7 in *Aging* series. New York: Raven Press, 1978, pp. 453–459.

67. DAVIES, P. "Neurotransmitter-Related Enzymes in SDAT," *Brain Research*, 171 (1979):319–327.

68. DAVIES, P., and MALONEY, A.J.R. "Selective Loss of Central Cholinergic Neurons in Alzheimer's Disease," *Lancet*, 2 (1976):1403.

69. DAVIES, P., and TERRY, R. D. "Cortical Somatostatin-Like Immunoreactivity in Cases of Alzheimer's Disease and Senile Dementia of the Alzheimer's Type," *Neurobiology of Aging*, 2 (1981):9–14.

70. DAVIES, P., and VERTH, A. H. "Regional Distribution of Muscarinic Acetylcholine Receptor in Normal and Alzheimer's Type Dementia Brains," *Brain Research*, 138 (1978):385–392.

71. DAVIS, B. M., et al. "Effects of Cholinergic Stimulation of Pituitary Hormonal Release," *Psychoneuroendocrinology*, 7 (1982):347–354.

72. DAVIS, K. L., and GOODNICK, P. J. "Acetylcholinesterase in Neuropsychiatric Disorders," in J. H. Wood, ed., *Neurobiology of Cerebrospinal Fluid*, vol. 2. New York: Plenum Press, 1983, pp. 197–203.

73. DAVIS, K. L., and MOHS, R. C. "Enhancement of Memory Processes in Alzheimer's Disease with Multiple Dose Intravenous Physostigmine," *American Journal of Psychiatry*, 139 (1982):1421–1424.

74. DAVIS, K. L., et al. "Physostigmine: Effects on Cognition and Affect in Normal Subjects," *Psychopharmacology (Berlin)*, 51 (1976):23–27.

75. DAVIS, K. L., et al. "Physostigmine: Improvement of Long-Term Memory Processes in Normal Subjects," *Science*, 201 (1978):272–274.

76. DAVIS, K. L., et al. "Cerebrospinal Fluid, Acetylcholine, Choline, and Senile Dementia of the Alzheimer Type," *Psychopharmacology Bulletin*, 18 (1982):193–195.

77. DAVIS, K. L., et al. "Biochemical Correlates of Dexamethasone Nonsuppression" (Abstract), American Psychiatric Association Annual Meeting, New York, 1983.

78. DAVIS, K. L., et al. "Hypercortisolemia in Alzheimer's Disease" (Abstract), Paper presented at the American Psychiatric Association Annual Meeting, New York, 1983.

79. DAVIS, K. L., et al. "Oral Physostigmine in Alzheimer's Disease," *New England Journal of Medicine*, 308 (1983):721.

80. DELFS, J. R., ZHU, C. H., and DICHTER, M. H. "Coexistence of Acetylcholinesterase and Somatostatin-Immunoreactivity in Neurons Cultured from Rat Cerebrum," *Science*, 223 (1984):61–63.

81. DEUTSCH, S. I., et al. "Acetylcholinesterase Activity in CSF in Schizophrenia, Depression, Alzheimer's Disease, and Normals," *Biological Psychiatry*, 18 (1983):1363–1373.

82. DIAMUKES, P. K., and RAHE, A. V. "Involvement of Biogenic Amines in Memory Formation," *Psychopharmacologia*, 23 (1972):17–25.

83. DRACHMAN, D. A. "Memory and Cognitive Function in Man: Does the Cholinergic System Have a Specific Role?" *Neurology*, 27 (1977):783–790.

84. DRACHMAN, D. A., and LEAVITT, J. "Human Memory and the Cholinergic System: A Relationship to Aging," *Archives of Neurology*, 30 (1974):113–121.

85. DRACHMAN, D. A., and SAHAKIAN, B. J. "Memory and Cognitive Functioning in the Elderly: A Preliminary Trial of Physostigmine," *Archives of Neurology*, 37 (1980):674–675.

86. DRACHMAN, D. A., and STAHL, S. "Extrapyramidal Dementia and Levodopa," *Lancet*, 1 (1975):809.

87. EARNEST, M. P., et al. "Cortical Atrophy, Ventricular Enlargement and Intellectual Impairment in the Aged," *Neurology*, 29 (1979):1138–1143.

88. EISDORFER, C., and COHEN, D. "Diagnostic Criteria for Primary Neuronal Degeneration of the Alzheimer's Type," *Journal of Family Practice*, 11 (1980):553–557.

89. ETIENNE, P., et al. "Clinical Effects of Choline in Alzheimer's Disease," *Lancet*, 1 (1978):508–509.

90. ETIENNE, P., et al. "Lecithin in Alzheimer's Disease," *Lancet*, 2 (1978):1206.

91. ETIENNE, P., et al. "Alzheimer's Disease: Lack of Effect of Lecithin Treatment for Three Months," *Neurology*, 31 (1981):1552–1554.

92. FARKAS, T., et al. "[18]F-2-Deoxy-2-Fluoro-D-Glucose as a Tracer in the Positron Emission Tomographic Study of Senile Dementia," *American Journal of Psychiatry*, 139 (1982):352–353.

93. FERNANDEZ, P. G. "Alpha and Methyldopa and Forgetfulness," *Annals of Internal Medicine*, 85 (1976):128.

94. FERRARI, E., et al. "Variations Circadiennes Des Effets D'une Substance Vagolytique Sur le Système ACTH-Secrétant Chez L'homme," *Annales d'Endocrinologie (Paris)*, 38 (1977):203–213.

95. FERRIS, S. H., et al. "Long-Term Choline Treatment of Memory-Impaired Elderly Patients," *Science*, 205 (1979):1039–1040.

96. FERRIS, S. H., et al. "Positron Emission Tomography in the Study of Aging and Senile Dementia," *Neurobiology of Aging*, 1 (1980):127–131.

97. FIBIGER, H. C. "The Organization and Some Projections of Cholinergic Neurons of the Mammalian Forebrain," *Brain Research*, 257 (1982):327–388.

98. FLEXNER, L. B., SEROTA, R. G., and GOODMAN, R. H. "Cycloheximide and

Acetoxycycloheximide: Inhibition of Tyrosine Hydroxylase Activity and Amnestic Effects," *Proceedings of the National Academy of Science USA,* 70 (1973):354–356.

99. FOLSTEIN, M. F., and BREITNER, J. C. S. "Language Disorder Predicts Familial Alzheimer's Disease," *Johns Hopkins Medical Journal,* 149 (1981):145–147.

100. FOLSTEIN, M. F., POWELL, D., and BREITNER, J.C.S. "The Cognitive Pattern of Familial Alzheimer's Disease," in R. Katzman, ed., *Biological Aspects of Alzheimer's Disease.* New York: Cold Spring Harbor Press, 1983, pp. 337–349.

101. FORD, C. V., and WINTER, J. "Computerized Axial Tomograms and Dementia in Elderly Patients," *Journal of Gerontology,* 36 (1981):164–169.

102. FORNO, L. "The Locus Coeruleus and Alzheimer's Disease," *Journal of Neuropathology and Experimental Neurology,* 37 (1978):614.

103. FORNO, L., and NORVILLE, R. L. "Synaptic Morphology in Human Locus Coeruleus," *Acta Neuropathologica (Berlin),* 53 (1981):7–14.

104. FOSTER, N. L., et al. "Alzheimer's Disease: Focal Cortical Changes Shown by Positron Emission Tomography," *Neurology,* 33 (1983):961–965.

105. FOVALL, P., et al. "Choline Bitartrate Treatment of Alzheimer-Type Dementias," *Communications in Psychopharmacology,* 4 (1980):141–145.

106. FRIEDLAND, R. P., et al. "Regional Cerebral Metabolic Alterations in Dementia of the Alzheimer Type: Positron Emission Tomography With ^{18}-F-Fluorodeoxy Glucose," *Journal of Computer Assisted Tomography,* 7 (1983):590–598.

107. FRIEDMAN, E., et al. "Clinical Response to Choline Plus Piracetam in Senile Dementia: Relation to Red-Cell Choline Levels," *New England Journal of Medicine,* 304 (1981):1490–1491.

108. FULD, P. A., et al. "Intrusions as a Sign of Alzheimer Dementia: Chemical and Pathological Verification," *Annals of Neurology,* 11 (1982):155–159.

109. GARCY, A. M., and MAROTTA, S. M. "Plasma Cortisol of Conscious Cats During Cerebroventricular Perfusion with Adrenergic, Cholinergic and Gabaner-gic Antagonists," *Neuroendocrinology,* 25 (1978):343–353.

110. GHONEIM, M. M., and MEWALDT, S. P. "Effects of Diazepam and Scopolamine on Storage, Retrieval, and Organizational Processes in Memory," *Psychopharmacologia,* 44 (1975):257–262.

111. ———. "Studies on Human Memory: The Interactions of Diazepam, Scopolamine and Physostigmine," *Psychopharmacology (Berlin),* 52 (1977):1–6.

112. GHOSH, S. K. "Methyldopa and Forgetfulness," *Lancet,* 1 (1976):202–203.

113. GLEN, A.I.M., et al. "Choline Uptake in Patients with Alzheimer's Pre-senile Dementia," *Psychological Medicine,* 11 (1981):469–476.

114. GO, R.C.P., TODOROV, A. B., and ELSTON, R. C. "The Malignancy of Dementias," *Annals of Neurology,* 3 (1978):559–561.

115. GOLDBERG, A. M. "The Interaction of Neuronal Activity and Choline Transport on the Regulation of Acetylcholine Synthesis," in S. Corkin, et al., eds., *Alzheimer's Disease: A Report of Progress in Research,* vol. 19 in *Aging* series. New York: Raven Press, 1982, pp. 327–330.

116. GONZALEZ, C. F., LANTIERI, R. L., and NATHAN, R. J. "The CT Scan Appearance of the Brain in the Normal Elderly Population: A Correlative Study," *Neuroradiology,* 16 (1978):120–122.

117. GOODIN, D. S., SQUIRES, K. C., and STARR, A. "Long Latency Event-Related Components of the Auditory Evoked Potential in Dementia," *Brain,* 101 (1978):635–648.

118. GOTTFRIES, C. G. "Biochemical Aspects of Dementia," in H. Van Praag et al., eds., *Handbook of Biologic Psychiatry,* vol. 4. New York: Marcel Dekker, 1980, pp. 417–438.

119. GOTTFRIES, C. G., et al. "Biochemical Changes in Dementia Disorders of the Alzheimer Type (AD/SDAT)," *Neurobiology of Aging,* 4 (1983):261–271.

120. GREENWALD, B. S., and DAVIS, K. L. "Experimental Pharmacology of Alzheimer's Disease," in R. Mayeux and W. G. Rosen, eds., *The Dementias.* New York: Raven Press, 1983, pp. 87–102.

121. GREENWALD, B. S., et al. "Cortisol in Alzheimer's Disease. II: Dexamethasone

Suppression, Dementia Severity and Affective Symptoms," *American Journal of Psychiatry,* in press.

122. GREENWALD, B. S., et al. "Red Cell Choline. I: Choline in Alzheimer's disease," in review.

123. GROSSBERG, S. "Processing of Expected and Unexpected Events During Conditioning and Attention: A Psychophysiological Theory," *Psychological Review,* 89 (1982):529–572.

124. HACHINSKI, V. C., et al. "Cerebral Blood Flow in Dementia," *Archives of Neurology,* 32 (1975):632–637.

125. HAGA, T., and NODA, H. "Choline Uptake Systems of Rat Brain Synaptosomes," *Biochimica et Biophysica Acta,* 291 (1973):564–575.

126. HALGREEN, E., et al. "Endogenous Potentials Generated in the Human Hippocampal Formation and Amygdala by Infrequent Events," *Science,* 210 (1980): 803–805.

127. HAMBURG, M. D., and KERR, A. "DDC-Induced Retrograde Amnesias Prevented by Injections of dl-DOPS," *Pharmacology, Biochemistry and Behavior,* 5 (1976):499–501.

128. HANIN, I., et al. "Red Cell Choline and Gilles de la Tourette Syndrome," *New England Journal of Medicine,* 301 (1979):661–662.

129. HANIN, I., et al. "RBC and Plasma Choline Levels in Control and Depressed Individuals: A Critical Evaluation," *Psychiatry Research,* 3 (1980):345–355.

130. HANIN, I., et al. "Blood Choline and Its Meaning in Psychiatric and Neurological Disease States," in G. Pepeu and H. Ladinsky, eds., *Cholinergic Mechanisms: Phylogenetic Aspects, Central and Peripheral Synapses, and Clinical Significance.* New York: Plenum Press, 1981, p. 901.

131. HAUBRICH, D. R., WANG, P. F. L., and WEDEKING, P. "Role of Choline in Biosynthesis of Acetylcholine," *Federation Proceedings,* 33 (1974):477.

132. HESTON, L. L., and MASTRI, A. R. "The Genetics of Alzheimer's Disease: Associations with Hematologic Malignancy and Down's Syndrome," *Archives of General Psychiatry,* 34 (1977):976–981.

133. HESTON, L. L., et al. "Dementia of the Alzheimer Type: Clinical Genetics, Natural History and Associated Conditions," *Archives of General Psychiatry,* 38 (1981):1085–1090.

134. HILLHOUSE, E. W., BURDEN, J., and JONES, M. T. "The Effect of Various Putative Neurotransmitters on the Release of Corticotrophin Releasing Hormone from the Hypothalamus of the Rat *In Vitro*: The Effect of Acetylcholine and Noradrenaline," *Neuroendocrinology,* 17 (1975):1–11.

135. HOKFELT, T., et al. "Peptidergic Neurones," *Nature,* 284 (1980):515–522.

136. HORVATH, T. B., et al. "The Late Components of the Cerebral Event Related Potential in Alzheimer's Dementia," in L. W. Poon, ed., *Handbook of Clinical Memory Assessment of the Older Adult.* Washington, D.C.: American Psychological Association, forthcoming.

137. HUCKMAN, M. S., FOX, J., and TOPEL, J. "The Validity of Criteria for the Evaluation of Cerebral Atrophy by Computed Tomography," *Radiology,* 116 (1975): 85–92.

138. HYMAN, B. T., et al. "Alzheimer's Disease: Cell-Specific Pathology Isolates the Hippocampal Formation," *Science,* 225 (1984):1168–1170.

139. JACOBY, R. H., and LEVY, R. "Computed Tomography in the Elderly. II: Senile Dementia: Diagnosis and Functional Impairment," *British Journal of Psychiatry,* 136 (1980):256–269.

140. JACOBY, R. H., LEVY, R., and DAWSON, J. M. "Computed Tomography in the Elderly. I: The Normal Population," *British Journal of Psychiatry,* 136 (1980): 249–255.

141. JERVIS, G. A. "Alzheimer's Disease," in J. Minckler, ed., *Pathology of the Nervous System,* vol. 2. New York: McGraw-Hill, 1971, p. 1385.

142. JOHNS, C. A., et al. "Effect of Combined Phosphatidylcholine (PPC)-Piracetam Therapy in Alzheimer's Disease (AD)," (Abstract), Paper presented at the meeting of the Society of Biological Psychiatry, Los Angeles, 1984.

143. JOHNS, C. A., et al. "Clinical Studies of the Cholinergic Deficit in Alzheimer's Disease," in I. Hanin, ed., *Dynamics of*

Cholinergic Function. New York: Plenum Press, forthcoming.

144. JOHNSTON, M. V., McKINNEY, M., and COYLE, T. J. "Neocortical Cholinergic Innervation: A Description of Extrinsic and Intrinsic Components in the Rat," *Experimental Brain Research,* 43 (1981):159–172.

145. JOPE, R. S., WRIGHT, S. M., and JENDEN, D. J. "Choline Flux in Human Erythrocytes," *Clinica Chimica Acta,* in press.

146. KANOF, P. D., et al. "Red Blood Cell Choline. II: Kinetics in Alzheimer's disease," submitted for review.

147. KATZMAN, R. "The Prevalence and Malignancy of Alzheimer's Disease," *Archives of Neurology,* 33 (1976):217–218.

148. KAY, D.W.K. "The Epidemiology and Identification of Brain Deficit in the Elderly," in C. Eisdorfer and R. O. Friedel, eds., *Cognitive and Emotional Disturbances in the Elderly.* Chicago: Year Book Medical Publishers, 1977, pp. 11–26.

149. KAYE, W. H., et al. "Modest Facilitation of Memory in Dementia with Combined Lecithin and Anticholinesterase Treatment," *Biological Psychiatry,* 17 (1982): 275–280.

150. KRIEGER, D. T., and KRIEGER, H. P. "Circadian Pattern of Plasma 17-Hydroxycorticosteroid: Alteration by Anticholinergic Agents," *Science,* 155 (1967):1421–1422.

151. KRISTENSEN, V., OLSEN, M., and THILGAARD, A. "Levodopa Treatment of Presenile Dementia," *Acta Psychiatrica Scandinavica,* 55 (1977):41–51.

152. KUHL, D. E. "Imaging Local Brain Function with Emission Computed Tomography," *Radiology,* 150 (1984):625–631.

153. LANCRANJAN, I., OHNHAUS, E., and GIRARD, J. "The Adrenoreceptor Control of Adrenocorticotropin Secretion in Man," *Journal of Clinical Endocrinology and Metabolism,* 49 (1979):227–230.

154. LUNDBERG, J. M., HEDLUND, B., and BARTFAI, T. "Vasoactive Intestinal Polypeptide Enhances Muscarinic Ligand Binding in Cat Submandibular Salivary Gland," *Nature,* 295 (1982):147–149.

155. LUNDH, H., and THESLEFF, S. "The Mode of Action of 4-Aminopyridine and Guanidine on Transmitter Release from Motor Nerve Terminals," *European Journal of Pharmacology,* 42 (1977):411–412.

156. McKINNEY, M., DAVIES, P. and COYLE, J. T. "Somatostatin Is Not Co-localized in Cholinergic Neurons Innervating the Rat Cerebral Cortex-Hippocampal Formation," *Brain Research,* 243 (1982): 169–178.

157. MALAMUD, N. "Neuropathology of Organic Brain Syndromes Associated with Aging," in C. M. Gaitz, ed., *Aging and the Brain.* New York: Plenum Press, 1972, pp. 63–87.

158. MANN, D.M.A., YATES, P. O., and HAWKES, J. "The Noradrenergic System in Alzheimer and Multi-infarct Dementia," *Journal of Neurology, Neurosurgery and Psychiatry,* 45 (1982): 113–119.

159. MANN, D.M.A., et al. "Changes in the Monoamine Containing Neurones of the Human CNS in Senile Dementia," *British Journal of Psychiatry,* 136 (1980):533–541.

160. MANN, J. J., et al. "Central Amine Metabolism in Alzheimer's Disease: *In vivo* Relationship to Cognitive Deficit," *Neurobiology of Aging,* 2 (1981):57–60.

161. MARSDEN, C. D., and HARRISON, M.J.G. "Outcome Investigation of Patients with Presenile Dementia," *British Medical Journal,* 2 (1972):249–252.

162. MESULAM, M., et al. "Alzheimer's Disease and the Cholinergic Innervation of Neocortex by the Nucleus Basalis of Meynert," in R. Katzman, ed., *Biological Aspects of Alzheimer's Disease.* New York: Cold Spring Harbor Press, 1983, pp. 79–94.

163. MEWALDT, S. P., and GHONEIM, M. M. "The Effects and Interaction of Scopolamine, Physostigmine and Methamphetamine on Human Memory," *Pharmacology, Biochemistry and Behavior,* 10 (1979):205–210.

164. MILLINGTON, W., and GOLDBERG, A. M. "Precursor Dependence of Acetylcholine Release from Rat Cortex *In Vitro,*" *Federation Proceedings,* 40 (1981):268.

165. MOHS, R. C., DAVIS, K. L., and LEVY, M. I. "Partial Reversal of Anticholinergic

Amnesia by Choline Chloride," *Life Sciences,* 29 (1981):1317–1323.

166. MOHS, R. C., ROSEN, W. G., and DAVIS, K. L. "Defining Treatment Efficacy in Patients with Alzheimer's Disease," in S. Corkin et al., eds., *Alzheimer's Disease: A Report of Progress in Research,* vol. 19 in *Aging* series. New York: Raven Press, 1982, pp. 351–356.

167. MOHS, R. C., et al. "Choline Chloride Treatment of Memory Deficits in the Elderly," *American Journal of Psychiatry,* 136 (1979):1275–1277.

168. MOHS, R. C., et al. "Choline Chloride Effects on Memory in the Elderly," *Neurobiology of Aging,* 1 (1980):21–25.

169. MOHS, R. C., et al. "Anticholinergic Dementia as a Model of Alzheimer's Disease," in L. W. Poon, ed., *Handbook of Clinical Memory Assessment of the Older Adult.* Washington, D.C.: American Psychological Association, forthcoming.

170. MOHS, R. C., et al. "Oral Physostigmine Treatment of Patients with Alzheimer's Disease," *American Journal of Psychiatry,* in press.

171. MURAMOTO, O., et al. "Effect of Physostigmine on Constructional and Memory Tasks in Alzheimer's Disease," *Archives of Neurology,* 36 (1979):501–503.

172. NAGUIB, M., and LEVY, R. "CT Scanning in Senile Dementia: A Follow-up of Survivors," *British Journal of Psychiatry,* 141 (1982):618–620.

173. NICKOLSON, V. J., and WOLTHIUS, O. L. "Effect of the Acquisition-Enhancing Drug Piracetam on Rat Cerebral Energy Metabolism: Comparison with Naftidrofuryl and Methamphetamine," *Biochemical Pharmacology,* 25 (1976): 2241–2244.

174. NORDBERG, A., et al. "Brain Enzymes and Acetylcholine Receptors in Dementia of the Alzheimer Type and Chronic Alcohol Abuse," in L. Amaducci, A. N. Davison, and P. Antuono, eds., *Aging of the Brain and Dementia,* vol. 13 in *Aging* series. New York: Raven Press, 1980, pp. 169–171.

175. OSTFIELD, A. M., and ARUGUETE, A. "Central Nervous System Effects of Hyoscine in Man," *Journal of Pharmacology and Experimental Therapeutics,* 137 (1962):133–139.

176. PALKOVITS, M., et al. "Selective Depletion of Somatostatin in Rat Brain by Cysteamine," *Brain Research,* 240 (1982):178–180.

177. PERRY, E. K. "The Cholinergic System in Old Age and Alzheimer's Disease," *Age and Aging,* 9 (1980):1–8.

178. PERRY, E. K., and PERRY, R. H. *Biochemistry of Dementia.* London: John Wiley & Sons, 1980.

179. PERRY, E. K., et al. "Necropsy Evidence of Central Cholinergic Deficits in Senile Dementia," *Lancet,* 1 (1977):189–191.

180. PERRY, E. K., et al. "Neurotransmitter Enzyme Abnormalities in Senile Dementia," *Journal of the Neurological Sciences,* 34 (1977):247–265.

181. PERRY, E. K., et al. "Correlation of Cholinergic Abnormalities with Senile Plaques and Mental Test Scores in Senile Dementia," *British Medical Journal,* 2 (1978):1457–1459.

182. PERRY, E. K., et al. "Neurochemical Activities in Human Temporal Lobe Related to Aging and Alzheimer-Type Changes," *Neurobiology of Aging,* 2 (1981):251–256.

183. PERRY, E. K., et al. "Neuropathological and Biochemical Observations on the Noradrenergic System in Alzheimer's Disease," *Journal of the Neurological Sciences,* 51 (1981):279–287.

184. PERRY, E. K., et al. "Intralaminar Neurochemical Distributions in Human Midtemporal Cortex: Comparison Between Alzheimer's Disease and the Normal," *Journal of Neurochemistry,* 42 (1984): 1402–1410.

185. PERRY, R. H., et al. "Neuropeptides in Alzheimer's Disease, Depression and Schizophrenia: A Postmortem Analysis of Vasoactive Intestinal Peptide and Cholecystokinin in Cerebral Cortex," *Journal of the Neurological Sciences,* 51 (1981):465–472.

186. PERRY, R. H., et al. "Extensive Loss of Choline Acetyltransferase Activity Is Not Reflected by Neuronal Loss in the Nucleus Basalis of Meynert in Alzheimer's Disease," *Neuroscience Letters,* 33 (1982):311–315.

187. PERRY, R. H., et al. "Cortical Cholinergic

Deficit in Mentally Impaired Parkinsonian Patients," *Lancet,* 2 (1983):789–790.

188. PETERS, B. H., and LEVIN, H. S. "Effects of Physostigmine and Lecithin on Memory in Alzheimer's Disease," *Annals of Neurology,* 6 (1979):219–221.

189. PETERSEN, R. C. "Scopolamine-Induced Learning Failures in Man," *Psychopharmacology* (Berlin), 52 (1977):283–289.

190. ———. "Scopolamine State-Dependent Memory Processes in Man," *Psychopharmacology* (Berlin), 64 (1979):309–314.

191. PHVAPRADIT, P., et al. "Bromocriptine in Presenile Dementia," *British Medical Journal,* 1 (1978):1052–1053.

192. PLUM, F. "Dementia, an Approaching Epidemic," *Nature,* 279 (1979):372–373.

193. PRADO DE CARVALHO, L., and ZORNETZER, S. F. "The Involvement of the Locus Coeruleus in Memory," *Behavioral Neurology and Biology,* 31 (1981): 173–186.

194. PRIBRAM, K. J., and McGUINESS, L. "Arousal, Activation and Effect in the Control of Attention," *Psychological Review,* 82 (1975):116–149.

195. QUARTERMAIN, D., and BOTWINICK, C. Y. "Role of Biogenic Amines in the Reversal of Cycloheximide-Induced Amnesia," *Journal of Comparative and Physiological Psychology,* 88 (1975):386–401.

196. RANDT, C. T., et al. "Norepinephrine Biosynthesis Inhibition: Effects on Memory in Mice," *Science,* 172 (1971):489–499.

197. RASKIND, M., et al. "Dexamethasone Suppression Test and Cortisol Circadian Rhythm in Primary Degenerative Dementia," *American Journal of Psychiatry,* 139 (1982):1468–1471.

198. RASKIND, M. A., et al. "Norepinephrine and MHPG Levels in CSF and Plasma in Alzheimer's Disease," *Archives of General Psychiatry,* 41 (1984):343–346.

199. RASMUSSON, D. D., and DUDAR, J. D. "Effect of Scopolamine on Maze Learning Performance in Humans," *Experientia,* 35 (1979):1069–1070.

200. REISINE, T. D., et al. "Pre- and Postsynaptic Neurochemical Alterations in Alzheimer's Disease," *Brain Research,* 159 (1978):477–481.

201. RENVOIZE, E. B., and JERRAM, T. "Choline in Alzheimer's Disease," *New England Journal of Medicine,* 301 (1979): 330.

202. ROBERTO, R. B., FLEXNER, J. B., and FLEXNER, L. B. "Some Evidence for the Involvement of Adrenergic Sites in the Memory Trace," *Proceedings of the National Academy of Sciences USA,* 66 (1970):310.

203. ROBERTS, M. A., and CAIRD, F. I. "Computerized Tomography and Intellectual Impairment in the Elderly," *Journal of Neurology, Neurosurgery and Psychiatry,* 39 (1976):986–989.

204. RON, M. A., et al. "Diagnostic Accuracy in Presenile Dementia," *British Journal of Psychiatry,* 134 (1979):161–168.

205. ROSEN, W. G., et al. "Pathological Verification of Ischemic Score in Differentiation of Dementias," *Annals of Neurology,* 7 (1980):486–488.

206. ROSSOR, M. N. "Neurotransmitters in CNS Disease: Dementia," *Lancet,* 2 (1982): 200–204.

207. ROSSOR, M. N., et al. "Arginine Vasopressin and Choline Acetyltransferase in Brains of Patients with Alzheimer Type Senile Dementia," *Lancet* 2 (1980): 1367–1368.

208. ROSSOR, M. N., et al. "Reduced Amounts of Immunoreactive Somatostatin in the Temporal Cortex in Senile Dementia of Alzheimer Type," *Neuroscience Letters,* 20 (1980):373–377.

209. ROSSOR, M. N., et al. "Reduced Cortical Choline Acetyltransferase Activity in Senile Dementia of Alzheimer Type Is Not Accompanied by Changes in Vasoactive Intestinal Polypeptide," *Brain Research,* 201 (1980):249–253.

210. ROSSOR, M. N., et al. "The Cholinergic Defect of the Frontal Cortex in Alzheimer's Disease Is Age Dependent," *Lancet,* 2 (1981):1422.

211. ROSSOR, M. N., et al. "A Post-mortem Study of the Cholinergic and GABA Systems in Senile Dementia," *Brain,* 105 (1982):313–330.

212. ROSSOR, M. N., et al. "Neurochemical Characteristics of Early and Late Onset Types of Alzheimer's Disease," *British Medical Journal,* 288 (1984):961–964.

213. ROSSOR, M. N., et al. "Patterns of Neuro-

peptide Deficits in Alzheimer's Disease," in R. J. Wurtman, S. H. Corkin, and J. H. Growdon, eds., *Alzheimer's Disease: Advances in Basic Research and Therapies.* N.P.: Center for Brain Sciences and Metabolism and Charitable Trust, 1984, pp. 29–38.

214. ROTH, M. "The Natural History of Mental Disorder Arising in the Senium," *Journal of Mental Science,* 101 (1955):281–301.

215. ROTH, M., and HOPKINS, B. "Psychological Test Performance in Patients Over Sixty: Senile Psychosis and Affective Disorders of Old Age," *Journal of Mental Science,* 99 (1953):439–538.

216. RUBERG, M., et al. "Muscarinic Binding and Choline Acetyltransferase Activity in Parkinsonian Subjects with Reference to Dementia," *Brain Research,* 232 (1982):129–139.

217. SACHAR, E. J., et al. "Dextroamphetamine and Cortisol in Depression," *Archives of General Psychiatry,* 37 (1980):755–757.

218. SAFER, D. J., and ALLEN, R. P. "The Central Effects of Scopolamine in Man," *Biological Psychiatry,* 3 (1971):347–355.

219. SAGAR, S. A., et al. "Depletion of Somatostatin-Like Immunoreactivity in the Rat Central Nervous System by Cysteamine," *Journal of Neurosciences,* 2 (1982):225–231.

220. SAJDEL-SULKOWSKA, E. M., and MAROTTA, C. A. "Alzheimer's Disease Brain: Alterations in RNA Levels and in a Ribonuclease-Inhibitor Complex," *Science,* 225 (1984):947–949.

221. SAJDEL-SULKOWSKA, E. M., et al. "*In Vitro* Protein Synthesis by Messenger RNA from the Alzheimer's Disease Brain," in R. Katzman, ed., *Biological Aspects of Alzheimer's Disease.* New York: Cold Spring Harbor Laboratory, 1983, pp. 193–200.

222. SELTZER, B., and SHERWIN, I. "A Comparison of Clinical Features in Early- and Late-Onset Primary Degenerative Dementia," *Archives of Neurology,* 40 (1983):143–146.

223. SIGNORET, J., WHITELEY, A. L., and L'HERMITTE, F. "Influence of Choline on Amnesia in Early Alzheimer's Disease," *Lancet,* 2 (1978):837.

224. SIM, M., and SUSSMAN, I. "Alzheimer's Disease: Its Natural History and Differential Diagnosis," *Journal of Nervous and Mental Disease,* 135 (1962):489–499.

225. SITARAM, N., WEINGARTNER, H., and GILLIN, J. C. "Human Serial Learning: Enhancement with Arecoline and Impairment with Scopolamine Correlated with Performance on Placebo," *Science,* 201 (1978):274–276.

226. SMITH, C. M., and SWASH, M. "Physostigmine in Alzheimer's Disease," *Lancet,* 1 (1979):42.

227. SMITH, C. M., et al. "Choline Therapy in Alzheimer's Disease," *Lancet,* 2 (1978):318.

228. SMITH, R. C., et al. "Cholinesterase Enzymes in the Blood of Patients with Alzheimer's Disease," *Life Sciences,* 30 (1982):543–546.

229. SOININEN, H., HALONEN, T., and RIEKKINEN, P. J. "Acetylcholinesterase Activities in Cerebrospinal Fluid of Patients with Senile Dementia of Alzheimer Type," *Acta Neurologica Scandinavica,* 64 (1981):217–224.

230. SOININEN, H., PURANEN, M., and RIEKKINEN, P. J. "Computed Tomography Findings in Senile Dementia and Normal Aging," *Journal of Neurology, Neurosurgery and Psychiatry,* 45 (1982):50–54.

231. SOLOMON, S., et al. "Impairment of Memory Function by Antihypertensive Medication," *Archives of General Psychiatry,* 40 (1983):1109–1112.

232. SPAR, J. E., and GERNER, R. "Does the Dexamethasone Suppression Test Distinguish Dementia from Depression?" *American Journal of Psychiatry,* 139 (1982):238–240.

233. SPILLANE, J. A., et al. "Selective Vulnerability of Neurons in Organic Dementia," *Nature,* 226 (1977):558–559.

234. SPOKES, E.G.S. "An Analysis of Factors Influencing Measurements of Dopamine, Noradrenaline, Glutamate Decarboxylase and Choline Acetylase in Human Postmortem Brain Tissue," *Brain,* 102 (1979):333–346.

235. STEINER, J. A., and GRAHAME-SMITH, D. G. "Central Pharmacological Control of Corticosterone Secretion in the Intact Rat: Demonstration of Cholinergic and Serotonergic Facilitatory and Adrener-

gic Inhibitory Mechanisms," *Psycho-pharmacology*, 71 (1980):213–217.

236. STRUBLE, R. G., et al. "Cholinergic Innervation in Neuritic Plaques," *Science*, 216 (1982):413–415.

237. SULLIVAN, E. V., et al. "Physostigmine and Lecithin in Alzheimer's Disease," in S. Corkin, K. L. Davis, and J. H. Growden, eds., *Alzheimer's Disease: A Report of Progress in Research*, (vol. 19 in *Aging* series.), New York: Plenum Press, 1982, pp. 361–368.

238. SUMMERS, W. K., et al. "Use of THA in Treatment of Alzheimer-like Dementia: Pilot Study in Twelve Patients, *Biological Psychiatry*, 16 (1981):145–153.

239. SYNDULKO, K., et al. "Long Latency Event-Related Potentials in Normal Aging and Dementia," in J. Courion, F. Mauguierer, and M. Revol, eds., *Clinical Applications of Evoked Potentials*. New York: Raven Press, 1981, pp. 279–285.

240. TAGLIAVINI, F., and PILLERI, G. "Neuronal Counts in Basal Nucleus of Meynert in Alzheimer's Disease and in Simple Senile Dementia," *Lancet*, 2 (1983):469–470.

241. TARBIT, I., et al. "Hippocampal Free Amino Acids in Alzheimer's Disease," *Journal of Neurochemistry*, 35 (1980): 1246–1249.

242. TERRY, R. D., and DAVIES, P. "Dementia of the Alzheimer's Type," *Annual Review of Neuroscience*, 3 (1980):77–95.

243. TERRY, R. D., and KATZMAN, R. "Senile Dementia of the Alzheimer Type," *Annals of Neurology*, 14 (1983):497–506.

244. THAL, L. J., and FULD, P. A. "Memory Enhancement with Oral Physostigmine in Alzheimer's Disease," *New England Journal of Medicine*, 308 (1983):720.

245. THAL, L. J., et al. "Choline Chloride Fails to Improve Cognition in Alzheimer's Disease," *Neurobiology of Aging*, 2 (1981):205–208.

246. THAL, L. J., et al. "Oral Physostigmine and Lecithin Improve Memory in Alzheimer Disease," *Annals of Neurology*, 13 (1983):491–496.

247. TOMLINSON, B. E., BLESSED, G., and ROTH, M. "Observations on the Brains of Non-Demented Old People," *Journal of the Neurological Sciences*, 7 (1968): 331–356.

248. ——. "Observations on the Brains of Demented Old People," *Journal of the Neurological Sciences*, 11 (1970):205–242.

249. TOMLINSON, B. E., IRVING, D., and BLESSED, G., "Cell Loss in the Locus Coeruleus in Senile Dementia of the Alzheimer Type," *Journal of the Neurological Sciences*, 49 (1981):419–428.

250. TORACK, R. M. *The Pathological Physiology of Dementia*, Berlin: Springer-Verlag, 1978.

251. TUNE, L., et al. "CSF Acetylcholinesterase in Dementia Syndromes," Paper presented at the American Psychiatric Association Annual Meeting, Los Angeles, 1984.

252. VAN WOERT, M. H., et al. "L-Dopa in Senile Dementia," *Lancet*, 1 (1970):573–574.

253. VIZI, E. S., VAN DIJK, J., and FOLDES, F. F. "The Effect of 4-Aminopyridine on Acetylcholine Release," *Journal of Neural Transmission*, 41 (1977):265–274.

254. VROULIS, G., et al. "Effects of Lecithin on Memory and Behavior in Alzheimer's Type Dementia," *Psychopharmacology Bulletin*, 17 (1981):127–128.

255. WECKER, L., DETTBARN, W. D., and SCHMIDT, D. E. "Choline Administration: Modification of the Central Actions of Atropine," *Science*, 199 (1978): 86.

256. WEINGARTNER, H., SITARAM, N., and GILLIN, J. C. "The Role of the Cholinergic System in Memory Consolidation," *Bulletin of the Psychoneurologic Society*, 13 (1979):9–11.

257. WELCH, M. J., MARKHAM, C. H., and JENDEN, D. J. "Acetylcholine and Choline in Cerebrospinal Fluid of Patients with Parkinson's Disease and Huntington's Chorea," *Journal of Neurology, Neurosurgery and Psychiatry*, 39 (1976):367–374.

258. WENK, H., BIGL, V., and MEYER, U. "Cholinergic Projections from Magnocellular Nuclei of the Basal Forebrain to Cortical Areas in Rats," *Brain Research Reviews*, 2 (1980):295–316.

259. WESSLING, H., and AGOSTON, S. "Effects of 4-Aminopyridine in Elderly Patients with Alzheimer's Disease," *New En-*

gland Journal of Medicine, 310 (1984): 988–989.

260. WHITALEY, A., et al. "Action de la Choline Sur les Troubles Mnesiques de la Maladie d'Alzheimer," *Revue Neurologique*, 135 (1979):475–565.

261. WHITE, P., et al. "Neocortical Cholinergic Neurons in Elderly People," *Lancet*, 1 (1977):668–671.

262. WHITEHOUSE, P. J., et al. "Alzheimer's Disease and Senile Dementia: Loss of Neurons in the Basal Forebrain," *Science*, 215 (1982):1237–1239.

263. WHITEHOUSE, P. J., et al. "Basal Forebrain Neurons in the Dementia of Parkinson Disease," *Annals of Neurology*, 13 (1983):243–248.

264. WILCOCK, G. K., and ESIRI, M. M. "Plaques, Tangles, and Dementia: A Quantitative Study," *Journal of the Neurological Sciences*, 56 (1982):343–356.

265. WILCOCK, G. K., et al. "Correlation of Cortical Choline Acetyltransferase Activity with the Severity of Dementia and Histological Abnormalities," *Journal of the Neurological Sciences*, 57 (1982):407–417.

266. WILSON, R. S., et al. "Computed Tomography in Dementia," *Neurology*, 32 (1982):1054–1057.

267. WINBLAD, G., et al. "Biogenic Amines in Brains of Patients with Alzheimer's Disease," in S. Corkin, et al., eds., *Alzheimer's Disease: A Report of Progress in Research*. New York: Raven Press, 1982, pp. 25–33.

268. WISNIEWSKI, H. M., and KOZLOWSKI, P. B. "Evidence for Blood-brain Barrier Changes in Senile Dementia of the Alz-heimer Type (SDAT)," in F. M. Sinek, and C. R. Merril, eds., *Alzheimer's Disease, Down's Syndrome, and Aging*. New York: Annals of the New York Academy of Science, vol. 396, 1982, pp. 119–129.

269. WOOD, P. L., et al. "Reduced Lumbar CSF Somatostatin Levels in Alzheimer's Disease," *Life Sciences*, 31 (1982):2073–2079.

270. WURTMAN, R. J., MAGIL, G. S., and REINSTEIN, D. K. "Piracetam Diminished Hippocampal Acetylcholine Levels in Rats," *Life Sciences*, 28 (1981):1091–1093.

271. YAKSH, T. L., et al. "Acetylcholinesterase Turnover in Brain, Cerebrospinal Fluid and Plasma," *Journal of Neurochemistry*, 25 (1975):853–860.

272. YAMAMURA, H. I., and SNYDER, S. "High-affinity Transport of Choline into Synaptosomes of Rat Brain," *Journal of Neurochemistry*, 21 (1973):1355–1374.

273. YATES, C. M., et al. "Dopamine in Alzheimer's Disease and Senile Dementia," *Lancet*, 2 (1979):851–852.

274. YATES, C. M., et al. "Noradrenaline in Alzheimer-type Dementia and Down's Syndrome," *Lancet*, 2 (1981):39–40.

275. YATES, C. M., et al. "Thyrotropin-Releasing Hormone, Luteinizing Hormone–Releasing Hormone and Substance P Immunoreactivity in Post-mortem Brain from Cases of Alzheimer-Type Dementia and Down's Syndrome," *Brain Research*, 258 (1983):45–52.

276. ZORNETZER, S. F., and GOLD, M. S. "The Locus Coeruleus: Its Possible Role in Memory Consolidation," *Physiology of Behavior*, 16 (1976):331–336.

CHAPTER 26

BIOLOGY, PATHOPHYSIOLOGY, AND THERAPY OF CHRONIC PAIN

John J. Bonica and C. Richard Chapman

The purpose of this chapter is to provide a discussion of some fundamental aspects and treatments of chronic pain—an objective that has been and continues to be one of the most important and pressing issues of the health care system of this and other industrialized countries throughout the world. This importance stems from the fact that chronic pain that requires therapy by physicians and other health professionals afflicts millions of persons annually, and in many (most?) patients, relief is inadequate.[9,22,30] Consequently, chronic pain is the most frequent cause of suffering and disability that seriously impairs the quality of life of millions of people throughout the world. Although accurate statistics from epidemiological studies are not available, data from various sources suggest that nearly a third of the population in industrialized countries have chronic pain, and of these, half to two-thirds are either partially or totally disabled for periods of days, weeks, and months, and some permanently. Consequently, chronic pain is a serious economic problem as well as a major health problem.

Convincing data to support these statements will be presented.

The material will be presented in four parts. First, brief mention will be made of anatomical, biochemical, physiological, psychological, and pathophysiological aspects of acute pain, and how these differ from those pertaining to chronic pain. A general consideration of chronic pain, including definition, prevalence, effects, mechanisms, and current status of therapy, will follow. Third, we will present an overview of basic principles of diagnosis of chronic pain and the therapeutic modalities currently available. And fourth, we will discuss some of the most important chronic pain syndromes. Considering the complexity of the subject and the limitation of space, many of these aspects will be covered rather superficially, with only "key" references cited. Detailed accounts and extensive bibliographies can be found in a number of books* and review articles.†

*See references 9, 11, 16, 30, 33, 57, 85, 98, 99, 132, 138, and 157.
†See references 4, 10, 18, 22, 25, 27, 31, 39, and 41.

¶ Acute Pain

Acute pain consists of a constellation of unpleasant perceptual and emotional experiences and certain associated autonomic, psychological, and behavioral responses provoked by tissue-damaging (noxious) mechanical, thermal, and/or chemical stimulation produced by injury or disease. The older concept of pain, which prevailed until two decades ago, suggested that the perception of pain was achieved via a simple, straight-through system consisting of peripheral nerves and spinothalamic fibers that transmitted nociceptive (pain) information to the brain without modification.[9,160] This assumed a one-to-one relationship between intensity of the stimulus and pain perception, and, although psychological, cognitive, and motivational factors were known to influence the "reaction to pain," they were relegated secondary roles.[160] However, extensive recent investigations provoked by the publication in 1965 of the Melzack-Wall theory of pain,[97] the founding and activities of the International Association for the Study of Pain and its journal, *PAIN*, and other factors,[25] have provided a vast amount of new information that clearly demonstrates that pain is a much more complex phenomenon than the aforementioned simple system suggested. Acute pain provoked by injury or disease is the net effect of many simultaneously interacting biochemical, physiological, and psychological mechanisms that involve activity in most parts of the nervous system concerned with sensory, motivational, and cognitive processes, and psychodynamic mechanisms. Limitations of space permit brief mention of only several aspects of the pain process.

Peripheral Nociceptive System

Tissue damage inherent in injury or disease causes cellular breakdown with liberation of intracellular biochemical substances, and also causes noxious stimulation. These substances activate specialized high-threshold receptors in "bare" nerve endings called nociceptors, which are endings of many small myelinated A delta and most unmyelinated C fibers that supply the skin, muscle, viscera, and other pain-sensitive body tissues. The chemical agents liberated by injury include potassium, H^+, lactic acid, serotonin, bradykinins, and prostaglandins, all of which apparently activate nociceptors either by direct action or indirectly by altering their microenvironment. The microenvironment consists of smooth muscles, blood capillaries, and efferent sympathetic nerve endings, which, in turn, sensitize nociceptors to respond to innocuous stimulation.[166] These algogenic (pain-producing) substances can also cause a marked increase in the tone of smooth muscles that results in pain (e.g., colic pain) and are probably operative in stimulating nociceptors in ischemic heart and skeletal muscles to produce pain.

The nociceptors transduce the stimuli into impulses that are transmitted from tissues below the head, via A delta and C fibers in spinal nerves, to the spinal cord dorsal horn, and from the head to the trigeminal nucleus caudalis. Upon reaching these structures, impulses are subjected to modulating influences that, in part, determine their further course. Some of the nociceptive impulses are transmitted to the anterior and anterolateral horn cells of the same and adjacent segments to produce segmental (nocifensive) reflex responses. Others stimulate the neurons, the axons of which make up ascending systems that transmit the nociceptive impulses to the brain stem to provoke suprasegmental reflex responses and to the brain to result in pain perception and other cortical responses. Recent data indicate that in addition to the spinothalamic tract, which traditionally was considered the primary (only) pain pathway, other ascending pathways are involved in the pain process. The anatomy of the nociceptive system is depicted in figures 26–1 and 26–2.

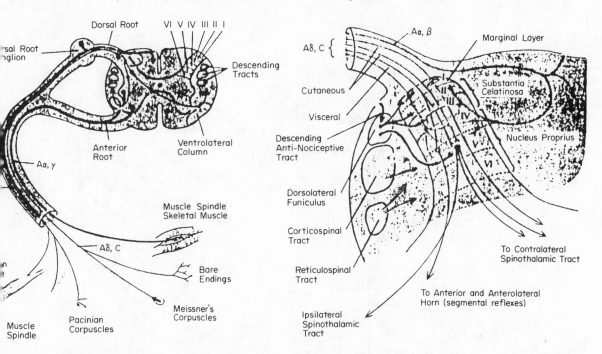

Figure 26–1. Disposition of nociceptive (and other afferent and efferent) pathways in typical spinal nerve (left) and the dorsal horn (right).
NOTE: Reprinted by permission from John J. Bonica, "Pathophysiology of Pain," *Current Concepts in Postoperative Pain,* January 1978, p. 7.

Modulation of Nociception and Pain

One of the most exciting areas of recent research concerns the various neural, biochemical, and psychophysiological mechanisms that participate in the modulation of nociceptive information from tissues to the brain. In the peripheral system, repeated stimulation or an inflammatory process consequent to injury or disease causes liberation of algogenic substances that lower the threshold of nociceptors, so that innocuous stimulation such as light touch produces pain and associated responses.[113] Moreover, the degree of nociceptive input from the periphery into the spinal cord is also influenced by sympathetic function, blood flow, and the chemical environment of the nociceptive afferent units in the injured tissue.[154] In damaged nociceptive afferents, as obtains in the postoperative period, these factors and the liberation of greater amounts of epinephrine and norepinephrine increase nociceptive input.[154] On the other hand, nonnoxious stimulation of the skin by rubbing, application of cold, or transcutaneous electrical stimulation increases activity in the large fibers. This in some way decreases the transmission of nociceptive impulses from the periphery to the central nervous system (CNS); perhaps at various levels of the neuraxis.

Nociceptive transmission in the dorsal horn is also affected by the activity and through interaction of local interneurons of the substantia gelatinosa[154] and supraspinal descending systems. Recent evidence suggests there are several descending systems that modulate pain, but the best studied is the one discovered in 1968 by Reynolds[117] and subsequently studied by many groups (see Fields[52]; Fields and Basbaum[53]; Liebeskind, Mayer, and Akil[83]; and Sherman and Liebeskind[123] for a review). These studies demonstrated that stimulation of certain neurons in the periaqueductal gray (PAG) and periventricular gray (PVG) matter of the

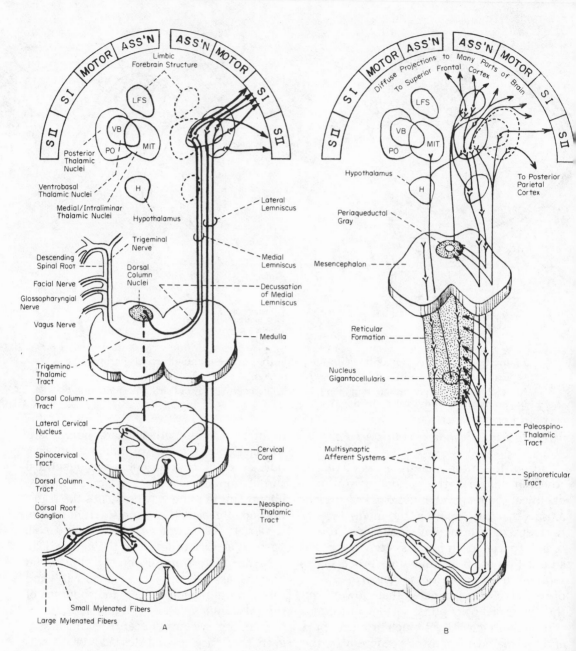

Figure 26–2.   The nociceptive system.

midbrain produces profound analgesia, apparently without interfering with motor function or with the animal's response to other sensory stimuli. The anatomy of the system is depicted in figure 26–3.

More recent studies suggest there are descending inhibitory systems that do not involve opioids.[82,100] The data acquired to date make it perfectly clear there are a number of mechanisms of pain inhibition, involving spinal mechanisms, supraspinal mechanisms, opioids, and/or centrifugal control on spinal nociceptive systems.

Psychological Factors

During the past quarter century, we have acquired much scientific data that impressively emphasize the importance of motivational, affective, cognitive, emotional, and other psychological factors on the individual's total pain experience.[99,133] Moreover, this new information has put in sharper focus the influence of perceptual factors, learning, personality, ethnic and sociocultural factors, and the environment, and has helped somewhat to clarify the dynamics of anxiety, depression, and attention and the significance of pain.[26,133,145]

Recent psychological studies have also provided impressive evidence that the medical model is not sufficient to explain the abnormal behavior manifested by some patients with chronic pain and requires inclusion of the behavioral model.[57] This emphasis on chronic pain behavior resulting primarily from reinforcing environmental influences, or so-called operant mechanisms, has had a favorable impact on the management of some patients with chronic pain.[25,57,98]

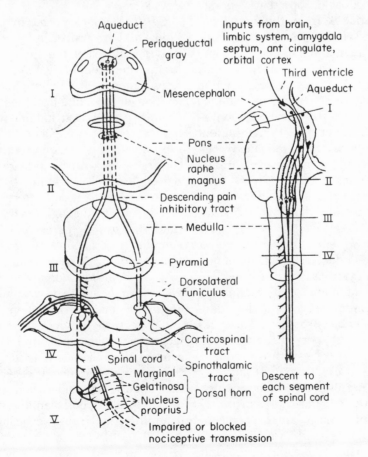

Figure 26–3. Nociceptive transmission in the dorsal horn.

Responses Associated with Acute Pain

Acute pain produces segmental, suprasegmental, and cortical responses that differ significantly from the physiological and psychological responses to chronic pain.[22,26] The responses to acute pain are intended to help maintain homeostasis, but as emphasized in the next section, they not infrequently become abnormal and produce deleterious effects.

Segmental reflex responses are the result of nociceptive stimulation of anterior horn cells and anterolateral horn cells and thus enhance nociception and produce alteration of ventilation, circulation, and gastrointestinal (GI) and urinary function.[9,22,26] Stimulation of somatomotor cells results in an increase in skeletal muscle tension that decreases chest wall compliance and initiates positive feedback loops that generate nociceptive impulses from the muscle.[166] Stimulation of sympathetic preganglionic neurons causes an increase in heart rate and stroke volume and, consequently, cardiac output, and also produces vasoconstriction that may progress to ischemia. The ischemia further contributes to the local pathophysiology and alters the chemical environment of nociceptors; both effects enhance nociceptive stimulation. Moreover, sympathetic hyperactivity causes a decrease in GI tone that may progress to ileus and a decrease in genitourinary function that results in urinary retention.[9,26]

Suprasegmental reflex responses result from nociceptive-induced stimulation of medullary centers of ventilation and circulation, hypothalamic autonomic (predominantly sympathetic) centers, neuroendocrine function, and some limbic structures. These responses consist of: (1) hyperventilation; (2) increased sympathetic tone, with consequent further increase in cardiac output and cardiac work, total peripheral resistance (which results in an increase in blood pressure), cardiac workload, metabolism, and oxygen consumption; and (3) increased hormonal secretion by the adrenal medulla and cortex and by the pituitary/hypothalamic axis, characteristic of the stress response.* The latter includes increased secretion of catabolically acting hormones, catecholamines, cortisol, adrenocorticotrophic hormone (ACTH), antidiuretic hormone (ADH), and glucagon and a decrease of anabolically acting hormones, insulin, and testosterone. The increased catecholamines further increase cardiac output and peripheral resistance and, together with other hormones, increase blood glucose, free fatty acid, plasma cyclic adenosine monophosphate (AMP), ketones, and lactates. These increase substrate mobilization from storages to central organs and traumatized tissue and lead to a catabolic state and a negative nitrogen balance. The degree and duration of these hormonal/metabolic changes are related to the degree of tissue damage, and many biochemical changes last for days.[5]

Cortical responses occur in the awake individual and are provoked by nociceptive impulses that reach the highest part of the brain, where they activate very complex systems concerned with integration and perception, or recognition, of the pain sensation. Cognitive, analytical, judgmental, and memory processes simultaneously interpret the type, quality, and meaning of the pain within the framework of the individual's learning, personality, culture, ethnic background, experience, motivation, interpersonal influences, and psychological condition at the time the pain is perceived. These highly complex interactions of sensory, motivational, and cognitive processes that produce pain act on the autonomic and somatic motor systems and initiate psychodynamic mechanisms of anxiety, apprehension, and fear and collectively produce the complex physiological, psychological, and behavioral responses that characterize the multidimensional pain experience. It deserves emphasis that anxiety, especially when severe, greatly enhances the hypothalamic response[69] and, in addition, may cause cortically induced in-

---

*See references 5, 9, 26, 78, 143, and 158.

creased blood viscosity[119] and clotting,[48] fibrinolysis,[108] and platelet aggregation.[164]

Biological Function

It has long been appreciated that acute pain of disease has the important biological function of warning the individual something is wrong and usually prompts him or her to seek medical counsel; it is also used by the physician as a diagnostic aid. Moreover, the physiological reflex responses usually help the organism cope with the disease or injury, thus helping to maintain homeostasis. What is not generally appreciated, however, is that severe acute pain in the postoperative period, or after burns or accidental injury, has no useful function. If not adequately relieved, it produces serious abnormal physiological and psychological reactions that often cause complications.* Similar deleterious effects result if, after it has served its biological function, severe pain of myocardial infarction, pancreatitis, and other acute pathological processes is not effectively relieved.[112] Even severe pain associated with certain physiological processes such as parturition, if allowed to persist, will produce deleterious effects.[28] The reflex responses are likely to become abnormal and cause serious complications, especially in patients with hypoxia, hypercapnia, hypovolemia, heart disease, or cachexia or who are otherwise in poor physical condition.

Although in many instances the injuries and/or disease that produce acute pain are properly managed, moderate to severe pain is inadequately relieved in all too many patients. Many patients with postoperative or posttraumatic pain or the pain of acute myocardial infarction, acute pancreatitis, or renal colic are given narcotics, which, while effective, are usually given in insufficient amounts, and as a result the pain remains partially or wholly unrelieved.[26,44,93,94] Moreover, even when properly administered, intramuscular or intravenous narcot-

*See references 4, 9, 22, 78, and 143.

ics frequently do not produce complete pain relief or decrease the abnormal segmental and suprasegmental reflex responses that aggravate the pathophysiology. Let us cite two examples of postinjury pain, two examples of pain associated with visceral disease, and the pain associated with the physiological phenomenon of human parturition.

POSTOPERATIVE PAIN

In the postoperative period, persistent noxious stimulation from the operative site often causes moderate to severe pain and abnormal reflex responses. Old and new data suggest that of nearly 25 million people who will undergo surgical operations in the United States in 1984, 30 percent will have mild or no pain; 30 percent will have moderate pain; and the rest will have severe pain (see Benedetti and Bonica[4] for review). Severe pain occurs more frequently following surgery of the upper abdomen, chest, back, major joints, and anorectal region. Following chest and intraabdominal surgery, nociceptive stimulation is produced by biochemical changes and surgical injury to the nerves in the skin, deep somatic tissue, and viscera. The incidence and severity of postoperative pain is also significantly influenced by the physical, psychological, emotional, and personality characteristics of the patient and the degree of preoperative and postoperative anxiety and fear (see Chapman[39] for review). All of these contribute to the pain and cause severe reflex muscle spasm and splinting, which decrease chest wall compliance; the sympathetic hyperactivity causes varying degrees of ileus and urinary retention. The decreased chest wall compliance, together with pain-induced voluntary splinting and other factors combine to produce decreased vital capacity, inspiratory capacity, and functional residual capacity. These frequently cause hypoxemia and microatelectasis, which, if untreated, develops into pulmonary complications. Such complications occur in 15 to 20 percent of patients after thoracic and upper abdominal surgery, 7 to 10 percent following lower intraabdominal surgery and back surgery, and 3 to 5 percent after other operations (see Benedetti and Bonica[4] for references). In addition, patients incur the risk of thrombus formation in the lower limbs if, because their pain is inadequately relieved, they consequently reduce physical activity. This process is enhanced by pain-induced anxiety and the consequent effects on blood clotting. Pain and reflex responses also markedly impair muscle metabolism and muscle function following major surgery on large joints. All of these complications prolong postoperative morbidity, disability, and hospitalization and greatly increase health care costs.

SEVERE POSTTRAUMATIC PAIN

Over 50 million accidental injuries occur annually in the United States. Of these, more than one-third are associated with moderate to severe pain; 400,000 patients incur partial or permanent disability; and over 100,000 die, usually from shock.[142] In many instances the pain is severe and the associated segmental and suprasegmental reflexes and the neuroendocrine and cortical responses are excessive; instead of normalizing the organism, they initiate and maintain the vicious circle of shock.[9,43] In such instances there is a persistent, grossly excessive vasoconstriction that produces tissue hypoxia and consequent biochemical and metabolic disturbances and toxic products. They, in turn, produce new nociceptive stimulation and widespread deleterious effects that further aggravate the physiopathology.[43] Vasoconstriction is most marked in the splanchnic vascular bed, and the resultant intestinal ischemia causes hypoxic tissue damage and consequent release of toxic substances that depress the cardiovascular system, particularly the myocardium (myocardial depressant factor [MDF]).[81] Like severe postoperative pain, severe posttraumatic pain is not always adequately relieved, and nothing is done to block the abnormal reflex responses. A few studies have shown that block of nociceptive and sympathetic pathways with local anesthetics prior to or soon after the injury will prevent, or promptly eliminate, the pain and abnormal reflex responses, with consequent improvement in cardiovascular function (see Bonica[22,26] for references). Unfortunately, although trauma has been the subject of intense biomedical research, the pain mechanisms associated with trauma and its adequate relief have received very little attention, and the beneficial effects of blockade have not been pursued.

PAIN OF ACUTE MYOCARDIAL INFARCTION

While initially the pain of acute myocardial infarction is useful because it prompts the patient to seek medical help, unless promptly relieved, it may aggravate the myocardial pathophysiology. Tissue damage from myocardial ischemia produces persistent noxious stimulation, with consequent segmental and suprasegmental reflex responses and pain.[9,20,22,112] In some patients the reflex responses consist of the Bezold-Jarisch effect of abnormal vagal reflex, consisting of bradycardia, atrioventricular block, peripheral vasodilation, and arterial hypotension that may progress to cardiogenic shock.[9,20,112,165] In other patients the reflexes consist of segmental and suprasegmental sympathetic hyperactivity, with an increase in cardiac output and myocardial oxygen consumption. Suprasegmental reflexes stimulate hypothalamic autonomic centers and invariably further increase general sympathetic tone and catecholamine release. Moreover, severe anxiety, which invariably develops in patients with acute myocardial infarction, markedly enhances the hypothalamic response. In addition, the emotional stress may cause the cortically mediated increased blood viscosity and clotting, fibrinolysis, and platelet aggregation.

Thus the combined effects of segmental and suprasegmental reflexes, anxiety, and stress greatly increase the workload of the heart and its oxygen consumption. By alteration of blood clotting, they may further decrease the already compromised arteriosclerotic coronary circulation, markedly increase the discrepancy between the oxygen supply and oxygen demand, and may cause extension of the infarct (see Bonica[20] and Pasqualucci[112] for references). One or more of these responses may be a critical factor that could cause a patient's death. It is therefore essential to promptly and effectively relieve the pain, anxiety, and mental stress and decrease the reflex responses primarily by blocking the sympathetic afferents and efferents with either local anesthetic or intraspinal narcotics. The value of this procedure is strongly suggested by old animal experiments that impressively demonstrated that sympathetic denervation of the heart significantly reduced the size of experimentally induced myocardial infarction and the mortality of the animals in the study group compared to a control group (see Bonica[9,16] for references). Moreover, in man, the use of beta-blocking agents eliminates serious cardiac arrhythmia consequent to acute myocardial infarction.[75]

Acute Pancreatitis

Acute pancreatitis produces severe excruciating pain as well as abnormal reflex responses provoked by the intense nociception arising from the pathophysiological process.[9,20,21,26,27] Associated with the pain is usually severe spasm and splinting of the muscles of the abdominal wall and chest, a rise and splinting of the diaphragm, reflex vasoconstriction of the splanchnic region, and marked ileus. Consequently, there is progressively severe hypoventilation that, unless aggressively treated, may end in death.[9,20,26] For this type of severe pain, narcotics, even when given in large doses intravenously, are often ineffective. They fail to relieve the pain and do nothing to the abnormal reflex responses. Interruption of nociceptive and efferent pathways with continuous segmental epidural block is the most practical method because it permits continuous pain relief and interruption of reflex responses for several days.[9,26] In addition, block of nociceptive impulses may decrease

the severity and duration of disease by interrupting reflex mechanisms that contribute to the pancreatic pathophysiology.[60]

Labor Pain

We cite labor pain because, even though it is the result of a physiological phenomenon, if unrelieved, it produces deleterious effects and because currently its control is the source of confusion and controversy and its relief is frequently and/or completely neglected.[12,21,28] Most proponents of natural childbirth claim that proper preparation decreases or completely eliminates the pain and that the experience of the delivery process is essential to the emotional well-being of the mother and the normal psychological and physiological development of the baby. However, a recent controlled study by Melzack and associates,[97] using the McGill Pain Questionnaire, showed that both primiparas and multiparas assessed their pain more severe than patients with low back pain, cancer pain, phantom limb pain, and postherpetic neuralgia, and that prepared childbirth reduced the pain intensity by only 10 to 15 percent even among the most motivated and well-prepared parturients. Although initially the pain of parturition has the important function of signaling the onset of labor, if it is not relieved when it becomes severe, it will result in residual maternal emotional and psychological problems and significant maternal and perinatal alterations (see Bonica[28] for literature review).

Human studies have shown the pains of uterine contractions cause: (1) a five- to twenty-fold increase in ventilation, with consequent severe respiratory alkalosis during contraction and alkalosis-induced hyperventilation between contractions; and (2) a marked increase in neurosympathetic tone and a two- to four-fold increase in catecholamines, cortisol, ACTH, and corticosteroids, which result in (3) a 5 to 150 percent increase in cardiac output, a 20 to 40 percent increase in blood pressure, a significant increase in metabolism and oxygen consumption, and a decrease in uterine blood flow and GI function.[12,28] All of these may have a deleterious effect on the mother, fetus, and newborn. The increased oxygen consumption that is added to that inherent in the work of labor, together with a loss of bicarbonate from the kidneys due to pain-induced respiratory alkalosis and, often, reduced carbohydrate intake, produces the progressive maternal metabolic acidosis that is transferred to the fetus.[28] The increased ventricular work is tolerated by the healthy parturient but may prove deleterious to the patient with heart disease, toxemia, hypertension, or diabetes. The decrease in GI and urinary activity caused by pain and anxiety markedly delays gastric emptying and thus causes the parturient to be at risk of vomiting and pulmonary aspiration if general anesthesia is given.

From the viewpoint of the fetus, a reduction of intervillous blood flow during the peak of contraction leads to a temporary decrease in placental gas exchange. This impairment is further increased by pain-induced severe hyperventilation, which, as previously mentioned, causes severe respiratory alkalosis that results in: (1) a shift to the left in the maternal oxygen association curve that diminishes transfer of oxygen from mother to the fetus, (2) maternal hypoxemia during uterine relaxation, and (3) uterine vasoconstriction with consequent decrease in umbilical blood flow. All of these factors result in a series of transient impairments of placental blood gas exchange, which is well tolerated by the normal fetus but may prove deleterious to a fetus at risk because of obstetric or maternal complications such as toxemia, heart disease, and diabetes. Moreover, metabolic acidosis makes the fetus vulnerable to the effects of intrauterine asphyxia caused by cord compression or prolapse.

Human studies have also shown that these alterations and their deleterious effects on the mother and the fetus[12,28] are eliminated in those parturients who obtain adequate or complete pain relief with continuous epidural analgesia. Several carefully carried out clinical studies have shown that parturients given no pain relief, or moderate pain relief

with narcotics, developed progressive metabolic acidosis, as did their fetuses, while mothers managed with epidural analgesia did not develop metabolic acidosis and their fetuses developed much less acidosis than the fetuses of the nonanalgesic group (see Bonica[28] for review).

¶ Chronic Pain

General Considerations

Chronic pain is defined as pain that persists beyond the usual course of an acute disease or a reasonable time for an injury to heal.[9,22] Although some clinicians use the arbitrary figure of six months to designate pain as chronic, this is not appropriate, because there are a number of acute diseases or injuries that heal in two, three, or four weeks. In such situations, if pain is still present three or four weeks after a cure should have been achieved, it must be considered chronic. This has important clinical implications because the earlier such chronic pain syndromes are effectively treated, the better the chances of cure. Chronic pain may be caused by chronic pathological processes in somatic structures of viscera, or by prolonged dysfunction of parts of the peripheral and/or central nervous system. In contrast with acute pain, it also can be caused by operant mechanisms and perhaps psychopathology. The suggestion of some clinicians[6] that the term chronic pain syndrome be limited to persistent pain caused by operant or psychological mechanisms is inappropriate and a source of confusion, and should be discontinued. Similarly, use of the term benign chronic pain to differentiate it from cancer pain is also inappropriate because chronic pain is *never* benign. The term noncancer or nonneoplastic chronic pain is more appropriate.

Because knowledge of the basic mechanisms of most chronic pain syndromes is meager, their diagnosis and therapy are more difficult than is the case with acute pain. Moreover, the physiological, affective, and behavioral responses to chronic pain are quite different from those to acute pain. Finally, in contrast to acute pain, in its chronic persistent form pain *never* has biological function, but is rather a malefic force that often imposes severe emotional, physical, economic, and social stresses on the patient and the family and is one of the most costly health problems for society.

PREVALENCE AND COST OF CHRONIC PAIN

Although the United States and many other medically advanced countries have the manpower, sophisticated equipment, and other resources to carry out large-scale national epidemiological studies on the incidence, prevalence, and economic impact of most disease states, unfortunately none have been carried out on the prevalence and cost of chronic pain. This lack of accurate statistics from national epidemiological studies prompted the senior author, some twenty years ago, to estimate the prevalence of chronic pain in the United States and other countries. For this purpose, he reviewed reports on numerous surveys on back pain, headache, arthritis, heart disease, and many other conditions in the United States, Britain, Scandinavia, Israel, and a number of other countries, as well as data published by the National Center for Health Statistics and other governmental bodies and by private agencies such as the Arthritis Foundation, the American Cancer Society, and the American Heart Association (see Bonica[22] for references). These were extrapolated to the American population, and the cost was estimated based on workdays lost and the cost of health care, compensation, litigation, and services by "quacks." The first report was published in 1972,[13] and since then the data have been updated at intervals of three to five years.* The estimates for 1983 suggest that some 90 million Americans had chronic pain, and of these, some 60 million were either partially or totally disabled for periods ranging from a few days (e.g., recurrent

*See references 15, 17, 22, 23, and 30.

headaches) to weeks, months, and years (e.g., low back pain), and some were permenently disabled (e.g., arthritis, low back pain, cancer pain). This caused a loss of some 750 million workdays. This loss of work productivity, together with health care costs and payments for compensation, litigation, and "quackery" totaled nearly $70 billion (see table 26-1).

EFFECTS OF CHRONIC PAIN

Even more important than the economic impact of chronic pain is the cost in terms of human suffering. It is a distressing fact that in this age of marvelous scientific and technological advances, millions of patients suffer persistent pain that produces serious physical, emotional, and affective disorders. Many patients with chronic pain undergo a *progressive physical deterioration* caused by disturbance in sleep and appetite, decrease in physical activity, and often excessive medication, all of which contribute to general fatigue and debility.[19,132,138] Sleep disturbance is one of the most common complaints of patients with chronic pain, who arise in the morning feeling unrested and tired. Many patients state they feel exhausted and drained of energy, not only due to lack of sleep but also because the continuous pain wears them down.[132] These factors, together with possible chronic depletion of serotonin and endorphins, may cause a decrease in pain tolerance, so that even minor injuries provoke major responses. A significant percentage of patients with chronic pain report a decrease or total loss of libido, but whether this is due to the pain or is a result of excessive medication is unclear.

The Psychological Effects. Many patients develop reactive depression, hypochondriasis, somatic preoccupation with disease conviction, somatic focusing, and a tendency to deny life problems unrelated to their physical problems.* This cluster of psychological effects, which Pilowsky and others[8,115] have labeled abnormal illness behavior, is characteristic of chronic pain regardless of etiology. As the patient goes from one doctor to an-

*See references 8, 57, 99, 115, and 132.

TABLE 26–1
1983 Estimated
Prevalence of Cost of Chronic Pain in the United States

Pathological Process/Type of Pain	Prevalence (in millions)	Disability (in millions)		Workdays Lost (in millions)	Total Cost ($ in billions)
		Partial	Total		
Back pain	23	10	3	220	23.0
Painful arthritis	21	6	2	180	17.0
Other musculoskeletal	6	4	0.5	16	2.0
Severe recurrent headaches					
Migraine	16	16		136	9.0
Other	20	20			
Cancer pain	0.8	0.6	0.2	?	0.5
Other chronic pain	?8–10	?4	?1	150	15.0
Neurologic					
Cardiac					
Visceral					
Orofacial, etc.					
Total	96.8	60.6		702	66.5

other and from one clinic to another, he or she repeatedly experiences hope and then disappointment and gradually becomes increasingly bitter and resentful toward doctors.

It deserves emphasis that psychological, emotional, and mental effects of persistent pain do not apply to the entire population of patients with chronic pain. There are thousands, and indeed millions, of patients with chronic painful arthritis, postherpetic and other forms of neuralgia, and other chronic painful disorders who do not have the severe depression, hypochondriasis, and other symptomatology just mentioned, and who lead useful and productive lives. Moreover, we have shown that the psychological profiles of one specialized university pain clinic population differed somewhat from those of another[115] and the psychological profiles of patients with chronic pain in a private practice setting differed from those in a university multidisciplinary pain center.[42] These studies indicate that the constellation of beliefs and attitudes held by patients with persistent pain set most of them apart from other patients commonly seen in a medical setting. However, broad statements about the psychological tendencies of pain patients must be made cautiously, since referral pain clinics and pain centers see only the psychological extremes of the national population of patients with chronic pain. A comprehensive review by Turner and Romano[149] found that overall rates of depression in chronic pain sufferers in a cross population were between 40 and 65 percent, and no significant depression was observed among the selected population of pain patients.

Behavioral changes. In some chronic pain patients, behavioral changes are produced by multiple medications, often prescribed in high doses by several physicians, which invariably lead to intoxication.[57,132] Some patients with chronic pain, especially that due to environmental and emotional factors, manipulate their families and coworkers, and manipulate their physicians to prescribe multiple drugs and even to perform useless operations. In addition to withdrawing from all social activity, many of these patients diminish their physical activities and spend much of their time in bed or lying down.[57,132]

Social effects. The social effects of chronic pain are equally devastating; many patients develop problems with their families and friends, decrease their social interactions, and are unable to work, or lose their jobs. Consequently, they no longer contribute to the well-being of society and instead are placed on the disability rolls, usually in early middle age, thus becoming an economic liability rather than an asset.[132] Many patients with chronic pain give up medical care and turn to "quacks," who may not only do no good but may also aggravate the problem. Some patients become so discouraged and desperate they contemplate or even commit suicide. Hendler[65] of the Johns Hopkins Medical Center has reported "70% of these people [with chronic pain] get divorced, and 20% attempt or contemplate suicide."

Mechanisms of Chronic Pain

The mechanisms of chronic pain are much more complex than those of acute pain and probably involve prolonged dysfunctions of the neurological and psychological substrates of pain. Since scientific data from humans with chronic pain are sparse, it is necessary to rely on speculations and hypotheses. From a therapeutic viewpoint, it may be useful to classify the suggested mechanisms of chronic pain in a simplistic fashion into "peripheral," "peripheral-central," "central," and "psychological" mechanisms.[9,17]

PERIPHERAL MECHANISMS

Peripheral mechanisms are probably responsible for chronic pain associated with chronic musculoskeletal, visceral, and vascular disorders such as arthritis, some forms of neoplasm, peptic ulcer, and coronary artery disease. Chronic pain may be due to persistent noxious stimulation of nociceptors or their sensitization or both. Persistent stimulation may be caused by chronic mechanical stimulation or, more frequently, by endogenous algogenic or algesic substances caused by cellular breakdown. These substances invariably cause sensitization so that innocuous stimulation caused by, for example, normal movement of the joint in patients with arthritis causes the nociceptors to fire with consequent pain. The algogenic substances may also stimulate nociceptors indirectly by influencing microcirculation and vascular permeability.[166]

Chronic increased muscle tension or spasm and/or sympathetic hyperactivity with vasoconstriction and possible ischemia through positive feedback mechanisms stimulate nociceptors and contribute to the pain.[17] Although the persistent nociceptive input into the neuraxis probably has a pathophysiological impact on the function of central neurons, this is eliminated with effective therapy. All of these have important clinical implications: If the pain is due to ischemia as obtained in coronary artery disease or chronic peripheral vascular disease, elimination of the ischemia by bypass surgery eliminates the chronic pain. Moreover, in conditions where chronic pain is due to persistent inflammation such as arthritis or cancer bone pain, the pain can be relieved by administering drugs that prevent the synthesis of prostaglandins and other algesic substances and /or agents that decrease inflammation, such as aspirin and indomethacin.

PERIPHERAL-CENTRAL MECHANISMS

The peripheral-central mechanisms are probably operative in chronic pain syndromes associated with partial or complete lesions of the peripheral nerves, dorsal roots, or dorsal ganglion cells. Such lesions produce abnormal activity in both the peripheral and central portion of the somatosensory system. These mechanisms are probably operative in causalgia and other reflex sympathetic dystrophy, phantom limb pain, postherpetic neuralgia, and cancer pain due to tumor-induced damage of the peripheral nerves or the sensory roots. Although many hypotheses have been proposed to explain these and other chronic pain states, only four will be mentioned here.

The "Vicious Circle" Mechanisms.   To explain the mechanisms of causalgia, phantom limb pain, and other related conditions, in 1943 Livingston[86] proposed that intense stimulation resulting from nerve and tissue damage activates fibers that project to internuncial neuron pools in the spinal cord, creating abnormal reverberatory activity in closed self-exciting neuron loops. This prolonged, abnormal activity bombards the spinal cord transmission (T) cells, which project to brain mechanisms that underlie pain perception. The abnormal internuncial activity also spreads to lateral and ventral horn cells in the spinal cord, activating the autonomic nervous system and motor system, respectively, and producing vasoconstriction, increased work of the heart, and skeletal muscle spasm. These, in turn, produce further abnormal input, thereby creating a "vicious circle." Brain activities such as fear and anxiety evoked by pain feed into and maintain the abnormal internuncial pool activity.

Sensory Interaction Theory.   In 1959 Noordenbos[107] proposed a sensory interaction theory that was derived from older studies and was subsequently included in Melzack and Wall's theory of pain.[97] He suggested that small-diameter, slowly conducting, somatic afferent fibers and small visceral afferents project into the cells in the dorsal horn of the spinal cord and that the summation of inputs from the small fibers produces the neural patterns that are transmitted to the brain to produce pain.[17] The large-diameter, fast-conducting fibers inhibit transmission of impulses from the small fibers and prevent summation from occurring. Diseases or injury that produce a selective loss of large fibers, such as diabetes, postherpetic neuralgia, toxic neuropathy, and perhaps trigeminal neuralgia, bring about a loss of inhibition and thereby increase summation and result in pain. He further proposed that one of the ascending systems that transmit pain signals is the short axon multisynaptic system in the core of the spinal cord.

Deafferentation Mechanisms.   To explain the pain, dysesthesia, and paresthesia that often accompany peripheral nerve section, whether caused by accidents or surgical interruption such as rhizotomy, Loeser and his associates,[88,89] Wall and associates,* and others[90,105] have proposed that loss of normal sensory input produces an abnormal firing pattern in the somatosensory system proximal to the deafferentation. In animal models, Loeser and Ward[88] found seizurelike abnormal firing patterns in deafferented dorsal root fibers and later the caudate nucleus, and Loeser, Ward, and White[89] noted similar findings in man. Similar abnormal firing patterns have been reported following trigeminal denervation consequent to tooth pulp extraction and section of the nerve.[1] Wall and colleagues (see Wall and Devor[156] for references) have shown that peripheral nerve section results in: (1) development of a neuroma that fires spontaneously abnormal patterns of impulses and that is very sensitive to touch, norepinephrine, and epinephrine; (2) the axons central to the injury lose conduction velocities, and the dorsal root ganglion cells and their terminals in the dorsal horn lose their peptide content; (3) minutes after the injury, spinal cord dorsal horn cells reorganize their receptive fields to emphasize (aggravate) messages from the area of injury; and (4) days later there is further reorganization of dorsal horn cells so that some of the cells that lost their input as a result of peripheral nerve section begin to respond to new inputs from nearby intact peripheral nerves. This conductivity appears to be associated with a loss of inhibition and is dependent on changes within the unmyelinated C afferent fibers caused by the transport of abnormal substances within those fibers to spinal dorsal horn cells. This loss of inhibition will permit transmission of pain messages to subsequent relay stations along the somatosensory projection system. Wall believes that these mechanisms are operative not only in some peripheral nerve lesions but also with root lesions, as occurs

*See references 98, 154, 155, 156, and 157.

with postherpetic neuralgia, arachnoiditis, and plexus avulsions.

Central Biasing Mechanism. A hypothesis somewhat related to the preceding two is that of Melzack,[95] by which he proposed to explain the pain of phantom limb, causalgia, and other peripheral nerve injuries. It is based on some recent data pertaining to the neural systems that exert powerful inhibitory influences on various parts of the neuraxis. According to this concept, a portion of the brain stem reticular formation acts as a "central biasing mechanism" by exerting a tonic inhibitory influence or bias on transmission at all synaptic levels of the somatosensory system, including the "gate" in the dorsal horn and at other levels of the neuraxis. This inhibitory function of the central biasing mechanism is dependent in part on a normal sensory input. Loss of input to the system, as occurs with peripheral nerve lesions and amputation, weakens inhibition, thus causing persistent pain. Emotional stress and certain drugs can also impair the efficacy of the biasing mechanism, thus aggravating the spontaneous pain. Contrarily, increased sensory input by mechanical stimulation or by direct electrical stimulation of the skin or nerve would increase the inhibition and decrease the pain.

Melzack has used this concept to explain the therapeutic efficacy of peripheral tactile or electrical stimulation in phantom limb pain and causalgia, in the mechanism of acupuncture analgesia, and of nerve blocks in the treatment of causalgia and other reflex sympathetic dystrophies. The nerve block permits temporary return to normalcy by breaking up the activity in the self-sustaining neuron pools, thus producing pain relief that may outlast the pharmacological effect of the block. After the block has worn off, stimulation again triggers sustained activity, but because of the time necessary for it to spread to a sufficiently large number of neurons within the pools, pain relief outlasts the local anesthetic action. Moreover, pain relief permits increased use of the limb, which produces patterned, temporarily dispersed inputs, particularly from muscles that are out of phase with the rhythmically firing neuron pools and that disrupt their activity. This delays resumption of self-sustaining firing.

CENTRAL PAIN MECHANISMS

Disease or injury of certain parts of the CNS often produces what is generally referred to as "central pain," characterized by spontaneous burning or aching pain, hyperalgesia, dysesthesia, and other abnormal sensations. Central pain often accompanies thalamic lesions (so-called thalamic pain) and accidental injury to the spinal cord as occurs in paraplegics, and may also be caused by surgical interruption of pain pathways as well as such disease states as tabes dorsalis, syringomyelia, and multiple sclerosis.

Paraplegic patients usually experience three types of pain: (1) root or "girdle" pain, localized at or near the level of the cord lesion; (2) visceral pain, which usually accompanies a distended bladder or bowel; and (3) phantom body pain felt in the areas of complete sensory loss. Melzack and Loeser[96] proposed that in paraplegics, massive loss of sensory input causes dorsal horn cells and other cells of the somatosensory projection system above the level of the spinal transsection to fire spontaneously in abnormal bursts for prolonged periods of time. The prolonged bursting activity generated by the deafferented neuron pools, which they called "pattern generating mechanisms," can be modulated by somatic, visceral, and autonomic inputs as well as by input from neural mechanisms that underlie personality and emotional variables and from brain stem descending inhibitory influences.

Loss of input leads to a decreased input to brain-stem mechanisms that normally exert inhibitory downstream influences on sensory transmission. The loss of descending inhibition would make it easier for nonnoxious input to trigger abnormal bursting patterns. Moreover, the neural substrates of memories of prior pain at spinal and supraspinal levels may become active and also trigger abnormal firing patterns. Thus the loss of inhibition, in addition to massive sensory deafferentation, allows unchecked abnormal bursting activity so that the pain persists for indefinitely long periods of time. The diminished inhibition would also allow recruitment of additional neurons into the abnormally firing pools and thus intensifies the pain and causes it to spread.

PSYCHOLOGICAL MECHANISMS

In addition to the important role psychological factors play in chronic pain produced by injury or disease, in a significant number of patients the chronic pain is primarily due to psychological factors. These factors can be arbitrarily subdivided into three categories: (1) psychophysiological mechanisms, (2) operant mechanisms, and (3) psychiatric mechanisms.

Psychophysiological (Psychosomatic) Mechanisms. Psychosomatic mechanisms are usually initiated by severe emotional stress, which, through psychophysiological (corticofugal) mechanisms, produces skeletal muscle spasm, local vasoconstriction, visceral dysfunction, liberation of pain substances, or a combination of these.[9,131] One or more of these produces peripheral noxious stimulation, with its consequences of pain, reflex responses, and affective reactions, all of which aggravate the emotional stress. This, in turn, provokes more psychophysiological impulses, thus sustaining the vicious circle of pain. This is probably the mechanism of tension headache and pain due to muscle spasm in the shoulder girdle, low back, and chest. The psychophysiological mechanism has also been invoked to explain migraine headache, in which emotional factors provoke the liberation of substances that produce the characteristic vasoconstriction and vasodilation. It has long been appreciated that this is the probable mechanism of coronary artery disease, peptic ulcer, and colitis, each of which is often accompanied by chronic pain.

Operant Mechanisms. Operant mechanisms, first proposed by Fordyce,[57] are operative in a significant number of patients in whom chronic pain behavior develops following a disease or injury of often a minor

nature. The initial injury provokes operant responses and pain behavior on the part of the patient, which are reinforced by favorable consequences or reactions on the part of those important to the patient. Thus a husband who for years has been inattentive to his wife becomes solicitous and concerned and gives her special attention when she sustains an injury—favorable consequences that reinforce her pain behavior. This concept involves well-established principles of operant conditioning, which state that behavior is subject to the influence or under the control of learning factors and is to a considerable degree governed by consequences in the environment. Chronic pain behavior continues as long as the consequences are favorable and eventually becomes independent of the underlying pathology, persisting even after the original pathogenic factor is gone. Under such conditions the patient has developed a *pain habit*, which is real and is readily accounted for by learning or conditioning. The important therapeutic implications are that to change the chronic pain behavior, it is necessary to eliminate the favorable consequences that act as positive reinforcers to pain behavior, rather than to seek out and try to eliminate underlying pathology.

Psychiatric Mechanisms. Patients with psychiatric disorders such as conversion hysteria (now termed somatization disorder) and neurotic (endogenous) depression not infrequently complain of persistent pain. The psychodynamics of these disorders are discussed by Mersky and Spear.[99]

¶ Therapies for Chronic Pain

General Considerations

The best pain therapy is to remove the cause by medical, surgical, or physical means; but, unfortunately, in many instances the cause cannot be eliminated and the pain itself must be treated. This is especially true when managing a number of nonmalignant chronic pain syndromes and in many patients with cancer-related pain. Analysis of past results reveals that many patients with chronic pain have not been relieved effectively.[22] This has been due to a number of reasons or deficiencies that can be arbitrarily grouped into three categories: (1) voids in knowledge of basic mechanisms of chronic nonmalignant and cancer-related pain due to insufficient or total lack of research by scientists in the past; (2) improper application of the available knowledge and therapies because physicians were not taught the basic principles of managing chronic pain; and (3) inadequate or total lack of communication among scientists of various basic science disciplines and between this group and clinical investigators and clinicians (see Bonica[22,30] for detailed review). Moreover, some chronic pain syndromes are such a complex array of physical, psychological, emotional, and social factors that it is difficult, if not impossible, for a single physician to effectively treat them. The usual consultation carried out in the isolation of each specialist's office and the consequent fragmented reports by each consultant inherent in traditional medicine have been found inefficient and often lead to wrong diagnosis and/or therapy.

The acquisition of much new knowledge and recent clinical experience have changed our concepts of and approaches to diagnosis and therapy of chronic pain (see Bonica[25] for review). Some of these will be elaborated in the discussion of specific therapies. Two advances in chronic pain therapy that Melzack and Wall[98] consider most important have been the activation of a number of multidisciplinary pain clinics/centers[34] and an increasing number of hospices for the treatment of terminally ill patients.[151]

The prolonged disability and risk of iatrogenic complications incurred by many patients with chronic pain can be obviated with proper management. This entails, among other things, early correct diagnosis and the institution of an effective therapeutic strategy. Although these are basic principles appreciated by all physicians, they are frequently neglected by some busy practi-

tioners who are unable to, or for other reasons are not capable of, devoting sufficient time and effort to obtain a detailed history, carry out a complete physical examination, and then develop the therapy. The following is a brief overview of the basic principles of management.

DIAGNOSTIC WORKUP

History of the Pain. The patient's pain history is taken first. The physician must obtain detailed information about the circumstances contributing to the cause of pain and its location, distribution, quality, intensity, and duration at the time of onset, during the interval, and at the present time. The patient must be questioned about factors that aggravate pain and those that relieve it. Specific details must be obtained about such associated phenomena as muscle spasm, muscle weakness, paresthesia, autonomic dysfunction, and local tenderness. The family and general personal history are as important, if not more so, in patients with chronic pain as in those with other disorders.

Psychosocial Evaluation. Complete psychological and social investigations into developmental history and current interactions of pain patients with their work and family environments are essential. These require clinical interviews by psychiatrists or psychologists and social workers that assess the impact and implications of pain on the lives of patients and their families, and psychological testing, such as the Minnesota Multiphasic Personality Inventory, the Illness Behavior Questionnaire developed by Pilowsky and associates,[114,115] and the Holmes-Rahe Schedule of Recent Events, which measures the patient's life changes over a three-year period.[67] These tests afford the pain team vital information regarding specific functional aspects of the chronic pain experience.

Information about intake of drugs, alcohol, and tobacco; the amount of daily physical activity; the impact of pain on sexual relations and social activities; family attitudes and responses; and what life stresses occurred at the time of the onset of the pain should be obtained. Information about the patient's social and cultural backgrounds and their impact on the patient's expression of pain is extremely important in helping the pain team make the correct diagnosis. It deserves emphasis that a diagnosis of "psychogenic" or "primarily psychologic" pain is not made by exclusion or lack of evidence of organic pathology, but rather by the presence of positive evidence of psychopathology. Further, this psychosocial analysis often indicates the necessity of behavioral or counseling therapy as an integral part of the total pain treatment and management plan.

Examination. Examination of the painful region and interpretation of the findings requires consideration of the mechanisms of pain. Frequently the pain is referred away from the site of the disease or injury. A general physical examination should follow examination of a painful region. Since many pain syndromes involve the musculoskeletal and nervous systems, complete neurological and orthopedic examinations are usually necessary.

Diagnostic Procedures. As with most other diagnostic problems, a clinical laboratory examination is often essential. In addition, special diagnostic procedures such as diagnostic blocks, thermography, and electromyography may provide valuable additional information. It deserves emphasis that these and other procedures intended to help in the differential diagnosis must be used as adjuncts to a thorough workup of the patient and the results obtained from the tests should be considered within the framework of all the other information obtained.

PRINCIPLES OF THERAPY

After a diagnosis has been established and the pain mechanism determined, treatment must be planned carefully. In patients for whom the cause and basic mechanisms can be removed by appropriate medical, surgical, and/or physical therapy, these are carried out by qualified physicians. In patients for whom the cause or mechanism is unknown, or it is known but cannot be eliminated, the therapy is directed to partially or completely relieving the pain (symptomatic

pain therapy). Currently the various therapies available for the symptomatic relief of chronic pain can be grouped into six categories, listed in the order of frequency of use, efficacy, incidence of adverse side effects, and availability: (1) systemic analgesics and related drugs; (2) neurostimulation techniques; (3) physical therapies; (4) psychological analgesic techniques; (5) regional analgesia; and (6) neurosurgical ablative or destructive procedures. To determine the best therapeutic modality or combination of therapies, it is essential to consider the causes, mechanisms, and characteristics of the pain; the age and social responsibilities of the patient; the chronology of the disease; its prognosis and previous therapy; and other aspects that can be ascertained only by a comprehensive evaluation of the patient and his or her problem.

With this background, let us now consider briefly the recent advances in the application of the various therapeutic modalities for chronic pain.

Systemic Analgesics and Related Drugs

Systemic analgesics, psychotropic drugs, anti-inflammatory agents, and hypnotics constitute the most practical and widely used agents for relieving cancer pain. These drugs are readily available, inexpensive, and simple to administer and, if properly used, are reasonably effective in relieving pain. Unfortunately, in many instances these drugs are not administered in the most effective way, and consequently the patient does not derive optimal benefit and, indeed, may suffer serious side effects.[64]

NONNARCOTIC ANALGESICS

The efficacy of aspirin and other nonnarcotic analgesics in relieving headache, arthritic pain, muscular pain, and mild to moderate pain caused by other conditions has been appreciated for nearly a century. Because in some individuals aspirin and other aspirinlike drugs produce adverse side effects such as dyspepsia, GI bleeding, and allergic reactions, other old and new compounds have been marketed in recent years. These include acetaminophen (paracetamol, Tylenol), ibuprofen, and nefopam. Although these produce fewer side effects, they are no more effective in relieving chronic pain and are much more expensive. Therefore, aspirin remains the best all-around nonnarcotic analgesic available at the present time. Most of these agents are now called nonsteroidal anti-inflammatory drugs (NSAIDs) and have the propensity to produce analgesia, reduce fever, and except for acetaminophen, they have an anti-inflammatory action.

Recent studies have revealed that most of these drugs produce analgesia by inhibiting the synthesis of prostaglandins, which, as previously mentioned, sensitize nociceptors to the action of bradykinin and other pain-producing substances.[153] During the past decade, NSAIDs have been proven to be especially effective in relieving severe bone pain due to cancer metastases (which produce prostaglandins) and to have some anti-tumor effects. Moreover, these drugs have been shown to potentiate the analgesic action of narcotics and are often given in combination with codeine to relieve moderate pain or with morphine or other potent narcotics for the relief of severe pain. For acute pain, NSAIDs are given as needed, but for chronic pain they should be *given at fixed intervals* to achieve and sustain effective analgesia for prolonged periods. The doses needed for chronic pain may be two to three times the recommended doses. For example, for cancer pain, doses of 650 to 975 mg given every four hours may be necessary.[27,55,150]

NARCOTICS

Morphine remains the best potent narcotic to treat severe pain and has long been considered the standard of reference against which all other narcotics are compared.[64] When given in equipotent doses, some two dozen narcotics in current use, whether they are semisynthetic derivatives of morphine or wholly synthetic compounds, produce similar degrees of pain relief; however, the duration of analgesia varies. Extensive clinical trials have shown that equivalent analgesic doses of various narcotics administered to the general population produce similar incidences of side effects, although some patients may be more sensitive to one or more of the side effects than the general population. Adverse side effects include constipation, excessive sedation, confusion, nausea and vomiting, and depression of respiration and circulation. Since pain is a powerful respiratory and circulatory stimulant, depression can be obviated by titrating the dose of the narcotic to the needs of each patient's pain. Moreover, all potent narcotics cause tolerance and physical dependence, which are normal pharmacological responses to prolonged narcotic administration. Tolerance is characterized by progressive resistance to the analgesic effects and other actions of the drug, while physical dependence is characterized by development of the abstinence syndrome on *prompt* withdrawal of the drug. Unfortunately, these pharmacological responses are often confused with addiction, or psychological dependence, which is characterized by: (1) an abnormal behavior pattern of drug abuse; (2) craving of a drug for reasons other than pain relief, (3) becoming overwhelmingly involved in the procurement and use of the drug, and (4) the tendency to relapse after withdrawal.

The fear of tolerance, physical dependence, and addiction among some physicians and nurses has caused them to prescribe and/or administer narcotics in insufficient doses, and consequently the patient's severe pain has persisted.[44,93,94] Indeed, some patients have received only one-third to one-fourth of the amount required to relieve severe pain.[93] In some instances, fear of addiction has caused patients not to take the prescribed doses. That these are not valid reasons for under-dosing narcotics has been clearly demonstrated by laboratory and clinical studies. For one thing, addiction *rarely* occurs in patients receiving narcotics for pain relief, even for as long as several months[77]; the psychologic profiles of these patients differ from those of drug abusers. For another, physical dependence does not occur in patients with acute pain given these drugs for several days; it requires three to four weeks of regular administration before clinically relevant physical dependence occurs.[3] In patients with severe pain due to metastatic advanced or terminal cancer who are likely to require narcotic therapy until death, addiction and physical dependence should not be considered valid reasons for withholding adequate amounts of these drugs. On the other hand, potent narcotics should *not* be prescribed for prolonged periods for patients with chronic malignant pain who are likely to live for years, because these patients do develop tolerance and physical dependence and may become disoriented as a result of chronic narcotic therapy.

One of the most important recent advances in pain therapy has been the recognition and full appreciation by some clinicians of the problem that patients with chronic nonmalignant pain are often prescribed many drugs by different physicians and, consequently, develop drug toxicity that impairs their ability to function and makes evaluation of the pain difficult. At the University of Washington Clinical Pain Service, we have found such patients will require the detoxification program that consists of the following steps[63]: Upon admittance to the hospital, all the drugs the patient has been taking are removed. The patient is instructed to ask for as much drug or combination of drugs as he or she has been taking and requires in order to remain comfortable. This procedure, which is called the "Drug Profile," is continued for forty-eight hours in order to obtain an idea of how much of each drug or drug combinations the patient requires. Following this, the patient is put on the "pain cocktail," in which are included the various components of the drugs used by the patient but translated into equivalents of phenobarbital for sedatives and methadone for narcotics. The various ingredients are mixed in a pleasant-tasting solution that is administered at regular intervals every four to six hours, depending on the needs of the patient, and reduced by 10 percent each day. This procedure usually permits patients to undergo progressive reduction of drug intake over a period of ten to twelve days without developing withdrawal symptoms.

For therapy of severe acute pain, narcotics are given intramuscularly or intravenously as needed. However, for cancer pain, they should be given by mouth and in ample doses administered at *fixed time intervals*, beginning with a lower dose and raising the dose until effective analgesia is achieved and sustained.

ADJUVANTS TO SYSTEMIC ANALGESICS

Adjuvant drugs that are used alone or in combination with systemic analgesics currently in use include: (1) *antidepressants*, such as amitriptyline hydrochloride (Elavil, Endep) and doxepin (Sinequan, Adapin), which in low doses produce an analgesic effect and decrease insomnia and in high doses decrease the depression that often is a consequence of chronic pain[54,91]; (2) *antihistaminics*, such as hydroxyzine hydrochloride, which potentiate the analgesic effects of narcotics[70]; (3) *anticonvulsants*,[54,140] such as carbamazepine (Tegretol) and phenytoin (Dilantin), which are effective in treating trigeminal neuralgia, postherpetic neuralgia, and other deafferentation pain syndromes; and (4) *corticosteroids*, which are potent anti-inflammatory agents that prevent the release of prostaglandins, stimulate appetite, and elevate mood, and are thus very useful in relieving severe pain caused by cancer infiltration of the brachial or lumbosacral plexus or soft tissue infiltration.[54,62]

Neurostimulation Techniques

The publication of the Melzack-Wall theory of pain and the information on intrinsic analgesic mechanisms prompted the introduction and the ever-increasing use of electrical stimulation applied to skin, peripheral nerves, the spinal cord, and deep parts of the brain (see Meyerson[101] for review).

Transcutaneous Electrical Nerve Stimulation

Transcutaneous electrical nerve stimulation (TNS), electroacupuncture, and even manual acupuncture, by stimulating peripheral nerves or nerve endings, in some way produce pain inhibition at dorsal horn and/or activate some of the supraspinal descending inhibitory systems.[98,101] Although manual acupuncture has been used for thousands of years for a variety of painful conditions and many reports have been published in western countries during the past decade, the literature in this area is disappointing. In a review of the area, Chapman[40] found that the published literature as a whole was of poor scientific quality and was inconclusive, because studies were inadequately designed, results were poorly analyzed, and the pain measurement techniques employed were so primitive that the outcomes often could not be interpreted. Nevertheless, there is widespread, if unaccounted, agreement that acupunctural methods can be of benefit for selected patients with chronic pain.

TNS has been widely used for a variety of acute and chronic pain syndromes, including cancer (see Meyerson[101] for review). The results in many thousands of patients suggest that this method produces significant short-term relief in 65 to 80 percent of the patients and long-term relief in 30 to 35 percent of patients.[49,101,116] It has been found useful in patients with chronic pain due to rheumatoid arthritis,[92] muscular spasm,[116] peripheral nerve injuries,[49] and postherpetic neuralgia,[106] among others. A review of the literature reveals that basically two types of stimulation can be effective: low-frequency, (2–20 Hertz [Hz]), high-intensity stimulation and high-frequency (20–100+ Hz), low-intensity stimulation. Swedish investigators have developed a procedure that combines these two methods by delivering brief bursts of stimulation at high intensities, with the bursts occurring at low frequencies.[9,49] TNS has the advantage that it can be self-administered by the patient after proper instruction. For many patients with chronic pain, prescription of a TNS unit is an excellent alternative to prescription of a potentially dangerous medication.

Peripheral nerve stimulation, which entails the implantation of an electrode on one of the major nerves supplying the upper or lower limb, such as the median or sciatic, has produced similar results to TNS, particularly in patients with peripheral nerve injuries and in those with cancer pain.[80,101,116]

Stimulation of the Spinal Cord

In the late 1960s and early 1970s this procedure, which was prompted by the publication of the Melzack-Wall theory of pain, was achieved via laminectomy and implantation of the electrode over the spinal cord.[101,121] However, in recent years the technique has been refined to avoid surgery; the electrode is placed on the dura over the spinal cord through a large needle that is introduced through the intact skin and advanced until its bevel (point) is in the epidural space—hence the long title of percutaneously implanted spinal cord epidural stimulation (PISCES). Published reports suggest that with this procedure there is significant short-term improvement in 70 to 80 percent of patients and long-term relief in 35 to 40 percent of patients.[92,101,116,152] Spinal stimulation is preferentially effective for the treatment of pain due to nerve injuries, but is not as effective in relieving very severe pain, especially that of visceral origin.

Deep Brain Stimulation

Deep brain stimulation, which produces stimulation-produced analgesia (SPA), is achieved by stereotactic placement of a stimulating electrode into the PAG or PVG, usually with patients under local anesthesia (see Meyerson[101] for review). Accurate placement of the electrode is achieved by means of stereotactic apparatus, fluoroscopic guidance, and a trial stimulation for one to two weeks before the wire is buried and connected to the induction receiver and external transmitter that allow self-stimulation by the patient for pain control. These techniques have been used mostly for patients with advanced cancer pain, although some have used it for nonmalignant chronic pain. The published data suggest that about 40 to 55 percent of patients derived excellent pain relief, 20 to 30 percent derived 50 to 75 percent relief, and the rest derived no benefit.[101,116] The data suggest that SPA is effective in patients with cancer pain due to persistent peripheral nociceptive stimulation and is ineffective in deafferentation pain. Stimulation of the thalamic somatosensory nucleus has been reported to produce prolonged relief of neuropathic pain.[147]

Physical Therapies

The large variety of physical therapeutic techniques that have been used for centuries remains an important method of pain relief. One or more of these procedures are usually combined with other modalities. The following is a partial list: (1) manual therapy in the form of massage or manipulation, (2) exercise, (3) mechanical therapy in the form of traction or compression, (4) superficial and deep heat, and (5) application of cold in the form of ice packs or ice massage or with the use of vapocoolant sprays. These procedures are used for mild to moderate pain caused by musculoskeletal disorders.

Despite the widespread use of these modalities, their mechanism of pain-relieving action is not known. It has been hypothesized that most of these procedures produce an increase in blood flow to the painful part and that this enhances the elimination of pain-producing substances and the repair of damaged tissue. However, Melzack and Wall[98] believe the most plausible hypothesis is that these procedures produce sensory inputs that ultimately inhibit pain signals by closing the gate. This effect may be achieved by activation of large fibers by gentle stimulation, which produces inhibition at segmental levels, or by strong stimulation of small fibers that project nociceptive signals to the brain stem, where they stimulate descending inhibitory mechanisms that close the gate at spinal cord and higher levels. Various procedures in physical medicine may be explained by either or both mechanisms.

Psychological Techniques

The recent knowledge acquired by psychological and behavioral studies has led to the development and widespread use of a number of techniques for the psychological control of pain, which Bonica calls "psychologic analgesia." The techniques include: (1) psychophysiological procedures, such as progressive muscular relaxation and biofeedback; (2) operant or external contingency-managing approaches; (3) hypnotic suggestion techniques; (4) the use of stratagems to distract attention or change the meaning of the pain; (5) social modeling techniques; and (6) a variety of other cognitive-behavioral interventions. Data from numerous reports suggest that all these techniques have some value in the treatment of pain in some patients, but there are meager data from controlled clinical trials (see Tan[139] and Turner and Chapman[148] for reviews).

PROGRESSIVE MUSCLE RELAXATION

The technique of progressive muscle relaxation has been widely used to relax tense muscles believed to cause pain, and beneficial results have been reported in patients with tension headache, migraine headache, low back pain, postoperative pain, temporomandibular dysfunction syndrome, and phantom limb pain. It has been suggested that this technique reduces pain not only by decreasing muscle tension but also by decreasing arousal. Decrease of arousal will minimize the increased release of catecholamines and the increase in blood pressure, heart rate, and metabolism. All of these are responses to psychological stress and, when present, feed into the nervous system to produce pain directly or indirectly by facilitating activity in neuron pools that project pain signals to the brain.

BIOFEEDBACK

Biofeedback has been widely used to treat a variety of painful disorders on the assumption that a physiological disorder underlies the pain and the patient can be taught to control and correct the underlying disorder when given feedback. Techniques currently used include: (1) electromyographic (EMG) feedback to reduce muscle tension; (2) skin temperature feedback intended to decrease the dilatation of extracranial vessels thought to be the cause of migraine headache; and (3) electroencephalogram (EEG) feedback to help the subject produce alpha brain activity, a relaxed state hypothesized to be incompatible with pain.[139] These techniques have been used primarily to treat tension headache, migraine headache, low back pain, and a few other types of chronic pain syndromes with variable success.[74,146] Indeed, several reports indicate that biofeedback is not superior to less expensive, less instrument-oriented treatment, such as relaxation and coping-skills training.[139] It has been suggested that biofeedback is a useful vehicle for distraction of attention, relaxation, and suggestion and for providing patients with a sense of control of their pain.[139]

Operant Conditioning

Operant conditioning strategies are very useful in patients with operant pain mechanisms previously described.[57] For such patients, the major therapeutic procedures are: (1) to place the patient in a controlled environment where the positive pain-behavior reinforcers are precisely identified; (2) to decrease pain behaviors by withdrawal of positive reinforcers, such as by ignoring the pain complaint and other pain behaviors and, at the same time, complimenting patient's well behaviors; (3) to progressively decrease pain behavior and drug intake (detoxification program); (4) to encourage increased physical activity and other types of well behavior by such positive reinforcements as complimenting and encouraging the improvement in exercise, walking, and other physical activities; and (5) to maintain the gain brought about in behavioral changes in the treatment program by modifying the consequences to pain behavior and well behavior at home and work.

Fordyce[57] and others[2,118,141] have reported improvement, as measured by increased activity, marked decrease or elimination of drug intake, return to some form of work, and in other ways leading normal lives, in 60 to 70 percent of the patients at follow-up, which has ranged from six months to seven years. While such results are very encouraging, it is important to realize that: (1) this obtains for a highly selected group, which in one study consisted of 29 percent of 130 patients referred to the program, and of the selected group, 74 percent achieved significant improvement (i.e., 19 percent of the 130 patients originally referred)[2]; (2) while the pain behavior is decreased or eliminated, many patients continue to feel pain but are simply conditioned not to manifest it overtly; and (3) the program as originally proposed entails hospitalization for six to eight weeks and is costly.[57] To minimize the cost, some clinicians conduct the program on an outpatient basis or use short hospitalization.[135] In any case, since most patients managed with the operant conditioning program have been disabled for many years and have cost society large amounts of money, the cost/benefit ratio is still favorable even when only 20 percent of the patients are rehabilitated.[57]

Hypnosis

Although hypnosis for the relief of pain has been used since ancient times and a number of isolated reports of hypnosis as an effective method of pain relief were published during the last half of the nineteenth and the first half of the twentieth century, its acceptance as an ethical form of medical practice and a legitimate subject for scientific study are recent developments.[66,122] During the past three decades a number of scientists have studied hypnosis, and many clinicians have reported its successful use in managing patients with a variety of pain syndromes (see Swanson, Maruta, and Swenson[135] for review). The advantage of the technique is that it reduces or eliminates pain without unpleasant or destructive side effects, and by reducing emotional stress and teaching autohypnosis, it can create life-enhancing attitudes in the patient. The disadvantages of the technique are that it requires the service of an experienced hypnotherapist, many techniques are time-consuming, and only about 20 to 25 percent of patients can achieve sufficient hypnotic depth to obtain complete relief of moderate to severe pain, although a larger percent can achieve partial relief of the pain.[135] To use this method effectively, it is necessary to determine the hypnotic susceptibility of the patient and his or her willingness to be hypnotized and ability to concentrate and to develop rapport with the therapist so the patient has no fear of hypnosis and has absolute confidence in the therapist.

OTHER COGNITIVE-BEHAVIORAL TECHNIQUES

Other cognitive-behavioral techniques aim to correct faulty conditions (attitudes, beliefs, and expectations) underlying emotional and behavioral disturbances.[148] With these procedures, patients learn to identify distorted beliefs and substitute more positive thoughts and are taught specific cognitive skills such as imagery, focused attention, distraction, relabeling of sensations, social modeling, and other strategies for coping with pain (see Tan[139] and Turner and Chapman[148] for reviews). These processes aim to increase the patient's awareness of events that aggravate the pain and actions that reduce it, so that the patient may better avoid or deal more effectively with pain-increasing events and use pain-relieving actions. A variety of cognitive-behavioral procedures have been given clinical trial. Although the results are encouraging, a precise role of these procedures for pain relief is not known and will require controlled clinical trials in patients with specific pain syndromes.[25,139,148]

Regional Anesthesia

For nearly a century analgesia limited to the painful part, achieved with local anesthetics or neurolytic agents, has been widely used for the treatment of acute and chronic painful conditions unrelated to a surgical operation (see Bonica[9,11] for reviews). Recently acquired knowledge has also prompted the application of narcotics into the spinal canal to produce regional analgesia for the relief of acute and chronic pain, including cancer pain.

REGIONAL ANALGESIA WITH LOCAL ANESTHETICS

Local anesthetics act by stabilizing the membrane of nerve fibers and thus prevent transmission of nociceptive and other impulses for periods ranging from minutes to hours, or even days, depending on the local anesthetic and technique used. Because the thinner the nerve fiber, the greater its susceptibility to local anesthetic, it is possible to preferentially block the A delta and C fibers involved in pain without significant interference of muscle function and touch sensation; hence the term regional *analgesia*. Using a higher concentration can produce loss of motor function and even touch sensation—or regional *anesthesia*. Regional analgesia with local anesthetics may be used for diagnostic, prognostic, and/or therapeutic purposes.[9,11,20,24]

Diagnostic Blocks. When properly applied, diagnostic blocks are very useful in helping to ascertain specific nociceptive pathways and to define the mechanisms of pain, and aiding in the differential diagnosis of the site of nociceptive input. For example, in a patient with pain in the low back and lower limbs from a herniated intervertebral disc, it is essential to determine which nerve root is involved; this can be achieved precisely by selective paravertebral somatic nerve block. Similarly, if after adequate examination there is still doubt whether pain in the chest or abdomen is caused by visceral disease or by disorders of the chest/abdominal wall, block of intercostal nerves will relieve the latter and not the former. In contrast, block of the visceral nociceptive afferents in the upper thoracic sympathetic chain will relieve thoracic visceral pain, while block of the celiac plexus (which contains the pain fibers from the abdominal viscera) relieves visceral pain but not chest/abdominal wall pain.

Prognostic Blocks. Prognostic blocks are useful to predict the analgesic efficacy and side effects of neurolytic blocks or neurosurgical operations and also afford the patient an opportunity to experience the numbness and other side effects that follow the long-term procedure.

Therapeutic Blocks. Blocks with local anesthetics are used to provide patients with prompt relief from severe excruciating pain for hours and days, and occasionally permanently. For example, continuous segmental epidural block of the affected spinal segments produces complete relief of postoperative or posttraumatic pain, the excruciating pain of a herniated disc, or severe cancer pain for a number of days or even a couple of weeks. Moreover, a series of local anesthetic infiltrations of trigger areas often permanently relieves myofascial pain syndromes, chronic low back pain due to muscle spasm, and chronic pain due to tendonitis or other disorders of the periarticular structures (see Bonica [9,11,29] for references). This procedure also may be useful in relieving painful scars. A series of blocks of the sympathetic supply to the upper or lower limb often produces prolonged pain relief in patients with causalgia and other reflex sympathetic dystrophy and occasionally in those with phantom limb pain and other chronic pain syndromes.[20] The mechanism of such action has already been mentioned in the discussion of the Melzack biasing mechanism.

Except for local infiltration of small amounts of local anesthetics, each technique carries the risk of adverse side effects and/or complications. These include systemic toxic reaction to the local anesthetic from injection of excessive amounts or accidental intravenous injection; hypotension from extensive vasomotor block associated with spinal or epidural block; total spinal anesthesia from accidental injection of large amounts of local anesthetic into the subarachnoid space; and pneumothorax from accidental puncture of the visceral pleura. Arterial hypotension can be minimized by limiting the extent of the block and by infusing fluids, while all of the other complications can be avoided with skillful administration.

INTRASPINAL NARCOTICS

The recently acquired knowledge on opiate receptors led to animal studies that clearly demonstrated that injection of small amounts of morphine or other narcotics into the subarachnoid or epidural space produced a block of nociceptive impulses from a region of the body *without* blocking other somatosensory, somatomotor, or sympathetic functions.[163] These findings promptly led to the use of intraspinal narcotics to produce regional analgesia in patients with severe acute and chronic pain, including cancer pain (see Jacobson[71] for review). In contrast to the duration of three to four hours achieved with intramuscular injection of morphine, subarachnoid or epidural injection of this drug produces pain relief for twelve to twenty-four hours.

To achieve relief for several days or weeks, a very small plastic catheter is introduced into the subarachnoid or epidural space through a special needle; the needle is then removed and the catheter taped to the patient's body. Usually 0.5 to 1 mg morphine injected into the subarachnoid space or 6 to 8 mg diluted in 6 to 8 ml saline injected into the epidural space every twelve to eighteen hours provides effective pain relief. In patients with cancer or other chronic pain syndromes that require prolonged administration, continuous implantable infusion systems are used to avoid the risk of infection inherent in repeated injections. A Silastic catheter is placed with its tip at the appropriate level of the epidural space; the catheter is then tunneled subcutaneously so its proximal end is in the anterior part of the body; it is then connected to an implanted infusion plant reservoir, which can be refilled percutaneously every ten to fifteen days.[45,71,109]

As with all other techniques, this procedure is associated with certain adverse side effects, the most important of which is respiratory depression, but fortunately the incidence is very low (see Jacobson[71] for review). Other side effects include diffuse pruritus, urinary retention, nausea and vomiting, and development of tolerance. Tolerance can be minimized by avoiding injection of large amounts. If it develops, injection of one or two doses of local anesthetic in some way eliminates it.

REGIONAL ANALGESIA WITH NEUROLYTIC AGENTS

Regional analgesia with neurolytic blocks, achieved by the injection of alcohol or phenol, involves the intentional destruction of a nerve or nerves for a period of time in order to produce interruption of nociceptive pathways for weeks, months, and sometimes permanently, depending on the site of the injection (see Bonica[9,11] for reviews). Neurolytic agents completely destroy nerve cell bodies or their connections to the CNS; these are not able to regenerate and consequently the interruption is permanent. In contrast, if the agent is injected into the nerve distal to the cell body, the nerve is capable of regeneration, and after several months the pain returns and a neuroma has formed that may itself produce pain. On the basis of these facts, neurolytic agents are injected primarily into the subarachnoid space to destroy sensory rootlets proximal to the cell bodies or into the gasserian ganglion to destroy many or all of the cell bodies of the trigeminal nerve. Only in rare cases have they been used to destroy peripheral nerves.

In the past, these procedures have been used primarily for patients with cancer pain but also for those with nonmalignant chronic pain. However, the recently acquired information that loss of peripheral sensory input produces long-term abnormal activity in the dorsal horn and other parts of the CNS dictates that neurolytic blocks should not be used in most patients with nonmalignant chronic pain. Moreover, the recent advent of refined neurosurgical procedures, neurostimulation techniques, and psychological methods has decreased the indication for neurolytic blocks even in cancer pain. Nevertheless, several neurolytic procedures remain useful, particularly in patients with severe advanced cancer pain who have a short life expectancy, are poor risks for major neurosurgical procedures, and cannot be relieved adequately with narcotics.

Subarachnoid Neurolysis.   Subarachnoid neurolysis entails the injection of alcohol or phenol into the subarachnoid space to achieve chemical sensory rhizotomy (destruction of sensory rootlets). It has been successfully used for the treatment of severe pain of advanced cancer in many thousands of patients (see Bonica,[9] Swerdlow,[137] and Wood[161] for reviews). Pain relief usually lasts for several months and sometimes even longer, although not infrequently it is necessary to do several blocks to achieve complete destruction of the rootlets. Available data suggest this procedure produces complete relief in about 50 to 60 percent of cancer patients, partial relief in about 20 to 25 percent, and no relief in the rest.[9,11,137,161] This procedure is particularly useful in relieving severe pain in the trunk because good analgesia can be achieved without significant adverse side effects. On the other hand, even when expertly carried out, subarachnoid neurolysis of the rootlets of the upper or lower limb will result in transient muscle weakness in 15 to 20 percent of patients; in 3 to 5 percent of these, weakness is prolonged.[9,137,161] Moreover, if the block is done for pain in the pelvis or lower limb, there is transient bladder and/or rectal sphincter dysfunction in 20 to 25 percent of patients due to interruption of the autonomic nerves, and this persists in 5 to 7 percent.

Other Neurolytic Techniques.   Block of the trigeminal sensory root or gasserian ganglion has been used for many years to effectively relieve severe trigeminal neuralgia and cancer pain in the anterior two-thirds of the head (see Bonica[9] and Bonica and Madrid[32] for review). Although the reintroduction of thermocoagulation of these structures has decreased the incidence for neurolytic block, there is still a definite place for these procedures in managing severe pain due to advanced or terminal cancer, particularly in localities where the neurosurgical technique is not available and there are physicians skilled in the block procedure. The same may be said of *celiac plexus block* achieved with either 50 percent alcohol or 7 to 10 percent aqueous phenol to relieve severe pain caused by cancer of the pancreas, stomach, or other abdominal viscera.[103] Both of these neurolytic procedures produce complete or almost complete relief of pain in 75 to 80 percent of patients until their death. For the reason just mentioned, neurolytic blocks of spinal nerves should *not* be carried out except in patients with severe excruciating pain not amenable to narcotics and in whom neurosurgery is contraindicated.

Neuroadenolysis of the Pituitary

Neuroadenolysis of the pituitary (NALP) is another procedure that has been found effective in relieving severe diffuse cancer pain in various parts of the body.[61,104] The procedure, introduced by Moricca,[104] entails the introduction of a needle through the nose and through the sphenoid bone under fluoroscopic control until its tip is in the center of the sella turcica, which contains the pituitary gland. Slow injection of small increments of absolute alcohol results in complete relief in about 50 to 60 percent of patients, partial relief in 25 to 35 percent, and no relief in the rest (see Gianasi[61] for extensive review). Adverse side effects include transient diabetes insipidus in about 60 percent of the patients, rhinorrhea for one or two days, and diplopia in 2 to 3 percent of the patients.[61]

Neurosurgical Operations

The studies that led to the wide acceptance of the specificity theory in the nineteenth and twentieth centuries suggested that in patients with severe intractable pain (the cause of which could not be eliminated), surgical section of the sensory pathways in peripheral nerves and spinal cord, or in the brain stem, should provide permanent relief.[157] These include: (1) section of sensory pathways in peripheral spinal or cranial nerves (neurotomy); (2) section of sensory pathways that supply viscera contained in sympathetic nerves (sympathectomy); (3) section of the sensory roots (rhizotomy) of spinal or cranial nerves; (4) section of the spinothalamic tract (cordotomy) in the upper thoracic or upper cervical region, the medulla, or the midbrain; and (5) lesions of the thalamus. All of these operations produce side effects and other disadvantages that, together with recently acquired knowledge, have prompted the abandonment of neurotomy and sympathectomy, greatly decreased the use of spinal dorsal rhizotomy and open spinothalamic tractotomy, and have led to the introduction of new and less destructive techniques. The role of these procedures will be briefly summarized. For detailed reviews, the reader is referred to the text by White and Sweet.[157]

SPINAL DORSAL RHIZOTOMY

Spinal dorsal rhizotomy is used only in highly selected patients with very severe pain involving one or a few spinal segments in the thorax and abdomen and in the perineum.[157] This procedure is rarely, if ever, indicated for the relief of extremity pain, because a section of all of the roots supplying the limb produces extensive deafferentation with loss of proprioception and consequently results in a virtually useless limb. To avoid this problem, "selective posterior rhizotomy" has been recently introduced[127]; with the aid of an operative microscope it is feasible to section only the fine afferent fibers in the lateral division of the dorsal root, thus leaving intact the larger afferents in the medial division that mediate touch and proprioception. In any case, this procedure should be reserved for patients with advanced cancer, because, as previously mentioned, chronic deafferentation produces long-term abnormal function in the CNS that may result in deafferentation pain.

CRANIAL SENSORY RHIZOTOMY

Section of the sensory root of the trigeminal nerve is still done for the relief of severe excruciating trigeminal neuralgia not relieved by drugs or other less destructive operations and is also used for severe excruciating pain in the anterior two-thirds of the head caused by advanced cancer.[157] In patients with cancer pain in the distribution of the trigeminal and other cranial nerves and the upper neck, section of the sensory root of cranial nerves V, VII, IX, and X and of the upper two or three cervical nerves is carried out through posterior craniotomy. The disadvantages of this operation are that it requires a major operation and produces loss of all sensation, it is often followed by very uncomfortable sensations (paresthesia), and it carries the risk of corneal ulcers due to loss of the conjunctival reflex.

These disadvantages have prompted the reintroduction and refinement of *percutaneous differential thermal rhizotomy* of the roots of ganglion of the fifth cranial nerve.[136,157] This procedure is performed with local anesthesia using a needle electrode that is introduced through the face and made to pass through the foramen ovale until its point is in the ganglion or root of the nerve; then a radio frequency is applied to permit differential thermocoagulation, with continuous monitoring of the patient to achieve the desired degree of analgesia. Since the unmyelinated and small myelinated nociceptive fibers are more sensitive to the destructive effects of heat, these fibers can be destroyed preferentially while sparing touch and sensation. Properly carried out, this procedure produces complete short-term pain relief in 80 to 90 percent of the patients and long-term relief in 50 to 60 percent.[126,136] A similar technique of percutaneous differential radio-frequency rhizotomy of the glossopharyngeal nerve for the relief of severe excruciating cancer pain in the throat recently has been described.[36]

SPINOTHALAMIC TRACTOTOMY

Section of the spinothalamic tract in the upper thoracic level has been used for more than half a century, and in the hands of a skilled neurosurgeon it produces almost complete pain relief in the lower part of the body in 75 to 90 percent of patients.[111,157] Unfortunately, the pain relief lasts only some twelve to sixteen months and rarely longer, despite the fact that the interruption produced by the lesion is permanent. This suggests that the nervous system finds other pathways for transmission of pain signals and that the procedure should be reserved only for patients with cancer predicted to live less than one to one and one-half years. Because the standard procedure requires a laminectomy to expose the cord and is thus associated with a mortality rate of 5 to 10 percent and morbidity in 15 to 20 percent of patients, it has been virtually replaced by percutaneous cervical cordotomy.[110]

Percutaneous cervical cordotomy entails the introduction of a needle through the skin and deeper tissues in the upper neck, which has been previously anesthetized with a local anesthetic (see Lipton[84] for review). The needle is made to pass through the C1 to C2 intervertebral space and advanced until its point is in the anterolateral part of the spinal cord. Precise location of the needle is ascertained by a stimulating technique that produces pain, tingling, and other signs; then a radiofrequency is applied in increments until there is ample analgesia in the contralateral half of the body. The procedure has the advantage of being a relatively minor operation with an extremely low operative and postoperative mortality and a very low incidence of complications, while at the same time producing good pain relief in 75 to 90 percent of patients for periods of several months. Because of these advantages, it has replaced not only open cordotomy but also subarachnoid alcohol or phenol blocks. Unfortunately, only a relatively small number of persons are skilled enough to carry out this procedure.

Medullary spinothalamic tractotomy is infrequently used because it carries a high risk of mortality and complications.[110,157] On the other hand, section of the descending trigeminal tract in the medulla interrupts the sensory fibers of cranial nerves V, VII, IX, and X and is highly effective in relieving pain in the face and the anterior two-thirds of the head. [110,157] The major disadvantage is that it requires a craniotomy.

CRANIAL STEREOTACTIC OPERATIONS

Mesencephalic tractotomy carried out under stereotactic control with local anesthesia interrupts the ascending systems in the midbrain and produces effective pain relief for six to twelve months. [110,157] Lesions of the hypothalamus and thalamus also have been shown to produce relief of severe cancer pain for periods of six to twelve months and are therefore indicated in patients with advanced cancer for whom other procedures are not available. [110,157] Unfortunately, only a few surgeons throughout the world have the skill to carry out these procedures accurately and effectively.

PSYCHOSURGERY

Prefrontal lobotomy, as originally proposed, produced pain relief but was accompanied by severe apathy, mental confusion, and loss of affect. [59] To diminish the side effects, White and Sweet [157] introduced gradual bilateral coagulation of the medial frontal white matter, achieved by implanting electrodes. This graduated lesion causes patients to be free from concern about pain or death. Another operation to achieve these objectives is cingulotomy [56]; this also produces affective changes, although to a much lesser degree than lobotomy. These operations should be reserved for patients with excruciating, intolerable cancer pain and with only a few months to live.

¶ Multidisciplinary Pain Clinics/Centers

Experience managing many patients with various pain syndromes in military hospitals during World War II led the senior author to the conviction that the diagnosis and therapy of complex problems required more knowledge and skill than was possessed by any individual physician. Consequently, he conceived and put into practice the idea that patients with complex pain problems could be more effectively managed by a multidisciplinary/interdisciplinary program, each member of which would contribute specialized knowledge and skills to the common goal of making a correct diagnosis and developing the most effective therapeutic strategy. Following sixteen years of favorable experience in the military and in a private community hospital, in 1961 Bonica developed such a facility in an academic environment. [14] During the ensuing two decades, the University of Washington Pain Clinic evolved into a group of over forty-five professionals representing a wide variety of medical specialties and basic sciences, and in 1980 it was designated as a center. [34] The clinical pain service of the center has since served as a prototype for hundreds of such facilities both in the United States and abroad. The structure of such facilities has been described by Bonica and associates, [34] Crue and co-workers, [46] and Lipton, [84] among others.

In general, a multidisciplinary center consists of: (1) an outpatient referral clinic, (2) an inpatient pain service with inpatient beds, (3) a multidisciplinary staff prepared to deal with both medical and psychological aspects of chronic pain, (4) a teaching program, and (5) an intrinsic or affiliated clinic with a basic research program. The clinical pain service usually manages patients referred to the center by family medicine practitioners and specialists who encounter complex pain problems. Each patient referred to the facility is assigned to a clinical algologist (pain specialist) who becomes the patient's manager and who has the responsibility of the initial evaluation and of coordination of the psychological and psychosocial evaluation with consultation by orthopedists, neurologists, and/or other relevant specialists as well as the use of specialized diagnostic procedures. This is followed by a multidisciplinary conference, attended by all physicians who have seen the patient, to determine a diagnosis and recommend a treatment plan, which usually includes both medical and psychological intervention and, if needed, vocational rehabilitation. In addition to providing services to patients, the close interaction of the team during their daily activities, and especially during the daily conferences, not only provides the patient with services but also constitutes an excellent forum for the exchange of information and is a highly effective educational program. Such a facility and its activities also encourages diffusion of information to physicians outside of the facility and, very importantly, encourages collaborative research relevant to the solution of major pain problems.

¶ Chronic Pain Syndromes

In this section we will briefly describe three chronic pain syndromes that have predominantly peripheral mechanisms, three syndromes with peripheral-central mechanisms, and one that is predominantly due to psychological mechanisms. The first category includes myofascial pain syndromes, low back pain, and cancer; the second category will include causalgia and other reflex sympathetic dystrophies and phantom limb pain; and the third category will include chronic pain predominantly due to operant mechanisms.

Myofascial Pain Syndromes

Myofascial pain syndromes constitute a group of disorders characterized by the presence of a very hypersensitive region, the so-called trigger area, in one of the muscles or in the connective tissue, together with a specific syndrome of pain, muscle spasm, tenderness, stiffness, limitation of motion, weakness, and, occasionally, autonomic dysfunction.* The pain may be in the region of the trigger areas or in an area of reference that is usually some distance from the trigger point. These disturbances have been previously described as, among other terms, myalgia, myositis, fibrositis, fibromyositis (or myofibrositis), fascitis, myofascitis, muscular

*See references 9, 10, 11, 129, and 144.

rheumatism, and muscular strains (see Bonica[9,11] and Travell and Simons[144] for reviews).

The management of myofascial pain syndromes constitutes one of the most important problems encountered in medical practice for three reasons: These disorders are among the most frequent causes of severe disabling pain and are the most common musculoskeletal disabilities of the shoulder girdle, neck, and low back; their peculiar symptomatology causes them to be often misdiagnosed and wrongly treated as bursitis, arthritis, and, occasionally, visceral disease; and they are relatively simple to manage, since most of the therapeutic procedures can be carried out in the physician's office and, when treatment is properly executed, prompt cure ensues.

ETIOLOGY

Myofascial pain syndromes are most frequently seen in middle-aged and elderly people and develop following an acute, sudden trauma to myofascial structures or they may be initiated by repeated microtraumata of daily work that requires repetitious activity of certain muscle groups in the upper or lower limb or low back, such as typewriting or screwdriving done all day long. They also follow chronic muscular strain, chilling or fatigue of muscles, arthritis, nerve injuries, neuromuscular disorders, cancer, and, in some instances, visceral pathology. The sudden severe or repetitious microtraumata produce "trigger areas" (synonymous with "trigger zones," "trigger points," or "myalgic spots") that are defined as small, circumscribed, hypersensitive regions in muscles or in connective tissue. Nociceptive impulses arise from trigger areas and are transmitted to the dorsal horn, particularly cells of lamina 5, onto which converge innocuous impulses from the skin to produce referred pain. The trigger area is so-called because its stimulation, like pulling the trigger of a gun, produces effects at another place (the target), called the "reference zone" or "area of reference." These conditions involve peripheral mechanisms because when the trigger area is temporarily eliminated by injection of a local anesthetic, the symptomatology disappears either temporarily or permanently. These abnormal foci of pain can be activated by pressure, motion that stretches the muscles or other structures containing them, or intense heat or cold.

SYMPTOMATOLOGY

During the early stage of the disorder, pain, tenderness, and muscle spasm are brought on only by active stimulation of the trigger areas; eventually the latter become so sensitive that they produce continuous pain and associated symptomatology, which may also include vasoconstriction, edema, and mild sweating. The pattern of the referred pain and associated phenomena is relatively constant and predictable, a fact that indicates that the nociceptive impulses concerned in the reference of somatic pain, like those of visceral pain, follow fixed anatomic pathways. However, unlike visceral pain, it does not follow a dermatomal pattern or nerve root distribution—a fact that has delayed the recognition of this group of disorders as clinical entities.

The referred pain is dull and continuous in character, and its intensity may vary from a low-grade discomfort to pain that is severe and incapacitating. The extent of the area of pain (and associated phenomena) apparently depends on the sensitivity of the trigger area. If it is very sensitive, there is a wide radiation of pain to include an essential zone of reference and a "spillover" zone, whereas if it is not very sensitive, pain is present in the "essential" zone only.

Diagnosis of these syndromes depends on identification of the trigger area by noting aggravation of pain when it is stimulated and elimination of pain when it is injected with a local anesthetic. Careful examination is required to differentiate these conditions from neurologic lesions. The distinction is relatively simple to make, since distribution of pain of myofascial syndromes is not segmental, nor does it fit a peripheral nerve distribu-

tion. Moreover, with myofascial pain syndrome there is usually no sensory deficit or reflex change, as occurs with herniated disc and other neurologic problems.

TREATMENT

The primary form of therapy is the injection of the trigger areas with a dilute solution of local anesthetic and, in patients who have chronic disorders, with a mixture of local anesthetic and long-acting corticoid compounds such as Depo-Medrol.[9,11,30] Some clinicians[129] use saline injection or dry needling—a form of acupuncture—and others a coolant spray on the trigger point.[144] Obviously it is necessary to have knowledge of the patterns of various syndromes and the locations of the trigger areas. After a detailed history has been taken, the patient is examined carefully for the presence of trigger areas. This may be best accomplished by palpating the suspected area with a finger or the end of a fountain pen, or any other dull object. Palpation should be systematic so that every square centimeter of the surface overlying the sensitive zone or the site from which the pain arises is palpated. Once the suspected spot has been found and marked with a skin pencil, palpation is varied and the patient is required to identify the particular spot repeatedly.

For the injection, the patient is placed in a recumbent position in order to prevent attacks of syncope. The injection is accomplished with a 25-gauge, 5-cm needle, which is inserted deliberately through the skin and advanced slowly until the trigger area is contacted, at which point the patient experiences unusual hypersensitivity and aggravation of the pain. Usually 5 ml of 0.25 percent bupivacaine hydrochloride (Marcaine) or equiactive concentrations of other local anesthetics will suffice. As previously mentioned, for patients with chronic syndromes we add a small dose of a long-lasting corticoid compound to the local anesthetic. Within five to eight minutes of the injection, there is prompt relief of pain and tenderness and often a decrease in muscle spasm. If no relief is obtained, it is most likely that the trigger point was not injected, requiring another trial.

The relief of pain, tenderness, muscle spasm, and other effects persists for several hours and sometimes a day, after which the pain is often exaggerated. The patient should be informed that such a reaction should not be considered unfavorable, because if the area is injected again, the postinjection pain will be much less and the secondary periods of relief will be longer and more encouraging. In acute cases, one treatment is sometimes sufficient, whereas in chronic cases a series of treatments is usually necessary. Physical therapy and active exercise are necessary adjuncts to local infiltration.

Low Back Pain

Low back pain is a serious health and economic problem that plagues all industrialized countries. As previously mentioned, based on data derived from numerous studies published in the United States, Britain, Sweden, Denmark, and Israel, the senior author estimates that in 1983 over 15 percent of the American adults (23 million) had chronic low back pain, and of these, eight million were partially or totally disabled for periods of weeks, months, and some permanently, causing a loss of over 225 million workdays. Moreover, about 225,000 operations were performed for low back pain, contributing to a total health care cost of over $8 billion. This cost, together with loss of work productivity, compensation payments, payments for litigation, and the services of "quacks," totaled in excess of $23 billion. This represents a third of the total cost of chronic pain in the United States.

ETIOLOGY

The pathophysiological bases of low back pain are not all well understood.[9,38,87] Fahrni[50] has stated that members of primitive societies who habitually squat rather than sit on chairs and never stand with a military posture have a zero incidence of low back pain and a very low incidence of x-ray evidence of disc collapse. In contrast, office workers and heavy laborers have an increasing incidence of x-ray changes with advancing age. Disc degeneration begins in childhood and is part of the aging process; yet only a small fraction of people have symptoms in spite of x-ray changes.

In a small percentage of patients with degeneration of the intervertebral disc, the annulus fibrosis ruptures or bulges.[47] The disc material mechanically compresses the nerve root to produce severe pain that radiates from the low back to the leg (sciatica) and is associated with sensory and motor deficits in the lower limb. Studies by Howe, Loeser, and Calvin[68] have clearly shown that chronically scarred axons can fire repetitively after mechanical compression, and thus have established a neurophysiological basis for radicular pain that characterizes "sciatica" caused by a ruptured disc.

Much more common causes of back pain are musculoskeletal derangements, including myofascial syndromes, muscle strains and sprains, and, possibly, facet joint dysfunction. Congenital abnormalities and trauma may play a role in some of these forms of low back pain. Recent evidence has pointed to the important roles of environmental and social factors in many patients with low back pain.[57] It seems certain that the etiological factors are multiple, hence no one form of therapy can be applied to all patients.[98]

THERAPY

A few principles for the management of low back pain may help to reduce the incidence of chronic pain and long-term disability. After all, every chronic pain patient began his or her career as a patient with an acute episode. The patient with acute low back pain deserves a careful history and physical examination. After infrequent causes such as infection, neoplasm, or abdominal/pelvic disease have been ruled out, the physician should focus on the evidence for muscle spasm, myofascial pain syndromes, disc protrusions, and psychological and social factors. A management strategy should be thoroughly explained to the patient and intensive, conservative therapy initiated.[9,38,87] Medications and bed rest should be prescribed for a reasonable period of time (a few weeks at most) and not allowed to become long-term therapies. If the pain process has an inflammatory component, aspirin, or another nonsteroidal anti-inflammatory drug should be used. Short-term use of narcotics, muscle relaxants, and sedatives is helpful in the patient with an acute back strain or sprain or in the conservative management of disc protrusion. The prolonged use of these drugs is contraindicated in patients with chronic low back pain.

Infiltration of local anesthetics is effective in the therapy of myofascial syndromes in the low back.[9,129] Some clinicians have reported good results with lumbar sympathetic blocks,[35] but the basis of such therapy is not clear. Many patients with acute and even chronic back pain obtain relief with massage, application of heat or cold, postural training, transcutaneous electrical stimulation, or acupuncture. In patients with acute low back pain and lower limb pain due to recent herniation of vertebral discs, some clinicians[159] have reported good results with extradural subarachnoid injection of corticoid compounds, which are said to decrease the edema of nerve roots injured by the extruded disc. Best results have been achieved in patients with a "virgin" back, that is, when no previous surgery has been done.

Surgical therapy should be restricted to those patients with clear-cut neurological and mechanical signs of disc rupture who have failed to improve with conservative therapy. In a review of 2,054 patients who had undergone discectomies, Spangfort[130] found a correlation between degree of pain relief and pathological findings. In patients for whom the exploration was negative, only 40 percent derived complete relief, while complete relief was derived by some 60 percent of those with bulging disc and 75 percent of those with incomplete or complete herniation of the disc. The reasons for lack of pain relief in the remainder of those who had evidenced pathology are not understood. It deserves reemphasis that only a small percentage of patients with low back pain have disc herniation. Moreover, removing a disc only relieves pressure on the nerve root; it does not restore normal back function. This requires aggressive physical therapy, including exercise. There is no good evidence that fusion of the spine is indicated in the management of back pain unless major trauma or congenital abnormality has occurred.[87]

The most difficult patient to manage is one who has failed to improve after surgery. Nerve root scarring and arachnoiditis are common after an unsuccessful operation, and they are essentially untreatable. Destructive operations such as rhizotomy or cordotomy rarely, if ever, are beneficial to the patient with chronic low back pain after discectomy. Facet rhizolysis has enjoyed popularity in the past, but this operation probably does not denervate the facet joint and lacks any statistically valid evidence for efficacy.[87] Similar comments can be made about the injection of papain, which is supposed to dissolve the disc.[120]

Patients with chronic low back pain due to operant mechanisms are usually depressed, have lifelong evidence of personal and social inadequacy, and unconsciously use their pain as the focal point of their lives. Environmental factors such as compensation for disability, avoidance of unpleasant and unsatisfactory jobs, and attention from family members because of pain behavior may all lead to continued symptoms in the absence of observable pathology. Traditional forms of psychotherapy have not been very effective, as these patients often lack the desire to change their life-styles. There is now some evidence that operant therapy strategies may help this type of patient learn more successful methods of coping with his or her world.[57] Patients must be helped to learn that increased activities, decreased medications, and reassessment of life goals and plans will decrease their disability. The combined physical therapies and operant therapy programs appear to offer the best chance of success in these patients.

Cancer

Among the many chronic pain syndromes, cancer pain is one of the most important because it afflicts nearly three-quarters of a million Americans annually. Sixty to 80 percent of those with advanced cancer have moderate or severe pain, while about 50 percent of those with the intermediate stage of the disease have significant pain. Moreover, some eighteen million patients worldwide have cancer pain.[27,31] Unfortunately, in many, if not most, instances, cancer pain is inadequately treated because, for reasons previously mentioned, many physicians underprescribe narcotics, do not use nonnarcotic analgesics sufficiently, and do not appreciate that in some patients, systematic analgesics produce insufficient pain relief and therefore must be combined with other therapeutic modalities (see Bonica[27] for review).

ETIOLOGY

In many, if not most, patients, cancer-related pain is due to several causes, including direct effect of the cancer, the result of anticancer therapy, and coincidental disorders.[54] The most important of these are listed in table 26–2.

EFFECTS OF CANCER PAIN

Usually the physiological and psychological impact of cancer pain on the patient is greater than that of noncancer chronic pain.[27,31] The physical deterioration is more severe because these patients have greater problems with sleep disturbance and with lack of appetite, nausea, and vomiting. Cancer patients also develop greater emotional reactions of anxiety, depression, hypochondriasis, somatic focusing, and neuroticism to pain than do patients with noncancer chronic pain. Woodforde and Fielding[162] examined cancer patients with and without pain using the Cornell Medical Index. They demonstrated that the former group was significantly more emotionally disturbed than the latter group, responded less well to treatment of their cancer, and died sooner. The main cause of emotional morbidity was found to be depression, although hypochondriasis and psychosomatic symptoms were recorded also. They commented that the combination of intractable pain and depression represents symptoms that indicate a state of helplessness or inability to cope with disease, damage to the body, and the threat to life; and this is a response to having a progressive and potentially fatal illness. Bond[8] found that cancer patients with pain had raised levels of hypochondriasis and neuroticism, while pain-free cancer patients had low levels. He further noted that the scores of patients with high levels of emotionality fell after the pain was relieved by percutaneous cordotomy. This led Bond[7] to conclude that personality factors are distorted by severe pain and that its relief results in restoration in the direction of normality.

The social effects of uncontrolled cancer pain are also more serious than those of noncancer chronic pain. Many patients develop interpersonal problems with members of their family, friends, and coworkers. The fact that most patients with advanced cancer have to stop working poses not only an economic but also an emotional stress and a feeling of dependency and uselessness. The physical appearance and behavior produced by the patient's pain and suffering stresses the family emotionally, which, in turn, is perceived by the patient, consequently aggravating his or her pain and suffering.[27,31]

TREATMENT

Most patients with cancer pain can be adequately managed with nonnarcotic and narcotic analgesics. As previously mentioned, nonnarcotic analgesics are highly effective in pain due to bone cancer or metastases and, when properly administered, are effective in relieving mild to moderate pain due to other forms of cancer. Usually two to three times the so-called optimal dose must be given at regular intervals in order to obtain analgesic ceiling effect. For example, aspirin must be given in doses of 650 to 975 mg every three to four hours, so the total daily dose is 4 to 5

TABLE 26–2

Pain Syndromes in Patients with Cancer

I. *Pain associated with direct tumor involvement.*
- A. *Tumor infiltration of bone*
  1. Base of the skull metastases
     - a. jugular foramen
     - b. clivus
     - c. sphenoid sinus
  2. Vertebral-body metastases
     - a. sublaxation of the atlas
     - b. C_7–T_1 metastases
     - c. L_1 metastases
     - d. sacral metastases
  3. Tumor or metastases of long bones
     - a. ribs
     - b. femur or humerus
- B. *Tumor infiltration of nerves*
  1. Peripheral neuropathy
  2. Brachial, lumbar, sacral plexopathy
  3. Meningeal carcinomatosis
  4. Epidural spinal-cord compression
- C. *Tumor obstruction of hollow viscus*
  1. Gastrointestinal tract
  2. Urinary tract
  3. Ducts of solid viscera
- D. *Obstruction of major vessels*
  1. Large veins → edema/pain
  2. Large artery → ischemia/pain
- E. Tumor of solid viscera → fascia distention
- F. Necrotic ulceration of mucous membrane

II. *Pain associated with cancer therapy*
- A. *Pain occurring postsurgery*
  1. Postthoracotomy pain
  2. Postmastectomy pain
  3. Postradical neck pain
  4. Phantom-limb pain
- B. *Pain occurring postchemotherapy*
  1. Peripheral neuropathy
  2. Postherpetic neuralgia
  3. Steroid pseudorheumatism
  4. Aseptic necrosis of bone
- C. *Pain occurring postradiation therapy*
  1. Radiation fibrosis of the brachial plexus and lumbar plexus
  2. Radiation myelopathy
  3. Radiation-induced peripheral-nerve tumors

III. *Pain unrelated to cancer or cancer therapy*
- A. Diabetic neuropathy
- B. Cervical- and lumbar-disc disease
- C. Rheumatoid arthritis

gm. Nonnarcotic analgesics may be combined with codeine or other mild narcotics to provide more effective relief. If this combination provides inadequate pain relief, the patient should be switched to a narcotic analgesic. It is best to start potent narcotics by mouth.

The dose of oral morphine required to achieve continuous pain relief may range from 5 to 200 mg every four hours.[31,54,150,151] In this regard, it is important to realize that oral equianalgesic doses of potent narcotics are two to five times that of intramuscular doses (e.g., the ratio is 2 for methadone and 3 to 6 for morphine). A baseline evaluation is carried out by noting the duration of each of the first two or three doses, and then the drug is prescribed at regular intervals of about half an hour shorter than the drug's average duration. This provides even analgesia and avoids the peaks-and-valleys effect that causes the patient to have intervals of pain and discomfort. To determine the optimum dose and frequency of administration, it is necessary to titrate the patient's pain with the drug over a period of days, and to monitor and evaluate carefully the analgesic action of each dose. This responsibility cannot be left to the nurse but must be assumed by the physician or pain therapist. Intramuscular or intravenous doses should be used only in patients who cannot take medication by mouth because of nausea, vomiting, or disturbed GI function.[31,54,150,151]

As previously mentioned, nonnarcotic and narcotic analgesics may be supplemented with corticosteroids, antidepressants, hydroxyzine, and/or phenothiazines, which are used to increase sedation, decrease nausea and vomiting, and possibly potentiate the analgesic action of narcotics.

Regional Analgesia. In patients whose condition or prognosis contraindicates major neurosurgical operations and for whom narcotic therapy is ineffective, therapeutic nerve blocks should be used.[9,11,19,31] Blocks with local anesthetics are used to provide patients with prompt relief of severe excruciating pain for hours or days, and occasionally for longer periods. For example, continuous segmental epidural block of the affected segments can be used for several weeks, and thus relieve patients of cancer pain while they are receiving radiation or other anticancer therapies. In some patients it may be desirable to combine a local anesthetic with a corticosteroid injected into the extradural space. Local anesthetic injection of trigger areas eliminates myofascial pain syndromes that frequently develop in association with cancer pain. Local anesthetic blocks of sympathetic pathways may help relieve the burning pain that is present in certain types of cancer of the head, chest, and abdomen. Moreover, repeated sympathetic blocks are effective in eliminating the symptomatology of reflex sympathetic dystrophy, which occasionally develops in cancer patients.

Epidural or subarachnoid injection of potent narcotics (intraspinal opiates) has been used widely for the treatment of cancer pain with significant success (see Jacobson[71] for review). Neurolytic blocks achieved by injection of alcohol or phenol have the best (and only) application in patients with inoperable cancer pain.[9,137,161] The value of subarachnoid neurolysis or chemical rhizotomy, neurolytic block of the gasserian ganglion or branches of the trigeminal nerve, and chemical hypophysectomy has already been stressed.

Other Therapies. Psychological techniques including relaxation, hypnosis, and even biofeedback have proven valuable adjuncts in patients with cancer pain. The role of various neurosurgical operations has been discussed in a preceding section (see Bonica and Benedetti[31] and Pagni[110] for reviews). Neurostimulation techniques, including transcutaneous nerve stimulation, dorsal column stimulation, and deep brain stimulation, have been used for cancer pain with some success (see Meyerson[101] and Ray, Burton,

and Litson[116] for reviews). These have been discussed in a previous section.

Causalgia and Other Reflex Sympathetic Dystrophies

Reflex sympathetic dystrophy, sometimes called sympathetic algodystrophy, is an all-inclusive term applied to a great variety of seemingly unrelated disorders that, in the past, were described separately under the names of major causalgia, minor causalgia, posttraumatic painful syndrome, posttraumatic spreading neuralgia, posttraumatic painful arthrosis, Sudeck's atrophy, sympathalgia, shoulder-hand syndrome, chronic traumatic edema, posttraumatic edema, and reflex dystrophy (see Bonica[9,18,30] and Livingston[86] for reviews). All of these are characterized by varying degrees of burning, aching pain; vasomotor, sudomotor, and other autonomic disturbances; and delayed recovery of function. If not properly treated, the patient undergoes progressive trophic changes. Moreover, if applied early, sympathetic interruption produces prompt pain relief and disappearance of the pathophysiological process.

ETIOLOGY
Causalgia, the most severe form of this group of disorders, is usually caused by incomplete severance of a major nerve in the upper or lower limb, usually above the elbow or knee, caused by high-velocity missiles.[18,19] Therefore, while it is seen most frequently during wartime, it is a rare complication occasionally seen in medical practice. In contrast, other reflex sympathetic dystrophies are usually due to trauma secondary to accidental injury and consequently are frequently seen in industrial, orthopedic, and traumatologic practices.[9,18] Injuries include fractures, sprains and dislocations, injury to small nerves due to laceration or a minor cut, traumatic amputation of fingers, and crush injuries of the fingers, hand, or wrist. There is no correlation between severity of the in-

jury and the incidence, severity, and cause of the disease. Indeed, most of these cases often follow minor injuries to those regions particularly rich in nerve endings, or there is minor injury to a peripheral nerve without significant neurological signs developing promptly after the injury. A number of reflex sympathetic dystrophies develop as iatrogenic complications of surgical or medical therapy, including amputations of hands and fingers, tight-fitting casts, and damage to peripheral nerves by injection of penicillin, alcohol, or other nerve irritants. Various visceral, neurological, and musculoskeletal disorders may also produce reflex sympathetic dystrophy. Outstanding among these is the shoulder-hand syndrome that not infrequently follows myocardial infarction.

In the early phase of the disorder, pain is produced by peripheral mechanisms; there is damage of the membranes of A delta and C fibers, which promptly develop hypersensitivity to circulating noradrenaline and to pressure and movement. As a consequence, these fibers fire spontaneously and in an abnormal fashion to produce pain. The peripheral pathophysiology has an immediate impact on the function of the CNS, probably by causing disinhibition or facilitation in the dorsal horn and other parts of the neuraxis, and consequently sets up abnormal firing patterns in closed self-exciting neuron loops in the CNS.[31,156] Initially this is reversible, because with effective therapy with a sympathetic block or intravenous guanethidine, the patient is promptly relieved of the pain and all of the clinical features and the pathophysiology disappear.[9,31,86,98] Moreover, a series of blocks is frequently followed by cure of reflex sympathetic dystrophy and often of causalgia, although sympathectomy may be necessary.[9,31,86] The efficacy for the beneficial effects of sympathetic interruption hypothesized by Melzack[95] was mentioned in the section on peripheral-central mechanisms. On the other hand, if causalgia and other sympathetic dystrophies do not improve spontaneously and the pathophysiological process is permitted to persist and

progress, the abnormal function in the CNS becomes self-sustaining and eventually becomes independent of the abnormal peripheral input. In such cases, block therapy or any other procedure intended to remove the peripheral input is no longer effective.

CLINICAL MANIFESTATIONS

Causalgia. Causalgia, first described by Mitchell, Moorehouse, and Kenn[102] during the Civil War, is characterized by excruciating burning pain that usually develops soon after the injury; is located superficially in the distal part of the limb; is intense, diffuse, and continuous, but subject to exacerbations; and tends to lead to profound emotional and behavioral changes. Moreover, the pain is almost always markedly aggravated by such physical factors as passive movements and touching or tapping the limb and by friction of clothing or bedclothes. It is also aggravated by visual and auditory stimuli such as loud noise, bright light, rattling of newspaper, noisy conversation, and so on, and by such emotional disturbances as anger, fear, excitement, and mental distress. Hyperalgesia, hyperesthesia, and/or hyperpathia are almost always present and are very prominent symptoms of causalgia. Vasomotor and sudomotor disturbances are almost always present, but there is variation among patients, with some showing signs of vasoconstriction, coldness, and sweating, while others have vasodilation, absence of sweating, and warmth. With time, the pain usually spreads proximally to the entire extremity and may even spread to other parts of the body or to the contralateral limb. Trophic changes affecting the skin, subcutaneous tissue, bones, and joints develop that eventually become irreversible.

Reflex Sympathetic Dystrophies. The early manifestations of lesser dystrophies are burning or aching pain, hyperalgesia, hyperesthesia, vasomotor and sudomotor disturbances, and skeletal muscle hypotonia.[9,31] Later features are weakness and atrophy, and trophic changes of the skin and its appendages and of the muscles, bones, and joints. The symptoms may be severe (grade 1), moderate (grade 2), or mild (grade 3). *Grade 1* is characterized by clinical features that are similar to classical causalgia. The pain is severe, burning, knifelike, or lancinating; is unrelieved by rest; is subjected to exacerbations by the slightest emotional or physical stimulation; and is associated with severe vasomotor and sudomotor disturbances. *Grade 2* is slower in onset and longer in duration and is characterized by a dull, throbbing, aching, diffuse pain, and by mild vasomotor and sudomotor disturbances. *Grade 3* is the mildest and perhaps the most common form, representing the border zone between the normal response of an extremity to trauma and the more severe disorders previously described. Because of the mildness of symptoms and paucity of physical signs, many patients in this category never receive the benefit of correct diagnosis and appropriate therapy.

The course of reflex sympathetic dystrophy also varies depending on the severity of the disorder and when proper treatment is instituted. Without treatment, the condition usually passes through three stages: the *first stage* is characterized by pain, hyperesthesia, hyperalgesia, localized edema, muscle spasm, and tenderness of the affected part of the limb. All of these are conducive to limitation of motion. During the early part of this stage the pain is usually localized in the distribution of one of the principal nerves and the skin is usually warm, dry, and red. Toward the end of this stage the pain spreads and the skin becomes cyanotic, cold, and moist. During this stage there are usually no radiographic changes of bones, but trophic changes of the hair, nails, and skin begin to appear. In patients with grade 3 and sometimes grade 2, the first stage lasts several weeks and then subsides spontaneously or responds rapidly to treatment. In severe cases that remain untreated, the symptoms become progressively worse.

The *second stage,* which develops in about three to six months in most untreated patients, is characterized by a gradual decrease of pain, spread of edema, increased thickness of the joint, and muscle wasting. The edema changes from a soft to a brawny type, with glazed overlying skin. The hair becomes scant and the nails become brittle, cracked, and heavily grooved. Early in the second stage, radiograms show spotty osteoporosis, but later these bony changes spread and eventually become indistinguishable from severe diffuse osteoporosis.

The *third stage* is characterized by marked trophic changes that eventually become irreversible. The hair becomes coarse; the skin becomes smooth, glossy, drawn, and pale or cyanotic; and skin temperature decreases. The nails become increasingly brittle and rigid with lateral arching. Subcutaneous tissue is very atrophied with marked decrease in fat pads, and the digits are thin and pointed. Atrophy of the muscles, particularly the interossei, is marked. The interphalangeal and other joints of the foot or hand are extremely weak, have limited motion, and finally become ankylosed. Contraction of the flexor tendons often occurs at this stage, and occasionally subluxations are produced. Bone atrophy becomes diffuse and marked.

TREATMENT

The patient should receive specific and aggressive treatment that consists initially of a series of sympathetic blocks or intravenous regional sympathetic blocks with guanethidine, and later sympathectomy if the blocks produce only transient relief of pain. Patients presenting with stage 2 or stage 3 of the disease should also have physical therapy, exercise and, if appropriate, psychotherapy. While some patients with mild posttraumatic reflex sympathetic dystrophy recover spontaneously or with the aid of very conservative measures, unfortunately many do not.

During the early stages of reflex sympathetic dystrophy, sympathetic blocks constitute the primary and most effective treatment of these disorders (see Bonica[9] and Bonica and Benedetti[31] for reviews). Provided it is properly executed, sympathetic block invariably provides prompt and dramatic response, with immediate relief of pain, increased warmth, disappearance of cyanosis, decrease in swelling over the next several hours, and improved function. The duration of the response varies from a few hours to several days. In some patients treated with sympathetic block promptly after the onset of the disorder, the pain is permanently relieved with the first or second block. With subsequent injections the relief of pain, hyperesthesia, and other symptomatology become progressively longer lasting than the duration of the drug action.

In patients in whom a series of sympathetic blocks produces complete but only temporary relief, sympathectomy should be considered. Whether this should be achieved chemically or surgically depends on the particular patient's physical condition, the severity of the disease, and the patient's attitude toward both techniques. Chemical sympathectomy with 6 percent aqueous phenol or 50 percent alcohol produces sympathetic interruption for several weeks to several months and is especially useful in older or poor-risk patients. In patients who are younger and in good physical condition, surgical sympathectomy is preferable.

Carron and McCue[37] reported that transcutaneous nerve stimulation is also a highly effective therapy for reflex sympathetic dystrophy. They claim that TNS, like sympathetic block, produces a cure in over 90 percent of the patients treated. Kaada[76] has reported that TNS can effect vasodilation and promote healing of chronic ulceration, suggesting the procedure causes sympathetic inhibition, thus increasing circulation in the extremity. Sympathetic inhibition may be the basis for the efficacy of TNS in reflex sympathetic dystrophy. If these results are confirmed, this method may replace blocks because it is simpler to apply and less stressful to the patient. However, more extensive clinical experience is needed before the efficacy of this method can be established.

In advanced cases of reflex sympathetic dystrophy, the sympathetic interruption (or TNS) should be supplemented with physical therapy, exercise, and psychotherapy. Without these adjuvants, optimal results are precluded. When organic changes, such as shortening of tendons, are present in advanced cases, orthopedic care is necessary for recovery of function after sympathectomy. In any case, it is important to consider and muster all possible therapeutic agents and neglect no useful adjuvant in treatment.

Pain After Amputation

When a limb or other body part (ear, nose, breast, or penis) is surgically amputated or denervated by trauma, 80 to 90 percent of patients report feeling a phantom sensation in the whole or part of the limb.[9,11,51] In some one-half of these cases, the phantom part is felt within the first twenty-four hours; in about one-quarter it appears between twenty-four and forty-eight hours; while in the remainder of patients, the phantom limb is felt within the first week or so.[73] One study showed that phantom sensation occurred in 86 percent of patients who had the right upper extremity amputated and in 75 percent of those who had lost the left upper limb.[125] In contrast, there was no laterality difference after lower limb amputation. In many patients this is not a distant or shadowy sensation but rather a startling, vivid perception of the limb as having a tingling feeling and a definite shape that resembles the real limb before amputation. In other cases the phantom becomes distorted and is felt to be shorter or longer and to be changed in volume.[73] Amputees also report a variety of other sensations such as pins and needles, warmth and coldness, and paresthesia. Many patients with phantom limb sense uncontrollable movements in the amputated part, irrespective of the site of amputation. For some this is uncomfortable or frankly painful.[125] In many patients the phantom fades with time, telescoping gradually until it has disappeared as if by contraction into the stump, although it may remain throughout the patient's life (see Bonica,[9] Jensen and Rasmussen,[72] and

Sherman, Sherman, and Parker[124] for reviews).

PHANTOM PAIN

Following amputation, a variable percentage of patients develop pain in the phantom limb or the stump, or both. The incidence of pain in the phantom has been reported to vary from zero to 100 percent,[9,72,134] but several recent detailed studies with follow-up[73,125] revealed that pain was experienced by 60 to 80 percent of the patients soon after surgery and by 40 to 67 percent of the patients six to twelve months after the amputation. The quality of the pain is variable and may be felt as knifelike, shooting, pricking, squeezing, throbbing, cramplike, or burning. In the experience of the senior author, two predominant types usually occur: a burning, throbbing pain, not unlike that of causalgia and other reflex sympathetic dystrophies, which the patient describes as if the hand or foot were held too close to a fire; and an extremely abnormal position of the phantom limb that is very uncomfortable. The sensations of abnormal posture and tension may vary from mild annoyance, which the patient often disregards, to almost unbearable discomfort, which interferes with rest, sleep, work, and play. The hand or foot may be felt in a painfully twisted, cramped, rigid, or flexed posture from which the patient is unable to release it. Some patients feel as if the nails of the fingers or toes have been pulled off or lifted from their nailbeds.

The location of the pain may vary, but in most instances is felt most intensely in the foot or hand, particularly in the instep, heel, or toes, or in the fingertips, knuckles, palms, or wrists. Fatigue, sleeplessness, persistent worry, and even the apprehension of knowing the stump is going to be examined may cause the pain to be worse. Exposure of the stump to cold very frequently aggravates the symptoms, and a considerable number of patients complain that changes in weather affect their condition. Pain may also be aggravated by cooling or warming the stump,

or even allowing it to hang. Some patients report that yawning, micturition, defecation, pressure on certain parts of the body, or visceral disease (e.g., renal colic) will temporarily exacerbate the pain. Trigger zones develop in many parts of the body, and when pressed upon will aggravate the pain in the phantom limb.

The long-term aspects of phantom limb pain have been studied by Sherman, Sherman, and Parker,[124] who sent questionnaires to 5,000 persons whose amputations were connected with military service. Fifty-five percent responded; 78 percent indicated they had experienced phantom limb pain. The average time since amputation was about twenty-six years for those who had phantom pain and thirty years for those not reporting pain. About half reported that the pain had decreased somewhat with time, while the others reported no change or an increase. The major factor causing exacerbation of the pain was weather change. These patients listed forty different treatments, but only a small percent indicated lasting benefits from therapy.

PAIN IN THE STUMP

Pain in the stump may also be present following amputation. Two predominant types are described: a constant, diffuse, burning, throbbing pain similar to that of reflex sympathetic dystrophies; and paroxysms of lancinating, shooting discomfort that has a segmental or peripheral nerve distribution. Some patients experience both types. Vasomotor and sudomotor disturbances are frequently manifested by coldness, cyanosis, edema, signs of vasoconstriction, and excessive sweating. The temperature of the skin of the stump may be as much as 10° C cooler than the opposite limb. The edema may be diffuse or localized, and the sweating may be profuse, so the stump is constantly clammy. In many painful stumps, with or without phantoms, the skin covering the end of the stump exhibits an abnormal sensibility. Usually both hyperesthesia and hyperpathia are present. If no previous neuromata have been resected and there is no evidence of additional nerve damage at higher levels, the hyperpathia is usually restricted to the scars and the most distal parts of the skin flaps. Typical delay overshooting and afterreaction can usually be demonstrated, and the sensations experienced may irradiate both into the phantom and the proximal end of the stump. The neuromata are very sensitive to pressure and, when squeezed, produce lancinating pain. Numerous trigger zones develop along the scar and elsewhere in the stump and at other body sites.

Wall and his associates[98,156,157] studied the pathophysiology and pharmacology of neuromata in an experimental rat model produced by cutting the rat's sciatic nerve and allowing the cut end to regenerate in a sealed polyethylene tube. Tiny electrodes were placed in the neuroma, the nerve, and the dorsal root to monitor the electrical activity of the neuroma. They found that the neuroma contained fine sprouts originating in small-diameter myelinated and unmyelinated fibers, but large fibers failed to penetrate the neuroma. They also found that normally silent fibers generated an ongoing barrage in the absence of stimulation. They noted that partially damaged nerve membranes and the sprouts of neuroma became extremely sensitive to norepinephrine applied locally or passing in the blood. This was stopped by the alpha-blocker phentolamine, but was unaffected by isoprenaline and other beta-agonists. The study also demonstrated that the firing of damaged or regenerating afferent nerve fibers was also influenced by temperature, local blood flow, chemical environment, previous stimuli, and high-frequency antidromic impulses, which, if allowed to penetrate the neuroma, silenced the nerve terminals, the effect lasting for a significant time. These findings explain the efficacy of sympathetic interruption and electrical counterstimulation in producing prolonged relief in many patients with peripheral nerve injuries or amputation stump pain.

THERAPY

Over the decades numerous therapies have been advocated and used to treat postamputation pain. The data by Sherman, Sherman, and Parker[124] suggest that only a small percent of patients with prolonged phantom limb pain derive benefit from various therapies. Nevertheless, the following have been reported to produce temporary and sometimes permanent relief of pain. Infiltration of trigger zones or nerves in the stump has been reported by Livingston[86] to stop pain for days, weeks, and sometimes permanently, even though the anesthesia wears off within hours. Successive blocks may produce increasingly longer periods of relief. It also is important to inject trigger areas in other parts of the body as part of the therapy.[9]

Sympathetic Blockade. In the experience of Livingston[86] and the senior author, patients who complain of burning, aching pain associated with vasomotor and sudomotor changes in the stump derive significant benefit from sympathetic interruption. This can be achieved by regional sympathetic block, by intravenous infusion of guanethidine during occlusion of the circulation (Bier block). Promptly after the onset of block, the patient feels partial or complete pain relief, warming of the extremity, and at times the cramped or twisted extremity seems to relax and assume a normal position. If the block affords complete or good relief of pain, it should be repeated on several occasions to confirm the results and also to ascertain the duration of pain relief. If relief is of progressively longer duration and significantly outlasts the duration of the block, surgical sympathectomy should be seriously considered. If the patient is in poor physical condition, chemical sympathectomy should be done.

COMMENTS

Several comments regarding the use of sympathetic interruption for postamputation pain as well as causalgia and other reflex sympathetic dystrophy should be made. First, the earlier the treatment, the better the prognosis for cure of the pain. Second, if the patient experiences relief, even if it is only partial, the sympathetic interruption should be repeated; sometimes when the first two or three blocks produce partial or no relief, subsequent blocks will relieve the pain. Finally, it is essential to ascertain that sympathetic interruption to the limb is complete. Bonica[9,31] has encountered a number of patients who had undergone surgical sympathectomy with only partial or no relief of burning pain in the phantom limb but who subsequently derived complete relief of pain with a local anesthetic sympathetic block. The reason for the discrepancy is that, while the local anesthetic solution diffused widely to involve the sympathetic chain and the anomalous sympathetic fibers (which often are present in lower cervical and upper thoracic chain and in the lumbar chain), the operation was not extensive enough and/or it did not include the anomalous pathways. In such patients a postsympathectomy block relieved the pain. Finally, the sympathetic interruption should be combined with local infiltration of trigger zones.

Procedures That Increase Sensory Input. These procedures include injection of a small amount of hypertonic saline into the interspinous tissue of amputees, which initially produces a sharp localized pain that radiates into the phantom limb, lasting about ten minutes; subsequently the patient experiences dramatic partial or total relief of pain for hours, weeks, and sometimes indefinitely. Vigorous vibration of the stump may also produce relief of phantom limb pain. The most recent of these techniques, inspired by the Melzack-Wall theory of pain, involves electrical stimulation applied to the stump, a procedure that has been reported to be effective in controlling pain in the phantom limb and the stump.[79] Similarly, electrical stimulation of the dorsal column of the spinal cord has been reported to be effective in relieving pain.[79,98]

Operant Mechanisms

It has been traditional in medicine to consider pain as a symptom of a disease state. If there is a stimulus such as a disease or injury, then there will be a response. Conversely, if there is pain—a response—there must be a stimulus—a disease or unhealed injury. Medical diagnosis is directed at finding that stimulus. Unfortunately, this model works poorly in some patients with chronic pain, and other explanations for why people who otherwise appear psychiatrically normal complain of pain must be considered.

Fordyce[57] and other behavioral psychologists[141] have pointed out that pain can be usefully construed as a pattern of behavior rather than as a response to a pathogenic stimulus. As Skinner[128] has emphasized, ongoing behavior is changed and controlled by the selective administration of rewards. Similarly, pain behavior may be maintained and supported by reinforcement from the patient's social environment. Elements of a typical chronic pain behavior pattern include grimacing, groaning, bracing or rubbing, requesting and ingesting medications, physician visits, bed rest, sitting or reclining time, and withdrawal from recreational or vocational activities. As chronicity progresses, complex patterns of such behaviors can emerge and produce elaborate suffering, recruiting of support from others, and medical help-seeking. These long-term behaviors may be related to the presence of organic disease only weakly, or not at all.

Our colleague Fordyce,[58] the primary developer of the behaviorist position in pain psychotherapy, has advocated and demonstrated the importance of identifying the unique operant factors that maintain chronic pain in the individual patient. In addition, he has pioneered the application of operant conditioning for pain therapy. For Fordyce, pain may be either respondent (under the control of a nociceptive stimulus) or operant (under the control of the patient's environment and the rewards for expressing pain in that environment). Operant factors are those elements in the social surroundings of the patient that yield gratifying responses when the patient expresses pain, displays pain or invalid behavior, or visits health care providers.

Within the Fordyce[57,58] framework, the developmental course of chronic pain is seen as a learning process. Pain states initiated by disease or injury may be exacerbated or prolonged by selective reinforcement of suffering behaviors. That is, if a patient carries out an action associated with pain, such as postural change or grimace, that action is more likely to occur if it has been followed by attention and sympathy than if it has been ignored. Over many months, repeated reinforcement of pain behavior may lead to well-entrenched habits of pain expression.

The patient who suffers chronically in the presence of an attentive and nurturing family may have serious stumbling blocks to recovery. In some cases, where life before injury or disease was unsatisfactory or lonely, sickness accompanied by pain may bring a patient new success at manipulating family members, friends, and employers, at obtaining attention and nurturance from others, and at getting time out from behaviors the patient would rather not engage in, such as work or sex. Moreover, the sick role brings some patients a well-defined and organized life-style that they have lacked in the past. The benefits associated with pain complaints and the sick role are known as secondary gains.

The behavioral model of chronic pain is not appropriate for all chronic pain patients. Indeed, in many, and perhaps the majority, of the pain patients seen in a private practice setting, operant mechanisms cannot be identified. For particularly difficult cases, however, the operant approach is highly effective in both the diagnosis and treatment of the patient. Inappropriate pain behavior can be corrected by identification and strategic control of reinforcers in a controlled hospital setting and in the patient's family and work environment. Operant therapies for chronic pain have proven valuable for pain patient rehabilitation programs.

TREATMENT

The details of the treatment methods employed in behavior modification are beyond the scope of this chapter. The following list provides Fordyce's basic principles of behavior modification for the rehabilitation of chronic pain patients.[58]

1. The principal target of treatment is to alter pain behaviors, because the evidence from evaluations of patients deemed appropriate for such an approach indicates that those pain behaviors are controlled by factors other than nociception.

2. Activity level and constraints on body movement are attacked by arranging that rest from activity becomes work-contingent, with incrementing quotas of work or exercise the method for expanding that activity level.

3. Where it is a problem, pain related to medication consumption is reduced by shifting from as needed to time-contingent medication regimens and systematically reducing active ingredients in the medications taken.

4. Social/interpersonal responses to pain behaviors by those around the patient are altered by systematic training of professional staff and family members in such a way that solicitous attention is withdrawn as a consequence to pain behaviors and interpersonal responsiveness becomes relatively work- or activity-contingent.

5. Systematic efforts are directed toward remediating whatever performance or behavioral problems appear to have been limiting the patient's ability to cope with being well and with the situational demands imposed by his or her circumstances.

6. Systematic efforts are directed toward promoting reengagement in work, if indicated, or social/leisure activities anticipated following treatment, which will serve to help sustain activity gains achieved in treatment.

Large-scale behavior modification programs for chronic pain, like the one established by Fordyce at the University of Washington, require that the patient be hospitalized in a controlled ward environment with behaviorally trained staff. Nevertheless, the principles on which this therapy is built can be usefully applied in the diagnosis and management of chronic pain patients in other settings. An awareness of operant mechanisms in chronic pain may help prevent the physician in private practice from undertaking surgical intervention, prescribing medication, or otherwise pursuing a potentially dangerous organic remedy for a problem that may be inherently behavioral.

¶ Bibliography

1. ANDERSON, L. S., et al. "Neuronal Hyperactivity in Experimental Trigeminal Deafferentation," *Journal of Neurosurgery,* 35 (1971):444–452.
2. ANDERSON, T. P., et al. "Behavior Modification of Chronic Pain: A Treatment Program by a Multidisciplinary Team," *Journal of Clinical Orthopaedics,* 129 (1977):96–100.
3. BALL, J. C., and Chambers, C. D. *The Epidemiology of Opiate Addiction in the United States.* Springfield, Ill.: Charles C Thomas, 1970.
4. BENEDETTI, C., and BONICA, J. J. "Postoperative Pain," in C. Benedetti, C. R. Chapman, and G. Moricca, eds., *Recent Advances in the Management of Pain— Advances in Pain Research and Therapy,* vol. 7. New York: Raven Press, 1984, pp. 373–406.
5. BESSMAN, F. P., and RENNER, V. J. "The Biphasic Hormonal Nature of Stress," in R. A. Cowley and B. F. Trump, eds., *Pathophysiology of Shock, Anoxia and Ischemia.* Baltimore: Williams & Wilkins, 1982, pp. 60–65.
6. BLACK, R. G. "The Chronic Pain Syndromes," *Surgical Clinics of North America,* 55 (1975):999–1011.
7. BOND, M. R. "Psychologic and Emotional Aspects of Cancer Pain," in J. J. Bonica and V. Ventafridda, eds., *Advances in Pain Research and Therapy,* vol. 2. New York: Raven Press, 1979, pp. 81–88.
8. ——. "The Suffering of Severe Intractable Pain," in H. W. Kosterlitz and L. Y. Terenius, eds., *Pain and Society.* Weinheim: Verlag Chemie, 1980, pp. 53–62.
9. BONICA, J. J. *The Management of Pain.* Philadelphia: Lea & Febiger, 1953.
10. ——. "Management of Myofascial Pain Syndromes in General Practice," *Journal of the American Medical Association,* 165 (1957):732–738.
11. ——. *Clinical Applications of Diagnostic and Therapeutic Nerve Blocks.* Springfield, Ill.: Charles C Thomas, 1959.
12. ——. *Principles and Practice of Obstetric Analgesia and Anesthesia,* vol. 1. Philadelphia: F. A. Davis Co., 1967.
13. ——. "New Progress Against Pain," *US News & World Report,* 77 (Dec. 30, 1974):46.
14. ——. "Organization and Function of a Pain Clinic," in J. J. Bonica, ed., *Advances in Neurology,* vol. 4. New York: Raven Press, 1974, pp. 433–443.
15. ——. Preface, in J. J. Bonica, ed., *Advances in Neurology,* vol. 4. New York: Raven Press, 1974, pp. vii–xi.
16. ——. Preface, in J. J. Bonica and D. G. Albe-Fessard, eds., *Advances in Pain Research and Therapy,* vol. 2. New York: Raven Press, 1976, pp. *xxvii–xxxix.*
17. ——. "Neurophysiologic and Pathologic Aspects of Acute and Chronic Pain," *Archives of Surgery,* 112 (1977):750–761.
18. ——. "Causalgia and Other Reflex Sympathetic Dystrophies," in J. J. Bonica, J. C. Liebeskind, and D. G. Albe-Fessard, eds., *Advances in Pain Research and Therapy,* vol. 3. New York: Raven Press, 1979, pp. 141–166.
19. ——. "Introduction to Nerve Blocks," in J. J. Bonica and V. Ventafridda, eds., *Advances in Pain Research and Therapy,* vol. 2. New York: Raven Press, 1979, pp. 303–310.
20. ——. *Blocks of the Sympathetic Nervous System,* vol. 1. Chicago: Frank J. Corbett, Inc., 1980.
21. ——. *Obstetric Analgesia and Anesthesia,* 2nd ed. Amsterdam: World Federation of Societies of Anesthesiologists, 1980.
22. ——. "Pain Research and Therapy: Past and Current Status and Future Needs," in J. J. Bonica and L.K.Y. Ng, eds., *Pain, Discomfort and Humanitarian Care.*

Amsterdam: Elsevier/North Holland, 1980, pp. 1–46.

23. ———. Editorial on Pain, *Triangle*, 20 (1981):1–6.

24. ———. "Management of Pain with Conduction Analgesia," *Bulletin Voor Regional Anesthesia*, 3 (1983):42–53.

25. ———. Presidential Address, in J. J. Bonica, U. Lindblom, and A. Iggo, eds., *Advances in Pain Research and Therapy*, Vol. 5. New York: Raven Press, 1983, pp. 1–36.

26. ———. "Biology, Pathophysiology and Treatment of Acute Pain," in S. Lipton and J. Miles, eds., *Persistent Pain*, vol. 5. London: Academic Press, forthcoming.

27. ———. "Importance of the Problem," in V. Ventafridda and K. Foley, eds., *Cancer Pain*. Hingham, Mass: MTP Publishers, forthcoming.

28. ———. "Labour Pain," in P. D. Wall and R. Melzack, eds., *Textbook of Pain*. London: Churchill Livingstone, 1984.

29. ———. "Local Anaesthesia and Regional Blocks," in P. D. Wall and R. Melzack, eds. *Textbook of Pain*, London: Churchill Livingstone, 1984, pp. 547–557.

30. BONICA, J. J., ed. *Advances in Neurology*, vol. 4. New York: Raven Press, 1974.

31. BONICA, J. J., and BENEDETTI, C. "Management of Cancer Pain," in A. R. Moossa, M. C. Robson, and S. C. Schimpff, eds., *Comprehensive Textbook of Oncology*. Baltimore: Williams & Wilkins, forthcoming.

32. BONICA, J. J., and MADRID, J. L. "Cancer Pain in the Head and Neck: Role of Nerve Blocks," in J. J. Bonica and V. Ventafridda, eds., *Advances in Pain Research and Therapy*, vol. 2. New York: Raven Press, 1979, pp. 537–542.

33. BONICA, J. J., and VENTAFRIDDA, V., eds. *Advances in Pain Research and Therapy*, vol. 2. New York: Raven Press, 1978.

34. BONICA, J. J., BENEDETTI, C., and MURPHY, T. M. "Functions of Pain Clinics and Pain Centers," in M. Swerdlow, ed., *Relief of Intractable Pain*. New York: Elsevier Science Publishers, 1983, pp. 65–84.

35. BRENA, S. F., et al. "Chronic Back Pain: Electromyographic, Motion and Behavioral Assessments Following Sympa-thetic Nerve Blocks and Placebos," *Pain*, 8 (1980):1–10.

36. BROGGI, G., and SIEGFRIED, J. "Percutaneous Differential Radio Frequency Rhizotomy of Glossopharyngeal Nerve in Facial Pain Due to Cancer," in J. J. Bonica and V. Ventafridda, eds., *Advances in Pain Research and Therapy*, vol. 2. New York: Raven Press, 1979, pp. 469–474.

37. CARRON, H., and McCUE, F. "Reflex Sympathetic Dystrophy in a Ten-year-old," *Southern Medical Journal*, 65 (1977): 631–632.

38. CARRON, H., and McLAUGHLIN, R. E., eds., *Management of Low Back Pain*. Bristol, England: John Wright and Sons, 1982.

39. CHAPMAN, C. R. "Pain Measurement and the Assessment of Acupuncture Therapy: Past Problems and New Directions," unpublished.

40. ———. "Psychological Factors in Postoperative Pain and Their Treatment," in B. Covino and G. Smith, eds., *Acute Pain*, vol. 1. London: Butterworths International Medical Review, forthcoming.

41. CHAPMAN, C. R., and BONICA, J. J. *Current Concepts of Acute Pain*. Kalamazoo, Mich.: The Upjohn Company, 1983.

42. CHAPMAN, C. R., SOLA, A., and BONICA, J. J. "Illness Behavior and Depression Compared in Pain Center and Private Practice Patients," *Pain*, 6 (1979):6–7.

43. CHIEN, S. "Role of the Sympathetic Nervous System in Shock," *Physiological Reviews*, 47 (1970):214–288.

44. COHEN, F. L. "Postsurgical Pain Relief: Patient's Status and Nurse's Medication Choices," *Pain*, 9 (1980):265–274.

45. COOMBS, D. W., et al. "Continuous Intraspinal Narcotic Analgesia. Technical Aspects of an Implantable Infusion System," *Regional Anesthesia*, 7 (1982):110–113.

46. CRUE, B. L., et al. "What Is a Pain Center?" in B. Crue, ed., *Chronic Pain*. New York: Spectrum Publications, 1978, pp. 3–12.

47. CYRIAX, J. *Textbook of Orthopaedic Medicine*, vol. 1. London: Bailliere Tindall, 1978.

48. DREYFUSS, F. "Coagulation Time of the

Blood, Level of Blood Uesinophyles and Thrombocytes Under Emotional Stress," *Journal of Psychosomatic Research,* 1 (1956):252–257.

49. ERIKSSON, M.B.E., SJOLUND, B. H., and NIELZEN, S. "Long-term Results of Peripheral Conditioning Stimulation as an Analgesic Measure in Chronic Pain," *Pain,* 6 (1979):335–347.

50. FAHRNI, W. H. "Conservative Treatment of Lumbar Disc Degeneration: Our Primary Responsibility," *Orthopedic Clinics of North America,* 6 (1975):93–103.

51. FEINSTEIN, B., LUCE, J. C., and LANGTON, J.N.K. "The Influence of Phantom Limbs," in P. Klopsteg and P. Wilson, eds., *Human Limbs and Their Substitutes.* New York: McGraw-Hill, 1954, pp. 79–138.

52. FIELDS, H. L. "Brainstem Mechanism of Pain Modulation," in L. Kruger and J. C. Liebeskind, eds., *Neural Mechanisms of Pain, Advances in Pain Research and Therapy,* vol. 6. New York: Raven Press, 1984, pp. 241–252.

53. FIELDS, H. L., and BASBAUM, A. I. "Brainstem Control of Spinal Pain-Transmission Neurons," *Annual Review of Physiology,* 40 (1978):217–248.

54. FOLEY, K. M. "The Management of Pain in Malignant Origin," in H. R. Taylor and D. M. Dawson, eds., *Current Neurology,* vol. 2. Boston: Houghton Mifflin, 1979, pp. 279–302.

55. FOLEY, K. M., and ROGERS, A. *Management of Cancer Pain,* vol. 2, *The Rational Use of Analgesics in the Management of Cancer Pain.* Nutley, N.J.: Hoffman-LaRoche, 1981.

56. FOLTZ, E. L., and WHITE, L. E. "Rostral Cingulotomy and Pain 'Relief,'" in R. S. Knighton and P. R. Dumke, eds., *Pain.* Boston: Little, Brown, 1966, pp. 469–491.

57. FORDYCE, W. E. *Behavioral Methods for Chronic Pain and Illness.* St. Louis: C. V. Mosby, 1976.

58. ———. "A Behavioral Perspective on Chronic Pain," in L.K.Y. Ng and J. J. Bonica, eds., *Pain, Discomfort and Humanitarian Care.* New York: Elsevier/North Holland, 1980, pp. 233–252.

59. FREEMAN, W., and WATTS, J. W. *Psycho-*

surgery in the Treatment of Mental Disorders and Intractable Pain. Springfield, Ill.: Charles C Thomas, 1950.

60. GAGE, I. M., and GILLESPIE, G. "Acute Pancreatitis Treatment," *Southern Medical Journal,* 44 (1951):769–776.

61. GIANASI, G. "Neuroadenolysis of the Pituitary (NALP)," in C. Benedetti, C. R. Chapman, and G. Moricca, eds., *Recent Advances in the Management of Pain—Advances in Pain Research and Therapy,* vol. 7. New York: Raven Press, 1984, pp. 647–678.

62. GILBERT, P. W., KIM, J. H., and POSNER, J. B. "Epidural Spinal Cord Compression from Metastatic Tumor: Diagnosis and Treatment," *Annals of Neurology,* 3 (1978):40–51.

63. HALPERN, L. M. "Substitution Detoxification and Its Role in the Management of Chronic Benign Pain," *Journal of Clinical Psychiatry,* 43 (1982):10–14.

64. HALPERN, L. M., and BONICA, J. J. "Analgesics," in W. Modell, ed., *Drugs of Choice.* St. Louis: C. V. Mosby, 1983.

65. HENDLER, N. Cited by Neff in "Pain Clinics: A Growth Industry," *Medical World News,* 17 (1976):54–56.

66. HILGARD, E. R., and HILGARD, J. *Hypnosis in the Relief of Pain.* Los Altos, Calif.: William Kaufman, 1975.

67. HOLMES, T. H., and RAHE, R. H. "The Social Readjustment Scale," *Journal of Psychosomatic Research,* 11 (1967):213–218.

68. HOWE, J. F., LOESER, J. D., and CALVIN, W. H. "Mechanosensitivity of Dorsal Root Ganglia and Chronically Injured Axons: A Physiological Basis for the Radicular Pain of Nerve Root Compression," *Pain,* 3 (1977):25–41.

69. HUME, D. M. "The Endocrine and Metabolic Response to Injury," in S. E. Schwartz, ed., *Principles of Surgery.* New York: McGraw-Hill, 1969.

70. HUPERT, C. "Treatment of Postoperative Pain—Analgesic Potentiation," *Hospital Practice* (Special Report), 13 (1978):27–31.

71. JACOBSON, L. "Intrathecal and Extradural Narcotics," in C. Benedetti, C. R. Chapman, and G. Moricca, eds., *Recent Ad-*

vances in the Management of Pain—
Advances in Pain Research and Therapy, vol. 7. New York: Raven Press,
1984, pp. 199–236.

72. JENSEN, T. S., and RASMUSSEN, P. "Amputation," in P. D. Wall and R. Melzack,
eds., *Textbook of Pain.* Edinburgh:
Churchill Livingston, 1984, pp.

73. JENSEN, T. S., et al. "Phantom Limb,
Phantom Pain and Stomach Pain in Amputees During the First Six Months Following Limb Amputation," *Pain,* 17
(1983):243–256.

74. JESSUP, B. A., NEWFIELD, R.W.J., and
MERSKEY, H. "Biofeedback Therapy for
Headache and Other Pain: An Evalua-
tive Review," *Pain,* 7 (1979):225–270.

75. JEWITT, D. E., MERCER, C. J., and SHIL-
LINGFORD, J. P. "Practolol in the Treatment of Cardiac Arrhythmias Due to
Acute Myocardial Infarction," *Lancet,* 2
(1969):227–230.

76. KAADA, B. "Promoted Healing of Chronic
Ulceration by Transcutaneous Nerve
Stimulation (TNS)," *Vasa,* 12 (1983):262–
269.

77. KANNER, R. M., and FOLEY, K. M. "Pat-
terns of Narcotic Drug Use in a Cancer
Pain Clinic," *Annals of the New York
Academy of Science,* 362 (1981):161–172.

78. KEHLET, H. "Modifying Effect of General
and Regional Anesthesia on the Endocrine Metabolic Response to Surgery,"
Acta Anaesthesiologica Scandinavica,
70 (1982):39–42.

79. KRAINICK, J. U., THODEN, U., and REI-
CHERT, T. "Pain Reduction in Amputees by Long-term Spinal Cord Stimulation," *Journal of Neurosurgery,* 52
(1980):346–350.

80. LAW, J., SWETT, J., and KIRSCH, W. M.
"Retrospective Analysis of 22 Patients
with Chronic Pain Treated by Peripheral Nerve Stimulation," *Journal of
Neurosurgery,* 52 (1980):482–485.

81. LEFER, A. M. "Role of Myocardial Depressant Factor in Pathogenesis of Circulatory Shock," *Federal Proceedings,* 29
(1970):1836–1847.

82. LEWIS, J. W., et al. "Neural, Neurochemical, and Hormonal Bases of Stress-
induced Analgesia," in L. Kruger and J.
C. Liebeskind, eds., *Neural Mechanisms*

of Pain—Advances in Pain Research
and Therapy, vol. 6. New York: Raven
Press, 1984, pp. 277–288.

83. LIEBESKIND, J. C., MAYER, D. J., and AKIL,
H. "Central Mechanisms of Pain Inhibi-
tion: Studies of Analgesia from Focal
Brain Stimulation," in J. J. Bonica, ed.,
Advances in Neurology. New York:
Raven Press, 1974, pp. 261–268.

84. LIPTON, S. "Current Views on the Management of a Pain Relief Center," in M.
Swerdlow, ed., *The Therapy of Pain,*
vol. 6. Philadelphia: J. B. Lippincott, p.
61.

85. LIPTON, S., and MILES, J., eds. *Persistent
Pain: Modern Methods of Treatment,*
vol. 3. New York: Grune & Stratton,
1981.

86. LIVINGSTON, W. K. *Pain Mechanisms.*
New York: Macmillan, 1943.

87. LOESER, J. D. "Low Back Pain," in J. J.
Bonica, ed., *Pain,* vol. 58. New York:
Raven Press, 1980, pp. 363–377.

88. LOESER, J. D., and WARD, A. A., Jr. "Some
Effects of Deafferentation on Neurons
of the Cat Spinal Cord," *Archives of
Neurology,* 17 (1967):629–636.

89. LOESER, J. D., WARD, A. A., Jr., and
WHITE, L. E. "Chronic Deafferentation
of Human Spinal Cord Neurons," *Journal of Neurosurgery,* 29 (1968):48–50.

90. LOMBARD, M. C., NASHOLD, B. S., Jr., and
PELISSIER, T. "Thalamic Recordings in
Rats with Hyperalgesia," in J. J. Bonica,
J. C. Liebeskind, and D. G. Albe-Fes-
sard, eds., *Advances in Pain Research
and Therapy,* vol. 3. New York: Raven
Press, 1979, pp. 767–772.

91. MALSEED, R. T., and GOLDSTEIN, F. J.
"Enhancement of Morphine Analgesia
by Tricyclic Antidepressants," *Neuropharmacology,* 18 (1979):827–829.

92. MANNHEIMER, C., and CARLSSON, C. A.
"The Analgesic Effect of Transcutane-
ous Electrical Nerve Stimulation (TNS)
in Patients with Rheumatoid Arthritis.
A Comparative Study of Different Pulse
Patterns," *Pain,* 6 (1979):329–334.

93. MARKS, R. M., and SACHAR, E. J. "Under-
treatment of Medical Inpatients with
Narcotic Analgesics," *Annals of Internal Medicine,* 78 (1973):173–181.

94. MATHER, L., and MACKIE, J. "The Inci-

dence of Postoperative Pain in Children," *Pain,* 15 (1983):271–282.

95. MELZACK, R. "Phantom Limb Pain: Implications for Treatment of Pathological Pain," *Anesthesiology,* 35 (1971):409–419.

96. MELZACK, R., and LOESER, J. D. "Phantom Body Pain in Paraplegics: Evidence for a Central 'Pattern Generating Mechanism' for Pain," *Pain,* 4 (1978): 195–210.

97. MELZACK, R., and WALL, P. D. "Pain Mechanisms: A New Theory," *Science,* 150 (1965):971–979.

98. ———. *The Challenge of Pain.* New York: Basic Books, 1982.

99. MERSKEY, H., and SPEAR, F. G. *Pain: Psychological and Psychiatric Aspects.* London: Balliere, Tindall, and Cassell, 1967.

100. MEYER, D. J., and WATKINS, L. R. "Multiple Endogenous Opiate and Nonopiate Analgesia Systems," in L. Kruger and J. C. Liebeskind, eds., *Neural Mechanisms of Pain—Advances in Pain Research and Therapy,* vol. 6. New York: Raven Press, 1984, pp. 277–288.

101. MEYERSON, B. A. "Electrostimulation Procedures: Effects, Presumed Rationale and Possible Mechanisms," in J. J. Bonica, ed., *Advances in Pain Research and Therapy,* vol. 5. New York: Raven Press, 1983, pp. 495–534.

102. MITCHELL, S. W., MOOREHOUSE, G. R., and KENN, W. W. *Gunshot Wounds and Other Injuries of the Nerves.* Philadelphia: J. B. Lippincott, 1864.

103. MOORE, D. C. "Celiac (Splanchnic) Plexus Block with Alcohol for Cancer Pain of the Upper Intraabdominal Viscera," in J. J. Bonica and V. Ventafridda, eds., *Advances in Pain Research and Therapy,* vol. 2. New York: Raven Press, 1979, pp. 357–371.

104. MORICCA, G. "Neuroadenolysis for the Antaglic Treatment of Advanced Cancer Patients," in J. J. Bonica, P. Procacci, and C. Pagni, eds., *Recent Advances on Pain.* Springfield, Ill.: Charles C Thomas, 1974, p. 313.

105. NASHOLD, B. S., Jr., and WILSON, W. E. "Central Pain. Observation in Man with Chronic Implanted Electrodes in the Midbrain Tegmentum," *Confinia Neurologica,* 27 (1966):30–34.

106. NATHAN, P. W., and WALL, P. D. "Treatment of Post-herpetic Neuralgia by Prolonged Electrical Stimulation," *British Medical Journal,* 3 (1974):645–647.

107. NOORDENBOS, W. *Pain.* Amsterdam: Elsevier Press, 1959.

108. OGSTON, D., McDONALD, G. A., and Fullerton, H. W. "The Influence of Anxiety in Tests of Blood Coagular Ability and Fibrinolytic Activity," *Lancet,* 2 (1962): 521–523.

109. ONOFRIO, B. M., YAKSH, T. L., and ARNOLD, P. G. "Continuous Low-dose Intrathecal Morphine Administration in the Treatment of Chronic Pain of Malignant Origin," *Mayo Clinic Proceedings,* 56 (1981):516–520.

110. PAGNI, C. A. "General Comments on Ablative Neurosurgical Procedures," in J. J. Bonica and V. Ventafridda, eds., *Advances in Pain Research and Therapy,* vol. 2. New York: Raven Press, 1979, pp. 405–423.

111. PAPO, I. "Open Cordotomy in the Treatment of Cancer Pain," in J. J. Bonica and V. Ventafridda, eds., *Advances in Pain Research and Therapy,* vol. 2. New York: Raven Press, 1979, pp. 449–452.

112. PASQUALUCCI, V. "Advances in the Management of Cardiac Pain," in C. Benedetti, C. R. Chapman, and G. Moricca, eds., *Recent Advances in the Management of Pain—Advances in Pain Research and Therapy,* vol. 7. New York: Raven Press, 1984, pp. 501–519.

113. PERL, E. R. "Afferent Basis of Nociception and Pain: Evidence from the Characteristics of Sensory Receptors and Their Projections to the Spinal Dorsal Horn," in J. J. Bonica, ed., *Pain.* New York: Raven Press, 1980, pp. 19–47.

114. PILOWSKY, I., and SPENCE, N. D. "Pain and Illness Behavior: A Comparative Study," *Journal of Psychosomatic Research,* 20 (1976):131–134.

115. PILOWSKY, I., CHAPMAN, C. R., and BONICA, J. J. "Pain, Depression and Illness Behavior in a Pain Clinic Population," *Pain,* 4 (1977):183–192.

116. RAY, C. D., BURTON, C. V., and LITSON, A. "Neurostimulation as Used in a Large

Clinical Practice," *Acta Neurochirurgica,* (Supplement 32) (1982).

117. REYNOLDS, D. V. "Surgery in the Rat During Electrical Analgesia Induced by Focal Brain Stimulation," *Science,* 164 (1969):444–445.

118. ROBERTS, A. H., and REINHARDT, L. "The Behavioral Management of Chronic Pain: Long-term Follow-up with Comparison Groups," *Pain,* 8 (1980):151–162.

119. SCHNEIDER, R. A. "The Relation of Stress to Clotting Time, Relative Viscosity and Certain Biophysical Alterations of the Blood in Normal Tensive and Hypertensive Subjects," in *Life Stresses and Bodily Disease.* Baltimore: Williams & Wilkins, 1950, pp. 818–831.

120. SCHWETSCHENAU, P. R., et al. "Double-blind Evaluation of Intradiscal Chymopapain for Herniated Lumbar Discs," *Journal of Neurosurgery,* 45 (1976):622–627.

121. SHEALY, C. N., MORTIMER, J. T., and RESWICK, J. "Electrical Inhibition of Pain by Stimulation of the Dorsal Column: Preliminary Clinical Reports," *Anesthesia Analgesia* (Cleveland), 46 (1967): 489–491.

122. SHEEHAN, P. W., and PERRY, C. W. *Methodologies of Hypnosis: A Critical Appraisal of Contemporary Paradigms of Hypnosis.* Hillsdale, N.J.: Lawrence Erlbaum Associates, 1976.

123. SHERMAN, J. E., and LIEBESKIND, J. C. "An Endorphinergic, Centrifugal Substrate of Pain Modulation: Recent Findings, Current Concepts, and Complexities," in J. J. Bonica, ed., *Pain.* New York: Raven Press, 1980, pp. 191–204.

124. SHERMAN, R. A., SHERMAN, C. J., and PARKER, L. "Chronic Phantom and Stump Pain Among American Veterans: Results of a Survey," *Pain,* 18 (1984):83–95.

125. SHUKLA, G. D., et al. "Phantom Limb: A Phenomenological Study," *British Journal of Psychiatry,* 141 (1982):54–58.

126. SIEGFRIED, J., and BROGGI, G. "Percutaneous Thermocoagulation of the Gasserian Ganglion in the Treatment of Pain in Advanced Cancer," in J. J. Bonica and V. Ventafridda, eds., *Advances in Pain Research and Therapy,* vol. 2. New York: Raven Press, 1979, pp. 463–468.

127. SINDOU, M., et al. "La Radicellotomie Posterieure Selective. Premiers Resultats dans la Chirurgie de la Douleur," *Neurochirurgie,* 20 (1974):391–408.

128. SKINNER, B. F. *Science and Human Behavior.* New York: Macmillan, 1953.

129. SOLA, A. E. "Myofascial Trigger Point Therapy," *Medical Times* (January) (1982):70–77.

130. SPANGFORT, E. V. "The Lumbar Disc Herniation," *Acta Orthopaedica Scandinavica,* 142 (Supplement) (1972):1–95.

131. STERNBACH, R. A. *Pain: A Psychophysiologic Analysis.* New York: Academic Press, 1968.

132. ———. *Pain Patients: Traits and Treatment.* New York: Academic Press, 1974.

133. STERNBACH, R. A., ed. *The Psychology of Pain.* New York: Raven Press, 1978.

134. SUNDERLAND, S. *Nerves and Nerve Injuries.* Edinburgh: Churchill Livingston, 1978.

135. SWANSON, D. W., MARUTA, T., and SWENSON, W. M. "Results of Behavior Modification in the Treatment of Chronic Pain," *Proceedings of the Staff Meetings of the Mayo Clinic,* 51 (1979):401–408.

136. SWEET, W. H. "Controlled Thermocoagulation of Trigeminal Ganglion and Rootlets for Differential Destruction of Pain Fibers: Facial Pain Other than Trigeminal Neuralgia," *Clinics of Neurosurgery,* 23 (1976):96–102.

137. SWERDLOW, M. "Subarachnoid and Extradural Neurolytic Blocks," in J. J. Bonica and V. Ventafridda, eds., *Advances in Pain Research and Therapy,* vol. 2. New York: Raven Press, 1979, pp. 325–337.

138. SWERDLOW, M., ed. *Relief of Intractable Pain,* 2nd ed. Amsterdam: Elsevier/ North Holland Biomedical Press, 1979.

139. TAN, F. Y. "Cognitive and Cognitive-Behavioral Methods for Pain Control: A Selective Review," *Pain,* 12 (1982):201–228.

140. TAUB, A. "Relief of Post-herpetic Neuralgia with Psychotropic Drugs," *Journal of Neurosurgery,* 39 (1973):235–239.

141. TAYLOR, C. B., et al. "The Effects of Detoxification, Relaxation, and Brief

Supportive Therapy on Chronic Pain," *Pain*, 8 (1980):319–329.

142. THAL, E. R., and SHIRES, G. T. "Post-traumatic Pain," in A. H. Gieseke, ed., *Anesthesia for the Surgery of Trauma*, vol. 11/12. Philadelphia: Davis Company, 1976.

143. THOREN, L. "Postoperative Pulmonary Complications. Observations on Their Prevention by Means of Physiotherapy," *Acta Chirurgica Scandinavica*, 107 (1954):193–205.

144. TRAVELL, J. G., and SIMONS, D. G. *Myofascial Pain and Dysfunction: The Trigger Point Manual*. Baltimore: Williams & Wilkins, 1983.

145. TURK, D. C., and GENEST, M. "Regulation of Pain: The Application of Cognitive and Behavioral Techniques for Prevention and Remediation," in P. C. Kendall and S. D. Hollon, eds., *Cognitive-Behavioral Interventions: Theory, Research, and Procedures*. New York: Academic Press, 1979, pp. 287–318.

146. TURK, D. C., MEICHENBAUM, D., and GENEST, M. *Pain in Behavioral Medicine: A Cognitive Behavioral Perspective*. New York: Gilford, 1983.

147. TURNBULL, J. M., SHULMAN, R., and WOODHURST, W. B. "Thalamic Stimulation for Neuropathic Pain," *Journal of Neurosurgery*, 52 (1980):486–493.

148. TURNER, J. A., and CHAPMAN, C. R. "Psychologic Interventions for Chronic Pain: A Critical Review," *Pain*, 12 (1982):1–46.

149. TURNER, J. A., and ROMANO, J. M. "Review of Prevalence of Coexisting Chronic Pain and Depression," in C. Benedetti, C. R. Chapman, and G. Moricca, eds., *Recent Advances in the Management of Pain—Advances in Pain Research and Therapy*, vol. 7. New York: Raven Press, 1984, pp. 123–130.

150. TWYCROSS, R. G. "Controlling Pain in Cancer Patients," *Modern Medicine* (London), 8 (1982):2–13.

151. TWYCROSS, R. G., and LACK, S. A. *Symptom Control in Far Advanced Cancer: Pain Relief*. London: Pitman Books, 1983.

152. URBAN, B. J., and NASHOLD, B. S. "Percutaneous Epidural Stimulation of the Spinal Cord for Relief of Pain," *Journal of Neurosurgery*, 48 (1978):323–328.

153. VANE, J. R. "Inhibition of Prostaglandin Synthesis as a Mechanism of Action for Aspirin-like Drugs," *Nature*, 231 (1971):232–235.

154. WALL, P. D. "The Role of Substantia Gelatinosa as a Gate Control," in J. J. Bonica, ed., *Pain*. New York: Raven Press, 1980, pp. 205–231.

155. ———. "Mechanisms of Acute and Chronic Pain," in L. Kruger and J. C. Liebeskind, *Neural Mechanisms of Pain—Advances in Pain Research and Therapy*, vol. 6. New York: Raven Press, 1984, pp. 95–104.

156. WALL, P. D., and DEVOR, M. "The Effects of Peripheral Nerve Injury on Dorsal Root Potentials and on Transmission of Afferent Signals into Spinal Cord," *Brain Research*, 209 (1981):95–111.

157. WHITE, J. C., and SWEET, W. H. *Pain and the Neurosurgeon. A Forty-Year Experience*. Springfield, Ill.: Charles C Thomas, 1969.

158. WILMORE, D. W., et al. "Stress in Surgical Patients as a Neurophysiologic Reflex Response," *Surgery, Gynecology and Obstetrics*, 142 (1976):257–269.

159. WINNIE, A. P., et al. "Pain Clinic II: Intrathecal and Extradural Corticosteroids for Sciatica," *Anesthesia Analgesia*, 51 (1972):990–999.

160. WOLFF, H. G., and WOLFF, S. *Pain*, 2nd ed. Springfield, Ill.: Charles C Thomas, 1958.

161. WOOD, K. M. "The Use of Phenol as a Neurolytic Agent: A Review," *Pain*, 5 (1978):205–229.

162. WOODFORDE, J. M., and FIELDING, J. R. "Pain and Cancer," in M. Weisenburg, ed., *Pain, Clinical and Experimental Perspectives*. St. Louis: C. V. Mosby, 1975, pp. 332–336.

163. YAKSH, T. L. "Spinal Opiate Analgesia: Characteristics and Principles of Action," *Pain*, 11 (1981):293–346.

164. ZAHAVI, J., and DREYFUSS, F. "Adenosine Diphosphate-induced Platelet Aggregation in Myocardial Infarction and Ischemic Heart Disease," Second Congress of the Society of Thrombosis and Hemostasis, Oslo, July 13, 1971.

165. ZANCHETTI, A., and MALLIANI, A. "Neu-

ral and Psychological Factors in Coronary Disease," *Acta Cardiologica,* 20 (Supplement) (1974):69–93.

166. ZIMMERMAN, M. "Peripheral and Central Nervous Mechanisms of Nociception Pain and Pain Therapy. Facts and Hypothesis," in J. J. Bonica, J. C. Liebeskind, and D. G. Albe-Fessard, eds., *Advances in Pain Research and Therapy,* vol. 3. New York: Raven Press, 1979, pp. 3–32.

CHAPTER 27

THE BIOLOGY AND EXPERIMENTAL TREATMENT OF ANOREXIA NERVOSA AND BULIMIA

Katherine A. Halmi

¶ **Introduction**

Comprehensive studies of the biology of anorexia nervosa are recent, occurring only in the last twenty years, with the greatest number in the last five years. Bulimia, a term that means binge eating, is also a DSM-III disorder. At the time the criteria were developed for bulimia, very little was known about this disorder. Therefore, the DSM-III criteria are merely descriptive and do not provide a clear distinction among the occasional behavior of binge eating, binge eating that occurs in anorexia nervosa, and the binge-eating disorder of persons in a normal weight range. In this chapter, the disorder bulimia will be referred to as bulimia nervosa to distinguish it from the behavior of binge eating, and the criteria presented in

table 27–1 will be used for anorexia nervosa and bulimia nervosa. Almost all the biological studies in this field use the criteria listed in the table, or a minor variation, for diagnoses of anorexia nervosa and bulimia. Most investigators agree that bulimia nervosa should be defined as a disorder in which patients have weight fluctuations within a 10 percent range of normal weight.

Anorexia nervosa patients can be subdivided into those who binge and purge and those who merely restrict food intake in order to lose weight. Bulimia nervosa patients can be subdivided into those who have had a previous history of anorexia nervosa and have returned to normal weight and those who have never had an episode of anorexia nervosa. In this discussion of the biology of these eating disorders, the physiological and metabolic changes associated with

TABLE 27–1
Diagnostic Criteria

Anorexia Nervosa

A. Intense fear of becoming obese, which does not diminish as weight loss progresses.
B. Body conceptualization disturbance—for example, claiming to "feel fat" even when emaciated.
C. Refusal to maintain body weight over a minimal normal weight for age and height.
D. Amenorrhea.

Bulimia Nervosa

A. Recurrent episodes of binge eating (rapid consumption of a large amount of food in a discreet period of time, usually less than two hours).
B. At least three of the following:
　1. Consumption of high-caloric, easily ingested food during a binge.
　2. Inconspicuous eating during a binge.
　3. Termination of such eating episodes by abdominal pain, sleep, social interruption, or self-induced vomiting.
　4. Repeated attempts to lose weight by several restricted diets, self-induced vomiting, or use of cathartics or diuretics.
　5. Frequent weight fluctuations greater than 10 lb due to alternating binges and fasts.
C. Awareness that the eating pattern is abnormal and fear of not being able to stop eating voluntarily.
D. Frequency of binge eating must be at least an average of once per week for three months.
E. Maintenance of body weight within 10 percent of a normal weight range for age, sex, and height.

---

bingeing and purging will not be divided into anorexia nervosa and bulimia nervosa sections, since the changes are qualitatively the same. The endocrine, neurotransmitter, and family studies unique to bulimia nervosa will be identified and compared with similar studies in anorexia nervosa. In the first section of this chapter, the physiology and metabolism, endocrinology, and genetic and familial studies will be presented and discussed. This will be followed by a section on the experimental treatment of anorexia and bulimia nervosa, since the treatment, for the most part, has emerged from the biological findings.

¶ Physiology and Metabolism

Most of the physiologic and metabolic changes found in anorexia nervosa or bulimia nervosa are also present in starvation states or are a direct result of purging behavior, and thus do not provide etiological clues for these disorders. When they are severely restricting their intake, most of these patients will preferentially take low-calorie dense foods and will take vitamin supplements. The starvation metabolic aberrations revert to normal with nutritional rehabilitation.

Hematopoiesis

Abnormalities in hematopoiesis, such as severe leukopenia and relative lymphocytosis, were described as early as 1959.[12] Later, Mant and Faragher[110] described a hypocellularity of the bone marrow with the presence of a large amount of gelatinous acid mucopolysaccharide that reversed with clinical improvement. They postulated that depletion of fat or the presence of background acid mucopolysaccharide adversely affected the local environment for normal hematopoiesis and that the increased mucopolysaccharide was a physiological response to starvation. Subsequently, several other investigators confirmed the finding of bone marrow hypoplasia in anorexia nervosa.[16,93,100] All these studies noted that bone marrow morphology reversed to normal after refeeding. Some investigators questioned whether there may be a direct influence of fat or carbohydrate depletion on the proliferation of hematopoietic cells.[100]

Decreased production of fibrinogen by the liver responding to the malnourished state was postulated to be the cause of low erythrocyte sedimentation rate (ESR) and low plasma fibrinogen levels measured in emaciated anorectic patients.[2] The low ESR values in anorectic patients may be a distinguishing physiological characteristic in differentiating the anorectic from a patient with weight loss due to occult malignancy, Crohn's disease, hyperthyroidism, and chronic infection.

The leukopenia observed in anorexia nervosa raises concern as to whether these patients are at an increased risk for infection. Two studies that have examined the immunocompetency in anorexia nervosa[8,50] found a generally depressed response to delayed hypersensitivity skin testing, and one study showed that the anergy was positively related to the severity of malnutrition.[133] Visceral proteins, such as serum albumin and transferrin, and total iron-binding capacity were not correlated with anergy. The *in vitro* response of lymphocytes to mitogenic stimulation was normal or increased in the anorectic patients, and there was a relatively normal percentage of T-lymphocytes.[50] The latter two findings are not typical of protein-calorie malnutrition and may be relevant to the peculiar dietary intake of the anorectic patients. Peripheral blood granulocytes from malnourished anorectics have a reduced rate of killing *Staphylococcus aureus* and *Escherichia coli* in two *in vitro* studies.[51,131] This finding reversed with weight gain. Although the granulocyte bactericidal capacity was reduced in these malnourished anorectic patients, its clinical significance was uncertain since none of the patients studied had recurrent or severe infectious diseases. The incidence of leukopenia and infection in anorexia nervosa was studied by Bowers and Eckert,[5] who reviewed sixty-eight cases of anorexia nervosa and found no more infection in the anorectic patients than in control subjects despite the patients' frequent and often severe leukopenia. Although the risk of infection seems to be no greater in anorectic patients than in control subjects, from the studies just described there is reason to be concerned that if the anorectic patient does develop an infection, the morbidity risk will be much greater than in a healthy person, since anorectic persons have a reduced bactericidal capacity to fight infection.

Fluids and Electrolytes

Both anorexia nervosa and bulimia nervosa patients who engage in self-induced vomiting or abuse purgatives and diuretics are susceptible to developing hypokalemic alkalosis.[115,142,174,178] In one study,[115] 49 percent of the patients had electrolyte abnormalities that included elevated serum bicarbonate, hypochloremia, hypokalemia, and, in a few cases, a low serum bicarbonate, indicating a metabolic acidosis. The latter was particularly true in laxative abusers. It is important to remember that fasting can promote dehydration, which results in volume depletion and which in turn can promote generation of aldosterone, which promotes further potassium excretion from the kidneys. Thus there can be an indirect renal loss of potassium as well as a direct loss through self-induced vomiting. Patients with electrolyte disturbances have physical symptoms of weakness, lethargy, and, at times, cardiac arrhythmias.

Renal Function

Impaired water diuresis was first noted by Russell in 1966.[151] He found that the impaired water diuresis was associated with a decreased glomerular filtration rate (GFR) and that this abnormality varied directly with the duration of malnutrition. It was not found in patients who had been ill for less than three years. The reduction of GFR was out of proportion to the reduction of para-aminohippuric acid (PAH) clearance as shown by a significantly lower filtration fraction in another study.[3] The authors thought the low filtration fraction could be attributed to reduced water permeability of the glomerular capillary. The urinary-concentrating capacity following fluid deprivation was moderately depressed both before and after administration of vasopressin. This indicates a renal origin for the concentrating defect. Of twenty anorectic patients with hypokalemic alkalosis reported by Wigley,[183] eleven showed some evidence of renal disorder. Autopsy findings on one of these patients showed renal tubal vacuolation.

Gastrointestinal System

It seems logical to start at the beginning of the gastrointestinal tract and discuss abnormalities in the mouth. Both anorexia nervosa and bulimia nervosa patients who binge and purge can be diagnosed by the dentist. Patients with anorexia and bulimia nervosa can have severe attrition and erosion of the teeth, causing an irritating sensitivity, pathologic pulp exposures, loss of integrity of the dental arches, diminished masticatory ability, and an unaesthetic appearance.[162] Hellstrom[74] believes the increase in cavities is caused by bingeing on carbohydrates and the erosion and abrasion are caused by self-induced vomiting. Reduced salivary secretion can produce a perimylolysis.

Parotid gland enlargement is another common physical sign in the patients who binge and self-induce vomiting.[72] Pancreatitis has been described both as a complication in the emaciated anorectic state and during refeeding.[17,157] Elevated serum amylase levels are often observed in patients who binge and purge.[115] In fact, the serum amylase level is an excellent way to follow reduction of vomiting in eating-disorder patients who deny purging episodes. Acute dilatation of the stomach is a rare emergency condition for patients who binge.[82,147] Acute gastric dilatation may be caused by a superior mesentary artery syndrome. The superior mesentary artery crosses in front of the duodenum, which it may compress, causing symptoms of partial obstruction. It is conceivable that severe weight loss, whether in anorexia nervosa or in other malnourished states, will cause a change in the amount of fat in the mesentary

and subsequently affect the position of the superior mesentary artery and its branches. Several cases of the superior mesentary artery syndrome have been reported in anorexia nervosa.[9,39]

Gastric emptying is delayed in emaciated anorexia nervosa patients.[26,77] In one study,[27] the administration of a parasympathetic agent, bethanechol chloride, produced only a partial restoration of gastric emptying and acid secretion in patients with anorexia nervosa. The investigators believe the defect in gastric emptying and acid secretion reflects the presence of inhibitory influences and not just impaired parasympathetic neurotransmission. Pharmacological treatment was sought to facilitate gastric emptying. Saleh and Lebwohl[154] demonstrated that gastric emptying returns to normal in patients using metoclopramide hydrochloride, which inhibits gastric relaxation produced by dopamine through blocking the dopaminergic receptors in the brain stem. This drug, however, has some neurological side effects; thus another drug that does not cross the blood-brain barrier and hence does not cause central neurological side effects was studied. This drug is domperidone, which enhances gastric peristalsis and has strong antiemetic properties. Although a double-blind study is now in process using this drug, a case report promises good results with subjective ratings of satiety and documented improvement of gastric emptying.[146]

It is not unusual for serum enzymes reflecting liver function to be elevated in anorexia nervosa. Serum glutamic-oxalacetic transaminase (SGOT), lactic dehydrogenase (LDH), and alkaline phosphatase are the enzymes most frequently elevated.[63] The elevation of these enzymes most likely reflects some fatty degeneration of the liver and is observed both in the emaciated anorectic phase and during refeeding. Total plasma protein and serum albumin levels are normal in anorectic patients.[63] Russell[148] reported that plasma aminograms were normal in nineteen anorexia nervosa patients and calculated the rate of degradation of labeled I^{131}-Albumin. He found a small but significant reduction in the breakdown of albumin in the anorectic patients compared to normal subjects.

There is a wide scatter of serum cholesterol and triglyceride levels in anorexia nervosa.[19,64] Nestel[123] found that the daily intake of cholesterol exceeded the total fecal excretion of steroids in anorectic girls with hypercholesterolemia. This indicated that dietary cholesterol was being retained. Bile acid excretion was markedly reduced in those patients. Nestel felt the hypercholesterolemia reflected the hypocaloric state in the anorectic patients. A more recent study[119] showed elevated cholesterol levels were due to an increase of low-density lipoprotein cholesterol. High-density lipoprotein and very low-density lipoprotein cholesterol levels were in the normal range. The authors postulated a diminished cholesterol turnover due to delayed low-density lipoprotein metabolism.

Carotenemia observed in malnourished anorectic patients was initially postulated to be due to a decreased catabolism of beta-lipoprotein, the major carrier of carotene in plasma.[139] More recently, significant elevation of serum beta-carotene, vitamin A esters, vitamin A alcohol, and vitamin A acid were found in anorexia nervosa patients compared to normal subjects, patients with cachexia from other causes, patients with ovarian failure, and patients with pituitary suppression.[141] The investigators hypothesized that an acquired but reversible error of metabolism of beta-carotene and vitamin A precursors occurs in anorexia nervosa.[141]

Cardiovascular Function

Malnourished patients with anorexia nervosa have cardiac abnormalities such as bradycardia, hypotension, tachycardia, and electrocardiographic changes.[165] The latter usually consists of irregularities of the T-wave, which is flat or inverted. Often there is a depression of the ST segments and at times a distinct U wave.[132] Thurston and Marks[165] noted that these electrographic changes are similar to those frequently observed in patients with head injuries. In acute intracranial disease, sympathetic centers are stimulated in the hypothalamus, and this results in release of catecholamines within the myocardium. The authors postulate that a similar phenomenon occurs in anorexia nervosa and that these catecholamines may cause damage to the contractile apparatus and to the cell membrane of the myocardial cells, resulting in the electrocardiographic abnormalities described. This opinion was also expressed by Palossy and Oo.[132] Another study investigating the myocardial function in anorexia nervosa[43] found that the undernourished anorectic patients had a lengthened preejection period, an increased electromechanical systole, and an increased ratio of the preejection period over the left ventricular ejection time. The authors also found increased systolic time intervals, which they thought was indicative of impaired left ventricular function. The latter, they postulated, was caused by decreased myocardial contractility. The oxygen transporting system was studied in twenty-eight anorectic patients who, during the emaciated state, had a low metabolic rate with bradycardia and hypotension at rest. The blood and heart volume was decreased proportionally to the weight loss. When patients were given a workload, the maximal aerobic power was lowered to the same extent as the resting metabolic rate. At maximal effort, however, the maximal aerobic power was reduced out of proportion to the circulatory dimensions and the maximal heart rate was low. The authors thought the main cause of the low maximal aerobic power was reduced muscle mass. After treatment, the heart volume and blood volume increased in proportion to the rise in body weight, and the lean body mass increased significantly in all patients. The authors felt the cardiovascular system was normalized after weight gain.[35,36] In a study that also showed decreased ventricular ectopy, relative hypotension, bradycardia, and blunted heart rate in response to exercise, mean left ventricular, left atrial, and aortic dimensions on echocardiogram were below normal adult values in the underweight state of anorectic patients.[52] All cardiac dimensions increased toward normal with weight gain, including left ventricular mass, and were accompanied by an increase in heart rate and blood pressure. The sudden deaths that have received the most publicity in eating-disorder patients have been in those patients who binge and purge, whether they are emaciated or within a normal weight range. Undoubtedly there are multiple mechanisms for cardiac arrhythmias in these patients. Recent investigations are showing that normal-weight bulimia nervosa patients who also have normal serum electrolytes can have severe cardiac rhythm disturbances.[187,188] These findings lend some support to the postulation made by Thurston and Marks[165] in 1974 that the electrocardiographic abnormalities in the eating disorders may be brought about by stimulation of sympathetic centers within the hypothalamus.

Injudicious rapid refeeding can cause heart failure in anorectic patients.[140] Unfortunately this fact was publicized in the lay press and influenced a large number of medically uneducated therapists to become dangerously cautious in seeking appropriate nutritional rehabilitation for their patients.

Skeletal and Bone Aberrations

Growth retardation has been observed in patients with anorexia nervosa.[99,144] Although this has been studied mainly in terms of growth hormone (GH) metabolism (to be discussed in the section on endocrinology), there has recently been some evidence that patients, especially those who have been self-inducing vomiting for several years, have osteoporosis.[63,108] In all cases, symptoms of pain led to appropriate x-rays, which showed rib fractures,[108] hip fractures,[63] and compression fractures of the vertebrae.[63] A preliminary report by Matthews and Lacey[113] indicates that serum levels of the bone isoenzyme of alkaline phosphatase are increased during refeeding of anorectic patients. In this preliminary study, the liver alkaline phosphatase isoenzyme serum levels did not change. Therefore the authors thought the increase in alkaline phosphatase was a sensitive measure for detecting changes in bone metabolism and growth due solely to an increase in nutrition.

Metabolic Changes with Weight Gain

There is great variability in the reported caloric requirements for weight gain in anorectic patients. However, it is of interest that in two studies the mean value of excess calories per kilogram was very similar.[148,173] Patients required 7,428 excess calories per kilogram in one study[173] and 7,500 in the other study.[148] The authors in one study noted that the mean calories required to gain a kilogram was lower in the initial part of treatment; in fact, this may be due to the fact that some of the subjects were dehydrated; part of the weight gain in the earlier period may have been in the form of water.[173] In this study, a highly significant correlation was present between the percent of standard weight gained during the first day of treatment and the excess calories required to gain a kilogram. Body composition studies have shown that higher excess caloric requirements are needed to form tissue containing a larger proportion of fat.[81,92] It is also likely that a dietary-induced thermogenesis occurs during the nutritional rehabilitation period. The significant correlations in the amount of weight to be gained and excess calories required to gain a kilogram could also be due to the differences in the type of tissue being formed and/or the fact that an increase in metabolic rate is part of an adaptive response as the patient nears target weight.

Changes in metabolism in anorexia nervosa also occur with lean body mass and skeletal muscles. Biopsy studies on anorectic patients showed all muscle fibers in the quadriceps femoris to be markedly atrophied during the emaciated state. In two patients studied after rehabilitation, the mean fiber area had increased by 40 percent.[31] In this study, during the emaciated state there was a complete absence of Type II B fibers. The authors noted that several months of regular endurance exercise will increase the proportion of Type II A fibers at the expense of Type II B fibers, while inactivity of the same duration increases the number of Type II B fibers. They also noted that the only situation in healthy subjects where no Type II B fibers are found is in extremely trained endurance muscle. They postulated that excessive exercising in the anorectic patients may account for this finding. Another study assessed the skeletal muscle function by the electrical stimulation of the ulnar nerve and the measurement of force of contraction, maximal relaxation rate, and muscle fatigue in the abductor pollicis muscle in anorectic patients during the emaciated and weight-recovered stages. There was a significant increase in the force of contraction, a slowing of maximal relaxation rate, and an increased muscular fatigue during emaciation. Although serum albumin was within normal range, patients had a low total body nitrogen and low creatinine-height index. During refeeding, body nitrogen increased only 13 percent and was still 19 percent below predicted normal total body nitrogen, whereas total body potassium increased by 32 percent and body fat by 46 percent. The authors concluded that normalization of muscle function may be related to restoration of muscle electrolyte rather than repletion of body nitrogen.[60] The role of trace metals in influencing metabolism in anorexia was studied with measures of plasma zinc, urinary zinc, and urinary copper, which were all found to be depressed in emaciated anorectics.[13] Total iron-binding capacity was also depressed, although plasma iron, ceruloplasmin, and folic acid were within normal range. In this study, although patients had hypercarotenemia, they had normal plasma vitamin A and normal retinol-binding protein levels. With weight gain, the plasma zinc, copper, and total iron-binding capacity levels increased. The authors suggested that the zinc and other micronutrients may be released from

catabolized tissue and, along with the patient's vitamin intake, may protect against more severe deficiency states in anorexia nervosa.

Neurological Investigation

Over the past ten years, occasional case reports have appeared in the literature describing patients who have been diagnosed as having anorexia nervosa and upon later investigation had hypothalamic tumors. There has been no single type of tumor in all of these reports, but all the tumors have been in the hypothalamic area. One report describes a polycystic craniopharyngioma compressing the optic chiasma and projecting to the midbrain region.[49] Another report described an ectopic pinealoma in the area of the hypothalamus.[75] A low-grade glioma with a large cystic mass was present in the floor of the third ventricle in another case.[182] A thirteen-year-old girl with anorexia nervosa was found to have an infiltrating tumor in the left hypothalamic area,[180] and in another case a fifty-five-year-old woman was diagnosed as having anorexia nervosa for six years before an extensive examination showed a tumor in the clivus extending into the anterior portion of the third ventricle.[34] These case reports provide indirect support for Russell's[149] hypothesis that anorexia nervosa is due to an impairment of hypothalamic function.

Severely malnourished anorectic patients may have neurological symptoms of vitamin deficiency, although this is uncommon. An unusual case of association of Wernicke's encephalopathy[71] was diagnosed in one patient with anorexia nervosa. Since there is a higher than expected prevalence of alcohol abuse in anorexia and bulimia nervosa patients, some neurological symptoms of alcohol abuse would not be unexpected, especially in the severely emaciated patients.[28]

Electroencephalographic abnormalities such as epileptiform dysrhythmias, 6-per-second spike and wave and 6- to 14-per-second spikes have been described in association with the malnourished state of anorexia nervosa and in association with bingeing and purging behavior irrespective of weight status.[18,94,160] Sleep studies in one investigation[98] showed less sleep and more restlessness in anorectic patients during the malnourished state. These symptoms were especially true in the last four hours of the night. During weight gain there was a significant increase in the length of sleep and rapid eye movement (REM) sleep. Another sleep investigation of seventeen anorectic patients during the malnourished state[122] found that only those patients with abnormal clinical electroencephalograms (EEGs) showed a decrease in tonic REM percent. Both normal and abnormal EEG subjects showed significant decreases in phasic REM sleep parameters, although the REM activity and REM density were found to be lower in the abnormal EEG patients. In this study, the authors divided the anorexia patients into those with primary anorexia nervosa and into a group that they labeled secondary anorexia nervosa. The latter group had other diagnoses, such as major depressive illness, phobic disorders, and so on. There were no differences in the occurrence of EEG abnormalities in these two groups. Nor was there a relationship between amount of weight loss and duration of illness with EEG pathology. Thus the authors felt it unlikely that starvation per se was responsible for the dysrhythmia. They did, however, find that patients who had bulimia and vomiting or were abusing laxatives and diuretics had greater EEG abnormalities. The authors did not feel this was necessarily due to electrolyte depletion or acid-base imbalance, since EEG abnormalities do not occur in other conditions with similar metabolic disturbances. They hypothesized that the abnormalities in the bulimia and vomiting subgroup may be due to retention of excessive fluid within the cranial vault or may represent a constitutional predisposition to the illness. The findings of this study are in agreement with an earlier study showing a high incidence of soft neurological signs and EEG abnormalities in intractable binge eaters.[53]

Cranial computed tomography (CT) in emaciated anorectic patients has shown abnormal enlargement of the cortical sulci, subarachnoid spaces, third ventricle, ventral horns, and sylvian fissures.[30,73] One study, in which fourteen patients with anorexia nervosa were examined, found only half had abnormal CT scans.[128] In another case report, reexamination of a patient after weight gain showed the "atrophy" abnormalities reverting to normal with nutritional rehabilitation.[124] Similar cerebral atrophy abnormalities were found in a patient with anorexia nervosa and in one with Cushing's syndrome.[73] These abnormalities reverted to normal with treatment of the disorders. The authors postulated that the mechanism responsible for the atropic changes was related to fluid retention and/or protein loss. There is no justification for routine CT scans in anorexia nervosa and bulimia nervosa patients, since treatment of these patients is not based on scan results unless a tumor is detected, and the latter is an extremely rare phenomenon. CT scans should be saved for those patients who have some atypical signs and symptoms or who are especially intractable to treatment.

A more recent area of neurological study in the eating disorders is that of the autonomic nervous system. In 1970 Wakeling and Russell[170] found a marked impairment of the temperature-regulating mechanism in anorectic patients who were malnourished. Their resting oral temperature was abnormally low and they had a reduced sensitivity of the central regulating mechanism, which responded to a heat load by inducing peripheral vasodilatation. An abnormally high rise in central body temperature was necessary for the peripheral response to occur, and when it did occur it was delayed and developed abnormally slowly. In response to a standard meal, the patients' central body temperature rose significantly, whereas in control subjects it remained constant. After refeeding there was still evidence of the same disorder of temperature regulation, although it was not as marked as in the malnourished state. This led the investigators to believe that a primary defective temperature regulation in anorexia may be linked with the feeding disorder characteristic of the illness. The disturbance of temperature regulation was indirectly confirmed in another study,[38] in which peripheral blood flow was found to be 50 to 60 percent lower in anorectic patients compared with normal controls, and the marked difference was maintained after a heat load. These investigators suggested a heat-conserving selective peripheral vasoconstriction was present in the anorectic patient. However, a study of thermoregulatory sweating showed a lower threshold for sweating and vasodilatation in patients with anorexia nervosa.[104] The onset of thermo-sweating occurred at a lower core and mean skin temperature in the patients with anorexia compared with controls. After ingesting a meal the patients had a significant increase in core temperature and a significant rise in peripheral blood flow, but the control subjects had no change in core temperature and no change in peripheral blood flow. The authors suggest that the finding of vasodilatation and sweating may be a contributory factor to the abnormally low core temperature of the anorectic patients and may explain their common complaint of warmth in their hands and feet after meals. Continued studies by the investigators showed that peripheral vessels in anorectic patients are unusually reactive to cold and that this increased cutaneous vasoreactivity to cold could contribute to the severe peripheral hypersuffusion observed in some anorectic patients.[106] In a water-immersion study, anorectic patients preferred temperatures that were significantly higher than those of control subjects, and these abnormally high preference responses persisted after a substantial weight gain had occurred. Elevation in deep body temperature produced a shift in preference toward a lower stimulus temperature in the control group, but in the patients who preferred the high-stimulus temperature, hyperthermia produced little change in their thermo-preference.[105] The authors proposed that there is an elevation in the set-point temperature for thermoregulation in some patients with anorexia nervosa,

and this may contribute to the distressing sense of cold that these patients experience.

Physiological evidence for separating anorectic patients into subgroups of those who restrict food intake and those who binge and purge was demonstrated in a study of autonomic arousal.[10] In this study there was no difference between the control groups and restricting anorectic patients in skin conductance level to 85 D tones. However, the patients with bulimia nervosa and anorectic patients who were bingeing and purging showed significantly fewer spontaneous skin conductance responses and were faster to habituate to the tone than either the controls or restricting anorectics. In analyzing all of the clinical variables in the groups, the authors thought it most likely that bingeing and vomiting could explain the difference between these groups. They did not find a higher manifest anxiety in the bingeing and vomiting patients. Explanations for the reduced spontaneous autonomic variability were drowsiness, boredom, inefficient processing of the information, or autonomic and cortical hypoarousal in bulimic subjects.

Although most of the physiological metabolic changes that have been described are attributable to malnutrition or bingeing and purging behaviors, some changes in cardiovascular function and neuroregulatory mechanisms suggest that a biological vulnerability for hypothalamic impairment may be present in anorexia nervosa and bulimia nervosa patients. This theme will be examined again after the endocrine aberrations in these eating-disorder patients have been presented.

¶ Endocrinology

The major issue with endocrine abnormalities seen in anorexia nervosa is whether these aberrations are due to the malnourished condition or whether they reflect a primary hypothalamic impairment. A more recent concern has been whether some of the endocrine abnormalities that are commonly seen in endogenous depression give support to the postulation that anorexia nervosa and bulimia nervosa are *forme frustes* of affective disorder. These issues will be discussed with each endocrine system.

Hypothalamic-Pituitary-Ovarian Axis

Since amenorrhea is a major diagnostic symptom of anorexia nervosa, extensive studies have been conducted on the hypothalamic-pituitary-ovarian axis in patients with this disorder. The question to be answered is whether the amenorrhea is a reflection solely of weight loss or whether it may indicate a primary impairment of hypothalamic function. There is evidence that amenorrhea occurs in many patients with anorexia nervosa before weight loss has occurred.[22,103] After treatment, the return of normal menstrual cycles lags behind the return to a normal body weight.[159] Resumption of menses in anorexia nervosa is associated with marked psychological improvement.[33,148] Early investigations showed that urinary excretion of estrogen was diminished in emaciated anorectic patients.[109] Both urinary excretion and plasma levels of gonadotrophins are decreased in anorexia nervosa.[125] In a study conducted by Brown and associates,[8] only 22 percent of the variance in luteinizing hormone (LH) levels was accounted for by the degree of weight loss or percentage below ideal body weight. Weiner[179] points out that if 78 percent of the variance in LH levels must be accounted for by factors other than weight loss, then there can be no simple relationship among weight loss, LH levels, and amenorrhea. In this excellent article, Weiner also points out that the amenorrheic runners in a study by Schwartz and coworkers[158] had increased LH levels when compared to exercising women who retain their menses. As evidence against a direct relationship between weight and gonadotrophin levels, Weiner[179] discusses the fact that women who lose weight but do not develop anorexia nervosa and have secondary amenorrhea can have normal LH levels. Some normal-weight bulimic patients have low LH and follicle-stimulating hormone (FSH) levels, and some patients with "psychogenic amenorrhea" have no weight loss but have low LH and FSH levels compared with normal controls. Postpubertal bulimic nervosa women with a normal weight can be amenorrheic and have age-inappropriate patterns of gonadotrophin secretion. Those women who exhibit full recovery of ideal body weight but the persistence of psychological symptoms of anorexia nervosa or bulimia nervosa still show age-inappropriate gonadotrophin secretion patterns.[88]

The positive feedback release of LH to estrogen stimulus was absent in nine of twelve weight-restored patients, indicating the hypothalamus was not able to respond normally to the estrogen.[172] A similar phenomenon was seen when clomiphene was tested in weight-restored anorectic patients.[171] The second LH peak after clomiphene administration was not present. This suggests a hypothalamic defect that is not related to the patient's nutritional status. Persistent exposure of anorectic women to gonadotrophin-releasing hormone (GnRH) produces the same changes in the pituitary of FSH and LH response that occur with restoration of weight.[125] This is further indication of a hypothalamic impairment. Although a recent study[137] has shown that normal women can assume prepubertal LH patterns when starved to 10 percent below normal body weight, this does not mean the age-inappropriate LH secretion pattern seen in anorexia nervosa is due solely to weight loss. Many factors influence the secretion of LH, and it is certainly plausible that "other factors" may be operating in the disorder anorexia nervosa. This entire discussion has given evidence that mere weight restoration does not change the inappropriate LH secretion in anorectic women.

There is a shift of estradiol metabolism from 16-alpha-hydroxylation to 2-hydroxylation in emaciated anorectic women, and consequently there is a disproportionate increase in catecholestrogens. Since the catecholestrogens have the potential of interacting with both catecholamine-mediated and estrogen-mediated systems in the central nervous system, these metabolites may influence catecholamine and dopamine metabolism in the brain, and this in turn may influence the development or maintenance of some of the behavioral signs and symptoms of anorexia nervosa.

Hypothalamic-Pituitary-Thyroid Axis

Most of the changes seen in thyroid function, such as low serum triiodothyronine (T_3) and a normal thyrotropin (TSH) reserve, are present in emaciated states and are not peculiar to anorexia nervosa.*

TSH responses to thyrotropin-releasing hormone (TRH) in anorexia nervosa patients tend to be delayed in about 70 percent of the cases studied.[40,47,171,174] In most of these studies, there was an abnormal GH response to TRH. In one study of bulimia nervosa patients, five of six responded normally to TRH with a prompt rise in TSH serum level.[114] In another study,[58] eight of ten bulimic patients showed a blunted TRH test. Most bulimic patients showed an abnormal GH response to TRH. The meaning of these results in bulimic patients is uncertain, and in anorectic patients the thyroid metabolism seems to reflect the metabolic state associated with the emaciation.

Hypothalamic-Pituitary-Adrenocortical Axis

The reduced metabolic clearance rate of cortisol and the incomplete suppression of adrenocorticotrophic hormone (ACTH) and cortisol levels by dexamethasone present in malnourished anorectic patients are also seen in protein-calorie malnutrition.[175,176] It is of interest that short-term administration of T_3 reversed such cortisol abnormalities as increased mean twenty-four-hour plasma cortisol concentration,[6] increased cortisol half-life, and increased tetrahydrocortisol/tetrahydrocortisone ratio in emaciated ano-

*See references 14, 21, 116, 121, and 169.

rectic patients. Presumably the increased adrenocortical activity is due to an increase in the pituitary secretion of ACTH, which in turn is responding to a rise in the release of corticotrophin-releasing factor from the hypothalamus. With weight recovery the adrenal secretory activity returns to normal.[66]

Dexamethasone nonsuppression is present in about one-half to two-thirds of the normal-weight bulimia nervosa patients tested.[79,114]

Growth Hormone

About one-third of malnourished anorectic patients have elevated basal GH levels.[155] Although this increase in serum GH is also found in protein-calorie malnutrition, the mechanism may be different for the increase in anorexia nervosa. Studies have shown that in order for serum GH to rise in protein-calorie malnutrition, severe protein deprivation was necessary and was associated with a drop in serum alanine and albumin levels.[136] However, these levels are normal in anorexia nervosa.[70] A decreased response of GH to levodopa and apomorphine has been observed even after weight recovery.[66] This suggests there may be a specific abnormality in dopaminergic regulation of GH secretion in anorexia nervosa. The adenohypophysis of an anorexia nervosa patient who was emaciated at the time of death was examined immunocytochemically and with a battery of differential stains.[61] The ACTH, GH, TSH, and prolactin cells stained with the same intensity as those in normal control pituitaries. The gonadotrophs immunostained for LH stained much more faintly in the anorectic patient's pituitary than in normal glands. These findings reflect a selective pituitary deficiency in the emaciated state of anorexia nervosa.

Neurotransmitter Studies

The first studies of neurotransmitters in anorexia nervosa were those measuring urinary 3-methoxy-4-hydroxy-phenylglycol (MHPG).[54,68] Urinary MHPG was decreased in all studies in emaciated anorectic patients and increased with weight recovery. There is some question as to whether the change in MHPG may also be related to change in depressive symptomatology. Plasma norepinephrine (NE) is decreased in malnourished anorectic patients and returns to normal levels with weight recovery,[54] and plasma dopamine-beta-hydroxylase is normal in both the malnourished and weight-recovered state. Studies of metabolites in the cerebrospinal fluid (CSF) are difficult to interpret. In one study, opioid activity was increased in the emaciated state and returned to normal with weight recovery,[89] and in another study beta-endorphin immunoreactivity was normal in underweight anorectic patients.[43,44] Gamma-aminobutyric acid (GABA)-CSF levels are also normal in emaciated anorectic patients. CSF-homovanillic acid (HVA), 5-hydroxyindoleacetic acid (5-HIAA), and tyrosine levels are decreased in the emaciated anorectic state and return to normal with weight recovery. Another study showed a reversal of the normal CSF/plasma ratio of arginine vasopressin.[48] This ratio corrects with weight gain. It is not yet possible to form a clear picture of the relationships of these various metabolites to each other in anorexia nervosa.

Impaired GH response to levodopa and impaired prolactin response to chlorpromazine[130] with decreased CSF-HVA suggests a disturbance in dopamine regulation, possibly at the postsynaptic receptor site.

A positive correlation between low urinary MHPG and failure to suppress cortisol[42] supports the idea of a hypothalamic disturbance in anorexia nervosa. Corticotrophin-releasing factor is disinhibited by low central nervous system NE. It is possible that significant changes occur after severe dieting to produce a state of self-stimulation with both dieting and/or bingeing behavior to maintain the abnormal eating behavior. There is some evidence that bingeing behavior releases anxiety. Anorexia nervosa and bulimia nervosa are truly heterogeneous disorders. This complicates researchers' ability to meaningfully interpret much of the data in the neurotransmitter studies.

Appetite and Satiety Mechanisms

There is substantial evidence from studies on animals that the metabolic processes that influence hunger and satiety also affect mood, activity level, and cognitive states. Identification of disturbances in the psychological processes of hunger, satiety, and taste could provide cogent clues for impaired central mechanisms in the eating disorders. These clues could be followed up more specifically with pharmacological perturbation tests, which in turn could provide the more pertinent information needed to develop effective treatment interventions for the primary eating disorders.

Based on the observation that animals with satiety center (paraventricular and medial hypothalamus) lesions overeat only when their food is palatable and become anorectic when its taste or other sensory properties are mildly aversive, Grossman[57] formulated the "hedonic disinhibition hypothesis." An impairment to the satiety center is associated with exaggerated affective reactions and exaggerated response to hedonic factors. Satiety is a relative rather than an absolute phenomenon that takes hedonic, as well as nutritive, considerations into account. Animal studies have shown that 5HT enhances satiety control and NE inhibits it. The eating behavior of underweight anorexia nervosa patients who exclusively starve and of underweight anorectic patients who alternate severe starving with binge eating provides a strong suspicion that there is a difference in detection of satiety in these two groups of patients. The normal-weight bulimia nervosa patients, despite their efforts at dieting, are unable to become emaciated. These patients have more effective control, most likely through purging mechanisms, over their body weight than obese patients. Differences in detection of hunger and satiety can be assessed with a test meal paradigm. In this paradigm, mood, food preferences, and taste preferences can also be assessed. These studies are currently in progress but are not completed or published. Animal studies with satiety center lesions have shown that affective disturbances can coexist with satiety disturbances. The 5HT agonist fenfluramine hydrochloride has already been shown in a preliminary study to reduce intake in a single meal in bulimic patients.[150] A double-blind study of imipramine hydrochloride in bulimic patients has shown that the drug was effective in reducing the number of bingeing episodes.[138] What is the mechanism for this? One could hypothesize that an increase in NE induced by the drug has the expected inhibitory effect on the satiety center. In this situation one would expect decreased control of satiety and/or bingeing behavior. It would be worthwhile to study the pharmacological mechanism behind the empirical observation that imipramine reduces bingeing episodes.

Food deprivation and food repletion in rats caused changes in alpha-adrenergic receptor binding in the lateral hypothalamus and paraventricular nucleus (PVN).[83] Decreased binding in the PVN is observed during deprivation, which could mean an increase in release of PVN-NE, resulting in receptor down-regulation and an inhibition of satiety. The opposite occurs in the lateral hypothalamus, where deprivation causes increased receptor binding, which could mean a suppression of NE release here and consequently a receptor proliferation or up-regulation.[102] Impairment in the regulation of receptor sites could account for differences in satiety in normal-weight bulimic, underweight anorectic, and underweight anorectic patients with bulimia. Clinically, it has been observed that restricting anorectic patients eat a small amount of food and are satiated. Bulimic anorectic patients begin eating, lose control—or rather do not experience satiety—and eat anywhere from 2,000 to 4,000 calories, purge, and then starve until the next starve-binge-purge episode. They stay emaciated. Normal-weight bulimic patients restrict intake but not as long or as

effectively as the anorectic bulimics. They will eat enough between purges to maintain a normal weight. It seems reasonable to suspect that the mechanism of satiety, which ends a meal, is different in these groups.

Beta-endorphin, morphine, and a long-acting enkephalin analog, all opiate agonists, induce feeding when injected into the PVN. The hypothalamic centers that mediate feeding and satiety also mediate reward and aversion. Self-stimulation rate decreases with gastric and metabolic factors that cause satiety.[143] Dopamine blockers, such as pimozide, can decrease intravenous self-injection, self-stimulation, or feeding.[76] There is evidence that both opiates and nonopiate peptides, such as neurotensin, activate dopamine neurons in the ventral thalamic area (VTA) and that the VTA integrates a number of opiate and nonopiate inputs in the control of reward processes.[46] Dopamine cells of the VTA project in the mesocortical pathway to limbic areas including the nucleus accumbens. It is this system that has a role in self-stimulation and self-injection. Complex feeding responses such as bulimia can easily be considered a self-administrative and a self-stimulation behavior. Many patients with bulimia are unable to stop their bingeing behavior and will describe the process of binge eating as alleviating anxiety. Bulimic patients develop an urge to binge that is similar to an addict's craving for drugs. At this time the most effective programs in stopping this behavior involve very restrictive environments, such as hospitalization, or five-day-a-week therapy sessions or antidepressant medications. No one has studied the mechanism of how antidepressant drugs may be reducing binge-eating behavior.

Multimodal sensory feature detection from the amygdala in multimodal sensory choices from the cortex go through the globus pallidus. This activates ascending thalamic pathways and extrapyramidal motor pathways, which potentiate sensori-motor arcs that bring the animal into mental or behavioral proximity with rewarding food. The dopaminergic systems are necessary for self-administration behaviors, and it seems reasonable to postulate that the dopaminergic self-administration system is a major link in the control of food as a reinforcer. The self-stimulating aspect to bulimic behavior suggests an impairment in satiety related to the dopaminergic system and possibly to opiates. It would be reasonable to test opiate or dopaminergic antagonists in a satiety test paradigm in primary-eating-disorder patients.

Satiety is also influenced by nonopiate peptides such as cholecystokinin, which is produced in the gut and is responsible for intestinal induced satiety.[161] Selective gastric vagotomy eliminates its feeding-suppressive effect. It is possible that a defect in this mechanism of producing satiety is present in bulimic patients.

Impairment of the mechanisms that normally provide satiety information could contribute to the symptom choice (binge eating) in anorexia nervosa patients with bulimia and in normal-weight bulimic patients. Central mechanisms that control satiety also affect mood, which is usually disturbed in patients with bulimia nervosa. Developing a model to study satiety in primary-eating-disorder patients may give a clue to areas with central impairment.

Impairment of central mechanisms regulating feeding behavior, satiety, and hunger may be reflected in taste preferences. We know from animal studies that some lateral hypothalamus cells alter their rate of firing in response to the taste of a palatable food and fire with a background rate that is correlated with food deprivation.[112] Lateral hypothalamus cells can fire during operant barpress responses to obtain food and fire discriminantly to food cues.[37] We can assume that these cells combine internal homeostatic information with external food cues to participate in appetitive behavior for food. Specific neurotransmitter systems can trigger specific appetites. For example, animal studies suggest that NE-induced feeding is preferential for carbohydrates.[76] Morphine-treated rats tend to select fatty foods, and naloxone

hydrochloride shifts food choice away from fat.[126] It is possible that the foods the patient selects to overeat may provide a clue to which neural system causes the overeating, and it is also possible that the effect of the diet on neurotransmitter levels may provide clues to an effective treatment for aberrant eating behavior. Massively obese patients have a taste preference for mixtures with a high percent of lipids when compared with normal-weight adults.[25] There is a high association of taste preferences with food intake. Anorexia nervosa patients refuse to eat carbohydrate-containing foods, but paradoxically some will binge on foods containing a high fat or sugar content. Patients who binge may well have taste preferences that are similar to obese patients. Although the attitudes anorectic patients have toward food may effectively suppress expected behavioral eating response, the restricting anorectic patient's taste preference might be a good predictor as to whether that patient will develop bulimia nervosa after weight recovery. Since there is evidence that central mechanisms can trigger specific taste preferences, it is then reasonable to assume that impairment in the central mechanisms may affect taste preferences. Specific taste preferences can be related to specific satiety impairments. Specific pharmacological interventions to treat bulimic behavior may well affect taste preference, and a measure of taste preferences could well be a predictor for treatment outcome. To date, appetite and satiety mechanisms in the eating disorders have been virtually unstudied.

¶ Genetic and Familial Studies

Although anorexia nervosa seems to be relatively common with a prevalence of about one in 200 girls in the age of risk between twelve and eighteen years,[20] the incidence of anorexia nervosa is actually rather low, between 0.37 and 0.45 per 100,000.[91,164] Because of its relatively low incidence in the general population, the methods used to determine whether an illness has a genetic component have not been feasible for studying anorexia nervosa. The ascertainment of this disorder, especially in its mild forms, is unreliable when the assessment is retrospective. This is a problem with most of the family history studies that have been conducted on the eating disorders. Comparison of monozygotic versus dizygotic twins for concordance rates, comparison of twins reared together with those reared apart for concordance rates, the study of genetic markers, and examination of the adopted-away offspring of an affected individual have not been used to study genetic factors in anorexia nervosa.

In a review of ninety-four anorectic females, Theander[164] found six probands with seven sisters who had anorexia nervosa. He calculated that the morbidity risk for a sister of an anorectic patient is about 6.6 percent, which greatly exceeds normal expectation. Single case reports of anorexia nervosa occurring in both a mother and child are present in the literature in large series surveys of anorexia nervosa. The mother-daughter combination has been reported in 1 to 3 percent of the cases.[86,164] Kalucy and associates[86] found that 16 percent of the anorectic mothers and 23 percent of the fathers had a definite history of "significantly low adolescent weight."

There are also problems in interpreting the reports of anorexia in monozygotic and dizygotic twins. In some cases, zygoticity was determined crudely, and in other cases the twinship was not followed beyond the age of risk. A review of the reported monozygotic cases in the literature (of course, this is a biased sample) shows a concordance rate of 52 percent.[62,127,167] About fifty cases of anorexia nervosa twins have been described in the American and European literature, and of these cases less than one-fifth are dizygotic.[127,167] The concordance rate for anorexia nervosa in monozygotic twins is considerably higher than in dizygotic twins (only one case has been reported); however, the numbers are small and the sample is obviously biased. Therefore, no interpretation

can be made about the genetic influence from these case reports.

Recent studies of first-degree relatives of anorexia nervosa patients have shown a higher prevalence of affective disorder compared with a control population.[11,184] In another study, the prevalence of affective disorder in the first-degree relatives of both anorexia nervosa and bulimia nervosa patients was similar to the prevalence found in the first-degree relatives of patients with bipolar disorder.[78] All of these studies are fraught with methodological problems, ranging from small numbers to inconsistent methods of interviewing. Two of the better-designed family history studies[45,163] showed a higher prevalence of affective disorder in the first-degree relatives of eating-disorder patients compared with a normal control sample; however, they did not find a higher prevalence of eating disorders in the first-degree relatives of affective disorder probands. Therefore the authors of both studies suggested that an independent predisposition to anorexia must be superimposed on a predisposition to affective disorders for anorexia to be manifest. Both papers stated that anorexia nervosa or bulimia nervosa is not supported as a manifestation of the tendency to affective disorders because there was no excess of anorectic and bulimic patients among relatives of affective disorder probands.

It is likely that a stronger familial association will be found between alcoholism and anorexia and bulimia nervosa. To date, several studies have shown well-documented alcoholism in 12 to 19 percent of the fathers and 2 percent of the mothers.[28,65] Studies of the prevalence of eating disorders in alcoholic probands are now in progress.

About twelve cases of anorexia nervosa in association with the 45-XO genotype and Turner's phenotype have been reported.[24] This may represent a higher than expected association between these two disorders. At present there is not enough evidence to suggest that subtle X chromosome abnormalities are associated with anorexia and bulimia nervosa.

¶ Experimental Treatment of Anorexia and Bulimia Nervosa

The only controlled treatment studies in the eating disorders have involved drug treatment or behavioral-cognitive therapies. Experimental treatments will be defined as those treatments derived from hypothetical or empirically based clear-cut rationale, with the use of systematic observations and assessment of outcome. Family treatment studies and psychodynamically oriented psychotherapy in the treatment of the eating disorders will not be discussed in this chapter, since they have not been assessed with systematic unbiased observations, nor have they been tested in any controlled studies.

Behavioral and Cognitive Therapy

The recognized clinical feature of the fear of becoming obese in the disorder anorexia nervosa has naturally led to the conceptualization of anorexia nervosa as an eating or weight phobia. Brady and Rieger[7] have explicitly stated

they [the patients] behave rather as though they suffer from an eating phobia—eating generates anxiety, and their failure to eat represents avoidance. In other words, their cessation of eating after ingesting a very small portion of a meal (or removing it from the body by self-induced vomiting) is reinforced by anxiety reduction. From such an analysis, two treatment procedures suggest themselves; deconditioning the anxiety associated with eating and/or shaping eating behavior (and hence, weight gain) by making access to powerful reinforcers contingent on eating. (P. 1)

Systematic desensitization,[185] a behavior therapy often used for treatment of phobias, tries to inhibit the anxiety evoked by a gradual series of imagined scenes with concurrent deep muscle relaxation. Leitenberg and coworkers[103] succinctly state

the assumption [with systematic desensitization] is that the desired behavioral changes in the real situation will automatically occur as anxiety dissipates in therapy sessions. The conditioning strategy, on the other hand, attempts to gradually change overt behavior, the assumption being that each behavioral step forward will reduce anxiety. In essence, the systematic desensitization strategy takes care of anxiety and lets overt behavior take care of itself, while the operant strategy takes care of behavior and lets anxiety take care of itself. (P. 3)

The use of systematic desensitization without operant conditioning has not been effective in treating anorectic patients.[60,101,185] The operant conditioning paradigm has been the most effective form of behavior therapy for the treatment of anorexia nervosa. Initially social reinforcements (attention, conversation, and praise) were made contingent upon eating behavior. Later, weight gain was enhanced by reinforcement deprivation and by making visits and activities contingent on satisfactory weight gain. Experimental control procedures have been used to study the operant conditioning paradigm. In a series of five single-case experiments, using the technique of systematic analysis, Agras and associates[1] were able to demonstrate a strong effect of regular feedback information regarding weight and calorie intake on the actual weight gain. Without the feedback information, positive reinforcement appeared to be relatively ineffective. In that study the effect of negative reinforcement associating leaving the hospital with weight gain was removed by contracting a patient for a twelve-week stay for "research purposes," whether or not the patient gained weight. Thus positive reinforcement was shown to contribute independently to weight gain. Pertschuk and coworkers[134] used a multiple baseline experimental design to show the efficacy of an operant conditioning therapy in anorectic patients. Each subject received the experimental behavioral treatment at a different time during hospitalization for a period of thirteen days. The outcome, weight gain, was evaluated using the Rn statistic for this multiple baseline approach. For the group, medium weight gain before behavioral treatment was 0.09 kg per day; the weight gain per day over the thirteen behavior therapy days was 0.32 kg. Another study[186] compared the efficacy of an operant conditioning form of behavior therapy with a program of strict isolation, appetite-stimulating drugs, and psychotherapy in sixteen anorectic patients. The latter program was not free of behavioral contingencies, since it contained a strong negative reinforcer of strict isolation. However, in this study the rate of weight gain was three times as great for those patients receiving an operant conditioning program.

The only randomly assigned, controlled treatment study evaluating behavior therapy was a collaborative study involving three hospitals.[29] Actually, this was a study designed to compare the effectiveness of behavior therapy and milieu therapy, and the drug cyproheptadine hydrochloride and placebo. Patients were randomly assigned to four treatment cells. The behavior therapy was an operant conditioning paradigm in which patients were followed for thirty-five days. In this study there was no overall significant difference in weight gain between the behavior therapy group and the milieu therapy group. Those receiving behavior therapy gained weight at a rate of 4.2 kg per month compared with a rate of 3.6 kg per month for milieu therapy. Explanations for the lack of efficacy of behavior therapy in this study were: constant reinforcers were used in all patients instead of individualized reinforcers; and a schedule of delayed reinforcers given only every fifth day might not have been as effective as a schedule of more immediate daily reinforcers; and the milieu program, which did involve some isolation, may have produced a maximal possible weight gain so that behavior therapy could not be expected to do any better. The authors felt that if these patients had been followed until they reached their target weight, there may have been a difference in the rate of weight gain in those receiving behavior therapy compared with those who had milieu therapy.

Response prevention is a technique that is currently being studied for the treatment of bulimia nervosa.[117,130] In hospitalized treatment programs response prevention is frequently used with bingeing and purging patients by requiring the patients to stay in an observed day room area for two to three hours after every meal. Very few patients vomit in front of other people, and thus the emesis response is prevented and, after a period of time, extinguished. In outpatient programs a response-prevention technique is used in a similar manner in that patients are either requested to bring in the foods they wish to binge on or are provided with those foods and then instructed to go ahead and eat as much as they wish. After the eating episode the therapist stays in the room until the patient's urge to vomit dissipates. Other techniques such as stimulus narrowing, self-reinforcement, and self-control relaxation are also being studied.[117] Five years from now we should have the result of randomly assigned controlled studies using many of these techniques.

Cognitive therapy techniques are being developed both for individual and group psychotherapy. The assessment of cognitions is the first step in cognitive therapy. Patients are often asked to write down thoughts on an assessment form so that the anorectic cognitions can be examined for systematic distortions in the processing and interpretation of events. This technique uses variations of Beck's cognitive behavior therapy.[4] Garner and Bemis,[41] in an excellent paper, describe the use of cognitive techniques such as operationalizing beliefs, decentering, the "what if" technique, evaluation of autonomic thoughts, prospective hypothesis testing, reinterpretation of body image misperception, examination of underlying assumptions, and modification of basic assumptions. Group therapies using both cognitive and behavioral treatment have been carefully designed,[15,32,95,96] but thus far no randomly assigned controlled treatment study has been completed. Preliminary open case studies show that these behavioral techniques should be effective.

Drug Treatment

Surprisingly, there are very few randomly assigned double-blind controlled drug studies in anorexia nervosa patients. The open drug trials are contaminated with concomitant use of psychotherapy and/or some type of behavioral contingency program. The first drug used in the treatment of anorexia nervosa was chlorpromazine.[23] This study was not a controlled treatment one; however, the authors did compare the rate of weight gain of patients on chlorpromazine with two other treatment groups; one had bed rest and one received insulin treatment. The average weight gain per week was significantly higher for chlorpromazine compared with either of the other groups, and the authors attributed the weight gain to the drug's overcoming the patient's resistance to food and panic at the time of eating. It is of interest to note that in this study more patients from the chlorpromazine-treated group developed a period of compulsive overeating compared with the group that had received only bed rest (45 percent compared with 12 percent). Chlorpromazine may stimulate weight gain through its dopamine antagonist action. However, since weight gain can be induced very effectively in anorexia nervosa without the use of any medication, it does not seem justified to use chlorpromazine except perhaps in those very severely agitated and anxious anorectic patients.

Anorexia patients have many depressive symptoms such as sleep disturbance, irritability, depressed mood, and difficulty concentrating.[67] Some biological signs found in depression, such as dexamethasone resistance, decreased MHPG secretion, and an impaired GH response to levodopa, are also present in anorectic patients. These observations have stimulated the treatment of anorectic patients with antidepressant medication. A recent double-blind study in which seventy-two anorectic patients were randomly assigned to amitriptyline hydrochloride, cyproheptadine hydrochloride, an antihistaminic drug, and placebo, showed that both cyproheptadine and amitriptyline had a marginal effect on decreasing the number of days necessary to achieve a normal weight. Cyproheptadine had an unexpected antidepressant effect demonstrated by a significant decrease on Hamilton Depression Ratings.[69] A differential drug effect was present on the bulimic subgroups of the anorectic patients, with cyproheptadine significantly increasing treatment efficiency for the bulimic patients when compared with the amitriptyline and placebo groups. The differential cyproheptadine effect on the anorectic-bulimic subgroups is the first pharmacological evidence for the validity of the subgroups.

Clomipramine hydrochloride given in a dosage of 50 mg at bedtime showed no main effect on weight gain in a randomly assigned double-blind controlled study with sixteen anorectic patients.[97] However, patients receiving clomipramine were more stable in their eating habits and maintained their weight better than those on placebo after completing the treatment study. Increased hunger and appetite as measured on analogue scales and caloric intake were associated with clomipramine. The authors thought the lack of increased weight may have been due to increased activity in the patients on the drug.

Lithium carbonate showed no overall effect on weight gain in a four-week double-blind study in sixteen anorexia nervosa patients.[55] There is little justification for using lithium in treating anorexia nervosa, since the risks of toxicity are high in patients who restrict fluid intake and who purge. Another double-blind crossover study compared eleven anorectic patients with delta[9]-tetrahydrocannabinol(delta[9]-THC) and eleven anorectic patients with an active placebo, diazepam. The drug had no overall effect on weight gain, and three of eleven patients experienced adverse reactions of paranoid ideation and feelings of loss of control.[56]

Naloxone hydrochloride was infused in anorexia nervosa patients to determine its effect on weight gain and lipolysis.[118] Some of these patients were on a behavior therapy program and others received amitriptyline. There was virtually no standardized methodology; the naloxone was administered in some patients for one week and in other patients for eleven weeks. Also, the naloxone was given at different periods in the hospital stay. Because the study was complicated with other treatments and had no systematic methodology, no conclusions can be made on the effect of naloxone in the treatment of anorexia nervosa.

Gastrointestinal symptoms such as postprandial epigastric pain, belching, vomiting, anorexia, and early satiety were significantly improved by the drug metoclopramide hydrochloride in a double-blind study.[154] This drug may be useful in a select group of anorectic patients with these gastrointestinal symptoms.

Because of the association of depressive symptomatology and the high prevalence of depression in first-degree relatives of patients with bulimia, antidepressants have also been used to treat this condition. In a randomly assigned, double-blind study with imipramine in twenty-two bulimic patients, the drug effect led to a reduced frequency of bingeing, decreased intensity of binges, decreased preoccupation with food, greater subjective global improvement, and decreased depression as measured by the Hamilton Depression Scale.[138]

In contrast to this study, mianserin hydrochloride, a tetracyclic piperazinoazepine, was found to have no effect on reducing bingeing behavior or depression in a randomly assigned, double-blind controlled study of fifty bulimic patients.[153]

In a recently reported study with a double-blind trial of twenty-two bulimic patients, desipramine produced a significant reduction in frequency and severity of bulimic symptoms while placebo produced no change.[80]

The mood disturbance of patients with bulimia has been equated to that of patients with atypical depression or depression with many symptoms of anxiety. Because of this observation, some clinicians have been treating bulimic patients with monoamine oxidase inhibitors (MAOIs). In a recent eight-week, double-blind study of phenelzine in twenty bulimic patients, the phenelzine-treated group had significantly fewer binges per week compared with the placebo group. No patients experienced a hypertensive reaction during this study, although they were carefully screened for compliance to a tyramine-free diet. The use of phenelzine is restricted to a biased population of patients who will not only comply with drug administration but will also adhere to a special diet. The effect of MAOIs on bulimia could be independent of their antidepressant activity.[177]

An anticonvulsant drug, phenytoin, has been studied in an open trial[53] and in a double-blind crossover trial in bulimic patients.[181] In the latter study of nineteen bulimic patients, there was a significant decrease in binges among subjects who received phenytoin preceding placebo. Phenytoin was effective in preventing binges at serum levels as low as 5 ug per ml. There was no association of EEG abnormalities and response to the medication. Another anticonvulsant drug, carbamazepine, was studied in six bulimic outpatients in a double-blind crossover trial over twenty weeks. Five patients had no drug response, but one with a history suggestive of bipolar disorder responded with complete cessation of binge eating.[87]

The immediate effects of methylamphetamine given intravenously under double-blind conditions was assessed in eight patients with bulimia. In laboratory conditions these bulimic patients reduced their food intake significantly more so on the drug compared with placebo. Also, none of the drug patients followed their meal with self-induced vomiting or purgation.[129]

Fenfluramine, studied by the same authors and in the same experimental paradigm, also suppressed the amount of food intake in patients with bulimia nervosa.[149] Two dopamine antagonist drugs, pimozide and sulpiride, have been studied in double-blind placebo crossover trials in anorexia nervosa patients. Each drug trial used eighteen patients and had a crossover period after three weeks. Pimozide[168] showed an almost significant effect on weight gain in the first period of the crossover trial, while sulpiride[166] also showed a tendency for increased daily weight gain during the first medication period. Thus the specific dopamine antagonist drugs did not have a dramatic effect on weight gain in the anorectic patients.

After considering all of these studies, recommendations to the clinician would be to use medications in the anorexia nervosa patients as an adjunct treatment. If an anorectic patient has a predominance of depressive symptomatology, a trial on amitriptyline or cyproheptadine is warranted. Behavioral contingencies are very useful in inducing weight gain and changing the patient's medical condition. With medical rehabilitation there is an associated improvement in the psychological state.[120] A bulimia nervosa patient with anxiety and depressive symptomatology may respond to phenelzine, imipramine, or desipramine, and some bulimic patients may respond with a reduction of bingeing episodes to phenytoin. Severely obsessive-compulsive, anxious, and delusional anorectic patients are likely to require chlorpromazine.

¶ Bibliography

1. AGRAS, S., et al. "Behavior Modification of Anorexia Nervosa," *Archives of General Psychiatry,* 30 (1974):279–286.
2. ANYAN, W. R. "Changes in Erythrocyte Sedimentation Rate and Fibrinogen During Anorexia Nervosa," *Journal of Pediatrics,* 85 (1974):525–527.
3. APERIA, A. "Renal Function in Anorexia Nervosa," *Acta Pediatrica Scandinavica,* 67 (1978):219–224.
4. BECK, A. T. *Cognitive Theory and Emotional Disorders.* New York: International Universities Press, 1976.
5. BOWERS, T. K., and ECKERT, E. "Leukopenia in Anorexia Nervosa: Lack of Increased Risk of Infection," *Archives of Internal Medicine,* 138 (1978):1520–1523.
6. BOYAR, R. N., et al. "Cortisol Secretion and Metabolism in Anorexia Nervosa," *New England Journal of Medicine,* 296 (1977):190–193.
7. BRADY, J. P., and RIEGER, W. "Behavior Treatment of Anorexia Nervosa," in *Proceedings of the International Symposium on Behavior Modification.* New York: Appleton-Century-Crofts, 1972, p. 1.
8. BROWN, G. M., et al. "Endocrine Profiles in Anorexia Nervosa," in R. A. Vigersky, ed., *Anorexia Nervosa.* New York: Raven Press, 1977, pp. 123–125.
9. BURRINGTON, J. D. "Superior-Mesentary-Artery Syndrome in Children," *American Journal Diseases of Children,* 130 (1976):1367–1370.
10. CALLOWAY, P., et al. "Autonomic Arousal in Eating Disorders," *British Journal of Psychiatry,* 142 (1983):38–42.
11. CANTWELL, D. P., et al. "Anorexia Nervosa, An Affective Disorder," *Archives of General Psychiatry,* 34 (1977):1087–1093.
12. CARRYER, H. M., et al. "Relative Lymphocytosis in Anorexia Nervosa," *Staff Meetings of the Mayo Clinic,* 34 (1959): 426–432.
13. CASPER, R. C., et al. "An Evaluation of Trace Metals, Vitamins and Taste Function in Anorexia Nervosa," *American Journal Clinical Nutrition,* 33 (1980): 1801–1808.
14. CHOPRA, I. A., et al. "Circulating Thyroid Hormones and Thyrotropin in Adult Patients with Protein-Calorie Malnutrition," *Journal of Clinical Endocrinology and Metabolism,* 40 (1975):221–227.
15. CINSIRIPINI, P. M., et al. "A Behavioral Program for the Management of Anorexia and Bulimia," *Journal of Nervous and Mental Disease,* 171 (1983):186–189.
16. CORNBLEET, P. J., et al. "A Histal Chemical Study of Bone Marrow Hypophlasia in Anorexia Nervosa," *Virchow's Archives of Pathology, Anatomy and Histology,* 374 (1977):239–247.
17. COX, K., et al. "Biochemical and Ultrasonic Abnormalities of the Pancreas in Anorexia Nervosa," *Digestive Diseases and Sciences,* 28 (1983):225–229.
18. CRISP, A. H., et al. "A Controlled Study of EEG in Anorexia Nervosa," *British Journal of Psychiatry,* 114 (1968):1149–1160.
19. CRISP, A. H., et al. "Aspects of Fat Metabolism in Anorexia Nervosa," *Metabolism* 17 (1968):1109–1118.
20. CRISP, A. H., et al. "How Common Is Anorexia Nervosa? A Prevalence Study,"

British Journal of Psychiatry, 128 (1976):549–556.

21. CROXSON, M. S., et al. "Low Serum Tri-iodothyronine and Hypothyroidism in Anorexia Nervosa," *Journal Endocrinology and Metabolism,* 44 (1977):167–174.

22. DALLY, P. J. *Anorexia Nervosa.* London: Heinemann, 1969.

23. DALLY, P. J., and SARGENT, W. "A New Treatment of Anorexia Nervosa," *British Medical Journal,* 1 (1960):1770–1773.

24. DOUGHERTY, G., et al. "Anorexia Nervosa in Treated Gonadal Dysgenesis: A Case Report and Review," *Journal of Clinical Psychiatry,* 44 (1983):219–221.

25. DREWNOWSKI, A., et al. "Taste Responses in Massively Obese Patients," *Proceedings of the Fourth International Congress on Obesity,* New York, 1983.

26. DUBOIS, A., et al. "Altered Gastric Emptying and Secretion in Primary Anorexia Nervosa," *Gastroenterology,* 77 (1979):319–323.

27. DUBOIS, A., et al. "Effect of Bethanechol on Gastric Functions in Primary Anorexia Nervosa," *Digestive Diseases and Sciences,* 26 (1981):598–600.

28. ECKERT, E. D., et al. "Alcoholism in Anorexia Nervosa," in R. W. Pikens and L. L. Heston, eds., *Psychiatric Factors and Drug Abuse.* New York: Grune & Stratton, 1979, pp. 283–294.

29. ECKERT, E. D., et al. "Behavior Therapy and Anorexia Nervosa," *British Journal of Psychiatry,* 134 (1979):55–59.

30. ENZMANN, D. R., and LANE, B. "Cranial Computed Tomography Findings in Anorexia Nervosa," *Journal of Computer Assisted Tomography,* 1 (1977):410–414.

31. ESSEN, B., et al. "Skeletal Muscle Fiber Types and Sizes in Anorexia Nervosa Patients," *Clinical Physiology,* 1 (1981):395–403.

32. FAIRBURN, C. "A Cognitive Behavioral Approach to the Treatment of Bulimia," *Psychological Medicine,* 11 (1981):707–711.

33. FALK, J. R., and HALMI, K. A. "Amenorrhea in Anorexia Nervosa: Examination of the Critical Body Hypothesis," *Journal Biological Psychiatry,* 17 (1982):799–806.

34. FIORILLO, A., and PELLTIERI, L. "Anorexia Nervosa—In a Patient with a Clivus Tumor," *Acta Neurologica,* 32 (1977):427–431.

35. FOHLIN, L. "Exercise Performance and Body Dimension in Anorexia Nervosa Before and After Rehabilitation," *Acta Medica Scandinavica,* 204 (1978):61–65.

36. ———. "Function and Dimension of the Circulatory System in Anorexia Nervosa," *Acta Pediatrica Scandinavica,* 67 (1978):11–16.

37. FRANKLIN, K. "Catecholamines and Self-Stimulation: Reward and Performance Effects Disassociated," *Pharmacology and Biochemistry of Behavior,* 11 (1979):71–75.

38. FREYSCHUSS, U., et al. "Limb Circulation in Anorexia Nervosa," *Acta Pediatrica Scandinavica,* 67 (1978):225–228.

39. FROESE, A. P., et al. "The Superior-Mesentary-Artery Syndrome," *Canadian Psychiatric Association Journal,* 23 (1978):325–327.

40. GARFINKEL, P., et al. "Hypothalamic-Pituitary Function in Anorexia Nervosa," *Archives of General Psychiatry,* 32 (1975):739–744.

41. GARNER, D. M., and BEMIS, K. M. "A Cognitive-Behavioral Approach to Anorexia Nervosa," *Cognitive Therapy and Research,* 6 (1982):123–150.

42. GERNER, R. H., and GWIRTSMAN, H. L. "Abnormalities of Dexamethasone Suppression Test in Urinary MHPG in Anorexia Nervosa," *American Journal of Psychiatry,* 138 (1981):650–653.

43. GERNER, R. H., and HARE, T. A. "CSF GABA in Normal Subjects and Patients with Depression, Schizophrenia, Mania and Anorexia Nervosa," *American Journal of Psychiatry,* 138 (1981):1098–1101.

44. GERNER, R. H., and SHARP, B. "CSF Beta-Endorphin-Immunoreactivity in Normal, Schizophrenic, Depressed, Manic and Anorexic Subjects," *Brain Research,* 237 (1982):244–247.

45. GERSHON, E. S., et al. "Anorexia Nervosa and Major Affective Disorders Associated in Families: A Preliminary Report", in S. B. Guze, F. J. Earles, and J. E. Barrett, eds., *Childhood Psychopathology and Development.* New York: Raven Press, 1983, pp. 279–287.

46. GLINCHER, P., et al. "Neurotensin: A New Reward Peptide," *Brain Research,* in press.

47. GOLD, M. S., et al. "TSH & GH Responses to TRH in Anorexia Nervosa," *International Journal of Psychiatry in Medicine,* 10 (1981):51–57.

48. GOLD, P. W. "Abnormalities in Plasma and Cerebral Spinal Fluid Arginine Vasopressin in Patients with Anorexia Nervosa," *New England Journal of Medicine,* 308 (1983):1117–1123.

49. GOLDNEY, R. "Craniopharyngioma Stimulating Anorexia Nervosa," *Journal of Nervous and Mental Disease,* 166 (1978):135–138.

50. GOLLA, J. A. "An Immunological Assessment of Patients with Anorexia Nervosa," *American Journal of Clinical Nutrition,* 34 (1981):2756–2762.

51. GOTSCH, F. M., "Reversible Granulocyte Killing Defects in Anorexia Nervosa," *Clinical and Experimental Immunology,* 21 (1975):244–249.

52. GOTTDIENER, J. S., et al. "Effects of Self-Induced Starvation on Cardiac Size and Function in Anorexia Nervosa," *Circulation,* 58 (1978):425–433.

53. GREEN, R. F., and RAU, J. H. "The Use of Diphenylhydantoin in Compulsive Eating Disorders," in R. A. Vigersky, ed., *Anorexia Nervosa.* New York: Raven Press, 1977, pp. 377–382.

54. GROSS, H. A., et al. "Catecholamine Metabolism in Primary Anorexia Nervosa," *Endocrinology and Metabolism,* 49 (1979):805–809.

55. GROSS, H. A., et al. "A Double Blind Controlled Trial of Lithium Carbonate in Primary Anorexia Nervosa," *Journal of Clinical Psychopharmacology,* 1 (1981): 376–381.

56. GROSS, H. A., et al. "A Double Blind Trial of TetrahydrocannabinolΔ^9-Tetrahydrocannabinol in Primary Anorexia Nervosa," *Journal of Clinical Psychopharmacology,* 3 (1983):165–171.

57. GROSSMAN, S. P. "The Biology of Motivation," *Annual Reviews of Psychology,* 30 (1979):209–242.

58. GWIRTSMAN, H. E., et al. "Neuroendocrine Abnormalities in Bulimia," *American Journal of Psychiatry,* 140 (1983): 559–563.

59. HALL, A. "Family Structure and Relationships of 50 Female Anorexia Nervosa Patients," *Australia and New Zealand Journal of Psychiatry,* 12 (1978):263–268.

60. HALLSTEN, E. A. "Adolescent Anorexia Nervosa Treated by Desensitization," *Behavior Research and Therapy,* 3 (1965):87–91.

61. HALMI, K. A. "Selective Pituitary Deficiency in Anorexia Nervosa," in E. J. Sachar, ed., *Hormones, Behavior and Psychopathology.* New York: Raven Press, 1976, pp. 285–289.

62. HALMI, K. A., and BRODLAND, G. "Monozygotic Twins Concordant and Discordant for Anorexia Nervosa," *Psychological Medicine,* 3 (1973):521–524.

63. HALMI, K. A., and FALK, J. R. "Common Physiological Changes in Anorexia Nervosa," *International Journal of Eating Disorders,* 1 (1981):16–27.

64. HALMI, K. A., and FRY, M. "Serum Lipids in Anorexia Nervosa," *Biological Psychiatry,* 8 (1974):159–167.

65. HALMI, K. A., and LONEY, J. "Familial Alcoholism in Anorexia Nervosa," *British Journal of Psychiatry,* 123 (1973):53–54.

66. HALMI, K. A., and SHERMAN, B. S. "Prediction of Treatment Response in Anorexia Nervosa," in Obiols et al., ed., *Biological Psychiatry Today.* Elsevier/North Holland Biomedical Press, 1979, Amsterdam: pp. 609–614.

67. HALMI, K. A., et al. "Pretreatment Evaluation in Anorexia Nervosa," in R. A. Vigersky, ed., *Anorexia Nervosa.* New York: Raven Press, 1977, pp. 45–54.

68. HALMI, K. A., et al. "Catecholamine Metabolism in Anorexia Nervosa," *Archives of General Psychiatry,* 35 (1978): 458–460.

69. HALMI, K. A., et al. "Anorexia Nervosa: Treatment Efficacy of Cyproheptadine and Amitriptyline," *Archives of General Psychiatry,* in press.

70. HALMI, K. A., et al. "Amino Acids in Anorexia Nervosa," in preparation.

71. HANDLER, C. E., and PERKIN, G. D. "Anorexia Nervosa and Wernicke's Encephalopathy," *Lancet,* 2 (1982):771–772.

72. HASLER, J. F. "Parotic Enlargement: A Presenting Sign of Anorexia Nervosa," *Oral Medicine,* 6 (1982):567–573.

73. HEINZ, E. R., et al. "Reversibility of Cerebral Atrophy in Anorexia Nervosa and Cushing's Syndrome," *Journal of Computed Assisted Tomography*, 1 (1977): 415–418.

74. HELLSTROM, I. "Oral Complications in Anorexia Nervosa," *Scandinavian Journal of Dental Research*, 85 (1977):71–76.

75. HERON, G. B., and JOHNSTON, D. A. "Hypothalamic Tumor Presenting as Anorexia Nervosa," *American Journal of Psychiatry*, 133 (1976):580–582.

76. HOEBEL, B. "Hypothalamic Self-Stimulation and Stimulation Escape in Relation to Feeding and Mating," *Federation Proceedings*, 38 (1979):2454–2461.

77. HOLT, S. E., et al. "Abnormal Gastric Emptying in Primary Anorexia Nervosa," *British Journal of Psychiatry*, 139 (1981):550–552.

78. HUDSON, J. I., et al. "Family History of Anorexia Nervosa and Bulimia," *British Journal of Psychiatry*, 142 (1983):133–138.

79. HUDSON, J. I., et al. "Hypothalamic-Pituitary-Adrenal Axis Hyperactivity in Bulimia," *Psychiatry Research*, 8 (1983):111–117.

80. HUGHES, P. L., et al. "A Controlled Trial Using Desipramine for Bulimia," Paper presented at the American Psychiatric Association Meeting, Los Angeles, May 5–11, 1984, Abstract # NR78.

81. JACKSON, A. A., et al. "The Energy Cost of Repleting Tissue Deficits During Recovery from Protein-Energy Malnutrition," *American Journal of Clinical Nutrition*, 32 (1979):1396–1400.

82. JENNINGS, K. P. "Acute Gastric Dilatation in Anorexia Nervosa," *British Medical Journal*, 2 (1974):477–478.

83. JHANWAR-UNIYAL, M., et al. "Impact of Food Deprivation on Hypothalamic Alpha-Adrenergic Receptor Activity and Norepinephrine Turnover in Rat Brain," *Abstracts of the Society of Neuroscience*, 8 (1982):711.

84. JOHNSON, C., et al. "Short Term Group Treatment of Bulimia," *International Journal of Eating Disorders*, 2 (1983): 199–208.

85. KALAGER, T., et al. "Cardiac Performance in Patients with Anorexia Nervosa," *Cardiology*, 63 (1978):1–4.

86. KALUCY, R. S., et al. "A Study of 56 Families with Anorexia Nervosa," *British Journal of Medical Psychology*, 50 (1977):381–395.

87. KAPLAN, A. S., et al. "Carbamazepine in the Treatment of Bulimia," *American Journal of Psychiatry*, 140 (1983):1225–1226.

88. KATZ, J. L., et al. "Weight and Circadian LH Secretory Pattern in Anorexia Nervosa," *Psychosomatic Medicine*, 40 (1978):549–567.

89. KAYE, W. H., et al. "Cerebrospinal Fluid Opioid Activity in Anorexia Nervosa," *American Journal of Psychiatry*, 139 (1982):643–646.

90. KAYE, W. H., et al. "Abnormalities in Central Nervous System Monoamine Metabolism in Anorexia Nervosa," *Archives of General Psychiatry*, 41 (1984):350–355.

91. KENDELL, R. E., et al. "The Epidemiology of Anorexia Nervosa," *Psychological Medicine*, 3 (1973):200–206.

92. KEYS, A., and BROZEK, J. "Body Fat in Adult Man," *Physiological Reviews*, 33 (1953):245–260.

93. KUBANEK, B., et al. "Hamatologische Veranderungen Ver Anorexia Nervosa," *Blut*, 35 (1977):115–124.

94. KUPFER, D. J., and FOSTER, F. G. "The Sleep of Psychotic Patients: Does It All Look Alike?" in D. X. Freedman, ed., *Biology of the Major Psychoses*. New York: Raven Press, 1975, pp. 143–164.

95. LACEY, J. H. "An Outpatient Treatment Program for Bulimia Nervosa," *International Journal of Eating Disorders*, 2 (1983):209–241.

96. ——— "Bulimia Nervosa, Binge Eating and Psychogenic Vomiting: A Controlled Treatment Study and Long-term Outcome," *British Medical Journal*, 286 (1983):1609–1613.

97. LACEY, J. H., and CRISP, A. H. "Hunger, Food Intake and Weight: The Impact of Chlorimipramine on a Refeeding Anorexia Nervosa Population," *Post Graduate Medical Journal*, 56 (1980): 79–85.

98. LACEY, J. H., et al. "Weight Gain and the Sleeping Electroencephalogram," *British Medical Journal*, 431 (1975):556–558.

99. LACEY, J. H., et al. "Weight and Skeletal

Maturation," *Post Graduate Medical Journal,* 55 (1979):38–55.

100. LAMPERT, F., and LAU, B. "Bone Marrow Hypoplasia in Anorexia Nervosa," *European Journal of Pediatrics,* 124 (1976): 65–71.

101. LANG, P. J. "Behavior Therapy with a Case of Anorexia Nervosa," in L. P. Ullmann and L. Krosner, eds., *Case Studies in Behavior Modification.* New York: Holt, Rinehart and Winston, 1965, pp. 35–41.

102. LEIBOWITZ, S. F. "Neurochemical Systems of the Hypothalamus: Control of Feeding and Drinking Behavior and Water-Electrolyte Excretion," in P. J. Morgan and J. Panksept, eds., *Handbook of the Hypothalamus,* vol. 3A, *Behavioral Studies of the Hypothalamus.* New York: Marcel Dekker, pp. 299–437.

103. LEITENBERG, H., et al. "A Sequential Analysis of the Effect of Selective Positive Reinforcement in Modifying Anorexia Nervosa," *Behavior Research and Therapy,* 6 (1968):211–218.

104. LUCK, P., and WAKELING, A. "Altered Thresholds for Thermoregulatory Sweating and Vasodilitation in Anorexia Nervosa," *British Medical Journal,* 281 (1980):906–908.

105. ———. "Set-Point Displacement for Behavioral Thermoregulation in Anorexia Nervosa," *Clinical Science,* 62 (1980): 677–682.

106. ———. "Increased Cutaneous Vasoreactivity to Cold in Anorexia Nervosa," *Clinical Science,* 61 (1981):559–567.

107. LUNDBERG, P. O., et al. "Effects of TRH on Plasma Levels of TSH in Anorexia Nervosa," *European Journal of Clinical Investigation,* 2 (1972):150–153.

108. MCARNARNEY, E. R. "Rib Fractures in Anorexia Nervosa," *Journal of Adolescent Health Care,* 4 (1983):40–43.

109. MCCULLAGH, E. P., and TUPPER, W. R. "Anorexia Nervosa," *Annals of Internal Medicine,* 14 (1940):817–838.

110. MANT, M. J., and FARAGHER, B. S. "The Hematology of Anorexia Nervosa," *British Journal of Hematology,* 23 (1972):737–749.

111. MARSHALL, M., and FRASER, T. R. "Amenorrhea in Anorexia Nervosa: Assessment and Treatment with Chlomi-phene Citrate," *British Medical Journal,* 4 (1971):590–592.

112. MARX-KAUFMAN, R., and KANAREK, R. B. "Modifications of Nutrient Selection Induced by Naloxone in Rats," *Psychopharmacology,* 74 (1981):321–324.

113. MATTHEWS, B. J., and LACEY, J. H. "Skeletal Maturation, Growth and Hormone and Nutritional Status in Anorexia Nervosa," *International Journal of Eating Disorders,* 2 (1983):145–150.

114. MITCHELL, J. E., and BANTLE, J. P. "Metabolic and Endocrine Investigations in Women of Normal Weight and the Bulimia Syndrome," *Biological Psychiatry,* 18 (1983):355–365.

115. MITCHELL, J. E., et al. "Electrolyte and Other Physiological Abnormalities in Patients with Bulimia," *Psychological Medicine,* 13 (1983):273–278.

116. MIYAI, K., et al. "Serum Thyroid Hormones and Thyrotropin in Anorexia Nervosa," *Journal of Endocrinology and Metabolism,* 40 (1975):334–338.

117. MIZES, J. S., and LOHR, J. M. "The Treatment of Bulimia," *International Journal of Eating Disorders,* 2 (1983):59–66.

118. MOORE, A., et al. "Naloxone in the Treatment of Anorexia Nervosa: Effect on Weight Gain and Lipolysis," *Journal of the World Society of Medicine,* 74 (1981):129–135.

119. MORDASINI, R., et al. "Secondary Type II Hyperlipal Proteinemia in Patients with Anorexia Nervosa," *Metabolism,* 27 (1978):71–79.

120. MORGAN, H. G., and RUSSELL, G. F. M. "Values of Family Background in Clinical Features of Predictors of Long-term Outcome in Anorexia Nervosa," *Psychological Medicine,* 5 (1975):355–371.

121. MOSHANG, T., et al. "Low Serum Triiodothyronine in Patients with Anorexia Nervosa," *Journal of Endocrinology and Metabolism,* 40 (1975):470–473.

122. NELL, J. F., et al. "Waking and All-Night Sleep EEGs in Anorexia Nervosa," *Clinical Electroencephalography,* 11 (1980): 9–15.

123. NESTEL, P. J. "Cholesterol Metabolism in Anorexia Nervosa and Hypercholesterolemia," *Journal of Clinical Endocrinology and Metabolism,* 38 (1974):325–328.

124. NEW, P. F. J., et al. "Computed Tomography in Cerebral Abscess," *Radiology,* 121 (1976):641–646.

125. NILLIUS, S. J., and WIDE, L. "Effects of Prolonged Luteinizing Hormone-Releasing Hormone Therapy on Follicular Maturation, Ovulation and Corpus Luteum Function in Amenorrheic Women with Anorexia Nervosa," *Upsala Journal of Medical Science,* 84 (1979):21–35.

126. NISHINO, H., et al. "Lateral Hypothalamic Neuron Activity During Monkey Bar Press Feeding Behavior: Modulation by Glucose, Morphine and Naloxone, in B. Hoebel and S. Novin, eds., *The Neural Basis of Feeding and Reward,* Brunswick, Maine: Haet Institute, pp. 355–372.

127. NOWLIN, N. S. "Anorexia Nervosa in Twins: Case Report and Review," *Journal of Clinical Psychiatry,* 44 (1983): 101–105.

128. NUSSBAUM, M., et al. "Cerebral Atrophy in Anorexia Nervosa," *Journal of Pediatrics,* 96 (1980):867–869.

129. ONG, Y. L. "Suppression of Bulimic Symptoms with Methylamphetamine," *British Journal of Psychiatry,* 143 (1983): 288–293.

130. OWEN, W. P., et al. "Dopamine Regulation in Anorexia Nervosa," *Psychopharmacology Bulletin,* 19 (1983):578–581.

131. PALMBLAD, J., "Anorexia Nervosa and Polymorphonuclear (PMN) Granulocyte Reactions," *Scandinavian Journal of Hematology,* (1977):334–342.

132. PALOSSY, B., and OO, N. "ECG Alterations in Anorexia Nervosa," *Advances in Cardiology,* 19 (1977):280–282.

133. PERTSCHUK, M. J. "Immunocompetency in Anorexia Nervosa," *American Journal of Clinical Nutrition,* 35 (1982):968–972.

134. PERTSCHUK, M. J., et al. "A Multiple Baseline Approach to Behavioral Intervention in Anorexia Nervosa," *Behavior Research and Therapy,* 9 (1978):368–376.

135. PIMSTONE, B. et al. "Studies on Growth Hormone Secretion in Protein Calorie Malfunction," *American Journal Clinical Nutrition,* 21 (1968):482–485.

136. PIMSTONE, B., et al. "TSH Response to Synthetic Thyrotropin-Releasing Hormone in Human Protein-Calorie Malnutrition," *Journal of Clinical Endocrinology and Metabolism,* 36 (1973): 779–783.

137. PIRKE, K. M., et al. "Hypothalamic Regulation of Gonadotropin Secretion in Anorexia Nervosa and in Starvation," *International Journal of Eating Disorders,* 2 (1983):151–158.

138. POPE, H., et al. "Bulimia Treated with Imipramine: A Placebo-Controlled Double-Blind Study," *American Journal of Psychiatry,* 140 (1983):554–558.

139. POPS, M. A., and SCHWABE, A. B. "Hypercarotenemia in Anorexia Nervosa," *Journal of the American Medical Association,* 205 (1968):121–122.

140. POWERS, P. S. "Heart Failure During Treatment of Anorexia Nervosa," *American Journal of Psychiatry,* 139 (1982):1167–1170.

141. ROBBOY, M. S., et al. "The Hypercarotenemia in Anorexia Nervosa: A Comparison of Vitamin A and Carotene Levels in Various Forms of Menstrual Dysfunction Protexia," *American Journal of Clinical Nutrition,* 27 (1974):326–327.

142. RODGER, M. W., and COLLYER, J. A. "Anorexia Nervosa with Concealed Hyperphagia and Self-Induced Vomiting, Hypokalemic Alkalosis and Normal Aldosterone Excretion," *Canadian Medical Association Journal,* 103 (1979):415–418.

143. ROLLS, E. T. "Feeding and Reward," in B. Hoebel and S. Novin, eds., *The Neural Basis of Feeding and Reward.* Brunswick, ME: Haet Institute, 1982, pp. 323–338.

144. ROOT, A. W. and POWERS, P. S. "Anorexia Nervosa Presenting as Growth Retardation in Adolescence," *Journal of Adolescent Health Care,* 4 (1983):25–30.

145. RUSSELL, D., et al. "A Comparison Between Muscle Function and Body Composition in Anorexia Nervosa: The Effect of Refeeding," *American Journal of Clinical Nutrition,* 38 (1983):229–237.

146. RUSSELL, D., et al. "Delayed Gastric Emptying and Improvement with Domperidone in Patients with Anorexia Ner-

vosa," *American Journal of Psychiatry,* 140 (1983):1235–1236.

147. RUSSELL, G. F. M. "Acute Dilatation of the Stomach in a Patient with Anorexia Nervosa," *British Journal of Psychiatry,* 112 (1966):203–207.

148. ———. "Metabolic, Endocrine and Psychiatric Aspects of Anorexia Nervosa," *Scientific Basis of Medicine Annual Review,* 14 (1969):236–255.

149. ———. Personal communication, 1984.

150. ———. Personal communication, 1984.

151. ———, and BRUCE, J. T. "Impaired Water Diuresis in Patients with Anorexia Nervosa," *American Journal of Medicine,* 40 (1966):38–48.

152. RUSSELL, G. F. M., and MEZEY, A. G. "An Analysis of Weight Gain in Patients with Anorexia Nervosa Treated with High Calorie Diet," *Clinical Science,* 23 (1962):449–461.

153. SABINE, E. J. "Bulimia Nervosa: A Placebo-Controlled Double-Blind Therapeutic Trial of Mianserin," *British Journal of Clinical Pharmacology,* 15 (1983): 195–202.

154. SALEH, J., and LEBWOHL, P. "Metoclopramide-Induced Gastric Emptying in Patients with Anorexia Nervosa," *American Journal of Gastroenterology,* 74 (1980):127–132.

155. SAMUEL, A. M., et al. "Growth Hormone Levels in Protein Calorie Malnutrition," *Journal of Clinical Endocrinology and Metabolism,* 35 (1972):863–867.

156. SCHNURER, A. T., and RUBIN, R. "A Systematic Desensitization of Anorexia Nervosa Seen as a Weight Phobia," *Journal of Behavior Therapy and Experimental Psychiatry,* 4 (1973):149–153.

157. SCHOETTLE, U. C. "Pancreatitis," *American Academy of Child Psychiatry,* 38 (1979):384–390.

158. SCHWARTZ, B., et al. "Exercise Associated Amenorrhea: A Distinct Entity?" *American Journal of Obstetrics and Gynecology,* 141 (1981):662–670.

159. SHERMAN, B. M., and HALMI, K. A. "The Effect of Nutritional Rehabilitation on Hypothalamic-Pituitary Function in Anorexia Nervosa," in R. A. Vigersky, ed., *Anorexia Nervosa.* New York: Raven Press, pp. 211–214.

160. SHIMODA, Y., and KITAGAWA, T. "Clinical and EEG Studies on Emaciation," *Journal of Neural Transmission,* 34 (1973): 195–204.

161. SMITH, J. P., et al. "Abdominal Vagotomy Blocks the Satiety Effect of Cholecystokinin in the Rat," *Science,* 213 (1981): 1036–1037.

162. STEGE, P. "Anorexia Nervosa: Review Including Oral and Dental Manifestations," *Journal of the American Dental Association,* 104 (1982):648–652.

163. STROBER, M. "Validity of a Bulimia-Restrictor Distinction in Anorexia Nervosa," *Journal of Nervous and Mental Disease,* 170 (1982):345–351.

164. THEANDER, S. "Anorexia Nervosa," *Acta Psychiatrica Scandinavica,* 214 (1970): 1–300.

165. THURSTON, J., and MARKS, P. "Electrocardiographic Abnormality in Patients with Anorexia Nervosa," *British Heart Journal,* 36 (1974):719–723.

166. VANDEREYCKEN, W. "Neuroleptics in the Short-Term Treatment of Anorexia Nervosa: A Double-Blind Placebo-Controlled Study with Sulpiride," *British Journal of Psychiatry,* 144 (1984):288–292.

167. VANDEREYCKEN, W., and PIERLOOT, R. "Anorexia Nervosa in Twins," *Psychotherapeutic and Psychosomatics,* 35 (1981):55–63.

168. ———. "Pimozide Combined with Behavior Therapy in the Short-Term Treatment of Anorexia Nervosa," *Acta Psychiatrica Scandinavica,* 66 (1982): 445–450.

169. VIGERSKY, R., et al. "Delayed Pituitary Hormone Response to LRF and TRF in Patients with Anorexia Nervosa," *Journal of Clinical Endocrinology and Metabolism,* 43 (1976):893–900.

170. WAKELING, A., and RUSSELL, G. F. M. "Disturbances in the Regulation of Body Temperature in Anorexia Nervosa," *Psychological Medicine,* 1 (1970): 30–39.

171. WAKELING, A., et al. "The Effects of Clomiphene Citrate on the Hypothalamic-Pituitary-Gonadal Axis in Anorexia Nervosa," *Psychological Medicine,* 6 (1976):371–388.

172. WAKELING, A., et al. "Assessment of the

Negative and Positive Feedback Effects of Administered Estrogen on Gonadotropin Release in Patients with Anorexia Nervosa," *Psychological Medicine*, 7 (1977):397–405.

173. WALKER, J., et al. "Calorie Requirements for Weight Gain in Anorexia Nervosa," *American Journal of Clinical Nutrition*, 32 (1979):1396–1400.

174. WALLACE, M., et al. "Persistent Alkalosis and Hypokalemia Caused by Surreptitious Vomiting," *Quarterly Journal of Medicine*, 148 (1968):577–588.

175. WALSH, T. B., et al. "Adrenal Activity in Anorexia Nervosa," *Psychosomatic Medicine*, 40 (1978):499–506.

176. WALSH, T. B., et al. "The Production Rate of Cortisol Declines During Recovery from Anorexia Nervosa," *Journal of Clinical Endocrinology and Metabolism*, 53 (1981):203–205.

177. WALSH, T. B., et al. "A Double-Blind Study of Phenelzine in Bulimia," Paper presented at the American Psychiatric Association Meeting, Los Angeles, May 5–11, 1984, Abstract #NR12.

178. WARRENT, S. E., and STEINBERG, S. M. "Acid-Base and Electrolyte Disturbances in Anorexia Nervosa," *American Journal of Psychiatry*, 136 (1979):415–418.

179. WEINER, H. "Hypothalamic-Pituitary-Ovarian Axis in Anorexia and Bulimia Nervosa," *International Journal of Eating Disorders*, 2 (1983):109–116.

180. WELLER, R. A., and WELLER, E. B. "Anorexia Nervosa in a Patient with an Infiltrating Tumor of the Hypothalamus," *American Journal of Psychiatry*, 139 (1982):824–825.

181. WERMUTH, B. M., et al. "Phenytoin Treatment of the Binge-Eating Syndrome," *American Journal of Psychiatry*, 134 (1977):1249–1253.

182. WHITE, J. H., et al. "Clinical Picture of Atypical Anorexia Nervosa Associated with Hypothalamic Tumor," *American Journal of Psychiatry*, 134 (1977):323–325.

183. WIGLEY, R. D. "Potassium Deficiency in Anorexia Nervosa, with Reference to Renal Tubular Vacuolation," *British Medical Journal*, 2 (1960):110–113.

184. WINOKUR, A., et al. "Primary Affective Disorder in Relatives of Patients with Anorexia Nervosa," *American Journal of Psychiatry*, 137 (1980):695–698.

185. WOLPE, J. *Psychotherapy by Reciprocal Inhibition.* Stanford, Calif.: Stanford University Press, 1958.

186. WULLIEMIER, F., et al. "La Therapie Comportementale de L'anorexie Nerveuse," *Journal of Psychosomatic Research*, 19 (1975):267–272.

187. YAGER, J. Personal communication, 1983.

188. ZUKER, S. "Disturbances in Cardiac Rhythm in Bulimia," Paper presented at the International Eating Disorder Meeting, New York, April 8–9, 1984.

CHAPTER 28

THE BIOLOGY AND EXPERIMENTAL TREATMENT OF OBESITY

Albert J. Stunkard

¶ Introduction

Obesity is a condition characterized by excessive accumulations of fat in the body. By convention, obesity is said to be present when body weight exceeds by 20 percent the standard weight listed in the usual height-weight tables.[11] This index of obesity, however, is only an approximate one at lesser degrees of overweight, since bone and muscle can make a substantial contribution to overweight. In the future, diagnosis will probably be based on newer and more accurate methods of estimating body fat. Skin-fold calipers have already gained acceptance because of their convenience and because half of body fat is localized in subcutaneous tissue. But for most clinical purposes the eyeball test is still the most reasonable: Anyone who looks fat is fat.

¶ Epidemiology

The prevalence of obesity is usually stated to be 35 percent of the male and 40 percent of the female population in the United States, but the criterion used to determine these figures is rarely given. More valid figures have been reported in 1983 by the National Center for Health Statistics, which utilized two criteria—"overweight" relative to an ideal weight and "obesity" as determined by skin-fold thickness.[1] Relative to ideal weight, 23 percent of men and 30 percent of women were classified as overweight, while 19 percent of men and 28 percent of women were classified as obese.

Three demographic factors are closely associated with obesity and, in fact, help to determine it. The first is gender; obesity is far more common among women than among men.[1]

The second major influence on obesity is age. There is a steady increase in the prevalence of obesity from childhood to age fifty, with a two- to threefold increase between the ages of twenty and sixty-four.

The third major influence on obesity is social factors. In many countries undernutrition limits the development of obesity. Where there is no shortage of food, as in an affluent American society, many ethnic groups show a marked increase in the prevalence of obesity in the first generation. Thereafter, a variety of social influences combine to radically reduce the prevalence of obesity. One study reported a drop of 24 percent to 5 percent between the first and fourth generation in the United States.[22]

The most striking antiobesity influence is that of socioeconomic status. Figure 28–1 shows that obesity is six times as common among women of low status as among those of high status in New York City.[22] A similar, though weaker, relationship was found among men. Two findings suggest that a causal relationship underlies these correlations. First, as figure 28–1 shows, the social class of an individual's parents is almost as closely linked to obesity as is the subject's own social class. Although obesity could conceivably influence a person's own social class, his or her obesity can hardly have influenced the social class of his or her parents. Furthermore, obesity is far more prevalent among lower-class children than it is among upper-class children; highly significant differences are already apparent by age six. Similar analyses have shown that social mobility, ethnic factors, and generational status in the United States also influence the prevalence of obesity.[22]

¶ Etiology

The Regulation of Body Weight

What causes obesity? In one sense, the answer is simple: Fat is accumulated when more calories are taken in as food than are expended as energy. In another sense, the answer is obscure. The regulation of body weight in normal-weight organisms is understood only poorly, and in obese organisms it is understood even less well. It does appear, however, that body weight is regulated even by many obese organisms. This idea that body weight may be regulated (even in obesity) rather than being the result of a number

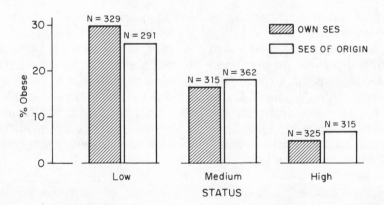

Figure 28–1. Decreasing prevalence of obesity with increasing socioeconomic status (SES) among women in a large American city. SES of origin is almost as strongly linked to obesity as is the person's own SES.

NOTE: Reprinted, by permission of the publisher, from P. B. Goldblatt, M. E. Moore, and A. J. Stunkard, "Social Factors in Obesity," *Journal of the American Medical Association,* 192 (1965): 1039, copyright 1965, American Medical Association.

of unconnected influences is relatively new. The evidence supporting it, however, is strong.[29]

It has been known for some time that the body weight of animals of normal weight is regulated. After the body weight of most experimental animals has been altered—lowered by starvation or raised by forced feeding—it returns promptly to baseline. More recently, however, it has become clear that animals suffering from a variety of forms of experimental obesity possess the same capacity for regulation.[29] Thus in animals, at least, obesity need not be due to a disorder in the regulation of body weight, as had been believed in the past. Instead, it can be due to an elevation in the level about which the regulation occurs, a level that has been viewed by some as a regulatory "set point."

Far less is known about the regulation of body weight in humans. Their weight tends to be the same year after year, despite the exchange of vast amounts of energy. For example, the average nonobese man consumes approximately one million calories a year; his body fat stores, however, remain unchanged during this time because he expends an equal number of calories. An error of no more than 10 percent either in intake or output would lead to a thirty-pound change in body weight within a year. There are only two studies of perturbation of this system in humans, and each supports the idea of regulation. Sims[41] found that normal-weight volunteers who were fattened by overfeeding and underactivity returned to their normal body weight without any special effort soon after they resumed their usual patterns of eating and activity. Keys's[30] classic study of experimental semistarvation showed that when subjects were permitted free access to food, their body weight also rapidly returned to normal. There are no similar studies of obese persons, and it is not known whether they regulate body weight. The evidence, however, suggests that they do not.

Lifetime weight histories of obese persons rarely show a level about which body weight appears to be regulated. How can this curious phenomenon be explained? Why should obese people be the only organisms that do not regulate body weight?

Nisbett has proposed an ingenious explanation for this apparent failure of regulation.[38] According to his theory, obese people may well have the capacity to regulate body weight. However, the set point about which their weight would be regulated, if only biological pressures existed, is higher than that which is tolerated by the society in which they live. As a result, such people go on reducing diets. And even if their weight does not fall to normal levels according to the height/weight charts, it still falls below what would be biologically normal for them. The result is the paradox of people who are statistically overweight and biologically underweight. Nisbett has described seven ways in which the biology and the behavior of obese people resemble that of people whose usually normal body weight has been reduced by starvation or other caloric restriction. In brief, they act as if they are hungry.

Nisbett's theory, attractive as it is, poses a major problem—it cannot be tested, at least not directly. Such a test would require, first, that obese people gain to their putative body-weight set point and, second, raise or lower their weight and then see if it would return to this (elevated) baseline. This test is unfeasible on theoretical as well as on ethical grounds, since the putative set point cannot be estimated.

Although Nisbett's theory cannot be tested directly, indirect tests are possible. One such test, to be described, supports the theory at least as far as some obese people are concerned. It is the results reported by Bjorntorp and associates[7] of the treatment of obese people who have a large excess number of fat cells.

The second test of Nisbett's theory has been carried out by Herman and Polivy.[26] They have shown that some obese people (and some nonobese people) who habitually exercise restraint in the amount they eat share psychological characteristics that distinguish them from persons who do not restrain their food intake. Such "restrained eaters," for example, may show "counter-regulation" of food intake and eat to excess when their habitual restraint is disinhibited. The range of such disinhibitors is impressive and includes dysphoric emotions such as anxiety and depression, alcohol, and even a high-calorie preload in a taste-testing experiment. Since this restraint may prevent obesity in persons of normal weight and mitigate its severity in those already obese, it suggests that the body weight of these people is below a biological set point. Bennett and Gurin provide a lucid account of this theory in their book *The Dieter's Dilemma.*[5]

A number of theories on the regulation of body weight have been proposed. Most ascribe this regulation to the regulation of a single nutrient. They start with the common-sense view that one stops eating at the end of a meal because of the repletion of some nutrient that had been depleted. And one becomes hungry again when the nutrient, which had been restored by the meal, is once again depleted. It seems reasonable that some metabolic signal, derived from food that has been absorbed, is carried by the blood to the brain, where it activates receptor cells, probably in the hypothalamus, to produce satiety. Hunger is the consequence of the decreasing strength of this metabolic signal, secondary to the depletion of the critical nutrient.

Four classical theories of the regulation of body weight have been based on this argument. They differ from each other only in the signal to which they ascribe primary importance. The thermostatic theory, for example, proposes that postprandial increases in hypothalamic temperature mediate satiety, with hunger resulting from a decrease in temperature at this site. Lipostatic, aminostatic, and glucostatic theories each assign the critical regulatory role to blood-borne metabolites of fat, protein, or carbohydrate, respectively.

Although each of these theories explains some of the many phenomena involved in the control of food intake, Mayer's[34] glucostatic theory has had the greatest influence on the field. According to this theory, depletion of carbohydrate stores decreases the amount of "available glucose" in the circulating blood; a fall in available glucose, signaled to hypothalamic glucoreceptors, becomes the stimulus for hunger. An increase in available glucose, with carbohydrate repletion, activates hypothalamic satiety areas and terminates eating. For more than twenty years this theory has exerted great organizational and heuristic power, and evidence for it continues to accumulate.

Despite the attractiveness of the glucostatic theory, it shares with all single-factor theories the general difficulty of encompassing the many events that are involved in the regulation of body weight. In addition to this difficulty, single-factor theories encounter two specific problems.

First, how can a mechanism of short-term, meal-to-meal control of food intake account for the remarkable stability of body weight over long periods of time and in the face of frequently marked short-term fluctuations? As a result of the problems of single-factor theories in modeling such stability, the newer theories of the regulation of body weight are multifactorial ones.[8,9] They are achieving increasing success in predicting food intake under a wide variety of conditions.

The second specific problem of single-factor, primarily physiological, theories is how they can explain the function of satiety. Satiety occurs so soon after the beginning of a meal that only a small proportion of the total caloric content of the meal can have been absorbed. If satiety were based solely on the limited information about food intake available at that time, it could contribute little or nothing to the regulation of food intake.

Although the nutritional value of meals plays little part in satiety in single-meal experiments, humans learn, as do other animals, to change food intake and even meal size in response to changes both in energy expenditure and in the nutritive value of the food.

Booth[8] has proposed that this learning is a special case of Pavlovian, or classical, conditioning. In this theory oral, gastric, and perhaps duodenal factors serve as conditioned stimuli; humoral factors absorbed from the gastrointestinal tract serve as the later, unconditioned stimuli. This sequence accounts both for the termination of eating early in the process of food absorption from the intestine and for the long-term adjustment of meal size to changing caloric needs. Booth[8,9,10] has extended this theory to encompass "conditioned hunger" as well as conditioned satiety. This learning of both hunger and satiety may serve as a bridge between the long-term physiological control of body weight based on humoral factors and the short-term control of hunger and satiety based on conditioning. If this view is even approximately correct, impaired learning may play a role in obesity and therapies based on classical conditioning may become feasible.

Determinants of Obesity

There are at least six known determinants of obesity. Social determinants have already been discussed. The other five determinants are genetic, developmental, physical activity, brain damage, and emotional.

Genetic Determinants

The existence of numerous forms of inherited obesity in animals and the ease with which adiposity can be produced by selective breeding make it clear that genetic factors can play a determining role in obesity. For years textbooks of biology and medicine have implied that a good deal is known about the topic and that genetic factors play an important part in human obesity. It therefore comes as a surprise to realize the extent of current ignorance about the heritability of human obesity. Not much research has been done and very little is known about it.

Animal models of obesity have helped to put into perspective the either/or controversy of nature versus nurture. These models show how each of several possible determinants can have its own particular interaction between genetic and environmental variables, and between different genes. Genetic influences, for example, may determine fat-

cell number in response to different diets at different periods of development, in regulating the efficiency of metabolic processes, and in establishing the sensitivity of different parts of the nervous system to nutrient depletion and repletion.[19] Already a few such interactions have been studied.

One of the most instructive examples of gene-gene interaction was effected by Mayer's[33] breeding the "waltzing gene" into genetically obese *(ob/ob)* mice. The increased physical activity of these mice prevented the development of obesity. An interesting example of gene-environmental interaction is the different responses to a high-fat diet of two different strains of mice.[19] The C3H or A strain became fat, while the C57BL or I strain remained thin or lost weight.

There are probably examples of single-gene obesity among humans that are comparable to the genetic obesity of the *ob/ob* mouse or the Zucker obese rat. But such single-gene obesity in humans, if it exists, seems confined to such rare conditions as the Laurence-Moon-Biedl and Prader-Willi syndromes.[19] Most human obesity is probably of polygenic origin and quite possibly encompasses a large number of different determinants. Efforts to study this problem have utilized three methods: the study of familial resemblance, of twins, and of adoptees.

Familial resemblance supports the familiar belief that obesity runs in families. But little progress has been made in determining whether this phenomenon is the result of genetic or environmental influences, and no progress has been made in determining genetic-environmental interactions. Garn and Clark's[20] quantitative studies have established a significant correlation between the skin-fold thicknesses of those parents and children who share common genes and environment ($r = 0.30$). However, the correlation coefficient between the skin-fold thicknesses of marital partners, who share only their environment, is almost as high ($r = 0.25$). These data have led Garn to propose that human obesity is primarily of environmental origin.

The study of twins, the second method of investigating human obesity, accords primary importance to genetic factors. Three studies estimated heritability via the difference between the intrapair resemblances of monozygotic and dizygotic twins. Estimates of heritability were high: 0.74 for 200 English twin pairs (meaning that 74 percent of the variance was accounted for by heredity); 0.88 for 100 Swedish twin pairs; 0.78 for 4,000 American twin pairs at the time of induction into the army; and 0.77 at a twenty-five-year follow-up.[19]

The results of the three major adoption studies, the third method of investigating human obesity, are in disagreement. Withers[58] reported findings that were originally interpreted as supporting a genetic origin of human obesity. In fact, however, these results are probably more supportive of an environmental origin. More recently, Garn and Clark[20] have posited a purely environmental origin on the basis of their finding that the correlation of skin-fold thickness between parents and adopted children was the same as that between parents and biological children. Biron, Mongeau, and Bertrand,[6] on the other hand, proposed that obesity is of genetic origin. They reported zero correlation between measures of obesity in parents and adopted children, and highly significant correlations between parents and their biological children.

DEVELOPMENTAL DETERMINANTS

A key to the understanding of obesity is provided by our growing knowledge of the anatomy of adipose tissue. It has become clear that the increased adipose tissue mass in obesity can result from an increase in fat-cell size ("hypertrophic obesity"), from an increase in fat-cell number ("hyperplastic obesity"), or from an increase in both size and number ("hypertrophic-hyperplastic obesity"). Johnson and Hirsch's study[28] of six forms of experimental obesity in rodents reveals that most are either hypertrophic or hypertrophic-hyperplastic, and it appears that obese humans also usually fall into one of

these two categories. These findings have important implications for prevention and treatment.

Most people whose obesity began in adult life suffer from hypertrophic obesity. When they lose weight it is solely by a decrease in the size of their fat cells; fat-cell number does not change. Salans, Horton, and Sims[40] have illustrated the dynamics of hypertrophic obesity in their study of human experimental obesity. When normal-weight men were induced to gain forty to sixty pounds, they did so solely through an increase in fat-cell size; when they lost the weight it was solely by a decrease in fat-cell size. Fat-cell number remained constant.

Persons whose obesity began in childhood are more likely to suffer from hyperplastic obesity, usually of the combined hypertrophic-hyperplastic type. They may have up to five times as many fat cells as persons of normal weight or those suffering from pure hypertrophic obesity. However, all of the reasons for the elevation in fat-cell number are still not known and at the present time the field is wracked with controversy. Recent research has challenged the old orthodoxy that fat-cell number cannot increase after early childhood and that events during a relatively brief "critical period" early in life are largely responsible for adipose tissue hyperplasia.[42] Instead, it has been proposed that fat-cell hypertrophy is a major stimulus for fat-cell hyperplasia and that it is this circumstance, and not a critical period, that accounts for the common association of hyperplastic adipose tissue and juvenile-onset obesity.[42]

This view is compatible with Stern and Johnson's[46] review that describes at least two periods when cellular proliferation is enhanced in normal-weight children. One is before the age of two years and the second is between the ages of ten and fourteen years. In obese, presumably overfed, children, however, the period of cell proliferation may extend well past two years of age, with consequent development of pronounced hypercellularity even early in life. Whether overnutrition alone can account for this prolonged period of cellular proliferation is not known; a genetic predisposition may also be required. Johnson and Hirsch's [28] studies of the genetically obese Zucker rat suggest the intriguing possibility that genetic factors may exert their influence by extending the period during which proliferation is particularly susceptible to the influence of overnutrition. The hypercellularity of the adipose tissue of these animals results from production of new fat cells well beyond the period of regulated proliferation found in their nonobese littermates. Whatever the final outcome of this research, enough is already known to single out the early years of life as particularly important in the genesis of hyperplastic obesity. The public health implications are clear. To the compelling psychological reasons for the prevention of childhood obesity must now be added these compelling anatomical reasons.

Our growing understanding of adipose tissue has clinical implications of equal importance. They are highlighted in a report by Bjorntorp and colleagues [7] on twenty-six outpatients who lost an average of thirty-three pounds on a dietary regimen. Body weight and body fat content at the end of treatment varied widely and had reached normal limits in only ten of the subjects. Individual fat-cell size, however, was quite similar in all patients at the end of treatment and had fallen to normal in twenty-three of them. Most patients stopped treatment just at the point when further weight loss could be achieved only by the reduction of their fat cells to subnormal size. It was as if fat-cell size (perhaps particularly certain events at the cell membrane) had set a biological limit to weight reduction. If this is the case, it would explain the difficulty that hyperplastic obese persons experience in reducing to normal body weight and their proclivity to regain the weight that they have lost. More speculatively, it also suggests that, for hyperplastic obese persons, the total of treatment should be reduction to a normal fat-cell size, not a normal body weight. Increased cell size, not increased body fat alone or increased cell number, appears responsible for the

malignant sequence of insulin resistance, hyperinsulinemia, and hyperlipidemia.

PHYSICAL ACTIVITY

Obesity is a rarity in most underdeveloped nations and not solely because of malnutrition. In some areas high levels of physical activity are at least as important in preventing obesity. The marked decrease in physical activity in affluent societies must surely contribute to the recent increase in the prevalence of obesity.

Experiments with genetically obese animals throw further light on the role of physical inactivity in promoting obesity and on the role of activity in controlling it. [45] When the tendency toward obesity is strong, as in the obese hyperglycemic mouse *(ob/ob)*, the obese Zucker rat *(fa/fa)*, and animals with large lesions in the ventromedial hypothalamus, exercise can lessen, although it cannot prevent, the development of obesity. When the tendency toward obesity is weaker, as in the yellow obese mouse *(Ay/a)* and in animals with small lesions in the ventromedial hypothalamus, exercise can often actually prevent the development of obesity.

Physical activity controls obesity by three mechanisms. [45] First, it increases caloric expenditure. Although the caloric expenditure produced by most forms of activity is small, the cumulative effects of continued activity are not negligible. Second, physical activity may actually *decrease* food intake among sedentary persons. Third, physical activity may affect obesity by increasing metabolic rate. One of the major effects of caloric restriction is a fall in basal metabolic rate. Physical activity can prevent or lessen this fall in metabolic rate, thereby obviating a major problem of dieting.

BRAIN DAMAGE

Brain damage can lead to obesity, although it probably does so only rarely in humans. Nevertheless, brain damage is of great theoretical interest in understanding obesity. The discovery, during the 1940s, that destruction of the ventromedial hypothalamus could produce obesity initiated the modern investigation of the condition. Subsequent work has delineated two broad anatomical systems mediating hunger and satiety—the former with special representation in the lateral hypothalamus, the latter in the ventromedial hypothalamus.

The way obesity is produced by ventromedial hypothalamic damage is particularly relevant to the thesis that obesity results from the level of regulation of body weight rather than from a disorder of regulation itself. Animals with such damage regulate body weight, but at a higher level. In the course of maintaining their new fat stores and body weight, such animals demonstrate interesting and potentially highly significant changes in behavior. Many of the features of this behavior in obese rats with hypothalamic lesions were described years ago by Miller, Bailey, and Stevenson in their report on the paradox of decreased hunger and increased food intake in hypothalamic obese rats.[35]

The cardinal feature of the rats' behavior was that they overate when food was freely available; but when an impediment was placed in the way of their eating, they not only decreased their food intake but actually decreased it to a far lower level than that of control rats without hypothalamic lesions. Furthermore, it seemed to make little difference what kind of impediment was used; motivation to work for food was impaired in every manner of task that could be devised. These rats seemed to be relatively unresponsive to all physiological cues concerning their nutritional state, and they responded imperfectly to signals both of satiety and of deprivation.

Nonetheless, the obese rats seemed hyperresponsive to the taste of food and to its availability. They increased their overeating when fat and sweet substances were added to their diet and radically restricted intake when the palatability of their food was decreased by the addition of quinine. Similar eating patterns have been reported in a wide variety of animals when they became obese for natural reasons—for example, in the genetically determined yellow obese mouse,

in the rat when it becomes obese with aging, and even in the dormouse during the hyperphagia that precedes its hibernation. Experimental obesity of various types in animals thus seems to possess some common behavioral correlates. Clinical research has revealed intriguing parallels to the behavior of obese humans.

In the exceptional case, obesity in humans results from hypothalamic damage from a strategically placed tumor or vascular lesion. Usually, however, the cause of the impaired satiety exhibited by many obese persons remains unknown. Such persons characteristically complain that it is difficult to stop eating; it is the unusual obese person who reports being driven by hunger or who eats in a ravenous manner. Instead, obese persons seem particularly susceptible to the palatability of foods and find it difficult to keep from eating if food is available.

Studying the problems of obese persons without brain damage, Bruch[14] has described their misperception of important visceral events. Some obese persons, who are also neurotic, have difficulty in identifying hunger and satiety and frequently seem unable to distinguish hunger from other kinds of dysphoria. Bruch has linked this "conceptual confusion" to severe deficits in identity and to feelings of personal ineffectiveness. She has convincingly described the need of these patients for external signals to tell them when to eat and when to stop eating. Support for Bruch's position has come from studies that show that neurotic obese persons have a strong response bias that impairs their perception of gastric motility.[23] Unfortunately, correction of the bias did not result in weight loss.

EMOTIONAL DETERMINANTS

Many obese persons report that they often overeat and gain weight when they are emotionally upset. But it has proven singularly difficult to proceed from this provocative observation to an understanding of the precise relationship between emotional factors and obesity. The most clear-cut evidence of how emotional factors influence obesity has come from two small subgroups of obese persons, each characterized by an abnormal and stereotyped pattern of food intake. [48,49]

When the first form of overeating, bulimia, occurs among obese persons, it is much like that which occurs among nonobese and anorexic persons, with one significant exception: Most obese bulimic persons do not vomit after bingeing. As a result, they do not obtain the relief that often accompanies vomiting, and the burden of an unwanted food intake is added to the depressed mood and self-deprecatory thoughts that regularly follow an eating binge. Obese bulimic persons (as well as bulimic persons of milder degrees of overweight) sometimes lose large amounts of weight by radically restrictive diets, but such efforts are almost always interrupted by a resumption of eating binges. Indeed, dieting may play a role in bulimia among obese persons as well as among those of normal weight. About 5 percent of obese persons may be bulimic. (See chapter 27.)

Another form of overeating is the night-eating syndrome, characterized by morning anorexia, evening hyperphagia, and insomnia. [49] The syndrome, which afflicts primarily women, appears to be precipitated by stressful life circumstances and may represent a form of depression. Attempts at weight reduction in persons suffering from night-eating appear to have a poor outcome and may even precipitate more severe psychological disturbance. About 10 percent of obese persons may be night-eaters.

¶ Complications

Physical Problems

Controversy has arisen in recent years by Andres's demonstration that the ill effects of milder degrees of obesity may have been overestimated and that the life expectancy of persons who are as much as 25 percent overweight may be as great as (or even greater than) that of thinner persons. [4] However this controversy is resolved, there is no debate about the ill effects of greater degrees of overweight. Drenick and associates have demonstrated a tenfold increase in mortality among young men who are 100 percent overweight. [18] Quite recently, another controversy about the ill effects of obesity has been resolved. There is now firm evidence that obesity is a *primary* risk factor, causing increased mortality by itself as well as by its *secondary* effects. [27]

This evidence of the direct effect of obesity on mortality is matched by evidence of its indirect effects. Even mild degrees of obesity often precipitate latent tendencies toward hypertension, diabetes, and hyperlipidemias. All three disorders are problems in their own right, and they make a major contribution to cardiovascular disease, the cause of more than half of the deaths in the United States. Fortunately, the effects of obesity on mortality are usually reversed by weight reduction.

In addition to obesity's contribution to mortality, a variety of physical manifestations of the disorder plague even persons suffering from relatively moderate degrees of overweight, and severe obesity impairs almost every organ system in the body. An excellent account of these problems is provided in Bray's volume on obesity. [11] As with mortality, these ill effects of obesity are usually reversed by weight reduction, which adds a sound medical argument to the usual cosmetic reasons for weight reduction.

Emotional Disturbances

Reports on emotional disturbances among obese people have flooded the literature in the past. The better the study, however, the less the evidence for such disturbance. The two most careful studies have shown little differences in psychopathology between obese and nonobese people. Moore, Stunkard, and Srole [37] reported slightly higher levels of psychopathology among obese people; Crisp and McGuiness [17] reported slightly lower levels. Even massively obese people do not seem to suffer undue psychiatric disability. The view that obese persons have a specific personality pattern is no longer held.

Although the differences in psychopathology are relatively small for the obese population as a whole, they may be quite significant for certain subgroups. Prominent among these are young women of upper and middle socioeconomic status. The reasons for the special vulnerability of these groups are of interest. Both obesity and emotional disturbances are common among persons of lower socioeconomic status;[22,44] any association between the two conditions in persons in this stratum is apt to be coincidental. Higher up on the socioeconomic ladder, however, obesity is far less prevalent, and the sanctions against it are far stronger. There is also far less emotional disturbance at this level. As a result, when obesity and emotional disturbance coexist in this group, the likelihood that they are associated is far greater. Among young, upper-class women, obesity is usually linked to neurosis. What is the nature of this linkage?

Of the various emotional disturbances to which obese persons are subject, only three are specifically related to their obesity. One is overeating, which has been discussed. The other two are disparagement of the body image and the complications of dieting.

Persons suffering from disparagement of the body image characteristically feel that their bodies are grotesque and loathsome and that others view them with hostility and contempt.[49] This feeling is closely associated with self-consciousness and impaired social functioning. While one may expect that all obese persons have derogatory feelings about their body, such is not the case. Emotionally healthy obese persons have no body-image disturbances, and, in fact, only a minority of neurotic obese persons have such disturbances. The disorder is confined to those who have been obese since childhood; and even among these juvenile-onset obese, less than half suffer from it. But in the group with body-image disturbances, neurosis is closely related to obesity, and this group contains a majority of obese persons with specific eating disorders.

The third form of emotional disturbance specific to obese persons is the complications of dieting. As many as half of all patients treated for obesity by family physicians experience mild anxiety and depression, and even higher percentages of severely obese people report these problems during their more rigorous diets.[53] Such emotional disturbances may arise from precisely the same mechanisms as in the case of a normal-weight person who tried to lose weight—starvation. If this be the case, it would be their proneness to dieting, not their proneness to emotional disturbance, that would distinguish emotionally disturbed obese persons.

¶ Treatment

Weight reduction confers such great benefits on obese persons and is apparently so simple that it might be expected to be a common occurrence. Perhaps the large number of women who try to reduce without medical assistance (following diets and advice from women's magazines) have more success. But most obese persons will not enter outpatient treatment of obesity; of those who do, most will not lose a significant amount of weight; and of those who do lose weight, most will regain it. Furthermore, these results are poor not because of failure to implement any simple therapy of known effectiveness, but because no simple or generally effective treatment exists. Obesity is a chronic condition, resistant to treatment and prone to relapse.

A recently proposed classification of obesity has made it easier to consider the treatment of this disorder.[21,51] An ideal classification of a disease is based on an understanding of its etiology and pathogenesis, and as yet such an understanding of obesity is still not available. Nevertheless, for the clinician the goal of classification is more limited—to know what to do when faced with a patient. For this purpose the classification is quite useful. It is a simple threefold one of mild, moderate, and severe obesity, based on body weights that are, respectively, 20 percent to 40 percent overweight, 41 percent to 100 percent overweight, and more than 100 percent overweight. Table 28–1 shows that the per-

TABLE 28–1

Classification of Obesity Together with Prevalence, Pathology, Complications, Anatomy, and Treatment of the Three Types

Type	Mild	Moderate	Severe
Percentage overweight	20–40	41–100	>100
Prevalence (among obese women) (%)	90.5	9.0	0.5
Pathology	Hypertrophic	Hypertrophic, hyperplastic	Hypertrophic, hyperplastic
Complications	Uncertain	Conditional	Severe
Treatment	Behavior therapy (lay)	Diet and behavior therapy (medical)	Surgical

centage of obese women in each of these categories is, respectively, 90.5 percent, 9 percent, and 0.5 percent. Comparable distributions for men are believed to be similar.

The table shows the nature of the treatment that is indicated for each of the three categories of obesity. Severe obesity is most effectively treated by surgical measures. Moderate obesity is probably best treated by behavior modification and diet under medical auspices; for mild obesity, behavior modification and diet under lay auspices are indicated.

Severe Obesity

The prevalence of severe obesity is no more than 0.5 percent of the *obese* population. This percentage, however, means that more than 200,000 persons in the United States suffer from severe obesity, and psychiatrists will encounter them in practice. It is, accordingly, important to recognize that the condition is both dangerous and potentially treatable. Twenty years of research and practice have given rise to surgical techniques that provide a reasonable option for the treatment of severe obesity.[32]

The first widely used surgical treatment of obesity, intestinal bypass, has been supplanted by gastric restriction procedures designed to radically reduce the volume of the stomach to as little as 50 milliliters and the passageway from this restricted stomach to no more than 1.2 centimeters in diameter. These operations are associated with the usual complications of major surgery, and are not to be performed casually or solely for cosmetic purposes. Nevertheless, for appropriately selected patients, they may provide major health benefits. Weight losses of 40 to 60 kg (about 90 to 130 lb) are achieved in the course of two years with relatively little difficulty, and they tend to be well maintained. Health benefits usually include alleviation of the complications attributable to severe obesity.

The benefits to physical health resulting from surgical treatment of severe obesity are paralleled by the benefits to mental health. These benefits were first described by Solow, Silverfarb, and Swift[43] in their report on the benign social and emotional course of many severely obese persons following the now-discontinued intestinal bypass surgery. This landmark report noted improvement in mood, self-esteem, interpersonal and vocational effectiveness, body image, and level of physical activity. Almost all subsequent accounts agree with this benign emotional course, irrespective of the type of surgery. The early studies, however, underestimated the benefits of this surgery. In assessing the emotional sequelae of surgery, they used an inappropriate control period—the time just before the surgery. The appropriate control period is previous times when the patient was losing weight by nonsurgical treatments. As has been noted, such times are often marked by complications of dieting. The more severe the obesity, the more severe the complications. In one study of severely obese persons, 15 percent reported severe depressive reactions during dieting and another 26 percent reported moderately severe depression.[24] Only a minority had not experienced some degree of depression, and fewer reported no anxiety, irritability, or preoccupation with food.

The emotional response of these same patients to gastric bypass surgery was far more benign, even though they lost far more weight. Half of them reported "much less" dysphoric mood following bypass surgery, and another 5 to 15 percent reported "less" dysphoria. The benefits of gastric bypass surgery extended also to an increase in positive emotions. Half of the patients reported "much more" elation and self-confidence, and 75 percent reported "much more" feelings of well-being.[24]

Surgery also improved the body-image disparagement that had afflicted 70 percent of the patients. After surgery no more than 4 percent reported severe disparagement, and nearly half were symptom-free. This result is particularly striking since it occurred before the patients had lost more than a small amount of weight and when they still appeared to others as grossly obese.

Another striking change in behavior involved food likes and dislikes.[25] Fifty percent of the patients reported that high-density fats and high-density carbohydrates were no longer enjoyable, and smaller percentages also reported lack of enjoyment of breads, high-fat meats, high-calorie beverages, eggs, cheese, and peanut butter. Not only did the patients develop a dislike of these foods, they also ate less of them.

Improvement in eating habits had been found earlier in the now-discontinued intestinal surgery.[12,36] Before surgery, most patients reported chaotic patterns of excessive food intake. After surgery, there was a marked decrease in binge eating, night-eating, excessive snacking, and difficulty in stopping eating. One finding of this study was particularly interesting. Before surgery, a very large percentage of these severely obese patients—as is true of such persons—ate no breakfast. Following surgery, and even while they were rapidly losing weight, these patients began to eat breakfast!

These changes in eating patterns were not only extensive but they occurred without voluntary effort on the part of the patients. Clearly this surgery must do far more than simply alter the functioning of the gastrointestinal tract; it must produce major changes in the biology of the organism. A parsimonious explanation of these changes is that surgery lowers the set point about which body weight is regulated.[24] Such an explanation helps to explain the infrequency of dysphoric reactions to weight loss, the normalization of eating patterns, and the minimal effort that suffices to ensure weight loss. With a lowered body-weight set point, patients need no longer struggle against biological pressures to support a higher weight and can easily limit their food intake until a new, lower set point is reached.

Moderate Obesity

Moderate obesity, from 41 to 100 percent overweight, afflicts about 9 percent of the obese population. The adipose tissue of these persons is usually of the hypertrophic type and may be, in addition, hyperplastic. Complications depend on the presence of conditions such as hypertension and diabetes, which can be precipitated or aggravated by obesity.

BEHAVIOR MODIFICATION

The treatment of moderate obesity consists of behavior modification and diet, conducted under medical auspices. A recent large-scale clinical trial has firmly established the efficacy of behavior modification in the treatment of obesity, particularly in helping patients to maintain weight losses.[16] This same trial has cast serious doubt on the usefulness of pharmacotherapy in the treatment of obesity.

One hundred forty-five persons with moderate obesity (60 percent overweight) were treated for six months, and follow-up information was obtained one year later on 99 percent of those who completed it. The three major treatments were (1) *behavior modifica-*

tion in groups; (2) *medication* (fenfluramine hydrochloride) administered to patients who also met in groups (to control for the effects of group contact in the behavior-modification condition); and (3) *combined treatment* of behavior modification and medication. In addition, there was a waiting-list control condition and a doctor's office medication condition designed to approximate the standard medical-office treatment of obesity, utilizing primarily medication and diet. During treatment, patients in the behavior-modification condition lost 10.9 kg (24 lb), perhaps the largest weight losses yet reported in a controlled clinical trial of this modality (see figure 28–2). The patients in the medication condition lost 14.5 kg (31.9 lb). Adding the two treatments

had no effect on weight loss: Patients in the combined treatment condition lost 15.0 kg (33 lb).

The results one year after the end of the treatment were strikingly different. The patients in the behavior modification condition maintained their weight losses quite well, regaining only 1.8 kg (4 lb). Those in the group medication condition, not unexpectedly, regained 8.6 kg (18.9 lb). The combined treatment group showed the most surprising and disappointing results. They regained no less than 9.5 kg (20.9 lb), ending the year weighing only 4.5 kg (9.9 lb) less than the weight at which they started treatment!

The major result of this study is to establish behavior therapy as an effective method for

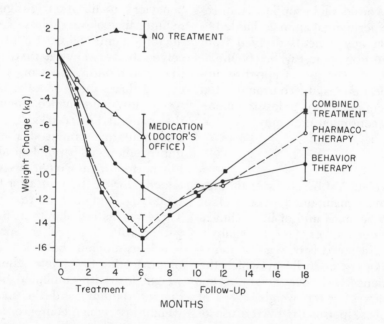

Figure 28–2. Weight changes during six-month treatment and twelve-month follow-up. The three major treatment groups lost large amounts of weight during treatment; behavior therapy (closed circles), 10.9 kg; pharmacotherapy (open circles), 14.5 kg; and combined treatment (squares), 15.3 kg. The behavior-therapy group continued to lose weight for two months and then slowly regained it; pharmacotherapy and combined-treatment groups rapidly regained weight. Among control groups, the no-treatment (waiting-list) group (closed triangles) gained weight; the physician's office medication group (open triangles) lost 6.0 kg. Patients in control groups received additional treatment at six months and so were not available for follow-up. Vertical lines represent one standard error of the mean.

NOTE: Reprinted, by permission of the publisher, from L. E. Craighead, A. J. Stunkard, and C. O'Brien, "Behavior Therapy and Pharmacotherapy for Obesity," *Archives of General Psychiatry*, 38 (1981):763, copyright 1981, American Medical Association.

helping obese patients to lose weight and to maintain their weight loss. A second result has been to cast doubt on the usefulness of current pharmacotherapy for the treatment of obesity. The immediate benefits of medication in increasing the rate of weight loss are more than outweighed by the deleterious effects of medication on the maintenance of this loss.

An appealing interpretation of the findings is that the medication acted by lowering a body-weight set point, thereby making it easier for patients to control their food intake.[50] The drug *did* suppress appetite. But this suppression of appetite appeared to be secondary to the lowering of a body-weight set point. When the drug was discontinued, set point rose and so did body weight. These findings, plus considerable support from research with experimental animals, has led to the belief that any benefits derived from *starting* medication are lost when the medication is *stopped*. The use of appetite-suppressant medication may be contraindicated in the treatment of obesity, unless the medication can be continued indefinitely.

DIET

Although weight lost by behavior therapy is relatively well maintained, such weight losses tend to be small and of little clinical significance. Even the loss of 10.9 kg (24 lb) in the program just noted is only a fraction of the 25 to 30 kg (55 to 66 lb) by which the average patient was overweight. One method of increasing the weight losses of moderately obese persons is by the use of "very-low-calorie diets." Extensive clinical experience has provided considerable information about these diets.[55]

Also called the "protein-sparing-modified fast," these diets provide from 400 to 700 calories, largely or exclusively protein, in the form of either formula or natural foods such as fish, fowl, or lean meat. They appear to be safe when administered under careful medical supervision for periods of up to three months. And weight losses achieved by these diets are striking. Patients lose 1.5 to 2.3 kg (3.3 to 5.1 lb) a week, the extent of weight loss depending on the initial amount of excess weight.

The big question in all dietary treatment of obesity is how well weight losses are maintained. Until recently the weight losses obtained with very-low-calorie diets have been poorly maintained.[55] The superior maintenance of weight loss achieved by behavior therapy suggests a combination of the two forms of treatment—behavior therapy and very-low-calorie diet. Wadden and associates have recently carried out such a combined treatment, with promising results.[56]

The study involved seventeen moderately obese (87.5 percent overweight) women, treated for six months with a combination of very-low-calorie diet (400 to 500 kcal) and behavior modification designed to assist maintenance of weight loss.[56] After an introductory month of treatment, patients received the very-low-calorie diet for no more than two months, following which they received three more months of training in weight-loss maintenance. Figure 28–3 shows that patients lost 20.5 kg (45.1 lb) during a treatment that produced also a significant improvement in psychological functioning. Furthermore, this weight loss was well maintained. During the year after treatment patients regained no more than 2.1 kg (4.6 lb). These results are shown in figure 28–3 together with those of the previous study, which combined behavior therapy with pharmacotherapy. Note the far greater weight loss with combined behavioral and dietary therapy, and the maintenance of weight loss, which compares favorably with that of the far smaller weight loss achieved with behavior therapy alone. This study gives grounds for optimism about combined treatment for moderate obesity, and such treatment is now under active investigation.

Mild obesity

Mild obesity, from 20 to 40 percent overweight, is by far the most common form of the disorder, afflicting more than 90 percent of obese persons. The adipose tissue of mildly

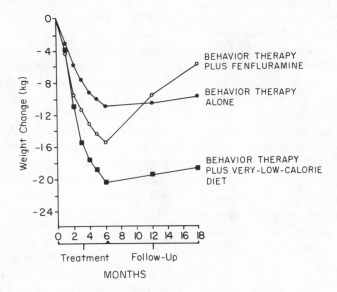

Figure 28–3. Weight loss (in kg) at the end of six months of treatment and one-year follow-up of patients treated with behavior therapy plus very-low-calorie diet. These results are contrasted with those obtained in an earlier study comparing the results of behavior therapy alone and behavior therapy plus fenfluramine.

SOURCE: T. A. Wadden et al., "Treatment of Moderate Obesity by Behavior Therapy and Very-Low-Calorie Diet: A Pilot Investigation," *Journal of Consulting and Clinical Psychology* 52 (1984) (fig. 1) [copyright 1984 by the American Psychological Association, adapted by permission], and L. E. Craighead, A. J. Stunkard, and C. O'Brien, "Behavior Therapy and Pharmacotherapy for Obesity," *Archives of General Psychiatry,* 38 (1981) (fig. 1).

obese persons is usually hypertrophic, and it is hyperplastic only in persons who maintain a lowered body weight by constantly dieting. The two types of treatment are the same as those for moderate obesity—diet and behavior modification—but with significant differences. The diet is far more moderate and the behavior modification is delivered by lay-led groups.

Diet

The very-low-calorie diet is *not* indicated for mildly obese persons. Instead they can choose from among a wide variety of diets. And there is a wide variety!

There are diets high in protein and low in protein, high in fat and low in fat, high in carbohydrates and low in carbohydrates, and, recently, a special diet from Beverly Hills that is high in papayas and mangos. A discussion of dietary treatment could easily fill this volume without exhausting the topic, but the general principle is simple—any diet that reduces calorie intake below caloric expenditure will produce weight loss. In this sense, all treatments for obesity are dietary. But diets today have become far more than simply a means of producing a caloric deficit. They have acquired all manner of magical properties in the minds of the lay public; consider the categories of diets just listed! How does one make a rational choice?

Perhaps one should not choose; the whole idea of dieting for mildly overweight persons may be unwise. *Going on* a diet implies *going off* it and resuming old eating habits. For this reason, the most effective diet may not be a diet at all but rather a gradual change in eating habits and a shift to foods that the patient can continue to eat indefinitely. This means increasing the intake of complex carbohydrates, particularly fruits, vegetables, and cereals, and decreasing the intake of fats and concentrated carbohydrates. This course of action probably gives the best chance of maintaining the weight that is lost, and it is an eminently safe one. A diet that consists primarily of sensible eating habits does not require medical monitoring and is particularly well suited for use by the lay organizations that are assuming the dominant role in the treatment of mild obesity.

BEHAVIOR MODIFICATION

Behavior modification programs were developed for the treatment of mildly obese persons, and they are admirably suited to this purpose. Furthermore, the key elements of behavior modification are easy to specify and therefore easy to learn. Many of them are readily packaged in easy-to-use treatment manuals. As a result, behavior modification has been administered by persons with progressively less formal training, even by those with no professional background. Behavior modification provides a technology that can promise modest weight losses at minimal risk. Although it is being applied by professional therapists, particularly psychologists, by far the largest number of obese persons is being treated under the auspices of lay-led groups. [47]

¶ Treatment Vehicles

Lay-led Groups

Lay-led groups for obesity antedate the development of behavioral weight control by several years. Prominent among them are TOPS (Take Off Pounds Sensibly), the largest of the nonprofit groups, and Weight Watchers, the largest commercial group. TOPS, founded in 1948, was the first self-help group for obesity, and it now enrolls more than 300,000 persons. [31] The key elements of TOPS are weekly meetings that provide group support, weigh-ins that are high points of the meeting, and policy supervision from the national headquarters. The membership of TOPS is almost exclusively female, middle-aged, and of lower-middle socioeconomic status; the average member is 60 percent overweight. Its effectiveness is difficult to assess because of the very high dropout rates.

Commercial weight-loss organizations appeal to much the same clientele as do the nonprofit ones, and with somewhat greater success—500,000 persons a week attend just one such organization, Weight Watchers. [47] The commercial organizations have added three important elements to the program pioneered by the nonprofit groups—behavior modification, inspirational lecturers drawn from successful members, and a carefully designed nutritional program. These programs are readily available to persons with even a casual interest in weight reduction. But they too suffer from high attrition rates: 50 percent of the members of one such group dropped out in six weeks and 70 percent in twelve weeks. [54] Dropout rates of this magnitude make it difficult to assess reports of weight lost by the survivors.

Despite these problems, the low cost and ready availability of lay-led groups make them an important resource for the control of mild obesity. Large numbers of persons can be reached by these groups, and their very low costs mean a favorable ratio of cost to effectiveness. For example, it costs far more to lose comparable amounts of weight in an exemplary university clinic than in a neighboring commercial program, even with its high dropout rate. [59] For the well-motivated person with mild obesity, commercial weight-loss programs are probably the treatment of choice.

Psychoanalysis

The results of a recent large-scale study of psychoanalysis suggest that this modality may be of more value in the treatment of obesity than we had believed. [39] The study involved eighty-four obese men and women treated by seventy-two psychoanalysts over a period of several years. Weight losses compared favorably with those achieved by other conservative measures. After a median duration of thirty-three months of treatment, weight losses averaged 4.5 kg (9.9 lb). At an eighteen-month follow-up, weight loss had increased to 9.5 kg (20.9 lb), and at a four-year follow-up, it had increased still further, to 11.6 kg (25.5 lb). Not only were significant amounts of weight lost during treatment, but these weight losses were well maintained at follow-up of as much as four years duration.

In addition to these unexpected results of the psychoanalysis of obese persons there were other, less surprising, ones. Notable among them was a marked reduction in the prevalence of severe body-image disparagement. At the beginning of treatment 39 percent of patients reported severe disparagement of the body image; this percentage had fallen to 18 percent at follow-up.

This study may reawaken interest in psychoanalytic psychotherapy of obese persons. Some general observations are therefore in order. First, there is no evidence that uncovering putative unconscious causes of overeating can alter the symptom choice of obese people who overeat in response to stress. Years after successful psychotherapy and successful weight reduction, persons who overate under stress continue to do so. Second, many obese people seem inordinately vulnerable to the overdependency on the therapist and to the severe regression that can occur in psychoanalytic therapy. Bruch[14] has provided excellent descriptions of measures designed to minimize such regression, to cope with the "conceptual confusion" described earlier, and to increase the patient's often seriously inadequate sense of personal effectiveness.

Although psychoanalysis and psychoanalytic therapy are very expensive ways to lose weight, they may be indicated for persons suffering from severe disparagement of the body image. They may also be indicated for treatment of bulimia, another particularly resistant condition. Furthermore, obese people may seek psychotherapy for reasons other than their obesity; helping them to cope with their obesity may help them to resolve other problems. I have noted that many obese people overeat under stress. If psychotherapy helps them to lead less stressful and more satisfying lives, then they are less likely to overeat. As a result, they may reduce and stay reduced. These benefits are no less significant for being nonspecific results of treatment.

¶ Obesity in Childhood

Obesity that begins in childhood shows a very strong tendency to persist. Long-term prospective studies in Hagerstown, Maryland, have revealed the remarkable degree to which obese children become obese adults. In the first such study,[2] 86 percent of a group of overweight boys became overweight men, as compared to only 42 percent of boys of average weight. Even more striking differences in adult weight status were found among girls: 80 percent of overweight girls became overweight women, as compared to only 18 percent of average-weight girls. A later study[52] showed that the few overweight children who reduced successfully had done so by the end of adolescence. The odds against an overweight child becoming a normal-weight adult, which were four to one at age twelve, rose to twenty-eight to one for those who did not reduce during adolescence. An even more recent study,[3] which used a longer interval (thirty-five years) and, unfortunately, different (more rigid) criteria for obesity, found the difference in adult-weight status continuing to grow; 63 percent of obese boys became obese men, as compared to only 10 percent of average-weight boys.

It is widely believed that obese children are very inactive and that their inactivity plays a major part in the development and maintenance of their obesity. Recent research suggests that excessive food intake is a far more important factor. At least four studies[57] that used objective measures of physical activity failed to reveal significant differences between obese and nonobese

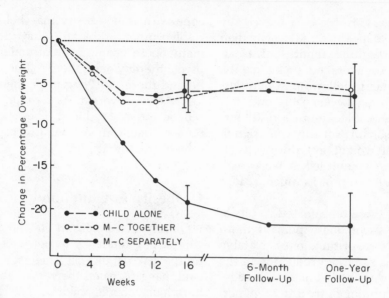

Figure 28–4. Mean changes in weight for three treatment conditions (Child Alone, Mother-Child Together, Mother-Child Separately) during treatment and one-year maintenance period.

Note: Reprinted, by permission of the publisher, from K. D. Brownell, J. H. Kelman, and A. J. Stunkard, "Treatment of Obese Children With and Without Their Mothers: Changes in Weight and Blood Pressure," *Pediatrics*, 71 (1983):518, copyright American Academy of Pediatrics 1983.

children, while only one study reported that obese children were less active.

A recent intensive study of energy intake and expenditure suggests that excessive food intake and not decreased physical activity maintains childhood obesity and may even produce it. Waxman and Stunkard directly measured food intake and energy expenditure in ten families that contained an obese and a nonobese same-sexed sibling whose ages were within two years of each other; four pairs were boys, six were girls.[57] Obese children consumed far more calories than did their nonobese siblings. Furthermore, when measures of physical activity were converted to calories, it was found that the obese children actually had higher levels of energy expenditure than did their nonobese siblings. This information is of value in the treatment of obese children.

Until recently, weight-reduction programs for children have been characterized by modest losses, poor maintenance of these losses, untoward emotional reactions, and high attrition rates.[15] The introduction of be-

havioral principles into the treatment of obese children has changed this gloomy picture, and nine recent studies suggest that behavioral weight reduction in children may be at least as effective as behavioral weight reduction in adults. The most promising of these studies was recently reported by Brownell, Kelman, and Stunkard.[13]

Forty-two children between the ages of twelve and sixteen were treated for four months for moderately severe obesity, averaging 55.7 percent overweight. Treatment was modeled on traditional behavioral principles, carried out in groups that met for periods of an hour. All children received the same treatment, with the exception of the type of parental involvement. In one treatment condition, the mother and child were treated separately (Mother-Child Separately); in the second, mother and child were treated together (Mother-Child Together); and in the third, the child was treated alone, without parental involvement (Child-Alone). The difference between the two Mother-Child conditions was that children and their mothers were either seen in groups together or were seen in separate groups that met at the same time but in different rooms.

Weight losses were as large as any reported in the pediatric literature. Children in the Mother-Child Separately condition lost 8.4 kg (18.5 lb), compared to 5.3 kg (11.7 lb) and 3.3 kg (7.0 lb) for the Mother-Child together and the Child-Alone conditions, respectively. The superiority of the Mother-Child Separately condition was maintained at the one-year follow-up, when children in this condition still showed a loss of 7.7 kg (17.0 lb), compared with a gain of 3 kg in the other two conditions. Even the children in the latter two conditions, however, maintained the decrease in their degree of obesity, despite their gain in weight. Figure 28–4 shows that there was no change in percentage overweight of any of the groups since increases in weight were offset by increases in height.

The surprisingly large weight losses and the excellent maintenance of these weight losses in the Mother-Child Separately condition may herald a new era in the treatment of childhood obesity. The fact that these results were obtained so early in the behavioral treatment of childhood obesity is grounds for optimism about even further progress.

¶ Bibliography

1. ABRAHAM, S. "Obese and Overweight Adults in the United States," National Center for Health Statistics, Vital and Health Statistics Series 11, No. 230. DHHS Pub. No. 83-1680, Public Health Service. Washington, D.C.: U.S. Government Printing Office, 1983.
2. ABRAHAM, S., and NORDSIECK, M. "Relationship of Excess Weight in Children and Adults," *Public Health Reports*, 75 (1960):263–273.
3. ABRAHAM, S., COLLINS, G., and NORDSIECK, M. "Relationship of Childhood Weight Status to Morbidity in Adults," *HSMHA Health Reports*, 86 (1971):273–284.
4. ANDRES, R. "Effect of Obesity on Total

5. Mortality," *International Journal of Obesity*, 4 (1980):381–386.
5. BENNETT, W., and GURIN, J. *The Dieter's Dilemma: Eating Less and Weighing More*. New York: Basic Books, 1982.
6. BIRON, P., MONGEAU, J. G., and BERTRAND, D. "Familial Resemblance of Body Weight and Weight/Height in 374 Homes with Adopted Children," *Journal of Pediatrics*, 91 (1977):555–558.
7. BJORNTORP, P., et al. "Effect of an Energy-Reduced Dietary Regimen in Relation to Adipose Tissue Cellularity in Obese Women," *American Journal of Clinical Nutrition*, 28 (1975):445–452.
8. BOOTH, D. A. "Satiety and Appetite are Conditioned Reactions," *Psychosomatic Medicine*, 39 (1977):76–81.
9. ———. "Acquired Behavior Controlling Energy Input and Output," in A. J. Stunkard, ed., *Obesity*. Philadelphia: W. B. Saunders Co., 1980, pp. 101–143.
10. BOOTH, D. A., ed. *Hunger Models: Computable Theory of Feeding Control*. New York: Academic Press, 1978.
11. BRAY, G. *The Obese Patient*. Philadelphia: W. B. Saunders Co., 1976.
12. BRAY, G. A., et al. "Factors Controlling Food Intake: A Comparison of Dieting and Intestinal Bypass," *American Journal of Clinical Nutrition*, 33 (1980):376–382.
13. BROWNELL, K. D., KELMAN, J. H., and STUNKARD, A. J. "Treatment of Obese Children With and Without Their Mothers: Changes in Weight and Blood Pressure." *Pediatrics*, 71 (1983):515–523.
14. BRUCH, H. *Eating Disorders: Obesity, Anorexia Nervosa, and the Person Within*. New York: Basic Books, 1973.
15. COATES, T. J., and THORESEN, C. E. "Treating Obesity in Children and Adolescents: A Review," *American Journal of Public Health*, 68 (1978):143–151.
16. CRAIGHEAD, L. W., STUNKARD, A. J., and O'BRIEN, R. M. "Behavior Therapy and Pharmacotherapy of Obesity," *Archives of General Psychiatry*, 38 (1981):763–768.
17. CRISP, A. H., and McGUINESS, B. "Jolly Fat: Relation Between Obesity and Psychoneurosis in General Population," *British Medical Journal*, 1 (1975):7–9.

18. DRENICK, E. J., et al. "Excessive Mortality and Causes of Death in Morbidly Obese Men," *Journal of American Medical Association*, 243 (1980):443–445.

19. FOCH, T. T., and McLEARN, G. E. "Genetics, Body Weight and Obesity," in A. J. Stunkard, ed., *Obesity*. Philadelphia: W. B. Saunders Co., 1980, pp. 48–71.

20. GARN, S. M., and CLARK, D. C. "Trends in Fatness and the Origins of Obesity," *Pediatrics*, 57 (1976):443–456.

21. GARROW, J. S. *Treat Obesity Seriously: A Clinical Manual*. London: Churchill Livingston, 1982.

22. GOLDBLATT, P. B., MOORE, M. E., and STUNKARD, A. J. "Social Factors in Obesity," *Journal of the American Medical Association*, 192 (1965):1039–1044.

23. GRIGGS, R. C., and STUNKARD, A. J. "The Interpretation of Gastric Motility, II. Sensitivity and Bias in the Perception of Gastric Motility," *Archives of General Psychiatry*, 11 (1964):82–89.

24. HALMI, K. A., STUNKARD, A. J., and MASON, E. E. "Emotional Responses to Weight Reduction by Three Methods: Diet, Jejunoileal Bypass, and Gastric Bypass," *American Journal of Clinical Nutrition*, 33 (1980):446–451.

25. HALMI, K. A., et al. "Appetitive Behavior After Gastric Bypass for Obesity," *International Journal of Obesity*, 5 (1981):457.

26. HERMAN, C. P., and POLIVY, J. "Restrained Eating," in A. J. Stunkard, ed., *Obesity*. Philadelphia: W. B. Saunders Co., 1980, pp. 208–225.

27. HUBERT, H. B., et al. "Obesity as an Independent Risk Factor for Cardiovascular Disease: A 26-Year Follow-Up of Participants in the Framingham Heart Study," *Circulation*, 67 (1983):968–977.

28. JOHNSON, P. R., and HIRSCH, J. "Cellularity of Adipose Depots in Six Strains of Genetically Obese Mice," *Journal of Lipid Research*, 13 (1972):2–11.

29. KEESEY, R. "Defense of the Body Weight Set Point: Metabolic Contributions," in A. J. Stunkard and E. Stellar, eds., *Eating and Its Disorders*, New York: Raven Press, 1984, pp. 87–96.

30. KEYS, A., et al. *The Biology of Human Starvation*, 2 vols. Minneapolis: University of Minnesota Press, 1950.

31. LEVITZ, L. S., and STUNKARD, A. J. "A Therapeutic Coalition for Obesity: Behavior Modification and Patient Self-Help," *American Journal of Psychiatry*, 131 (1974):423–427.

32. MASON, E. E. *Surgical Treatment of Obesity*. Philadelphia: W. B. Saunders Co., 1981.

33. MAYER, J. "Decreased Activity and Energy Balance in the Hereditary Obesity-Diabetes Syndrome of Mice," *Science*, 117 (1953):504–505.

34. ———. "Some Aspects of the Problem of Regulation of Food Intake and Obesity," *New England Journal of Medicine*, 274 (1966):610 ff.

35. MILLER, N. E., BAILEY, C. J., and STEVENSON, J. A. F. "Decreased Hunger and Increased Food Intake in Hypothalamic Obese Rats," *Science*, 112 (1950):256–259.

36. MILLS, M. J., and STUNKARD, A. J. "Behavioral Changes Following Surgery for Obesity," *American Journal of Psychiatry*, 133 (1976):527–531.

37. MOORE, M. E., STUNKARD, A. J., and SROLE, L. "Obesity, Social Class and Mental Illness," *Journal of the American Medical Association*, 181 (1962):962–966.

38. NISBETT, R. E. "Hunger, Obesity and the Ventromedial Hypothalamus," *Psychological Review*, 79 (1972):433–453.

39. RAND, S. W., and STUNKARD, A. J. "Obesity and Psychoanalysis: Treatment and Four-Year Follow-Up," *American Journal of Psychiatry*, 140 (1983):1140–1144.

40. SALANS, L. B., HORTON, E. S., and SIMS, E. A. H. "Experimental Obesity in Man: The Cellular Character of the Adipose Tissue," *Journal of Clinical Investigation*, 50 (1971):1005–1011.

41. SIMS, E. A. H. "Experimental Obesity, Diet-induced Thermogenesis and Their Clinical Implications," *Clinics in Endocrinology and Metabolism*, 5 (1976):377–395.

42. SJÖSTRÖM, L. "Fat Cells and Body Weight," in A. J. Stunkard, ed., *Obesity*. Philadelphia: W. B. Saunders Co., 1980, pp. 72–100.

43. SOLOW, C., SILVERFARB, P. M., and SWIFT, K. "Psychosocial Effects of Intestinal Bypass Surgery for Severe Obe-

sity," *New England Journal of Medicine*, 290 (1974):300–304.

44. SROLE, L., et al. *Mental Health in the Metropolis: The Midtown Manhattan Study.* New York: McGraw-Hill, 1962.

45. STERN, J. "Is Obesity a Disease of Inactivity?" in A. J. Stunkard and E. Stellar, eds., *Eating and Its Disorders.* New York: Raven Press, 1984, pp. 131–140.

46. STERN, J. and JOHNSON, P. R. "Size and Number of Adipocytes and Their Implications," in H. Katzer and R. Mahler, eds., *Advances in Modern Nutrition*, vol. 2. New York: John Wiley & Sons, 1978, pp. 303–340.

47. STUART, R. B. "Self-Help Group Approach to Self-Management," in R. B. Stuart, ed., *Behavioral Self Management.* New York: Brunner/Mazel, 1977, pp. 278–305.

48. STUNKARD, A. J. "Eating Patterns and Obesity," *Psychiatric Quarterly*, 33 (1959):284–294.

49. ———. *The Pain of Obesity.* Palo Alto: Bull Publishing Company, 1976.

50. ———. "Minireview: Anorectic Agents Lower a Body Weight Set Point." *Life Sciences*, 30 (1982):2043–2055.

51. ———. "The Current Status of Treatment for Obesity in Adults," in A. J. Stunkard and E. Stellar, eds., *Eating and Its Disorders.* New York: Raven Press, 1984, pp. 157–174.

52. STUNKARD, A. J., and BURT, V. "Obesity and the Body Image II. Age at Onset of Disturbances in the Body Image," *American Journal of Psychiatry*, 123 (1967):1443–1447.

53. STUNKARD, A. J., and RUSH, A. J. "Dieting and Depression Reexamined: A Critical Review of Reports of Untoward Responses During Weight Reduction for Obesity," *Annals of Internal Medicine*, 81 (1974):526–533.

54. VOLKMAR, F. R., et al. "High Attrition Rates in Commercial Weight Reduction Programs," *Archives of Internal Medicine*, 141 (1981):426–428.

55. WADDEN, T. A., STUNKARD, A. J., and BROWNELL, K. D. "Very Low Calorie Diets: A Critical Review," *Annals of Internal Medicine*, 99 (1983):675–684.

56. WADDEN, T. A., et al. "Treatment of Moderate Obesity by Behavior Therapy and Very Low Calorie Diet: A Pilot Investigation," *Journal of Clinical and Consulting Psychology*, 52 (1984):692–694.

57. WAXMAN, M., and STUNKARD, A. J. "Caloric Intake and Expenditure of Obese Boys," *Journal of Pediatrics*, 96 (1980): 187–193.

58. WITHERS, R. F. J. "Problems in the Genetics of Human Obesity," *Eugenics Review*, 56 (1964):81–90.

59. YATES, B. T. "Improving the Cost-Effectiveness of Obesity Programs. Three Basic Strategies for Reducing the Cost Per Pound," *International Journal of Obesity*, 2 (1978):249–266.

CHAPTER 29

THE BIOLOGY AND
TREATMENT OF DRUG ABUSE

Philip A. Berger and Meredith J. Dunn

¶ Introduction

Almost all cultures throughout every era have sought ways to alter consciousness by ingesting psychoactive, or mind-altering, substances. Alcohol has always been the most widely used psychoactive substance. Drugs such as hashish, opium, and naturally occurring hallucinogens have always been used in limited ways by certain cultures, but psychoactive drug use has not been a major health problem until recently; psychoactive compounds are currently consumed by most cultures. A significant amount of humankind's time and energy is spent on the production, distribution, and consumption of psychoactive drugs, and modern chemistry and psychopharmacology have increased the varieties, quantity, and availability of such drugs.[12] By 1894 the use of drugs of all types was so prevalent that Sir William Osler suggested, somewhat seriously, that man had an inborn craving for medicine. More recently, Andrew Weil[191] has argued that the widespread use of psychoactive drugs in most societies suggests that the drive and desire for altered states of consciousness are a natural part of human nature.

The popularity and use of psychoactive drugs causes many philosophical, social, and ethical controversies. For example: Has the heavy reliance of overworked physicians on prescription medications created a "drug-dependent society"? In a democratic society, shouldn't individuals be able to ingest whatever psychoactive drug they choose as long as their drug use does not infringe on the rights of others? Are stringent legal controls of psychoactive drugs needed to prevent an epidemic of drug use that could seriously threaten social order? Is it not inconsistent to advertise and allow easy access to such dangerous substances as alcohol and tobacco, while severely restricting the use of what may be less dangerous psychoactive drugs such as benzodiazepines and marijuana? Has the fragmentation of our society and the decreasing importance of the extended family and traditional religious values left a gap that only psychoactive drugs can fill? Can the altered states of consciousness produced by some psychoactive drugs give individuals better insight into their own psychological problems or perhaps even lead to insights or perspectives that might benefit society? Why has research on the risks and benefits of psychoactive drug abuse been given such a low priority when the problem is considered to be a threat to both individuals and society? These controversies suggest that the use of psychoactive drugs is as much a social and ethical problem as it is a medical problem. [12,14]

This chapter focuses primarily on the medical aspects of psychoactive drug use and abuse and is divided into sections based on the major pharmacological classes of abused substances. Each section contains a brief history of a class of psychoactive drug, a description of its pattern of use, a discussion of the reasons for its use, and a description of the medical management of both the acute and chronic adverse reactions to its use. When appropriate, each section ends with a brief summary of the hypothesized mechanisms of action of that class of psychoactive drug. The chapter includes a discussion of the increasing phenomenon of polydrug abuse and its treatment, which requires knowledge of the interactions between classes of psychoactive drugs. Finally, the chapter ends with a brief summary of the long-term treatment and rehabilitation of users of psychoactive drugs of abuse.

Dividing psychoactive drugs into ten pharmacological classes offers a convenient classification scheme. This chapter discusses nine of these: opioids; psychostimulants; phencyclidine (PCP); inhalants; anticholinergics; classical hallucinogens, methylated amphetamines, and cannabis; sedative-hypnotics; tobacco; and caffeine. Since a discussion of the problem and treatment of alcoholism can be found in chapter 30, this most common psychoactive drug of abuse is not discussed in this chapter. Table 29–1 presents examples of psychoactive drugs from each pharmacological category.

¶ Opioids

History of Opioids

The earliest written record of opium use is Sumerian and may date from 4,000 B.C.; however, opium use predates written history. Methods of collection are used today that were described by the Assyrians more than three thousand years ago. The unripened seed capsule of the opium poppy *(Papaver somniferum)* is incised, and after the sap has oozed and dried, it is scraped off the incisions as raw opium. In the Science Museum of London, there are Bronze Age ceramic jugs from Cyprus shaped like opium poppy capsules and with stylized incision marks. These jars were probably used to hold opium dissolved in wine or water for export to Egypt. Artistic representations of the opium poppy are found in Egyptian art; on ancient Greek coins, pottery, and jewelry; and on Roman statuary and tombs. In Homer's *Odyssey,* Helen of Troy mixes a potion containing opium "to quiet all pain and strife and bring forgetfulness of every ill." It has been suggested that the "vinegar mingled with gall" offered to Christ on the Cross (Matthew 27:34) contained opium, since the ancient Hebrew word for gall, *rosh,* means "opium." [12,142]

Opium was used by Greek physicians, including Galen, who combined it with alcohol for medicinal purposes. Opium was introduced to China by the Arabs, probably in the ninth century. In 1530 the great physician Paracelsus dissolved opium in alcohol in the same manner as Roman physicians, and the resulting analgesic mixture, called laudenum, was widely used throughout the world until the twentieth century. In 1803 F. W. A. Serturner, a German pharmacist, isolated the pure alkaloid base from opium and named it morphine after Morpheus, the Greek god of dreams. Morphine is still considered by many physicians to be the most important drug in medicine; it is the analgesic standard against which all other pain medications are judged. In 1874 synthesized

TABLE 29-1
Pharmacological Classification of Abused Substances

Substance Class	Representative Substances	Problems Requiring Treatment
Alcohol (ethanol)	See chapter 30	See chapter 30
Opioids (narcotic analgesics)	Heroin (diacetylmorphine), morphine, pethidine (meperidine), methadone, opium, codeine, and others	*Organic Mental Disorders* intoxication withdrawal *Substance Use Disorder* abuse dependency
Psychostimulants	Cocaine, amphetamine, dextroamphetamine, methamphetamine, methylphenidate, phenmetrazine, diethylproprion, fenfluramine, phentermine, chlorphentermine, and others	*Organic Mental Disorders* intoxication delirium delusional syndrome
Phencyclidine (PCP) and related arylcyclohexylamines	Phencyclidine (PCP), ketamine	*Organic Mental Disorders* intoxication delirium mixed organic syndrome *Substance Use Disorder* abuse
Inhalants	Glues, cleaning solutions, solvents, lighter fluids, paint and paint thinners, aerosols, and other petroleum products containing toluene, acetates, hexane, benzene, xylene, acetone, gasoline, chloroform, naphtha, nitrous oxide, ether, isoamyl and isobutyl nitrite, and others	*Organic Mental Disorders* intoxication delirium delusional syndrome hallucinosis amnestic syndrome mixed organic brain syndrome *Substance Use Disorder* abuse
Anticholinergics	Many nonprescription substances for insomnia and anxiety (scopolamine and methapyrilene), colds, hayfever, asthma, motion sickness, and acid-peptic disease. Tricyclic antidepressants, neuroleptics, and antiparkinsonian agents, *Datura stramonium* (jimsonweed), Ditran (JB-329)[a]	*Organic Mental Disorders* intoxication delirium delusional syndrome hallucinosis amnestic syndrome mixed organic brain syndrome
Classical Hallucinogens and Methylated Amphetamines	Lysergic acid diethylamide (LSD-25), psilocybin, dimethyltryptamine (DMT), diethyltryptamine (DET), mescaline, 2, 5-dimethoxy-4-methylamphetamine (DOM or STP), methylenedioxyamphetamine (MDA), methylenedeoxymethamphetamine (MDMA), and others	*Organic Mental Disorders* hallucinosis delusional syndrome affective syndrome *Substance Use Disorder* abuse

TABLE 29–1 *(Continued)*

Substance Class	Representative Substances	Problems Requiring Treatment
Cannabis	Marijuana, hashish, tetrahydrocannabinol (THC)	*Organic Mental Disorders* intoxication delusional syndrome *Substance Use Disorder* abuse
Sedative-hypnotics	Barbiturates, barbiturate substitutes such as glutethimide, methaqualone; benzodiazepines including anxiolytic and sedative-hypnotic benzodiazepines	*Organic Mental Disorders* intoxication withdrawal *Substance Use Disorder* abuse dependency
Tobacco	Cigarette, cigar, pipe, or chewing tobacco	*Organic Mental Disorders* withdrawal *Substance Use Disorder* use
Caffeine	Coffee, tea, cola drinks, caffeine-containing pills (NoDoz®, Vivarin®, Zoom (Quarana), and others	*Organic Mental Disorders* caffeinism

[a]See tables 29–2 and 29–3.

diacetylmorphine, or heroin, was first suggested as a cure for morphine addiction.[12]

In the nineteenth century the use of opium preparations was widespread in Europe and the United States. The general public could purchase opium preparations from grocery and general stores and could order them through mail-order catalogues from stores such as Sears and Roebuck. Labeled "pain killers," "cough mixtures," "women's friends," and "consumption cures," laudenum was also used by factory workers to quiet crying babies while they worked. A popular drink called Godfrey's Cordial contained opium mixed with molasses and sassafras flavoring. Morphine- and, later, heroin-containing preparations became even more popular after the American Civil War for the same purposes. The hypodermic syringe, invented in 1853, was first widely used during the Civil War to administer morphine.[12]

Despite the fact that opium use was legal in the nineteenth century, it was considered by many to be disreputable, if not immoral, and in a class with alcohol use. The first laws against opium use banned the "opium dens"

and increased tariffs on opium imports. British and American transport of opium from India to China was extremely lucrative and was the major source of financial support for the British navy. Chinese resentment of the increase in opium addiction and the enormous expense of buying opium from the British, led to the two "opium wars" fought between Britain and China. Consequently, international efforts to regulate the opium trade were instigated and ultimately led to the regulation of opium in the United States. The 1906 Pure Food and Drug Act required that medicines state their contents on the label if they contained drugs such as the opiates; the Harrison Narcotic Act of 1914 restricted legal distribution of opiates to physicians.[3,16]

The relief of pain has been a primary task of physicians throughout history. Thus opiates and synthetic narcotic analgesics remain one of the most important drug categories in medicine. The development of specific narcotic antagonists, the identification of the opiate receptors, and the discovery of endogenous substances with opiate-like activity (endorphins) characterize the recent history of this important pharmacological class. [3,12]

Patterns of Opioid Use

In the United States a significant percentage of opiate users prior to World War II were white and from the Southern states, and female users were commonplace. Since then an increasing number of opiate users have been urban black, Puerto Rican, and Chicano males, who primarily use intravenous heroin. These groups may account for about half of the opiate users today. The number of individuals in the United States who regularly use heroin has stabilized during the last few years to about 600,000. There was a tenfold increase in regular heroin use between 1960 and 1969, from about 60,000 to more than 600,000, followed by a slight decline and then leveling off during the late 1970s and 1980s. [12,14]

Urban users typically belong to a drug subculture and obtain daily supplies of illegally synthesized and imported heroin from a "dealer" or "connection." Many enter the heroin subculture with intermittent parenteral heroin injections called chipping or skin-popping, which gradually escalate to daily intravenous injections. Opioid users within the medical profession use preparations manufactured by drug companies, such as morphine sulfate, oxycodone hydrochloride, methadone, pethidine (meperidine hydrochloride), and codeine. [13,14,29]

Recently heroin users have been using a combination of pentazocine hydrochloride (Talwin) and the antihistamine tripelennamine hydrochloride (Pyribenzamine, or PBZ). [23] This combination is known on the street as T's and blues, and users report a euphoric rush similar to that from heroin; however, the claim is anecdotal. The pharmacological properties, including the toxicity of this opiate/antihistamine combination, are not yet fully known. Users have been reported to have seizures, strokes, central nervous system (CNS) infections, hepatic failure, and encephalopathies. [23] However, much of this toxicity may be related to intravenous drug use rather than a direct pharmacological complication of the drugs themselves. The recent addition of the opioid antagonist naloxone hydrochloride to the formulation of pentazocine (Talwin-NX) may decrease its intravenous abuse. Naloxone counteracts the intravenous effect of pentazocine but not the intended oral effect, since naloxone is not well absorbed from the gastrointestinal (GI) tract. [156]

The combination of glutethimide (Doriden) and codeine has been used orally as a heroin substitute. [171] Although this combination was reported more than sixteen years ago, current users refer to the combination as loads. [158] The term frequently refers to a packet containing two 500 mg tablets of glutethimide and four tablets of codeine No. 4, which equals 60 mg. Thus the user will ingest 1 gm glutethimide and 240 mg codeine. This combination is alleged to produce euphoria equal to that of heroin without the stigma associated with intravenous drug use, and effects lasting for six to eight hours. The use of loads is dangerous because patients have been reported to use three to twelve loads per day, corresponding to a daily intake of 3 to 12 gm glutethimide and 720 to 2,880 mg codeine. These amounts can easily produce sudden death. [171]

Another fad among opioid users are so-called designer drugs. These drugs are created by underground chemists who modify the molecular structure of illegal opiates to produce variants that are not specifically banned by federal law. One of these "designer" opiates is a methylated derivative of the opiate anesthetic fentanyl, which is many times more potent than heroin. A major problem with these modified opiates is their increased potency and therefore their increased tendency to cause death by overdose. To date, at least six fentanyl derivatives, one of them a thousand times more potent than heroin, have been identified as street opioids of abuse. By 1985, it is estimated that these designer opioids have been responsible for at least ninety cases of fatal overdose. [37]

All opioid users, like other psychoactive

drug users, claim that euphoria is the primary reason for their drug use.[12,119] The euphoria produced by intravenous opiates immediately after injection is described as an intense, orgasmic sensation known as a rush, followed by a peaceful withdrawal from one's physical and psychological environment into a state of quiet bliss, "like floating on a cloud." After repeated intravenous injections, tolerance develops, and users require increasing amounts of opiates to prevent withdrawal reactions and even for everyday functioning. At this stage, the intravenous use is no longer described as euphoric, and the user is involved in a daily struggle to maintain an expensive addiction. Martin[119] suggests that much drug abuse, including opioid abuse, is an attempt to reverse hypophoria, a state characterized by a poor self-image—that is, feeling like a failure, unpopular, inept, and not respected or appreciated. The peaceful, oblivious euphoria described by opiate addicts who use intravenous preparations may be one method of reversing hypophoria.

Acute Opioid Toxicity

Heroin users have a higher mortality rate than that of their age-matched peers: sixteen deaths per 1,000 users per year for addicts under thirty, thirty per 1,000 per year in older addicts. The increased mortality rate is due in part to acute toxicity of heroin or adulterants. The heroin user is often unaware of the purity and hence of the dose of heroin injected, and users vary considerably in their level of tolerance to opioids at any time. After withdrawal, users who had a high degree of prewithdrawal tolerance might become acutely toxic with their usual prewithdrawal dose. Children of heroin users on methadone maintenance may unknowingly swallow a toxic amount of methadone dissolved in fruit juice or flavored syrup and stored in the refrigerator for weekend use.[12,13,14]

Sixty milligrams morphine or the equivalent dose of another opioid may be dangerous for an adult; 240 mg can be fatal. In one

report, 60 mg morphine was fatal; however, with careful medical management, recovery from a dose of 760 mg morphine has also been reported. The elderly, children, and patients with hypothyroidism or respiratory disease have increased sensitivity to opioid toxicity.[14]

A recent investigation of an epidemic of heroin-related deaths in Washington, D.C., sheds new light on the factors that contribute to regional increases in opioid toxicity.[151] Deaths associated with intravenous injection of illegal heroin increased substantially between April 1979 and December 1982; and in 1981 the population-based mortality rate in Washington was 17.4 per 100,000, which is possibly the highest ever reported. A case-controlled investigation based on postmortem blood analysis suggested that increased concentrations of heroin were a substantial risk factor, as would be expected. However, the investigation also indicated that increased concentrations of ethanol were a substantial risk factor. During the Washington epidemic, there was more heroin in individual packages sold on the street and it was available for a lower price, which suggests that when inexpensive heroin of higher concentration is available, former heroin addicts who are currently abusing alcohol may return to recreational heroin use, with a resulting increase in mortality. Finally, there was some evidence in the Washington epidemic that quinine, which is a well-documented street heroin adulterant, may also have contributed to the deaths.[151]

The acute opioid toxicity syndrome includes respiratory distress, which often presents as apnea with cyanosis, areflexia, and pupillary miosis, unless anoxia has caused them to dilate. Intoxicated patients are often unresponsive, but the coma is characteristically light relative to the degree of respiratory depression. Evaluation of cardiopulmonary function can reveal hypotension, tachycardia, and at times pulmonary edema. Seizures occur but are rare. Acute heroin toxicity usually represents the combination of opioid toxicity and an allergic or hypersensitivity reaction to the adulterants used to dilute the heroin. The opioid toxicity syndrome is relatively uniform among natural and synthetic opioids; however, pethidine may cause dilated pupils and muscular tremors, while both it and dextropropoxyphene more frequently cause seizures.[12,13,14]

These clinical characteristics are usually sufficiently obvious to make the diagnosis of acute opioid toxicity a relatively straightforward one. Sometimes persons accompanying the patient to the hospital can specify the time of administration of heroin, and for a child with opioid toxicity from methadone, the dose can often be determined. In addition, many users of illegal opioids have distinct areas of hyperpigmented needle tracks from vein scarring, which result from repeated drug injection in nonmedical settings.

Management of Opioid Toxicity

Cardiorespiratory resuscitation is the first task in the management of the patient with acute opioid toxicity. After the upper respiratory passages have been cleared of obstructions, mouth-to-mouth or mouth-to-oral airway resuscitation should be given to the patient who is apneic or cyanotic. If the patient has no pulse, external cardiac massage must be given simultaneously. If the patient remains apneic or is vomiting, intubation with a cuffed endotracheal tube may be needed to prevent aspiration. To evaluate the efficacy of the resuscitation efforts, arterial blood oxygen, carbon dioxide, and pH should be monitored. A large intravenous (IV) line is needed and sometimes requires a "venous cutdown" because of scarred surface veins. To correct for the possibility that hypoglycemia has exacerbated the coma, 50 ml of 50 percent glucose should be administered through the IV line.*

The appropriate pharmacological agent for the management of acute opioid toxicity is the narcotic antagonist naloxone, since it causes no respiratory suppression. Naloxone 0.4 mg to 1.0 mg (1 ml or 1 ampoule of standard preparation Narcan equals 0.4 mg naloxone) is given to both adults and children. If no response is seen in the first five minutes, 2 mg naloxone (5 ml Narcan) can be given. Intravenous naloxone is so safe that it could be used routinely as a diagnostic test in any comatose patient on the chance that opioid toxicity is contributing to the coma. Naloxone can be administered through the femoral vein in adults or the external jugular vein in children before the IV line is established. Physical restraints are often placed on the patient before naloxone is administered. This is advisable, because when the drug is effective, patients often wake up disoriented, angry, and assaultive, with severe opioid withdrawal symptoms. Naloxone commonly reverses symptoms of opioid toxicity within minutes, and dilation of the pupils is often the first sign of a positive response.*

Since naloxone has a short duration of pharmacological activity, opioid-induced respiratory depression can return within two to four hours. Thus patients with opioid toxicity require continued monitoring of respiratory status. Following a heroin overdose, one or two doses of naloxone are often sufficient. However, the child with an overdose of methadone will probably require repeated injections of naloxone and constant observation over the next twelve to twenty-four hours.†

Attempts to revive the illegal opioid user "on the street" may complicate the medical treatment of the toxicity syndrome. Well-meaning friends often try to revive heroin addicts with facial slaps or by squeezing or applying ice to nipples or testicles. Street myths have suggested that intravenous amphetamine, milk, or saline can reverse heroin overdoses. Regrettably, amphetamine can precipitate seizures in patients with hypoxia; milk can cause lipoid pneumonia; and saline, probably the safest of the three, may disturb the electrolyte balance. Any unsterilized injection can introduce infection.[14]

*See references 12, 13, 14, 67, and 68.

*See references 12, 13, 14, 67, and 68.
†See references 12, 13, 14, 67, and 68.

MPTP Toxicity and Parkinson's Disease in Heroin Addicts

In an effort to evade the laws against opioids, the illegal synthesis of new compounds with opiate activity is an increasingly common practice. Recently this activity led to a tragic story of drug toxicity.[32,110,176] A synthetic opioid, 1-methyl-4-phenyl-1,2,5,6-tetrahydropyridine (MPTP), was produced in a northern California laboratory and sold illegally in the San Jose area. MPTP is rapidly oxidized to the 1-methyl-4-phenylpyridinium ion (MPP+), and this oxidation produces an extremely toxic intermediate chemical that selectively kills specific brain cells. The cells that are selectively affected are those of the substantia nigra, and a syndrome with clinical symptoms that are identical to Parkinson's disease can result. The disease can be severe enough to cause permanent disability.[32,76,110] A team of investigators from the Centers for Disease Control in Atlanta has determined that more than three hundred people in the state of California have used MPTP and that as of April 1985, the drug was still being sold.

The identification of MPTP as the toxic agent responsible for an outbreak of Parkinson's disease among young heroin users in California is one of the most remarkable stories of recent medical history. It involved careful observation and follow-up by a Stanford neurologist, L. William Langston, who located a team at the National Institute of Mental Health (NIMH), including Drs. Glenn Davis, Sanford Markey, Stanley Burns, and Irwin Kopin, who were already investigating the case of a graduate student who developed a parkinsonlike condition after using 1-methyl-4-phenyl-proprionoxy-piperidine (MPPP) that was probably contaminated with MPTP.[110]

The ultimate connection between the toxic opiate MPTP and Parkinson's disease was probably simultaneously made by both the Stanford group led by Langston and the NIMH team of investigators. This important investigation has also recently revealed that the monoamine oxidase (MAO) inhibitor deprenyl inhibits the metabolism of MPTP. When given as a pretreatment to nonhuman primates before MPTP administration, it can prevent the development of the parkinsonian symptoms. The investigation has also stimulated a renewed interest in research in classical and atypical Parkinson's disease. Researchers are looking for a history of exposure to chemical toxins in patients with the classical form. They are also searching for toxins in one rural area in Canada, where the incidence of Parkinson's disease is five times higher than that of the general population, and on the island of Guam, where until 1965 one out of five deaths was due to an atypical form of the disease.[32,76,110]

While this story may shed light on Parkinson's disease, it remains tragic for those heroin users exposed to MPTP. Of 150 MPTP users examined by researchers from the Center for Disease Control, as many as half had early and subtle signs of Parkinson's disease. Since cell death in the substantia nigra is part of the normal aging process, many of these individuals may develop more serious parkinsonian symptoms as they get older.[110]

Management of Opioid Withdrawal with Opioids

The opioid abstinence syndrome is less serious and easier to manage than the withdrawal syndromes of alcohol or sedative-hypnotics. Eight to twelve hours after the last dose of morphine or heroin, the syndrome begins with restlessness, anxiety, and sometimes drowsiness. Brief and disturbed sleep can follow. Lacrimation, nasal discharge, sweating, yawning, and deep sighing respirations appear as agitation increases. After twenty-four to thirty-six hours, the patient usually has insomnia, anorexia, severe anxiety, waves of "goose-flesh," and alternating periods of chills and warmth, often accompanied by fevers of 38° C to 39° C. Muscle and joint pains are common, as are abdominal cramps, vomiting, and diarrhea. Tachycardia and hypertension may be found on physical examination. The severe symptoms usually subside after seventy-two hours, while weakness, anxiety, and disturbed sleep may persist for weeks or even months.[12]

The withdrawal syndrome from opioids other than heroin is similar, differing only in intensity and time course. Codeine and pethidine (meperidine, Demerol) produce mild withdrawal syndromes; the symptoms of codeine withdrawal are slow to appear, while those of pethidine withdrawal appear early. Methadone withdrawal lasts about two weeks and is mild, but can include deep muscle and bone pain.[13,14]

There are really two parts to the opioid abstinence syndrome. The first part is the physiological/psychological syndrome just described. The second part is the elaboration or exaggeration of symptoms that abusers frequently use in their desire to obtain more opioids. It is often hard to distinguish between these two, and heroin users are expert at creative complaining, stealing, forging prescriptions, and conning other patients and staff. For this reason, treatment of the opioid withdrawal syndrome requires an inpatient or outpatient unit with adequate security and an experienced, skeptical, and hypervigilant staff.[12]

Patients withdrawing from opioids require a complete medical and drug abuse history. They also need a careful physical examination and a routine clinical blood evaluation, including screening tests for common substances of abuse. One standard method of detoxification begins with 20 mg methadone *per os* (PO). If this dose causes gross intoxication, the patient will probably not require gradual opioid withdrawal. If the patient develops withdrawal symptoms during the next twelve to twenty-four hours, a second 20 mg oral dose of methadone should be given. For most opioid addicts, two 20 mg methadone doses (40 mg) PO on the first day will prevent severe withdrawal symptoms. Only drug dealers or patients withdrawing from methadone maintenance commonly require higher doses of methadone on the first day of abstinence. After two or three days on a stable dose, methadone can be reduced by 5 or 10 mg each day, leading to complete detoxification in four to ten days. Diazepam can be given if the anxiety is severe, while any benzodiazepine hypnotic can be used for insomnia. Massage and Jacuzzi baths can be useful for muscle and bone pain.[12,13,14]

The children born to opioid-using mothers can develop a syndrome that probably represents opioid withdrawal. Within forty-eight hours after delivery, these infants may become extremely irritable and hyperactive. The hyperactivity can cause extreme irritation on the skin of the face, elbows, and knees. They may also develop fever, coarse tremors, anorexia, and vomiting. Respiratory disturbances such as tachypnea, a shrill, high-pitched "catlike" cry, and seizures have also been reported.[14]

The treatment of these infants is more urgent than the treatment of the adult abstinence syndrome; infants with respiratory distress and seizures will require immediate attention. The maintenance of fluid and electrolyte balance may require intravenous feedings, and a careful diagnostic evaluation should be carried out. One pharmacological treatment for this syndrome is Paregoric (camphorated tincture of opium), three to ten drops every four hours. The dose can be titrated to decrease hyperactivity, irritability, and other symptoms without causing oversedation. Dosage should be tapered gradually over four to five days.[12,117]

Management of Opioid Withdrawal with Clonidine or Lofexidine

The discovery of the effects of clonidine in opiate withdrawal was a result of studies on the activity of the locus coeruleus in nonhuman primates.[57] Electrical or pharmacological activation of the locus coeruleus was reported to produce changes in animals similar to those seen with opiate withdrawal.[54,143,144] Morphine and clonidine hydrochloride inhibited the effects of this electrical and pharmacological activation of the locus coeruleus. This suggested that opioid withdrawal may be due in part to increased norepinephrine (NE) neuronal activity in areas such as the locus coeruleus. Studies of the locus coeruleus have shown it to contain receptors for both opiates and alpha-2 adrenergic compounds such as clonidine. Both opioids and clonidine seem capable of reducing locus coeruleus activation through independent receptors. This hypothesis has subsequently been supported by the use of clonidine and other alpha-2 adrenergic agonists as treatments for opioid withdrawal in human subjects.[54,57,143,144]

Clonidine has been used as an experimental treatment for the withdrawal of patients on methadone maintenance or patients who are addicted to other opioids. Two groups of investigators have reported the drug's utility in inpatient withdrawal from methadone addiction.[56,187,188] One method[57] for clonidine withdrawal begins with a test dose of 6 μg per kg PO. If the patient's withdrawal symptoms are reduced, detoxification proceeds using clonidine in a dose of 17 μg per kg for an additional ten to fourteen days—7 μg per kg at 8:00 A.M., 3 μg per kg at 4:00 P.M., and 7 μg per kg at 10:00 P.M. This dosage schedule is followed for ten days. From day 10 through 13, the dose is reduced by 50 percent daily, and then clonidine is discontinued. To minimize the risk of additional hypotension, the opiate should be discontinued as soon as the clonidine is started. An alternative to this method[181] gives a greater dose of clonidine at bedtime, when the increased sedative effects can improve sleep and when orthostatic hypotension is less of a problem because the patient is supine.

This regimen was used successfully in a fourteen-day inpatient study of one hundred methadone addicts. The total dose of opioid per day for methadone addicts is usually higher than the street dose of opioid used by a patient addicted to illegal heroin. However, such a regimen seems to be safe and effective for most subjects on an inpatient basis. Major side effects of clonidine are sedation and hypotension, and they are serious enough to make outpatient detoxification hazardous. The drowsiness and dizziness induced by clonidine can interfere with normal daily activities. However, the drug does not produce euphoria and is not an opioid, and clonidine withdrawal, if it exists at all,

has not yet been reported in human detoxification studies.[55,181]

When clonidine is used to treat patients addicted to opiates other than methadone, the dose can be modified. For some individuals, 20 μg per kg per day may be necessary to prevent withdrawal symptoms from a high dose of methadone or another opiate. For some opiates, the duration of the withdrawal syndrome is shorter than that of methadone. Thus pethidine withdrawal may require only six days of clonidine treatment, since pethidine has a shorter half-life, while the ten- to fourteen-day withdrawal regimen just described is necessary for patients addicted to methadone, which has a longer half-life.[181]

While clonidine has generally proven to be effective when used to treat withdrawal symptoms on inpatients addicted only to opiates, a recent case report suggests that it must be used cautiously in patients with mixed drug dependencies.[85] In such cases, clonidine may obscure some common early signs of the more dangerous sedative-hypnotic withdrawal syndrome such as tachycardia, hypertension, perspiration, and tremor (see section entitled "Management of the Sedative-hypnotic Withdrawal Syndrome"). The absence of these warning signs in a patient addicted to both opiates and sedative-hypnotics may allow the withdrawal state from sedative-hypnotics to go unrecognized until the more serious psychotic syndrome develops.[85] In addition, the hypotensive effects of clonidine are frequently severe enough to preclude its use in outpatient detoxification.[106]

Lofexidine is a structural analogue of clonidine that has milder sedative and hypotensive effects. Recently the same two groups of investigators who introduced the technique of using clonidine in opioid withdrawal have reported successful detoxification of opioid addicts using lofexidine.[58,189] Lofexidine appeared to be approximately as efficacious as clonidine in reducing the symptoms of opioid withdrawal and, in these preliminary open trials, produced less sedation and hypotension than clonidine.[58,189]

One regimen began with a test dose of

lofexidine of 3 μg per kg PO. This was followed by lofexidine 20 μg per kg per day in divided doses for at least ten additional days. Thus a 60 kg patient would receive 1.2 mg per day. In the other investigation, the dose of lofexidine varied from 0.6 mg to 1.6 mg across ten subjects, with an average dose of 1.2 mg. The major complaint of the patients was difficulty in falling or staying asleep. Withdrawal symptoms were not completely suppressed, and using higher doses of lofexidine to suppress all withdrawal symptoms may produce hypotension and/or sedation. Nevertheless, these two investigations suggest that lofexidine may prove to be even safer and therefore more clinically useful than clonidine, especially in outpatient detoxification.[58,189]

Both inpatient and outpatient treatment of the opioid abstinence syndrome are an important part of the management and rehabilitation of opioid addicts. Treatment centers now appear to have the option of using either methadone substitution and withdrawal or a withdrawal program that uses an alpha-2 adrenergic agonist such as clonidine or lofexidine. Both withdrawal procedures seem satisfactory. The major determinant of future drug use by detoxified opioid addicts seems to be based on relapse to opioid use after detoxification rather than on the method of detoxification.[12] However, future investigations that include direct comparisons of methadone detoxification versus lofexidine or clonidine withdrawal are needed to determine the safest and most efficacious detoxification method.

Medical Disorders Complicating Opioid Abuse

Opioid abusers have an increased incidence of medical complications, some of which are directly related to the method of opioid abuse and others that are more a function of the users' life-style. Unsterile conditions cause an increased incidence of hepatitis; thrombophlebitis; subcutaneous abscesses; infective endocarditis that may involve the right, left, or both sides of the heart; lung abscesses; septic pulmonary emboli; and osteomyelitis. The use of contaminated syringes and needles and the substance of abuse itself can transmit tetanus, acquired immune deficiency disease (AIDS), and rarely, malaria. Pulmonary fibrosis, acute and chronic polyneuropathy, glomerulonephritis, nephrotic syndrome, and transverse myelitis have all been reported in users of illegal opioids. In addition, pneumonia, tuberculosis, urinary tract infections, and venereal diseases are more commonly seen in opioid abusers than in the general population. Finally, some have other injuries or illnesses such as teeth abscesses, appendicitis, or an injury whose pain has been masked by the analgesic effect of the opioid they abuse.[12,14]

The opioid overdose syndrome sometimes includes pulmonary edema. However, pulmonary edema sometimes occurs at lower doses of opioids, particularly when the opioid is injected illegal heroin. This pulmonary edema may represent a hypersensitivity or an allergic phenomenon. The opioid abuser with pulmonary edema will require a chest x-ray and arterial blood gas determinations. If the patient is found to be hypoxic, the situation is life-threatening. The patient may have to sit up and receive such emergency treatments as oxygen, diuretics, digitalis, aminophylline, and rotating tourniquets.[12,14]

Mechanism of Action of Opioids

The understanding of the mechanism of actions of the opioid narcotic analgesics was greatly facilitated by the discovery of opioid receptors and endogenous opioid peptides. These discoveries, which were not serendipitous, may be the most exciting advances in the recent history of neurobiology. The high degree of structural specificity and stereospecificity of many of the effects of opioid drugs led some investigators to suggest as early as the 1940s that these drugs acted through specific opioid receptors.[11,15] A vigorous search for these receptors began in the 1970s, after Avram Goldstein proposed a paradigm for the search.[60] In 1973 three groups of investigators reported highly specific opioid receptors in mammalian brain.[135,164,178] Following this discovery, numerous investigators suggested that brain opioid receptors must be the target of a naturally occurring, or endogenous, opioid substance.[11,15]

A second observation also led to the search for endogenous opioid compounds. In 1972 Akil, Mayer, and Liebeskind[4] reported that the analgesia produced by electrical stimulation of certain brain areas in the rat could be partially reversed by the potent opioid antagonist naloxone. This observation suggested that electrically stimulated analgesia was mediated in part by a natural substance with actions like those of morphine, an endogenous opioid.[11,15]

The first endogenous opioids discovered were two small peptides of five amino acids, named methionine enkephalin (met-ENK) and leucine enkephalin (leu-ENK) by their discoverers, Hughes and Kosterlitz.[84] Since then numerous opioid peptides have been discovered and characterized in mammalian brain. There has also been an explosion of research on the possible role of these numerous endorphins or endogenous opioids. Recent studies suggest that there are at least three completely different opioid peptide families whose precursors have now been defined as three distinct proteins, each with a molecular weight from around 28,000 to 30,000 daltons. The precursor for beta-endorphin also produces adrenocorticotropin (ACTH) and is known as pro-opiomelanocortin. The precursor of met-ENK and leu-ENK is produced by a protein known as proenkephalin, which occurs in mammalian brain and adrenal gland. Finally, a third precursor known as prodynorphin/neoendorphin produces the endorphins dynorphin A and B and alpha- and beta-neoendorphin. Each of the major protein precursors has been fully characterized and sequenced. However, many years of research will be required to determine the physiological role of these three opioid peptide families.[11]

The task is even more complex because of the existence of multiple opioid receptors. The first evidence for the existence of multiple opioid receptors was reported by Martin and coworkers,[51,120] who performed classical pharmacological studies in dogs. Based on their results, three types of opioid receptors were postulated, which Martin named for the prototype drugs used in the studies: mu from morphine, kappa from ketocyclazocine, and sigma from SKF 10047.[15,163]

Subsequent to the work of Martin and associates, Kosterlitz and colleagues provided the first evidence of an additional opiate receptor that prefers enkephalins.[114] Since this receptor appeared to be the predominant receptor type present in the mouse vas deferens, which is an important *in vitro* bioassay system for opioids, it was named the delta receptor (for "deferens"). The other *in vitro* bioassay system, the guinea pig ileum, was found to have mainly the Martin's mu receptor.[163] Recent studies suggest that morphine and beta-endorphin show high affinity for both mu and delta receptors. Dynorphin seems to bind to kappa receptors, while the enkephalins show the highest affinity for delta receptors. Although this is a gross oversimplification, it gives some idea of the complications of trying to determine the role of opioid receptors and endogenous opioids both in normal and abnormal physiology and in the pharmacological actions of opioids.[15,163]

The best evidence for a role of the endogenous opioids is in the area of pain modulation. Much of this evidence is based on investigations of the antagonism by naloxone of a variety of non-drug-induced analgesias. In addition, a number of studies show that the release of enkephalins or endorphins increases dramatically during stress and analgesia.[15,163]

Thus, to date, the most important consequence of research into the complex system of endogenous opioids and their multiple receptors is the knowledge that they exist. However, future research will probably demonstrate that the mechanism of action of exogenous opioids, which are used as substances of abuse, is through some alteration of the endogenous opioid system and its receptors. Research on the endogenous opiates and their receptors should eventually add to our understanding of the mechanisms of opioid addiction.[11] Such research could also lead to better medical methods for controlling pain, memory disorders, mood and appetite abnormalities, and perhaps other psychiatric disorders.

¶ Psychostimulants

History of Cocaine

Cocaine is an alkaloid of the leaves of the *Erythoxylon coca* plant, which grows on the mountain and central slopes of Central America. Chewing coca leaves was probably common prior to the great conquest by the Inca tribe, after which its use was reserved for the nobility and priesthood. The Incas believed that the plant was a divine gift from the sun god. When the Spanish, led by Pizarro, conquered the Inca Empire, they learned of the benefits ascribed to chewing coca leaves, and the use of coca leaves among the Indians again became widespread. Mild mood elevation, alertness, a feeling of increased energy, and decreased appetite are the common effects of chewing these leaves. The leaves were brought to Spain during the sixteenth century and to Vienna, Austria, where Albert Nieman isolated the cocaine alkaloid in the mid-nineteenth century.[12,16,128]

Although the chewing of coca leaves was relatively uncommon in Europe or the United States, small amounts of coca extract were added to various "medicinal" drinks. Vin Mariani coca wine was popular in Europe in the late nineteenth century and was endorsed by world-famous people, including members of European royal families. An American drink containing coca extract was introduced in 1886 by J. S. Pemberton of Atlanta. Pemberton combined the extracts of the kola nut, which contains caffeine, and coca leaves, labeling the syrup Coca-Cola®. However, by the early 1900s Coca-Cola was made from coca leaves from which the cocaine had been removed.[16]

In addition to oral use, coca-leaf smoking was also part of the culture of the Indians of the Andes. Coca and tobacco were often mixed both for chewing and smoking. In 1787 the Peruvian physician Antonio de Julia suggested that coca-leaf smoking was safer than tobacco-leaf smoking. In 1885 the Parke-Davis company manufactured coca cigarettes and a cocaine inhalant that was suggested to be useful in the treatment of hayfever, opium addiction, respiratory complaints, bronchitis, asthma, hoarseness, influenza, snoring, croup, and headache.[12,16,128,161]

Pure cocaine isolated by Merck Laboratories was given to Bavarian soldiers by Theodore D. Aschenbrandt in 1884, who reported that it decreased fatigue. Sigmund Freud, who was then a young neurologist in Vienna, read this report and began experimenting with cocaine. He described his personal euphoric experiences with the drug in the July 1884 issue of *Zentral Blatt fur die gesammte Therapie*. In this and subsequent papers, Freud recommended the drug for hysteria, depression, hypochondria, and digestive disorders and as a cure for morphine and alcohol addiction. Freud sent cocaine to his fiancée and gave some to his colleague, Ernst von Fleischl-Marxow, who was addicted to morphine because of painful neuromata. Von Fleischl-Marxow began his treatment with small doses of cocaine and gradually increased the dosage. Within a year he was taking at least a gram a day, more than twenty times the dose Freud occasionally used for his depressions. As a result, von Fleischl-Marxow developed cocaine psychosis, a syndrome that resembles acute paranoid schizophrenia. Because of this tragic incident, Freud abandoned his personal use of cocaine and eliminated all mention of his cocaine studies from his autobiography. Unfortunately, Freud was so dismayed by his experiences with cocaine research that he stopped all psychopharmacological investigations.*

In the late nineteenth century Karl Koller

---

*See references 12, 16, 20, 128, and 161.

discovered the local anesthetic properties of cocaine and described its use for ophthalmic surgery. The primary medical use of cocaine today is as a local anesthetic in otolaryngological surgery not only because of its anesthetic properties but also because of its vasoconstrictive action.[161] The use of cocaine as a vasoconstrictor had been known since the nineteenth century, when Europeans described Cobo Indians in Peru and Bolivia inhaling the vapors of burning coca seeds as a treatment for nosebleeds.[161]

History of Amphetamines

An excellent description of the discovery of amphetamines is given by Chauncey Leake.[7] K. K. Chen, a colleague of Leake's at the University of Wisconsin in the 1920s, went to China to begin a systematic investigation of the ancient Chinese drug classification. The desert plant Ma Huang *(Ephedra vulgaris)* was commonly recommended for asthma in several areas of China. In 1925 Chen and Carl Schmidt rediscovered the active alkaloid, ephedrine, which is still used as a treatment for asthma.[7,12]

In the 1930s Gordon Alles, in his attempt to find a synthetic substitute for ephedrine, collaborated with Leake, then at the University of California, San Francisco, in testing several related phenylethylamines for biological activity. The most active compound of their first series of ephedrine analogues was d,l-phenyl-isopropyl-amine (amphetamine or benzadrine). The dextro-rotated isomer of amphetamine, dextroamphetamine (Dexedrine), was clinically tested in the 1930s. Increased alertness, improved physical and mental performance, euphoria, and decreased appetite similar to but longer-lasting than the effects of cocaine were observed and reported.[7,12]

During World War II both the Allied and Axis forces made extensive use of amphetamines. Postwar Japan placed large supplies of amphetamines on the open market. This led to an epidemic of amphetamine abuse and numerous cases of amphetamine psychosis. Other epidemics of amphetamine abuse have occurred in Sweden and the United States. It is ironic that the amphetamine epidemic in the Haight-Ashbury district of San Francisco in the late 1960s took place six blocks from the San Francisco Medical Center where Alles and Leake had first synthesized amphetamine forty years earlier.

Patterns of Cocaine Use

Cocaine is a highly valued psychoactive substance that strongly reinforces its own use. Cocaine use continues to increase, and it is currently believed that more than 22 million Americans have used the drug. However, many users take cocaine sporadically, probably due to its high cost and unpredictable supply. While cocaine of 90 to 100 percent purity was frequently available on the illicit market several years ago, today the purity has dropped to between 30 to 50 percent. Of the current substances of abuse, cocaine holds the highest status among middle- and upper-class young people, many of whom consider it the most desirable of the psychoactive substances. Cocaine use is popular among musicians, artists, and athletes.[12]

The salt cocaine hydrochloride is usually inhaled as a dry powder through a thin tube inserted into the nostril to the nasal mucosa. It can also be dissolved in water and injected intravenously and can be mixed with other psychoactive agents such as heroin. The combination of heroin and cocaine became popular with the American forces during the Korean war, when the combination was known as a speedball. This combination of a psychostimulant and an opioid continues to be popular.[12]

Both intravenous and nasal administration of cocaine rapidly produce high plasma levels and a clinical syndrome of short duration requiring frequent administration to sustain the effects of the drug. Cocaine users claim they experience a euphoria that is different from that described after the use of opiates or hallucinogens.

A recent trend in cocaine use is the smoking of cocaine "freebase." Cocaine hydrochloride salt is soluble in water (1 gm will dissolve in less than 1 ml), making it suitable for intravenous injection and for dissolving on the nasal mucous membrane. When cocaine hydrochloride is dissolved in water and the pH is changed to alkaline, followed by extraction into ether or chloroform, which is then evaporated, the result is the volatile "freebase" (its melting point is 98°C), which is more suitable for smoking. The freebase is not very water soluble (1 gm will dissolve in 600 ml), and this makes it impossible to use intranasally or intravenously. Smoking freebase brings the compound to the large surface of the lungs for absorption, which produces as rapid an elevation of plasma level as intravenous injection or intranasal application.[12]

Cocaine euphoria is reported to be exhilarating, sometimes enabling the user to feel creative, energetic, articulate, talkative, attractive, excited, motivated, and capable of performing difficult and sometimes grandiose tasks. Cocaine users frequently use metaphors of energy, power, and sexual orgasm to describe this ecstasy. A subjective sense of improved mental and physical abilities and decreased appetite are also reported. All of these effects rapidly dissipate, and cocaine must be taken frequently to maintain them. Negative effects include restlessness, agitation, anxiety, hyperexcitability, irritability, and hostility.[136] Chronic negative effects include slurred speech, muscle pains, tremulousness, weight loss, chest pain, urination difficulty, respiratory problems, edema, seizures, insomnia, and paranoid psychosis.[12,136,161]

Patterns of Amphetamine Use

There are several common legal and illegal patterns of use of amphetamines and related substances. These psychostimulants accounted for almost 17 million prescriptions in 1977.[29] Oral amphetamine users include those who believe they require its stimulant qualities to prevent sleep or fatigue for periods of sustained activity, those desiring to lose weight, and those who desire improved athletic or mental performance. Long-dis-

tance truck drivers, individuals holding two jobs, students preparing for or taking examinations, and athletes in almost every sport are among those who use amphetamines or amphetaminelike substances. The syndrome produced by oral amphetamine use is similar to that described for cocaine, but is generally of longer duration and can be milder if lower dosages of amphetamine are used. A second pattern of amphetamine use involves the intravenous administration of the drug in rapidly increasing doses over a period of days in what is called a speed-run; this intravenous use usually stops after four to six sleepless days and nights when the user falls asleep, or "crashes."[12,14,43,180]

Thus the clinical symptoms produced by cocaine and amphetamines are remarkably similar. For example, the chronic use of both drugs can produce symptoms that are nearly identical to those of acute paranoid schizophrenia.[43,167] However, amphetamine and amphetaminelike substances generally have a longer duration of action than cocaine, and amphetamine rapidly produces tolerance. True tolerance to the chronic use of cocaine has been demonstrated in animal studies but has not been reported in human users.[43]

The Psychostimulant Intoxication Syndrome

There are two major adverse reactions to cocaine, amphetamines, and amphetaminelike compounds. These are the paranoid psychosis that can result from chronic psychostimulant use and the acute and potentially fatal reaction that results from an overdose. Psychostimulant paranoid psychosis[43,167] generally occurs with high concentrations of amphetamines and amphetaminelike drugs. After repeated use, tolerance to amphetamines develops, and the dose is increased. Alternatively, high blood-plasma levels may result from repeated intravenous injections of large doses of amphetamines. These high plasma concentrations or a sudden increase in plasma concentrations can produce paranoid psychosis.[12]

The psychostimulant psychotic syndrome

is characterized by suspiciousness, aggression, persecutory delusions, and visual and auditory misperceptions or hallucinations. The psychosis can also include hyperactivity and repetitive compulsive behavior that is reminiscent of animal stereotypy. Psychostimulant psychosis sometimes includes tactile hallucinations of small insects crawling on or just under the skin (parasitosis, formication).[43,167] Unfortunately, individuals experiencing an amphetamine-induced paranoid state have the potential for assaultiveness and violent behavior because of their suspiciousness and delusions of persecution. Clinically, case reports have described a cocaine psychosis syndrome that is nearly identical and in fact may be indistinguishable from amphetamine psychosis.[12,14]

Extremely high doses of either amphetamine or cocaine can cause death by suppressing cardiac function or, more commonly, by suppressing respiratory function. Death through psychostimulant overdose can occur rapidly in a patient and is caused by cardiorespiratory failure, hyperpyrexia, and seizures. Hypertension complicates the clinical presentation of amphetamine or cocaine overdose.* Cocaine deaths have been reported after inhalation, ingestion, or intravenous use of cocaine; the number of deaths due to cocaine overdose has increased dramatically in the United States in the last few years.[140]

Management of Psychostimulant Toxicity

Psychostimulant toxicity is treated using the same general principles as those used for treating toxicity of other psychoactive substances. The highest priority is to secure the safety of the patient and the treatment staff. For patients with amphetamine or cocaine psychosis, this may require arranging for someone to stay with them constantly and the use of physical restraints to control combative or self-destructive behaviors.

A working diagnosis should be made

after the safety of the patient and staff has been ensured. The diagnosis can often be made on the basis of direct questions to the patient or friends about the use of psychostimulants. The drugs need to be mentioned, not only by their generic or trade names but also by their common "street" names: speed, diet pills, uppers, whites, bennys, crystal, crank, hearts, double crosses, and others for amphetamines, and coke, snow, toot, blow, freebase, base, rocks, and others for cocaine.

Physical examination can reveal a variety of symptoms that characterize adverse reactions to psychostimulants and should be performed because of the numerous illnesses associated with psychostimulant use. For example, psychostimulant users can have high blood pressure and excessive sweating. Chronic psychostimulant users may look emaciated because of the appetite suppressing activity of amphetamine and cocaine. Some users will have cutaneous excoriations from skin picking. Urinary tests can be useful, but not all amphetaminelike stimulants are detected in standard toxic screening tests.[12,43]

When a working diagnosis has been made, the patient's surroundings can be arranged to decrease superfluous or threatening stimuli. The treating staff should not position themselves too close to or immediately behind the patient. The paranoid individual can feel overwhelmed by too many staff members and confined by limited space. A paranoid psychostimulant abuser is always capable of unprovoked and unpredictable assault. The psychostimulant user will often improve with supportive nonpharmacological methods; however, some patients will need more active intervention.[14,43]

If paranoid behavior is present or if the blood pressure, pulse rate, or temperature is rising, and it is reasonably certain that psychostimulants were the only drugs taken, the patient can be given an antipsychotic agent such as haloperidol. Antipsychotic drugs block dopamine (DA) receptors and therefore antagonize the effects of psychostimulants. Two to 10 mg haloperidol can be given

*See references 12, 14, 43, 128, and 136.

either orally or intramuscularly (IM). Subsequent doses can be titrated to control both behavior and vital signs. The dosage schedule is also determined by the time course of peak antipsychotic drug effects. To avoid excessive sedation, further doses should not be given until the maximal effect has been observed. Monitoring body temperatures may be useful in determining subsequent doses; rising temperatures suggest that the toxicity is dangerous and that larger doses of antipsychotic medications are necessary. Hyperpyrexia can be treated with cooling blankets, fans, and alcohol and sponge baths. Aspirin with or without acetaminophen can also reduce the fever. Hydration and acidification of the urine to a pH below 5 accelerates the excretion of amphetamines. Urine can be acidified by giving 500 mg to 1 gm ammonium chloride every three to five hours orally or through a nasogastric tube until the urine pH is below 5.[12,14]

Severe hypertension is rare but dangerous when produced by psychostimulant toxicity. Immediate treatment is necessary when the systolic blood pressure is above 200 mm Hg or there are premonitory signs of a cerebral vascular accident, such as visual disturbances or other transient neurological symptoms or signs. Intravenous infusion containing 1 to 5 mg phentolamine should be given over five to ten minutes while the blood pressure is being monitored. The systolic blood pressure should be reduced to 160 to 170 mm Hg, but this must be done slowly to avoid precipitating hypotension.[14]

When the toxic syndrome is due to psychostimulants plus unknown psychoactive substances or when the symptoms are less severe, the use of an antipsychotic drug can be hazardous. There is a narrow margin between effective behavioral sedation with antipsychotic drugs and excessive sedation. The possible interaction of the anticholinergic activity of an antipsychotic agent such as chlorpromazine with the anticholinergic activity in the psychoactive substance can also be a problem. If the intoxication is not life-threatening and blood pressure, pulse, and temperature are not rising, reassurance may suffi-

ciently calm the patient. If agitation and behavioral disturbances continue, benzodiazepines, such as 10 to 30 mg diazepam PO, are useful and safe.

Persistent paranoid psychosis and unstable vital signs despite vigorous treatment are indications for hospitalizing the psychostimulant abuser. Since suicidal ideation sometimes follows the discontinuation of psychostimulants, suicide risk must be carefully assessed; if the risk is high, admission to a security facility with suicide precautions is recommended. Hospitalization is also necessary if markedly impaired perceptions or cognitive function persists and if the numerous medical problems that can be associated with drug abuse are present. If hospitalization is unnecessary, patients should be discharged with a responsible relative or friend, who should observe them closely over the next few days.

Irritability, weakness, lethargy, and depression are often seen when psychostimulants are discontinued, and these symptoms can be predicted in advance.[14,143] In addition to the multidisciplinary approaches to the treatment of psychostimulant abuse including behavioral, group, and psychodynamic therapies, a recent investigation suggests that tricyclic antidepressants may also be useful, at least in cocaine abuse.[48,107]

Gawin and colleagues at Yale have recently offered evidence suggesting that the tricyclic antidepressant desipramine hydrochloride may be effective in the treatment of cocaine abusers with or without depression and that patients with a history of cyclothymia and cocaine abuse might respond to lithium carbonate.[48] The conclusion that desipramine is effective is preliminary; it is based on a retrospective report that ten of fifteen cocaine abusers treated with the drug stopped using cocaine whether they were depressed or not. The conclusion was also bolstered by a preliminary nonblind, nonplacebo-controlled investigation with sixteen patients randomly assigned to desipramine, lithium, or a nonmedication group. Six desipramine-treated patients had a complete remission of cocaine abuse by the end of the third week and were cocaine-free during three further months of tricyclic treatment. Three of the six lithium-treated cocaine abusers also stopped using cocaine by week 12, but all three of these patients had a diagnosis of cyclothymia in addition to cocaine abuse. The three noncyclothymic lithium-treated patients and three of the four patients in the nonmedication group were still using cocaine by week 12. While these results are encouraging, prospective placebo-controlled trials are needed to determine the role of tricyclic antidepressants and lithium in the treatment of cocaine abuse.[107] Further investigations are also needed to determine the possible utility of tricyclic antidepressants and lithium in amphetamine and other psychostimulant abuse.

Mechanisms of Action of Amphetamine and Cocaine

The striking similarity between the behavioral effects of cocaine and amphetamine suggest that they may share a common mode of action. Amphetamine exhibits a wide range of pharmacological activity, the most important of which involves the catecholamines. Amphetamine inhibits the catecholamine metabolizing enzyme MAO, blocks the neuronal uptake of catecholamines, and causes the release of catecholamines from nerve terminals. It may also act directly on postsynaptic catecholamine receptors. The net effect of these actions is to increase catecholaminergic activity. In addition to its effects on catecholamine neuronal activity, amphetamine also alters serotonin (5HT) neuronal activity.

The relative importance of the particular catecholaminergic and serotonergic neurons in amphetamines' actions seems to depend on the behavior being studied. Thus depletion of the catecholamines or destruction of catecholaminergic pathways blocks both stereotyped behaviors and hyperactivity in animals. In contrast, selective depletion of NE alone reduces motor activity but does not prevent the appearance of stereotyped behaviors.[22,134]

¶ PCP

History of PCP

PCP (phencyclidine) is an unusual drug, with unique pharmacological activity and a strange history. There are four distinct phases in the twenty-five-year history of this substance. Animal studies on PCP, one of a number of arylcyclohexylamines, were performed by Parke-Davis in the 1950s. PCP was found to be a highly potent but relatively nontoxic animal anesthetic, even when administered intravenously. The second phase of the history of PCP involved observation of patients and human volunteers, which eventually led to the discovery that the drug is not an ideal human anesthetic agent. Even in low doses, PCP is a uniquely potent psychotomimetic, causing disorientation, delirium, and hallucinations as its anesthetic effects dissipate. PCP was therefore withdrawn as a human anesthetic agent in 1965.[12]

Between 1965 and 1973, in the third phase of its history, PCP was used as a substitute or an adulterant for lysergic acid diethylamide (LSD), mescaline, psilocybin, N, N-dimethyltryptamine (DMT), tetrahydrocannabinol (THC), and other drugs. Users accustomed to other psychoactive substances were so negative about the effects of PCP that they had to be duped into using it. In the fourth phase of its history, which continues today, PCP is used for its inherent properties, a tragic phenomenon quite unexpected considering the numerous negative effects of its intoxication syndrome.[12,137,138]

Patterns of PCP Use

The popularity of PCP as a drug of choice is difficult to explain. Its intoxication syndrome is both variable and unique. The ratio of euphoria to dysphoria is probably lower for PCP than for other substances of abuse, and even confirmed and repeated users agree that disturbing and negative experiences with the drug are common. Several patterns of PCP use have emerged over the past few years. Many users report smoking a cigarette containing PCP, which as a powder is placed on parsley, tobacco, marijuana, or other leafy mixtures. This practice may enable the user to better titrate the dose. PCP can also be inhaled through the nostrils as is cocaine. Street names for PCP include sherman, sherm, sherm-joint, angel dust, dust, crystal, elephant or horse tranquilizer, hog, super or killer weed, mist, and KJ or KW.[137,138]

Approximately half the number of present users of PCP average at least one dose per week. The mean age for the beginning of continuous use of PCP is approximately fifteen years. PCP is used in social settings, and users frequently use other drugs. In fact, in several surveys every PCP user abused additional drugs. The PCP user is more likely to be frequently intoxicated with alcohol, to have more arrests for offenses related to substance abuse, and to have more episodes of drug overdose. Several sources of evidence suggest that PCP use is increasing; more PCP has been confiscated by police departments, more patients intoxicated with PCP are being seen in emergency rooms, and there is an increasing number of referrals by family members, friends, and the criminal justice system for the treatment of PCP abusers.[28,137,138]

PCP abusers describe the drug as producing a syndrome that is different from that of other psychoactive substances. Users describe a "dream world" or a "perfect escape." The drug is reported to have a pronounced effect on thinking, time perception, sense of reality, and mood. Thoughts are perceived as sped up, the mind going faster while time is slowed down, with "no more reality." Experiences assume new perspectives and events seem more dramatic, a fantasy world where wishes are fulfilled and where everything appears more complete and more beautiful. A profound sense of "oneness" with others and with animals is reported, and religious and philosophical thoughts and experiences are described.[137,138]

Intense and euphoric mood states can occur, although almost every PCP user has also experienced severe depression and therefore describes the drug as bringing one to either "the heights or the depths." Feelings of endurance, power, energy, and floating are described. Visual hallucinations are unusual. Effects are said to begin within one to five minutes after smoking and peak after five to thirty minutes. Users describe staying "loaded" or "high" for four to six hours, followed by a "come-down," which lasts from six to twenty-four hours. Nasal insufflation (snorting) leads to a more rapid onset of thirty seconds to one minute, but otherwise is said to produce a clinical syndrome of similar type and duration.[12]

The PCP Intoxication Syndrome

PCP and related arylcyclohexylamines such as ketamine are difficult to classify pharmacologically. The clinical syndrome produced includes pharmacological properties that are shared with psychostimulants, hallucinogens, sedative-hypnotics, alcohol, analgesics, and general anesthetics. PCP has sympathomimetic properties causing increased heart rate and elevated blood pressure.[137]

The negative aspects of the PCP syndrome include disorientation, mental confusion, anxiety, irritability, paranoia, and violent, aggressive, or assaultive behavior. Furthermore, chronic users are reported to have flattened affect, depression, and, sometimes, agitation. Hostility, belligerence, and a proclivity for violence remain long after one would expect the pharmacological effects from the drug to have dissipated; and chronic users may develop a persistent schizophreniclike psychotic syndrome that may last for some months after abstinence. This syndrome can resemble chronic schizophrenia more closely than any other syndrome that is presumed to be drug-induced.[82,137,138]

PCP-related deaths can result from both its pharmacological and behavioral effects.

Because PCP users exhibit bizarre, unpredictable, and assaultive behavior and are often severely agitated and confused, dangerous or life-threatening situations are possible. In California drowning is a major cause of death for individuals who are intoxicated with PCP. Automobile accidents, falls, fires, and other accidents are also reported in PCP-related fatalities.[29,137]

Pharmacological overdose of PCP can also be fatal because of its effects on the cardiovascular system. Unlike LSD, psilocybin, and mescaline, PCP produces cardiopulmonary depression. Less severe overdoses present with variable signs, including dramatic psychosis, ataxia, assaultiveness, vertical and horizontal nystagmus, catatonic staring, analgesia or anesthesia, increased heart rate and blood pressure, and sometimes, seizures. PCP psychosis can last from several days to several weeks and can include symptoms such as paranoia, violent behavior, depression, and suicidal ideation.

Management of the PCP Intoxication Syndrome

Patients with PCP overdose who present in coma and with cardiopulmonary depression require cardiopulmonary resuscitation and treatment for seizures. The general methods for treatment of the overdose syndrome described in the section on polydrug abuse later in this chapter should also be used for the PCP overdose. In addition, acidifying the urine may hasten the excretion of PCP. The urine can be acidified with 500 mg to 1 gm ammonium chloride every three to five hours PO or through a nasogastric tube until the urine pH is below 5.[12]

As the PCP coma recedes, the patient may be delirious, disoriented, paranoid, and assaultive. Patients who are less intoxicated with PCP may initially present with this psychotic state and often require physical restraints. There are no specific pharmacological antagonists for the toxic effects of PCP. However, some procedures have been reported to be useful for the symptomatic

treatment of the hypertension and psychosis. Some clinicians use 5 mg haloperidol IM, given hourly if needed, to control both the psychosis and the assaultive behavior. Other physicians use 10 to 30 mg diazepam PO or IM to lessen violent behavior. Phenothiazine neuroleptics should be avoided because of the possibility of potentiating PCP anticholinergic effects. Both diazoxide and hydralazine have been suggested to treat the hypertensive crisis that can occur with PCP intoxication. The hypertension usually responds quite rapidly. PCP psychosis has a characteristically slow response, sometimes lasting for weeks. Even as the psychosis resolves, unpredictable reemergence of psychotic symptoms or the appearance of suicidal ideation, depression, anxiety, hostility, or belligerence may complicate the recovery.[137,138]

The Mechanism of Action of PCP

The mechanism of action of PCP has been intensely investigated during the last ten years; nevertheless, it remains poorly understood. There is considerable evidence that PCP interacts with a variety of neurotransmitters in the central and peripheral nervous systems. For example, PCP has been shown to interact with acetylcholine (ACh)-, NE-, and DA-containing neurons in mammalian brain.[40,41,97,122]

Recently PCP receptors in mammalian brain have been described and characterized. This discovery suggests the extraordinary possibility that there may be an endogenous ligand for the PCP receptor that is either psychotomimetic or antipsychotomimetic. However, the true nature and even the existence of the PCP receptor has been questioned, and further study is clearly needed.[40,185,197]

Thus at the present time, there are no specific antidotes for PCP and related compounds analagous to naloxone for the opiates. In addition, a general explanation for the widespread pharmacological activity of PCP remains to be discovered.[41]

¶ Inhalants

History of Inhalants

As a method for using psychoactive substances, the efficiency of absorption of gases, smoke, and volatile liquids has been recognized by humankind for centuries. The surface area of the pulmonary epithelium is large and absorption is rapid. A further advantage of inhalation is that the inhaled psychoactive substance reaches the brain directly without first passing through the liver with its complex system of detoxifying enzymes. In the past, smoked substances have included opium, cannabis, DMT and related methylated indoleamines, and cocaine.

Ether, chloroform, and nitrous oxide were inhaled recreationally before they were discovered to be useful as general anesthetics. Use of nitrous oxide for recreational purposes, primarily by medical, pharmacy, and dental students, continues today. Nitrous oxide causes a brief, giddy, dissociated euphoria. It presents a danger when inhaled without sufficient oxygen, which is fairly common since it is difficult to get a sufficient plasma concentration of this weakly psychoactive substance without inhaling the pure gas. [12,30,159]

The inhalants described in this section are different from the psychoactive substances mentioned earlier in that they are readily available to consumers and are inexpensive. Glue sniffing may have begun in California in the early 1950s, where it was discovered accidentally by adolescents working on model airplanes. Eventually large numbers of volatile compounds were found to possess intoxicating ingredients and were subsequently used as inhalants. These include cements, glues, adhesives, paints, lacquers and their thinners, dry cleaning fluids, spot removers, liquid waxes and shoe polishes, lighter fluids, degreasers, refrigerants, transmission and brake fluids, gasoline, and others substances. Aerosol sprays from supermarkets were found to be intoxicating and thus became popular. They contain conventional solvents as well as Freons (chlorinated and fluorinated substituted methane or ethane derivatives), which are also capable of producing psychoactive intoxication. Aerosol "whipped cream" frequently contains nitrous oxide. Other aerosols used for intoxication include glass chillers, nonstick frying pan sprays, cold weather car starters, air sanitizers, window cleaners, insecticides, deodorants, hair sprays, and spray paints, especially gold and bronze. The psychoactive ingredients in inhalants include a wide variety of solvents from several chemical classes such as aliphatic and aromatic hydrocarbons, halogenated hydrocarbons, Freons, ketones, esters, alcohols, and glycols. [12,30,159]

Patterns of Inhalant Use and Clinical Syndrome

Psychoactive inhalant use is faddish. In one community a specific inhalant, such as bronze paint, will be used by the young for a period of time and then will lose popularity as the attractions of another inhalant (for example, one brand of nonstick frying pan spray) are extolled. Generally, inhalant use is a phenomenon of young, poor, white or Chicano males. It is more common among underprivileged Chicanos and native Americans than among blacks or whites. Inhalants are the only psychoactive substances more frequently used in grade or junior high schools than in high schools or colleges. The extent of inhalant use is difficult to determine. However, data from a national survey suggests that approximately 8 percent of all youths, but 25 percent of Chicano youths in Los Angeles, have experimented with inhalants; about 1 percent of all youths and 13 percent of Chicano youths in Los Angeles are currently using inhalants. [12,30,159]

Inhalant abuse occurs in peer-oriented and peer-perpetuated social settings. Young inhalant users choose these substances because they are cheaper than other psychoactive intoxicants and readily available in a convenient and legal package. A small can of varnish remover costing two dollars can be legally carried in the pocket of a twelve-year-old and can intoxicate more individuals than a gallon of cheap wine.[30,159]

The syndrome produced by inhaling solvents is reported to resemble alcohol intoxication but is of shorter duration and with only a minor hangover. Inhalant users describe the state as a "floating euphoria" that eradicates the unpleasant events of life. The intoxicated state enables these youths to escape temporarily from their chaotic, depressing, and often hopeless home environment, to escape from performance pressure at school, and, temporarily, to correct their personal sense of inadequacy. Sadly, as is the case with alcohol, inhalant intoxication can also release aggressive impulses and therefore lead to violent behavior.[12,30,159]

The volatile nitrites produce an intoxication syndrome and a pattern of abuse that is different from solvent inhalants. Amyl nitrite is used clinically to dilate the coronary arteries during an episode of angina pectoris. Isobutyl nitrite is a nonprescription compound with similar pharmacological activity. When either of these substances is used prior to orgasm, a subjective sense of sustained and enhanced sensitivity is described. The popularity of these compounds to enhance sexual activity probably occurred first among homosexuals and subsequently spread to heterosexual adults.

In addition, the volatile nitrites are being used to produce a brief "altered state of consciousness," which is probably secondary to the dilation of cerebral blood vessels. The volatile nitrites, called poppers or snappers, are frequently legally sold in adult bookstores under such brand names as Locker Room, Jac Aroma, Rush, Kick, Bullet, Toilet Water, and Vaporole. These preparations frequently contain isobutyl nitrite, isobutyl alcohol, and isopentyl nitrite. The clinical syndrome produced is clearly different from that of the solvent inhalants. They are used by a different population and very little is known of the adverse effects of chronic use. One survey found that 19 percent of regular cocaine users also reported the use of volatile nitrites.[12,29,162]

Management of Inhalant Intoxication Syndromes

Users of solvent inhalants are seen infrequently by medical personnel because the acute state ends rapidly either with complete recovery or, very rarely, with death. There are two common causes of sudden death in individuals using solvent inhalants. The first is asphyxiation resulting from the method of self-administration of these inhalants. These substances are placed on a rag, sponge, or article of clothing or in a paper or plastic bag, which the user holds against the nose and/or mouth before breathing deeply. The use of a plastic bag is most dangerous since the user may lose consciousness and suffocate. Sudden death during inhalant use can also be caused by cardiac arrest, probably due to cardiac arrhythmias that are induced either directly by the inhaled solvent or by a combination of the toxic effects of the solvent and hypoxia.[30,159]

Recently a number of cases of CNS and other systemic toxicities have been reported in solvent abusers. For example, inhalation of toluene, a common organic solvent found in paints and glue, can cause hypokalemia and other metabolic abnormalities such as renal tubular acidosis, coma, ataxia, convulsions, and encephalopathies.[38,186] Reversible respiratory arrest has been reported, as well as sudden death from toluene secondary to cardiac arrhythmias and severe electrolyte imbalance.[34,103] Inhalation of the organic solvent 1,2-dichloropropane, which is used as a spot remover, can cause acute kidney failure, hemolytic anemia, and disseminated intravascular coagulation.[113]

Death due to ventricular fibrillation has been reported following inhalation of bromochlorodifluoromethane (BCF), a compound used to extinguish fires.[172] Asthma aerosol medication containing fluorocarbon propellants can produce grand mal seizures.[179] Inhaling gasoline has been reported to cause organic lead encephalopathy, peripheral neuropathy, and sometimes acute myopathy or myoglobinuria.[108] Cardiac arrhythmias, coma, and death have been reported following inhalation of 1,1,1-trichloro-ethane, perchloroethylene, and trichloroethylene found in Scotchgard™ glue, and typewriter correction fluids such as Liquid Paper®.[102] The management of these rare but dangerous syndromes due to organic solvent abuse requires the expertise and interaction of several medical specialties. Sadly, most patients who die from solvent inhalation are never seen by health professionals.

Adverse reactions to amyl, butyl, and isobutyl nitrites include dizziness, headache, tachycardia, syncope, hypotension, acute psychosis, increased intraocular pressure, methemoglobinemia, coma, and rarely, sudden death.[25]

For the episodic inhalant user who comes to the emergency room acutely intoxicated, some of the treatments described for abusers of hallucinogens or psychostimulants are appropriate. If the patient is agitated and assaultive, physical restraints may be necessary. When the patient is primarily anxious and confused, oral doses of a benzodiazepine, such as 10 to 30 mg diazepam, can be helpful.[12]

The chronic abuser of solvent inhalation is more likely to be seen by a medical professional. A preliminary study of thirty-seven chronic solvent abusers (average number of inhalations in excess of 7,000) using the Halstead Reitan Neuropsychological Battery found that 40 percent scored in the brain-damaged range on impairment indices in comparison to none of the control subjects.[159] These results must be interpreted cautiously, since some of the inhalant abusers may have been neuropsychologically impaired prior to solvent abuse. It is unclear whether solvent use itself or other factors, such as hypoxic episodes or abuse of other drugs, contribute to the deficits seen. Further study is needed to determine the natural course and long-term reversibility of these putative solvent inhalant-induced neuropsychological impairments.[12]

The chronic toxicity syndrome may vary from solvent to solvent, and only some solvents produce chronic organic brain syndrome. Toluene, perhaps one of the more common solvents of abuse, has not been shown to produce chronic organic brain syndrome. However, its chronic use may produce kidney and bone marrow disorders. Chronic use of other solvents may produce peripheral neuropathy, kidney damage, liver disease, and bone marrow suppression. Unfortunately, much of our information on these potential toxic effects is based on single-case reports or on attempts to extrapolate from chronic industrial exposure to the same solvents. An accurate assessment of the toxic consequences of repeated self-administration of solvent inhalants requires reliable and careful epidemiological study.[12,30,159]

Mechanisms of Action of Solvent Inhalants

There is no systematic pharmacological or biochemical information on the mode of action of the heterogeneous group of substances classified as volatile organic solvents. These organic solvents have one major characteristic in common, which is their great lipid solubility, and this explains their rapid transport across biological membranes. The extraordinary lipophilia of these compounds may also be a key to the global effects of these compounds in the brain.

¶ Anticholinergics

History of Anticholinergics

Descriptions of anticholinergic intoxication appear in early written history. The toxic anticholinergic plants have been specifically mentioned in many historical documents. *Datura stramonium* (locoweed, jimsonweed, thorn apple, devil's apple, devil's trumpet, stinkweed, apple of Peru) is described by Homer in *The Odyssey* as a poison. Cleopatra allegedly used it in her seduction of Caesar. In A.D. 38, the troops of Mark Antony partook of the same plant in their retreat from Parthia and suffered the dire consequences of stupor, confusion, and death. [12,59,96]

The name jimsonweed stems from an incident at Jamestown during Bacon's Rebellion in 1676. British troops, sent to halt the rebellion, used *Datura stramonium* in the preparation of a meal. Many soldiers suffered the anticholinergic intoxication syndrome as a result. A description from *Beverly's History of Virginia* states how "some ate plentifully of it, the effect of which was a very pleasant comedy, for they turned natural fools upon it for several days: one would blow up a feather in the air, another would dart straws at it with much fury, and another, stark naked, was sitting in a corner like a monkey." The plant became known as Jamestown weed, and over the years the term has been condensed to "jimsonweed." The use of jimsonweed was also mentioned by Omar Khayyam, Henry Thoreau, and others. [12,59,96]

Patterns of Anticholinergic Use

Anticholinergic agents are used as psychoactive substances in spite of their obvious psychological and physiological toxicity. Frequently they are used unintentionally. They are commonly used as adulterants in other psychoactive substances, such as hallucinogens. Thus the buyer of what is sold as LSD may, in fact, purchase and ingest the combination of LSD and scopolamine, or perhaps atropine or scopolamine alone. [14]

However, some substance abusers knowingly use anticholinergic compounds. For example, the anticholinergic stromonium, an ingredient in the antiasthma preparation Asthmador®, had a brief period of popularity as an intoxicating agent. It was said to produce euphoria and altered states of consciousness that allowed the user to withdraw from the stresses and boredom of everyday reality into a dreamlike state. In California, prisoners who work outside the prison walls fighting fires or repairing roads bring jimsonweed back to the prison. They then brew a tea from it and ingest it to produce the same altered state of consciousness sought by the users of Asthmador. Some prisoners and psychiatric patients have discovered that trihexyphenidyl (Artane) and other anticholinergic antiparkinsonian agents can also produce this syndrome. If the dose is carefully titrated, Artane has been described by some users to produce a feeling of comfort and well-being without the accompanying severely altered state of consciousness. Thus Artane abuse is now a problem for some psychiatric patients and prisoners. Unfortunately, the incidence, prevalence, and consequences of intentional and unintentional anticholinergic abuse are largely unknown, because these substances have not been recognized as a separate category of substances of abuse until recently.*

Anticholinergic compounds are found in drugs used for a variety of indications. Drugs used to treat the common cold, allergies, asthma, motion sickness, peptic ulcer disease, insomnia, depression, schizophrenia, menstrual symptoms, and Parkinson's disease can have anticholinergic activity. Medications used by ophthalmologists, a wide variety of toxic plants, and hallucinogens with anticholinergic activity can also produce the anticholinergic intoxication syndrome. [96] A comprehensive list of substances with anticholinergic activity is found in tables 29–2 and 29–3.

The Anticholinergic Intoxication Syndrome

Both physiological and psychological symptoms characterize the anticholinergic intoxication syndrome. The physiological symptoms include widely dilated and unreactive pupils, blurred vision, flushed face, warm and dry skin, dry mouth and throat, difficulty in swallowing, foul breath, diminished or absent bowel sounds, urinary retention, tachycardia, hypertension, increased respiratory rate, and fever. The psychological symptoms include disorientation, incoherence, hallucinations, delusions, bizarre motor behavior, fluctuating levels of awareness, and, at times, profound delirium.

*See references 12, 14, 59, 62, and 96.

TABLE 29–2

Examples of Prescription Medications with Anticholinergic Activity

Tricyclic Antidepressants

Amitriptyline (Elavil)	Imipramine (Tofranil)
Desipramine (Norpramin)	Nortriptyline (Aventyl)
Doxepin (Sinequan)	Protriptyline (Vivactil)

Antipsychotic Neuroleptics
Phenothiazines, especially chlorpromazine (Thorazine) and thioridazine (Mellaril)

Antiparkinsonian Medications

Benztropine (Cogentin)	Procyclidine (Kemadrin)
Biperiden (Akineton)	Trihexyphenidyl (Artane)
Ethopropazine (Parsidol HCl)	

Antihistamines with Anticholinergic Activity

Chlorpheniramine (Teldrin, Chlor-Trimeton, Ornade)	Phrilamine (Histalon)
Cyclizine (Marezine)	Promethazine (Phenergan, a phenothiazine
Dimenhydrinate (Dramamine)	antihistaminic)
Diphenhydramine (Benadryl)	Tripelennamine (Pyribenzamine)
Methapyrilene (Histadyl)	and many others
Orphenadrine (Disipal)	

Antispasmodics for the Gastrointestinal Tract

Adiphenine (Trasentine)	Isopropamide (Darbid)
Anisotropine (Valpin)	Mepenzolate (Cantil)
Belladonna alkaloids (Belladenal and others)	Methantheline (Banthine)
Clidinium (Quarzan and in Librax)	Methixene (Trest)
Dicyclomine (Bentyl)	Methscopolamine (Pamine)
Diphemanil (Prantal)	Oxyphencyclimine (Daricon, Enarax)
Glycopyrrolate (Robinul)	Oxyphenonium (Antrenyl)
Hexocyclium (Tral)	Propantheline (Pro-Banthine)
Homatropine (Matropinal)	Tridihexethyl Chloride (in Milpath with meprobamate)
Hyoscyamine, Atropine, and Hyoscine (in Donnatal)	

Ophthalmic Preparations

Atropine 1% ophthalmic solution	Eucatropine (Euphthalmine)
Cyclopentolate (Cyclogyl)	Tropicamide (Mydriacyl)

Severe impairment of recent memory is a pathognomonic symptom of the anticholinergic intoxication syndrome. Intoxicated patients who have not been unconscious but who are unable to recall events in the immediately preceding half hour or to remember where or who they are should be strongly suspected of anticholinergic intoxication.

A massive overdose of an anticholinergic substance can occasionally produce coma. Comatose patients with anticholinergic toxicity often exhibit the peripheral physiological symptoms just described and may have clonic movements, upgoing plantar reflexes (a positive Babinski's sign), and hyperreflexia.[14,59,62,96]

The cardiac complications of the anticholinergic intoxication syndrome are complex. Toxic levels of anticholinergics cause tachycardia and directly suppress the myocardium. Cardiac conduction disturbances similar to those produced by quinidine toxicity result from enhanced re-entrant excitation secondary to reduced conduction velocity. This can cause widening of the QRS complex, prolonged QT intervals, and ST segment depression.[59,62,96]

Management of Anticholinergic Toxicity

Physical examination, electrocardiogram (EKG), laboratory evaluation, and psychological assessment are basic preliminary proce-

TABLE 29–3
**Plants and Over-the-Counter Medications with Anticholinergic
Activity**

Over-the-Counter-Tranquilizers and Hypnotics

Alva Tranquil	Quietabs
Asper-Sleep	Quiet World
Compoz	Rexall Sleep Capsules
CVS Sleep Capsules	Rexall Sleep Tablets
Devarex	Sedacaps
Dormin	Seda Tabs
Dormirex	Seedate
Dormutol	Sleep-Aid
Dozar	Sleep Eze
Ex Tension	Sleeping Pill-Professional
Masons Timed Sleeping Capsules	Sleeprin
McKesson Sleep Tablets	Slumba-Plus Time Capsules
Neo Nyte	Slumba-Tabs
Nite Rest	Somets
Nytol	Sominex Capsules
Osco Sleep Tablets	Somnicaps
Paradorm	Sta-Kalm

Many other similar preparations also contain anticholinergics. Listed
medications contain either methapyrilene or scopolamine or both.

Other Over-the-Counter Medications
Cold remedies: Allerest, Coricidin, Flavihist, Romilar, Sine-Off, Contac,
Sinutabs, and many others.
Analgesics with anticholinergic activity: Excedrin PM, Cope, and others.
Menstrual products: Codurex and others.
Asthma medications: Asthmador and others.

Plants with Anticholinergic Activity
Datura stramonium (jimsonweed and many other names)
Hyoscyamus niger (henbane)
Atropa belladonna (deadly nightshade and belladonna)
Lycium halimifolium (matrimony vine)
Cestrum nocturnum (night-blooming jessamine)
Solanum dulcamara (woody nightshade, bittersweet and others)
Solanum nigrum (common nightshade and others)
Solanum tuberosum (common potato)
Solanum pseudocapsicum (Jerusalem cherry and silver leaf nightshade
and many others)
Lycoperisicon esculentum (tomato)
Solandra species (trumpet flower, chalice vine)
Physalis heterophylla (ground cherry)

dures in the treatment of the anticholinergic intoxication syndrome. Patients who are severely agitated and assaultive may require physical restraints. While patients may be unable to cooperate by describing or naming the ingested substance, family members or friends may be of help.

Supporting vital functions is the first priority of treatment for the patient with anticholinergic toxicity. Cardiopulmonary resuscitation may be required immediately since the anticholinergic syndrome can sometimes include respiratory or cardiac arrest. When vital functions are stable but the diagnosis of anticholinergic toxicity is in doubt, diazepam can be given PO or IM for sedation. The patient should not be treated with phenothiazine neuroleptics, even in the presence of obvious psychosis, since these compounds, particularly thioridazine hydrochloride and chlorpromazine, can exacerbate the anticholinergic toxicity because of their anticholinergic activity.[14,59,62,96]

Physostigmine, up to 2 mg IV given slowly, should be reserved for a patient with the classical symptoms of the anticholinergic toxicity syndrome who also has a fever or is profoundly delirious, severely agitated, or comatose. Physostigmine is used because, unlike other reversible acetylcholinesterase inhibitors, it is a tertiary rather than quaternary ammonium salt; therefore, it is unique in crossing the blood-brain barrier. A second dose of 1 to 2 mg physostigmine IV can be given fifteen minutes later. Vital signs should be monitored with care, and the patient should be connected to a cardiac monitor and observed for cardiac arrhythmias. A decrease in heart rate is good evidence that physostigmine is counteracting the anticholinergic toxicity. Because physostigmine has a short duration of action, it is sometimes necessary to readminister the drug in two or three hours, or even more frequently.[96]

Physostigmine must be given cautiously, however, to avoid cholinergic toxicity. Too much can cause a cholinergic crisis with bradycardia, increased salivation, diarrhea, and occasionally seizures and respiratory arrest. Atropine, 0.5 to 1.0 mg IV, can reverse cholinergic crisis, but it is better to give physostigmine with caution and prevent the crisis. Relative medical contraindications to physostigmine administration include a history of heart disease, asthma, peptic ulcer, diabetes, mechanical obstruction of the bowel or bladder, hyperthyroidism, pregnancy, or a history of a previous allergic reaction to it. Not every patient with anticholinergic toxicity will need physostigmine. Many patients can be treated with diazepam and nonpharmacological methods, including the supportive reassurance that is also used for the management of adverse reactions to hallucinogens.[14,62,96]

The patient with anticholinergic toxicity may also need further medical procedures. The comatose patient will require a urinary catheter to avoid urinary retention, 50 cc of 50 percent glucose IV in case hypoglycemia has contributed to the coma, and 0.4 mg naloxone IV to counteract the possibility that opioids have contributed to the coma. Physostigmine is useful only for the supraventricular tachycardia caused by the anticholinergic overdose; it is not helpful for the cardiac conduction defects or ventricular tachyarrhythmias. For these problems, intravenous fluids and alkalinization with sodium bicarbonate or sodium lactate can be helpful. If the arrhythmias do not respond to alkalinization, lidocaine hydrochloride, phenytoin, and propranolol hydrochloride may be useful; quinidine gluconate or procainamide hydrochloride is contraindicated. Finally, psychiatric evaluation and treatment should be offered to the patient who has attempted suicide with anticholinergic agents or who abuses anticholinergics for their psychoactive effects.[14,59,62,96]

Mechanisms of Action of Anticholinergics

The anticholinergic compounds have a clearly understood molecular mechanism of action. They block muscarinic-cholinergic receptors in the CNS. Although the anticholinergics are defined by the pharmacology of the receptor they block and are treated accordingly, there is so little information about the anatomy of the ACh system in the brain that a true understanding of the mechanisms that translate muscarinic receptor blockade into a toxic psychosis must await a better understanding of the anatomy of brain ACh neurons.

One part of the toxic psychosis produced by the anticholinergics is relatively unique for this group of compounds: The amnesia they produce is more profound than with any other psychoactive substance. Recent evidence suggests this anticholinergic amnesia is probably related to altered cholinergic function in the hippocampus. Similar but more permanent alterations of cholinergic function are probably a biochemical basis for some of the symptoms of Alzheimer's disease (see chapter 25).

¶ Classical Hallucinogens, Methylated Amphetamines, and Cannabis

History

Hallucinogens derived from natural substances have been used by numerous cultures for many centuries: the hemp plant, *Cannabis sativa,* in China, India, and Italy; the mushroom, *Amanita muscaria* (fly agaric) in Europe; and the *Psilocybe mexicana* mushroom, peyotl cactus, and *Rivea corymbose* (morning glory) seeds in pre-Columbian America. The psychological syndromes produced by these substances were central elements in religious ceremonies and healing rituals as well as for predicting the future. The substances were also used in warfare. The word assassin derives from *Hashshashian,* the name of a group that terrorized Persia during the eleventh century. This group allegedly committed murder under the influence of hashish, derived from *Cannabis sativa.* The Viking Berserkers are thought to have prepared for battle by using the mushroom *Amanita muscaria.*[7,12]

The discovery of lysergic acid diethylamide-25 (LSD-25) begins the modern history of hallucinogens. In the 1930s in Basel, Switzerland, Albert Hofmann was working at Sandoz with ergot alkaloids, which are active in smooth muscle tissue and are therefore of interest to medicinal chemists. Hofmann participated in a project that obtained the lysergic acid nucleus from ergot alkaloids by alkaline hydrolysis. He and his associates modified the lysergic acid nucleus in an attempt to obtain more smooth muscle activity. To this end, Hofmann combined lysergic acid with amines in a protein linkage. LSD-25, synthesized in 1938, was one of the products of this effort but was not tested until April 16, 1943, when Hofmann, seeking to examine the compound, accidentally ingested a small amount. Hofmann described a classical psychedelic experience in his diary, a description as vivid as any that followed.[7,12]

The fact that LSD was active in doses of 100 to 250 µg (5,000 to 10,000 times more active than mescaline) was of great scientific interest to pharmacologists and psychiatrists. It now seemed more feasible that undetected traces of a psychoactive substance produced by the body itself could cause schizophrenia. The first synthetic hallucinogen, LSD-25, is unique because of its potency, not its clinical syndrome. The syndrome was also produced by natural substances such as mescaline and psilocybin.[7,12,160]

The Spanish naturalists who accompanied Hernando Cortez described a number of plants possessing psychoactive characteristics that were known in Mexico but unknown in Europe. The three main groups of plants were peyotl cacti (peyote), teonanacatl mushrooms, and ololiuqui or the seeds of bind weeds, now called morning glory.[160]

Peyote was the first of these compounds to be studied. In 1924 Louis Lewin, a brilliant plant pharmacologist, wrote about it in his monograph *Phantastica.* The peyotl cactus is named *Anhalonium lewinii* in honor of his isolation of mescaline in 1896. In 1919 E. Spaeth determined the structure of mescaline (3,4,5-trimethoxyphenylethylamine, structurally related to DA) and synthesized it. This led to a period of pharmacological research on mescaline that was summarized in 1920 by K. Beringer in *Der Meskalinrausch,* published in 1927.[7,12,160]

Mescaline is the prototype of a class of "ring substituted" or methylated phenylethylamines or amphetamines that produce a syndrome ranging from the classical LSD-like syndrome to one identical to that produced by cocaine or amphetamine. These compounds were first synthesized at the beginning of the twentieth century and continue to be manufactured illegally by chemists for an ever-increasing market. The goal of these chemists is to produce a stimulating hallucinogen that produces a syndrome with a mixture of amphetamine and classical hallucinogenic symptoms. In California in the 1960s, two methylated amphetamines, DOM or STP (4-methyl-2,5-dimethoxyamphetamine) and MDA (3,4-methylenedioxyamphetamine), were the primary methylated amphetamines used by the "hippie" culture. More recently, MDMA (3,4-methylenedioxymethamphetamine) and bromo-DMA (4-bromo-2,5-dimethoxyamphetamine) have become popular in the United States and Australia, respectively.

Richard Schultes, a distinguished botanist from Harvard, learned in 1936 that the naturalists who followed Cortez had been correct; mushrooms were still being used for their hallucinogenic properties in Mexico. In 1955 Gordon Wasson was the first outsider to ingest the "holy" mushrooms. Wasson sent samples to R. Heim of the National Natural History Museum of Paris, who classified the mushrooms and cultivated them in his laboratory. Wasson also sent them to Albert Hofmann in Basel who, after evaluating them, ate 2.4 gm of the *Psilocybe mexicana* and consequently had another remarkable psychedelic experience.[12,160]

Shortly after, the psychoactive compounds psilocybin and psilocin (phosphorylated N,N-dimethyl-4-hydroxytryptamine and N,N-dimethyl-4-hydroxytryptamine, both structurally related to 5HT) were elucidated, and Hofmann and his group synthesized these substances. In 1963 Hofmann took synthetic psilocybin in pill form to Mexico and gave the pills to the Indians who had originally supplied the mushrooms. They were delighted and could not distinguish between the effects of the mushrooms and the synthetic psilocybin.[7,12,160]

Ololiuqui was first described in 1570 by Francisco Hernandez, who was sent by Philip II of Spain to study the flora and fauna of Mexico. He wrote a scholarly description of the morning glory plant *(Rivea corymbosa)* and mentioned that its seeds induced "a thousand visions and satanic hallucinations." Shultes described an unsuccessful attempt to isolate the active principle in 1937.[160] In 1955 Canadian psychiatrist Humphrey Osmond took 800 *Rivea corymbosa* or morning glory seeds and had a hallucinatory experience. Wasson sent some of these seeds to Hofmann, and Hofmann found a relative of LSD, lysergic acid 1-hydroxyethylamide, in the seeds. The syndrome induced by this psy-choactive substance is different from that of LSD-25 and mescaline. Morning glory seeds are described as producing tiredness, apathy, and feelings of mental depression, unreality, and meaninglessness.[7]

Amanita muscaria, the hallucinogenic mushroom from Europe, has proved to be more difficult to characterize pharmacologically. For many years it was assumed that the mushroom's active ingredient was the potent and often toxic muscarine, a cholinergic agonist. However, recently the gamma-aminobutyric acid (GABA) agonist muscimol was also isolated from *Amanita muscaria* and found to be a hallucinogen. Further study is needed to determine whether muscimol alone is responsible for *Amanita muscaria*'s hallucinogenic activity.[12,160]

The early history of cannabis can be traced through references to hemp, a plant that yields both a psychoactive drug and a useful fiber. Such references have been found in the earliest writings from India, Assyria, and China. The ancient Greeks used alcohol instead of cannabis as an intoxicant, but there are passages in ancient Greek (Herodotus, Dioscorides, and others) and Hebrew writings that describe the cultivation and use of cannabis in neighboring cultures. The references are frequent enough to confirm that throughout Asia and the Near East, cannabis was grown from the earliest known times to the present, both for its fiber and for its psychoactive properties. Cannabis currently remains the fourth most popular psychoactive substance worldwide, preceded only by caffeine, nicotine, and alcohol.[12,160]

Patterns of Use of Classical Hallucinogens, Methylated Amphetamines, and Cannabis

LSD and other classical hallucinogens are most frequently used by middle- and upper-class youths, often college students. The classical hallucinogens were most widely used in the mid-1960s. By 1972 the use had decreased, and a survey found that somewhat less than 5 percent of youths over twelve years of age have ever used hallucinogens.

Since 1970 their use has remained relatively stable. Daily use is not common because of the rapid tolerance that develops and because the psychoactive effects are believed to produce a powerful and important experience that consumes both psychological and physical energy.[12]

Advocates of hallucinogenic drug use claim these substances produce a very special kind of euphoric experience. Rather than the peaceful withdrawal produced by opioids or the exhilaration produced by the psychostimulants amphetamine and cocaine, the classical hallucinogens produce an experience that has been variously described as mystical, religious, and philosophical. The experience is commonly described as providing users with new insight and greater understanding of themselves or some aspect of reality.[14,29,82]

Hallucinogenic amphetamines or methylated amphetamines are also used by middle- and upper-class youths and by medical practitioners, often psychiatrists or psychotherapists. In the 1960s MDA was considered a classical hallucinogen and used as a substitute for or with other such classical hallucinogens as LSD or mescaline. However, MDMA, which is distinct from classical hallucinogens, has been recently used in three distinct patterns. It is touted by psychotherapists who use it to facilitate individual and couples' therapy; individuals eager for "personal growth" use MDMA without supervision to achieve alleged insights and to increase their sense of trust; and young users have recently discovered that when taken frequently— that is, five to fifteen times per day—MDMA produces the classical central and peripheral sympathomimetic syndrome commonly associated with amphetamine and cocaine. Recently MDMA, which was previously uncontrolled legally, was placed under an emergency ban by the Drug Enforcement Administration (DEA) for one year from July 1, 1985. The DEA also plans to include MDMA as a schedule I drug, the most stringent classification of the Federal Controlled Substances Act, reserved for drugs with high abuse potential and no accepted medical use.

Marijuana is the most commonly used of all the nonlegal psychoactive drugs.[46] In 1979 more than 50 million persons had tried cannabis as marijuana at least once: 68.2 percent of young adults (eighteen to twenty-five), but only 19.6 percent of individuals twenty-six and older. There was a 45 percent increase in marijuana use between 1970 and 1980; currently the most significant increase in use by young adults is among males, whites, high school nongraduates and people in the Southern United States and in nonurban areas. Among older adults, college graduates have shown the greatest increase.[124] Males are daily users at almost twice the rate of females.[8,98]

Marijuana is most commonly smoked in hand rolled cigarettes called joints, reefers, or roaches. Marijuana itself is commonly referred to as pot, grass, or weed, and is sometimes ingested in baked goods or raw with or without other food.[145]

Clinical Syndrome—Classical Hallucinogens

The clinical syndrome produced by classical hallucinogens such as LSD or mescaline includes perceptual, somatic, and psychological symptoms. Perceptual symptoms can include changes in colors and shapes, increased auditory acuity, difficulty in focusing on objects, and, occasionally, synesthesia, the appearance of sensations in one sensory modality caused by a stimulus in another. For example, the user of mescaline may report "seeing" a sound. Somatic symptoms include drowsiness, dizziness, paresthesias, weakness, tremors, and nausea.[14,32,82]

The symptoms of classical hallucinogen intoxication are quite variable and influenced by personality predispositions. Symptoms of intoxication can include profound but labile alterations in mood, difficulty in expressing thoughts, distorted time sense, dreamlike feelings, and, at times, visual hallucinations. What is perceived is intensified and seems to have greater significance. There is a decrease in logical thought patterns and a tendency to reach nonlogical or nonlinear conclusions that are believed by the user to be more valid than conclusions reached by everyday logic. There are reports of feeling a sense of "universal insight" or an emotional connection to all other people or other living things. Advocates of hallucinogens such as LSD, psilocybin, and mescaline see these aspects of the syndrome as positive. Hallucinogens are described as profoundly attractive euphoriants that can give users new insights into themselves and the universe.

The classical hallucinogen user, however, may also experience unpleasant, frightening images or disturbing, even paranoid thoughts. Just as hallucinogens give a feeling of universal knowledge, they can also give a feeling of hopeless dysphoria and of being irretrievably lost and alone. Loss of control of motor coordination, emotions, or intellectual function may lead from confusion to anger or panic. [14,32,82]

Tragic results can follow the brief aberrant behavior caused by classical hallucinogens. Drug-induced feelings of omnipotence can cause fatal leaps from high places or attempts to stop moving cars. Severe panic can also lead to injury when a user tries to escape terrifying thoughts or sensations. While such phenomena are reported to occur, they are probably not as common as the lay press frequently suggests. Prolonged reactions with persisting psychosis, depression, clouded thinking and judgment, and deficient social functioning are also reported. These reactions have not been shown to be direct pharmacological effects of the classical hallucinogens. In some areas, the mixing of less expensive psychoactive agents such as anticholinergic medications with expensive hallucinogens is a common practice. The so-called chronic effects of hallucinogen drug abuse may also be intensified by existing personality problems. [14]

The clinical symptoms caused by LSD, psilocybin, and mescaline are reported as being virtually indistinguishable by users. DMT produces a syndrome with similar symptoms to the classical hallucinogens, but this syndrome is of shorter duration, and visual distortions are more commonly reported.

Clinical Syndrome—Hallucinogenic or Methylated Amphetamines

Several structural analogues of amphetamine produce a clinical syndrome that can have characteristics of both the classical hallucinogenic syndrome and the syndrome produced by the psychostimulants amphetamine and cocaine. These amphetamine analogues are methylated amphetamines, and at least twenty-six of such compounds have been characterized. The use of these compounds is faddish and one or another methylated amphetamine has been popular in certain areas at certain times. In the 60s and 70s, STP, also known as DOM, and MDA were popular hallucinogens. In addition, bromo-DMA is a methylated amphetamine used as a hallucinogen that also has amphetaminelike pharmacological activity. [18] More recently, attention has focused on MDMA, also called ecstacy, XTC, or Adam.

MDMA has been described as having effects that are different from classical hallucinogens. Users say it does not destroy one's ability to distinguish between reality and fantasy. Rather than producing perceptual distortions, the drug is described as having the capacity to make people trust one another, to banish jealousy, and to break down barriers that exist between married couples, a parent and child, or a therapist and patient. A number of psychiatrists in northern California have used the substance to facilitate individual or couples' therapy. Many of these physicians and their patients describe the drug as providing new insights and allowing patients and therapists to view problems from new and more helpful perspectives. The drug is described as helpful for recalling important events from the past, decreasing phobias, increasing energy and self-esteem, and giving patients the strength to use less alcohol and benzodiazepines.

Unfortunately, these anecdotal reports have not been confirmed by any investigations that use even the minimal standards of modern psychopharmacological research. Many other substances, including heroin and PCP, were initially described in anecdotal reports as useful or therapeutic. There are already reports of some problems with MDMA. Individuals who take multiple doses of MDMA in one day are said to experience an amphetaminelike high that can include amphetaminelike side effects, such as elevated blood pressure and increased pulse rate.

The DEA emergency ban has generated controversy. A number of therapists and physicians have criticized it and hope that rigidly controlled psychopharmacological research can be conducted to evaluate the putative potential clinical utility of MDMA as an adjunct to individual and couples' therapy.

The chronic and acute toxicity of hallucinogenic or methylated amphetamines is largely unknown. A few investigations suggest that amphetamines themselves may have some toxicity to brain DA and 5HT neurons in animal investigations.[147] One recent animal investigation found possible damage to 5HT nerve terminals following MDA administration.[148] The relevance of these animal toxicity studies of amphetamines and methylated amphetamines to human use is unknown. Because of differences in species, dose, frequency, and route of administration, as well as in the ways in which rodents and humans metabolize amphetamines, it would be premature to derive any conclusions about methylated amphetamine neurotoxicity in humans.[148] In general, the human dose of MDA is lower than the dose that produces animal toxicity.[148] However, the possibility of human toxicity of amphetamines and methylated amphetamines should be investigated.

Clinical Syndrome—Cannabis

"Cannabis" is the term given to psychoactive compounds derived from the hemp plant *Cannabis sativa*. A variety of terms are used for these preparations, which contain the THCs. The concentration of THC and therefore the potency varies considerably in different preparations of cannabis. "Marijuana" is one term for a relatively weak preparation of cannabis that is smoked or eaten; "hashish" refers to a preparation with a higher concentration of THC.[72,123]

Cannabis produces psychoactive effects that depend on the concentration of the active pharmacological substances, the THCs, in the preparation that is used. Users describe a biphasic sequence of initial stimulation and euphoria followed by sedation and tranquility. Distortion of time sense, altered thought patterns, an initial giddiness, increased appetite, heightened sensory awareness, a tendency toward thoughtful reflection, and a comfortable, warm feeling are some of the positive aspects of marijuana intoxication described by users. Stronger preparations of cannabis, such as hashish, can produce the mystical, philosophical, and insightful euphoria that is similar to the syndrome described by users of the classical hallucinogens such as LSD.[73,123]

Cannabis, like the classical hallucinogens and the methylated amphetamines, may produce panic reactions. Adverse cannabis reactions can include anxiety, fear, and a sense of helplessness and loss of control. Delusions, including paranoid thoughts, confusion, depersonalization, temporary amnesia, emotional lability, and hallucinations may also be present, particularly at high levels of intoxication. These more serious adverse psychological reactions are similar to the "bad trips" that are often associated with the use of the classical hallucinogens. However, adverse reactions to cannabis occur less frequently and are often of shorter duration than those involving such hallucinogens as LSD, mescaline, and psilocybin.

While adverse reactions to cannabis are often associated with high doses, they can occur with any dose in someone who fears adverse reactions or is unprepared for the psychoactive effects. Individuals with a prior history of a personality or psychiatric disorder have been reported to have intensification of their underlying pathology following cannabis use. Disagreement exists as to whether these reactions should be attributed to individual premorbid pathology or to a direct pharmacological effect of cannabis.[14,73,123]

Numerous other adverse effects have been attributed to cannabis. There have been reports of chromosomal damage, fetal malformations in the children of cannabis users, depressed immune responsiveness, brain atrophy, decreased male sexual function, and the so-called amotivational syndrome. Marijuana has also been described as producing precancerous changes in the lungs of marijuana smokers.[129]

The claims of adverse effects led to large investigations in an attempt to confirm the potential dangers of cannabis. If such serious adverse effects were occurring in American marijuana smokers, these effects should be present even more severely in cannabis users from other cultures where the THC content of cannabis preparations is usually higher and the average rate of consumption greater than in the United States. Thus the mental and physical status of heavy users of cannabis was compared to nonusers in the same age range and occupational and educational status in Greece, Jamaica, Costa Rica, and Egypt.[28,168,169,173]

In these investigations, cannabis users consumed an average of five to ten marijuana cigarettes a day, for periods ranging from five to twenty years. The THC content of the marijuana was generally 2 to 5 percent compared to the 1 percent average THC content in a typical American marijuana cigarette. Importantly, the incidence of mental illness and of abnormalities of mood, thinking, and behavior was not different between chronic heavy marijuana smokers in Jamaica when compared to nonsmokers. In both the Jamaican and Greek studies, chest x-rays, EKGs, blood and plasma chemistry tests, liver and kidney function tests, and chromosome analyses were no different in smokers and nonsmokers.[28,168,173] In one study of long-term hashish users in Egypt, heavy users did show a tendency to be psychologically dependent on the drug and appeared to be slower learners with decreased work capacity.[169] However, the Egyptian study is difficult to interpret, since most of the hashish users also used other psychoactive substances, especially opium.[168,169]

While tolerance to the effects of cannabis has been demonstrated in both animals and humans, it disappears at an extremely rapid rate.[99] Physical dependence is extremely mild, never life-threatening, and similar in many respects to the mild withdrawal syndrome produced by low doses of sedative-hypnotics. Withdrawal symptoms include restlessness, irritability, mild agitation, insomnia, and sleep electroencephalogram (EEG) disturbances.[99]

One of the great uncertainties about marijuana smoking is its potential for causing lung cancer. There is no reliable data available concerning the incidence of carcinoma of the lungs and upper respiratory passages in long-term users of cannabis.[145] Long-term observations of human subjects who smoke only marijuana and not tobacco are needed to settle this important scientific and public health question.

There is no persuasive evidence that cannabis use causes morphological changes in the brain. Computed tomography scan studies on users of marijuana reveal no evidence of gross changes in brain structure.[145]

A variety of studies have confirmed that marijuana and other derivatives of cannabis have reversible suppressive effects on testicular function in male animals and men. This suppression is primarily due to a decrease in spermatogenesis.[145] However, there was no evidence of changes in testosterone levels in the Costa Rican or the Greek study.[28,173] There is no evidence of an effect of cannabis on female reproductive function, and there is no conclusive evidence in young women of reproductive age of any teratogenic effects of high frequency or consistent association with cannabis.[145] Some subtle developmental effects such as reductions in birth weight and height and CNS abnormalities have been reported but will require further investigation.[145]

Habitual cannabis users are said to develop an "amotivational syndrome" characterized by passivity, decreased motivation, and a preoccupation with drug-taking. The pharmacological role of cannabis in this syndrome is controversial. There are numerous case reports of individuals who appear to be satisfied with a lower level of motivation and /or performance after chronic marijuana use. However, this evidence could not be substantiated by the studies from Greece and Jamaica, where marijuana use is even heavier than in the United States.[28,173] Consistent evidence that cannabis induces permanent organic brain damage does not exist. However, preexisting personality traits, social factors, and other drug use, together with regular cannabis use, could conceivably cause some personality changes, particularly during the formative period of adolescence. Further study in this area is important as cannabis use becomes more widespread.[73,123]

Management of Adverse Reactions to Classical Hallucinogens, Methylated Amphetamines, and Cannabis

The common name given to adverse reactions to hallucinogens is "bad trips." Fatal overdoses of classical hallucinogens such as LSD, psilocybin, and mescaline are probably rare, but a fatal outcome can occur when the classical hallucinogen has been mixed with adulterants, such as sedative-hypnotics or anticholinergics. The management of the anticholinergic intoxication syndrome is described earlier in this chapter. When used in repeated high doses or in an overdose, the methylated amphetamines can produce all of the toxic reactions of amphetamine and cocaine. Thus, unlike LSD, methylated amphetamines have been reported to cause deaths from overdose. The management of the psychostimulant intoxication syndrome is discussed earlier in this chapter. The general principles for the treatment of "bad trips" associated with classical hallucinogenic drugs, methylated amphetamines, and cannabis are similar to those for the treatment of adverse reactions that result from PCP, solvent inhalants, and CNS stimulants and from combinations of these substances.[14,66]

A careful physical examination can help determine the diagnosis. Specific physical findings should be sought because the classical hallucinogens are frequently mixed with other drugs. LSD, mescaline, and psilocybin classically produce mydriasis and hyperactive reflexes; cannabis does not produce mydriasis but can cause dilation of conjunctival blood vessels. Signs of other drug effects, such as anticholinergic, sedative-hypnotic, or psychostimulant toxicity, may also be present. The physician should reduce the toxic effects of the drug and manage behavioral disturbances as the diagnosis is established. Nonpharmacological interventions are preferable to pharmacological ones when the diagnosis is unclear.[14]

The environment for the patient should be arranged to avoid either too little or too much sensory input, since both can cause the hallucinogen user to become more anxious. Rapid or sudden movements can be frightening to the intoxicated patient; therefore, an uncrowded room with moderate light and sound can be helpful. A treatment technique called the "talk down" can be very useful for "bad trips" and cannabis panic reactions. The treating staff should talk to patients in a soothing, parental manner. Patients are told they are experiencing a drug reaction that is transient and are reassured that disturbing thoughts and feelings will gradually disappear. Some patients are calmed by being repeatedly oriented to the environment. Others find it helpful to verbalize experiences, thus giving them a greater sense of control.[14,66]

The treating staff should be flexible and find and pursue any topic of conversation that reduces anxiety. As the toxic reaction diminishes, patients can often experience an ebb and flow of disturbing symptoms. This phenomenon should be anticipated and described by the treating staff, who should not conclude that the adverse reaction has passed, since patients may be experiencing a transient improvement.

Classical hallucinogen-, methylated amphetamine-, or cannabis-induced adverse reactions usually require only clarifying and supportive treatment. However, in the busy emergency ward, there is usually insufficient staff or time for the "talk down" procedure.

In these circumstances, medication is necessary to control anxiety and agitation. Antianxiety agents such as diazepam (20–30 mg PO if possible, or IM) or other benzodiazepines, which have a wide margin of safety, may be used.[24,49] These medications are best given in the lowest dose sufficient to reduce anxiety and as infrequently as possible (e.g., every three to six hours) to reduce agitation to manageable levels without altering and depressing vital signs or causing oversedation.[14]

Phenothiazines or other antipsychotic agents should be avoided in the treatment of adverse reactions to hallucinogens, cannabis, or multiple psychoactive drugs. Anticholinergic drugs, which may have been taken by the drug user in the form of an adulterant, can interact with phenothiazines to induce anticholinergic toxicity. The use of antipsychotic drugs for sedation is questionable for any clinical disorder in which the untreated course is usually benign. Antipsychotic agents may also mask a schizophrenic psychosis that could otherwise be diagnosed and treated appropriately. Finally, the frequent extrapyramidal reactions are distressing and may exacerbate the patient's feelings of loss of control and helplessness.[14]

Uncomplicated adverse reactions to hallucinogens, methylated amphetamines, and cannabis rarely require hospitalization. Hospitalization is needed when impaired cognitive functions or perceptions last for more than four to six hours despite medication. If there is no need for hospitalization, patients can be discharged into the care of a responsible person as soon as their cognitive functions and vital signs are stable. Patients who live alone should be assisted in finding a place with relatives or friends for at least twenty-four hours. Lethargy, irritability, and depression can sometimes characterize recovery from an adverse hallucinogenic drug reaction. These symptoms should be explained to the patient and friends or relatives, and a psychiatric evaluation or a drug treatment program should also be offered.[14]

It has recently been suggested that children who accidentally ingest cannabis are best treated with emetics and/or gastric lavage because the syndrome of marijuana intoxication can be a traumatic experience for children and vomiting may reduce the amount of the THC that is ingested.[192]

"Flashbacks" is the term given to spontaneous recurrences of thoughts, feelings, and perceptions originally experienced during acute hallucinogenic drug intoxication. The mechanism of these flashbacks is not clear, but they are probably psychological in origin. They can occur months after the last drug ingestion, when the pharmacological actions of the drug would not be expected. Flashbacks are usually triggered by fairly specific psychological factors, such as specific emotions, thoughts, or environmental events. They rarely require treatment. A patient with flashbacks should be advised to refrain from the use of hallucinogens or other psychoactive drugs that may contribute to the problem. Flashbacks can be diminished by avoiding the precipitant factors that trigger the phenomenon. Patients can be reassured by the fact that for most people, flashbacks gradually become less intense and frequent and eventually they disappear altogether, usually within one year. For some individuals with flashbacks, it may be helpful to use antianxiety medications such as a benzodiazepine.[1,14]

Mechanisms of Action of Cannabis

The neurochemical mechanism of action of cannabis is poorly understood. There is no major neurotransmitter hypothesis that can account for the actions of THC. However, there are some suggestions that indoleamines and catecholamine neurotransmitters may be involved.[182] For example, cannabis causes a small decrease in brain NE concentration and turnover, while 5HT concentrations are increased with a decrease in turnover. The alterations produced by cannabis in 5HT are similar to those seen with LSD and other classical hallucinogens and suggest a common mode of action. Cannabis seems to interfere with ACh activity in hippocampal and limbic structures, which may be the mechanism for the reported effects of cannabis on memory and concentration.[42] A third type of evidence suggests that cannabis may directly affect nerve conduction. THC is reported to produce a dose-related decrease in the action potential of nonmyelinated nerve fibers in the rabbit.[21] Thus, while the mode of action of cannabis is not understood, there are some intriguing clues that will stimulate further investigation.

Mechanisms of Action of Classical Hallucinogens and Methylated Amphetamines

Classical hallucinogens have been proposed to act through 5HT neurons. LSD, for example, preferentially inhibits serotonergic cell firing by binding to presynaptic receptors while sparing postsynaptic 5HT receptors. Nonpsychoactive analogues of LSD show no preference for these 5HT receptors. This suggests that there are at least two different conformations of 5HT receptors, one of which has a higher affinity for LSD. 5HT is generally an inhibitory transmitter; therefore, when its activity is decreased, the neuron it connects to is freed from inhibition and becomes activated. The 5HT system is intimately involved in the control of sensation, sleep, attention, and mood. Thus it may be possible to explain the actions of LSD and other classical hallucinogens by their disinhibition of the 5HT control of these critical brain functions.[2,190]

In addition to its effects on 5HT, several investigators have demonstrated that LSD has effects on DA neurons. The methylated amphetamines have also been hypothesized to act by stimulating brain dopaminergic activity. However, the effect of classical hallucinogens on DA systems has yet to be integrated with their effects on 5HT to produce a comprehensive theory of their mechanism of action.[36]

¶ Sedative-hypnotics

History of Sedative-hypnotics

Sedative-hypnotics are synthetic chemicals that are all relatively new. Chloral hydrate, probably the first sedative-hypnotic, was synthesized in 1832 and was first used clinically as a hypnotic in 1869.[112] Barbiturates, the largest family of sedative-hypnotics until the development of the benzodiazepines, are derivatives of barbituric acid (malonylurea). The barbiturates were probably named because barbituric acid was first synthesized from uric acid by the chemist Adolf Von Baeyer on St. Barbara's day. Barbital, which was synthesized by the organic chemist Emil Fischer in collaboration with Josef Von Mering, was the first barbiturate used in clinical medicine, in 1903. The trade name for barbital, Veronal, probably derives from the fact that Von Mering was in Verona when he learned of barbital's synthesis in a telegram from Fischer. Barbital was immediately recognized to be a sleep-inducing hypnotic and to have some antianxiety effects when used during the daytime.[121]

Barbital became popular in clinical medicine immediately after its introduction in 1903. The next important barbiturate, phenobarbital, was introduced in 1912. Phenobarbital was commonly used until recently as an antianxiety agent, and it remains one of the most important pharmacological treatments for epilepsy.[141] The systematic search for shorter-acting barbiturates led to the synthesis of pentobarbital and secobarbital in 1930. These two barbiturates are still widely used as sleep-inducing medications and are also the most commonly abused barbiturates. The synthesis of amobarbital in 1923 led to the use of the "amytal interview" as a diagnostic and therapeutic procedure in psychiatry, while the synthesis of thiopental in 1935 produced a barbiturate with an extremely short duration of action for intravenous anesthesia for surgery and dentistry.[141]

Meprobamate, one of the first popular nonbarbiturate antianxiety agents, was developed by the combination of serendipity and careful observation that is so common in the history of science. In 1945 Frank Berger was searching for a chemical that would kill the gram negative bacteria that were resistent to penicillin. Berger and his colleagues decided to modify a phenylglycol ether that was marketed as a disinfectant. They gave these modified pheny glycol ethers to rodents to determine toxicity. One of these substances, mephenesin carbamate, produced profound muscle relaxation in rats without producing total paralysis. It also seemed to quiet the animals.

Mephenesin was soon marketed as a muscle relaxant. Several physicians noted that the compound seemed to decrease anxiety, although the effect was brief and required high doses. Over the next five years, Berger and his colleagues attempted to increase the duration of mephenesin's antianxiety effects by systematic alterations of the molecule. The group produced meprobamate, a propanediol dicarbamate compound with no obvious structural relationship to mephenesin unless each step in its chemical development is described. Thus what began as a search for a new antibiotic resulted in the first modern antianxiety agent.[9]

The most widely used antianxiety agents are the benzodiazepines. In the 1930s Leo Sternbach, who would eventually discover the benzodiazepines, was a postdoctoral research student at the University of Cracow in Poland. He was interested in the theoretical rather than the medical or pharmacological aspects of chemistry and synthesized several heptoxdiazines. Twenty years later Sternbach, who was then a medicinal chemist at Hoffman-La Roche laboratories in the United States, followed a procedure common to much of medicinal chemistry. Because he was familiar with compounds from his work in Poland, he decided to screen the heptoxdiazines for biological activity. He soon discovered that the compounds were not heptoxdiazines with seven-member rings but rather quinazolone-3-oxides with six-member rings. This finding led to the synthesis of forty derivatives, all of which were tested and found to have no pharmacological activity. The last compound in the series, a quinazolone treated with methylamine, was not tested. Instead the compound was labeled RO 5–0690 and shelved because of other pressing research studies.

During a cleanup of the laboratory in May 1957, one of Sternbach's chemists found RO 5–0690 sitting on a shelf and suggested they test the compound for pharmacological activity. Pharmacologist Lowell Randall was excited to discover that RO 5–0690 was similar to, but two to five times more potent than meprobamate in cats. The compound was 1,4-benzodiazepine—chlordiazepoxide hydrochloride, or Librium—the first benzodiazepine to be marketed. Chlordiazepoxide is not a quinazolone-3-oxide derivative without biological activity, as were the forty inactive compounds. Methylamine caused an unexpected ring enlargement, forming a seven-member ring. An additional year of work was required to determine the structure of chlordiazepoxide because of this unexpected chemical reaction. Thus its introduction was delayed for a year.

Since then several hundred benzodiazepine derivatives have been synthesized and their muscle relaxant, antianxiety, sleep-inducing, and anticonvulsant properties have been widely used. The benzodiazepine diazepam (Valium) is currently the most widely used antianxiety agent in the world except for alcohol. The recent discovery of endogenous benzodiazepine receptors and the search for the endogenous benzodiazepine ligand are the most recent chapter in the history of these important compounds. These developments may lead to a better understanding of the biochemical basis of anxiety and sleep. A more detailed discussion of the impact of the discovery of the benzodiazepine receptor and the search for the endogenous ligand can be found in chapter 21.

Patterns of Sedative-hypnotic Use

Sedative-hypnotic abuse occurs at all ages and in all social classes but is slightly more common in women than in men. The abuse may be chronic, episodic, or acute. Chronic users include two distinct groups.[157] One group is composed of middle-aged, often middle-class, Caucasians between thirty and fifty years of age. These individuals initially receive sedatives or hypnotics for anxiety or sleep disturbances and then continue daily use for these purposes, slowly increasing the dose as tolerance develops until a physically addicting dose is reached. Such individuals often have conventional appearance and social adjustment, which masks the addiction and facilitates acquisition of multiple prescriptions and repeated refills. Many of these individuals do not realize they are physically addicted until they attempt to decrease or stop their consumption.

The second major group are younger people, including teenagers, who use sedative-hypnotics either to obtain an alcohollike intoxication or as part of their use of a variety of psychoactive substances. Many of these young people use sedative-hypnotics only when their preferred drug is not available. For example, these individuals may use intravenous barbiturates or oral diazepam when they are unable to purchase heroin. The goal of this second group of sedative-hypnotic users is to produce altered states of consciousness. These users experience disinhibition euphoria, a paradoxical excitement and exhilaration produced by CNS depressants in moderate to low doses. This exhilaration is often accompanied by increased confidence and a sense of improved performance, similar to the disinhibition euphoria associated with alcohol use. Violent behavior may occur and is more common among the young members of more violent subcultures.

The most dangerous form of sedative-hypnotic abuse is the intravenous injection of these drugs, most commonly barbiturates, to produce a "rush," an intensely pleasurable sensation of warmth, escape, and drowsiness. Intravenous use is dangerous because the margin between an intoxicating dose and a fatal dose is dangerously narrow. Additional medical complications of intravenous injections are listed in table 29–4.

Another group of sedative-hypnotic abusers are those caught in a stimulation-sedation cycle, using sedative-hypnotics to counteract the effects of amphetamine or cocaine, which are then used to overcome the effects of the sedatives. Others use sedative-hypnotics to combat the effects of alcohol or opioid withdrawal. In the drug subculture, sedative-hypnotics are sold as treatments for both withdrawal symptoms and for such psychiatric symptoms as hallucinations and intense anxiety. The individuals who self-administer sedative-hypnotics include health professionals, especially physicians, nurses, and pharmacists.

Sedative-hypnotic Toxicity

Suicide attempts are the most common cause of acute sedative-hypnotic toxicity. Severe depression is common among sedative-hypnotic abusers, and they are at high risk both for intentional and unintentional overdoses. The overdose syndrome is most often seen in individuals between thirty and fifty years of age and is more common in women than in men.[13]

Mild-to-moderate barbiturate intoxication closely resembles alcohol intoxication. Symptoms of mild intoxication include garrulousness, emotional lability, confusion, and ataxia. Moderate intoxication includes sensory and motor impairment, depressed tendon reflexes, lateral nystagmus, and constricted pupils. Severe intoxication can cause hypotension, apathy, and drowsiness, which can lead to coma, respiratory depression, and death.[13]

The intoxication syndrome produced by other sedative-hypnotics is essentially identical to that for barbiturates. However, the sedative-hypnotics do vary widely in their capacity to cause respiratory depression and death. Thus while meprobamate and glu-

Table 29–4
Some Medical Complications of Intravenous Drug Abuse

Local infection	Skin abscess, thrombophlebitis, skin cellulitis and folliculitis
Distant infection	Septicemia; bacterial endocarditis; osteomyelitis; lung, bone, and kidney abscess; malaria; acquired immune deficiency syndrome (HTLV-III infection, AIDS); serum hepatitis; tetanus
Foreign-body lung emboli	Cotton, talc, starch, and other substances
Chronic tissue destruction	Pulmonary fibrosis, acute and chronic polyneuropathy, glomerulonephritis, nephrotic syndrome

tethimide are a cause of fatal overdoses, oral doses of benzodiazepines are rarely, if ever, implicated as the sole cause of death.[13]

Management of Sedative-hypnotic Toxicity

The general principles for the management of sedative-hypnotic intoxication are the same as for the treatment of the intoxication syndromes produced by other psychoactive drugs. A detailed description of the management of acute toxic drug reactions appears in each section of this chapter and in the polydrug abuse section. Unfortunately, a specific antagonist, such as naloxone for opioid toxicity, is not yet available for the treatment of sedative-hypnotic overdose. However, the series of new compounds that has been synthesized to act on the benzodiazepine receptor may soon yield a clinically useful antagonist to the benzodiazepine toxicity syndrome (see chapter 21). Patients with sedative-hypnotic toxicity should nevertheless receive both naloxone and glucose, since these treatments are safe, and one can never be sure whether opioid toxicity or hypoglycemia has contributed to a coma that is presumed to be caused by sedative-hypnotic overdose.

Once the acute toxicity syndrome has been treated and vital signs are stable, patients who are comatose and who require continued respiratory assistance must be admitted to an intensive care unit and managed by a team experienced in the treatment of drug overdoses. If the intoxicating drug or drugs are dialyzable, hemodialysis may hasten recovery.

Glutethimide intoxication presents a particular problem during the recovery phase since patients can improve, only to relapse later into a deep and sometimes fatal coma. This phenomenon, which can occasionally occur with drugs other than glutethimide, has been ascribed to the release of glutethimide from lipid stores, to delayed absorption from the GI tract, or to excretion in the bile followed by reabsorption. Whatever the cause, this potential for relapse demands increased vigilance by the treating medical staff.[10,13,65,83]

Some patients develop a toxic psychosis as they recover from the acute effects of an overdose of barbiturates or other sedative-hypnotics. Patients who are hospitalized for sedative overdose have often taken the overdose in an attempt to end their life and therefore may have a depression syndrome. Thus psychiatric evaluation should commence as soon as the patient recovering from a sedative-hypnotic overdose is no longer confused and is able to communicate.

Management of the Sedative-Hypnotic Withdrawal Syndrome

The prototype withdrawal syndrome for sedative-hypnotics was described for pentobarbital.[87] In the study performed by Isbell, chronic users of 400 mg per day pentobarbital had only mild withdrawal symptoms; those taking 600 mg per day often developed anxiety, tremulousness, and feelings of weakness. Abrupt discontinuation of more than 800 mg per day pentobarbital led to seizures and psychosis in the majority of patients. This prototype barbiturate abstinence syndrome is a medical emergency and should almost always be treated in the hospital.

The withdrawal syndrome from sedative-hypnotics has both minor and major components. Minor components include insomnia, anxiety, sweating, anorexia, nausea, vomiting, muscular weakness, postural hypotension, and coarse tremors that worsen with anxiety or voluntary movement.[59] The major components of the sedative-hypnotic abstinence syndrome include grand mal seizures, fever, and toxic psychosis. The grand mal seizures usually begin on the second or third day after the abrupt cessation of pentobarbital use, while the psychosis can appear any time from the third to the eighth day. This toxic psychosis is virtually indistinguishable from the psychosis that accompanies the alcohol abstinence syndrome known as delirium tremens. Hyperpyrexia is less frequent than seizures and psychosis, but the appearance of fever is an ominous sign.

The abstinence syndrome is somewhat variable, depending on the sedative hypnotic. Table 29–5 lists the approximate chronic daily doses that have been reported to produce severe abstinence syndromes with sedative-hypnotics other than barbiturates. Sedative-hypnotics with long half-lives of elimination such as phenobarbital and diazepam may produce a prolonged abstinence syndrome, with the onset of seizures and psychosis delayed for as long as seven to fourteen days after abrupt cessation of the medication. The danger and severity of the sedative-hypnotic abstinence syndrome produced by such compounds as methaqualone, benzodiazepines, and other drugs is often underappreciated, and there are many people who help maintain the myth that these substances are "nonaddictive."

Treatment of the severe sedative-hypnotic abstinence syndrome will frequently require hospitalization and careful medical management. Treatment begins with a complete medical and substance abuse history, a complete physical examination including a mental status examination and a neurological evaluation, a urinary or plasma screen for substances of abuse, a routine battery of clinical laboratory tests, and an EKG.

Unfortunately, even fully cooperative patients who are daily users of sedative-hypnotics may have difficulty estimating the extent of their tolerance to these substances. Daily intake is highly variable for some sedative-hypnotic abusers and is generally remembered as the number of pills or capsules usually ingested. The problem of estimating tolerance is further complicated by the use of "street drugs" of unknown strength and purity. Thus it is frequently necessary to determine the degree of tolerance empirically.

Several tests of tolerance have been recommended in the literature. The first recommended test suggests giving the alert and asymptomatic sedative-hypnotic-abusing patient 200 mg pentobarbital PO. A more recent formulation of the same test recommends a single oral dose of 60 mg phenobarbital to the nonintoxicated supine patient. Both tests suggest that the patient be observed for the hour following the test dose. The following estimates of tolerance can then be made:

Minimal: Patient is asleep or grossly intoxicated with slurred speech, nystagmus, and ataxia. The abstinence syndrome should be mild.

Moderate: Patient is comfortable, has normal speech, exhibits no ataxia, and shows only a fine lateral nystagmus. Abstinence syndrome can be prevented with 200 to 300 mg phenobarbital per day.

Strong: Patient shows no response to the test dose or shows signs of withdrawal. Prevention of the abstinence syndrome will require from 300 to 500 mg of phenobarbital per day.

While the pentobarbital or phenobarbital tolerance test is frequently recommended in textbooks, it is not as easy or as practical as it sounds in a busy hospital emergency service. Many experienced emergency room physicians prefer to determine the degree of tolerance empirically as the patient is treated. One technique involves the administration of 30 mg phenobarbital PO every hour until patients with withdrawal symptoms are asymptomatic. Following this, the total amount of phenobarbital required to reduce

TABLE 29–5
Abstinence Syndromes with Nonbarbiturate Sedative-Hypnotics

Drug	Threshold Dose (g/day)	Comments
Chlordiazepoxide (Librium)	0.3	Seizures may occur as late as the twelfth to fourteenth day.
Diazepam (Valium)	0.12	Seizures may occur as late as the twelfth to fourteenth day.
Ethchlorvynol (Placidyl)	2.0	
Ethinamate (Valmid)	13.0	
Glutethimide (Doriden)	2.5	Seizures appear as late as the sixth day.
Meprobamate (Miltown)	3.2–6.4	Death in one patient receiving greater than 10 g per day.
Methaqualone (Quaalude)	1.8–2.0	
Methyprylon (Noludar)	2.4	Death in one patient taking 7.5 to 12 g per day.

SOURCES: P. A. Berger, "The Addict in the Emergency Room," in C. P. Rosenbaum and J. Beebe, eds., *An Introduction to Treatment in Psychiatry: Crisis Clinic and Consultation* (New York: McGraw-Hill, 1975), pp. 161–171; P. A. Berger and J. R. Tinklenberg, "Treatment of Abusers of Alcohol and Other Addictive Drugs," in J. D. Barchas et al., eds., *Psychopharmacology: From Theory to Practice* (New York: Oxford University Press, 1977), pp. 355–385; C. F. Essig, "New Sedative Drugs That Can Cause States of Intoxication and Dependence of the Barbiturate Type," *Journal of the American Medical Association*, 196 (1966):714–717; and L. E. Hollister, "Diazepam in Newly Admitted Schizophrenics," *Diseases of the Nervous System*, 24 (1963):746–775.

or abolish the withdrawal symptoms is then given over twenty-four hours in four equal doses at six-hour intervals. During the first forty-eight hours of treatment, adjustments in the dosage of phenobarbital can be made by looking for withdrawal signs just before each dose or for signs of severe intoxication one hour after each dose. The patient should be kept mildly intoxicated.[10,13,166,195]

The sedative-hypnotics are cross-tolerant and any of them could be theoretically used in place of phenobarbital at the proper dosage. Based on prospective studies, there is no evidence of either significant advantages or significant disadvantages to using the drug upon which the patient originally became dependent. However, many emergency room physicians are more comfortable using a drug with which they are familiar, such as phenobarbital or a benzodiazepine with a long half-life (i.e., diazepam).

Once the patient is stabilized for two or three days with phenobarbital or another long-acting sedative-hypnotic and after careful medical evaluation, the dose of phenobarbital can be reduced by 30 mg every other day. If withdrawal symptoms are a problem, the reduction can proceed more slowly. For addiction to sedative-hypnotics with a short half-life, the reduction may proceed more rapidly. Seizures should not occur on this reduction schedule; but if a convulsion does occur, 100 to 150 mg phenobarbital IM can be administered to reintoxicate the patient.

Benzodiazepines are becoming increasingly popular in the treatment of severe sedative-hypnotic withdrawal syndromes. The principles of this treatment are the same as for the use of phenobarbital. One common regimen involves loading doses of diazepam given either intravenously or orally. For example, patients can be given 20 mg diazepam PO every hour until they are no longer experiencing sedative-hypnotic withdrawal symptoms. Patients unable to take oral medications can be given 20 mg diazepam IV every hour until they are asymptomatic. Patients can then be withdrawn slowly from the diazepam over a period of days that approximates the usual duration of the sedative-hypnotic withdrawal syndrome. For a short-acting sedative-hypnotic, a five-day withdrawal regimen would probably be sufficient. A longer-acting sedative-hypnotic may require up to two weeks of gradual withdrawal.[101,112]

Because of the long duration of action of phenobarbital and diazepam, an alternative method of withdrawal involves phenobarbital or diazepam loading followed by no additional medication. This procedure takes advantage of these medications' long half-lives of administration. Martin and colleagues[118] describe giving phenobarbital to patients in clinical withdrawal from sedative-hypnotics as a slow continuous intravenous infusion at the rate of 0.04 mg per kg per minute or in equivalent hourly oral doses of 2.4 mg per kg until the patient exhibits marked nystagmus and at least two other signs of intoxication (asleep but arousable, dysarthric, ataxic, or emotional changes). According to these investigators, additional phenobarbital is seldom needed.[118] A drawback of this method is the necessity of monitoring the phenobarbital serum concentration to identify the occasional patient who requires additional phenobarbital because of elimination of the rapid-loading dose. However, Martin and colleagues state that this rapid elimination occurs only rarely. Their recommendation is based on a seven-patient study and will need to be confirmed.[118]

Diazepam loading has been described as a simplified method for treating alcohol withdrawal that should also be effective in treating sedative-hypnotic withdrawal. Sellers and colleagues[154] describe a procedure that involves intoxicating withdrawing alcoholic patients with either intravenous or oral diazepam given at the rate of 20 mg per hour. In a double-blind study with thirty-three consenting inpatients withdrawing from alcohol, the diazepam loading was effective in suppressing initial symptoms; there were no adverse effects, and no further drug treatment was required. These authors conclude that intravenous or oral loading-dose administration of diazepam is a simple, rapid, and effective treatment for alcohol withdrawal. Further investigation is needed to see if this treatment will be safe and useful in sedative-hypnotic withdrawal.

The use of phenytoin in the sedative-hypnotic abstinence syndrome is controversial. Some clinicians attempt to make a case for its prophylactic use. A loading dose of 750 to 1,000 mg phenytoin given intravenously at the rate of 50 mg per min will rapidly establish a therapeutic blood level of 20 μg per ml.

A maintenance dose of 300 to 400 mg PO per day will maintain this plasma level.[13,14]

Of course, the patient with a sedative-hypnotic abstinence syndrome has other needs in addition to pharmacological treatment. A low bed with padded side rails can prevent injuries in an agitated patient with psychosis. Patients who are unable to eat will require intravenous fluids, restoration and maintenance of electrolyte balance, and vitamin supplementation. Like the opioid addict, the user of sedative-hypnotics may have associated medical illnesses and will require a careful medical evaluation. Finally, and most important, once the patient has recovered from the abstinence syndrome, follow-up psychiatric treatment should be offered to prevent the all-too-common relapse to the addictive state.

Mechanisms of Action of Sedative-hypnotics

An important advance in the understanding of the mechanism of action of sedative-hypnotic drugs came in 1977, when two groups of investigators reported the presence of benzodiazepine receptors in rat brain.[126,170] These receptors have subsequently been shown to be part of a molecular complex associated with CNS GABA receptors. Since GABA is a major inhibitory neurotransmitter in the brain that may be present in from 20 to 30 percent of all brain neurosynapses, the association of the benzodiazepine receptor with GABA may explain the antianxiety activity of the benzodiazepines.

Recently other sedative-hypnotics, including barbiturates, meprobamate, and even ethanol, have been reported to interact with the benzodiazepine-GABA receptor complex in a manner different from the benzodiazepines but in one that offers a possible explanation for the parallel antianxiety action of many sedative-hypnotics.[165] Further details on the mechanism of action of the benzodiazepines and other sedative-hypnotics can be found in chapter 21.

¶ Tobacco

History of Tobacco

Almost five hundred years after its controversial introduction to Europe, tobacco use remains a topic of considerable debate. The inclusion of tobacco in this chapter is evidence of a recent change in attitude toward tobacco use and smoking. There is recent evidence suggesting that tobacco qualifies for inclusion as a psychoactive substance of abuse despite that fact that the criteria used for such a classification remain controversial.

Tobacco use is centuries old; tobacco smoking was traditionally a religious, medicinal, and ceremonial custom of the Americas of the New World. The earliest evidence of tobacco use is in the depiction of a Mayan shaman in the Palenque ruins in Mexico, which dates from the fifth century A.D.[80] Tobacco was a integral part of North American tribal life. Many varieties of tobacco were available; several were mixed together for flavor or taste, and specific varieties were used by individual tribes. Tobacco was wrapped in corn husks and smoked by the Tainos of Hispanola, placed in hollow reeds by the Aztecs of Mexico, or placed in elbow-shaped pipes by the Plains tribes in Minnesota. While the most common method of tobacco use was smoking, the leaves could be chewed, eaten, drunk as juice as in South America, or snuffed, as is still the custom in the Amazon.[80]

Columbus may have been responsible for the introduction of tobacco from the Americas to Europe after 1493.[89] Smoking became very popular in Spain, spread rapidly across Europe, and brought in its wake a storm of controversy. The appearance in London of Sir Walter Raleigh's treasure of pipes, tobacco, and leaves from the Americas brought a vehement condemnation from James I in 1604.[89] Both rulers and religious leaders were wary of the "foreign substance" and denounced the practice of smoking as a source of political unrest, moral decadence, unwarranted pleasures, and a fire hazard. In Turkey and Germany, public display of smoking was punishable by death, and in Russia, castration was the threatened punishment for smoking.[16,33]

In 1885 the New York *Times* editorialized, "The decadence of Spain began when the Spaniards adopted cigarettes and if this pernicious habit obtains among adult Americans the ruin of the Republic is close at hand."[17] Between 1895 and 1921, fourteen states banned the use of cigarettes, and all the remaining states except Texas had strict laws that regulated the use of cigarettes and their possession by minors. These and other attempts to control tobacco use through the legal system were as ineffective as the efforts of previous governments.[74]

The warnings and punishments were mostly ignored despite increasing evidence of medical hazards. Tobacco use spread rapidly through every class in most European and American cultures, where its use was reported to be and is currently experienced as pleasurable and relaxing and a fashionable accoutrement to social functions. The cigarette break was as much a part of military life and private sector employment as the annual vacation. The popularity of tobacco and its widespread social acceptance stimulated competitive industry, technology, agriculture, and the economy. The appearance of the modern slim, mass-produced cigarette and more mild varieties of tobacco made smoking easily accessible and available.[33] The cigarette is now one of the most efficient and least expensive devices for self-administration of tobacco. Industry, employment, and taxes on the import and export of tobacco helped to boost tobacco into the position of a source of economical and political power. In the United States tobacco remains a $16 billion a year industry, and tobacco sales yield more than $8 billion a year in tax revenues.[183]

Patterns of Tobacco Use

Smoking tobacco is a popular and commonly accepted and practiced social act among almost all societies and by people of all races and social classes. It is a behavior recognized as a sign of sophistication and a symbol of companionship, acceptance, and attainment of maturity. Thus the image of adulthood, maturity, and freedom currently includes casual but regular use of tobacco, often combined with alcohol (and other drugs).

Currently, more than 4,000 cigarettes are smoked per person each year in the United States.[31] The principal users until recently have been men; however, the advent of the women's liberation movement has changed the female role and attitudes toward women. The stigma of cigarette smoking for women has been lifted, and a rapidly increasing proportion of women smoke as much as men. Smokers constitute 41 percent of the adult population in the United States, and 25 percent of adults smoke more than one pack of twenty cigarettes per day.[88]

Most smokers begin experimentation with smoking in adolescence, a developmental stage characterized by a vulnerability to image-conforming behaviors. Many teenagers are reported to be regular users of tobacco. They begin tobacco use in response to the influence and smoking habits of friends, family, and significant others and their own changing self-concept, perception of reality, and personality. There is evidence to show that children of parents who smoke, who are less educated, and who work part-time are more likely to smoke.[88] Adolescents who smoke are likely to have friends, siblings, and parents who smoke.[45] Tobacco smokers appear to be more extroverted, impulsive, and antisocial.[89]

Personality characteristics, the effect of local environment, peer and social pressure, and perhaps innate drug-seeking behavior are all factors that potentially contribute to and influence the extent and frequency of tobacco use. What proportion or combination of each of these factors determines such behaviors as light, medium, and heavy smoking is at present in doubt. As important as an understanding of the factors that lead to smoking is an understanding of the factors that lead most smokers to attempt to quit and then to relapse.

Reasons for Tobacco Use/Abuse

Tobacco is a paradoxical substance of abuse, since it seems to act as a treatment for seemingly opposite psychological and physiological states. Smoking can provide stimulation for those who are fatigued or bored; it has subjectively been reported and also clinically demonstrated to improve coordination in activities such as routine methodical tasks. Tobacco use has been shown to enhance performance on tasks involving speed, reaction time, vigilance, and concentration.[193] Conversely, studies reveal that smoking acts to "calm the nerves" and as a muscle relaxant during periods of stress, allowing individuals under long-term pressure and tension to perform better than average;[89] thus tobacco can reduce responsiveness to stressful stimuli and enhance mood.[50] Tobacco has also been reported to reduce aggressive responses in experimental situations.[26] Finally, smoking acts as an anorectant in three ways.* First, smoking tobacco decreases the efficiency with which food is metabolized.[52,152] Second, tobacco smoking specifically has been reported to reduce appetite for foods containing simple carbohydrates (sweets).[72] Third, smoking nonspecifically reduces the eating that occurs in times of stress.[19]

Tobacco smoking not only lowers anxiety levels in experimental situations,[50] but is also reported to allay anticipated tension in social functions. The social ritual of taking a cigarette, lighting it, and inhaling occupies the hands and is an acceptable introductory behavior. It is often also used as a rebellious gesture, one easily available to teenagers.

However, for many people, smoking is a pleasurable act in itself. Smoking tobacco is an easy habit to acquire, uphold, and maintain, as there is subjective as well as external reinforcement. Unlike other substances of abuse, tobacco is inexpensive, readily available, and an attractive alternative to the other

*See references 19,47,53,72,79,105, and 152

psychoactive substances that impair muscle function and coordination. Tobacco smoking also has fewer immediate negative medical or psychological consequences or side effects. Physiological effects of tobacco smoking in a novice include vasoconstriction, increased blood pressure, tremor, tachycardia, nausea, and increased GI activity.[89]

The reasons for smoking just discussed suggest some degree of conscious control, flexibility, and choice on the part of the smoker. However, recent investigations also show evidence that tobacco contains a chemical substance or substances that trigger the desire, need, or craving for regular and continued self-administration of that substance.[74] Most studies show nicotine to be the basic pharmacological reinforcer in smoking.*

Recent investigations suggest that nicotine is an addictive substance and that tobacco smoking is a form of drug dependence. Several lines of investigation and reasoning have led the U.S. Public Health Service to classify cigarette smoking as a form of drug dependence in which nicotine is the critical abuse-producing drug.[184] The first line of evidence is indirect and based on the observation of the many commonalities of cigarette smoking and known forms of psychoactive drug use and dependence. Since the prototypic form of psychoactive drug abuse is the use of opioids, opioid dependence is the standard by which cigarette smoking has been evaluated.[74]

As with many drugs of abuse, attempts to eliminate tobacco use from any culture into which it has been introduced have been as unsuccessful as attempts to eliminate opioid abuse. As is the case with opioids, the major problem does not seem to be a specific withdrawal syndrome; rather opioid users and cigarette smokers frequently completely quit their substance of abuse only to relapse a short time later. Tolerance and physiological dependence has been demonstrated with both opioids and tobacco smoking.[39] Following several hours of deprivation, tolerance is diminished and a person is more sensitive to

the effects of nicotine.[100] Both opioids and nicotine lead to orderly patterns of administration that transcend individual and even species differences. As is the case with opioids, when relatively unrestricted, people and nonhuman primates smoke in orderly patterns from day to day.[5,70] Deprivation of both opioids and nicotine increases the tendency for the substance to be used when available.[70] Thus the commonalities among the phenomena associated with the use of tobacco and opioids provide compelling, yet circumstantial and indirect, evidence that smoking tobacco is an addictive form of behavior. The missing element from this argument is direct evidence that the use of nicotine specifically reinforces further use.

A large number of investigations have demonstrated the tendency to maintain a consistent level of nicotine in the body despite changes in the nicotine concentration of cigarettes, the use of nicotine preloading, or the administration of nicotine antagonists.[71,116,127] Three recent exhaustive reviews of the investigations of nicotine regulation have been published in the last three years.[71,116,127] Almost all of these investigations demonstrate increases in smoking as cigarette nicotine content decreases and decreases in smoking when cigarette nicotine content is unusually high. Additional studies demonstrate compensatory increases in smoking behavior when smoke is filtered or diluted. Both oral and intravenous nicotine administration decreases subsequent cigarette smoking in experimental settings, and nicotine gum reduces cigarette smoking rates in smoking treatment programs. The nicotine antagonist mecamylamine, which is a centrally acting nicotinic ACh receptor blocker, increases smoking rates in experimental subjects.[95,133] Thus, there is strong evidence that smoking rate is a behavior whose goal is to maintain a relatively consistent level of nicotine in the body.[71,116,127]

Another major line of evidence confirming nicotine's classification as a psychoactive drug leading to dependence comes from classical pharmacological studies, such as single-dose studies of abuse potential and self-

*See references 33,74,88,89,90, and 131.

administration studies.[74] Recent investigations demonstrate that nicotine can be readily distinguished from placebo when given intravenously or when smoked.[93] Using two instruments developed for assessing the abuse potential of a compound administered in a single dose, the Liking Scale (Single Dose Questionnaire) and the Morphine Benzedrine Group Scale of the Addiction Research Center Inventory, nicotine has been shown to produce positive or euphoric responses similar to those of more commonly studied drugs of abuse, such as morphine and d-amphetamine.[74,93]

Self-administration studies can establish whether the pharmacological activity of the drug is sufficient to maintain the drug-seeking behavior. In recent human and nonhuman studies under a variety of experimental conditions, nicotine has been found to be a highly efficacious reinforcer of self-administration.[75,78]

The implications of the single-dose abuse potential studies and the self-administration studies provide direct evidence that in doses delivered by cigarette smoking, nicotine is a drug that can produce psychoactive drug dependence.[74] This means that nicotine meets the critical criteria of being psychoactive, producing euphoriant effects, and serving as a pharmacological reinforcer of its own use.[74]

Tobacco: Long-term Effects

Recent research has demonstrated a strong correlation between heavy tobacco smoking and major medical disorders such as respiratory diseases, including emphysema; cancer of the lung, larynx, and mouth; and coronary atherosclerosis.[16,90] Heavy smokers are at high risk for developing serious medical diseases, and many are disturbed by their inability to refrain from smoking. Currently three out of four smokers express a desire to quit smoking.

The medical risks of chronic and heavy smoking are confirmed and are well publicized in the reports of investigations of respiratory types of cancer as well as other lung and blood vessel diseases.[90] However, to many these negative consequences are relatively remote—perhaps thirty to forty years in the future. This is indeed unfortunate considering the immediate positive reinforcement and reward of pleasure that smoking provides.

Medical Management of Both Acute and Chronic Adverse Reactions to Nicotine

While psychological, physiological, and behavioral reactions of varying intensities are experienced following the cessation of smoking, these symptoms do not appear to comprise a clear-cut, recognizable withdrawal syndrome. Symptoms include mild or severe disturbances in sleep, GI distress, nausea, irritability, restlessness, headache, anxiety, difficulty in concentration and psychomotor coordination, weight gain, and changes in heart rate, blood pressure, and pulse. The syndrome is experienced within either hours or days after cessation of smoking and may last up to several months. Toxicity is rarely seen among chronic cigarette smokers because of their tolerance to nicotine.

Toxicity is common in nonsmokers who attempt to smoke. Symptoms of this toxicity include diarrhea, vomiting, increased salivation, abdominal cramps, sweating, dizziness, and occasionally faintness and shock; nonsmokers may also demonstrate an allergic reaction.[89]

Withdrawal symptoms of tobacco may be physiological responses to the interruption of nicotine consumption or may represent psychological reactions to the change in habitual behaviors. Yet the fact that these symptoms disappear completely and relatively quickly upon resumption of smoking or on chewing nicotine gum[74] supports the existence of a physiological withdrawal syndrome. Severity of this syndrome correlates with the intensity and frequency of smoking.[74,88,89,90]

The high relapse rate among smokers is the major problem in the treatment of the tobacco use disorder. Selecting a compatible group for treatment is difficult. Individuals have differing levels of motivation, different levels of knowledge of the medical consequences, different accompanying medical problems, disparate degrees of addiction to nicotine, and differing levels of dependence on and tolerance to nicotine. Variability exists in individual withdrawal patterns, because the withdrawal syndrome is a complex interaction of tobacco and nicotine ingestion, personality, environmental factors, and stress-response.*

There are three major approaches to the management of tobacco use disorder. Substitution therapy, which is analogous to the methadone maintenance program for heroin addicts, provides nicotine in a more manageable and less harmful form such as nicotine gum. Blockade therapy, which is analogous to the naltrexone treatment of heroin addicts, uses a compound that blocks the effects of nicotine, such as mecamylamine. Finally, nonspecific or supportive therapies have been found to be essential as an adjunct to pharmacological treatments, and supportive treatments can occasionally be successful without pharmacological intervention.

A variety of putative nicotine substitutes have been used as experimental treatments for tobacco use disorder. Some have contained lobeline, which is a partial nicotinic receptor agonist that has not yet been demonstrated to be useful in the treatment of tobacco use disorder.[153] Substitution of other stimulants for nicotine has not been useful. In fact, administration of amphetamine to smokers appears to enhance the pleasure of smoking and increases the rate of nicotine consumption.[76]

In 1984 the Food and Drug Administration approved a nicotine-delivering chewing gum for use in the treatment of tobacco use disorder.[74] The gum was demonstrated to increase the rate of success in cigarette smoking treatment programs under a wide variety of conditions. Nicotine gum reduces the desire to smoke in most individuals but

rarely eliminates the desire completely.[92] It also reduces but does not eliminate the nicotine abstinence or withdrawal syndrome for most individuals. As is the case in methadone maintenance treatment of opioid addiction, nicotine gum treatment of smoking is most efficacious when used in conjunction with nonspecific supportive therapies. It is also important to note that there are individuals who do not inhale cigarette smoke and who therefore absorb very little nicotine. These individuals are not addicted to nicotine but are dependent on the behavioral aspects of smoking and should not be treated with nicotine gum.

Nicotine blockade treatment with mecamylamine may be a useful treatment for a subpopulation of smokers, just as naltrexone is useful for some but certainly not all opioid addicts. A preliminary trial of mecamylamine was modeled after successful naltrexone treatment programs for opioid addiction. In this investigation of tobacco use, seven of fourteen subjects quit smoking within two weeks of initiation of mecamylamine treatment, and these subjects reported reduced tobacco craving.[177] These results are extremely preliminary, and it is too early to tell whether mecamylamine will prove useful for the treatment of tobacco use disorder.

Many nonpharmacological or supportive treatments for the prevention of smoking are currently being used and studied. Behavioral modification techniques include aversive conditioning, desensitization, and covert desensitization; and therapeutic techniques include[86,88,90,150] educational therapy, group therapy, individual therapy, and hypnotherapy. Other treatments include confrontation, rapid smoking methods, and a combination of one or two of the previously mentioned treatments with drug therapy. Many of these treatments are somewhat successful. Interestingly, the success rate in abstinence after cessation of smoking is higher in men than women. The success rate depends on motivation, willpower, motivation for medical reasons, method of treatment, and the

*See references 74,86,90,91,131, and 150.

compatibility of the subject with the method of treatment.

There is no "cure" for nicotine addiction; however, the most impressive results are seen when nicotine gum is combined with supportive therapies.* Treatment on a short-term basis is more effective, with an approximate 70 percent success rate after the completion of an average six-week course. However, the percentage of individuals who remain abstinent declines with time. After twelve months 80 percent of smokers revert to their original habit with respect to quantity and time spent smoking. Approximately 20 percent of previous smokers remain non-smokers. [131]

Motivation is a major problem, and research is needed to find more effective methods or combinations of methods of treatment. The problem with many of the behavioral treatments for the cessation of smoking is that motivation is either too low or is very difficult to sustain, since the social aspects of smoking are so comforting. [90,150] An additional obstacle to successful treatment is the social opinion of smoking. In contrast to the attitude to heroin abuse, the common social acceptance of and tolerance in attitude toward smoking make it more difficult for the would-be abstainer. However, in the last five years public attitudes toward smoking have changed dramatically and have led to a number of laws banning smoking in public places.

Finally, there is an ethical dilemma for the treating physician who smokes. Members of society, including both patient and physician, are aware of the image, social prestige, and the sometimes unjustified influence on public opinion that physicians currently possess. It is crucial for physicians, as well as other educators and influential persons, to critically reevaluate the effects their smoking habit and behaviors may have on their patients and to avoid any double standards with regard to the dangers and consequences of cigarette smoking.

*See references 33,86,88,90, and 131.

The Mechanism of Action of Tobacco

The mechanism of action of tobacco remains poorly understood despite the enormous amount of research on the toxicity of its active ingredient, nicotine. One of the problems in understanding the mechanism of action of nicotine as a psychoactive substance is its poorly defined psychoactive effects. While there is considerable evidence from both animal and human studies that nicotine has effects on the CNS, these effects are clearly less dramatically psychoactive than any of the other substances of abuse discussed in this chapter. [74]

On the one hand, the mechanism of action of nicotine is precisely defined. Nicotine is an agonist at the ACh-nicotinic receptors in the peripheral nervous system and in the brain. However, the anatomy and function of central nervous nicotinic receptors are so poorly understood that it is not possible even to speculate on the precise way that a nicotinic agonist could cause psychoactive pharmacological effects and the extreme dependence that large numbers of individuals have on nicotine use. [77,175]

¶ Caffeine

History of Caffeine

Caffeine in the form of coffee, tea, cocoa, and "cola" beverages is currently the most widely used psychoactive substance, followed by nicotine and alcohol. Yet, like these substances, the initial reaction to coffee in Europe and the Americas was one of rejection and opposition. This was no doubt a response to the alleged "intoxicating" and "hazardous" behavioral effects exhibited by users of the new beverages.

The explorers of the fifteenth and sixteenth centuries returned from their voyages with ships richly laden with caffeine-containing commodities. From Arabia and Turkey came the first samples of coffee, originally from Ethiopia and North Africa. From China came ships laden with tea; from West Africa, the ships brought the kola nut, from which caffeine was later added to the cola drinks; while from Mexico and the Central Americas, the ships brought the nuts of the cocoa tree. The ilex plant, the source of the caffeine drink *maté,* was brought back from Brazil. In North America, the Europeans discovered cassine, the tea plant or Christmas berry tree, from which Native Americans made a caffeine brew.[16]

The first written description of coffee was by the Arabian physician Avicenna in the tenth century. In the following centuries coffee, with its stimulant properties, was paradoxically revered and ceremoniously used by Moslem Arabs in religious all-night vigils, while being thoroughly condemned by pious European priests and respectable European citizens as "intoxicating" and giving rise to unseemly, overexcited, and blasphemous behavior.[80]

The coffee habit endured and prospered despite warnings, prohibitions, and punishment. Humankind has long searched for natural stimulants, so coffee became popular and was valued socially for its ability to stimulate with its mellow yet piquant flavor. The introduction of sugar and its combination with coffee added to the beverage's fast-growing popularity as consumers responded enthusiastically to the pleasing mixture. There were strong demands for import to maintain a constant supply of coffee beans. In 1554 coffee houses appeared, first in Constantinople. Later, coffee groups, such as the Bohemians of the 1840s, became popular, their members drinking coffee while discussing political and philosophical issues in stimulating debates.[16]

The honor and ceremony given to tea and its consumption in China in A.D. 350, and much later in England, bears witness to the central role of this beverage in these countries. Descriptions of the "aphrodisiac" properties of cocoa and chocolate date from as early as 3,000 years ago. One famous story describes the Aztec ruler Montezuma consuming fifty cups of "chocolatl" in prepara-tion for a lively evening with many of his 700 wives.[80] Of all the caffeine-containing beverages, chocolate caused the greatest suspicion, as it was considered to incite lustful energy and immoral behavior.[16,80]

Another major category of caffeine-containing substances is the many over-the-counter medications for headaches and colds and certain nonprescription stimulants. In addition, a substance derived from the Brazilian herb guarana, which contains caffeine and possibly other psychoactive substances, can be bought at certain health food stores as a natural stimulant called Zoom and other names.

The popularity, social acceptance, and extensive use of caffeine-containing beverages may be seen as proof of humankind's need for stimulating substances. As a stimulant, coffee is also comparatively inexpensive. Caffeine in coffee, tea, carbonated cola drinks, and chocolate has been thoroughly incorporated into the average daily life-style. There is still debate as to whether caffeine should be categorized as a drug of abuse, despite its clinically obvious pharmacological activity. Many consumers protest and deny they are "addicted" to caffeine-containing beverages.

Patterns of Caffeine Use

Coffee, tea, cocoa, cola drinks, and over-the-counter medications with caffeine content are so widely used that a household without one or more of these beverages would be rare indeed. Considering that most caffeine in the United States is imported and that coffee constitutes the most common source of caffeine, it is not surprising to discover that in 1972, the United States spent $1.2 billion for 2.8 billion pounds of coffee.[196] In addition, in the same year, approximately 34 million pounds of caffeine were consumed.[61]

Since coffee is the most easily available source of caffeine, and as the average cup of coffee contains 85 mg caffeine (range of 50–120 mg, excluding decaffeinated coffee) and the average consumption is three cups a day, the average daily intake of caffeine is

255 mg. Combined with caffeine from other dietary sources and medications, this results in an average daily per capita intake of approximately 275 mg caffeine. This figure varies between 140 and 600 mg. Naturally, the technique of brewing, coffee bean chosen, and number of cups per day varies widely among individuals according to mood, activity, and personality characteristics, such as caffeine dependency and personal habits.[61]

Throughout the world, caffeine-containing beverages are an essential part of most life-styles and cultures. Caffeine drinks and tobacco are a central element of daily meals and ritual intake. Caffeine is used in the morning to awaken, to sustain individuals at midmorning and during the work day, and to give a sophisticated sense of closure after the evening meal. Coffee and tea are an acquired taste, since most children dislike the bitterness of these beverages. Paradoxically, many parents forbid their children's consumption of tea and coffee yet encourage the use of caffeine-containing cola drinks. Chocolate milk and hot cocoa are still acceptable drinks for children, although they contain a small amount of caffeine and a large amount of theobromine, a chemical closely related to caffeine.

The daily consumption of caffeine rises with age during childhood and adolescence, with initial intake beginning as young as six to eleven months. Adults are the heaviest consumers, as are "extroverted" personalities and those involved in successful, fast-paced professions. Heavy users are often achievers, obsessive-compulsive personalities, individuals having anxiety and/or depression, and those whose active life-styles require sustained periods of concentration and performance. Heavy caffeine users are frequently users of other psychoactive substances of abuse, such as alcohol and tobacco. Housewives compose a large proportion of regular users of caffeine-containing beverages, just as students, shift workers, and long-distance truck drivers ingest large amounts of coffee and over-the-counter caffeine-containing stimulants.[16]

Reasons for Caffeine Use

Caffeine, theophylline, and theobromine are structurally related methylated xanthines that occur naturally and are available in synthetic form. They act as CNS and cardiac stimulants, although their intensity and effect on specific organs differ. Pharmacologically, caffeine is the more potent CNS stimulant, theophylline is used as a bronchial and coronary artery dilator and as a diuretic, and theobromine, with the least stimulating activity, is used as a diuretic. Physicians prescribe caffeine for the treatment of asthma, respiratory problems, headache (including migraine) pain, and fatigue. The "C" in the formerly ubiquitous "APC" stands for caffeine. A common pharmacological dose of caffeine is about 200 mg.[109]

Oral caffeine is absorbed twice as rapidly as intramuscular caffeine and is evenly distributed throughout the body (including the placenta and fetus) in proportion to tissue water content. In humans, caffeine possesses a half-life of three hours and is almost entirely excreted by the kidney, leaving no residue in plasma and thus no day-to-day accumulation.[61,109] Caffeine must be regularly administered to sustain its pharmacological effects. Chronic long-term use of even large amounts seems to be relatively safe and nontoxic compared to other substances of abuse.[109] Acute toxicity, however, does occur and can produce hazardous consequences.

Caffeine's effects are well known from personal experience. In our performance- and success-oriented society, the stimulant properties of caffeine are highly valued and appreciated. These include the subjective increase in concentration, energy, alertness, wakefulness, and work capability and the alleviation of fatigue and boredom. Arousal and alteration of mood can occur without changes in the perception of reality.[109]

Given these relatively mild and pleasant effects, coffee use is a welcome habit used to allay dysphoria and low energy levels. Due to its short half-life, dependency results from efforts to sustain the stimulant effects. Tolerance and psychological dependency develop over time, and most people admit their need for the early morning "pick-me-up" and the later "keep awake" properties. These properties explain why caffeine is used widely by long-distance drivers, office workers, students, and others who feel the need for pharmacological stimulation.[16]

The countless number of over-the-counter stimulating tablets, headache and pain remedies, and allergy relief tablets containing caffeine attest to the popularity and need for this compound. These nonprescription drugs include Bromoquinine, Sinarest, Dristan, Cope, Excedrin, Anacin, NoDoz, Vivarin, and others. Caffeine can also be found in foods such as coffee-flavored ice cream, chocolate, and chocolate-flavored foods.

Thus the need for caffeine and the withdrawal symptoms at some dosage levels are evidence of the dependency that develops to caffeine and hence the reason for its inclusion in the category of drugs of abuse. In nonusers, caffeine ingestion causes a syndrome characterized by nervousness, irritability, sleep disturbance, headache, dysphoria, and anxiety. These pharmacological effects are almost identical to those experienced as withdrawal symptoms by regular and/or heavy users. High caffeine intake is associated with high levels of anxiety. It is unclear whether the high levels of anxiety are the result of caffeine excess or whether anxiety stimulates the need for caffeine and motivates regular coffee ingestion.[16,61,109]

Withdrawal Symptoms and Toxicity

The symptoms of caffeine withdrawal are directly related to dosage, potency, individual sensitivity to caffeine, and the combination of caffeine with other drugs. Withdrawal symptoms are relatively mild and can include irritability, anxiety, and headache, all of which spontaneously disappear after a few hours.[109] Caffeine toxicity can occur after extreme and prolonged excessive ingestion of caffeine, usually at doses of approximately 600 to 1,000 mg.[174] The symptoms include headache, sleep disturbance, GI distress, restlessness, irritability, palpitations, arrhythmia, tremor, vertigo, agitation, and anxiety. Extreme cases of acute toxicity can cause convulsions, vomiting, and occasionally hallucinations as in "caffeine-induced delirium."[109,174]

Moderate use of caffeine may be safe and even useful for some individuals when sleep is not possible. However, there is a narrow margin between comfortable, desirable, and efficient caffeine intake and excessive intake or abuse. Stimulant caffeine tablets are readily available, and many people may be hovering close to the point where hazardous complications may arise, such as while driving. Self-prescription and increased usage of the combination of coffee and caffeine stimulant tablets in times of stress may be harmful. Caffeine overdose can occasionally produce hypomanic or severely agitated states that can require brief hospitalization.[16] In rare cases, as few as five 200 mg caffeine tablets are reported to have caused an agitated delirious state.[174]

Medical Management

Caffeine toxicity is rarely reported by physicians. However, there may in fact be more cases than is first apparent. Caffeine toxicity due to chronic heavy caffeine use can be easily misdiagnosed as acute or chronic anxiety and occasionally can mimic some of the symptoms and signs of diabetic ketoacidosis.[115] A detailed history can reveal heavy consumption of caffeine and should include reference to additional sources of caffeine, such as over-the-counter medications.

Decreasing the caffeine intake or recommending abstinence will allow the symptoms of toxicity to completely disappear within forty-eight hours. Mild withdrawal symptoms will spontaneously improve after four to six hours. Pharmacological intervention is rarely necessary, except for the patient with extreme agitation and anxiety, for whom 10 to 30 mg diazepam PO can be useful. To relieve severe withdrawal headaches when agitation is not a problem, 150 mg caffeine can be helpful.

The interaction of caffeine use and affective disorders is a relatively unstudied area. Some bipolar depressed patients are reported to increase their caffeine intake during depressive episodes.[132] When combined with tricyclic antidepressants and MAO inhibitors, caffeine may cause increased nervousness, irritability, and anxiety.[63,132] Caffeine, in coffee, seems a natural choice of beverage to alleviate the side effects of increased thirst, dry mouth, and sedation of some tricyclic antidepressants. However, it can exacerbate mixed depression-anxiety states and increase the likelihood of panic attacks.[63,196]

The physician should consider the possibility of an overdose of over-the-counter caffeine stimulants by children. For example, if a three-year-old takes twenty-five NoDoz tablets, the child can experience emesis, altered states of consciousness, palpitations, photophobia, muscle twitching, miosis, and elevated blood sugar.[115] Finally, caffeinism should be considered in the differential diagnosis of anxiety syndromes, particularly among students, intellectuals, entertainers, long-distance truck drivers, waiters or waitresses, and night workers.

It is ironic that the most commonly used psychoactive substance has received so little attention from medical researchers. Psychiatric inpatients consume vast amounts of coffee, as it is one of the few stimulating substances available to them. There is some evidence that caffeine may have some, as yet undefined, effects on severe psychiatric disorders, such as schizophrenia.[63,196] Studies are needed to define interactions between caffeine use and psychopathology as well as the interactions between caffeine and other psychoactive compounds.

Mechanisms of Action of Caffeine

The mechanism of the action of caffeine has recently been related to its action on the brain neurotransmitter adenosine. In electrophysiological studies, adenosine inhibits the spontaneous firing of most central neurons and inhibits transsynaptic potentials through interaction with specific extracellular receptors. In behavioral studies, adenosine and adenosine analogues have marked depressant effects. In biochemical investigations, adenosine inhibits adenylate cyclase by acting through a "high" affinity receptor (A_1) and activates adenylate cyclase by acting through a "low" affinity receptor (A_2). The A_1 and A_2 receptors show differing profiles for activation by various adenosine analogues. Radioactive N_6-cyclohexyladenosine appears to bind selectively to the A_1 receptor.[35]

One major class of adenosine antagonists has been identified for the adenosine receptors. The alkylxanthines, which include caffeine and theophylline, act as antagonists at the adenosine receptor. Theophylline and caffeine have several behavioral effects that are probably correlated with their blockade of adenosine receptor mechanisms. The doses of caffeine and theophylline that markedly increase exploratory behavior in animals yield brain levels of these compounds that would be very effective in blocking brain adenosine receptors. This is consistent with the hypothesis that the central stimulatory action of caffeine is due in large part to its antagonism of central adenosine receptors. Thus further investigation of caffeine stimulatory action will probably be most productively directed toward studies of alkylxanthine actions on adenosine receptors.[35]

¶ Polydrug Abuse

Most substance abusers use more than one psychoactive agent for recreational purposes, and this polydrug abuse is increasing.[29] Many polydrug abusers have a regular pattern of substance abuse; for example, psychostimulants in the morning, antianxiety agents during the day, and sedative-hypnotics or alcohol in the evening. Other polydrug abusers take whatever psychoactive agents are available or least expensive when their preferred substance of abuse is not available. The general principles for the acute management of severe toxicity or overdose in the polydrug abuser are the same as those for abusers of specific psychoactive agents.

In the management of drug overdose, four basic medical procedures are major priorities: to secure the safety of the patient and treatment staff, to establish a tentative working diagnosis, to reduce toxic physiological effects, and to manage acute concomitant behavioral disturbances and problems.[12,14,180]

The safety of the patient and the treatment staff is the first priority. The patient should not be left alone while awaiting medical attention or during diagnostic procedures. Assaultive, severely disoriented, or extremely agitated patients who show signs of self-destructive behavior should be placed in physical restraints. Vital signs (blood pressure, pulse, temperature, and EKG) should be taken immediately so that rapid intervention can start for patients with fever or with cardiovascular or EKG abnormalities. Vital signs are also important for following the longitudinal course of intoxication.[12,14,180]

When initial safety is ensured and vital signs are stabilized, a tentative or working diagnosis should be established. Information about the possible combination of drugs involved in the toxic reaction should be obtained from as many sources as possible. Those who accompany the intoxicated patient can often give information on the substance or substances that were used as well as describe the reactions of others who took the same drug. Comparing the patient's reactions with those of other users can yield information about doses and possible idiosyncratic or allergic reactions. Friends may also be helpful in determining the approximate doses, the method of administration, the time the drug was taken, and whether any other drugs were used by the patient.

Well-meaning friends may have given or the patient may have taken another drug in an attempt to treat the adverse reaction. Accompanying friends sometimes give misleading information, either because they also are intoxicated or because they are fearful of legal reprisals. Many emergency wards have lists of drugs currently used in the community that have been assessed by a chemical analysis service. These lists specify the alleged content and the actual content of the drug and include a description of the substances locally available and in fashion. This information is helpful but must be up-to-date, since drug availability and street drug names change rapidly.[12,14,180]

A working diagnosis should be based on the results of a physical examination integrated with information obtained from taking a medical history. Because of polydrug abuse and drug adulteration or contamination, specific physical symptoms should be sought. The common clinical findings associated with each of the major classes of substances of abuse are described earlier in this chapter.

In stabilizing vital signs, the immediate treatment of disturbed cardiopulmonary function has the highest priority, and cardiopulmonary resuscitation is the first treatment for a comatose patient with depressed respiration and cardiac function. Arrhythmias also require immediate intervention. Every comatose patient should be intravenously injected with 0.4 to 1.0 mg of the opioid antagonist naloxone. If no response is seen in the first five minutes, 2 mg naloxone (5 ml) can be given. Naloxone will reverse respiratory and CNS depression due to opioids and is harmless if opioids are not involved in the toxic reaction. Fifty ml of a 50 percent glucose solution should be intravenously infused in case hypoglycemia has contributed to the coma. More detailed information on the action and administration of naloxone is found in the section on the management of opioid toxicity.

Preventing further gastric absorption of the ingested drug is a useful strategy in patients with toxic drug reactions. Induction of emesis, gastric lavage, activated charcoal, and a cathartic should be utilized for this purpose. Emesis should be induced (with ipecac syrup or apomorphine intravenous injection) only if the patient is fully conscious. Gastric lavage (after placement of a cuffed endotracheal tube to prevent aspiration) is not as efficient at removing undigested drugs as induced emesis but is the only safe procedure if the patient is not fully conscious. When the gastric contents have been evacuated, a normal saline solution should be infused and withdrawn until the fluid is clear. Gastric lavage is effective for most drugs within four hours of ingestion except for alcohol, heroin, and LSD, which are rapidly absorbed. However, lavage should be attempted in every case, since anticholinergic adulterants may delay the absorption of any substance of abuse. Following gastric lavage, 50 to 100 gm activated charcoal can be administered through the gastric tube. A purgative such as 30 gm sodium sulfate or sorbitol (70 percent solution, 30–50 ml) can be given at the same time as the activated charcoal. The purgative should be used repeatedly until diarrhea develops. For the patient who continues to demonstrate unstable vital signs or remains comatose, admission to an intensive care unit is essential.[13,14,67,180] The techniques used by the specialized treatment teams who manage complicated drug toxicity and overdose in intensive care units is beyond the scope of this chapter.

Withdrawal syndromes may develop as the patient recovers from acute toxicity. The management of the withdrawal syndromes for each specific drug category is described earlier in this chapter. Patients withdrawing from the combination of alcohol or one of the sedative-hypnotics and an opioid should have the alcohol/sedative-hypnotic withdrawal managed first, while they are maintained on a stable dose of methadone.

The use of anticonvulsant medications in the treatment of polydrug withdrawal syndromes is controversial. Some clinicians argue for the prophylactic use of phenytoin. A loading dose of 750 to 1000 mg phenytoin given at the rate of 50 mg per min IV will rapidly establish a therapeutic blood level of 20 μg per ml. A maintenance dose of 300 to 400 mg PO per day will maintain this plasma level.[13,14]

¶ Long-term Treatment and Rehabilitation of Substance Abusers

Psychoactive substance abuse does not respond well to long-term treatment; users have a high relapse rate regardless of the treatment used. However, some general principles apply to the long-term treatment of substance abusers. The physician must always consider the possibility that the patient may be taking the psychoactive substance in an unsupervised attempt to treat a psychiatric disorder. For example, a patient with mania may try to reduce hyperactivity with a CNS depressant such as a barbiturate, while a depressed individual may use psychostimulants such as cocaine or amphetamine in an attempt to relieve dysphoria.[14] However, most substance abusers do not have psychiatric problems that would respond to specific treatments, but rather have the relatively permanent maladaptive patterns of behavior that are classified as character or personality disorders. For some of these patients, hospitalization or at least separation from their drug-taking environment can be helpful in treatment.[14]

Treatment approaches should include some focus on the improvement of interpersonal skills, since substance abusers are frequently deficient in social functioning and in their personal relationships. A combination of group and individual psychotherapy is sometimes helpful. Programs and workshops that teach the development of vocational skills can be effective, as are treatment methods that emphasize the development and modeling of coping skills for future anticipated problems. These methods can include behavioral modification techniques or traditional insight-oriented therapies. The use of groups that emphasize confrontation or Gestalt techniques have yielded mixed results and can be detrimental for some participants. The successful transfer of interpersonal skills from these therapy sessions to real-life situations is rare.

The most comprehensive treatment programs available for substance abusers are for opioid abusers, mainly heroin addicts. This is an unfortunate and mysterious bias of American society. On the positive side, these programs and their relative success rates may pave the way for the development of programs for abusers of other substances. There are at least five major treatment programs for the opioid abuser: methadone maintenance, maintenance with the opioid antagonist naltrexone, therapeutic communities, drug-free programs, and detoxification programs. Most treatment centers use a combination of several approaches. Others offer opioid abusers a choice of more than one treatment method. No single treatment technique has proven to be successful for the majority of opioid abusers who apply for or who are recommended for treatment.[14,125]

Methadone maintenance[104,125] is the most successful drug treatment for opioid abusers. A biochemical hypothesis of relapse to opioid use led to the introduction of methadone maintenance in the mid-1960s by Vincent Dole and Marie Nyswander.[12] These investigators stated that a return to opioid use was due to a biochemical defect that resulted from chronic opioid use and led to "narcotics hunger." Methadone corrected this hypothesized biochemical defect and thus prevented the "narcotics hunger."

The cross-tolerance between methadone and opioids can also explain its success. Methadone in high oral doses has been shown to reduce or even prevent opioid-induced euphoria from an additional opioid.[14,64,104] Long-term studies of patients on methadone maintenance have not revealed any serious consequences to chronic methadone use.[14,64,104] Levo-alpha-acetyl-methadol (LAAM) is a long-acting (two to three days) congener of methadone that has a pharmacological action similar to methadone with a longer duration of activity, which may make it more clinically practical.[111]

Critics of methadone maintenance charge that it merely substitutes one addiction for another. The illegal use of intravenous methadone can produce a euphoric experience similar to intravenous heroin or morphine. Thus the theft of methadone from methadone programs is also a problem. Attempts to make methadone insoluble and therefore difficult to administer intravenously are often countered illegally by chemists who continue to develop techniques to restore the methadone to an injectable form. In addition, the investigations that claim to show methadone maintenance to be successful for many opioid abusers have been criticized for using techniques that artificially inflate the success rate.[125] However, for many former heroin addicts, the use of clinically supervised oral methadone leads to a safer and more healthy life than the use of illegal, expensive, and impure heroin.

Maintenance with opioid antagonists such as naltrexone is based on a conditioning theory of opioid dependence and relapse.[194] Former opioid abusers experience classically conditioned abstinence symptoms, even though they have not recently used opioids, when they return to environments where they have experienced pharmacological withdrawal symptoms in the past. The relief from "conditioned" withdrawal symptoms produced by intravenous heroin is a powerful motivation for the former addict to relapse. Thus the classically conditioned withdrawal syndrome rather than a biochemical defect may be the basis for so-called narcotics hunger. If opioid use and relapse to opioid use are conditioned behaviors, then they should respond to deconditioning. Therefore, opioid use should be extinguished or gradually decline if opioid injection no longer relieves the conditioned withdrawal symptoms and no longer produces euphoria.[194] An opioid antagonist taken daily can prevent both the euphoria and the relief of conditioned withdrawal symptoms of the former opioid abuser.[146]

Cyclazocine, naloxone, nalorphine, and naltrexone have all been used as opioid antagonists in experimental treatment programs. Cyclazocine has some agonist activity, has a slight withdrawal syndrome, and causes dysphoria and is therefore less than ideal. Nalorphine also produces dysphoria and has proved to be unacceptable.[52] Naloxone is a pure opioid antagonist, but unfortunately, when taken orally, it is poorly absorbed.

Naltrexone is nearly a pure opioid antagonist, is well absorbed orally, and may play a role in the treatment of opioid addiction. Numerous investigations have demonstrated that naltrexone is pharmacologically effective. Naltrexone antagonizes the actions of illegal American street opioids for forty-eight to seventy-two hours after an oral dose, in spite of the fact that the half-life of the parent compound and major metabolite would suggest a shorter duration of action. Naltrexone may be effective because American street opioids are weak. Naltrexone is a competitive antagonist, which means it does not completely block exogenous opioids.

In spite of a large number of controlled investigations, it is difficult to demonstrate that naltrexone is effective in placebo-controlled investigations. Many investigators argue that the placebo-controlled paradigm is not a valid test of the efficacy of naltrexone, just as it is not a valid test of the disulfiram treatment for alcohol addiction. Thus while it is difficult to demonstrate the efficacy of naltrexone in classical pharmacological trials, most researchers agree that it is a useful treatment for some opioid addicts.

Naltrexone is almost never effective as a sole treatment. It seems to work best in individuals who have high motivation to end their addiction, such as job jeopardy or threatened incarceration. Some of the best results have been with populations of addicted middle-class business people or physicians who are jeopardizing their careers with continued drug use. Psychotherapy, family therapy, behavioral therapies, job counseling, and group therapy are often successfully combined with naltrexone maintenance. Urine testing for opioids is a common feature of successful naltrexone treatment programs. Relapses are fairly common in these programs, and when patients relapse, they should not necessarily be considered treatment failures. Many individuals require several courses of treatment to remain abstinent.

In general, naltrexone maintenance is not as successful for many individuals as methadone maintenance. However, since the treatment of opioid addiction is characterized by high relapse rates, poor compliance, and difficulty in initial motivation, naltrexone maintenance may be an alternative to methadone maintenance for a subgroup of opioid addicts who do not wish to use methadone because it is an addicting substance or who are required to remain free of addictive substances.[139]

Naltrexone is a relatively nontoxic compound. Dysphoria has been reported by some individuals with acute doses, but chronic former addicts who are gradually introduced to naltrexone rarely report dysphoria. No clinically significant long-term endocrine changes, carcinogenic effects, or effects on reproductive function that are clinically relevant have been reported. Recent concern has been raised because abnormalities in liver function tests have been reported in some former addicts using naltrexone. The extent and clinical significance of this possible liver toxicity is a subject of considerable debate. Further investigations are needed to determine if the possible liver toxicity of naltrexone will be a problem for its use as one treatment modality for opioid addiction.[6,27,69,149]

Buprenorphine is a mixed opioid agonist-antagonist that has been proposed for potential use in treating narcotic addiction. It appears to be acceptable to addicts, is long-acting, produces a low level of physical dependence allowing for easy detoxification, and, most important, antagonizes the effects of injected opioids. This potentially useful compound deserves a trial as a maintenance treatment for abusers of opioids.[94]

Therapeutic communities are usually full-time residential programs that emphasize group therapies, peer pressure, patient confrontation, and patient government. Their goal is to reeducate the former opioid abuser to more adaptive attitudes and more mature and successful patterns of behavior. Such programs include Odessey House, Daytop, Phoenix House, and other private agencies for the rehabilitation of opioid addicts. The duration of therapeutic community treatment in these facilities varies from short-term programs that last for weeks to programs that take a year or longer. A continuing problem for therapeutic communities of this type is the large number of opioid abusers who fail to complete the required program or who use opioids during the program.[12,125,155]

Drug-free outpatient treatment programs are an alternative frequently offered to opioid and nonopioid substance abusers. These programs vary widely in philosophy as well as in program content, processes, goals, and duration of treatment. At one end of the spectrum are the relaxed programs that offer informal group discussions, recreational activities, and help with social and vocational problems on request. At the other end are rigorously structured resocialization programs that are similar to daytime therapeutic communities. Outpatient drug-free programs are even less successful than inpatient therapeutic communities.[12,155]

Detoxification programs are short-term programs whose goal is to withdraw the patient from opioids in relative comfort and, therefore, terminate the opioid abuser's physiological dependence on opioids. Common programs include seven- to twenty-one-day inpatient detoxification treatments using oral methadone, clonidine, or lofexidine. Some detoxification programs provide a limited amount of counseling, although this is not a primary goal. Outpatient detoxification of opioid abusers with these drugs is an experimental treatment without demonstrated efficacy.[12] Outpatient detoxification programs are frequently less rigorous and of longer duration than inpatient programs.[155] However, outpatient detoxification with clonidine or lofexidine may be more dangerous, since patients' vital signs cannot be carefully monitored.

Comparison of the various treatment regimens for opioid abusers is difficult because of methodological issues. Even within each of these treatment regimens, there is considerable variation in treatment goals, treatment processes, staffing, physical facilities, demand on patient time and effort, duration of treatment, discipline and use of sanctions, degree of individual responsibility allowed to the patient, and use of patient influence in treatment. Other variations in programs include the use of ancillary rehabilitation services such as vocational training, job placement, family counseling, personal counseling, educational programs, recreational programs, medical services, and individual and group psychotherapy. Therefore, it is extremely difficult to compare the successful rehabilitation rate and method of one program with another. Long-term follow-up is a necessary but formidable task to determine whether a former opioid abuser has been successfully treated. Finally, in comparison to well-designed trials of psychopharmacological agents for anxiety, depression, and schizophrenia, random-assignment studies in substance abuse rehabilitation are extremely rare.[12,155]

Given these methodological problems, the outcomes of methadone maintenance and therapeutic communities seem to be most favorable for opioid abusers. Drug-free regimens are probably more suited to nonopioid substance abusers. When used as the sole method of treatment, detoxification programs seem to be the least effective. Detoxification is best used as an entry procedure for drug-free treatment or as a means of recruitment for other treatment modalities. While there is some evidence that at least two types of treatment have some efficacy in the long-term rehabilitation of opioid abusers, even these treatments are effective in less than half of the patients who participate in these programs. The majority of opioid abusers relapse to their former opioid use either during or after completing the treatment program. The relapse rate for users of other psychoactive substances is even greater than that for former opioid abusers.[12,155]

¶ Conclusion

Abuse disorders cause profound problems for society and are a continuing challenge to the medical profession. Careful emergency medical management of patients with substance abuse disorders often yields dramatic recoveries. The acute organic brain syndromes produced by intoxication with or withdrawal from psychoactive substances of abuse usually respond rapidly to treatments based on knowledge of and clinical experience with the pharmacological properties of these psychoactive substances.

Sadly, long-term treatment and rehabilitation programs for patients with substance abuse disorders are far less successful than treatments of their acute toxic reactions. Most substance abusers revert rapidly to the dangerous patterns of drug self-administration that initially caused the acute toxic reactions. The most widespread substance abuse disorder, tobacco use disorder, almost never produces an acute toxic reaction that requires treatment by physicians. Yet the long-term effects of this disorder, such as increased risk for respiratory system cancer and cardiac disease, make tobacco use disorder one of the most serious threats to the health of humanity. Medical research is urgently needed to develop new treatment approaches for the chronic maladaptive and self-destructive behaviors of substance abusers.

¶ Acknowledgements

Supported by the Medical Research Service of the Veterans Administration and the National Institute of Mental Health Specialized Research Center Grant MH 30854. The authors thank Christie Price and Pamela Elliott for help in preparing this chapter.

¶ Bibliography

1. ABRAHAM, H. D. "Visual Phenomenology of the LSD Flashback," *Archives of General Psychiatry*, 40 (1983):884–889.

2. AGHAJANIAN, G. K., and HAIGLER, H. J. "Hallucinogenic Indoleamines: Preferential Action Upon Presynaptic Serotonin Receptors," *Psychopharmacology Communications* 1 (1975):619–629.

3. AKIL, H. "Opiates: Biological Mechanisms," in J. D. Barchas et al., eds., *Psychopharmacology: From Theory to Practice.* New York: Oxford University Press, 1977, pp. 293–305.

4. AKIL, H., MAYER, D. J., and LIEBESKIND, J. C. "Comparison Chez le Rate Entre l'Analgesic Induite par Stimulation de la Substance Grise Periaqueducale et l'Analgesie Morphinique," *CR Comptes Rendus Hebdomadaires des Séances de L'Academie Des Sciences* (Paris), 274 (1972):3603.

5. ANDO, K., and YANAGITA, T. "Cigarette Smoking in Rhesus Monkeys," *Psychopharmacology*, 72 (1981):117–127.

6. ATKINSON, R. L. "Endocrine and Metabolic Effects of Opiate Antagonists," *Journal of Clinical Psychiatry*, 45 (1984):20–24.

7. AYD, F. J., and BLACKWELL, B., eds. *Discoveries in Biological Psychiatry.* Philadelphia: J. B. Lippincott, 1970, pp. 218–219.

8. BACHMAN, J. G., JOHNSTON, L. D., and O'MALLEY, P. M. "Smoking, Drinking, and Drug Use Among American High School Students: Correlates and Trends, 1975–1979," *American Journal of Public Health*, 71 (1981):59–69.

9. BERGER, F. M. "Anxiety and the Discovery of Tranquilizers," in F. J. Ayd and B. Blackwell, eds., *Discoveries in Biological Psychiatry.* Philadelphia: J. B. Lippincott, 1970, pp. 115–129.

10. BERGER, P. A. "The Addict in the Emergency Room," in C. P. Rosenbaum and J. Beebe, eds., *An Introduction to Treatment in Psychiatry: Crisis Clinic and Consultation.* New York: McGraw-Hill, 1975, pp. 161–171.

11. ———. "Endorphins," in B. Wolman, ed., *International Encyclopedia of Psychiatry, Psychology, Psychoanalysis, and Neurology.* New York: Aesculapius Publishers, 1984, pp. 121–125.

12. BERGER, P. A., and DUNN, M. J. "Substance Use Disorders: Diagnosis and

Treatment," in J. Greist, J. Jefferson, and R. Spitzer, eds., *Treatment of Mental Disorders.* New York: Oxford University Press, 1982, pp. 78–142.

13. BERGER, P. A., and TINKLENBERG, J. R. "Treatment of Abusers of Alcohol and Other Addictive Drugs," in J. D. Barchas, et al., eds., *Psychopharmacology: From Theory to Practice.* New York: Oxford University Press, 1977, pp. 355–385.

14. ———. "Medical Management of the Drug Abuser," in A. M. Freeman, R. L. Sack, and P. A. Berger, eds., *Psychiatry for the Primary Care Physician.* Baltimore: Williams & Wilkins, 1979, pp. 359–380.

15. BERGER, P. A., et al. "Investigating Opioid Peptides in Schizophrenia and Depression," in J. Martin and J. Barchas, eds., *Neuropeptides: Implications for Neurologic and Psychiatric Diseases.* New York: Raven Press, forthcoming.

16. BRECHER, E. M., and the editors of Consumer Reports. *Licit and Illicit Drugs.* Boston: Little, Brown, 1972.

17. BROOKS, J. E. *The Mighty Leaf: Tobacco Through the Centuries.* Boston: Little, Brown, 1952.

18. BUHRICH, N., MORRIS, G., and COOK, G. "Bromo-DMA: The Australasian Hallucinogen," *Australia–New Zealand Journal of Psychiatry,* 17 (1983):275–279.

19. BURSE, R. L., et al. "Increased Appetite and Unchanged Metabolism upon Cessation of Smoking with Diet Held Constant," *Physiologist,* 18 (1975):157.

20. BYCK, R., ed. *Cocaine Papers, by Sigmund Freud.* New York: Stonehill Publishing Co., 1978.

21. BYCK, R., and RITCHIE, J. M. "Delta-9-tetrahydrocannabinol: Effects on Mammalian Nonmyelinated Nerve Fibers," *Science,* 180 (1973):84–85.

22. CALDWELL, J., and SIEVER, P. S. "The Biochemical Pharmacology of Abused Drugs. I. Amphetamines, Cocaine, and LSD," *Clinical Pharmacology & Therapeutics,* 16 (1974):625–628.

23. CAPLAN, L. R., THOMAS, C., and BANKS, G. "Central Nervous System Complications of Addiction to 'T's and Blues,' " *Neurology,* 32 (1982):623–628.

24. CASTELLANI, S., GIANNINI, A. J., and

25. CENTERS FOR DISEASE CONTROL. *Morbid and Mortal Weekly Report* 32 (1983):457.

26. CHEREK, D. R. "Effects of Smoking Different Doses of Nicotine on Human Aggressive Behavior," *Psychopharmacology,* 75 (1981):339–345.

27. CHRISTIAN, M. S. "Reproductive Toxicity and Teratology Evaluations of Altrexone," *Journal of Clinical Psychiatry,* 45 (1984):7–10.

28. COGGINS, W. J. "The Costa Rica Cannabis Project: An Interim Report on the Medical Aspects," in M. C. Braude and S. Szara, eds., *The Pharmacology of Marijuana.* New York: Raven Press, 1976, pp. 667–670.

29. COHEN, S. "Trends in Substance Abuse," *Drug Abuse and Alcoholism Newsletter,* 7(1978).

30. ———. "Inhalants," in R. I. Dupont, A. Goldstein, and J. O'Donnell, eds., *Handbook on Drug Abuse.* Washington, D.C.: U.S. Government Printing Office, National Institute on Drug Abuse, DHEW, 1979, pp. 213–220.

31. ———. "The Hallucinogens, *Drug Abuse and Alcoholism Newsletter,* 13 (1984).

32. ———. "A Matter of Quality Control: Manufactured Drugs of Abuse," *Drug Abuse and Alcoholism Newsletter,* 13 (1984).

33. COHEN, S., ed. "On the Smoking of Cigarettes," *Drug Abuse and Alcoholism Newsletter,* 8 (1979).

34. CRONK, S. L., BARKLEY, D.E.H., and FARRELL, M. F. "Respiratory Arrest After Solvent Abuse," *British Medical Journal;* 290 (1985):897–898.

35. DALY, J. W., Bruns, R. F., and Snyder, S. H. "Adenosine Receptors in the Central Nervous System: Relationship to the Central Actions of Methylxanthines," *Life Sciences,* 28 (1981):2083–2097.

36. DAPRADA, M., et al. "Lysergic Acid Diethylamide: Evidence for Stimulation of Cerebral Dopamine Receptors," *Brain Research,* 94 (1975):67–73.

37. "Death by Design." *Time.* 8 April 1985, p. 61.

38. DEVATHASAN, G., et al. "Complications of

ADAMS, P. M. "Physostigmine and Haloperidol Treatment of Acute Phencyclidine Intoxication," *American Journal of Psychiatry,* 139 (1982):508–510.

Chronic Glue (Toluene) Abuse in Adolescents," *Australia and New Zealand Journal of Medicine,* 14 (1984):39–43.

39. DOMINO, E. F. "Behavioral, Electrophysiological, Endocrine and Skeletal Muscle Actions of Nicotine and Tobacco Smoking," in A. Remond and C. Izard, eds., *Electrophysiological Effects of Nicotine.* Amsterdam: Elsevier, 1979, pp. 78–92.

40. DOMINO, E. F. "Phencyclidine and Analogues—Future Directions," in E. F. Domino, ed. *PCP (Phenycyclidine): Historical and Current Perspectives.* Ann Arbor, Mich.: NPP Books, 1981, pp. 515–528.

41. DOMINO, E. F., ed. *PCP (Phencyclidine): Historical and Current Perspectives.* Ann Arbor, Mich.: NPP Books, 1981.

42. DREW, W. G., and MILLER, L. L. "Cannabis: Neural Mechanisms and Behavior—A Theoretical Review," *Pharmacology,* 11 (1974):12–32.

43. ELLINWOOD, E. H., JR. "Amphetamines/Anorectics," in R. I. Dupont, A. Goldstein, and J. O'Donnell, eds., *Handbook on Drug Abuse.* Washington, D.C.: U.S. Government Printing Office, National Institute on Drug Abuse, DHEW, 1979, pp. 221–231.

44. ESSIG, C. F. "New Sedative Drugs That Can Cause States of Intoxication and Dependence of the Barbiturate Type," *Journal of the American Medical Association,* 196 (1966):714–717.

45. EVANS, R. I., and RAINES, B. E. "Control and Prevention of Smoking in Adolescents: A Psychosocial Perspective," in T. J. Coates, A. C. Petersen, and C. Perry, eds., *Adolescent Health Promoting.* New York: Academic Press, 1982, pp. 146–152.

46. FISHBURNE, P. M., ABELSON, H. I., and CISIN, I. *National Survey on Drug Abuse: Main Findings: 1979.* Washington, D.C.: U.S. Government Printing Office, DHHS Publication No. (ADM) 80–976, 1980.

47. GARVEY, A. J., "Smoking, Weight Change, and Age," *Archives of Environmental Health,* 28 (1974):327–329.

48. GAWIN, F. H., and KLEBER, H. D. "Cocaine Abuse Treatment," *Archives of General Psychiatry,* 41 (1984):903–909.

49. GIANNINI, A. J., et al. "Comparison of Haloperidol and Chlorpromazine in the Treatment of Phencyclidine Psychosis," *Journal of Clinical Pharmacology,* 24 (1984):202–204.

50. GILBERT, D. G. "Paradoxical Tranquilizing and Emotion-reducing Effect on Nicotine," *Psychological Bulletin,* 86 (1979):643–662.

51. GILBERT, P. E., and MARTIN, W. R. "The Effects of Morphine and Naloxphine-like Drugs in the Nondependent, Morphine-dependent and Cyclazocine-dependent Chronic Spinal Dog," *Journal of Pharmacology and Experimental Therapeutics,* 198 (1976):66–82.

52. GINZBURG, H. M., and GLASS, W. J. "The Role of the National Institute on Drug Abuse in Development of Naltrexone," *Journal of Clinical Psychiatry,* 45 (1984): 4–6.

53. GLAUSER, S. C., et al. "Metabolic Changes Associated with the Cessation of Cigarette Smoking," *Archives of Environmental Health,* 20 (1970):377–381.

54. GOLD, M. S., and REDMOND, D. E., JR. "Pharmacological Activation and Inhibition of Noradrenergic Activity Alter Specific Behaviors in Non-human Primates," *Neuroscience Abstracts,* 3 (1977): 250.

55. GOLD, M. S., REDMOND, D. E., JR. and KLEBER, H. D. "Clonidine Blocks Acute Opiate-withdrawal Symptoms," *Lancet,* 2 (1978):599–602.

56. GOLD M. S., et al. "Clonidine and Opiate Withdrawal," *Lancet,* 2 (1980):1078–1079.

57. GOLD M. S., et al. "Opiate Withdrawal Using Clonidine: A Safe, Effective and Rapid Non-opiate Treatment," *Journal of the American Medical Association,* 243 (1980): 343–346.

58. GOLD M. S., et al. "Lofexidine, a Clonidine Analogue Effective in Opiate Withdrawal," *Lancet,* 1 (1981):992–993.

59. GOLDFRANK, L., and MELIEK, M. "Locoweed and Other Anticholinergics," *Hospital Physician,* 8 (1979):18–39.

60. GOLDSTEIN, A., LOWNEY, L. I., and PAL, B. K. "Stereospecific and Nonspecific Interactions of the Morphine Cogener

Levorphanol in Subcellular Fractions of Mouse Brain," *Proceedings of the National Academy of Science* (USA), 68 (1971): 1742–1747.

61. GRAHAM, D. M. "Caffeine—Its Identity, Dietary Sources, Intake and Biological Effects," *Nutrition Reviews,* 36 (1978): 97–102.

62. GRANACHER, R. P., BALDESSARINI, R. J., and MESSNER, E. "Physostigmine Treatment of Delirium Induced by Anticholinergics," *American Family Physician,* 13 (1976):99–103.

63. GREDEN, J. F., et al. "Anxiety and Depression Associated with Caffeinism Among Psychiatric Inpatients," *American Journal of Psychiatry,* 135 (1978): 963–966.

64. GREEN, A. I., MEYER, R. E., and SHADER, R. I. "Heroin and Methadone Abuse: Acute and Chronic Management," in R. I. Shader, ed., *Manual of Psychiatric Therapeutics: Practical Psychopharmacology and Psychiatry.* Boston: Little, Brown, 1975, pp. 203–210.

65. GREENBLATT, D. J., and SHADER, R. I. "Drug Abuse and the Emergency Room Physician," *American Journal of Psychiatry,* 131 (1974):559–562.

66. ———. "Bad trips," in R. I. Shader, ed., *Manual of Psychiatric Therapeutics: Practical Psychopharmacology and Psychiatry.* Boston: Little, Brown, 1975, pp. 185–192.

67. ———. "Psychotropic Drug Overdosage," in R. I. Shader, ed., *Manual of Psychiatric Therapeutics: Practical Psychiatry and Psychopharmacology.* Boston: Little, Brown, 1975, pp. 237–267.

68. GREENE, M. H., and DUPONT, R. L. "The Treatment of Acute Heroin Toxicity," in P. G. Bourne, ed., *A Treatment Manual for Acute Drug Abuse Emergencies.* Washington, D.C.: U.S. Government Printing Office, DHEW, 1974, pp. 11–16.

69. GREENSTEIN, R. A., et al. "Naltrexone: A Clinical Perspective," *Journal of Clinical Psychiatry,* 45 (1984):25–28.

70. GRIFFITHS, R. R., and HENNINGFIELD, J. E. "Experimental Analysis of Cigarette Smoking," *Federation Proceedings,* 41 (1982):234–240.

71. GRITZ, E. R. "Smoking Behavior and Tobacco Abuse," in N. K. Mello, ed., *Advances in Substance Abuse.* Greenwich, Conn.: JAI Press, 1980, pp. 57–68.

72. GRUNBERG, N. E., and MORSE, D. E. "Cigarette Smoking and Food Consumption in the United States," *Journal of Applied Social Psychology,* in press.

73. HARRIS, L. S. "Cannabis: A Review of Progress," in: M. A. Lipton, A. DiMascio, and K. F. Killam, eds., *Psychopharmacology: A Generation of Progress.* New York: Raven Press, 1978, pp. 1565–1574.

74. HENNINGFIELD, J. E. "Pharmacologic Basis and Treatment of Cigarette Smoking," *Journal of Clinical Psychiatry,* 45 (1984):24–32.

75. HENNINGFIELD, J. E., and GOLDBERG, S. R. "Nicotine as a Reinforcer in Human Subjects and Laboratory Animals," *Journal of Clinical Psychiatry,* 45 (1984):989–992.

76. HENNINGFIELD, J. E., and GRIFFITHS, R. R. "Cigarette Smoking and Subjective Responses: Effects of d-amphetamine," *Clinical Pharmacology and Therapeutics,* 30 (1981):497–505.

77. HENNINGFIELD, J. E., and JASKINSKI, D. R. "Human Pharmacology of Nicotine," *Psychopharmacology Bulletin,* 19 (1982):413–415.

78. HENNINGFIELD, J. E., MYASATO, K., and JASINKSKI, D. R. "Cigarette Smokers' Self-administered Intravenous Nicotine," *Pharmacology, Biochemistry and Behavior,* 19 (1983):887–890.

79. HEYDEN, S. "The Workingman's Diet," *Nutr Meta,* 20 (1976):381–386.

80. *High Times Encyclopedia of Recreational Drugs.* New York: Stonehill Publishing Company, 1978.

81. HOLLISTER, L. E. "Diazepam in Newly Admitted Schizophrenics," *Diseases of the Nervous System,* 24 (1963):746–775.

82. ———. *Chemical Psychoses.* Springfield, Ill.: Charles C Thomas, 1968.

83. ———. "Overdoses of Psychotherapeutic Drugs," in C. P. Rosenbaum and J. E. Beebe, eds., *Psychiatric Treatment: Crisis, Clinic, and Consultation.* New York: McGraw-Hill, 1975, pp. 145–154.

84. HUGHES, J., et al. "Identification of Two Related Pentapeptides from the Brain

with Potent Opiate Agonist Activity,"
Nature 258 (1975):577–579.

85. HUGHES, P. L., and MORSE, R. M. "Use of
Clonidine in a Mixed Drug Detoxifica-
tion Regimen: Possibility of Masking
Clinical Signs of Sedative Withdrawal,"
Mayo Clinic Proceedings, 60 (1985):47–
49.

86. HUNT, W. A., and BESPALEC, D. A. "An
Evaluation of Current Methods of
Modifying Smoking Behavior," *Journal
of Clinical Psychology*, 30 (1974):431–
438.

87. ISBELL, H. "Addiction to Barbiturates and
the Barbiturate Abstinence Syndrome,"
Archives of General Medicine, 33
(1950):108.

88. JAFFE, J. H., and JARVIK, M. E. "Tobacco
Use and Tobacco Use Disorder," in M.
A. Lipton, A. DiMascio, and K. F. Kil-
lam, eds., *Psychopharmacology: A Gen-
eration of Progress*. New York: Raven
Press, 1978, pp. 1665–1676.

89. JARVIK, M. E., and GRITZ, E. R. "Nicotine
and Tobacco," in M. E. Jarvik, ed., *Psychopharmacology in the Practice of
Medicine*. New York: Appleton-Century-Crofts, 1977, pp. 481–495.

90. JARVIK, M. E., et al., eds. *Research on
Smoking Behavior*. Washington, D.C.:
U.S. Government Printing Office,
NIDA Research Monograph Series No.
17, DHEW, 1977.

91. JARVIK, M. E., et al. "Can Cigarette Size
and Nicotine Content Influence Smoking and Puffing Rates?" *Psychopharmacology* 58 (1978):303–306.

92. JARVIS, M. "The Treatment of Cigarette
Dependence," *British Journal of Addiction*, 78 (1983):125–130.

93. JASINSKI, D. R., JOHNSON, R. E., and HEN-
NINGFIELD, J. E. "Abuse Liability Assessment in Human Subjects," *Trends
in Pharmacological Sciences*, 5 (1984):-
196–200.

94. JASINSKI, D. R., PEVNICK, J. S., and GRIF-
FITH, J. D. "Human Pharmacology and
Abuse Potential of the Analgesic Buprenorphine," *Archives of General Psychiatry*, 35 (1978):501–516.

95. JASINSKI, D. R., et al. "Progress Report
from the ARC, Baltimore, MD.," in L. S.
Harris, ed., *Problems of Drug Depen-*

dence, Washington, D.C., U.S. Government Printing Office, NIDA Research
Monograph Series No. 49, 1984.

96. JOHNSON, A. L., HOLLISTER, L. E., and
BERGER, P. A. "The Anticholinergic Intoxication Syndrome: Diagnosis and
Treatment," *Journal of Clinical Psychiatry*, 42 (1981):313–317.

97. JOHNSON, J. M., and VICKROY, T. W. "The
Effects of Phencyclidine and Two
Metabolites on Synaptosomal Dopa-
mine Synthesis, Uptake and Release," in
E. F. Domino, ed., *PCP (Phencyclidine):
Historical and Current Perspectives*.
Ann Arbor, Mich.: NPP Books, 1981, pp.
191–206.

98. JOHNSTON, L. D. "Frequent Marijuana
Use: Correlates, Possible Effects, and
Reasons for Using and Quitting," Paper
presented at a conference on treating
the marijuana-dependent person,
American Council on Marijuana and
Other Psychoactive Drugs. Bethesda,
Md., May 4, 1981.

99. JONES, R. T. Cited in Report of an Addiction Research Foundation/ World
Health Organization (ARF/WHO)
Scientific Meeting on Adverse Health
and Behavioral Consequences of Cannabis Use. Toronto: ARF/WHO, 1981.

100. JONES, R. T., FARRELL, T. R., and HERN-
ING, R. I. "Tobacco Smoking and Nicotine Tolerance," in N. A. Krasnegor, ed.,
*Self-Administration of Abused Sub-
stances: Methods for Study*. Washington, D.C.: U.S. Government Printing
Office, NIDA Research Monograph Series No. 20, 1978.

101. KHANTZIAM, E. J., and MCKENNA, G. J.
"Acute Toxic and Withdrawal Reaction
Associated with Drug Use and Abuse,"
Annals of Internal Medicine, 90 (1979):
361–372.

102. KING, G. S., SMIALEK, J. E., and TROUT-
MAN, W. G. "Sudden Death in Adolescents Resulting from the Inhalation of
Typewriter Correction Fluid," *Journal
of the American Medical Association*,
253 (1985):1604–1606.

103. KIRK, L. M., ANDERSON, R. J., and MAR-
TIN, K. "Sudden Death from Toluene
Abuse," *Annals of Emergency Medi-
cine*, 13 (1984):119–120.

104. KISSIN, B., LOWINSON, J. H., and MILL-MAN, R. B., eds. *Recent Developments in Chemotherapy of Narcotic Addiction,* vol. 311. New York: New York Academy of Sciences, 1978.

105. KITTEL, F., et al. "Psycho-socio-biological Correlates of Moderate Overweight in an Industrial Population," *Journal of Psychosomatic Research,* 22 (1978):145–158.

106. KLEBER, H. D. "Clonidine in Outpatient Detoxification from Methadone Maintenance," *Archives of General Psychiatry,* 42 (1985):391–394.

107. KLEBER, H. D., and GAWIN, F. H. "The Spectrum of Cocaine Abuse and Its Treatment," *Journal of Clinical Psychiatry,* 45 (1984): Sect. 2.

108. KOVANEN, J., SOMER, H., and SCHROEDER, P. "Acute Myopathy Associated with Gasoline Sniffing," *Neurology,* 33 (1983):629–631.

109. LEVENSON, H. S., and BICK, E. C. "Psychopharmacology of Caffeine," in M. E. Jarvik, ed., *Psychopharmacology in the Practice of Medicine.* New York: Appleton-Century-Crofts, 1977, pp. 451–463.

110. LEWIN, R. "Trail of Ironies to Parkinson's Disease," *Science,* 224 (1984):1083–1085.

111. LING, W., and BLAINE, J. D. "The Use of LAAM in Treatment," in R. I. Dupont, A. Goldstein, and J. O'Donnell, eds., *Handbook on Drug Abuse.* Washington, D.C.: U.S. Government Printing Office, National Institute on Drug Abuse, DHEW, 1979, pp. 87–96.

112. LISKOW, B. "Substance Induced and Substance Use Disorders: Barbiturates and Similarly Acting Sedative Hypnotics," in J. H. Greist, J. W. Jefferson, and R. L. Spitzer, eds., *The Diagnosis and Treatment of Mental Disorders.* New York: Oxford University Press, 1982, pp. 62–77.

113. LOCATELLI, F., and POZZI, C. "Relapsing Haemolytic-uraemic Syndrome After Organic Solvent Sniffing," *Lancet,* 2 (1983):220.

114. LORD, J. A. H., et al. "Endogenous Opioid Peptides: Multiple Agonists and Receptors," *Nature* (London) 267 (1977):495–499.

115. MACE, J. "Toxicity of Caffeine," *Journal of Pediatrics,* 92 (1978), 345–346.

116. MCMORROW, M. J., and FOXX, R. M. "Nicotine's Role in Smoking: An Analysis of Nicotine Regulation," *Psychological Bulletin,* 93 (1983):302–327.

117. MAHENDER, R. A. "The Management of the Narcotic Withdrawal Syndrome in the Neonate," in P. G. Bourne, ed., *A Treatment Manual for Acute Drug Abuse Emergencies.* Washington, D.C.: U.S. Government Printing Office, DHEW, 1974, pp. 27–28.

118. MARTIN, P. R., et al. "Intravenous Phenobarbital Therapy in Barbiturate and Other Hyposedative Withdrawal Reactions: A Kinetic Approach," *Clinical Pharmacology and Therapeutics,* 2 (1979):256–264.

119. MARTIN, W. R., HAERTZEN, C. A., and HEWETT, B. B. "Psychopathology and Pathophysiology of Narcotic Addicts, Alcoholics, and Drug Abusers," in J. A. Lipton, A. DiMascio, and K. F. Killam, eds., *Psychopharmacology: A Generation of Progress.* New York: Raven Press, 1978, pp. 1591–1602.

120. MARTIN, W. R., et al. "The Effects of Morphine- and Nalorphine-like Drugs in the Nondependent and Morphine-dependent Chronic Spinal Dog," *Journal of Pharmacology and Experimental Therapeutics,* 197 (1976):517–532.

121. MAYNERT, E. W. "Sedative and Hypnotics, II: Barbiturates," in J. R. DiPalma, ed., *Drill's Pharmacology in Medicine.* New York: McGraw-Hill, 1965, pp. 188–209.

122. MELTZER, H. Y., et al. "Phencyclidine as an Indirect Dopamine Agonist," in E. F. Domino, ed., *PCP (Phencyclidine): Historical and Current Perspectives.* Ann Arbor, Mich.: NPP Books, 1981, pp. 207–242.

123. MEYER, R. E. "Behavioral Pharmacology of Marihuana," in M. A. Lipton, A. DiMascio, and K. F. Killam, eds., *Psychopharmacology: A Generation of Progress.* New York: Raven Press, 1978, pp. 1639–1652.

124. MILLER, J. D. and CISIN, I. H. *Highlights from the National Survey on Drug Abuse: 1979.* Washington, D.C.: U.S. Government Printing Office, DHHS Publication No. (ADM) 80–1032, 1980.

125. MIRIN, S. M., and MEYER, R. E. "Treat-

ment of Substance Abusers," in W. G. Clark and J. del Guidice, eds., *Principles of Psychopharmacology*. New York: Academic Press, 1978, pp. 701–720.

126. MOHLER, H., and OKADA, T. "Benzodiazepine Receptor: Demonstration in the Central Nervous System," *Science*, 198 (1977):849–851.

127. MOSS, R. A., and PRUE, D. M. "Research on Nicotine Regulation," *Behavior Therapy*, 13 (1982): 31–46.

128. MULE, S. J. "The Pharmacodynamics of Cocaine Abuse," *Psychiatric Annals*, 14 (1984):724–728.

129. NAHAS, G. G. *Marijuana, Deceptive Weed*. New York: Raven Press, 1973.

130. National Clearing House for Drug Abuse Information. *DOM (STP)*. Series 17, No. 1, May 1973.

131. National Institute on Drug Abuse Report. *Technical Review on Cigarette Smoking as an Addiction*. September 1979.

132. NEIL, J. F., et al. "Caffeinism Complicating Hypersomnic Depressive Episodes," *Comprehensive Psychiatry*, 19 (1978):377–385.

133. NEMETH-COSLETT, R., et al. "Effects of Mecamylamine on Cigarette Smoking and Subjective Response," Paper presented at the 92nd annual meeting of the American Psychological Association, Toronto, August 24–28, 1984.

134. PATRICK, R. L. "Amphetamine and Cocaine: Biological Mechanisms," in J. D. Barchas, et al., eds., *Psychopharmacology: From Theory to Practice*. New York: Oxford University Press, 1977, pp. 331–340.

135. PERT, C. B., and SNYDER, S. H. "Opiate Receptor: Demonstration in Nervous Tissue," *Science* 179 (1973):1011–1014.

136. PETERSEN, R. C., and STILLMAN, R. C., eds., *Cocaine: 1977*. Washington, D.C.: U.S. Government Printing Office, NIDA Research Monograph No. 13, DHEW, May 1977.

137. ———. *Phencyclidine (PCP) Abuse: An Appraisal*. Washington, D.C.: U.S. Government Printing Office, NIDA Research Monograph 21, DHEW, August 1978.

138. PITTEL, S. M., and OPPEDAHL, M. C. "The Enigma of PCP," in R. I. Dupont, A. Goldstein, and J. O'Donnell, eds., *Handbook on Drug Abuse*. Washington, D.C.: U.S. Government Printing Office, National Institute on Drug Abuse, DHEW, 1979, pp. 249–254.

139. PITTS, F. ed., "A New Approach to the Management of Opioid Dependence: Naltrexone, An Oral Antagonist," *Journal of Clinical Psychiatry*, 45 (1984): 1–57.

140. POLLIN, W. "The Danger of Cocaine," *Journal of the American Medical Association*, 254 (1985):98.

141. RAESE, J. "Sedative Hypnotics: Biological Mechanisms," in J. D. Barchas, et al., eds., *Psychopharmacology: From Theory to Practice*. New York: Oxford University Press, 1978, pp. 308–317.

142. RAYMER, S. "The Poppy," *National Geographic*, 167 (1985):143–188.

143. REDMOND, D. E., JR., GOLD, M. S., and HWANG, Y. H. "Enkephalin Acts to Inhibit Locus Coeruleus Mediated Behaviors," *Neuroscience Abstracts*, 4 (1978): 413.

144. REDMOND, D. E., JR., HWANG, Y. H., and GOLD, M. S. "Anxiety: The Locus Coeruleus Connection. *Neuroscience Abstracts*, 3 (1977):258.

145. RELMAN, A. S., ed. *Marijuana and Health Report of A Study of the Institute of Medicine*. Washington, D.C.: National Academy Press, 1982.

146. RESNICK, R. B., SCHUYTON-RESNICK, E. S., and WASHTON, A. M. "Treatment of Opioid Dependence with Narcotic Antagonists: A Review and Commentary," in: R. I. Dupont, A. Goldstein, and J. O'Donnell, eds., *Handbook on Drug Abuse*. Washington, D.C.: U.S. Government Printing Office, National Institute on Drug Abuse, DHEW, 1979, pp. 97–104.

147. RICAURTE, G. A., SCHUSTER, C. R., and SEIDEN, L. S. "Long-term Effects of Repeated Methylamphetamine Administration on Dopamine and Serotonin Neurons in the Rat Brain: A Regional Study," *Brain Research*, 193 (1980):153–163.

148. RICAURTE, G. A., et al. "Hallucinogenic Amphetamine Selectively Destroys Brain Serotonin Nerve Terminals," *Science* 229 (1985):986–988.

149. ROSENKRANTZ, H. "Physiologic and Morphologic Changes and Incidence of Neoplasms in Mice and Rats Fed Naltrexone HCl for 24 Months," *Journal of Clinical Psychiatry*, 45 (1984): 11–14.

150. RUSSELL, M.A.H. *Smoking Problems: An Overview*. Washington, D.C.: U.S. Government Printing Office, NIDA Research Monograph No. 17, DHEW, December 1977.

151. RUTTENBERG, A., et al. "Heroin-related Deaths: New Epidemiologic Insights," *Science*, 226 (1984):14–20.

152. SCHECHTER, M. D., and COOK, P. G. "Nicotine-induced Weight Loss in Rats Without an Effect on Appetite," *European Journal of Pharmacology*, 38 (1976):63–69.

153. SCHWARTZ, J. L. "A Critical Review and Evaluation of Smoking Control Methods," *Public Health Report*, 84 (1969): 483–506.

154. SELLERS, E. M., et al. "Simplifying Treatment of Alcohol Withdrawal: Diazepam Loading," *Clinical Pharmacology and Therapeutics*, 1 (1982):262–263.

155. SELLS, S. B. "Treatment Effectiveness," in R. I. Dupont, A. Goldstein, and J. O'Donnell, eds., *Handbook on Drug Abuse*. Washington, D.C.: U.S. Government Printing Office, National Institute on Drug Abuse, DHEW, 1979, pp. 105–118.

156. SENAY, E. C. "Clinical Experience with T's and B's," *Drug and Alcohol Dependence*, 14 (1985):305–311.

157. SHADER, R. I., CAINE, E. D., and MEYER, R. E. "Treatment of Dependence on Barbiturates and Sedative Hypnotics," in R. I. Shader, ed., *Manual of Psychiatric Therapeutics: Practical Psychopharmacology and Psychiatry*. Boston: Little, Brown and Company, 1975, pp. 195–202.

158. SHAMOAIN, C., and SHAPIRO, A. "Abuse of an Euphoretic Combination," *Journal of the American Medical Association*, 207 (1969): 1919.

159. SHARP, C. W., and BREHM, M. L., eds. *Review of Inhalants: Euphoria to Dysfunction*. Washington, D.C.: U.S. Government Printing Office, NIDA Research Monograph 15, DHEW, October 1977.

160. SHULTES, R. E., and HOFFMANN, A. *Plants of the Gods, Origins of Hallucinogenic Use*. Maidenhead, U.K.: McGraw-Hill, 1979.

161. SIEGEL, R. K. "Cocaine Smoking Disorders: Diagnosis and Treatment," *Psychiatric Annals*, 14 (1984):728–732.

162. SIGELL, L. T., et al. "Popping and Snorting Volatile Nitrites: A Current Fad for Getting High," *American Journal of Psychiatry*, 135 (1978):1216–1218.

163. SIMON, E. J. "Opiate Receptor Update: Recent Studies on Opiate Receptors: What We Know and What We Know We Don't Know," *Roche Receptor* 1 (1984):1–6.

164. SIMON, E. J., HILLER, J. M., and EDELMAN, I. "Stereospecific Binding of the Potent Narcotic Analgesic [³H] Etorphine to Rat-brain Homogenate," *Proceedings of the National Academy of Science* (USA), 70 (1973):1947–1949.

165. SKOLNICK, P., and PAUL, S. M. "New Concepts in the Neurobiology of Anxiety," *Journal of Clinical Psychiatry*, 44 (1983):12–19.

166. SMITH, D. E., and WESSON, D. R. "Phenobarbital Technique for Treatment of Barbiturate Dependence," *Archives of General Psychiatry*, 24 (1971):56–60.

167. SNYDER, S. H. "Catecholamines in the Brain as Mediators of Amphetamine Psychosis," *Archives of General Psychiatry*, 27 (1972):169–179.

168. ——. *Biological Aspects of Mental Disorder*. New York: Oxford University Press, 1980.

169. SOUEIF, M. I. "Long-term Effects of Cannabis," *Bulletin of Narcotics*, 23 (1971): 17–28.

170. SQUIRES, R. F., and BRAESTRUP, C. "Benzodiazepine Receptors in Rat Brain," *Nature*, 266 (1977): 732–734.

171. SRAMEK, J. J., and KHAJAWALL, A. "Loads," *New England Journal of Medicine*, 305 (1981):231.

172. STEADMAN, C., et al. "Abuse of a Fire-extinguishing Agent and Sudden Death in Adolescents," *Medical Journal of Australia*, 141 (1984):115–117.

173. STEFANIS, C., BOULOUGOUIS, J., and

LIAKOS, A. "Clinical and Psychophysiological Effects of Cannabis in Long-term Users," in M. C. Braude and S. Szara, eds., *The Pharmacology of Marijuana*. New York: Raven Press, 1976, pp. 659–665.

174. STILLNER, V., POPKIN, M. K., and PIERCE, C. "Caffeine-induced Delirium During Prolonged Competitive Stress," *American Journal of Psychiatry*, 135 (1978): 855–856.

175. STOLERMAN, I. P., et al. "Influencing Cigarette Smoking with Nicotine Antagonists," *Psychopharmacologia*, 28 (1973): 247–259.

176. "Surprising Clue to Parkinson's." *Time*, 8 April 1985, p. 61.

177. TENNANT, F. S., TARVER, A. L., and RAWSON, R. A. "Clinical Evaluation of Mecamylamine for Withdrawal from Nicotine Dependence," in L. S. Harris, ed., *Problems of Drug Dependence*. Washington, D.C.; U.S. Government Printing Office, NIDA Research Monograph Series No. 49, 1984.

178. TERENIUS, L. "Characteristics of the 'Receptor' for Narcotic Analgesics in Synaptic Plasma Membrane Fraction from Rat Brain," *Acta Pharmacologica et Toxicologica* 33 (1973):377–384.

179. THOMPSON, P. J., DHILLON, P., and COLE, P. "Addiction to Aerosol Treatment: The Asthmatic Alternative to Glue Sniffing," *British Medical Journal*, 287 (1983):1515–1516.

180. TINKLENBERG, J. R., and BERGER, P. A. "Treatment of Abusers of Non-addictive Drugs," in J. D. Barchas, et al., eds., *Psychopharmacology: From Theory to Practice*. New York: Oxford University Press, 1977, pp. 387–403.

181. TRAUB, S. L. "Clonidine for Opiate Withdrawal," *Hospital Formulary*, 21 (1985): 77–80.

182. TRUITT, E. B., and ANDERSON, S. M. "Biogenic Amine Alterations Produced in the Brain by Tetrahydrocannabinols and Their Metabolites," *Annals of the New York Academy of Science*, 191 (1971):68–72.

183. U.S. DEPARTMENT OF HEALTH AND HUMAN SERVICES. *Smoking, Tobacco and Health (A Fact Book)*. Washington, D.C.: U.S. Government Printing Office, 1980.

184. U.S. Department of Health and Human Services. *Why People Smoke Cigarettes*. USPHS Publication PHS-83-50195. Washington, D.C.: U.S. Government Printing Office, 1983.

185. VINCENT, J. P., et al. "Receptor Sites for Phencyclidine in Mammalian Brain and Peripheral Organs," in E. F. Domino, ed., *PCP (Phencyclidine): Historical and Current Perspectives*. Ann Arbor, Mich.: NPP Books, 1981, pp. 83–104.

186. VOIGTS, A., and KAUFMAN, C. E., Jr., "Acidosis and Other Metabolic Abnormalities Associated with Paint Sniffing," *Southern Medical Journal*, 76 (1983): 443–452.

187. WASHTON, A. M., RESNICK, R. B., and RAWSON, R. A. "Clonidine for Opiate Outpatient Detoxification," *Lancet*, 1 (1980):1078–1079.

188. ———. "Clonidine Hydrochloride: A Nonopiate Treatment for Opiate Withdrawal," *Psychopharmacology Bulletin*, 16 (1980):50–52.

189. WASHTON, A. M., et al. "Lofexidine, a Clonidine Analogue Effective in Opiate Withdrawal," *Lancet*, 1 (1981):991–992.

190. WATSON, S. J. "Hallucinogens and Other Psychotomimetics: Biological Mechanisms," in J. D. Barchas, et al., eds., *Psychopharmacology: From Theory to Practice*. New York: Oxford University Press, 1977, pp. 341–354.

191. WEIL, A. *The Natural Mind*. Boston: Houghton Mifflin, 1972.

192. WEINBERG, D., et al. "Intoxication from Accidental Marijuana Ingestion," *Pediatrics*, 71 (1983):848–849.

193. WESNES, K., and WARBURTON, D. M. "Smoking, Nicotine and Human Performance," *Pharmacology and Therapeutics*, 21 (1983):189–208.

194. WIKLER, A. "Conditioning Factors in Opiate Addiction and Relapse," in D. M. Wilner and G. G. Kassebaum, eds., *Narcotics*. New York: McGraw-Hill, 1965, pp. 85–100.

195. ———. "Diagnosis and Treatment of Drug Dependence of the Barbiturate Type," *American Journal of Psychiatry*, 125 (1968):758–765.

196.   WINSTEAD, D. K. "Coffee Consumption Among Psychiatric Inpatients," *American Journal of Psychiatry,* 133 (1976): 1447–1450.

197.   ZUKIN, S. R., and ZUKIN, R. S. "Identification and Characterization of [^{3}H] Phencyclidine Binding to Specific Brain Receptor Sites," in E. F. Domino, ed., *PCP (Phencyclidine): Historical and Current Perspectives.* Ann Arbor, Mich.: NPP Books, 1981, pp. 105–130.

CHAPTER 30

THE BIOLOGY AND TREATMENT OF ALCOHOLISM

Marc A. Schuckit

¶ **Introduction**

This chapter presents a clinically oriented discussion of the diagnosis and treatment of patients with severe and persistent alcohol-related life problems. Because no single chapter can cover all relevant material, current references to further readings in specific areas of importance are offered as a source of additional information.

It is best to begin a consideration of alcoholism by giving up several myths.[25] The first myth is that most alcoholic persons live on "skid row." Only 5 percent to 10 percent do so; the average alcoholic individual is likely to appear in clinical settings in a sober state, looking well groomed, having no smell of alcohol about him or her, and lacking many of the other traits we may associate with the stereotype of the alcoholic. He or she will complain of a variety of medical and emotional problems, which must be properly diagnosed if the clinician hopes to avoid unexpected calls in the middle of the night

and ill-advised treatments that should never have been given to alcoholic patients in the first place (e.g., sleeping pills). The typical alcoholic patient has a job and financial resources, close friends and relatives (a network of "significant others"), a history of alternation between periods of heavy problematic drinking and abstinence, and limited times when drinking is carried out in moderation.

A second important myth is that alcoholic individuals are not likely to respond to treatment. This idea comes from observations of the skid-row alcoholic who presents with severe intoxication or withdrawal and end-stage organ damage (e.g., advanced cirrhosis). Many physicians, who encounter this obvious alcoholic while working in central city hospitals, have concluded that the extremely bleak prognosis for these patients applies to alcoholic patients in general. However, the average alcoholic individual (with his or her job and extended family group) has perhaps a 60 percent to 70 percent chance of achieving and maintaining abstinence after treatment.[44]

Alcoholism is of great importance to psychiatrists because, as is described in detail later, alcohol-related problems can mimic almost any major psychiatric disorder, and alcohol is likely to intensify preexisting psychopathology.[64] The high prevalence of alcoholism in our society, coupled with the fact that alcoholism is frequently associated with psychopathology, means that it is often the psychiatrist who is the gatekeeper to treatment for this group. Patients presenting with alcohol-related insomnia, depression, psychotic symptoms, or anxiety must be properly diagnosed and treated. The incorrect diagnosis of primary affective disorder or primary schizophrenia can lead to improper care and problems for both patient and physician. The first section of this chapter presents background information on the diagnosis and nature of alcoholism, its prevalence, and its natural history. The second section of this chapter describes the treatment of alcoholism.

¶ The Nature of Alcoholism

The Pharmacology of Alcohol

Understanding the structure and metabolism of ethanol (beverage alcohol) is not essential for identifying and treating alcohol-related life problems. Therefore, this section will be brief; readers wishing a more detailed discussion of this topic are referred to an excellent text by Lieber.[38]

Ethanol has a simple chemical structure. The predominant mode of ethanol metabolism occurs through the enzyme alcohol dehydrogenase, which is found in many places in the body and especially in the liver. The first breakdown product of ethanol, acetaldehyde, is highly toxic (it is a relative of formaldehyde) and capable of causing intoxication by itself, even at very low concentrations.[74] While alcohol dehydrogenase is producing acetaldehyde from alcohol at a fairly slow rate, the enzyme that breaks down acetalde-

hyde, aldehyde dehydrogenase, acts swiftly to convert this substance to acetylcoenzyme A, which then enters the citric acid cycle yielding carbon dioxide and water.

Alcohol is readily absorbed from the lining of the digestive tract, especially in the stomach and the proximal portion of the small intestine. Only 5 to 15 percent is excreted directly through the lungs, sweat, and urine, with the remainder being metabolized in the liver at the rate of about 7 g of ethanol per hour, with 1 g equaling 1 ml of 100 percent ethanol (approximately one drink per hour).

From the clinical standpoint, it is important to recognize that ethanol is one of a group of drugs that, at the usual doses taken, decreases nervous tissue activity.[66] These related substances are called central nervous system (CNS) depressants and include (in addition to alcohol) all prescription sleeping pills and all prescription antianxiety drugs or minor tranquilizers (e.g., the benzodiazepines).[66] All these substances are capable of producing an ethanollike intoxication; are physically addicting; demonstrate various levels of cross-tolerance; and are capable of inducing symptoms of depression, hallucinations and/or paranoia, anxiety, and insomnia. A more detailed discussion of the CNS depressants and associated medical and psychiatric problems can be found in the monograph by this author[66] and in chapter 29 of this volume.

The intoxication achieved with these drugs depends on the unique attributes of the individual, is most intense while blood alcohol concentrations (BACs) are rising and less intense when they are falling back toward zero, and is most pronounced when high levels in the blood are reached relatively quickly. Despite these contingencies, it is possible to see a general correlation between levels of impairment and BACs, as given in table 30–1.

Individuals who are otherwise physically healthy (e.g., have no evidence of brain or liver damage) and have been increasing their level of alcohol intake will demonstrate three kinds of tolerance. These include *metabolic tolerance* (i.e., they will have induced liver

TABLE 30-1

The Usual Expected Effects of Ethanol by Blood Alcohol Concentration for the Average Person Without Alcohol Tolerance

Rising Blood Alcohol Level in mg/100 ml Blood (mg/dl)	Usual Expected Effect
20–99	Impaired coordination, euphoric
100–199	Ataxia, decreased mentation, poor judgment, labile mood
200–299	Marked ataxia and slurred speech, poor judgment, labile mood, nausea and vomiting
300–399	Stage I anesthesia, memory lapse, labile mood
400 and above	Respiratory failure, coma, death

NOTE: Reprinted, by permission of the publisher, from M. A. Schuckit, *Drug and Alcohol Abuse: A Clinical Guide to Diagnosis and Treatment* (New York: Plenum Press, 1984), p. 51.

enzymes that will more rapidly metabolize the ethanol), *behavioral tolerance* (i.e., they will have learned how to function better and appear less intoxicated at a given BAC), and *cellular tolerance* (i.e., brain cells will have changed so that they are less sensitive to the effects of ethanol). Each of these will shift the balance shown in table 30-1 upward so that, for instance, ataxia might not be noticed until 200 mg of ethanol per 100 ml of blood (mg per deciliter [mg per dl]) has been reached, and some patients might even be able to walk and talk at 400 mg per dl.[28]

Finally, a clinical consideration of the pharmacology of alcohol must recognize that there is no clear antidote for the effects of this drug. General stimulants including caffeine can increase overall levels of alertness but do not effectively reverse the direct actions of ethanol on the CNS. Infusions of fructose can increase the rate of metabolism of ethanol by as much as 25 percent but may create a dangerous acid-base imbalance. Therefore, treatment of severe intoxication follows the conservative guidelines of giving life supports and allowing the body to metabolize the ethanol.[59] The next section introduces the concept of severe persistent life problems related to alcohol, the disorder we call *alcoholism.*

The Diagnosis of Alcoholism

Alcoholism is a disorder for which there is a known prognosis and important informa-

tion regarding treatment.[21,66,82] This label is important to the health care deliverer because it outlines a clinically useful entity that must be considered as part of the differential diagnosis of psychiatric (as well as medical) disorders, a syndrome worthy of diagnosis because the label imparts information about the probable course and available options for treatment. Whether labeled a syndrome, a disorder, or a disease, alcoholism is a useful and important diagnosis.

It would be easier to place alcoholism into a semantic niche if the cause of this disorder were known. As is true with most syndromes in psychiatry (e.g., major affective disorder and schizophrenia), it is unlikely that there is one single necessary and sufficient cause. Rather, the clinical picture appears to be the result of the interaction of multiple biological and environmental factors.[67,69]

For example, there is much data supporting the importance of genetic factors in the genesis of alcoholism. These include *family* studies (alcoholism runs strongly in families), *animal* investigations (showing that genetic factors influence whether an organism chooses to continue to drink after the first taste), and *twin* studies (demonstrating a significantly higher risk for alcoholism in the identical twin of an alcoholic than in a fraternal twin).[59] The strongest support for a genetic influence in alcoholism lies with the demonstration that sons and daughters of alcoholic persons adopted at birth and raised without knowledge of their biological parents' problem have a four times higher risk for alcoholism than children of nonalcoholic individuals adopted and raised by nonbiological parents. [11,22,59,76] Being reared by an alcoholic parent or experiencing a broken home prior to the age of sixteen appears to add nothing to this risk. Finally, a series of investigations has begun to identify unique attributes of sons of alcoholic persons who are drinking but have not yet had major life problems from alcohol. These higher-risk young men appear to develop higher levels of acetaldehyde after drinking, [74] may evidence lower amplitude of a brain wave that is generated in response to an expected but random stimulus—the P300, [7] and may demonstrate less intoxication at a given BAC. [68]

Diagnostic Criteria for Alcoholism

There are many diagnostic criteria for alcoholism. Different schemes outline slightly different but overlapping populations. [12,66] Each approach has inherent assets and liabilities, and the final choice depends on the goals and biases of the clinician.

One approach is to diagnose alcoholism by observing how much someone drinks; however, it may be difficult to accurately establish drinking practices, especially for the heaviest drinkers, who may be experiencing memory impairment at their highest BACs. [15] A second possible diagnostic technique assesses psychological dependence by observing a life-style centered around alcohol (i.e., drinking at work or in the morning, taking drinks before going to a party, hiding alcohol, etc.), but this approach is too subjective and thus of limited use. [25] A diagnosis based on evidence of physical addiction (i.e., the occurrence of an abstinence syndrome when alcohol is decreased [78,79] is too restrictive, as only 5 to 15 percent of alcoholic individuals actually go through clinically obvious withdrawal. [66,85]

The technique of greatest use to the clinician evaluates the occurrence of significant alcohol-related life problems, gathered as part of the usual social history. Once a pattern of problems has been established,

the next step is to determine whether alcohol has contributed significantly to these difficulties. Thus alcoholism is diagnosed with a history of any of the following: a marital separation or divorce related to alcohol; multiple arrests related to drinking; physical evidence that alcohol has harmed health; or a job loss or layoff related to drinking. [66] This shorthand version of diagnosis, seen in figure 30–1, has been shown to accurately predict individuals who are likely to continue to have persistent and pervasive alcohol-related problems.

Table 30–2 outlines a more formal way of approaching this diagnosis, as given in the American Psychiatric Association's *Diagnostic and Statistical Manual of Mental Disorders,* 3rd edition (DSM-III). [2] Here the syndrome is subdivided into *alcohol abuse* (305.0X) and *alcohol dependence* (303.9X). The former is based on a pattern of alcohol use approaching what might be called psychological dependence (e.g., need for daily alcohol for adequate functioning, efforts to control or reduce excess drinking), occasional heavy consumption (e.g., a fifth of spirits or its equivalent in wine or beer), alcoholic blackouts, and/or a continuation of drinking despite serious problems and impairment in social or occupational functioning due to alcohol. Alcohol dependence, on the other hand, results in similar impairment, along with evidence of increased tolerance or signs of physical withdrawal from alcohol. The shorthand definition given in figure 30–1 incorporates much of the DSM-III criteria. In addition, the DSM-III labels are more cumbersome and, as yet, there is little data available on the prognostic meaning of alcohol abuse versus alcohol dependence.

One difficulty with these approaches to the diagnosis of alcoholism is that they fail to identify individuals before alcohol has caused serious problems. Unfortunately, a diagnosis of alcoholism relying upon a single drunk-driving arrest, arguments with friends, or alcoholic blackouts is likely to identify up to 40 or 50 percent of men in our society, most of whom will learn from their alcohol-related problems and spontaneously

THE DIAGNOSIS OF ALCOHOLISM

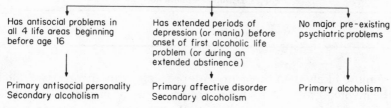

Figure 30–1.   The diagnosis of primary and secondary alcoholism.

NOTE: Reprinted, by permission of the publisher, from M. A. Schuckit, *Drug and Alcohol Abuse: A Clinical Guide to Diagnosis and Treatment* (New York: Plenum Press, 1984), p. 47.

and permanently decrease intake and associated difficulties.[15,82,83] Thus, while it is clinically useful to relate less severe life problems to alcohol, a diagnosis using only these problems is not specific enough to be of clinical use.

Primary Versus Secondary Alcoholism

No matter what definition of alcoholism is used, if the purpose of diagnosis is to predict a future course and select treatment, it makes sense to distinguish between a primary and secondary disorder.[65,66] Therefore, as outlined in figure 30–1, *primary* (or uncomplicated) alcoholism indicates serious alcohol problems occurring in an individual with no preexisting major psychiatric disorder. *Secondary* (or complicated) alcoholism is an alcoholic syndrome beginning after another major psychiatric disorder has developed.[55,56] A series of investigations has shown that between 60 and 70 percent of alcoholic inpatients meet rigorous criteria for primary alcoholism.[56,77] Of those who demonstrate preexisting psychiatric disorders (i.e., have secondary alcoholism), the

most common diagnoses are antisocial personality and primary affective disorder.

As used here, the *antisocial personality* (301.70) is defined as having serious antisocial problems in all major life areas (family, peers, police, and school) beginning prior to the age of fifteen and before the first major life problem stemming from alcohol or drugs.[50,55] The DSM-III divides life problems into those with onset prior to the age of fifteen (e.g., problems with school, police, home, and peers), as well as problems since age eighteen (e.g., difficulties with work, inability to function as a responsible parent, repeated legal difficulties, evidence of aggressiveness, recklessness, etc.).[2] Thus all alcoholics should be asked about their pattern of problems with school, peers, family, and police *antedating* their first major life problem from alcohol.

This syndrome is seen in at least 20 percent of groups of male alcoholic patients entering either a private or a public alcoholic treatment facility and in at least 5 percent of such female alcoholic patients.[66] Secondary alcoholics with primary antisocial personalities carry a bleak prognosis for alcohol-related

TABLE 30–2

Schematic Representation of DSM-III "Alcoholism" Definitions

305.OX Alcohol Abuse

A.	Pattern of Pathological Alcohol Use, e.g. Daily use; Efforts to control; Binges; Blackouts; Occasional very heavy consumption
B.	Impaired Social/Occupational Functioning, e.g. Violence; Job loss; Arrests; Arguments
C.	Duration One Month

303.9 Alcohol Dependence

A + B	above *plus*
C.	Tolerance or Withdrawal

life problems, are more likely than the average alcoholic to be involved with drugs, have a greater likelihood of serious police problems after treatment, and are more difficult to manage in a therapeutic situation.[75]

Major affective disorders antedate the first major life problems from alcohol in perhaps 15 percent of female alcoholic and 5 percent of male alcoholic individuals. These people should be given the diagnosis of primary affective disorder with secondary alcoholism.[46,56] For example, a third of patients with no preexisting major life problems from alcohol who undergo a severe depression (primary affective disorder) increase their drinking during the affective episode. The same increase in alcohol intake is seen in up to half of manic patients. Patients with either affective disorder might be mislabeled as primary alcoholics. Many of these primary affective disorder patients with secondary alcohol abuse will require treatment with antidepressants or lithium carbonate, as described in chapter 13 of this volume.

To make the proper primary versus secondary diagnosis, a history of the age of onset of major life problems related to alcohol and a careful history of the time course of major affective episodes must be gathered from both the patient and a reliable resource person.[64] A corroborative history is needed, because in the midst of heavy drinking, 60 percent or more of primary alcoholics will report serious sadness, insomnia, and feelings of guilt. As alcohol-induced secondary

depressions can incorporate all the symptoms seen in primary affective disorders, these primary alcoholics are sometimes mislabeled as having primary depressive disease. This is unfortunate, because alcohol-induced secondary depressions almost always clear within two days to two weeks *without* antidepressant medications. Even these patients with primary alcoholism and a temporary secondary affective disorder must be carefully evaluated for suicidal ideation and may need to be hospitalized for their depression for several days to several weeks, until the clinical syndrome improves.[56]

Other major psychiatric disorders are rarely seen as primary disturbances in cases of secondary alcoholism. While hallucinations and/or delusions can be seen in the midst of primary alcoholism (but clear spontaneously within several days to several weeks of abstinence), psychotic thought disorders beginning before the onset of alcoholism are found in less than 5 percent of alcoholic patients coming to alcohol treatment programs.[64,66] Also, symptoms of anxiety are common during alcoholic withdrawal, but the primary anxiety syndromes of panic disorder (300.02) account for less than 5 percent of alcoholic individuals.[60,66]

The Prevalence of Alcoholism

Alcoholism and alcohol-related problems are common in our society. Between 5 and 10 percent of the adult male population and between 2 and 5 percent of adult women will meet the criteria for alcoholism at some time in their lives.[25] An additional 40 percent or more of young men will also demonstrate isolated alcohol-related life problems of limited severity that, while not indicative of alcoholism, can have negative consequences for society and the individual.[15,25] Thus clinicians in industrial counseling or police work, as well as those in private practices, must recognize alcohol-related problems as an important factor in their patients' lives.

Because alcohol so adversely affects most body systems, the rate of alcoholism is even higher in medical and psychiatric patients than in the general population. Between 15 and 30 percent of such patients meet the criteria for alcoholism.[6,43,65] Thus one out of every five men and women walking into any mental health treatment setting is experiencing serious enough alcohol-related pathology to be labeled as alcoholism, and a significant additional percentage demonstrate temporary alcohol-related life problems of a less severe nature.

These patients are likely to resemble the average patient seen in any setting, as alcoholism can exist in patients of either sex, any socioeconomic stratum, and any age. Identification can be helped by looking for the pattern of emotional problems most likely to be associated with alcoholism (e.g., insomnia, anxiety, and depression) and by observing the pattern of physical signs and symptoms more likely to be seen in alcoholic patients than in the general population. These latter include mild elevations in blood pressure, evidence of repeated bruising, or recurrent and otherwise unexplained infections (e.g., pneumonias). Also, in the presence of heavy drinking, blood tests are likely to show a mildly elevated mean corpustular volume (e.g., greater than 100), a gamma glutamyl transferase higher than 40 units, a mildly elevated uric acid, or an elevation in any of the more usually observed liver function tests.[51,71,89]

In summary, clinicians must be alert to the high prevalence of temporary alcohol-related problems that can negatively influence mental health and be aware of the high prevalence of alcoholism itself. Accurate diagnosis depends on suspecting that any patient is a candidate for either primary or secondary alcoholism; gathering a thorough history of life problems and the possible role of alcohol in precipitating or exacerbating these problems; and observing physical findings and laboratory tests, which are likely to be abnormal in the alcoholic patient.

The Natural History of Alcoholism

The most probable course of primary alcoholism is as predictable as the usual course of adult-onset diabetes or atherosclerotic heart disease. One cannot be certain of the exact incidence and time course of problems, but it is possible to make some educated estimates. Of course, cases of alcoholism occurring secondary to another major preexisting psychiatric disorder (such as the major affective disorders or the antisocial personality disorder) are likely to run a complex course that is heavily influenced by the primary diagnosis.

If the definition of primary alcoholism based on major life problems related to alcoholism is used, there are a number of predictable milestones as outlined in table 30–3.[66,82] Average alcoholic persons demonstrate their first drink and first intoxication, as well as the first relatively minor life problem related to alcohol, at the same age as the general population. The first major life problem related to alcohol is likely to occur in the late twenties to mid-thirties, with treatment often beginning in the forties (although only 10 percent or so of alcoholic individuals actually enter care and receive a diagnosis). The life span is shortened by about fifteen years, even when one controls for socioeconomic stratum.[52,54] The leading causes of death, in approximate decreasing order, are heart disease, cancer, accidents, and suicide, with the latter related to the temporary but severe alcohol-induced depressions that have already been discussed.[66]

One important aspect of the course of alcoholism is its fluctuating nature. In any given

TABLE 30-3
The Natural History of Primary Alcoholism

1.	Age of first drink[a]	12–14
2.	Age first intoxicated[a]	14–18
3.	Age first minor alcohol problem[a]	18–25
4.	Usual age of onset First major problem	23–33
5.	Usual age entering treatment	40
6.	Usual age of death Leading causes: heart disease cancer accidents suicide	55–60
7.	In any year, abstinence alternates with active drinking. "Spontaneous remission" rate or response to nonspecific intervention	25–33%

NOTE: Reprinted, by permission of the publisher, from M. A. Schuckit, *Drugs and Alcohol Abuse: A Clinical Guide to Diagnosis and Treatment* (New York: Plenum Press, 1984), p. 59.
[a]These ages are about the same in the general population.

month after treatment, approximately one-half of alcoholic patients report abstinence, with a mean of four months of being "dry" in the one and one-half years following release from therapy.[4] Thus usual alcoholic patients do not begin drinking in their late teens and continue to imbibe until they die, but rather demonstrate periods of abstinence and marked decreases in drinking that can be expected to alternate with periods of heavier drinking.[82,83]

Finally, 10 to 30 percent of primary alcoholic individuals learn to abstain or seriously limit their alcohol intake without treatment.[31,36,83] This phenomenon has been documented through follow-ups of individuals in treatment who did not initially seem to respond, comparisons of those who entered to those who were denied care, and information on alcoholic persons and the general population who never received therapy.

Most readers are already conversant with some of the major medical problems that can be expected in the course of alcoholism and that account for the inordinately high level of medical expenditures and missed work time seen for the average alcoholic per-

son.[4,66] In short, digestive system problems include cirrhosis (seen in only about 15 percent of identified alcoholics), pancreatitis (seen in 10 percent or less), high rates of cancers of all areas of the digestive tract—especially the esophagus and stomach,[26] high rates of ulcer disease,[29] and elevated risk for gastritis.[37] Cardiovascular problems include elevations in blood pressure[33] and blood lipids,[16] as well as direct destruction of heart muscle[95] at high doses of alcohol (even though one or two drinks per day in healthy nonalcoholic individuals may help prevent atherosclerotic heart disease).[18] The elevated risk for cancers of the digestive tract extends to malignant neoplasms of the head and neck; in one series, over 50 percent of individuals presenting with such cancers above the epiglottis met criteria for alcoholism.[40] There is also a general vulnerability of striated muscles to heavy doses of alcohol in some alcoholic persons, with a resulting skeletal muscle deterioration labeled alcoholic myopathy.[27,34]

These brief comments would not be complete without mention of the neurological system. Perhaps the most common alcohol-related disorder is peripheral neuropathy of the skin and muscles in the hands and feet, which is noted in 10 percent of alcoholic patients.[8] Rapidly developing confusion can be caused by simple intoxication, especially in elderly individuals or those with brain damage from trauma.[54,58,64,97] An important, but uncommon, confused state associated with a thiamine deficiency is Wernicke-Korsakoff's syndrome, which, while likely to improve with adequate vitamin supplementation, may become permanent.[39,87] In addition, the majority of alcoholic patients presenting for detoxification show some signs of intellectual impairment and 40 to 70 percent show an increased brain ventricular size.[39,90] Not all investigators agree that there is a correlation between this ventricular enlargement and the level of neuropsychological impairment, and it is probable that most alcoholic individuals will recover in both parameters after several months of abstinence.[90]

¶ The Treatment of Alcoholism

This section discusses the treatment of alcoholism, including confrontation of the identified alcoholic, detoxification, general treatment philosophy, and rehabilitation. Until evidence to the contrary develops, alcohol problems that do not meet diagnostic criteria for alcoholism are probably best approached with education and general counseling. Alcohol intake complicating primary psychiatric disorders is best addressed through education and counseling in conjunction with treatment of the primary disease. The focus of this section is on the treatment of primary alcoholic individuals.

Confrontation of Alcoholic Patients

The process of helping individuals recognize their problems and the need for care can be termed confrontation. In a disorder like alcoholism, where patients have been unable or unwilling to consciously admit the role that alcohol might have in their life problems, this first step can be difficult.

There is no single best way to confront alcoholic individuals. One approach is to use patients' presenting complaints as the entree to the subject of alcohol, sharing concerns and educating them about the problems that can be expected unless drinking ceases. Patients might be told that it appears as if they have reached a point in life where alcohol is causing significant problems (note: the term alcoholism might not have to be used at this stage). For instance, individuals coming in for insomnia or anxiety might be told that these are important symptoms, the laboratory tests and physical findings could be shared, and they might be told that alcohol appears to have contributed to their complaint and is making them a high risk for further medical and psychological problems. The physician might then share information about the course of alcoholism and explore possible avenues of attacking the problem.

The process of confrontation is rarely accomplished in one session. It is helpful to let patients know that they alone are responsible for their actions and that the decision to quit drinking rests entirely with them. For patients who refuse to recognize the problem and stop drinking at the first confrontation, a logical goal is to "keep the door open" by encouraging them and their families to maintain contact, while being careful to keep the responsibility for cessation of drinking in the patients' hands.

At the same time, the families may benefit from some counseling or referral to a self-help group, such as Alanon (the Alcohol Anonymous–related group for family members) and Alateen (the group for teenage children). When patients refuse to stop drinking at the first confrontation, it is wise to establish future meetings, so that while they are learning to cope with the life problems associated with alcohol, help is available when the crises escalate. One hopes that patients will agree to stop drinking in the future.

Those patients who refuse to stop but who admit that they might "cut down" should be reminded that the average alcoholic individual successfully cuts back scores of times but eventually escalates drinking. Patients who absolutely refuse to stop might be offered guidelines telling them that they cannot drink more than two drinks (e.g., 4 oz. of wine, 12 oz. of beer, *or* 1.5 oz. of 80-proof beverage equals one drink) in any twenty-four-hour period. In order to do this adequately, it is important to work with both patients and "significant others" so that they all understand that this is not an adequate approach. This increases the likelihood that they will come back when the next crisis occurs as the drinking escalates.

The education of family and friends can be carried a step further, advising them of their option of gathering all significant others together at one time to confront the patient. In effect, each individual would say to the alcoholic person, "I love you, but I must tell you what I think alcohol is doing to you. It is very important that you stop drinking." This approach has been suggested by some clinicians, but it has inherent dangers.[81] While it might result in patients getting treatment, there is also the possibility that they will choose to ignore the help, take offense by confrontation, and become isolated from their support group. Therefore, the family should prepare for this possibility. Perhaps this more intensive intervention is best reserved for those individuals whose drinking has caused a crisis point in their lives (e.g., those whose medical problems are likely to result in high risk of death in the future and /or those who are about to lose their major support systems).

In summary, the first step in treating alcoholic patients is to help them recognize that alcohol is the major problem and that the treatment rests with abstinence. There is no single best way to confront alcoholic patients, but the clinician can be guided by the goals of: (1) keeping the door open to the patient even if the first confrontation fails and (2) emphasizing that the decision to stop drinking rests with the patient. Confrontation can be helped through outreach to the family and significant others who must learn to understand alcoholism in order to participate in the confrontation process and to make their own plans. Once the patient has agreed to stop drinking, the clinician is faced with the decision about whether active detoxification treatment is required.

Detoxification of Alcoholic Patients

Adequate detoxification of alcoholic patients must be supervised by a knowledgeable physician, be it a psychiatrist, family practitioner, or internist. Because alcoholics are at high risk for serious medical problems and because the alcohol withdrawal syndrome, as well as the withdrawal syndrome from sedative-hypnotic drugs that are crosstolerant to alcohol, is so potentially dangerous, it may be best to hospitalize patients.[66,78] Outpatient detoxification should be reserved for those individuals with no prior history of withdrawal seizures and little evidence of withdrawal signs and symptoms

despite low BACs, those in good physical condition, and those who are not abusing other drugs in addition to alcohol.[66]

The average alcoholic individual who is going through withdrawal experiences signs and symptoms that are the opposite of the acute effects of ethanol in healthy individuals. Autonomic nervous system dysfunction predominates with evidence of tremors, labile blood pressure, elevated body temperature, rapid pulse and respirations, and sweating, along with signs of anxiety, insomnia, and a strong drive to drink.[78,79] Only about 5 percent of withdrawing alcoholic patients experience withdrawal seizures. There is usually only a single seizure, often unrelated to any general seizure diathesis. Approximately 5 percent of withdrawing alcoholic patients experience hallucinations or serious confusion (as discussed later). The remaining 95 percent or more of withdrawing alcoholic patients have a less complicated withdrawal that, if uncomplicated by serious medical problems, can be treated fairly easily. However, it is essential that any associated medical disorders (e.g., pneumonias, anemias, internal bleeding, heart failure, diabetes, etc.) be recognized and treated, as the rigors of withdrawal added to preexisting major medical disorders can be a lethal combination. Therefore, the first step in adequate detoxification is to take a good medical history (including information on abuse of other drugs) and to conduct a thorough physical examination.

General supports in alcoholic withdrawal include vitamins, rest, adequate food, and oral liquids. Intravenous fluids should be avoided unless there has been bleeding or prolonged vomiting or diarrhea, as the average alcoholic patient tends to be overhydrated rather than dehydrated.[35] It is especially important to prescribe 100 mg thiamine orally for at least five days; this vitamin is not stored well in the body and alcohol may interfere with its absorption from the small intestine, causing a thiamine deficiency in many heavy drinkers, including well-nourished ones.[19,87]

These general supportive measures do not

address the physiological causes of depressant drug withdrawal. The activities just described will do little for the anxiety, convulsions, insomnia, and psychosis that can be part of the withdrawal syndrome. These symptoms occur because the brain is physiologically dependent on a CNS depressant. Drug withdrawal causes overactivity of the CNS. Therefore, the pharmacologically correct treatment is a depressant drug that is cross-tolerant to alcohol, such as prescription sedative hypnotics or antianxiety drugs. These drugs are administered in high enough doses to abolish symptoms and then decreased slowly, usually over five days. A common approach utilizes antianxiety drugs such as chlordiazepoxide (Librium) or diazepam (Valium), because these have relatively low rates of respiratory and blood pressure depression and yet long enough half-lives to allow for a gradual decrease in blood levels and subsequent mild withdrawal symptoms. Most physicians administer between 100 and 200 or more mg chlordiazepoxide on the first day, with the specific dose adjusted for the individual patient depending on degree of addiction (as can be gauged from autonomic nervous system symptoms such as pulse rate at low blood alcohol levels) and degree of alertness. Patients are not given drugs if they are already sleeping or heavily sedated.[78] After establishing the dose needed to alleviate symptoms on the first day, the dose is decreased by about 20 percent of the original dose each day and depressant medication stopped on the fourth or fifth day. This requires careful patient management, using the patient's level of alertness and autonomic nervous system functioning (e.g., pulse and blood pressure) to avoid overmedication. An alternate approach is to use a benzodiazepine with a shorter half-life, such as lorazepam (Ativan), to avoid accumulation of the drug.[24] The danger here is that the short half-life results in marked fluctuations in blood levels, with a possible increased risk for convulsions.

Two aspects of withdrawal are of special importance to the psychiatrist. The agitated confusion seen in 5 percent or so of alcoholic patients undergoing withdrawal can present a psychiatric emergency, with the patient so out of contact with reality that one-to-one observations or (rarely) physical restraints might be required. This state of agitated confusion with the possible concomitance of convulsions or hallucinations/delusions (psychosis) is often referred to as delirium tremens or DTs. Once DTs begin, there are few data on adequate treatment. The goal may be to give the patient general supports over the three to five days required for the syndrome to disappear. This can be accompanied with benzodiazepines, using high enough doses to control the symptoms described earlier. Some physicians use antipsychotic medications (e.g., thioridazine [Mellaril] or haloperidol [Haldol]); however, these medications can increase the likelihood of seizures. No matter what medication is used, it is likely that the symptom complex known as the DTs will continue for four or five days. Of course, the occurrence of seizures or significant confusion also requires a special physical evaluation to rule out physical disorders such as electrolyte abnormalities or trauma (e.g., subdural hematomas), which, if present, must be addressed immediately.

Finally, in the midst of withdrawal (and some clinicians feel even when there are no signs and symptoms of withdrawal), alcoholic patients can present with auditory hallucinations and/or paranoid delusions. When this state of paranoia and/or hallucinosis occurs in the midst of the autonomic dysfunction expected during withdrawal, it can be considered part of the abstinence syndrome and treated as just described.

However, paranoid delusions or auditory hallucinations may occur in a clear sensorium, in which case the clinical picture may appear identical to paranoid schizophrenia.[63,64,86] There is a debate in the literature as to whether alcoholic paranoia and alcoholic hallucinosis, which frequently occur together, are related to withdrawal or are separate phenomena. In any event, it is important to consider this alcohol-induced schizophreniclike syndrome, with its relatively benign prognosis (symptoms disappear within several days to several weeks of abstinence), in all patients presenting with an acute-onset psychotic disorder. The differential diagnosis of primary alcoholism with secondary hallucinosis and/or delusions versus primary schizophrenia is usually made by gathering a careful chronological history. For example, schizophrenia is diagnosed when the hallucinations and/or delusions in a clear sensorium and without insight are noted prior to the onset of major life problems related to alcohol or independent of the drinking history.

Treatment of the alcohol-related psychotic state involves giving general support, hospitalizing patients, if necessary, to avoid significant embarrassment or danger to self or others, and observing their condition over the several days or several weeks required for the syndrome to resolve. Judicious use of antipsychotic medications (e.g., thioridazine or haloperidol) may be helpful in controlling symptoms acutely but is not required for symptomatic remission, and the clinician must remember to stop the antipsychotic medication when patients recover.

Rehabilitation of Alcoholic Patients

GENERAL PHILOSOPHY

Once patients have been identified as alcoholic, the diagnosis of primary versus secondary alcoholism established, major medical problems identified and treated, and detoxification carried out if required; alcoholic rehabilitation must be initiated. There is no best way to rehabilitate alcoholic patients, and current approaches focus on general supports that meet commonsense guidelines. Treatment programs for alcoholic individuals suffer from a lack of controlled studies carefully documenting the effectiveness of therapy through: (1) random assignment of patients to maximal versus minimal care or (2) treatment versus no rehabilitation. Until these are carried out, it is possible only to outline an approach that makes sense rather

than to document one that has shown to be effective.[70]

The bias presented here is that, in light of the lack of data on efficacy, it is best to keep treatment interventions as simple, safe, and inexpensive as possible. Reviewing the literature on the treatment of alcoholism and visiting various alcohol treatment programs leaves the impression that almost all maneuvers in rehabilitation fall into two general categories. First are those efforts that attempt to help alcoholics achieve and maintain a high level of motivation toward abstinence through education about alcoholism for patients and their family, helping significant others to stop protecting alcoholics from the problems caused by alcohol, use of disulfiram (Antabuse) to help alcoholics avoid returning to drinking on the spur of the moment, and behavioral treatments (e.g., aversive conditioning) to remind alcoholics that they should be refusing a drink when it is offered. The second series of maneuvers helps patients to readjust to life without alcohol and reestablish a functional life-style through psychotherapy or counseling, vocational rehabilitation when needed, and family and sexual counseling or therapy.

A major area of concern for the psychiatrist may be whether or not to address the underlying psychopathology that might have contributed to the development of alcoholism. Because the etiology of alcoholism is unknown (except for genetic factors already described) and because there is an absence of evidence that any personality constellation is uniquely related to alcoholism,[72] most clinicians choose to deal with only the alcoholism for the first six months or so of treatment. It may take this long to establish which, if any, forms of psychopathology are secondary to the alcohol and which appear to be more stable personality attributes that may require therapeutic attention. Premature efforts to deal with more in-depth psychotherapy may also divert patients' attention from the need to stop drinking while increasing their level of anxiety to a point where they may find it impossible to abstain.

With these thoughts in mind, it is possible to give a brief overview of the usual components that must be considered in alcoholic rehabilitation. The following section deals with some basic issues of the optimal setting for rehabilitation.

THE BEST SETTING FOR REHABILITATION

There is no convincing evidence that inpatient rehabilitation is any more effective for the average primary alcoholic individual than outpatient care.[65] In an outpatient setting, patients have the opportunity to learn lessons in a real-life setting and do not face the problems of "reentry readjustment" seen after release from an inpatient facility. While the inpatient treatment offers the advantage of forced abstinence, it has disadvantages, not the least of which is the greater expense. Therefore, until better data are available, it is probably wise to attempt to use outpatient rehabilitation whenever possible.

The decision to hospitalize alcoholic persons for rehabilitation can be based on a series of patient preferences and characteristics. These include the practitioner's opinion of what is best for each patient, the preferences of the individual and his or her family, financial considerations, and prior experiences with this individual. Valid reasons for considering inpatient care include the following:

1. Serious medical problems that make functioning outside a hospital difficult for the alcoholic individual.
2. Psychiatric syndromes of severe depression, psychosis, or organicity that accompany the alcoholism.[56,64]
3. Secondary alcoholism when the primary major psychiatric disorder represents a danger (e.g., primary affective disorder with suicidal ideations).
4. Severe life crises that make outpatient treatment difficult.

If inpatient care is needed, what type of facility might be best for that specific patient? The average clinician will end up using the hospital that is most convenient and appropriate for his or her training. It is possible to carry out good inpatient alcoholic rehabilitation in a general psychiatric facility. As is true for medical facilities, this benefits the institution by boosting the census and, with adequate staff preparation, alcoholic rehabilitation can be carried out without an increase in patient problems over that expected of any psychiatric patient. The psychiatric hospital is especially appropriate if the patient is suicidal (e.g., primary alcoholism with secondary depression) or demonstrates confusion, alcoholic hallucinosis, or paranoia. One danger of such a setting is that the patient's medical needs might not be adequately met, although this problem is easily solved by medical consultation. An additional problem is the tendency to carry out more intensive psychotherapy with patients in this setting even though the cost of this added treatment may not be justified for the average alcoholic patient. Alcoholic rehabilitation can be carried out in almost any type of facility, although freestanding alcoholic programs (i.e., not part of an inpatient hospital) may be the most cost effective.

Finally, the optimal period of inpatient or outpatient rehabilitation must be determined. Alcohol problems have probably been going on for at least ten years before the patient is confronted, a fact consistent with the idea that the recovery process is likely to occur over a relatively long and difficult period.[66] The general approach to care is to establish an extended period of interaction with the patient through aftercare; inpatient treatment, if used at all, should be viewed as only the first stage in any rehabilitation process. Involvement in aftercare should be for a minimum of six months—the time during which the patient is most likely to relapse. It is difficult to establish an optimal inpatient stay, but it may be best to be guided by the dictum of "keep it short unless you've got good reasons to make it longer."[49,91] Comparison of short-term inpatient treatment (usually two weeks or less) with longer treatment (usually three to six weeks) reveals that the shorter treatment appears to be as effective as the longer. There is little data to guide the clinician on when to make exceptions to the short inpatient stay, but common sense indicates longer inpatient care for patients who have not yet benefited from the shorter term treatment and those whose medical or emotional conditions have not been adequately resolved.

In summary, the biases of this chapter are toward avoiding patient risks or unnecessary expenditures in the absence of adequate data. Therefore, most alcoholic rehabilitation can be carried out in an outpatient setting or after a relatively short term (i.e., two weeks or so) of inpatient care, which is then followed by aftercare. Whichever approach is used, the higher probability of relapse within the first six months of care justifies the commonsense conclusion that outpatient contact should be maintained for at least this period of time.

SUITABLE PSYCHOTHERAPY OR COUNSELING

As is true with all therapeutic approaches, therapists are likely to choose that approach with which they themselves feel most comfortable, an observation that may be especially true for a disorder for which no one specific mode of treatment has been shown to be better than any other. No matter which regimen is used, it is probably best to remember the overriding principle presented in this chapter: Keep it simple. There is no evidence that those treatments aimed at finding deep psychological meanings for drinking or those that require high levels of therapist training are any more effective[9,17,20,66] than "day-to-day" discussions. In these day-to-day discussions, most therapists deal with patients' attempts to stop alcohol-related difficulties, their "new" and changed interactions with their family, the difficulties encountered on the job, their self-concept, and the physiological as well as behavioral problems occurring during recovery. Sessions can also be used to educate patients about their "disease" and give

them some idea of the risks of continued drinking.

Group therapy may be an excellent forum for this relatively superficial approach.[14] Comparisons of group and individual settings for the primary alcoholic demonstrate that the former is at least as effective but costs less.[9,20] Some authors believe that group therapy has specific advantages, as it allows patients to share feelings with a number of other people with similar problems and teaches them social skills; however, there is little hard evidence based on clinical research for or against this suggestion.

During the typical group session, the therapist can help the group of patients focus on the problems of the "here and now." Topics can include stresses at work and at home that tend to increase the desire to drink, mechanisms for learning how to "say no" when alcohol is offered, the possible need to establish a new cadre of abstinent friends, the best manner for filling in the large amounts of free time that can be generated by abstinence, and vocational hints for finding work where alcohol is not so tempting. Many therapists choose to reach out to the family through either groups or individual family sessions with a similar emphasis on the "here and now," which offers insights into maladaptive behavior and the opportunity to "ventilate" past resentments and injustices.

Individual therapists have found many types of psychotherapy useful. Two frequently cited in the literature are psychodrama and transactional analysis.[23,66] While role playing and improved insights into communication and stereotyped behavior may be beneficial, there is no evidence that these approaches are required in alcoholism therapy. Nor are there data to support the importance of psychodynamic psychotherapy in treating alcoholic patients.[9] While it is difficult to deny that the opportunity to "work through" needed areas of personality development and to gain greater self-understanding would certainly appear to be beneficial, the high cost and anxiety provocation inherent in these approaches make them of limited value for the average alcoholic individual in the absence of specific data justifying their use.

One "special" case for alcoholism treatment may be behavior modification.[13] Behavioral approaches such as relaxation training, biofeedback, and meditation can be useful in helping alcoholic persons to learn to cope with their anxiety and insomnia, symptoms that can be expected to persist for three to six months or more after abstinence.[1] In addition, some alcoholism treatment programs have incorporated aversive conditioning as an adjunct to the usual counseling to give patients an additional edge when the desire to drink becomes strong.[44] Adversive conditioning requires a series of sessions (usually three times a week for two weeks) during which patients are given an injection that makes them feel nauseated coupled with the smell and taste of their favorite alcoholic beverage. As a result, the next time they see, smell, or taste alcohol, they are likely to feel nauseated and to vomit. To be maximally effective, this approach must be coupled with a series of "refresher" courses, in which patients undergo an additional short series of aversive sessions every three months or so over the following year. After conditioning, patients who very much want to return to drinking can do so by gulping down alcohol quickly enough to become intoxicated, which will break the aversion. On the other hand, individuals who wish to stop drinking can use the nausea as a reminder and a motivation builder that might add to their chances for abstinence.

Finally, a mode of intervention that requires further mention is Alcoholics Anonymous (AA). This approach offers the patient a self-help discussion group that is available at no cost twenty-four hours a day.[45,83] While this should not be viewed as formal therapy, a commonsense approach to rebuilding a life without alcohol is offered by individuals who can serve as models for recovery and who can offer an abstinence-oriented peer group. Any self-help approach has the inherent dangers of a too-rigorous acceptance of a rigid dogma and a rejection of other modes of help, but for AA, the potential benefits out-weigh the potential risks. Patients must be advised to choose their specific group carefully, since certain individuals will feel more comfortable in groups of blue-collar workers, while others may prefer groups with a high percentage of women. Yet others might feel it most appropriate to participate in groups of highly educated people. For patients whose problems extend to the misuse of other substances in addition to alcohol, a referral to a local Narcotics Anonymous (NA) group may be appropriate.

The "psychotherapies" used in alcoholic rehabilitation are general helping mechanisms. There is little evidence to suggest that one treatment is any better than another. Most therapists choose to take advantage of their specific mode of training, which they adapt to the alcoholic individual's situation and place an emphasis on day-to-day life readjustment without alcohol. While it is possible that a specific type of patient may respond preferentially to a specific mode of therapy, no reliable methods have yet been devised for making this kind of selection. It may be possible to maximize the treatment efficiency by using group therapy that emphasizes day-to-day life adjustment in discussions about problems of readjustment to life without alcohol.

MEDICATIONS APPROPRIATE TO ALCOHOLIC REHABILITATION

Spontaneous remissions in alcoholism are common.[82] As a result, any treatment given to a group of alcoholic patients may have an inflated level of apparent success. The crucial step is to show that the therapeutic regimen *caused* the outcome and that it was not just the result of a spontaneous remission or nonspecific response to intervention. Therefore, it is not surprising that without controlled studies many medicinal treatments such as metronidazole (Flagyl) and LSD have, in the past, been erroneously touted as new "cures" for alcoholism.[42,66]

In dealing with alcoholic patients, it is sometimes what is *not* done that is as important as what is done. Only in rare instances is there justification for treating alcoholic persons with medication after detoxification has been completed.

There is no evidence that average primary alcoholic patients have a better chance of achieving and maintaining abstinence if they take lithium, antidepressant medication, or antipsychotic drugs.[66] Nor are there data to date that justify the extended use of antianxiety medications in alcoholic rehabilitation. Even though these drugs have the apparent benefit of decreasing anxiety, which might increase ease of readjustment to life without alcohol, there is a risk of creating physical dependence by escalating doses in these patients who have already shown themselves to be unable to control the use of ethanol and other CNS depressants. Therefore, with the exception of research occurring as part of carefully controlled studies, most psychotropic drugs should not be used during alcoholic rehabilitation.[66,84]

Disulfiram (Antabuse) is one of the few promising drugs used to treat alcoholic patients, although it too has risks.[5,32,48] This medication does not decrease the drive to drink, but, because the effects of the medication last up to seventy-two hours or more after the drug is taken, the rate of abstinence is enhanced by decreasing the chance that patients will go back to drinking on the spur of the moment.[61,65,94] The drug is usually given orally in a dose of 250 mg per day and is maintained for three months to a year depending on the patient's risk for returning to drink. While controlled studies comparing disulfiram with no additional treatment make this drug look promising, comparisons of the effect of the usual doses versus placebos show few differences and raise the possibility that psychological deterrence is more important than the pharmacological effects of the drug. A number of evaluations have looked at longer-acting subcutaneous implants, but none developed to date maintain blood levels high enough to be of use.[10,93]

Disulfiram does have inherent dangers and cannot be given to patients with serious medical disorders. These restrictions are based on the commonsense assumption that because an alcohol-disulfiram reaction involves vomiting and a rapid drop in blood pressure, it should not be given to patients with a history of serious heart disease, strokes, or diabetes, or to patients with esophageal varices who may experience severe bleeding with vomiting. In addition, the drug can cause feelings of fatigue in perhaps 50 percent of patients, a metallic taste in the mouth, skin rash, and, rarely, the more dangerous complications of seizures, confusion, neuritis, and psychosis.[61]

There is no perfect treatment for the alcohol-disulfiram interaction. Most clinicians recommend symptomatic therapy in which dangerous hypotension is treated conservatively with the Trendelenburg position and oxygen, and antihistamines are used to block histamine release. Ascorbic acid may be helpful in speeding up acetaldehyde metabolism.[61]

The pharmacologic approach to treating alcoholic patients once detoxification has ceased is fairly straightforward. As was discussed in the sections on detoxification, vitamins, especially thiamine at 100 mg per day, might be continued for many months if confusion persists. This section has reviewed the possible roles for disulfiram in the otherwise healthy recovering alcoholic patient. However, there is no evidence that the use of other psychotropic medications is justified in treating the average primary alcoholic patient.

MANAGING PSYCHIATRIC SYNDROMES IN THE MIDST OF ALCOHOLISM

Inherent in the proper treatment of alcoholism is the distinction between primary and secondary disorder.[21,64,66] This chapter has emphasized rehabilitation of the *primary* alcoholic. However, even in primary disease, alcoholic patients can present with temporary problems of severe anxiety (e.g., during withdrawal), obvious confusion (e.g., through a vitamin deficiency, trauma, or the direct effects of ethanol), depression, or psychosis in a clear sensorium. In each of these instances (with the possible exception of long-lasting confused states), treatment involves recognizing the primary alcoholic individual and offering general supports during the several days to several weeks necessary for the clinical syndrome to resolve. During that time a thorough physical evaluation must be carried out, medical problems must be adequately treated, and detoxification begun. After the serious psychopathology has cleared, the patient may be considered a candidate for rehabilitation. Confused states that persist beyond the two weeks (as might be seen in Wernicke-Korsakoff's syndrome) may require adequate nursing care, and such patients may not be appropriate for rehabilitation until clearer thought processes are established.

Secondary alcoholic patients may require detoxification if there is evidence of physical addiction. Alcoholic rehabilitation may be needed to address the possibility that patients have two primary disorders; and continued alcohol-related problems could also jeopardize treatment of the primary disorder. However, severe depression or psychosis may make it difficult for patients to function adequately in an alcoholic rehabilitation program. The decision to begin alcoholic rehabilitation in the adequately treated schizophrenic or affective disorder patient, therefore, must be made on a case-by-case basis.

Primary antisocial personality/secondary alcoholic patients present another therapeutic dilemma. As opposed to primary affective disorder, there is no known psychotherapy or medication that has been shown to alter reliably the course of the antisocial personality. It is probable that heavy drinking will undercut any chances for recovery in these impulsive, violent patients. Therefore, many therapists believe it is appropriate to treat primary antisocial personality/secondary alcoholic patients for their alcohol abuse using the same rehabilitation maneuvers that are invoked in primary alcoholics. When this is done, it is necessary to recognize the greater likelihood that such patients will misuse other substances, attempt to undercut staff authority, stir up patients against each other and against staff, and carry a significantly worse prognosis for the year after treatment.[55,75] In treating these men and women, it is probably best to establish clear rules for acceptable and unacceptable behaviors and to not tolerate behavior that undermines the safety or treatment milieu of other patients.

APPLICATION OF THESE GENERAL RULES TO PATIENT SUBGROUPS

The foregoing discussion of rehabilitation has made little note of the heterogeneity within primary alcoholic patients. The chapter offers only general treatment guidelines that must be specifically modified for the particular case. For instance, while group therapy appears to be cost effective for the average patient, the individual who is extremely shy or who has great difficulty verbalizing in front of others may find this too stressful.

The need to recognize individual characteristics is underscored by the importance of these factors in predicting one-year abstinence treatment. For example, the skid-row alcoholic, while only representing 3 to 5 percent of alcoholic individuals,[25] definitely carries the worst prognosis and has the greatest incidence of physical disease. Programs aimed primarily at these patients should justify their actions through the medical and psychological help they give and not expect an impressive rate of abstinence. On the other hand, the middle-class working man or woman who does not actively abuse other substances, has few police problems unrelated to alcohol, and has an interested family has a 60 to 70 percent chance of abstinence no matter what style of rehabilitation is used.

The interventions involved in alcoholic rehabilitation are so general that it is not surprising that few programs have convincing evidence that different treatments should be used for women, the elderly, minority groups, or other special populations. Rather, it is a reflection of our current state of knowledge that the same general helping mechanisms are used for all of these groups, but with good commonsense adaptions for the needs of that specific population.[3,66]

Once one controls for the socioeconomic class and primary versus secondary diagnosis, it does not appear that the course of alcoholism is significantly different for men and women.[73] However, therapists need to consider the higher risk women have for primary affective disorder (perhaps 15 percent), the effects that alcohol may have on moods as they relate to the menstrual cycle, the unique roles of women in the family[47] and society,[92] and special child-care needs.[30,47,92] Program personnel should also recognize that female alcoholics might prefer to work with a female therapist and should recognize possible special vocational treatment needs.[57] Special medical problems can include a possible higher risk for cirrhosis[53] and the need to consider pregnancy in alcoholic women and the possible effect alcohol might have on the developing fetus.[79] It is advisable to use the general treatment guidelines offered in earlier sections of this chapter and carry out commonsense modifications while recognizing the unique medical difficulties, the higher risk for primary affective disorder, and the need for discussion groups dealing with the problems of women.

Another group with special needs is the elderly. Their rate of alcoholism may be as high as younger groups, but they may be more difficult to identify because they look so different from the public stereotype of the alcoholic.[58,97,98] Actively drinking elderly alcoholic individuals are less likely to drink daily and tend to have fewer social problems but more medical and interpersonal difficulties related to their heavy drinking than younger alcoholics. In addition to alcoholic rehabilitation, adequate treatment probably requires referral to special facilities in the community to serve older citizens' medical and social needs. Once again, the same general approach to treatment is used in this population, but special commonsense modifications are added to help deal with the unique medical needs and requirements for therapy groups addressing special problems in this population.

Minority groups also have unique problems, but data in this area are limited. Within these special groups (for example, Native Americans),[88] drinking may have a special meaning, and behavior while under the influence of alcohol must be understood in a social context. The same may be true for Hispanic and Black Americans.[25,65,66] While there are no good guidelines, a possible approach to treatment utilizes the same basic rehabilitation techniques given earlier but employs some understanding of the stresses experienced by each specific population. One should consider using counselors of relevant ethnic groups, and, in some instances, actual referral to an ethnically oriented facility may be beneficial.

This discussion of special groups of alcoholic patients is far from exhaustive. What is important is to have a general treatment approach in mind and to recognize the relevant areas of possible modifications for members of subgroups.

¶ Summary and Conclusions

An introduction to alcoholism can fill an entire text (and frequently has). By necessity, this chapter is a compromise. The goal has been to present psychiatrists and other mental health professionals with clinically relevant information on the single most prevalent mental health disorder in the Western world.

The information presented here has three emphases. *First,* the practicing psychiatrist must understand something about the drug, alcohol, and must also learn about the disorder, *alcoholism.* A clinically relevant distinction has been made between information about the drug itself, the (economically important) occurrence of limited problems in 40 percent or so of men in our societies, and the persistent and pervasive alcohol-related problems that might be labeled alcoholism. The latter is a highly prevalent problem affecting 10 percent of men at some time during their life and 2 to 5 percent of women. Because this disorder is associated with high levels of both physical and mental pathology, one in five of neatly dressed and highly functional psychiatric patients present to the psychiatrist with psychopathology related to alcoholism. Because only 5 percent of alcoholics fit the skid-row stereotype, one problem faced by practitioners is to overcome myths and to recognize that the average alcoholic individual fits the characteristics of the average patient being seen for depression, anxiety, confusion, or temporary psychoses.

The *second* emphasis has been a presentation of various criteria for alcoholism. While emphasis has been placed on the DSM-III, a clinically relevant shorthand approach emphasizing major life problems related to alcohol has also been presented. Once a label of definite or probable alcoholism has been established, the proper prognosis and selection of treatment rests with accurate distinction between primary and secondary disease. Alcohol-related life problems occurring in the midst of a preexisting schizophrenia, a long-established pattern of antisocial life problems antedating alcoholism (i.e., primary antisocial personality with secondary alcoholism), or severe alcohol-related difficulties occurring only in the midst of major affective episodes is best termed secondary alcoholism. In each of these instances, the prognosis and treatment is complicated by the major preexisting psychiatric disorder. Therapeutic efforts must not only deal with the alcohol-related life problems but also aggressively address and treat the preexisting or primary disorder (e.g., antidepressants for primary unipolar affective disorder or antipsychotics for primary preexisting schizophrenia).

The third emphasis has been placed upon treatment of primary alcoholism. This disorder is characterized by a fluctuating course with alternation between periods of abstinence, limited periods of apparent controlled drinking, and severe alcohol-related life problems. Primary alcoholism can result in temporary but severe psychoses, states of confusion, and depressions (each of which tends to clear within several days to several weeks of abstinence without more aggressive treatment). Therefore, the psychiatrist frequently serves as the gatekeeper in identifying and referring the alcoholic patient for adequate therapy. The first step in treatment involves repeated confrontations with both the patient and the family members. This is followed by addressing whether or not clinically significant withdrawal symptoms are likely to occur and treating these symptoms, if necessary. The final step involves the general helping mechanisms that serve as the basis of rehabilitation. This last step is frequently carried out in an outpatient setting by offering patients a number of maneuvers aimed at increasing their motivation toward abstinence and then helping them to readjust to a life without alcohol.

¶ Acknowledgments

This work was supported by the Veterans Administration Research Service, NIAA Grant #05526, and a grant from Joan and Ray Kroc.

¶ Bibliography

1. ADAMSON, J., and BURDICK, J. "Sleep of Dry Alcoholics," *Archives of General Psychiatry*, 28 (1973):146–149.
2. American Psychiatric Association. *Diagnostic and Statistical Manual of Mental Disorders*, 3rd ed. (DSM-III). Washington, D.C.: American Psychiatric Association, 1980.
3. ARMOUR, D., POLICH, J., and STAMBUL, H. "Alcoholism and Treatment." Prepared for National Institute of Alcohol and Alcohol Abuse, Report R–1739–NIAAA.
4. ASHLEY, M. "The Physical Disease Characteristics of Inpatient Alcoholics," *Journal of Studies on Alcohol*, 42 (1981): 1–11.
5. BAEKELAND, F., et al. "Correlates of Outcome in Disulfiram Treatment of Alcoholism," *Journal of Nervous and Mental Disorders*, 153 (1971):1–9.
6. BARCHHA, R., STEWART, M., and GUZE, S. "The Prevalence of Alcoholism Among General Hospital Ward Patients," *American Journal of Psychiatry*, 125 (1968):133–136.
7. BEGLEITER, H. "Subjects at Risk for Alco-

holism: Recent Findings," Paper presented at the 14th Annual Medical Scientific Conference of the National Alcoholism Forum, Houston, Texas, April 14–17, 1983.

8. BEHSE, F., and BUCHTHAL, F. "Alcoholic Neuropathy: Clinical Electrophysiological and Biopsy Findings," *Annals of Neurology,* 2 (1977):95–110.

9. BERGER, F. "Alcoholism Rehabilitation: A Supportive Approach," *Hospital and Community Psychiatry,* 34 (1983):1040–1043.

10. BERGSTROM, B., et al. "Is Disulfiram Implantation Effective?" *Lancet,* 1 (1982):-49–50.

11. BOHMAN, M., SIGVARDSSON, S., and CLONINGER, R. "Maternal Inheritance of Alcohol Abuse," *Archives of General Psychiatry,* 38 (1981):965–969.

12. BOYD, J., DERR, K., and GROSSMAN, C. "Different Definitions of Alcoholism," *American Journal of Psychiatry,* 140 (1983):1314–1317.

13. BRIDDELL, D., and NATHAN, P. "Behavior Assessment and Modification with Alcoholics: Current Status and Future Trends," *Progress in Behavior Modification,* vol. 2. New York: Academic Press, 1976.

14. BROWN, S., and YALOM, I. "Interactional Group Therapy with Alcoholics," *Journal of Studies on Alcohol,* 38 (1977):-426–456.

15. CAHALAN, D. *Problem Drinkers.* San Francisco: Jossey-Bass, 1970.

16. CAMERON, J., ZUIDEMA, G., and MARGOLIS, S. "A Pathogenesis for Alcoholic Pancreatitis," *Surgery,* 77 (1975):754–763.

17. COSTELLO, J., BIEVER, P., and BAILLARGOON, J. "Alcoholism Treatment Programming: Historical Trends and Modern Approaches," Paper presented at the National Council on Alcoholism, 7th Annual Medical-Scientific Conference, Washington, D.C., May 1976.

18. Editorial. "Alcoholic Heart Disease," *Lancet,* 1 (1980):961–962.

19. EISENSTEIN, A. "Nutritional and Metabolic Effects of Alcohol," *Journal of the American Dietetic Association,* 81 (1982):247–251.

20. EMRICK, C. "A Review of Psychologically Oriented Treatment of Alcoholism, II," *Journal of Studies on Alcohol,* 36 (1975):88–108.

21. GOODWIN, D., and GUZE, S. *Psychiatric Diagnosis.* New York: Oxford University Press, 1979.

22. GOODWIN, D., et al. "Alcohol Problems in Adoptees Raised Apart From Alcoholic Biological Parents," *Archives of General Psychiatry,* 28 (1973):238–243.

23. GORAD, S., McCOURT, W., and COBB, J. "A Communications Approach to Alcoholism," *Quarterly Journal of Studies on Alcoholism,* 32 (1971):651–668.

24. GREENBLATT, D., and SHADER, R. "Prazepam and Lorazepam," *New England Journal of Medicine,* 299 (1978):1342–1344.

25. HAGLUND, M., and SCHUCKIT, M. "The Epidemiology of Alcoholism," in N. Estes and E. Heinemann, eds., *Alcoholism: Psychological and Physiological Basis.* St. Louis: C. V. Mosby Company, 1982, pp. 32–48.

26. HAKULINEN, R., LEHTIMAK, L., and LENTONEN, M. "Cancer Morbidity Among Two Male Cohorts," *National Cancer Institute,* 52 (1974):1711–1717.

27. HALLER, R., and DRACHMAN, D. "Alcoholic Rhabdomyolysis: An Experimental Model in the Rat," *Science,* 208 (1980):412–414.

28. HAMMOND, K., RUMACK, B., and RODGERSON, D. "Blood Ethanol: A Report of Unusually High Levels," *Journal of the American Medical Association,* 226 (1973):63–64.

29. IBER, F. "Alcohol and the Gastrointestinal Tract," *New England Journal of Medicine,* 61 (1971):120–123.

30. JONES, B., and JONES, M. "Women and Alcohol," in M. Greenblatt and M. A. Schuckit, eds., *Alcohol Problems in Women and Children.* New York: Grune & Stratton, 1976, pp. 103–136.

31. KENDELL, R., and STATON, M. "The Fate of Untreated Alcoholics," *Quarterly Journal of Studies on Alcoholism,* 27 (1966):30–41.

32. KITSON, T. "The Disulfiram-ethanol Reaction; A Review," *Journal of Studies on Alcohol,* 38 (1977):96–113.

33. KLATSKY, A., et al. "Alcohol Consumption and Blood Pressure, Kaisere-Per-

manente Multiphasic Health Examination Data," *New England Journal of Medicine*, 296 (1977):1194–1200.

34. KNOCHEL, J. "Hypophosphatemia in the Alcoholic," *Archives of Internal Medicine*, 140 (1980):613–615.

35. KNOTT, D., and BEARD, J. "A Diuretic Approach to Acute Withdrawal from Alcohol," *Southern Medical Journal*, 62 (1969):485–489.

36. LEMERE, F. "What Happens to Alcoholics," *American Journal of Psychiatry*, 109 (1953):674–676.

37. LIEBER, C. "Alcohol and Malnutrition in the Pathogenesis of Liver Disease," *Journal of the American Medical Association*, 233 (1975):1077–1082.

38. ———. *Medical Disorders of Alcoholism*. Philadelphia: W. B. Saunders, 1982.

39. LISHMAN, W. "Cerebral Disorder in Alcoholism Syndromes of Impairment," *Brain*, 104 (1981):1–20.

40. LOWRY, W. "Alcoholism in Cancer of the Head and Neck," *Laryngoscope*, 85 (1975):1257–1280.

41. LUDWIG, A. "On and Off the Wagon," *Quarterly Journal of Studies on Alcoholism*, 33 (1972):91–96.

42. LUDWIG, A., LEVINE, J., and STARK, L. *A Clinical Study of Treatment Efficacy*. Springfield, Ill.: Charles C Thomas, 1970.

43. MOORE, R. "The Prevalence of Alcoholism in Medical and Surgical Patients," in B. Locke, ed., *Monograph in Psychosocial Epidemiology*, vol. 5, forthcoming.

44. NEUBUERGER, O., et al. "Replicable Abstinence Rates in an Alcohol Treatment Program," *Journal of the American Medical Association*, 248 (1982):960–963.

45. OGBORNE, A., and GLASER, F. "Characteristics of Affiliates of Alcoholics Anonymous: A Review of Literature," *Journal of Studies on Alcohol*, 42 (1981):661–675.

46. O'SULLIVAN, K., et al. "Alcoholism and Affective Disorder Among Patients in a Dublin Hospital," *Journal of Studies on Alcohol*, 40 (1979):1014–1022.

47. POLIT, D., NUTTALL, R., and HUNTER, J. "Women and Drugs," *Urban Social Change Review*, 9 (1976):9–16.

48. RAINEY, J. "Disulfiram Toxicity and Carbon Disulfide Poisoning," *American Journal of Psychiatry*, 134 (1977):371–378.

49. RAVENSBORG, M., and HOFFMANN, J. "Program Versus Time: Length of Stay Patterns in Alcoholism," *Drug Alcohol Dependency*, 1 (1975–76):51–56.

50. ROBINS, L. N. *Deviant Children Grown Up*. Baltimore: Williams & Wilkins, 1966.

51. RYBACK, R., ECHARDT, M., and PUTLER, C. "Biochemical and Hematological Correlates of Alcoholism," *Research Communications in Chemical Pathology and Pharmacology*, 27 (1980):533–550.

52. SANDBY, P. *Alcoholism and Mortality*. Oslo: Universitetsforlaget.

53. SAUNDERS, J., DAVIS, M., and WILLIAMS, R. "Do Women Develop Alcoholic Liver Disease More Readily than Men?" *British Medical Journal*, 282 (1981):1140–1143.

54. SCHMIDT, W., and POPHAM, R. "Heavy Alcohol Consumption and Physical Health Problems: A Review of the Epidemiological Evidence," *Drug and Alcohol Dependence*, 1 (1975–76):27–50.

55. SCHUCKIT, M. "Alcoholism and Sociopathy: Diagnostic Confusion," *Quarterly Journal of Studies on Alcoholism*, 34 (1973):157–164.

56. ———. "Alcoholism and Depression: Diagnostic Confusion," in D. W. Goodwin and C. O. Erickson, eds., *Proceedings of Alcoholism and Affective Disorder*. New York: Spectrum Publications, 1977, pp. 9–20.

57. ———. "Alcoholism in Women: A Report to the President's Commission on Mental Health." Submitted to the President's Commission on Mental Health, August 1977.

58. ———. "Geriatric Alcoholism and Drug Abuse," *Gerontologist*, 17 (1977):168–174.

59. ———. "Biological Markers: Metabolism and Acute Reactions to Alcohol in Sons of Alcoholics," *Pharmacology Biochemistry & Behavior*, 13 (Supplement 1) (1980):9–16.

60. ———. "Current Therapeutic Options in the Management of Typical Anxiety,"

Journal of Clinical Psychiatry, 42 (1981):15–24.

61. ———. "Disulfiram (Antabuse) and the Treatment of Alcoholic Men," *Advances in Alcoholism*, 2 (1981):1–5.

62. ———. "Peak Blood Alcohol Levels in Men at High Risk for the Future Development of Alcoholism," *Alcoholism: Clinical and Experimental Research*, 5 (1981):64–66.

63. ———. "The History of Psychotic Symptoms in Alcoholics," *Journal of Clinical Psychiatry*, 43 (1982):53–57.

64. ———. "Alcoholism and Other Psychiatric Disorders," *Hospital and Community Psychiatry*, 34 (1983):1022–1026.

65. ———. "Treatment of Alcoholism in Office and Outpatient Settings," in J. H. Mendelson and N. K. Mello, eds., *Diagnosis and Treatment of Alcoholism*. New York: McGraw-Hill, 1983, pp. 229–256.

66. ———. *Drug and Alcohol Abuse: A Clinical Guide to Diagnosis and Treatment*. New York: Plenum Press, 1984.

67. ———. "Genetic and Biochemical Factors in the Etiology of Alcoholism," in L. Grinspoon, ed., *Psychiatric Update: American Psychiatric Association. Annual Review*, vol. 3. Washington, D. C.: American Psychiatric Press, 1984, pp. 320–327.

68. ———. "Subjective Response to Alcohol in Sons of Alcoholics and Controls," *Archives of General Psychiatry*, 41 (1984):-879–884.

69. ———. "Trait and State Markers in Psychobiology," in L. L. Judd and P. Groves, eds., *Psychobiology Foundations of Clinical Psychiatry*, Philadelphia: J. P. Lippincott, forthcoming.

70. SCHUCKIT, M., and CAHALAN, D. "Evaluation of Alcoholism Treatment Programs," in W. J. Filshead, J. J. Rossi, and M. Keller, eds., *Alcohol and Alcohol Problems: New Thinking and New Directions*. Cambridge, Mass.: Ballinger Publishing Company, 1976, pp. 292–267.

71. SCHUCKIT, M., and GRIFFITHS, J. "Gamma-Glutamyltransferase Values in Nonalcoholic Drinking Men," *American Journal of Psychiatry*, 139 (1982): 227–228.

72. SCHUCKIT, M., and HAGLUND, R. "Etiological Theories on Alcoholism," in M. R. Riley, ed., *Alcoholism—Development, Consequences, and Interventions*. St. Louis: C. V. Mosby, 1982, pp. 16–31.

73. SCHUCKIT, M., and MORRISSEY, E. "Alcoholism in Women: Some Clinical and Social Perspectives with an Emphasis on Possible Subtypes," in M. Greenblatt and M. Schuckit, eds., *Alcohol Problems in Women and Children*. New York: Grune & Stratton, 1976, pp. 5–36.

74. SCHUCKIT, M., and RAYSES, V. "Ethanol Ingestion: Differences in Blood Acetaldehyde Concentrations in Relatives of Alcoholics and Controls," *Science*, 203 (1979):54–55.

75. SCHUCKIT, M., and WINOKUR, G. "A Short-term Follow-up of Women Alcoholics," *Disorders of the Nervous System*, 33 (1972):672–678.

76. SCHUCKIT, M., GOODWIN, D., and WINOKUR, G. "A Study of Alcoholism in Half Siblings," *American Journal of Psychiatry*, 128 (1972):1132–1136.

77. SCHUCKIT, M., et al., "Alcoholism," *Archives of General Psychiatry*, 20 (1969): 301–306.

78. SELLERS, E., and KALANT, H. "Alcohol Intoxication and Withdrawal," *New England Journal of Medicine*, 294 (1976): 757–762.

79. SELLERS, E. M., NARANJO, C. A., and PLACHY, J. E. "Drugs to Decrease Alcohol Consumption," *New England Journal of Medicine*, 305 (1981):1255–1261.

80. STREISSGUTH, A. "Fetal Alcohol Syndrome: An Epidemiologic Perspective," *American Journal of Epidemiology*, 107 (1978):467–478.

81. TWERSKI, A. "Early Intervention in Alcoholism: Confrontational Techniques," *Hospital and Community Psychiatry*, 34 (1983):1027–1030.

82. VAILLANT, G. *The Natural History of Alcoholism*. Cambridge, Mass.: Harvard University Press, 1983.

83. VAILLANT, G., and MILOFSKY, E. "Natural History of Male Alcoholism," *Archives of General Psychiatry*, 39 (1982):127–133.

84. VIAMONTES, J. "Review of Drug Effectiveness in the Treatment of Alcoholism,"

American Journal of Psychiatry, 128 (1972):120–121.

85. VICTOR, M. "Treatment of Alcoholic Intoxication and the Withdrawal Syndrome," *Psychosomatic Medicine,* 28 (1966):636–649.

86. VICTOR, M., and HOPE, J. "The Phenomenon of Auditory Hallucinations in Chronic Alcoholism," *Archives of General Psychiatry,* 126 (1955):451–481.

87. VICTOR, M., ADAMS, R., and COLLINS, G. *The Wernicke-Korsakoff Syndrome.* Philadelphia: F. A. Davis Company, 1971.

88. WESTEREMEYER, J. "Research on Treatment of Drinking Problems, Importance of Cultural Factors," *Journal of Studies on Alcohol,* 9 (1981):44–59.

89. WHITEFIELD, J., et al. "Some Laboratory Correlates of Drinking Habits," *Annals of Clinical Biochemistry,* 15 (1978):297–303.

90. WILKINSON, D. "Examination of Alcoholics by Computed Tomographic (CT) Scans: A Critical Review," *Alcoholism: Clinical and Experimental Research,* 6 (1982):31–44.

91. WILLENS, P., LETEMENDIA, F., and ARROYAVE, F. "A Two-year Follow-up Study Comparing Short with Long Stay Inpatient Treatment of Alcoholics," *British Journal of Psychiatry,* 122 (1973):637–648.

92. WILSNACK, C. "The Impact of Sex Roles and Women's Alcohol Use and Abuse," in M. Greenblatt and M. Schuckit, eds., *Alcohol Problems in Women and Children.* New York: Grune & Stratton, 1976, pp. 37–64.

93. WILSON A., DAVIDSON, W., and BLANCHARD, R. "Disulfiram Implantation: A Trial Using Placebo Implants and Two Types of Controls," *Journal of Studies on Alcohol,* 41 (1980): 429–436.

94. WILSON, A., DAVIDSON, W., and WHITE, J. "Disulfiram Implantation: Placebo, Psychological Deterrent, and Pharmacological Deterrent Effects," *British Journal of Psychiatry,* 129 (1976):277–280.

95. WU, C. F., SUDHAKAR, M., and JAFERI, G. "Preclinical Cardiomyopathy in Chronic Alcoholics: A Sex Difference," *American Heart Journal,* 91 (1976):281–286.

96. ZELAZOWSKI, R., et al. "Relationship of Cerebral Ventricular Size to Alcoholics' Performance on the Luria-Nebraska Neuropsychological Battery," *Journal of Studies on Alcohol,* 42 (1981):749–756.

97. ZIMBERT, S. "The Elderly Alcoholic," *Gerontologist,* 14 (1974):221–224.

98. ———. "Evaluation of Alcoholism Treatment in Harlem," *Quarterly Journal of Studies on Alcoholism,* 35 (1974):550–557.

CHAPTER 31

THE PSYCHOLOGICAL PRESENTATIONS OF SOMATIC DISORDERS

Thomas B. Horvath

¶ Introduction

The last decade witnessed several related events in the behavioral sciences. The rise of biological and descriptive approaches to mental disorders paralleled the professional remedicalization of psychiatry. The practical, medically oriented psychiatric consultation process[114,125] proved to be ascendant over the more psychodynamic and pedagogic liaison model in general hospital practice.[336,337] The psychiatrist is increasingly expected to function as a medical subspecialist and to develop a repertoire of diagnostic and therapeutic recommendations based on the psychobiological pathophysiology of medical disorders.[209,210,211]

This chapter attempts to provide an overview of an area of knowledge essential for contemporary general hospital psychiatrists: the diagnosis of medical diseases heralded by psychological symptoms or disturbed behavior. This borderland of medicine and psychiatry is virtually ignored by the textbooks of internal medicine and neurology, and it fares only a little better in most textbooks of psychiatry. On the other hand, several recent monographs provide extensive coverage on the neuropsychiatric presentations and features of medical diseases and the psychological consequences of cerebral disorders.* While the chapter covers this ground, it cannot adequately deal with two related areas: the diagnosis of abnormal illness behavior and of psychosomatic disorders.

The tasks of diagnosis are twofold[280,345]: (1)

*See references 27,28,127,167,199,200, and 218.

the scientific, objective evaluation of symptoms, signs, and laboratory tests to determine the pathophysiological processes common to a group of patients (i.e., the study of *disease*); and (2) the evaluation of the consequences of the pathological processes and their interactions with the unique life history of specific individuals (i.e., the study of illness).[184] Adolf Meyer's influence on American psychiatry ensured the generation of a large literature on the latter area of individual reactions to illness.* This has been conceptualized lately in the biopsychosocial framework introduced by Engel[90,91] and bolstered by studies of human development and adaptive/defensive styles.[40,319] Social scientists refer to this topic under the rubric of normal and abnormal illness behavior,[239] or coping and adaptation to stress and illness.[249]

The second area this chapter cannot deal with is what used to be known as psychosomatic medicine, then as psychophysiological reactions, and which is now classified in the third edition of the *Diagnostic and Statistical Manual of Mental Disorders* (DSM-III)[8] as "psychological factors affecting physical conditions." Here a relationship is postulated between environmental stimuli and physical conditions, where the stimuli are both psychologically meaningful and temporally related to the initiations or exacerbations of the condition.[153,197,253] Coping with major medical transitions calls on the patient's life experience and adaptive and defensive skills.[135,249] Lipowski[215] has provided a conceptual overview, and Weiner[374] has published a magisterial review of the main disorders: asthma, peptic ulcer, hypertension, thyrotoxicosis, rheumatoid arthritis, and ulcerative colitis, with a review of psychobiological contributions to disease development.

Some of the psychological symptoms discussed in this chapter are ubiquitous. Anxiety, depression, irritability, and expansive mood are everyday experiences. Even in their more severe forms, large numbers of people admit to experiencing them[255]: In

several communities, the six-month prevalence of depression was 8 percent among women and 5 percent among men; combined states of anxiety and depression affected 12 percent of the population. At such high rates of prevalence, chance associations between these symptoms and some medical disorders must be common. Furthermore, the limits of normality of mood variation are difficult to agree on.

Other psychological symptoms are less common and are more easily seen as abnormal: hallucinations, delusions, thought disorder, disorientation, and amnesia. At any one time, 1 percent of the population may show psychotic symptoms and 1 percent appear demented.[255] Other, more subtle manifestations of the disorder easily escape notice: changes in attention and vigilance and decline in cognitive efficiency and emotional modulation. There is a 5 percent prevalence of minor cognitive changes.[255]

Behavioral aberrations are readily observable, but it is difficult to agree on their significance, as they depend on social conventions. Alterations of personality occasioned by illness may not come to light in a low-expectation, permissive atmosphere, but only under the demands of the workplace or under social stress.

This review of the literature revealed three clusters of reports, not necessarily equal in practical importance or theoretical relevance. First, there was a group of common medical disorders that numbered specific mental changes among their defining features (thyrotoxicosis and anxiety,[113] hypothyroidism and lassitude,[166] hepatic failure and confusion,[254] etc.). Second, there were the common disorders occasionally complicated by psychological symptoms (digitalis and propranolol hydrochloride intoxication and hallucinations,[104,315] epilepsy and delusions,[322] cancer and depression,[179] etc.). Finally, there was a large collection of obscure, rare medical diseases with puzzling presentations that often ended up in psychiatrists' consulting rooms—or even on their old-fashioned couches (myasthenia gravis,[177,309] Wilson's disease,[295] atrial myx-

*See references 125,182,280,336, and 337.

oma,[382] porphyria,[21] vitamin A intoxication,[167] pheochromocytoma,[163] "carcinoid,"[167] etc.).

Reports in the psychiatric literature were often thin in medical or physiological detail. Medical reports, on the other hand, dealt superficially with psychological and behavioral observations. The literature generally predated the recent introduction of operational definitions for psychological symptoms and signs;[8] thus the terminology was inaccurate and variable. (The term schizophrenia was often misapplied to affective psychoses or to organic episodes with prominent delusions; depressive disorder was often diagnosed when only isolated dysphoric mood was present; etc.)

The emphasis of this review is necessarily on the experience of medical practice in contemporary developed countries. Such experience is dominated by the degenerative disorders, cardiovascular disease, neoplasia, and the pathologies of aging.[30,175,395,397] Diseases are more often multisystemic and at least partly treatment-resistant. Iatrogenic contributions to pathogenesis are significant, and drug side effects[199] and complex homeostatic interactions[200] may be as important as the original pathogen. On the other hand, in underdeveloped countries (and in Europe during the lifetime of the great psychiatric systematizers), the main medical causes of aberrant mental state ("exogenous psychosis of Bleuler")[27] were trauma, malnutrition, and infections.[212]

From the practical, clinical point of view, it is most useful to focus on frequent psychological symptoms and common medical disorders, especially if the discovery of early or prominent psychological symptoms may lead to an early diagnosis or avoidance of misdiagnosis.[64,351,367,390] However, at times it will be useful to discuss those clinical curiosities whose examination may throw light on certain aspects of brain function and that therefore have heuristic, if not pragmatic, usefulness. Encyclopedic collections of psychological signs and symptoms due to medical disease are available.[368] A pathophysiological approach that emphasizes the mechanisms of symptom production is more useful, however.[270]

¶ Epidemiology and Importance to Medical Practice

The association of physical illness with psychiatric disorders is not uncommon.[87,88] Maguire and Granville-Grossman[231] and Marshall[237] detected a high frequency of medical problems (from 33 to 44 percent) among psychiatric patients. In half of the cases, the illness was unknown to the patient or his or her family doctor.[231] Herridge[147] noted physical illness in half of over two hundred consecutive psychiatric admissions. In 25 percent of these, the disease contributed to the onset of psychological symptoms, while in 8 percent, it was the psychiatric illness or its treatment that caused the medical problem. In the majority of cases, however, the medical and psychiatric disorders were incidental to each other and ran parallel courses. The coexistence of medical and psychiatric problems frequently leads to diagnostic confusion in an emergency room setting.[198]

A more recent, detailed clinical and laboratory study of a lower-socioeconomic class, state hospital population revealed an 80 percent incidence of medical illness.[133] Almost 50 percent of the psychiatric patients experienced an exacerbation or even causation of their symptoms by medical illness. Koranyi's review of the literature[191] suggests that the prevalence of physical morbidity in psychiatric populations ranges from 30 to 60 percent, with somatopsychic etiological connection in 10 to 40 percent.

Less severely disturbed patients are similarly afflicted.[48] Davies[79] found a 58 percent prevalence of medical disease in psychiatric outpatients and judged 42 percent to be etiologically relevant. Koranyi[189] attributed half of the twenty-eight deaths experienced by a large mental health outpatient population to medical illness. An extension of this study[190] found 43 percent of 2,000 outpatients to be medically ill, where the mental illness was medically caused in 20 percent and aggravated in 50 percent. Half the medical problems detected in these and similar surveys [147,189,190,231] were previously unknown.

Hall and his group [131] prospectively studied a group of subjects presenting for psychotherapy. This group was more representative of the clients seen in private practice settings than some of the earlier cohorts, which were composed of chronic mental patients. The study patients had exclusively psychological presentations, and in only a few was an organic mental syndrome diagnosed; yet a medical etiology was eventually found for 9 percent of the psychiatric presentations. Cardiovascular, endocrine, pulmonary, infectious, gastrointestinal, and hematological disorders; malignancies; and some neurological diseases were responsible for the medical problems, none of which was rare or esoteric. Detailed systems reviews and screening blood studies were more useful than routine physical examinations, even when performed by the patient's own physician.

Hall and associates [134] recommend a screening multiple-panel blood analysis, complete blood count, electrocardiogram, and a sleep-deprived electroencephalogram (EEG) in addition to a careful history, physical, mental state, and neurological examination for all psychiatric admissions. Chest x-ray, serology, thyroid tests, lupus cell preparations, and antinuclear antibodies, B_{12} and folate determinations, and urine toxicology were also proposed. Screening tests are said to be particularly important, as there is little correlation between specific somatic symptoms and the underlying organic diseases in patients presenting with psychological symptoms. [150] Surveys found routine screening useful, detecting a 14 percent prevalence for anemia, 1 percent for B_{12} deficiency, 22 percent for folate deficiency, 3 percent for diabetes, 0.5 percent for hypothyroidism, and 0.7 percent for hyperthyroidism. [69,191] Thomas, [349] on the other hand, argues that extensive screening incurs a high cost for a low rate of true positive findings with clinical significance. Hendrie [144] argues that tests be performed only when there is a high level of clinical suspicion, rather than as a "screening procedure."

The presence of a number of the following factors suggests organic disease, [144] but their absence does not rule it out: presentation of psychiatric problems (especially conversion symptoms) after age sixty; change in the clinical syndrome with time; diurnal fluctuation and confusion; episodes of urinary or fecal incontinence; absence of family history; absence of psychogenesis; failure to respond to indicated biological treatment; and the development of unusual side effects or mental confusion to such treatment.

The concept of "screening" readily leads to controversy among epidemiologists, public health advocates, and cost-conscious administrators. The clinician may find more practical utility in a diagnostic algorithm that proceeds through a hierarchical series of investigations from the simple and inexpensive to the costly and dangerous. [96] Fauman's [96] level I evaluation includes a validated description of the current episode; a medical, psychiatric, and drug history; a mental state examination; and vital signs. Level II includes the physical examination and those laboratory tests that assess the adequacy of the major organ systems. Level III tests, generally more expensive and invasive, are directed toward specific problems tentatively identified earlier on, while level IV tests attempt to gain structural confirmation in selected cases. Prospective studies are needed in order to assess the clinical and monetary cost effectiveness of the various steps in similar algorithms.

The cost and burden of undiagnosed—and untreated—organically induced mental disturbances may be quite high. Patients presenting with a delirium eventually had a higher mortality than patients with the same disease and with the same apparent severity, but without mental changes. [276] The behavior was not the prime cause of morbidity; rather, it was the underlying medical disorder. Among behaviorally disturbed geriatric patients, those with organic mental syndromes had a higher mortality than those with "functional" disorder, [359] yet the mental changes indicative of physical pathology were often not noted by the primary care physicians and nurses.[186] Saraway and Koran[302] speculated that some misdiagnoses could be traced to the staff's unconscious wish to discontinue clinical responsibility in situations that threatened their self-esteem. Hoffman and Koran[150] later broadened their analysis of misdiagnosis to disease-, patient-, and physician-related factors.

Medical diseases share symptoms with mental disorders, and their psychiatric symptoms often precede the physical signs.[238] Psychiatric patients are often uncooperative or incapable of providing accurate information. Physicians may fail to perform a truly comprehensive evaluation, depend excessively on consultant's advice, fail to recognize unusual variants of medical disorders, and attribute unusual behaviors to ubiquitous psychosocial stressors. Physicians still confuse symptoms and syndromes at a semantic level: "Depression" is often diagnosed in the presence of dysphoric mood without the other symptoms of the syndrome of depression.

¶ Definitions: Presenting Syndromes of Organic Origin

Psychological symptoms of cerebral or systemic disease do not occur in scattered isolation. They tend to cluster into specific syndromes, which in turn have been grouped into three main categories by Lipowski.[213] He noted several types of *global* impairment of mental function (delirium, dementia, and reversible dementia), a variety of *focal* neuropsychological disturbances (amnesia, aphasia, apraxia, etc.), and a group of syndromes that resembled *functional* psychiatric disorders (schizophreniform, affective, and personality disorders).

Physicians are accustomed to having mental confusion and fluctuating disorientation complicate the more advanced stages of a variety of medical disorders, especially in the elderly.[30] Acute confusional state,[338] delirium,[212] metabolic encephalopathy,[272] and

acute organic brain[145] or mental syndrome[218] are terms that are often used interchangeably for this cluster of symptoms, which include clouding of consciousness, disorders of attention, disorientation, memory impairment, perceptual and psychomotor aberrations, incoherent speech, and a disturbed sleep-wake cycle.[8]

The more insidious development of amnesia, intellectual decline with a variety of cortical neurological signs, and the personality deterioration that characterizes the dementias[379] or the chronic organic syndromes[313,376,380] can appear in a variety of systemic disorders, as well as in the traditional degenerative and vascular primary cerebral diseases. Focal neurological syndromes affecting higher cortical or subcortical functions can complicate medical illness and can at times lead to spurious functional presentations (i.e., dressing apraxia, cortical blindness with denial, jargon aphasia, etc.).[364,365,366]

The introduction into formal classification of a group of syndromes that resemble functional disorders but are organically caused has not been without controversy.[8,27] The common denominators include evidence from history, physical examination, and laboratory tests of a specific organic factor etiologically related to the disturbance; and absence of the criteria for delirium, dementia, or focal neurological syndromes.

Comprehensive phenomenological descriptions are still missing, but several syndromes seem present:

1. Psychotic syndromes dominated by one or more of: delusions, hallucinations, incoherence, illogicality, poverty of content of thought, and/or bizarre or catatonic behavior. These "exogenous psychoses"[27] may take on a distinct schizophreniform flavor.[80,282]

2. Affective syndromes present with depressed, irritable, or expansive moods, often with associated vegetative, behavioral, and cognitive signs.[127,185,194]

3. Irrational anxiety (beyond that to be expected from the psychological consequences of disease and iatrogenic stress)

may present in a persistent generalized form with motor tension, autonomic hyperactivity, and apprehensive expectation, or as a panic attack.[127,228,258]

4. Aggressive, violent, defiant, oppositional, or frankly antisocial behavior may also emerge in the course of medical illness. Less dramatic changes in personality include carelessness, lack of foresight, and loss of social judgment.[33,127]

5. Loss of mental sharpness, fatigue, and subtle accentuation of preexisting personality features, often ascribed to "neurosis," may also herald early cerebral or systemic illness.[65] Less commonly, specific "neurotic" symptoms (i.e., conversion, dissociation, obsessions and compulsions, depersonalization, and/or body image distortions) may emerge in the course of medical diseases.[220,240,321]

6. In patients with preexisting psychiatric illness, the stress of a superimposed medical condition can exacerbate the typical signs of the functional mental disorder. Such organic accentuation of psychological symptoms can easily lead to diagnostic delays.[123,302] The problem is compounded by the fact that the life-style of many chronic psychiatric patients predisposes them to medical problems: malnutrition, self-neglect, substance abuse, and iatrogenic drug side effects.[134]

The practical relevance of this group of pseudofunctional disorders[129,266] is that these mental changes generally prompt referral to psychosocially oriented professionals. Even if a psychiatrist is involved, the tendency is to focus on interpersonal and intrapsychic inquiries and to limit medical evaluation and laboratory tests.[302]

Fatigue and Loss of Mental Sharpness: Early and Nonspecific Symptoms

Vague, subjective symptoms are common presentations of disease[150] and may account for the misapplied label of neurosis for undiagnosed medical problems.[133] Early studies of fatigue did indeed find a high incidence of anxiety and depressive disorders.[6,316] However, 20 percent of fatigued patients had medical problems: neurological illness (amyo-

trophia lateral sclerosis, myasthenia, parkinsonism, and multiple sclerosis [MS]), chronic infections (tuberculosis, brucellosis, and subacute bacterial endocarditis), metabolic disturbance (diseases of the thyroid, parathyroid, and adrenal gland and diabetes), heart-lung disease, anemia, and renal disease (uremia) being the leading causes. Malnutrition can also present with fatigue, and so can occult malignancy.

Fatigue of medical origin is not relieved by sleep and is followed, rather than preceded, by anxiety.[6] Manfred Bleuler's[27] review of the early European literature on "exogenous psychosis" (i.e., organic mental syndrome) shows fatigue and weakness to be among its premonitory symptoms, along with mood lability, perceptual difficulties, hypersensitivity to stimuli, and increased vivid dreaming. Lipowski[212] notes that the early symptoms of intoxication with industrial and environmental contaminants include decreased alertness, concentration, and vigilance; mild cognitive impairment; apathetic but irritable mood; and a sense of fatigue.

The loss of mental sharpness seems to be the cognitive counterpart of the physical symptom of fatigue. Among the subtle sequelae of brain damage,[206] fatigue, perplexity, and distractibility lead the way, followed by a reduced capacity for new skills, imagery, and associations and an inability to time-share and alternate between different activities. Chapman and Wolf, in their classic studies[65] of the nonfocal effects of brain damage, noted several levels of impairment. It was the amount of tissue lost and the rate of the damage that determined the functional level, although premorbid personality and intellect and environmental supports played a part. The loss of 30 to 60 grams of cortical tissue led to difficulties with concentration and effort, a loss of sparkle and creativity, and reduced frustration tolerance. At 60 to 90 grams of tissue loss, the patients were slow, self-absorbed, and irritable. They exhibited much anxiety and primitive defenses. At 90 to 120 grams of loss, there was a perception by others that something was "radically wrong." These patients were inert, lethargic, and mentally very slow. They exhibited very little anxiety and very little self-control or self-monitoring. With over 120 grams of tissue loss, the patients appeared frankly demented, with disorientation, left-right confusion, confabulations, and perseverations. The time when fatigue and loss of mental sharpness become manifest in a specific case depends not only on the presence of other defect symptoms but on the restitutive responses of the total organism.[117] The nature of the pathology determines the rate of progress and the extent of the damage but provides no further clinical indicators. Thus a tumor, an infarct, or a demyelination can produce the same type of direct psychological defects and restitutive responses.

Delirium: Syndromes of Fluctuating Global Impairment

The presenting symptom of delirium is often a change in mood. This may evolve in reaction to cognitive loss or in response to the stressful environment, but it may also represent a primary neurophysiological change. Dysphoric, irritable, and anxious moods predominate, but brief episodes of agitation and euphoria may occur.[145]

The characteristic cognitive failure is one of environmental integration;[212] there is earlier and more extensive temporal than spatial disorientation, while personality identity is well-preserved. Attention is distractible and exhibits spontaneous fluctuations. There is a reduced ability to select, maintain, and shift cognitive focus.[208]

Thinking is characterized by an increase in associative thought and unconscious imagery, while goal-directed thinking, concept formation, and abstractions are reduced.[212] Transient delusions occur in 40 percent of cases. Memory is impaired, and there is reduced registration, defective transfer from short- to long-term memory, and difficulty in retrieval. Confabulations occur in 15 percent of cases.[212]

Perceptual abnormalities start with sensory hypersensitivity, perceptual distortions, and minor changes in body image. Visual illu-sions are particularly common. In more severe cases, visual, auditory, and tactile hallucinations may dominate, especially in association with hyperactivity.[338,340] Psychomotor activity is always altered; lethargy and retardation may alternate with agitation and indiscriminate overactivity. Advanced states of delirium may be accompanied by a coarse tremor, asterixis, myoclonic jerking, dysarthria, and ataxia.[272]

As long as the presentation of delirium is one of acute confusion or of diurnal variation of mental lucidity ("sundowning"), general physicians seem to have little trouble diagnosing it, especially in the elderly.[214] If the patient presents, however, with aberrant behavior, psychotic experience, or marked disturbances of mood, all of which can be superimposed on the basic cognitive defect, the mistaken diagnosis of the functional psychoses or affective disorder is often made.[367] The formal DSM-III criteria for delirium emphasize the cognitive aspects of the disorder and imply a uniformity of presentation not often seen in practice (see table 31–1). The next revision of the DSM-III may consider the establishment of operational criteria to subtype the basic delirium syndrome, so that the physiological correlates of a delirium accompanied by psychotic features or by a vegetative syndrome could be studied. The identification of a delirium by DSM-III criteria should be followed by an estimation of its cognitive severity (e.g., through the Folstein Mini Mental State Examination[106]) and by an assessment of its behavioral impact (e.g., through the Brief Psychiatric Rating Scale[264]).

The pathophysiology and etiology of delirium has precipitating, predisposing, and sustaining elements.[212] These act at different times and on different systems at different levels. Delirium is usually precipitated by a significant deterioration in the metabolic integrity of the neuron or synaptosome (through substrate deficiency or enzyme or cofactor defect) or by alteration in membrane stability or ionic balance.[272] The dominant notion has been one of basic neuronal or glial metabolic impairment or "brain fail-

TABLE 31–1
Diagnostic Criteria for Delirium

A. Clouding of consciousness (reduced clarity of awareness of the environment), with reduced capacity to shift, focus, and sustain attention to environmental stimuli.
B. At least two of the following:
    (1) perceptual disturbance: misinterpretations, illusions, or hallucinations
    (2) speech that is at times incoherent
    (3) disturbance of sleep-wakefulness cycle, with insomnia or day-time drowsiness
    (4) increased or decreased psychomotor activity
C. Disorientation and memory impairment (if testable).
D. Clinical features that develop over a short period of time (usually hours to days) and tend to fluctuate over the course of a day.
E. Evidence, from the history, physical examination, or laboratory tests, of a specific organic factor judged to be etiologically related to the disturbance.

NOTE: Reprinted, by permission of the publisher, from American Psychiatric Association, *Diagnostic and Statistical Manual of Mental Disorders*, 3rd ed. (Washington, D.C.: APA, 1980), p. 107.

ure."[92] Evidence has been accumulating, however, that delirium could occur at levels of metabolic disturbance that fail to derange the basic metabolic processes in isolated tissue slices.

A hypothesis has been emerging that a specific impairment of transmitter synthesis in the synaptosomes of cholinergic neurons was responsible for the symptoms of delirium. The choline acetyl transferase system has been shown to be exquisitely sensitive to hypoxia, hypoglycemia, and thiamine deficiency.[30] Elderly patients, substance abusers, and subjects with previous cerebral damage are predisposed to delirious states.[212,218] The presence of psychological stress, sleep deprivation, immobilization, and sensory overload or deprivation will facilitate and sustain the development of the clinical syndrome, provided sufficient metabolic precipitants act on the predisposed brain.[212] This hypothesis would predict exacerbation of delirium by anticholinergic agents, and this is certainly supported by clinical experience with antidepressants and anticholinergics. The isolated reports of improvement of deliria by cholinomimetics are also consistent with this notion.[30]

There are two levels of etiological understanding of the complex and multifactorial state of acute brain failure, or delirium: a level of empirical associations established by observational studies of natural history and a level of experimentally determined pathophysiological causation. At each of these levels, distinctions need to be made among *predisposing*, *precipitating*, and *sustaining* conditions or factors. An ideal, all-inclusive etiological statement would draw from each of the six cells of this matrix. For example, the empirical association of delirium tremens and pneumonia in a middle-aged alcoholic patient in an intensive care unit environment is a common event. To give a balanced account of the respective *predisposing* roles of increased sedative tolerance, receptor and membrane changes, neuronal loss, cortical atrophy, chronic obstructive pulmonary disease, and cigarette smoking; to describe the multiple *precipitating* causes of hypoxia, rebound locus coeruleus activation, and circulating bacterial toxins; and to include the *sustaining* effects of sleep deprivation, sensory overload, and fear in a strange environment is a more challenging but, from the therapeutic point of view, necessary task. One can of course "muddle through" with an empirical regime of detoxification and antibiotics. The more rational approach of correcting and monitoring each disordered pathophysiological factor is a more demanding task and one that becomes necessary in more complicated cases.

The common empirical associations of medical disorders and delirium depend on the setting and on the age of the patient.[30,212]

Emergency rooms[198] will see a disproportionate number of street drug or industrial
toxicities, acute infections, and sudden de-
compensations of organ failures, often with
single, major precipitants. Hospital wards
and nursing homes are witnesses to the gradual, multifactorial deteriorations of system
functions, compounded by iatrogenic side
effects,[276] or the multisystem effects of malignancy.[245]

Lipowski[212] devotes considerable attention to age as an empirical sorting factor. In
childhood, the common precipitants of delirium include infectious diseases, accidental
ingestion of drugs and household toxins, epilepsy, head injury, and salt/water disturbance. In underdeveloped countries, malnutrition and infestations loom large. In the
adolescent age group, use of deliriogens and
acute sedatives, alcohol intoxications, head
injuries and complications of automobile accidents, and postoperative and infectious
episodes need to be taken into account.

Several neurological disorders first come
to light in early *adulthood*: systemic lupus,
MS, and certain primary tumors. In *middle
age*, the withdrawal effects—and acute or
chronic intoxications—from alcohol and
sedatives and the emerging organ damage
caused by them begin to take center stage.
Endocrine disorders (especially diabetic
complications), organ failures (hepatic, renal,
and respiratory), nutritional deficiencies, and
the emergence of cardiovascular diseases (especially the complications of myocardial infarction and cardiac failure) are important
middle-age issues. The long-term effects of
head injury, epilepsy, demyelinating disease,
and chronic alcohol abuse, first sustained in
young adulthood, are likely to come to light
at this age.

Old age is the province of cerebrovascular
accidents and metabolic encephalopathies.
These are often superimposed on early Alzheimer changes. Organ failures, often multiple, dominate the picture, and cancer raises
multiple metastatic and nonmetastatic
events. Head injuries now precipitate quietly
enlarging subdural hematomas. There is a
high incidence of iatrogenic episodes, since

the aging brain seems peculiarly susceptible
to the direct and indirect neurological side
effects of therapeutic agents.[199] (Direct
effects are caused by anticholinergics, antiadrenergic hypotensives, digitalis, aspirin,
cimetidine, sedatives, anticonvulsants, and
steroid and nonsteroid antiinflammatory
agents; while indirect effects are caused by
diuretics, lithium, anticoagulants, etc.)* Attempts at more encyclopedic lists can be
found in the major monograph and some
chapters.[212,214,338,340] A more discriminating,
hierarchically stepwise approach is suggested by others.[96]

Once the suspicion of a delirium is raised
by the presence of clinical mental state criteria in association with one of these medical
disorders, two diagnostic steps need to be
taken. First, there is often the need to
confirm the presence of an acute brain failure and to distinguish it from functional psychoses. While the clinical examination is
often sufficient, the difficult case or the skeptical consultee requires direct evidence of
brain dysfunction, and currently, this is best
reflected in the EEG.[259,275,341]

Remarkably little has changed since Engel
and Romano's studies in the 1940s that established a relationship between the clinical severity of deliria and the amount of slowing of
the dominant EEG frequencies.[92] The earliest and mildest of deliria are associated with
slowing and disorganization of the alpha
waves and the beginning of sporadic theta
waves. At the other extreme, severe deliria
show large amounts of delta activity. The exception to this rule is not only of empirical,
but of theoretical, interest as well: In delirium tremens, there is much fast beta activity,
and this may be an index of the rebound activation of the cortex by the noradrenergic
locus coeruleus system. There may be a need
to go beyond an exclusively cortical interpretation of the EEG in other instances as well.
In cases of hepatic encephalopathy, there are
episodic bursts of bilaterally synchronous
delta activity, which may represent a thalamic dysfunction. Computer-averaging of

*See references 37, 130, 314, 315, and 373.

the EEG signal to derive event related potentials shows a reversible delay of a late component, the P300, in deliria. This wave is probably generated partly in the hippocampus and is cholinergically mediated.[160] The increasing availability of EEG small computers may make frequency analysis, evoked potentials (EPs), and even topographic brain electrical activity mapping (BEAM) ready tools for the demonstration of cerebral metabolic dysfunction.[160]

The second diagnostic question, the cause of delirium, can be broken into two distinct sets of inquiries. First, there are those laboratory tests that prove the presence of a disease but which, in themselves, do not measure the factors that directly influence brain function. Chest x-ray; sputum, urine or blood cultures; determination of liver enzymes; tests for antinuclear antibody; lupus cell preparations; cerebrospinal fluid (CSF) protein, glucose, and cell levels; and complete blood counts with differential white counts are commonly applied to the diagnostic problems posed by delirium.[272]

The other set of diagnostic tools measures physiological variables that directly affect brain function (blood gases, pH, electrolytes, calcium and magnesium concentrations, vitamin—thiamine, B_{12}, and folate—levels, drug toxicology, and hormone levels). There are also biological variables that covary with the actual toxins for which no convenient measurement exists. (Blood urea nitrogen is a proxy for phenols and aromatic acids; CSF gamma globulin is a measure of demyelinating activity.) The detection of focal cerebral lesions is also a critical direct diagnostic step, with the proviso that the computed tomographic, radionucleide, or angiographic determination of these lesions may not adequately measure the full extent of their metabolic effects on neighboring tissues.[272]

Dementia: Syndromes of Progressive Cerebral Deterioration

The study of dementia,[20,176,353,379] hitherto neglected, is enjoying a major scientific renaissance. It is now clear that the majority of cases of dementia, even in old age, show the pathological picture of neurofibrillary tangles and extracellular plaques described in Alzheimer's disease.[348] A unified theory is emerging, one that ascribes this disease to a retrograde degeneration of nucleus basalis cholinergic neurons.[72] Alzheimer's disease patients present with primary memory and cognitive problems, but are usually in a state of reasonable physical health. Although in its late phases Alzheimer's is associated with significant physical morbidity (weight loss, malnutrition, and terminal infections), only occasionally does it present in the context of a medical disease. It differs in this sense from the other causes of dementia.

Multi-infarct dementia[124] and alcoholic brain damage[292] vie for second place in frequency,[313] and both usually evolve from longstanding, though often neglected, health problems. Most individuals with multi-infarct dementia suffer from hypertension or extracranial vascular disease, often with other stigmata and risk factors of atherosclerosis (smoking, diabetes, and/or hyperlipidemia). The dementia itself is built from a mosaic of discrete ischemic cerebral events with transient focal and persistent cognitive effects,[124] but there are rare diffuse forms as well.[54]

Brain damage in alcoholism is usually a late complication[77,158] and seems to be related to the total lifetime alcohol consumption and the usual amounts consumed on individual occasions.[89] Its presentation is so insidious that it is first dismissed as an indication of psychosocial or personality deviance, or as a by-product of medical deterioration (liver disease, head trauma, chronic obstructive pulmonary disease [COPD], and/or malnutrition). The amnestic variety associated with untreated thiamine deficiency (Wernicke-Korsakoff's syndrome) may have a more dramatic entrance,[363] as might the pellagrinous type. Brain damage is very much part of the late course of the natural history of alcoholism, although neuropsychological testing may be required to fully explore its impact on cognitive function.[265] About 10 percent of alcoholic subjects manifest frank dementia, but many others demonstrate relatively asymptomatic cerebral atrophy.[45,158] It is likely that this predisposes them to delirious episodes.[212] As alcoholism is associated with a large number of medical disorders[207] (cirrhosis, peripheral neuropathy, cardiomyopathy, tuberculosis, megaloblastic anemia, pancreatitis, and even peptic ulcer and hypertension), the presence of delirium or dementia with any of these should lead to a careful inquiry into drinking and nutritional habits. Intoxication and withdrawal modify the basic clinical picture.[312]

The absence of neurosyphilis from a discussion of leading causes of dementia is probably the major success of primary prevention in psychiatry.[120] In Kraepelin's day it was so common that other, emerging mental disorders were compared and contrasted to general paresis for descriptive purposes.[137] A further small fraction of the cases of dementia are due to rare degenerative disorders (Huntington's chorea, Wilson's disease, Jakob-Creutzfeldt's disease, subacute sclerosing panencephalitis, and Pick's disease). These attract attention in proportion to their pathological, rather than their public health, importance.[376,379]

About 20 percent of patients presenting with the clinical syndrome of dementia do not have primary degenerative cerebral problems but rather have largely reversible metabolic, inflammatory, or space-occupying disorders.[26,376] Until the development of really effective treatments for Alzheimer's disease, the practical task confronting the physician caring for demented patients is the identification of these "reversible dementias."[211,213] The limitations of the catchword "reversible" should be noted, however. Delay in the treatment of subdural hematomas, vitamin deficiency, or chronic meningitis may leave the patient with significant cognitive defects. In Larson's series[195] the "reversible" cases improved, but rarely reverted to normal. On the other hand, energetic medical treatment of concurrent disorders improved the mental state of Alzheimer's patients,[195,378] cessation of drinking arrested and perhaps even reversed

the course of alcohol dementia,[55,77] and treatment of hypertension and other cardiovascular risk factors and the use of platelet anti-sticking agents or carotid endarterectomy have been shown to prevent the further accumulation of cognitive deficits in multi-infarct dementia.[51]

In DSM-II, chronic organic brain syndrome[376] was defined by the symptoms of impaired orientation, memory, intellectual functions, and judgment, and a labile, shallow affect. Chronicity was used as a term for irreversibility. It is not clear that the current description[8] (DSM-III) is much of an improvement on this, except for deletion of any reference to reversibility and a reference to cortical signs (see table 31–2). The separation of the more focal syndrome of amnesia from dementia is of some theoretical, rather than practical, use (see table 31–3).

More detailed descriptions await the development of validated rating instruments and their application in extended prospective studies in a variety of dementias.[72] Until that time, however, certain predictions about clinical features and etiology may be made from the dominant distribution of lesions and the neurological defects associated with damage to those areas. The association between a certain type of amnesia (difficulty of transferring from short- to long-term memory and the absence of new declarative memories) and lesions of the hippocampal and mamillo-thalamic areas is well-substantiated. This is the basis of the amnesic syndrome of the Wernicke-Korsakoff type, of herpes simplex encephalitis, of certain strokes in the posterior cerebral artery distribution, and of transient global amnesia.[28] It is likely that postconcussion anterograde amnesia, alcohol blackouts, anoxia, prolonged seizure activity, and hypoglycemia also affect the hippocampus with relative selectivity, as these can lead to the classical amnesic syndrome.[28]

The further distinction between cortical and subcortical dementias is more controversial. The concept of subcortical dementia was introduced to account for some of the cognitive features of progressive supranuclear

TABLE 31–2
Clinical Diagnostic Criteria for Dementia

A. A loss of intellectual abilities of sufficient severity to interfere with social or occupational functioning.
B. Memory impairment.
C. At least one of the following:
    (1) impairment of abstract thinking, as manifested by concrete interpretation of proverbs, inability to find similarities and differences between related words, difficulty in defining words and concepts, and other similar tasks
    (2) impaired judgment
    (3) other disturbances of higher cortical function, such as aphasia (disorder of language due to brain dysfunction), apraxia (inability to carry out motor activities despite intact comprehension and motor attention), agnosia (failure to recognize or identify objects despite intact sensory function), "constructional difficulty" (e.g., inability to copy three-dimensional figures, assemble blocks, or arrange sticks in specific designs)
    (4) personality change, i.e., alteration or accentuation of premorbid traits
D. State of consciousness not clouded (i.e., does not meet the criteria for Delirium or Intoxication, although these may be superimposed).

NOTE: Reprinted, by permission of the publisher, from American Psychiatric Association, *Diagnostic and Statistical Manual of Mental Disorders*, 3rd ed. (Washington, D.C.: APA 1980), p. 111.

TABLE 31–3
Clinical Diagnostic Criteria for the Amnestic Syndrome

A. Both short-term memory impairment (inability to learn new information) and long-term memory impairment (inability to remember information that was known in the past) are the predominant clinical features.
B. No clouding of consciousness, as in Delirium and Intoxication, or general loss of major intellectual abilities, as in Dementia.

NOTE: Reprinted, by permission of the publisher, from American Psychiatric Association, *Diagnostic and Statistical Manual of Mental Disorders*, 3rd ed. (Washington, D.C.: APA 1980) p. 113.

palsy[5] but it has been extended not only to Parkinson's disease,[62,244,375] Huntington's chorea,[227] normal-pressure hydrocephalus,[101,174,261,286] and the lacunar syndrome[100] but also to the metabolic dementias and the dementia of depression.[26,273] The alleged features include a disheveled, perplexed appearance; psychomotor retardation; stooped, twisted posture; and unsteady, ataxic gait. Chorea, tremors, and dystonia are common, and the speech is marked by dysarthria and hypophonia. Such patients are emotionally apathetic or labile; they have difficulty in retrieving information but have a relatively normal, though slowed, ability to learn; they demonstrate normal language skills; and they have no cortical neurological signs. Benson[26] urges an exhaustive search for reversible factors in the clinical syndrome.

Luria's[221] distinctions between anterior and posterior cortical functions may lead to a further clinical differentiation. General paresis,[82,218] alcoholism,[74] blunt head injuries,[28] and the rare Pick's disease[218] preeminently affect the frontal lobes, and thus they tend to leave language, praxis, and gnostic skills intact. Indeed, a marked personality deterioration takes place, memory retrieval is affected, the ability to plan future courses of action is impaired, and socially inappropriate behavior emerges. The results of formal Wechsler Adult Intelligence Scale (WAIS) testing may look better than the actual behavior of these patients, as mostly posterior dysfunctions are elicited there, and a cognitive structure is provided.

A final diagnostic dilemma concerns the concept of pseudodementia. At least two syndromes are graced with this term. Post[273] described elderly patients with major affective illness who demonstrated cognitive decline both in clinical and psychometric testing, but who recovered upon the treatment of their depression. Some workers call this the "dementia of depression," but Benson[26] noted that the resemblance was to subcortical dementias rather than to Alzheimer's disease. Wells,[377] on the other hand, described a clinical syndrome that is distinguishable from dementia by a careful history and mental state exam. Pseudodemented patients have less objective signs of impairment, show more dependent behavior than expected, exhibit more emotional reactivity, and appear to try less. Their premorbid personality is marked by dependent or histrionic features, and they do not usually meet criteria for major depression. It seems that Wells's description approximates the DSM-III category of a factitious mental disorder superimposed on an abnormal personality, while Post describes a truly reversible dementia. These patients more often had a history of depression than Alzheimer's patients, and the onset of their illness was marked by depressed mood, self-blame, hopelessness, somatic delusions, and decreased appetite. Their dementia was phenomenologically similar to that of Alzheimer's patients, although cortical signs were not present, and it was milder.

The etiology of reversible dementia outside of primary neuronal degeneration is as varied as that for delirium. However, the rate of development is slower, so both physiological and psychological adaptations can occur and modify the presentation. More rapidly evolving pathophysiology is likely to lead to more dramatic pictures. The degree of pathophysiological deviation cannot be as extreme as in severe deliria, as in those cases stupor, semicoma, and finally coma are the end results.[272]

There are a number of conditions associated with gradually developing aberrations of moderate intensity, and these give rise to the clinical syndrome that resembles primary degenerative dementia. The medical illness itself, however, will manifest its specific features, or it will induce other neurological signs that ease the differential

diagnostic problem. Medical interventions, on the other hand, are likely to complicate the diagnostic problem. First, almost all common drugs have central nervous system (CNS) side effects, especially when taken in various combinations over long periods of time. The overall presentation can be dementiform rather than delirious.[199,314,315] Drugs with CNS side effects include sedatives, heterocyclic antidepressants, neuroleptics, other agents with central anticholinergic side effects, anticonvulsants, and antiadrenergic hypotensive agents. The second iatrogenic confound is the half-completed or inadequate treatment. Patients on dialysis, cirrhotic patients with porto-caval shunts, and COPD subjects maintained with low arterial oxygen levels may not show overt features of their organ failures, but have just enough cerebral impairment to show up as a mild to moderate dementia. Third, the advances of technology may induce new syndromes: dementia dialytica, opportunistic meningeal infections in immune-suppressed patients, organophosphate poisoning in agriculture, and nitrobenzene and industrial hydrocarbon exposure in the workplace.

Of the vitamin deficiencies, thiamine's role in amnesic syndromes is well documented,[363] and B_{12} deficiency is a well-known cause of dementia.* Pellagra is virtually unknown now, although it was responsible for a veritable epidemic of dementias in the South earlier this century.[167] The role of folate deficiency in causing mental disorders is less clear and the evidence for depression is stronger than for dementia.†

Among the endocrine disorders, hypothyroidism presents a requirement for thyroid screening, as its clinical signs are elusive until late in the course.[271] Acute hypoglycemia presents a picture resembling intoxication or delirium, although repeated or prolonged severe episodes may lead to dementia.[236] The other endocrinopathies are less common and more likely to mimic affective disorders.[94]

*See references 139, 152, 224, 318, and 389.
†See references 39, 56, 58, 161, 306, and 343.

Space-occupying lesions that grow slowly and intrude only on "silent" areas of the brain (frontal, posterior parietal, and/or inferior temporal) are likely to show a dementing picture.[64,180,181] Meningiomas[311] and subdural hematomas[342] are the likely candidates. Metastatic cancer usually has a more dramatic or more focal manifestation. The nonmetastatic, distant effects of malignancy[42,66] in promoting multifocal leucoencephalopathy, limbic encephalopathy,[43,73] and endocrine and calcium metabolic changes may present, however, as a rapidly evolving dementia. Severe brain injury by trauma, hypoxia, or massive metabolic insult can lead to a chronic, irreversible mental syndrome, but the circumstances make the diagnosis obvious. At times, however, the insults may have been repeated over a period of time,[78] and even forgotten, or emerge after a period of delayed demyelination, as in dementia pugilistica,[168] carbon monoxide poisoning,[324] and post-hypoglycemic encephalopathy.[236]

Finally, dementias complicate the later stages of several chronic CNS disorders, parkinsonism,[244,374] and MS.[356] There are usually so many other disabilities to contend with that the cognitive decline is often disregarded. The dementia can be the presenting feature of Wilson's disease[303,369] and Huntington's disease,[227] although aberrant movements should have been detected by careful observers, and personality deviations usually precede the cognitive changes.[227,295]

¶ Selective Organic Mental Disorders: Medical Conditions That Mimic Functional Disorders

The frank clinical syndromes of delirium and dementia, once recognized, generally prompt an extended search for medical causes. The occult presentation of a medical disorder with "functional" psychiatric symptoms, on the other hand, will often divert attention from the biomedical to the psychosocial sphere. Taylor,[347] in a book written for the nonmedical human service professional, points to several sources of error: confusing a symptom with a disorder (i.e., the dysphoric mood "depression" is not always caused by the major affective disorder "depression," but possibly by an occult malignancy, hypercalcemia, or Cushing's disease, etc.); listening without fully considering the total context (i.e., exploring the psychological impact of the dysphoric mood without considering its possible biological etiology); equating psychosis with schizophrenia (i.e., delirious states have florid psychotic symptoms); and relying on a single information source (i.e., usually the mildly organic patient is not able to give a full account of his or her symptomatology).

Taylor[347] recommends that certain alerting clues for the presence of underlying medical disease be looked for: mental changes first appearing after fifty-five, with no similar past history, without psychological precipitants, or in the context of chronic disease or excessive exposure to street, over-the-counter (OTC), or prescription drugs. The presence of any of the following should be regarded as presumptive evidence of a cerebral disorder: recent head injury, change in headache pattern, visual disturbances, speech problems, movement disorders, change in vital signs, and/or alteration in consciousness. Even without these warnings, subtle changes in attention, orientation, recent memory, abstract reasoning, and sensory discrimination should be looked for.

Taylor[347] recommends that patients be asked to write a sentence, draw a clock, and copy a three-dimensional figure. Similar tasks are incorporated in the Mini Mental State Examination,[106] and a detailed higher nervous system examination is described by Strub and Black.[339] It is possible that such careful evaluation would elicit subtle cognitive disorders in the conditions that mimic affective, schizophreniform, neurotic, and personality disorders, although the more crude clinical criteria for delirium, dementia, or amnesia would not be met. Neuropsychological evaluations come into their own in these difficult diagnostic problems,[99,116,204] as do careful neurological, electroencephalographic, and radiological examinations.* Exacerbation of subtle cognitive defects by intravenous sodium amylobarbitone has been proposed as a useful provocative test, but there is an incidence of both false negatives and false positives.[256,298,371]

The "Exogenous" Psychoses

The term psychosis has had so many partially overlapping meanings during the last twenty years that it is difficult to know what is reported in articles claiming associations between psychoses and medical disorders. Articles claiming high frequency[46] may use criteria as loose as "altered reality testing" or "regressed behavior" and fail to differentiate between organic and functional psychoses.[46] This accounts for associations[282] that include viral encephalitis; temporal lobe epilepsy; systemic lupus; tumors, infarcts, or abscesses in the parietal and temporal areas; Cushing's disease; myxedema; pancreatitis; uremia; hepatic encephalopathy; porphyria; B_{12} deficiency; and Wilson's disease. The list of drugs is almost as long: sympathomimetics, central anticholinergics, alcohol, bromide, cannabis, hallucinogens, procaine penicillin, xanthine bronchodilators, exogenous steroids, cimetidine, organophosphates, and PCP.

Some of these psychoses run a recurrent, cyclic course dictated by the natural history of the medical disease causing them. The common disorder of MS[356] will infrequently present with recurrent psychotic symptoms. The clinical manifestations of the more uncommon pheochromocytoma[163] and porphyria[1,21] often include such symptoms. Pancreatitis is often complicated by hallucinations and delusions.[307] Its recurring nature and its complications are due to alcoholism. Systemic lupus[14,97,123] is classically recurrent, as is the controversy about the relative contribution of steroids to the clinical picture.[202] Other medically caused psychoses are more schizophreniform both in manifestation and in progressive course. Some au-

thors[282] define schizophrenia in very wide, Bleulerian terms and claim an impressive list of medical causes (epilepsy, brain injury, neurosyphilis, cerebral neoplasm, cerebral toxoplasmosis, Huntington's chorea, myxedema, Cushing's disease, porphyria, homocystinuria, Klinefelter's syndrome, Turner's syndrome, Kartagener's syndrome and drugs, such as sympathetic stimulants, bromide, and alcohol). If more restrictive criteria[87,119] depending on specific symptoms had been applied, or if poor premorbid function had been included as well, a smaller number of positive case reports would have surfaced.

It is more helpful at times to focus on a single, well-defined syndrome, as Gelenberg did with catatonia,[112] defined as muscular rigidity, posturing, negativism, and mutism. If structural lesions were involved, these generally affected the limbic system or its immediate connections. Causes of structural lesions include viral encephalitis, frontal or third-ventricle tumors, Wernicke's encephalopathy, head injury with orbitofrontal contusions, and neurosyphilis. However, there are reports of generalized electrical (petit mal and narcolepsy) or metabolic (diabetic acidosis, hypercalcemia, pellagra, porphyria, and drug intoxication) disturbances leading to catatonia. The pharmacological precipitants of instances of catatonia (PCP, mescaline, amphetamine, and phenothiazines) suggest a certain neurotransmitter-based specificity. In particular, modulations of the catecholaminergic system have found a central place in modern theories of schizogenesis, supported in part by reports of drug side effects.*

Visual hallucinosis in other than delirious states and hallucinogen intoxications or flashbacks[156] have been reported in epilepsy, migraine, retinal disorders, and temporal arteritis.[127] (In seizure disorders, an occipital locus is associated with simple visual phenomena, while a temporal lobe ictus may evoke scenes and panoramas.[251]) Auditory hallucinosis is experienced in salicylate intox-

*See references 154,177,287,367, and 380.

*See references 16,22,61,171,183,250, and 315.

ication, middle ear disease, acoustic neuroma, and seizure disorders[127] and, at times, in chronic alcoholism.[362] Migraine and partial complex epilepsy have also been associated with somatic and olfactory hallucinosis.[127] Acute pancreatitis[307] and systemic lupus[14] are often complicated by hallucinations, but usually in a delirious context.[167] An interplay of environmental, perceptual, and neurochemical changes seems necessary for organic hallucinosis to take place.[165,320,381]

Delusions have been described in temporal lobe epilepsy,[80,322] in the aftermath of encephalitis lethargica, in systemic lupus, in Huntington's chorea, in tuberous sclerosis, and in endocrinopathies as different as thyrotoxicosis, myxedema, and Cushing's disease. There were some clinical differentiations: Delusions in the endocrine disorders seem to rise from affective changes; in Huntington's chorea, from dementia; in systemic lupus, from deliria.[167] Delusions previously thought unique to schizophrenia have been seen in organic states.[141,225] Only in the interictal delusions of temporal lobe epilepsy, in the psychic symptoms of limbic tumors, and in limbic-encephalitic states was there a strong resemblance to schizophrenia.[31,84,149,232]

Davison and Bagley[80] came to the conclusion that medical diseases of the temporal lobes and diencephalon are associated with an increased incidence of phenomenologically defined schizophrenia. These "schizophrenics" have no genetic loading, however, and their illness comes on at ages atypical for schizophrenia. Psychotic phenomenology figured prominently in Mulder and Daly's study[251] of one hundred temporal lobe epileptics: olfactory, gustatory, and auditory hallucinations, and auditory and frequently complex visual memories. Déjà-vu experiences, perceptual illusions, forced thoughts, dreamy states, and automatic behaviors also suggest psychosis, especially when accompanied by inexplicable mood changes.[252] The paroxysmal autonomic changes, the stereotyped lip smacking and chewing movements, and, of course, the frequently attendant generalized seizures suggest the correct diagnosis.[31] The rich variety of ictal psychotic experiences are at times followed by episodes of postictal confusion and automatism, often interpreted as psychotic.[34] More prolonged confusional psychoses may be the result of excessive anticonvulsants or, more rarely, petit mal or temporal lobe status epilepticus.[31]

It is the schizophreniform interictal psychosis of temporal lobe epilepsy that has attracted most interest.[32,80,322] It occurs in a clear state of consciousness and may alternate with flurries of seizure activity. The psychosis develops after more than a decade of indifferently controlled seizures and is superimposed on the interictal personality change.[17,18,19,33] The patients generally have deeper and more appropriate affect than process schizophrenics, and they do not show the deterioration or the development of negative symptoms of schizophrenia. It has been noted that primary delusions are uncommon in these epileptic psychoses, even though Schneiderian first-rank symptoms do occur.

Ferguson and Rayport's recent review of this area[32] implicated subtle ongoing seizure activity in the production of several related psychotic states: acute episodes, chronic psychoses, dysphoric-paranoid states, paranoid-aggressive states, and affective psychoses. The schizophreniform designation was seen as inaccurate and not in keeping with the finding of intensive seizure monitoring, stereo-EEG, and clinical-EEG correlations.

It seems difficult to conclusively demonstrate the existence of psychoses that closely mimic functional states. Perhaps the effort is misguided, and what is needed are careful phenomenological studies in parallel with explorations of brain states.

Organic Affective Disorders

The term depression is used in several different ways in medical reports. Perhaps the simplest misunderstanding is the use of this term for sedation, as in "barbiturates as depressant drugs." This misunderstanding is perpetuated when a high frequency of depression is described following the use of central hypotensive and beta-blocking agents.[325,385] Second, patients will often use the term depression to describe the inexplicable fatigue and tiredness that accompanies many serious physical diseases. It may be that the depression said to follow infectious hepatitis and mononucleosis, tuberculosis, cardiac failure, and metastatic cancer is simply this feeling of fatigue.[6]

A more complex set of cognitive and mood disturbances follows catastrophic or mutilating events.[195] Depressed, sad, and pessimistic mood is coupled with a negative evaluation of the future, of caregivers, or of one's capacity to improve or recover. This demoralization is not usually accompanied by vegetative symptoms, cognitive decline, marked changes in psychomotor activity, or psychotic symptoms. Thus it meets only the criteria for adjustment disorder with depressed mood, although in some cases it seems continuous with a longstanding dysthymic disorder. While demoralization is often a therapeutic challenge, it poses few diagnostic questions; it comes after the full impact of a given disease has been felt. It is seen after major traumas: burns, spinal cord injury, amputation, ileostomy and colostomy, and mutilative head and neck surgery.[192] It follows the diagnosis of life-threatening disorders: ischemic heart disease, cerebrovascular disease, and malignancy.[47,127,201,386] It also develops in the course of chronic painful or disabling diseases, especially when patients are poorly managed without education or participation: complicated diabetes, rheumatoid arthritis, epilepsy, renal dialysis, and sickle cell disease.[248,294]

Occasionally the "demoralization" label may misdirect the physician's attention away from relevant organic factors. Depression in COPD may also be due to a hypoxia-induced decline in catecholamine production.[173] Dysphoric mood in uremic[13] and dialysis patients[393] may be a reflection of impaired cerebral metabolism, as shown by slow waves on the EEG.[272,393] In the aftermath of cerebrovascular accidents (CVAs), not only demoralization but also endogenomorphic

depressions may emerge.[289] While it is often the discovery, rather than the biology, of hypertension that causes symptoms,[290] and while the question of sedation versus true depression in the course of antihypertensive treatment is not fully settled,[16,37,325,385] occasionally iatrogenic psychotic depressions can be seen.[203]

A full depressive syndrome, with dysphoric mood, psychomotor and cognitive changes, and biological vegetative symptoms, may indeed be the harbinger of underlying medical disorders, especially in those late-middle-age patients who had good adjustments to life and who have not experienced recent psychosocial stress. Kerr[179] found five of twenty-eight older males who presented with depression developed a malignancy within four years. Their depression had an insidious onset, no precipitants, and only transient therapeutic responses in a course of slow deterioration. In a group of depressed, paranoid elderly patients, half had significant medical diseases.[359] Other series show a high incidence of hearing loss.[71] In investigations of pancreatic cancer,[109] depression preceded the diagnosis and even the onset of pain and was present in 75 percent of cases. In similarly advanced cases of carcinoma of the colon, only 20 percent of subjects had a depression. The depression of cancer of the pancreas was not marked by guilt, delusions, paranoia, suicide, or cognitive loss. It did present at times with episodes of marked, unexplained anxiety.

It is not surprising that endocrine disorders often present with depression, since the brain is a sensitive end-organ and will manifest changes prior to those in skin, adipose tissue, or blood pressure control.[59,300] The absence of thyroid hormone has devastating effects on the developing brain (cretinism), but even in the adult, it produces a range of serious disturbances,[257,271] from apathetic depression[352] to subcortical dementia[354] to a full-blown "myxedema madness."[10,86] The latter resembles melancholia with psychotic features.[94,140] Hyperthyroidism usually presents with anxiety, but its apathetic form in the elderly may be diagnosed as a depression complicated at times by cardiac arrhythmias.[9,346,350]

Two-thirds of patients with Cushing's disease may meet Research Diagnostic Criteria for a major affective disorder,[140] and even the vegetative signs of depression may precede the obesity, hirsutism, and striae.[326] The paranoid delusions that emerge in severe cases do so from affective rather than schizoid context.[94] Addison's disease is accompanied by depressive symptoms.[85] The extent of remission of these symptoms is not complete after treatment with electrolytes, even though the fatigue and hypotension disappear without steroid replacement. Pituitary deficiency may mimic depression or other psychiatric disorders: Simmond's disease used to be in the differential diagnosis of anorexia nervosa.[93]

In disorders of the parathyroid, there does not seem to be a CNS need for a given parathormone effect, only a requirement for a carefully controlled calcium level.[267] (The latter is understandable given the central role calcium plays in neurotransmitter release.) Mental changes covary with serum calcium above 12;[267,283,323] mEq per l calcium levels between 12 and 16 are often associated with depression, which merges into delirium with calciums above 16 mEq per l. While about 40 percent of patients with hyperparathyroidism have mental symptoms, in only 12 percent are they the presenting feature.[172] The many other causes of hypercalcemia also induce mental changes (metastatic malignancy, sarcoidosis, osteoporosis with immobilization, and vitamin D intoxication). In hypocalcemia, tetany and neuromuscular twitching can present as anxiety; primary hypoparathyroidism is associated with basal ganglia calcification and some cognitive loss, and cases of hypomania and depression have been described.[81,305]

The hypoglycemia of exogenous or endogenous insulin excess usually induces an agitated, intoxicated state, but gradually developing neuroglycopenia may imitate some of the symptoms of depression, especially fatigue, and headache.[236,284] The development of depression in the carcinoid syndrome is mostly of theoretical interest; the tumor may act as a tryptophan-sink.[167] The relationship of sex hormones and mood is controversial, especially concerning the issues of menopausal precipitation of psychiatric disorders and the validity of the premenstrual tension syndrome. It is clear, however, that oral contraceptives can precipitate major affective disorders in a small percentage of women.[103]

An ingenious theory has been proposed to explain depression in hypoxic states.[173] Tyrosine hydroxylase activity is reduced at levels of anoxia that leave the rest of the metabolic activity of the neuron intact. Reduced availability of norepinephrine is, of course, one of the hypotheses for depression. If indeed catecholaminergic neurons and especially their synapses are more sensitive to metabolic disturbances than other neural elements, then the frequent appearance of depression in a variety of deficiency disorders (thiamine deficiency,[363] pellagra,[218] B_{12} deficiency,[335] and low folate levels[285]) is more understandable, since many vitamins function as cofactors in metabolic pathways. Lassitude, fatigability, and depression regressed with folate replacement in folate-deficient patients.[39,285] The suggestion of a final common metabolic pathway to organic depression through reduced catecholaminergic transmission is analogous to the hypocholinergic theory for deliriogenesis.[30] Major organ failure may act through this mechanism: Depression is common in COPD, congestive cardiac failure, uremia, and liver disease.*

Certain pharmacological agents have a direct effect on noradrenergic neurons[17,314,315] (antihypertensives, beta-blockers, aliphatic phenothiazines, Antabuse, isoniazid, cycloserine, and ethambutol). The use of central adrenergic stimulants (caffeine, amphetamines, and cocaine) may be followed by rebound depressions.[16,130,314,315]

Membrane stability also plays a critical role in neurotransmission. Depression associated with calcium disorders was mentioned under parathyroid disorders. In sodium/water dis-

*See references 3, 98,242,277,279,330, and 357.

orders[372] the initial mental alteration is depression,[301] with delirium with psychotic features[49] emerging if the sodium falls below 120 mEq per l and seizures likely at 110 mEq per l.[209] On the other hand, hypokalemia appears to cause a sense of fatigue through a peripheral mechanism of muscle weakness, rather than a true depression through a cerebral effect.[127] Magnesium deficiency, especially in alcoholic patients, presents with irritability and depression.[128] Fatigue, rather than a true depression, seems to be the complication of anemia and iron deficiency.

The mechanism of depression in infectious disease is a comparable mix of peripheral and central effects.[308] Tuberculosis and brucellosis induce a great deal of tiredness, and recovery from viral hepatitis is prolonged partly due to enforced bed rest, but there is a possibility that influenza and infectious mononucleosis[52,126] might have specific cerebral effects. There are major affective changes, of course, after recovery from encephalitis.[84,149,392] The mental changes in the course of acquired immune deficiency syndrome (AIDS) are yet to be worked out, but both reactive and organic components are present.

Depression is a common complication of cerebral lesions. In MS, it seems to conform to an adjustment disorder, since patients with multiple, extensive cerebral demyelination develop a shallow euphoric mood with cognitive deficits, and the mostly spinal patients with good insight are depressed.[356] There is frequently a reactive depression to the knowledge of brain tumors.[151,327] However, tumors around the third ventricle, including pituitary tumors, can present with depression.[70,233,383] In the late stages of primary and secondary tumors, when increased intracranial pressure occurs, depression, psychomotor retardation, and apathy are common.[181,218] Subdural hematomas may also cause depression.[4,342] The motor manifestations of basal ganglia disorders tend to overshadow their specific affective changes.[155] Immobile, depressive facial expression is common in parkinsonism, but there is also a true depression.[247] Wilson's disease and Huntington's disease may both present with an affective disorder. Lack of effort, poor motivation, and psychomotor retardation are the main features of depression in basal ganglia disorders.[164,227,369,375]

Mood disorders can be a specific complication of strokes.[107,118] The incidence of major depression in a six-month period following a stroke is 34 percent, while dysthmic symptoms occur in a further 26 percent.[291] The positive dexamethasone suppression test in many post-CVA depressed patients indicates a relationship to an endogenous or melancholic depression and a hypothalamic dysfunction and predicts a response to tricyclic antidepressants. The suggestion that cerebral lateralization may play a part connects this issue with the notion of a nondominant hemispheric contribution to the regulation of affect.[18,105]

Two of the vascular inflammations affecting the CNS are complicated by depression. Systemic lupus has protean neuropsychiatric manifestations, including depressive affect and even psychotic depression.* It is difficult to differentiate such depression from steroid psychosis.[132,202] (Steroid psychosis emerges in 18 percent of patients treated for any disorder with daily prednisone dosage exceeding 80 mg.[38]) Tapering the steroids and electroconvulsive therapy (ECT) helped some patients with affective disorders secondary to steroids, while tricyclics did not.[202] In elderly patients, the temporal arteritis-polymyalgia-rheumatica complex often presents with dysphoria, headache, and aches and pains, and prompt treatment with steroids will prevent blindness and the possible onset of a delirium.[299,361] Periarteritis nodosa also has psychiatric complications, usually delirium.[108]

A provocative review by Himmelhoch[148] suggests that as many as 10 percent of affective disorder patients may have a subictal convulsive disorder. Their clinical presentation may be more dramatic, their mood may

*See references 15,23,24,44,68,110,169,229, and 260.

fluctuate or cycle more, and they may not do well on tricyclic antidepressants and neuroleptics but may improve with carbamazepine. Careful EEG studies with temporal lobe recordings are needed in order to clarify this issue.

Secondary mania in medical illness[194] is less common than depression, and its incidence may reflect the true organic contribution to affective disturbances in the absence of psychological grief reactions to the presence of a disability. Hepatic encephalopathy[279] goes through a disinhibited, euphoric stage; MS patients with cerebral demyelination[356] and patients with neurosyphilis[82] are often euphoric, irresponsible, and disinhibited. Increased sympathetic activity in hypoglycemia,[236] hyperthyroidism,[388] and porphyria[115] mimic hypomania. Exogenous steroids are associated with mood elevation, while similar levels of endogenous steroids appear to be mood depressants.[94] Perhaps other psychoactive agents include adrenocorticotrophic hormone (ACTH) and corticotrophin-releasing factor (CRF), as Cushing's syndrome originating from a hypothalamic problem is more often complicated by depression than is the primary adrenal variety.[94] It is possible, therefore, that the secondary reduction of CRF and ACTH by exogenous steroids is the event responsible for the development of euphoria.

Lesions of the orbitofrontal aspects of the frontal lobe are associated with disinhibited, shallow euphoric and impulsive behavior that may mimic hypomania. Dorsolateral lesions produce retardation and apathy and may mimic depression.[33]

Is There an Organic Anxiety Disorder?

Anxiety, in the sense of worry over unpleasant possibilities, is a ubiquitous response to illness. It occurs after an initial denial and cognitive clarification, and it may lead into a period of depression.[249] In a more extensive, syndromal sense, it occurs in two forms: generalized and paroxysmal.[8] Generalized anxiety has persistent symptoms in the motor sphere (tension and restlessness), in the autonomic system (sweating, vasoconstriction, and diarrhea), in cognitive processing (distractibility and hypervigilance), and in cognitive content (rumination and anticipation of problems). Panic anxiety comes on in paroxysms of fear, dyspnea, palpitations, chest discomfort, hyperventilation, dizziness, depersonalization, fear of death, and a sense of impending doom. It is clear in the hierarchical diagnostic system of DSM-III that if anxiety occurs in the context of delirium, dementia, psychoses, or affective disorders, as is the case often enough, those diagnoses are made without independent reference to anxiety. On the other hand, primary anxiety disorders have so many somatic symptoms that these may overshadow the mental components and may masquerade as "spastic colon," "cardiac neurasthenia," "tension headaches," "battle fatigue," or "hyperventilation syndrome."[167]

The early recognition of anxiety or a state of hyperarousal and the role of the ascending reticular formation[159] has recently been complemented by discoveries concerning a noradrenergic system from the locus coeruleus[67] balanced by a GABA (gamma-aminobutyric acid)-ergic inhibitory system, where an endogenous benodiazepinelike ligand may play a part. Anxiety as a sympathomimetic state is a useful concept to link caffeinism[121] and overuse of sympathomimetic amines and amphetamines[135] with such endogenous evocations of sympathetic activity as hypoxia, hypoglycemia, hyperthyroidism, and pheochromocytoma.*

The presenting state of hyperthyroidism mimics generalized anxiety quite closely, including all the symptoms just described. In rare cases, the state may progress to exhilaration, manic episodes, and agitated delusional syndromes.[354] Panic episodes are not common, except as nocturnal awakenings in a terror state with tachycardia. In thyroiditis, there may be rapid mood changes as well.

*See references 83,94,236,272, and 354.

The rare syndrome of pheochromocytoma, on the other hand, tends to present as panic attacks.[163]

Hypoxia and hypoglycemia act as focal points to a variety of very different disorders and thereby bring order into what appeared to be a list of random associates.[272] Hypoxia (arterial oxygen tension less than 60 mm Hg) is seen in pulmonary embolization, pneumonia, atelectasis, asthma, fat emboli, COPD /emphysema, and adult respiratory distress syndrome, among other conditions. Hypoglycemia (glucose less than 30 mg/dl) is seen not only after insulin and oral antidiabetics, but also in a reactive manner after subtotal gastrectomy, in early diabetes, and after large carbohydrate loads and, spontaneously, especially with fasting, in islet tumors of the pancreas, cirrhosis, Addison's disease, and hypopituitarism.[236] (Despite this strong connection between hypoglycemia and anxiety, the majority of people diagnosed as "hypoglycemic" by fad nutritionists probably suffer from primary anxiety and psychological maladjustment.)

There are specific cerebral ways of evoking anxiety, perhaps the most dramatic of which is the terror and sudden sinking feeling that accompanies some partial complex seizures from the temporal lobe (uncinate fits).[76,138,230] Subacute encephalitis can present as a state of marked agitation.[149] Transient ischemic attacks (TIAs) involving some of the "silent" areas of the brain may show up as puzzling anxiety attacks with vague neurological signs, as can episodes of MS, but anxiety with TIAs has a time frame of hours rather than minutes. In the early stages, cerebral tumors, Wilson's disease, or Huntington's chorea can present with progressive mood lability and periodic anxiety before specific neurological symptoms emerge.* Peripheral neuromuscular excitability may add to whatever central nervous stimulation exists in the hypocalcemia of hypoparathyroidism or in hyperventilation.[81,167,305]

Anxiety is also described in Cushing's disease and other cases of hypercortisolemia and in the milder degrees of hypercalcemia. It is likely, however, that the anxiety in these disorders is part of a larger depressive syndrome.

Anxiety is part of a syndrome of dizziness, mood lability, and headache that follows head injury.[241] The inverse correlation between the severity of this "postconcussion" syndrome and actual brain tissue loss led to a belief of psychogenic etiology.[216,217] Tissue loss, however, is not a good measure of the extent of blunt trauma, which may have a major impact on the limbic and upper mesencephalic areas. Affective changes and attentional problems may be the only indicators of this real pathology.[28]

Headache and anxiety are common complications of high blood pressure. Careful studies in medical clinics have demonstrated, however, that while 75 percent of known hypertensives complained of anxiety and headache, only 16 percent of patients ignorant of their diagnosis and with equally severe high blood pressure did so.[332]

Anxiety is common in heart disease,[125,317] where much of it is clearly reactive. However, panic disorder and anxiety are thought to be associated with the mitral valve prolapse syndrome (MVPS)[102] and a hyperbetaadrenergic state, and treatment with propranolol has been proposed.[167] However, as both anxiety and the presence of a *systolic* click and murmur are common in the general population, the association of MVPS and anxiety may be a chance correlation.

The instances of anxiety in hypoglycemia, hypertension, MVPS, and head injury indicate the very great care necessary in sorting out psychogenic anxiety from the proposed "organic anxiety syndrome."[228] A final complication is that many patients with medical disease are habituated to sleeping pills, sedatives, benodiazepines, or alcohol. This habituation may be denied or perhaps not even noticed by the subject, family, and physician. Emergence of anxiety, insomnia, and tremor in such cases results from a withdrawal reaction and probably represents the most common instance of organic anxiety syndrome.[228]

*See references 35,36,164,227,262, and 295.

"Personality Disorder": The Problems of Negligent, Oppositional, Difficult, and Aggressive Patients with Brain Dysfunction

A good percentage of psychiatric consultations arise from the physician's difficulty in getting along with a patient or the patient's problems in adhering to the medical regime. Interpersonal difficulties are the stuff of literature and everyday living and not yet of science. There are, however, individuals who have a minimum of medical symptoms and a paucity of formal psychiatric signs, yet whose modes of perceiving reality and attempts to adjust to it are significantly altered by the presence of medical disease, as it affects the brain. (We will not discuss here the way medical disease affects behavior through the psychosocial mechanism of illness behavior.[329])

The clinical features of organic personality syndrome in DSM-III[8] include at least one of the following behavioral changes: (1) emotional lability, (2) impaired impulse control, (3) apathy and indifference, and (4) suspicions or paranoid ideation. As these changes are common in other major organic mental syndromes, the central features characterizing those should be largely absent, though mild cognitive impairment or irritability may be present. Lezak's[205,206] list is similar: (1) emotional alteration to apathy, silliness, lability, irritability, and changes in sex drive; (2) impaired impulse control, restlessness, and impatience; and (3) decreased behavioral initiative, difficulty in planning, and social dependence due to stimulus-bound behavior. She adds two features: (4) impaired capacity for social perceptiveness, with loss of self-reflective and self-critical attitude; and (5) inability to profit from experience in social contacts, even when the ability to absorb new information is intact.

Goldstein[117] contrasted these general responses of the organism to the specific neuropsychological effects of focal lesions. Head injury (both blunt and penetrating), cerebrovascular accidents, primary cerebral tumors and neurosurgical resections, systemic disorders that metastasize to the brain (cancer of the lung, breast, and ovaries; bacterial endocarditis, and septicemia), brain abcesses, and systemic diseases with multiple cerebrovascular involvement manifest these symptoms during the early part of their course.* All of these have the capacity to precipitate later delirium or to render the patient demented.

Subtle forms of slowly developing metabolic encephalopathies may present the same characterological picture. The irascible personality of the uremic patient, the facile, irresponsible cirrhotic patient, and the indifferent hypothyroid patient are well-known clinical presentations.[166,254,330]

More specific behavioral alterations are associated with relatively focal brain lesions in the absence of neurological signs. (These "silent areas" of the brain do speak eloquently to the observer equipped with the right tools of observation—not the reflex hammer.) The *International Classification of Diseases*, ninth edition (ICD 9),[82] formally recognizes a frontal lobe syndrome[142] consisting of diminution of self-control, foresight, creativity, and spontaneity; and emotional dullness, lack of drive, slowness or impulsiveness, outbursts, and fatuous humor. DSM-III[8] also alludes to two forms of personality change in frontal lobe damage: one of emotional lability and loss of impulse control and one of apathy and indifference. Blumer and Benson[33] make a case for relating the former "pseudopsychopathic" picture to lesions of the orbital surface, and the latter "pseudodepressed" form to lesions of the dorsal lateral convexity. As most lesions (especially the infectious or toxic types) are not so clearly restricted, mixed forms are more common.

The functions of the frontal lobe have been extensively explored by Luria,[221,222] Pribram,[274] and European psychiatrists (Kleist, Goldstein, and Oppenheim). Yet there are no "frontal lobe tests" in routine psychometric evaluation (WAIS, Wechsler Memory, etc.) that are thus likely to turn up false negatives. The Halsted Categories Test or Wisconsin Card Sorting Task should be specifically re-

*See references 7,11,170,193, and 340.

quested to demonstrate the difficulty in shifting conceptual sets characteristic of frontal lobe damage.[204]

Neurosyphilis used to be the prime example of frontal lobe type psychopathology.[9,137] The moody, egocentric man who lost his social refinement as well as his insight might soon develop grandiose delusions and increasing psychosis and then degenerate to a demented, vegetative existence. Nowadays, the common cause of a less rapidly progressive frontal lobe damage is chronic alcoholism.[74,77] The early organic personality changes are generally and inaccurately attributed to a preexistent character defect, although studies show a correlation between lifetime alcohol consumption and subtle indices of brain damage.[89,158] The potential reversibility of neuropsychological and even anatomical features of alcoholic brain damage[55] indicates a need to detect this disorder in its organic personality disorder phase, before it progresses to a full-blown dementia, when it has a poor prognosis.[158]

Blunt head injury has been shown to lead to frontal lobe contusions and demyelination in the white matter and the brain stem tegmentum.[28] Careful psychometric testing[122] and the use of brain stem auditory EPs and electronystograms[296] have demonstrated physiological brain stem disturbances and subtle cognitive deficits in the postconcussive syndrome.[241] Doubt is thrown on the former identification of this syndrome with "accident neurosis."[243] ICD 9[8] does list a postconcussion syndrome characterized by features of a frontal lobe lesion or of any of the neurotic disorders, but in which, in addition, headache, giddiness, fatigue, insomnia, and subjective mental impairment are prominent. It is claimed that the syndrome is more common in subjects with previous psychological difficulties or where there is a possibility of compensation. One wonders, however, whether the level of functional disability associated with *any* organic disorder is not likewise affected by past problems or future hopes.

Alexander's review of the effects of blunt head trauma implicates specific neuro-anatomical lesions with specific psychological problems.[28] Fronto-polar features include decreased judgment and problem-solving ability and an apathetic attitude. Orbitofrontal syndromes include impulsive, socially irresponsible behavior. Anterior temporal lobe damage involves memory loss and impaired new learning. Brain stem tegmentum demyelination is associated with decreased attention, vestibular dysfunction, and subtle cerebellar, pyramidal, and extrapyramidal signs. Diffuse white matter lesions are associated with motor, cognitive, and concentration problems.[28] Subtle brain damage may follow open heart surgery[391] or prolonged heart block.[78] Other causes of personality changes due to brain damage include subarachnoid hemorrhage,[333,334] which gives rise to a frontal lobe type of picture, an amnesic syndrome, or frank dementia.

Psychiatrists have long observed a variety of personality changes with epilepsy.[32,105,310] Kraepelin remarked on the intellectual slowness, persistence, and circumstantiality of epileptics; their religiosity; and their deep-running, angry irritability. Under the influence of psychoanalysts, many of these traits were given a dynamic interpretation. Geschwind and other neurologists[18,19,27,28] recently began to emphasize, however, a specific biological relationship between persistent, repetitive, partial complex seizures from the anterior temporal lobes and the development of a "hyperconnection" syndrome. While the frontal syndromes are due to a "disconnection" and while the Kluver-Bucy syndrome is the temporal lobe variety of disconnection, the increased, repetitive electrical activity in the limbic system seems to induce a "hyperconnection," a partial inverse of the Kluver-Bucy syndrome. Such patients demonstrate viscosity, circumstantiality, hypergraphia, verbosity, increased emotional depth, irritability and anger, mood swings, a decrease in sexual interests, and arousal. There are deep philosophical and religious interests and a strong sense of justice combined with an almost awkward, helpful attitude. Bear[18,19] was able to distinguish temporal lobe epileptics from a control group based on a questionnaire developed from these observations.

Subtle differences were apparent between groups of patients with left- and right-sided lesions. In one, the "tarnishers," the subjects found faults and responded negatively to their problems, while the "polishers" minimized their difficulties and wished to appear better than expected.[18] The Boston group regards these personality changes as the milder and earlier part of a continuum leading to atypical affective disorders and "epileptic" psychoses.[32] It would seem appropriate to follow Blumer's[32] suggestion and engage in careful prospective phenomenological and electrophysiological studies to delimit the syndromes, rather than to squeeze them into a preexistent classification (i.e., "schizophreniform" or "nonspecific organic personality"). Bear's[18] observation should also be heeded; perhaps the majority of patients with recurrent partial-complex seizures develop these personality traits, but perhaps only a minority will allow them to dominate their life to the extent that a formal personality disorder can be diagnosed. Thus the prevention of the personality disorder would require both meticulous pharmacology to reduce the incidence of ictal events and kindling and educational psychotherapy to help the patient monitor and control a propensity for viscosity, hyperemotionality, and self-righteousness.[32]

The practical problems associated with the diagnosis of organicity in patients presenting with personality disorders can be illustrated by three controversial disorders: MS, Wilson's disease, and episodic dyscontrol.

The early notion[53,356] that MS was a psychosomatic disorder in the sense that personality factors and psychic trauma played a part in its etiology has been rejected.[218] The diagnostic trap of attributing some early symptoms of MS to hysteria is now well known.[2] The personality changes that develop with this chronic, disabling disorder can very naturally be attributed to reactive factors. However, careful psychometric and postmortem studies suggest that two different personality

changes exist with different etiologies.[268,344] Extensive cerebral demyelination leads to a euphoric, careless, cognitively impaired state,[293] while the relative preservation of cerebral white matter in conjunction with severe spinal demyelination often leads to depression and pessimism, based probably on demoralization and failure of psychological defenses. Whitlock and Siskind's[387] study even showed a higher incidence of "endogenous" depression in patients with MS who were not demented than in patients with other CNS disorders matched for the severity of their disabilities. That this is not a simple mechanism of increased general psychopathology is suggested by the observation that the association of MS and psychosis is only a chance concurrence.[80]

Wilson's disease[370] is a rare condition, but it can be dramatically misdiagnosed in its early phases.[295,369] Over half the patients have psychological abnormalities, and these are the presenting symptoms in 25 percent. These include emotional lability, explosiveness, immaturity, feelings of anxiety and despondence, and, occasionally, delusional ideas.[164,303]

The issues in MS and Wilson's disease are different. Personality change is late in MS and does not lead to medical diagnostic confusion; it has important bearing, however, on the type of psychotherapeutic techniques used. In Wilson's disease, the psychiatric presentation can significantly delay the necessary medical diagnosis and intervention; psychotherapy is not necessary if effective copper chelation takes place.

Even the very existence of the third disorder, episodic dyscontrol syndrome, is controversial.[12] While the episodes are described as "seizurelike," preceded by a period of impending tension and followed by remorse, headache, and drowsiness, there is usually no evidence of seizure activity. Soft neurological signs and abnormal EEGs are reported in about half of these cases, and there is often a history of "hyperkinetic" disorder of childhood. On the other hand, the subjects usually come from the lower socioeconomic classes, have witnessed a good deal of violence, and have family histories of alcoholism, violence, and sociopathy. While the majority of subjects are reported to respond to phenytoin, the lack of double-blind conditions and longer follow-ups reduces the strength of the argument. While it is important to bear in mind the biological causes of violence[235] in a cultural atmosphere that espouses psychodynamic and social explanations, one should not prematurely establish syndromes based on single features (see intermittent explosive disorder in DSM-III) that may not be separable from other disorders or other concomitants of violent antisocial behavior.

A final note of caution applies to the very diagnosis of a personality disorder and concerns the distinction between state and trait features. Recurrent, rather than persistent, behavioral changes may well be due to unrecognized or hidden repeated intoxications, either by alcohol, sedatives, marijuana, stimulants, or solvent inhalants or by industrial toxins (heavy metals, organophosphates, or fumes).[187,212,340] Dramatic state changes may occur with acute exposure, and there may be a subtle, long-lasting behavioral deterioration as well. A careful, chronological history from family and employer is more important than the patient's own biased or confused account.

"Neurotic Disorders": Mistaken Invitations to Psychotherapy

In the older literature, there are many case reports of medical disorders presenting with "neurotic symptoms." Careful reading would reveal that the majority of these referred to anxiety disorders, depression, and fatigue[226,234] (in the guise of neurasthenia). There remain, however, the conversion symptoms and the dissociative reactions of hysteria, as well as that perennial semantic confound, the demonstrative histrionic personality who overreacts to illness and becomes mislabeled as a "hysteric." There is also the ever-present danger of an unusual set of organic symptoms being labeled "hysterical" by the uninitiated. Compulsions, intrusive obsessional thoughts, body-image distortion, and hypochondriasis are other neurotic symptoms evoked by physical disease.

Once again, it should be made clear that the stress of disease can evoke any number of psychological defenses by chronic psychodynamic neurotic processes; other life stresses lead to disease stimulation and confabulation.[29,57] This section deals with a different, less common situation: when the biological disease process itself provokes the apparent neurotic phenomena.

Slater's seminal article[321] demonstrated that about a quarter of the patients confidently diagnosed as "hysteric" at a leading neurological institute go on to reveal the more classical symptoms of their initially unrecognized physical disease. Hysteria seems to presage organic brain disease, and the incidence of conversion symptoms is greater than that of other neurotic symptoms in patients with a history of brain damage.[240,384] Other disorders with a high frequency of pseudohysterical presentations include MS,[41,269] myasthenia gravis,[177] Wilson's disease,[295] porphyria,[1] and spinal root or cervical cord compression.[177]

The common denominator seems to be the patient's subjective complaint of a neurological symptom unaccompanied by easily detectable or classical neurological signs. In this context, several other, more common disorders may be misdiagnosed as hysteria: transient ischemic attacks, early peripheral neuropathy, and Ménière's disease.[127] The sometimes profound muscular weakness in hypokalemia[246] and Addison's disease[328] and the episodic weakness and confusion evoked by hypoglycemia[236] due to insulin, islet cell tumor, or postgastrectomy have been ascribed to hysteria. Certain syndromes may not be recognized by the nonspecialist: language disorders in dominant-hemisphere lesions,[25,95] dressing and other apraxias in the parietal lobe syndromes[75,157] (including those caused by tumor and CVAs), and movement disorders in rheumatic disease, early Huntington's chorea, and Wilson's disease.[380] The distinction between seizures and pseudoseizures[288] becomes progressively more difficult with the sophistication of the patients and their exposure to the seizures of fellow patients or family members. However, as most pseudoseizures seem to occur in people with real seizures as well, this becomes a management issue rather than a dichotomizing diagnostic point.

Sudden, reversible amnesic episodes due to bilateral hippocampal dysfunction[28] can closely mimic hysterical fugue states: transient global amnesia, drug intoxication (anticholinergics and benzodiazepines), chemical poisoning (organophosphates), unrecognized hypoglycemic episodes, and transient metabolic encephalopathies, especially anoxia.[28] Postconcussion confusion can be followed by a period of apparently normal behavior during which the anterograde amnesia continues.[218] Depersonalization and derealization are common features of partial complex seizure disorder from temporal lobe foci[138] and may be the first, transient symptoms of other limbic lobe disorders: viral encephalitis, limbic encephalopathy associated with systemic cancer, and limbic tumors. These dissociative symptoms and transient body-image distortions also occur in severe migraine. Compulsions were common in postencephalitic parkinsonism,[304] and EEG spiking in the anterior aspects of frontal lobe has been described in some obsessive patients. Finally, narcolepsy[279,396] is often misdiagnosed by inexperienced observers as a psychogenic disorder. Sleep attacks, hypnagogic hallucinations, catalepsy, and sleep paralysis can appear in various strange combinations, complicated by adjustment difficulties and personality changes.[380]

¶ The Medically Ill Mental Patient: Double Jeopardy

Chronic mental patients are handicapped in the area of physical health care by a variety of psychological and social factors.[134] Conceptual disorganization leads to lack of self-observation; social ineptitude leads to difficulty in getting care; and intermittent lapses in reality-testing lead to lack of compliance and difficulty in health education. Many such patients live in poverty and isolation and suffer from neglect or malnutrition. Others pursue unhealthy life-styles with lack of exercise, consumption of "junk food," smoking, and alcohol and drug misuse. In the asylums of past years, tuberculosis, hepatitis, and gastroenteritis were endemic, and there were epidemics of pellagra. Today's revolving-door patient comes in with infestations, neglected skin infections, and cracked or blistered feet. There is an increased incidence of tuberculosis, bronchopneumonia, and chronic obstructive pulmonary disease. Malnutrition not infrequently results in scurvy, thiamine deficiency, and low folate levels.[56,162] Both obesity and cachexia are common. Poor compliance with complicated and sustained medical treatment makes the management of epilepsy, diabetes, and hypertension very difficult. Even during medical hospitalization, chronic mental patients may end up getting inferior care; due to miscommunication with health care personnel, interpersonal difficulties, and unusual personal habits, there may be pressures to discharge these patients prematurely, or they may leave against medical advice or reject needed diagnostic or therapeutic interventions.

Patients in long-term psychotherapy fare much better, but certain aspects of the therapeutic process mitigate against the early recognition of a newly emerging disease. Therapist and client alike are likely to focus on the symbolic meaning and personal significance of symptoms rather than on their physiological origin. The problem is intensified if the therapist is a nonmedical professional.

There are multiple biological reasons for somatic illness in psychiatric patients as well. Prolonged immobility leads to deep-vein thrombosis and pulmonary emboli, which may present as anxiety. Agitation requiring restraints or multiple intramuscular injections can result in myoglobinuria and renal failure, causing a confusional state. Psychogenic polydipsia and inappropriate antidiuretic hormone secretion[167] can cause dilutional hyponatremia, presenting as depression, apathy, and confusion.

The most potent biological causes of somatic symptoms are the medications and nonmedicinal psychoactive substances and OTC drugs ingested by patients.[17,111,127] Tricyclic antidepressants, anticholinergics, aliphatic phenothiazines, and some OTC sleep medications, frequently taken in combination, will cause the central anticholinergic syndrome. Noradrenergic blockade (tricyclics, phenothiazines) can lead to postural hypotension and intermittent weakness and confusion. Tricyclics may lead to heart block, bradycardia, and intermittent disorientation. The sedative effects of major and minor tranquilizers and antidepressants are at times misinterpreted as depressogenic by patients and families. On the other hand, the insomnia and rebound restlessness and anxiety following prolonged sedative-hypnotic use is often not attributed to the agents and leads to unnecessary medical investigations.

The extrapyramidal manifestation of the high-potency neuroleptics includes not only Parkinson's disease and acute dystonic reactions, but also an akathisic-restless syndrome that presents with increased anxiety and even exacerbated psychotic symptoms. Further use of neuroleptics to reduce these symptoms of course only makes them worse. Neuroleptics impair temperature regulation and may help to induce both hypothermia and malignant hyperthermia. Psychotropic drug use is occasionally associated with hyponatremia due to inappropriate secretion of antidiuretic hormone,[301] which may present with weakness, lethargy, or increased intensity of psychotic symptoms. Lithium can cause some subtle effects. The polyuria of lithium is well recognized, as is the difficulty in concurrently using diuretics. Mild goiter formation is not uncommon and hypothyroidism can develop so insidiously that its symptoms of lassitude may be attributed to an emerging depression.[331]

Alcohol abuse is common among psychiatric patients and is associated with intoxication and withdrawal, liver disease, pancreatitis, gastrointestinal bleeding, nutritional deficiencies, peripheral neuropathy, proximal myopathy, cardiomyopathy, nutritional and chronic toxic effects on the cerebrum or cerebellum, increased incidence of trauma, subdural hematomas, and seizure disorders.[207,312] Several of these disorders or frank deliria (liver failure, pancreatitis, and malnutrition) can present with increased anxiety, or depression. Others (Wernicke's syndrome, alcoholic cerebral atrophy, and subdural hematoma) present with global mental disorders with amnesia, confabulation, and gradual confusion. Yet others may be dismissed as hysterical if the examiner does not recognize the gait of cerebellar atrophy, which coexists with normal finger-nose and even heel-shin tests; the syndrome of alcohol-tobacco amblyopia; or the focal neuropathies so easily evoked by pressure on nutritionally deficient peripheral nerves.

Intravenous (IV) drug abuse has a well-known morbidity involving the skin, peripheral veins, and introduced infections of bacterial endocarditis and hepatitis.[263] Liver damage may also be sustained from the circulating impurities. However, liver failure seems an uncommon complication. The kidney is affected by the glomerulonephritis of endocarditis, the secondary effects of viral hepatitis, occasional myoglobinuria, and necrotizing angiitis; there is an increasing incidence of renal failure requiring dialysis. IV-drug-using psychiatric patients can thus present with the mental symptoms of uremia (personality change, depression, and delirium), with embolic manifestations from the endocarditis, or with delirium from septicemia or other systemic infections. One of the challenges in looking after medically sick addicts is to separate the behavioral disturbances of their psychological makeup and sociocultural background from the toxic and withdrawal symptoms of their polysubstance use on the one hand and the neuropsychiatric complications of their medical disorders on the other.

The recent emergence of AIDS was accompanied by both severe psychosocial complications to the news of a fatal, debilitating, sexually and intravenously transmissible disease and a plethora of neuro-psychiatric symptoms, from abcesses and meningitis caused by opportunistic infections to septicemia, pneumonia, and metabolic disorders.

Hoffman and Koran[150] review the reasons for potential misdiagnosis of medical disease in mental patients: The symptoms of the physical and mental disease may overlap and may be easily misattributed; the patient may be confused, difficult, or just a poor witness; and the physician may be systematically prone to error. Physician-related factors include incomplete assessments; acceptance of plausible but incorrect assumptions; and reliance on inadequate consultation, "routine physicals," and "medical clearances." To correct some of these problems, a medical screening using algorithms and laboratory tests has been devised.[188]

¶ Management of Patients Whose Psychological Symptoms May Have Organic Origin

The diagnostic literature[127,192,218] reviewed so far gives a sense of the empirical associations between psychiatric and medical syndromes. The literature on the pathophysiology of symptoms is just emerging from a dominance of naturalistic studies in the context of medical pathology[167] and from the shadow of psychoanalytic speculations.[60] There are some promising beginnings in a neuroscience-based pathophysiology,[17] but it is yet to be integrated into medical thinking.

The literature on management, however, is weaker than that on diagnosis or pathophysiology. There are only a few controlled studies. Clinical need necessitates the combination of medical interventions, psychopharmacologic treatment, and even psychosocial maneuvers, with the subsequent difficulty in apportioning the improvement among the different factors.

Some fundamental questions remain unanswered: Will a depression secondary to a medical illness respond to antidepressants alone, or to medical treatment, or to a combination of both? Post-CVA depression and depression in cancer would provide our affirmative to the first question,[291] folate or B_{12} deficiency depression[343] and depression in hyperparathyroidism[172,267] to the second. Does psychotherapy play a similar role in the treatment of secondary psychiatric disorders as in the management of their primary counterpart? Does the phenomenological resemblance of a medical disorder to a psychiatric syndrome imply a similar response to psychotropic medications?

The currently prevailing symptomatic approach to treatment is based more on clinical experience than on formalized studies. It is supported in a suggestive rather than a definitive manner by the "final common pathway" hypotheses for anxiety, depression, and psychoses and the mechanism of drug action in these syndromes.[17,67] If anxiety is fueled by locus coeruleus overactivity from a variety of causes, then benzodiazepine-induced facilitation of GABA inhibition of that system or direct inhibition by a postsynaptic beta-blocker or a presynaptic alpha-agonist will be effective. Likewise, if the full depressive syndrome (precipitated by a variety of biopsychosocial factors) is a behavioral and vegetative counterpart of reduced limbic and hypothalamic catecholaminergic and/or serotonergic activity, then antidepressants, ECT, or lithium should reverse it. Finally, to the extent that the florid symptoms of a psychosis are a reflection of increased dopaminergic activity triggered by a range of etiologies, dopaminergic blockade by antipsychotics will reverse them.

The use of these psychotropic agents in the context of a medical disease is complicated by age, frailty, pharmacokinetic problems, potential drug-drug interactions, and the impact of unintended side effects on other disease-affected systems (especially potential anticholinergic effects on a dysfunctional brain). The dangers of an untreated psychiatric complication may be greater, however, than those from well-defined and predictable drug side effects, especially with careful monitoring of plasma levels and target organ effects.[278,360] Antidepressant treatment seems helpful in post-CVA depression,[218] organic emotionalism,[196] post-myocardial infarct depression,[278,360] and depression in cancer.[46] Prophylactic lithium reduced the psychiatric complications from ACTH treatment.[167] On the other hand, tricyclics were not useful in steroid-induced depression,[132] and ECT has been used in delusional depression complicating Cushing's disease.[167] In frail, elderly patients, amphetamine-type psychostimulants have been used instead of the more risky tricyclics for moderate apathy and depression, with good results.[178]

The psychotic complications of delirium and aspects of the organic delusional syndrome are currently best treated by haloperidol.[212] Relatively small doses (2 to 10 mg/day) seem to suffice in the frail and elderly, and parenteral titration to a behavioral end point is possible without inducing drowsiness or cardiovascular or respiratory side effects. In hepatic failure, the use of renally excreted benzodiazepines that put few demands on the liver in their metabolism is more advised (oxazepam and lorazepam).

Only the principles of medical management can be commented on here, but they are perhaps useful for psychiatrists, since they are often in a position to coordinate the efforts of several subspecialists who are likely to forget these basic, general suppositions. Acute treatment is often directed to the main precipitating pathogen (e.g., antibiotics for pneumonia) without necessarily attending to the predisposing causes (e.g., immune deficiency or repeated inhalations) or to the sustaining or contributing factors (hypoxia contributing to restlessness and lack of cooperation). Medical treatment itself may lead to psychiatric complications, but the debate over the status of steroid psychosis should give pause before recommending the withdrawal of a biologically necessary regime.

The psychosocial management of the global cognitive disorder (delirium and/or dementia) encompasses attention to the regulation and timing of sensory input, provision of familiar and orienting helpers and objects, reduction of stress, help and simplification of cognitive tasks, and regulation of sleep and daytime activities.[212,397] Cognitive retraining regimes have been designed for amnesia and the effects of focal brain injury.[63] The literature is largely silent on specific psychosocial approaches to mood and behavior disorders that result directly from biological factors. Lezak[205] provides an approach based on the subtle cognitive deficits that underlie "characterological" changes, and N. L. Mace and P. V. Rabins, in their book *The 36 Hour Day* (1981), describe a family-based regime. It is likely that the increased interest in the integrative approach by geriatric and geropsychiatric medicine, dealing as it does with aging complicated by disease processes, may lead to the development of more specific psychotherapeutic, environmental engineering, and health education techniques.[50]

¶ Conclusion

The critical knowledges and skills necessary for the psychiatrist in the management of physical diseases presenting with psychological symptoms include a knowledge of psychiatric phenomenology, an understanding of the biopsychological pathophysiology of such symptoms, familiarity with the wide variety of presentations of common medical disorders, an acquaintance with the range of unusual but not unlikely diseases, an ability to use psychotropic agents in conjunction with medical therapies, and a facility to communicate clearly with the patient, family, nursing staff, and medical consultants. All these skills depend on a fundamental attitude of seeing oneself as a medical subspecialist or, even more centrally, as a primary care provider. Seen in this light, the remedicalization of psychiatry is not a tactical move, nor just a response to recent advances in the neurosciences, but a return to our roots in clinical medicine in the best Hippocratic tradition.

¶ Bibliography

1. ACKNER, B., et al. "Acute Porphyria: A Neuropsychiatric and Biochemical Study," *Journal of Psychosomatic Research,* 6 (1962):1–24.

2. ADAMS, D. K., SUTHERLAND, J. M., and FLETCHER, W. B. "Early Clinical Manifestations of Disseminated Sclerosis," *British Medical Journal,* 2 (1950): 431–436.

3. ADAMS, R. D. "Neurological Manifestations of Chronic Pulmonary Insufficiency," *New England Journal of Medicine,* 257 (1957):579–590.

4. ALARCON, R. D., and THWEATT, R. W. "A Case of Subdural Hematoma Mimicking Severe Depression with Conversion-like Symptoms," *American Journal of Psychiatry,* 140 (1983):1360–1361.

5. ALBERT, M. L., FELDMAN, R. G., and WILLIAMS, A. L. "The 'Subcortical Dementia' of Progressive Supranuclear Palsy," *Journal of Neurology, Neurosurgery and Psychiatry,* 37 (1974):121–130.

6. ALLAN, F. N. "Differential Diagnosis of Weakness and Fatigue," *New England Journal of Medicine,* 231 (1944):414–418.

7. ALPERS, B. J. "Relation of Hypothalamus to Disorders of Personality," *Archives of Neurology and Psychiatry,* 38 (1937): 291–303.

8. AMERICAN PSYCHIATRIC ASSOCIATION. *Diagnostic and Statistical Manual of Mental Disorders,* 3rd ed. (DSM-III). Washington, D. C.: American Psychiatric Association, 1980.

9. ARNOLD, B. M., CASAL, G., and HIGGINS, H. P. "Apathetic Thyrotoxicosis," *Canadian Medical Association Journal,* 3 (1974):957–958.

10. ASHER, R. "Myxedematous Madness," *British Medical Journal,* 2 (1949):555–562.

11. AVERY, T. L. "Seven Cases of Frontal Tumor with Psychiatric Presentation," *British Journal of Psychiatry,* 119 (1971): 19–23.

12. BACH-Y-RITA, G., et al. "Episodic Dyscontrol: A Study of 130 Violent Patients," *American Journal of Psychiatry,* 127 (1971):1473–1478.

13. BAKER, A. B., and KNUTSON, J. "Psychiatric Aspects of Uremia," *American Journal of Psychiatry,* 102 (1946):683–687.

14. BAKER, M., "Psychopathology in Systemic Lupus Erythematosis," *Seminars in Arthritis and Rheumatism,* 3 (1973):95–110.

15. BAKER, M., et al. "Psychopathology in Systemic Lupus Erythematosis, II," *Seminars in Arthritis and Rheumatism,* 3 (1973):111–126.

16. BANT, W. P. "Antihypertensive Drugs and Depression: A Reappraisal," *Psychological Medicine,* 8 (1978):725.

17. BARCHAS, J. D., et al., eds. *Psychopharmacology: From Theory to Practice.* New York: Oxford University Press, 1977.

18. BEAR, D. M. "The Temporal Lobes: An Approach to the Study of Organic Behavioral Changes." in M. Gazzaniga, ed., *Handbook of Behavioral Neurobiology,* vol. 2, *Neuropsychology.* New York: Plenum Press, 1979, pp. 75–95.

19. BEAR, D. M., and FEDIO, P. "Quantitative Analysis of Interictal Behavior in Temporal Lobe Epilepsy," *Archives of Neurology,* 34 (1977):454–467.

20. BECK, J. C. "Dementia in the Elderly: The Silent Epidemic," *Annals of Internal Medicine,* 97 (1982):231–241.

21. BECKER, D. M., and KRAMER, S. "The Neurological Manifestations of Porphyria: A Review," *Medicine,* 56 (1977):411–423.

22. BELL, D. S. "Comparison of Amphetamine Psychosis and Schizophrenia," *British Journal of Psychiatry,* 111 (1965): 701–707.

23. BENNAHUM, D. A., and MESSNER, R. P. "Recent Observations on Central Nervous Systemic Lupus Erythematosis," *Seminars in Arthritis and Rheumatism,* 4 (1975):253–256.

24. BENNETT, R., et al. "Neuropsychiatric Problems in Systemic Lupus Erythematosis," *British Journal of Medicine,* 4 (1972):342–345.

25. BENSON, D. F. "Psychiatric Aspects of Dysphasia," *British Journal of Psychiatry,* 123 (1973):555–556.

26. ———. "The Treatable Dementias," in D. F. Benson and D. Blumer, eds., *Psychiatric Aspects of Neurologic Disease.*

New York: Grune & Stratton, 1982, pp. 123–148.

27. BENSON, D. F., and BLUMER, D. eds. *Psychiatric Aspects of Neurologic Disease.* New York: Grune & Stratton, 1975.

28. ———. *Psychiatric Aspects of Neurologic Disease,* vol. 2. New York: Grune & Stratton, 1982.

29. BERLYNE, N. "Confabulation," *British Journal of Psychiatry,* 120 (1972):31–39.

30. BLASS, J. P., and PLUM, F. "Metabolic Encephalopathies in Older Adults," in R. Katzman and R. Terry, eds., *The Neurobiology of Aging.* Philadelphia: F. A. Davis, 1983, pp. 189–220.

31. BLUMER, D. "Temporal Lobe Epilepsy and Its Psychiatric Significance," in D. F. Benson and D. Blumer, eds., *Psychiatric Aspects of Neurological Disease,* New York: Grune & Stratton, 1975, pp. 171–198.

32. BLUMER, D., ed. *Psychiatric Aspects of Epilepsy.* Washington, D.C.: American Psychiatric Press, 1984.

33. BLUMER, D., and BENSON, D. F. "Personality Changes with Frontal and Temporal Lobe Lesions," in D. F. Benson, and D. Blumer, eds., *Psychiatric Aspects of Neurological Disease.* New York: Grune & Stratton, 1975, pp. 151–170.

34. ———. "Psychiatric Manifestations of Epilepsy," in D. F. Benson and D. Blumer, eds., *Psychiatric Aspects of Neurological Disease,* vol. 2. New York: Grune & Stratton, 1982, pp. 25–47.

35. BLUSTEIN, J. E. "Further Observations on Brain Tumors Presenting as Functional Psychiatric Disturbances," *Psychiatric Journal of the University of Ottawa,* 197 (1976):21–26.

36. BLUSTEIN, J. E., and SEEMAN, M. V. "Brain Tumors Presenting as Functional Psychiatric Disturbances," *Canadian Psychiatric Association Journal,* 17 (1972):55–59.

37. BOSTON COLLABORATIVE DRUG SURVEILLANCE PROGRAM. "Psychiatric Side Effects of Non-psychiatric Drugs." *Seminars in Psychiatry,* 3 (1971):406.

38. ———. "Acute Adverse Reaction to Prednisones in Relation to Dosage," *Clinical Pharmacology,* 13 (1972):694–697.

39. BOTEZ, M. I., and REYNOLDS, E. H., eds.

Folic Acid in Neurology, Psychiatry and Internal Medicine. New York: Raven Press, 1979.

40. BOWDEN, C. L., and BURSTEIN, A. G. *Psychosocial Basis of Medical Practice,* 2nd ed. Baltimore: Williams & Wilkins, 1979.

41. BRAIN, W. R. "Critical Review: Disseminated Sclerosis," *Quarterly Journal of Medicine,* 23 (1930):343–391.

42. BRAIN, W. R. and NORRIS, F. H., eds. *The Remote Effects of Cancer on the Nervous System.* New York: Grune & Stratton, 1965.

43. BRENNAN, L. V. and CRADDOCK, P. R. "Limbic Encephalopathy as a Nonmetastatic Complication of Oat Cell Lung Cancer," *American Journal of Medicine,* 75 (1983):518–520.

44. BRESNIHAN, B. "CNS Lupus," *Clinical Rheumatic Disease,* 8 (1982):183–195.

45. BREWER, C., and PERRETT, L. "Brain Damage Due to Alcohol Consumption: An Airencephalographic, Psychometric and Electroencephalographic Study," *British Journal of Addiction,* 66 (1971): 170–182.

46. BRODSKY, L., and BRODSKY, V. "Reconciling Silent Psychoses Accompanying Medical or Surgical Problems," *Psychosomatics,* 25 (1984):191–196.

47. BUKBERG, J., PENMAN, D., and HOLLAND, J. C. "Depression in Hospitalized Cancer Patients," *Psychosomatic Medicine,* 46 (1984):199–212.

48. BURKE, A. W. "Physical Disorder Among Day Hospital Patients," *British Journal of Psychiatry,* 133 (1978):22–27.

49. BURNELL, G. M., and FOSTER, T. A., "Psychosis with Low Sodium Syndrome," *American Journal of Psychiatry,* 128 (1972):133–134.

50. BUTLER, R. N., and LEWIS, M. I. *Aging and Mental Health,* 2nd ed. Saint Louis: C. V. Mosby, 1977.

51. BYER, J. A., and EASTON, J. D. "Therapy of Ischemic Cerebrovascular Disease," *Annals of Internal Medicine,* 93 (1980): 742–756.

52. CADRE, M., NYE, F. J., and STOREY, P. "Anxiety and Depression After Infectious Mononucleosis," *British Journal of Psychiatry,* 128 (1976):559–561.

53. CAPLAN, L. R., and NADELSON, T. "Multi-

ple Sclerosis and Hysteria," *Journal of the American Medical Association,* 243 (1980):2418–2421.

54. CAPLAN, L. R., and SCHOENE, W. C. "Clinical Features of Subclinical Cortical Arteriosclerotic Encephalopathy (Binswanger Disease)," *Neurology,* 28 (1978):1206.

55. CARLEN, P. L., et al. "Reversible Cerebral Atrophy in Recently Abstinent Chronic Alcoholics Measured by Computed Tomography Scans," *Science,* 200 (1978): 1076–1078.

56. CARNEY, M.W.P. "Serum Folate Values in 423 Psychiatric Patients," *British Journal of Medicine,* 4 (1967):512–516.

57. CARNEY, M.W.P., and BROWN, J. P. "Clinical Features and Motives Among 42 Artifactual Illness Patients," *British Journal of Medical Psychology,* 56 (1983):57–66.

58. CARNEY, M.W.P., and SHEFFIELD, B. F. "Serum Folic Acid and B_{12} in 272 Psychiatric Inpatients," *Psychological Medicine,* 8 (1978):139–144.

59. CARROLL, B. J. "Mood Disturbances and Pituitary-adrenal Diseases," *Psychosomatic Medicine,* 39 (1977):54.

60. CAVENAR, J. O., and BRODIE, H.K.H., eds. *Signs and Symptoms in Psychiatry.* Philadelphia, J.B. Lippincott, 1983.

61. CELESIA, G. G., and BARR, A. N. "Psychosis and Other Psychiatric Manifestations of Levodopa Therapy," *Archives of Neurology,* 23 (1970):193–200.

62. CELESIA, G. G., and WANAMAKER, W. M. "Psychiatric Disturbances in Parkinson's Disease," *Diseases of the Nervous System,* 33 (1972):577–583.

63. CERMAK, L. S. *Improving Your Memory.* New York: McGraw-Hill, 1976.

64. CHAMBERS, W. R. "Neurosurgical Conditions Masquerading as Psychiatric Diseases," *American Journal of Psychiatry,* 112 (1955):387–389.

65. CHAPMAN, L. F., and WOLF, H. G. "Diseases of Neopallium," *Medical Clinics of North America,* 42 (1958):677–690.

66. CHARATAN, F. B., and BRIERLEY, J. B. "Mental Disorder Associated with Primary Lung Carcinoma," *British Medical Journal,* 1 (1956):765–768.

67. CHARNEY, D. S., HENINGER, G. R., and

BREIER, A. "Noradrenergic Function in Panic Anxiety," *Archives of General Psychiatry,* 41 (1984):751–763.

68. CLARK, E. C., and BAILEY, A. A. "Neurological and Psychiatric Signs Associated with Systemic Lupus Erythematosus," *Journal of the American Medical Association,* 160 (1956):455–457.

69. COHEN, K. L., and SWIGAR, M. E. "Thyroid Function in Screening in Psychiatric Patients," *Journal of the American Medical Association,* 242 (1979):254–257.

70. COHEN, L. M., GREENBERG, D. B., and MURRAY, G. B. "Neuropsychiatric Presentation of Men with Pituitary Tumors (the Four A's)," *Psychosomatics,* 25 (1984):925–928.

71. COOPER, A. F., KAY, D.W.K, and CURRY, A. R. "Hearing Loss in Paranoid and Affective Psychoses of the Elderly," *Lancet,* 2 (1974):851–854.

72. CORKIN, S., et al. *Alzheimer's Disease: A Report of Progress in Research.* New York: Raven Press, 1982.

73. CORSELLIS, J.A.N., GOLDBERG, G. J., and NORTON, A. R. "Limbic Encephalitis and Its Association with Carcinoma," *Brain,* 91 (1968):481–496.

74. COURVILLE, C. B. *Effects of Alcohol on the Nervous System of Man.* Los Angeles: San Lucas Press, 1955.

75. CRITCHLEY, M. "Psychiatric Symptoms and Parietal Disease: Differential Diagnosis," *Proceedings of the Royal Society of Medicine,* 57 (1964):422–428.

76. CURRIE, S., et al. "Clinical Course and Prognosis of Temporal Lobe Epilepsy: A Survey of 666 Patients," *Brain,* 94 (1971): 173–190.

77. CUTTING, J. "Alcoholic Dementia," in D. F. Benson, and D. Blumer, eds., *Psychiatric Aspects of Neurologic Disease,* vol. 2, New York: Grune & Stratton, 1982, pp. 149–165.

78. DALESSIO, D. J., BENCHIMOL, A., and DIMOND, E. G. "Chronic Encephalopathy Related to Heart Block," *Neurology,* 15 (1965):499–503.

79. DAVIES, D. W. "Physical Illness in Psychiatric Outpatients," *British Journal of Psychiatry,* 11 (1965):27–33.

80. DAVISON, K., and BAGLEY, C. R. "Schi-

zophrenia-like Psychoses Associated with Organic Disorders of the Central Nervous System," in R. N. Herrington, ed., *Current Problems in Neuropsychiatry. British Journal of Psychiatry.* Special Publication No. 4. Kent: Headley Bro., 1979.

81. DENKO, J. D., and KAELBING, R. "The Psychiatric Aspects of Hypoparathyroidism," *Acta Psychiatrica Scandinavica,* 38 (Supplement 164). (1962):1–70.

82. DEWHURST, K. "The Neurosyphilitic Psychoses Today: A Survey of 91 Cases," *British Journal of Psychiatry,* 115 (1969):31–38.

83. DOUST, B. C. "Anxiety as a Manifestation of Phaeochromocytoma," *Archives of Internal Medicine,* 102 (1958):811–815.

84. DRACHMAN, D. A., and ADAMS, R. D. "Herpes Simplex and Acute Inclusive Body Encephalitis," *Archives of Neurology,* 7 (1962):45–63.

85. DRAKE, F. R. "Neuropsychiatric-like Symptomatology of Addison's Disease; a Review," *American Journal of Medical Science,* 234 (1957):106–113.

86. EASSON, W. M. "Myxedema with Psychosis," *Archives of General Psychiatry,* 14 (1966):277–283.

87. EASTWOOD, M. R., and TREVELYAN, M. H. "Relationship Between Physical and Psychiatric Disorder," *Psychological Medicine,* 2 (1972):363–372.

88. EASTWOOD, M. R., MINDHAM, R.H.S., and TENNENT, T. G. "The Physical Status of Psychiatric Emergencies," *British Journal of Psychiatry,* 116 (1970):545–550.

89. ECKHARDT, M. J., et al. "Relationship Between Neuropsychological Performance and Alcohol Consumption in Alcoholics," *Biological Psychiatry,* 13 (1978):551–556.

90. ENGEL, G. L. "The Need for a New Medical Model: A Challenge for Biomedicine," *Science,* 196 (1977):129.

91. ———. "The Clinical Application of the Biopsychosocial Model," *American Journal of Psychiatry,* 137 (1980):535–544.

92. ENGEL, G. L., and ROMANO, J. "Delirium: A Syndrome of Cerebral Insufficiency," *Journal of Chronic Disease,* 9 (1959): 260–277.

93. ESCAMILLA, R. F., and LISSER, H. "Simmonds Disease: A Clinical Study with Review of the Literature, Differentiation from Anorexia Nervosa by Statistical Analysis of 595 Cases, 101 of Which Were Proved Pathologically Ill," *Clinical Endocrinology,* 2 (1942): 65–96.

94. ETTIGI, P. G., and BROWN, G. M. "Brain Disorders Associated with Endocrine Dysfunctions," in H. C. Hendrie, ed., *Psychiatric Clinics of North America,* 1 (1978):117–136.

95. FABER, R., et al. "Comparison of Schizophrenic Patients with Formal Thought Disorder and Neurologically Impaired Patients with Aphasia," *American Journal of Psychiatry,* 140 (1983):1348–1351.

96. FAUMAN, M. A.: "The Emergency Psychiatric Evaluation of Organic Mental Disorders," *Psychiatric Clinics of North America,* 6 (1983):233–257.

97. FEINGLASS, E. J., et al. "Neuropsychiatric Manifestations of Systemic Lupus Erythematosus: Diagnosis, Clinical Spectrum, and Relationship of Other Features to Disease," *Medicine,* 55 (1976):323–339.

98. FERRER, M. I. "Mistaken Psychiatric Referral of Occult Serious Cardiac Disease," *Archives of General Psychiatry,* 18 (1968):112–113.

99. FILSKOV, S. B., and BOLL, T. J. *Handbook of Clinical Neuropsychology.* New York: John Wiley & Sons, 1981.

100. FISHER, C. M. "Lacunes: Small Deep Cerebral Infarcts," *Neurology,* 15 (1965): 774–784.

101. ———. "Communicating Hydrocephalus," *Lancet,* 1 (1978):37–40.

102. FLANNERY, J. G., and SZMUILOWICZ, J. "Psychiatric Implications of the Mitral Valve Prolapse Syndrome (MVPS)," *Canadian Journal of Psychiatry,* 24 (1979):740–743.

103. FLEMING, O., and SEAGER, C. P. "Incidence of Depressive Symptoms in Users of the Oral Contraceptives," *British Journal of Psychiatry,* 132 (1978):431–440.

104. FLEMINGER, R. "Visual Hallucinations and Illusions with Propranolol," *British Medical Journal,* 1 (1978):1182.

105. FLOR-HENRY, P. "Psychosis and Tempo-

ral Lobe Epilepsy," *Epilepsia,* 10 (1969): 363–395.

106. FOLSTEIN, M. F., FOLSTEIN, S. E., and McHUGH, P. R. "Mini-mental State," *Journal of Psychiatry Research,* 12 (1975):189–198.

107. FOLSTEIN, M. F., MAIBERGER, R., and McHUGH, P. R. "Mood Disorder as a Specific Complication of Stroke," *Journal of Neurology, Neurosurgery and Psychiatry,* 40 (1977):1018–1021.

108. FORD, R. G., and SIEKERT, R. G. "Central Nervous System Manifestations of Periarteritis Nodosa," *Neurology,* 15 (1965): 114–122.

109. FRAS, L., LITIN, E. M., and PEARSON, J. S. "Comparison of Psychiatric Symptoms of Carcinoma of the Pancreas with Those in Some Other Intra-abdominal Neoplasms," *American Journal of Psychiatry,* 123 (1967):1553–1562.

110. GANZ, V. H., et al. "The Study of the Psychiatric Symptoms of Systemic Lupus Erythematosus," *Psychosomatic Medicine,* 34 (1972):207–220.

111. GARDNER, E. R., and HALL, R. C.W. "Psychiatric Symptoms from Over-the-counter Drugs," *Psychosomatics,* 23 (1982):186–190.

112. GELENBERG, A. J. "The Catatonic Syndrome," *Lancet,* 1 (1976):1339–1341.

113. GIBSON, J. G. "Emotions and the Thyroid Gland: A Critical Appraisal," *Journal of Psychosomatic Research,* 6 (1962):93–116.

114. GLICKMAN, L. S. *Psychiatric Consultation in the General Hospital.* New York: Marcel Dekker, 1980.

115. GOLDBERG, A. "Acute Intermittent Porphyria: A Study of 50 Cases," *Quarterly Journal of Medicine,* 28 (1959):183–209.

116. GOLDEN, C. J., et al. *Clinical Neuropsychology.* New York: Grune & Stratton, 1983.

117. GOLDSTEIN, K. "The Effect of Brain Damage on the Personality," *Psychiatry,* 15 (1952):245–260.

118. GOODSTEIN, R. K. "Overview: Cerebrovascular Accident and the Hospitalized Elderly—A Multidimensional Clinical Problem," *American Journal of Psychiatry,* 140 (1983):141–147.

119. GOODWIN, D. W., and GUZE, S. B. *Psychi-* *atric Diagnosis,* 3rd ed., New York: Oxford University Press, 1984.

120. GOWARDMAN, M. G. "Problems of Diagnosis and Management of Neurosyphilis in Psychiatric Hospital: Report of 10 Cases," *New Zealand Medical Journal,* 72 (1970):178–182.

121. GREDEN, J. "Anxiety or Caffeinism? A Diagnostic Dilemma," *American Journal of Psychiatry,* 131 (1974):1089–1092.

122. GRONWALL, D., and WRIGHTSON, P. "Delayed Recovery of Intellectual Function After Minor Head Injury," *Lancet,* 2 (1974):605–609.

123. GUZE, S. B. "The Occurrence of Psychiatric Illness in Systemic Lupus Erythematosus," *American Journal of Psychiatry,* 123 (1967):1562–1570.

124. HACHINSKI, V. C., LASSEN, N. A., and MARSHALL, J. "Multiinfarct Dementia: A Cause of Mental Deterioration in the Elderly," *Lancet,* 2 (1974):207–210.

125. HACKETT, T. P., and CASSEM, N. H. *Massachusetts General Hospital Handbook of Hospital Psychiatry.* St. Louis: C. V. Mosby, 1978.

126. HAFSTROM, T. "Neurological Complications of Mononucleosis," *Acta Neurologica Scandinavica,* 39 (1963): 69–81.

127. HALL, R.C.W., ed. *Psychiatric Presentations of Medical Illness: Somatopsychic Disorders.* New York: Spectrum Publications, 1980.

128. HALL, R.C.W., and JOFFE, J. R. "Hypomagnesia," *Journal of the American Medical Association,* 224 (1978):1749–1751.

129. HALL, R.C.W., GRUZENSKI, W. P., and POPKIN, M. K. "Differential Diagnosis of Somatopsychic Disorders," *Psychosomatics,* 20 (1979):381–389.

130. HALL, R.C.W., STICKNEY, S. K., and GARDNER, E. R. "Behavioral Toxicity of Nonpsychiatric Drugs," in R.C.W. Hall, ed., *Psychiatric Presentations of Medical Illness.* New York: SP Medical and Scientific Books, 1980, pp. 337–405.

131. HALL, R.C.W., et al. "Physical Illness Presenting as a Psychiatric Disease," *Archives of General Psychiatry,* 35 (1978): 1315–1320.

132. HALL, R.C.W., et al. "Presentation of the

Steroid Psychosis," *Journal of Nervous and Mental Disease,* 167 (1979):229–236.

133. HALL, R.C.W., et al. "Physical Illness Manifesting as Psychiatric Disease," *Archives of General Psychiatry,* 37 (1980): 989–995.

134. HALL, R.C.W., et al. "The Medical Care of Psychiatric Patients," *Hospital and Community Psychiatry,* 33 (1982):25–34.

135. HAMBURG, D. A., and ADAMS, J. E. "A Perspective on Coping Behavior: Seeking and Utilizing Information in Major Transitions," *Archives of General Psychiatry,* 17 (1967):277–284.

136. HAMMERSTEN, J. F., and SMITH, W. O. "Symptomatic Magnesium Deficiency in Man," *New England Journal of Medicine,* 256 (1957):897–899.

137. HARE, E. H. "The Origin and Spread of Dementia Paralytica," *Journal of Mental Science,* 105 (1959):594–626.

138. HARPER, M., and ROTH, M. "Temporal Lobe Epilepsy and the Phobic Anxiety-depersonalization Syndrome, Parts 1 and 2," *Comprehensive Psychiatry,* 3 (1962):129–151, 215–226.

139. HART, R. J., and McCURDY, P. R., "Psychosis in Vitamin B-12 Deficiency," *Archives of Internal Medicine,* 128 (1971): 596–597.

140. HASKETT, R. F., and ROSE, R. M. "Neuroendocrine Disorders and Psychopathology," *Psychiatric Clinics of North America,* 4 (1981):239–252.

141. HAYMAN, M. A., and ABRAMS, R. "Capgras' Syndrome and Cerebral Dysfunction," *British Journal of Psychiatry,* 130 (1977):68–71.

142. HECAEN, H., and ALBERT, M. L. "Disorders of Mental Functioning Related to Frontal Lobe Pathology," in D. F. Benson and D. Blumer, eds., *Psychiatric Aspects of Neurologic Disease.* New York: Grune & Stratton, 1975, pp. 137–149.

143. HEINE, B. E. "Psychiatric Aspects of Systemic Lupus Erythematosis," *Acta Psychiatrica Scandinavica,* 45 (1969):307–326.

144. HENDRIE, H. L., ed. "Brain Disorders: Clinical Diagnosis and Management," *Psychiatric Clinics of North America,* 1 (1978).

145. HENKER, F. O. "Acute Brain Syndromes," *Journal of Clinical Psychiatry,* 40 (1979):117–120.

146. HERKERT, E. E., WALD, A., and ROMERO, O. "Tuberous Sclerosis and Schizophrenia," *Diseases of the Nervous System,* 33 (1972):439–445.

147. HERRIDGE, C. "Physical Disorders in Psychiatric Illness," *Lancet,* 2 (1960):949–951.

148. HIMMELHOCH, J. M. "Major Mood Disorders Related to Epileptic Changes," in D. Blumer, ed., *Psychiatric Aspects of Epilepsy.* Washington, D.C.: American Psychiatric Press, 1984, pp. 271–294.

149. HIMMELHOCH, J. M., et al. "Subacute Encephalitis: Behavioral and Neurological Aspects," *British Journal of Psychiatry,* 116 (1970):531–538.

150. HOFFMAN, R. S., and KORAN, L. M. "Detecting Physical Illness in Patients with Mental Disorders," *Psychosomatics,* 25 (1984):654–660.

151. HOLMES, G. "Discussion on the Mental Symptoms Associated with Cerebral Tumors," *Proceedings of the Royal Society of Medicine,* 24 (1931):65–67.

152. HOLMES, J. M. "Cerebral Manifestations of Vitamin B_{12} Deficiency," *British Medical Journal,* 2 (1956):1394–1398.

153. HOLMES, T. H. "Life Situations, Emotions and Disease," *Psychosomatics,* 19 (1978):747–754.

154. HOLT, R. E., et al. "Computed Tomography of the Brain and the Psychiatric Consultation," *Psychosomatics,* 23 (1982):1007–1009.

155. HORN, S. "Some Psychological Factors in Parkinsonism," *Journal of Neurology, Neurosurgery and Psychiatry,* 37 (1974):27–31.

156. HOROWITZ, M. J. "Flashbacks: Recurrent Intrusive Images After LSD," *American Journal of Psychiatry,* 126 (1969):565–569.

157. HORTON, P. C. "Personality Disorder and Parietal Lobe Dysfunction," *American Journal of Psychiatry,* 133 (1976):782–785.

158. HORVATH, T. B. "Clinical Spectrum and Epidemiological Features of Alcohol Dementia," in J. G. Rankin, ed., *Alcohol, Drugs and Brain Damage.*

Toronto: Addiction Research Foundation, 1975, pp. 1–16.

159. ———. "Arousal and Anxiety," in A. D. Burrows and B. Davies, eds., *Handbook of Studies on Anxiety.* Amsterdam: Elsevier/North Holland, 1980, pp. 89–109.

160. HORVATH, T. B., et al. "The Late Components of the Cerebral Event Related Potential in Alzheimer's Dementia," in L. W. Poon, ed., *Handbook of Clinical Memory Assessment of the Older Adults.* Washington, D.C.: American Psychological Association, in press.

161. HUNTER, R., et al. "Serum B$_{12}$ and Folate Concentrations in Mental Patients," *British Journal of Psychiatry,* 113 (1967):1291–1295.

162. HURDLE, A.D.F., and PICTON-WILLIAMS, T. C. "Folic Acid Deficiency in Elderly Patients Admitted to Hospital," *British Medical Journal,* 2 (1966):202–205.

163. HUTCHINSON, G. B., EVANS, J. A., and DAVIDSON, D. C. "Pitfalls of the Diagnosis of Phaeochromocytoma," *Annals of Internal Medicine,* 48 (1958):300–309.

164. INOSE, T. "Neuropsychiatric Manifestations in Wilson's Disease," *Birth Defects,* 4 (1968):74–77.

165. JACOBS, B. L. "Dreams and Hallucinations: A Common Neurochemical Mechanism Mediating Their Phenomenological Similarities," *Neuroscience Biobehavioral Review,* 2 (1978):59.

166. JAIN, V. K. "Affective Disturbances in Hypothyroidism," *British Journal of Psychiatry,* 119 (1971):279.

167. JEFFERSON, J. W., and MARSHALL, J. R. *Neuropsychiatric Features of Medical Disorders.* New York: Plenum Press, 1981.

168. JOHNSON, J. "Organic Psycho-syndromes Due to Boxing," *British Journal of Psychiatry,* 115 (1969):45–53.

169. JOHNSON, R. T., and RICHARDSON, E. P. "The Neurological Manifestations of Systemic Lupus Erythematosus," *Medicine,* 47 (1968):337–369.

170. JONES, H. R., SIEKERT, R. G. and GEVACI, J. E. "Neurological Manifestations of Bacterial Endocarditis," *Annals of Internal Medicine,* 71 (1969):21–28.

171. KANE, F., and FLORENZANO, R. "Psychosis Accompanying the Use of Broncho-

dilator Compounds," *Journal of the American Medical Association,* 215 (1971):2116.

172. KARPATI, G., and FRAME, B. "Neuropsychiatric Disorders in Primary Hyperparathyroidism," *Archives of Neurology,* 10 (1964):387–397.

173. KATZ, L. R. "Is There a Hypoxic Affective Syndrome?" *Psychosomatics,* 23 (1982): 846–853.

174. KATZMAN, R. "Normal Pressure Hydrocephalus," in C. E. Wells, ed., *Dementia.* Philadelphia: F. A. Davis, 1977, pp. 69–92.

175. KATZMAN, R., and TERRY, R. D. *The Neurology of Aging.* Philadelphia: F. A. Davis, 1983.

176. KATZMAN, R., TERRY, R. D., and BICK, K. L., eds. *Alzheimer's Disease: Senile Dementia and Related Disorders.* New York: Raven Press, 1978.

177. KAUFMAN, D. M. *Clinical Neurology for Psychiatrists.* New York: Grune & Stratton, 1981.

178. KAUFMAN, M. W., MURRAY, G. B., and CASSEM, N. H. "Use of Psychostimulants in Medically Ill Depressed Patients," *Psychosomatics,* 23 (1982):817–819.

179. KERR, T. A., SCHAPIRA, K., and ROTH, M. "The Relationship Between Premature Death and Affective Disorders," *British Journal of Psychiatry,* 115 (1972):1277–1282.

180. KERSCHNER, M., BENDER, M. B., and STRAUSS, I. "Mental Symptoms in Cases of Tumor of the Temporal Lobe," *Archives of Neurology and Psychiatry,* 35 (1936):572–596.

181. ———. "Mental Symptoms Associated with Brain Tumor: A Study of 530 Verified Cases," *Journal of the American Medical Association,* 110 (1938):714–718.

182. KIMBALL, C. P. *The Biopsychosocial Approach to the Patient.* Baltimore: Williams & Wilkins, 1981.

183. KLAWANS, H. L. "Levo-dopa Induced Psychosis," *Psychiatric Annals,* 1 (1978):19–29.

184. KLEINMAN, A., EISENBERG, L., and GOOD B. "Culture, Illness and Care," *Annals of Internal Medicine,* 88 (1978):251–258.

185. KLERMAN, G. L. "Depression in the Medi-

cally Ill," *Psychiatric Clinics of North America,* 4 (1981):301–317.

186. KNIGHTS, E. B., and FOLSTEIN, M. F. "Unsuspected Emotional and Cognitive Disturbance in Medical Patients," *Annals of Internal Medicine,* 87 (1977): 723–724.

187. KOLANSKY, H., and MOORE, W. T. "Toxic Effects of Chronic Marihuana Use," *Journal of the American Medical Association,* 222 (1972):35–41.

188. KORAN, L. M., SOX, H. C., and MARTON, K. I. "Mobile Medical Screening Teams for Public Programs," *Hospital and Community Psychiatry,* 35 (1984):1151–1152.

189. KORANYI, E. K. "Physical Health and Illness in a Psychiatric Outpatient Department Population," *Canadian Psychiatric Association Journal,* 17 (supplement) (1972):109–116.

190. ———. "Morbidity and Rate of Undiagnosed Physical Illness in a Psychiatric Clinic Population," *Archives of General Psychiatry,* 36 (1979):414–419.

191. ———. "Somatic Illness in Psychiatric Patients," *Psychosomatics,* 21 (1980):887–891.

192. KORANYI, E. K., ed. *Physical Illness in the Psychiatric Patient.* Springfield, Ill.: Charles C Thomas, 1982.

193. KOZOL, H. L. "Pretraumatic Personality and Psychiatric Sequelae of Head Injury," *Archives of Neurology and Psychiatry,* 56 (1946):245–275.

194. KRAUTHAMMER, C., and KLERMAN, G. L. "Secondary Mania," *Archives of General Psychiatry,* 35 (1978):1333.

195. LARSON, E. B., et al. "Dementia in Elderly Outpatients: A Prospective Study," *Annals of Internal Medicine,* 100 (1984): 417–423.

196. LAWSON, I. R., and MACLEOD, R. D. M. "The Use of Imipramine and Other Psychotropic Drugs in Organic Emotionalism," *British Journal of Psychiatry,* 115 (1969):281–285.

197. LAZARUS, R. S. "Psychological Stress and Coping Adaptation and Illness," *International Journal of Psychiatry in Medicine,* 5 (1974):321–333.

198. LEEMAN, C. P. "Diagnostic Errors in Emergency Room Medicine: Physical Illness in Patients Labeled 'Psychiatric'

and Vice Versa," *International Journal of Psychiatry in Medicine,* 6 (1975):533–540.

199. LEVENSON, A. J., ed. *Neuropsychiatric Side-effects of Drugs in the Elderly.* New York: Raven Press, 1979.

200. LEVENSON, A. J., and HALL, R. C. W., eds. *Neuropsychiatric Manifestation of Physical Disease in the Elderly.* New York: Raven Press, 1981.

201. LEVINE, P. M., SILBERFARB, P. M., and LIPOWSKI, Z. J. "Mental Disorders in Cancer Patients: A Study of 100 Psychiatric Referrals," *Cancer,* 42 (1978):1385–1391.

202. LEWIS, D. A., and SMITH, R. E. "Steroid-induced Psychiatric Syndromes—A Report of 14 Cases and a Review of the Literature," *Journal of Affective Disorders,* 5 (1983):319–332.

203. LEWIS, W. H. "Iatrogenic Psychotic Depressive Reaction in Hypertensive Patients," *American Journal of Psychiatry* (1971):152–153.

204. LEZAK, M. D. *Neuropsychological Assessment.* New York: Oxford University Press, 1976.

205. ———. "Living with the Characterologically Altered Brain-Injured Patient," *Journal of Clinical Psychiatry,* 39 (1978):592–598.

206. ———. "Subtle Sequelae of Brain Damage," *American Journal of Physical Medicine,* 57 (1978):9–15.

207. LIEBER, C. S., ed. *Medical Disorders of Alcoholism.* Philadelphia: W. B. Saunders, 1982.

208. LIPOWSKI, Z. J. "Delirium, Clouding of Consciousness and Confusion," *Journal of Nervous and Mental Disease,* 145 (1967):227–255.

209. ———. "Review of Consultation Psychiatry and Psychosomatic Medicine. Part II, Clinical Aspects," *Psychological Medicine,* 24 (1967):201–224.

210. ———. "Consultation-liaison Psychiatry: An Overview," *American Journal of Psychiatry,* 131 (1974):623–630.

211. ———. "Psychiatry of Somatic Diseases: Epidemiology, Pathogenesis, Classification," *Comprehensive Psychiatry,* 16 (1975):105–124.

212. ———. *Delirium.* Springfield, Ill.: Charles C Thomas, 1980.

213. ———. "A New Look at Organic Brain Syndromes," *American Journal of Psychiatry*, 137 (1980):674–678.

214. ———. "Transient Cognitive Disorders (Delirium, Acute Confusional States) in the Elderly," *American Journal of Psychiatry*, 140 (1983):1426–1436.

215. LIPOWSKI, Z. J., LIPSIT, D. R., and WHYBROW, P. L. *Psychosomatic Medicine*. New York: Oxford University Press, 1977.

216. LISHMAN, W. A. "Brain Damage in Relation to Psychiatric Disability After Head Injury," *British Journal of Psychiatry*, 114 (1968):373–410.

217. ———. "The Psychiatric Sequelae of Head Injury: A Review," *Psychological Medicine*, 2 (1973):304–318.

218. ———. *Organic Psychiatry*. London: Blackwell Science Publishers, 1978.

219. LOGOTHETIS, J. "Psychotic Behavior as the Initial Indicator of Adult Myxedema," *Journal of Nervous and Mental Disease*, 136 (1963):561–568.

220. LUDWIG, A. M. "Hysteria—A Neurobiological Theory," *Archives of General Psychiatry*, 27 (1972):771–777.

221. LURIA, A. R. *Higher Cortical Functions in Man*. London: Tavistock Publishers, 1966.

222. ———. *The Working Brain: An Introduction to Neuropsychology*. New York: Basic Books, 1975.

223. LURIA, A. R., et al. "Restoration of Higher Cortical Function Following Local Brain Damage," in P. J. Vinken and G. W. Bruyn, eds., *Handbook of Clinical Neurology*, vol. 3, *Disorders of Higher Nervous Activity*. Amsterdam: North Holland Publishers, 1969, pp. 368–434.

224. MCALPINE, D. "A Review of the Nervous and Mental Aspects of Pernicious Anemia," *Lancet*, 2 (1929):643–647.

225. MACCALLUM, W. A. G. "Capgras Syndrome with an Organic Basis," *British Journal of Psychiatry*, 123 (1973):639–642.

226. MCEVEDY, C. P., and BEARD, A. W. "A Controlled Follow-up of Cases Involved in an Epidemic of 'Benign Myalgic Encephalomyelitis,'" *British Journal of Psychiatry*, 122 (1973):141–150.

227. MCHUGH, P. R., and FOLSTEIN, M. F. "Psychiatric Syndromes of Huntington's Chorea," in D. F. Benson and D. Blumer, eds., *Psychiatric Aspects of Neurological Disease*. New York: Grune & Stratton, 1975, pp. 267–286.

228. MACKENZIE, T. B., and POPKIN, M. K. "Organic Anxiety Syndrome," *American Journal of Psychiatry*, 140 (1983): 343–344.

229. MACNEILL, A., et al. "Psychiatric Problems in Systemic Lupus Erythematosus," *British Journal of Psychiatry*, 128 (1976):1365–1369.

230. MACRAE, D. "Isolated Fear: A Temporal Lobe Aura," *Neurology*, 5 (1954):497–505.

231. MAGUIRE, G. P., and GRANVILLE-GROSSMAN, K. L. "Physical Illness in Psychiatric Patients," *British Journal of Psychiatry*, 114 (1968):1365–1369.

232. MALAMUD, N. "Psychiatric Disorder with Intracranial Tumors of Limbic System," *Archives of Neurology*, 17 (1967):113–123.

233. ———. "Organic Brain Disease Mistaken for Psychiatric Disorder: A Clinicopathologic Study," in D. F. Benson, and D. Blumer, eds., *Psychiatric Aspects of Neurological Disease*. New York: Grune & Stratton, 1975, pp. 287–307.

234. MALETZKY, B. M. "The Episodic Dyscontrol Syndrome," *Diseases of the Nervous System*, 34 (1978):178–185.

235. MARKS, V. H., and ERVIN, F. R. *Violence and the Brain*. New York: Harper & Row, 1970.

236. MARKS, V. H., and ROSE, F. C. *Hypoglycemia*. Philadelphia: F. A. Davis, 1965.

237. MARSHALL, H. "Incidence of Physical Disorders Among Psychiatric Inpatients," *British Medical Journal*, 2 (1970):468–470.

238. MARTIN, M. J. "A Brief Review of Organic Diseases Masquerading as Functional Illness," *Hospital and Community Psychiatry*, 34 (1983):328–332.

239. MECHANIC, D. *Medical Sociology*, 2nd ed. New York: Free Press, 1978.

240. MERSKEY, H., and BUHRICH, N. A. "Hysteria and Organic Brain Disease," *British Journal of Medical Psychology*, 48 (1975):359–366.

241. MERSKEY, H., and WOODFORDE, J. M. "Psychiatric Sequelae of Minor Head Injury," *Brain*, 95 (1972):521–528.

242. MEYENDORF, R. "Psychopathology in

Heart Disease Aside from Cardiac Surgery: A Historical Perspective of Cardiac Psychosis," *Comprehensive Psychiatry,* 20 (1979):4.

243. MILLER, H. "Accident Neurosis," *British Medical Journal,* 1 (1961):919–925.

244. MINDHAM, R. H. S. "Psychiatric symptoms in Parkinsonism," *Journal of Neurology, Neurosurgery and Psychiatry,* 33 (1970):188–191.

245. MITCHELL, W. E. "Etiological Factors Producing Neuropsychiatric Syndromes in Patients with Malignant Diseases," *International Journal of Neuropsychiatry,* 3 (1967):464–468.

246. MITCHELL, W. E., and FELDMAN, F. "Neuropsychiatric Aspects of Hypokalemia," *Canadian Medical Association Journal,* 98 (1968):49–51.

247. MJONES, H. "Paralysis Agitans: A Clinical and Genetic Study," *Acta Psychiatrica et Neurologica,* 54 (Supplement) (1949): 1–195.

248. MOFFIC, H. S., and PAYKEL, E. S. "Depression in Medical Inpatients," *British Journal of Psychiatry,* 126 (1975):346–353.

249. MOOS, R., ed. *Coping with Physical Illness.* New York: Plenum Press, 1977.

250. MOSKOWITZ, C., MOSES, H., and KLAWANS, H. L. "Levodopa-induced Psychosis: A Kindling Phenomenon," *American Journal of Psychiatry,* 135 (1978):669–675.

251. MULDER, D. W., and DALY, D. "Psychiatric Symptoms Associated with Lesion of Temporal Lobe," *Journal of the American Medical Association,* 150 (1952):173–176.

252. MULDER, D. W., BICKFORD, R. G., and DODGE, H. W. "Hallucinatory Epilepsy: Complex Hallucinations and Focal Seizures," *American Journal of Psychiatry,* 113 (1957):1100–1102.

253. MURPHY, E., and BROWN, G. W. "Life Events, Psychiatric Disturbance and Physical Illness," *British Journal of Psychiatry,* 136 (1980):326–338.

254. MURPHY, T. L., et al. "Hepatic Coma: Clinical and Laboratory Observations on Forty Patients," *New England Journal of Medicine,* 239 (1948):605–612.

255. MYERS, J. K., et al. "Six-month Prevalence of Psychiatric Disorders in Three Communities," *Archives of General Psychiatry,* 41 (1984):959–970.

256. NAPLES, M., and HACKETT, T. P. "The Amytal Interview," *Psychosomatics,* 19 (1978):98–105.

257. NICKEL, S. N., and FRAME, B. "Neurological Manifestations of Myxedema," *Neurology,* 8 (1958):511–517.

258. NOYES, R., et al. "Anxiety Neurosis and Physical Illness," *Comprehensive Psychiatry,* 19 (1978):407–413.

259. OBRECHT, R., OKHOMINA, F. O. A., and SCOTT, D. F. "Value of EEG in Acute Confusional States," *Journal of Neurology, Neurosurgery and Psychiatry,* 42 (1979):75–77.

260. O'CONNOR, J. F., and MUSHER, D. M. "Central Nervous System Involvement in Systemic Lupus Erythematosus," *Archives of Neurology,* 14 (1966):157–164.

261. OJEMAN, R. G., et al. "Further Experience with the Syndrome of 'Normal' Pressure Hydrocephalus," *Journal of Neurosurgery,* 31 (1969):279–294.

262. OLIN, H. S., and WEISMAN, A. D. "Psychiatric Misdiagnosis in Early Neurological Disease," *Journal of the American Medical Association,* 189 (1964):533–538.

263. OSTOR, A. G. "The Medical Complications of Narcotic Addiction," *Medical Journal of Australia,* 1 (1977):410–415.

264. OVERALL, J. E., and GORHAM, D. R. "The Brief Psychiatric Rating Scale," *Psychological Reports,* 10 (1962):799–812.

265. PARSONS, O. "Cognitive Dysfunction in Alcoholics and Social Drinkers," *Journal of Studies on Alcohol,* 41 (1980):105–118.

266. PETERSON, H. W., and MARTIN, M. J. "Organic Disease Presenting as Psychiatric Syndrome," *Postgraduate Medicine,* 54 (1973):78–82.

267. PETERSON, P. "Psychiatric Disorders in Primary Hyperparathyroidism," *Journal of Clinical Endocrinology,* 28 (1968):1491–1495.

268. PEYSER, J. M., EDWARDS, K. R., and POSER, C. M. "Psychological Profiles in Patients with Multiple Sclerosis," *Archives of Neurology,* 37 (1980):437–440.

269. PEYSER, J. M., et al. "Cognitive Function in Patients with Multiple Sclerosis," *Archives of Neurology,* 37 (1980):577–579.

270. PINCUS, J. H., and TUCKER, G. J. *Behav-*

ioral Neurology, 2nd ed. New York: Oxford University Press, 1978.

271. PITTS, F. N., and GUZE, S. B. "Psychiatric Disorders and Myxedema," *American Journal of Psychiatry,* 118 (1961):142–147.

272. PLUM, F., and POSNER, J. B. *The Diagnosis of Stupor and Coma,* 3rd ed. Philadelphia: F. A. Davis, 1980.

273. POST, F. "Dementia, Depression, and Pseudodementia," in D. F. Benson and D. Blumer, eds., *Psychiatric Aspects of Neurological Disease.* New York: Grune & Stratton, 1975, pp. 99–120.

274. PRIBRAM, K. H., and LURIA, A. R. *Psychophysiology of the Frontal Lobes.* New York: Academic Press, 1973.

275. PRO, J. D., and WELLS, C. E. "The Use of the Electroencephalogram in the Diagnosis of Delirium," *Diseases of the Nervous System,* 318 (1977):804–808.

276. RABINS, V. P., and FOLSTEIN, M. F. "Delirium and Dementia: Diagnostic Criteria and Fatality Rates," *British Journal of Psychiatry,* 140 (1982):149–153.

277. RASKIN, N. H., and FISHMAN, R. A. "Neurologic Disorders in Renal Failure," *New England Journal of Medicine,* 294 (1976):143–148.

278. RASKIND, M., et al. "Cardiovascular and Antidepressant Effects of Imipramine in the Treatment of Secondary Depression in Patients with Ischemic Heart Disease," *American Journal of Psychiatry,* 139 (1982):114–117.

279. READ, A. E., et al. "Neuropsychiatric Syndromes Associated with Chronic Liver Disease and Extensive Portal Systemic Collateral Circulation," *Quarterly Journal of Medicine,* 36 (1967):135–150.

280. READING, A. "Illness and Disease," in A. Reading and T. N. Wise, eds., "Psychiatry in Internal Medicine," *Medical Clinics of North America,* 66 (1977): 703–711.

281. REICH, P., et al. "Unrecognized Organic Mental Disorders in Survivors of Cardiac Arrest," *American Journal of Psychiatry,* 140 (1983):1194–1196.

282. REID, A. A. "Schizophrenia—Disease or Syndrome?" *Archives of General Psychiatry,* 28 (1973):863–869.

283. REILLY, E. L., and WILSON, W. P. "Mental Symptoms in Hyperparathyroidism," *Diseases of the Nervous System,* 26 (1965):361–363.

284. RENNIE, T. A. C., and HOWARD, J. E. "Hypoglycemia and Tension Depression," *Psychosomatic Medicine,* 4 (1942):273–282.

285. REYNOLDS, E. H., et al. "Folate Deficiency in Depressive Illness," *British Journal of Psychiatry,* 117 (1970):287–292.

286. RICE, E., and GENDELMAN, S. "Psychiatric Aspects of Normal Pressure Hydrocephalus," *Journal of the American Medical Association,* 223 (1973):409–412.

287. RICKLER, K. C. "Neurological Diagnosis in Psychiatric Disease," *Psychiatric Annals,* 13 (1983):408–411.

288. RILEY, T. L., and ROY, A., eds. *Pseudoseizures.* Baltimore: Williams & Wilkins, 1982.

289. ROBINS, A. H. "Are Stroke Patients More Depressed than Other Disabled Subjects?" *Journal of Chronic Disease,* 29 (1976):479–482.

290. ROBINSON, J. O. "Symptoms and the Discovery of High Blood Pressure," *Journal of Psychosomatic Research,* 13 (1969):157–161.

291. ROBINSON, R. G., STARR, L. B., and PRICE, T. R. "A Two-year Longitudinal Study of Mood Disorders Following Stroke," *British Journal of Psychiatry,* 144 (1984):256–262.

292. RON, M. A. "Brain Damage in Chronic Alcoholism," *Psychological Medicine,* 7 (1977):103–112.

293. ROSS, A. T., and REITAIN, R. M. "Intellectual and Affective Functions in Multiple Sclerosis," *Journal of Nervous and Mental Disorders,* 153 (1971):218–224.

294. ROTH, M., and KAY, D. W. K. "Affective Disorder Arising in the Senium. II: Physical Disability as an Aetiological Factor," *Journal of Mental Science,* 102 (1956):141–150.

295. ROUECHÉ B. "Annals of Medicine: Live and Let Live," *The New Yorker.* 16 July 1979, pp. 82–87.

296. ROWE, M. J., and CARLSON, C. "Brainstem Auditory Evoked Potentials in Post-concussion Dizziness," *Archives of Neurology,* 37 (1980):679–683.

297. ROY, A. "Psychiatric Aspects of Narco-

lepsy," *British Journal of Psychiatry*, 128 (1976):562–565.

298. ROY, A., BYRNE, P., and EDELSTEIN, C. "Identifying Organic Brain Disease by Amobarbital Sodium Interview: Diagnostic Pitfalls," *Psychosomatics*, 23 (1982):1069–1075.

299. RUSSELL, R. W. R. "Giant Cell Arteritis: A Review of 35 Cases," *Quarterly Journal of Medicine*, 28 (1959):471–489.

300. SACHAR, E. J., ed. *Hormones, Behavior and Psychopathology*. New York: Raven Press, 1976.

301. SANDIFER, M. G. "Hyponatremia Due to Psychotropic Drugs," *Journal of Clinical Psychiatry*, 44 (1983):301–303.

302. SARAWAY, S. M., and KORAN, L. M. "Organic Disease Mishandled, Diagnosed as Psychiatric," *Psychosomatics*, 18 (1977):6–11.

303. SCHEINBERG, I. H., STERNLIEB, I., and RICHMAN, J. "Psychiatric Manifestations in Patients with Wilson's Disease," *Birth Defects*, 4 (1968):85–87.

304. SCHILDER, P. "The Organic Background of Obsessions and Compulsions," *American Journal of Psychiatry*, 94 (1938):1397–1413.

305. SCHNEIDER, A. B., and SHERWOOD, L. M. "Pathogenesis and Management of Hypoparathyroidism and Other Hypocalcemic Disorders," *Metabolism*, 24 (1975):871–898.

306. SCHULMAN, R. "The Present Status of Vitamin B_{12} and Folic Acid Deficiency in Psychiatric Disease," *Canadian Psychiatric Association Journal*, 17 (1972):205–216.

307. SCHUSTER, M. M., and IBER, F. L. "Psychosis with Pancreatitis: A Frequent Occurrence Infrequently Recognized," *Archives of Internal Medicine*, 116 (1965):228–233.

308. SCHWAB, J. J. "Psychiatric Illnesses Produced by Infection," *Hospital Medicine*, 5 (1969):98–108.

309. SCHWAB, J. J., and PERLO, V. P. "Syndromes Simulating Myasthenia Gravis," *Annals of the New York Academy of Sciences*, 135 (1966):350–366.

310. SCOTT, D. F. "Psychiatric Aspects of Epilepsy," *British Journal of Psychiatry*, 132 (1978):417–430.

311. SELECKI, B. R. "Intracranial Space Occu-

pying Lesions Among Patients Admitted to Mental Hospital," *Medical Journal of Australia*, 1 (1965):383–390.

312. SELLERS, E. M., and KALANT, H. "Alcohol Intoxication and Withdrawal," *New England Journal of Medicine*, 294 (1976): 757–762.

313. SELTZER, B., and SHERWIN, I. "Organic Brain Syndromes," *American Journal of Psychiatry*, 135 (1978):13–21.

314. SHADER, R. I. "Psychiatric Effects of Nonpsychiatric Drugs," *Seminars in Psychiatry*, 3 (1971):401–492.

315. SHADER, R. I., ed. *Psychiatric Complications of Medical Drugs*. New York: Raven Press, 1972.

316. SHANDS, H. C., FINESINGER, J. E., and WATKINS, A. L. "Clinical Studies on Fatigue," *Archives of Neurology and Psychiatry*, 60 (1948):210–217.

317. SHINE, K. I. "Anxiety in Patients with Heart Disease," *Psychosomatics*, 25 (Supplement) (1984):27–31.

318. SHULMAN, R. "Psychiatric Aspects of Pernicious Anaemia," *British Journal of Medicine*, 3 (1967):266–270.

319. SIMONS, R. C., and PARDES, H., eds. *Understanding Human Behavior in Health and Illness*, 2nd ed. Baltimore: Williams & Wilkins, 1981.

320. SLADE, P. "Hallucinations," *Psychological Medicine*, 6 (1976):7–13.

321. SLATER, E. "Diagnosis of Hysteria," *British Medical Journal*, 1 (1965):1395–1399.

322. SLATER, E., BEARD, A. W., and CLITHERO, E. "The Schizophrenia-like Psychoses of Epilepsy," *British Journal of Psychiatry*, 109 (1963):95–150.

323. SMITH, C. K., et al. "Psychiatric Disturbance in Endocrinologic Disease," *Psychosomatic Medicine*, 34 (1972):69–86.

324. SMITH, J. S., and BRANDON, S. "Morbidity from Acute Carbon Monoxide Poisoning at Three Year Follow-up," *British Medical Journal*, 1 (1973):318–321.

325. SNAITH, R. P., and McCOUBRIE, M. "Antihypertensive Drugs and Depression," *Psychological Medicine*, 4 (1974):393–398.

326. SOFFER, L. J., IANNACCONE, A., and GABRILOVE, J. L. "Cushing's Syndrome," *American Journal of Medicine*, 30 (1961):129–146.

327. SONIAT, T. L. L. "Psychiatric Symptoms

Associated with Intracranial Neoplasms," *American Journal of Psychiatry,* 108 (1951):19–22.

328. SORKIN, S. A. "Addison's Disease," *Medicine,* 28 (1949):371–425.

329. SPILLANE, J. D. "Nervous and Mental Disorders in Cushing's Syndrome," *Brain,* 74 (1951):72–94.

330. STEINBACK, A., and HAAPANEN, E. "Azotemia and Psychosis," *Acta Psychiatrica Scandinavica,* 197 (Supplement) (1967): 1–65.

331. STERNBACH, H. A., et al. "Identifying Depression Secondary to Lithium-induced Hypothyroidism," *Psychosomatics,* 25 (1984):864–866.

332. STEWARD, I. McD. G. "Headache and Hypertension," *Lancet,* 1 (1953):1261–1266.

333. STOREY, P. B. "Psychiatric Sequelae of Subarachnoid Hemorrhage," *British Medical Journal,* 3 (1967):261–266.

334. ———. "Brain Damage and Personality Change After Subarachnoid Hemorrhage," *British Journal of Psychiatry,* 117 (1970):129–142.

335. STRACHAN, R. W., and HENDERSON, J. G. "Psychiatric Syndromes Due to Avitaminosis B_{12} with Normal Blood and Marrow," *Quarterly Journal of Medicine,* 34 (1965):303–317.

336. STRAIN, J. *Psychological Interventions in Medical Practice.* New York: Appleton-Century-Crofts, 1978.

337. STRAIN, J., and GROSSMAN, B. eds. *Psychological Care of the Medically Ill: A Primer in Liaison Psychiatry.* New York: Appleton-Century-Crofts, 1975.

338. STRUB, R. L. "Acute Confusional State," in D. F. Benson, and D. Blumer, eds., *Psychiatric Aspects of Neurologic Disease,* vol. 2. New York: Grune & Stratton, 1982, pp. 1–25.

339. STRUB, R. L., and BLACK, F. W. *The Mental Status Examination in Neurology.* Philadelphia: F. A. Davis, 1977.

340. ———. *Organic Brain Syndromes.* Philadelphia: F. A. Davis, 1981.

341. STRUVE, F. A. "The Necessity and Value of Screening Routine Electroencephalograms in Psychiatric Patients," *Clinical Electroencephalography,* 7 (1976): 115–130.

342. STUTEVILLE, P., and WELCH, K. "Subdural Hematoma in the Elderly Person,"

Journal of the American Medical Association, 168 (1958):1445–1449.

343. SULLIVAN, L. W. "Differential Diagnosis and Management of the Patient with Megaloblastic Anemia," *American Journal of Medicine,* 48 (1970):609–617.

344. SURRIDGE, D. "Investigation into Some Psychiatric Aspects of Multiple Sclerosis," *British Journal of Psychiatry,* 115 (1964):749–764.

345. TAYLOR, D. "The Component of Sickness: Diseases, Illnesses and Predicaments," *Lancet,* 2 (1979):1008–1010.

346. TAYLOR, J. W. "Depression in Thyrotoxicosis," *American Journal of Psychiatry,* 132 (1973):552–553.

347. TAYLOR, R. L. *Mind or Body.* New York: McGraw-Hill, 1982.

348. TERRY, R. D., and DAVIES, P. "Dementia of the Alzheimer's Type," *Annual Review of Neuroscience,* 3 (1980):77.

349. THOMAS, C. J. "The Use of Screening Investigations in Psychiatry," *British Journal of Psychiatry,* 135 (1979):67–72.

350. THOMAS, F. B., MAZZAFERRI, E. L., and STILLMAN, T. G. "Apathetic Thyrotoxicosis: A Distinctive Clinical and Laboratory Entity," *Annals of Internal Medicine,* 72 (1970):679–685.

351. TISSENBAUM, M. J., HARTER, H. M., and FRIEDMAN, A. P. "Organic Neurological Syndromes Diagnosed as Functional Disorders," *Journal of the American Medical Association,* 147 (1951):1519–1521.

352. TONKS, C. M. "Mental Illness in Hypothyroid Patients," *British Journal of Psychiatry,* 110 (1964):706–710.

353. TORACK, R. M. *The Pathologic Physiology of Dementia.* New York: Springer-Verlag, 1978.

354. TREADWAY, C. R. "Mental Changes Accompanying Thyroid Gland Dysfunction," *Archives of General Psychiatry,* 20 (1969):48–63.

355. TRETHOWAN, W. H., and COBB, S. "Neuropsychiatric Aspects of Cushing's Syndrome," *Archives of Neurology and Psychiatry,* 67 (1952):283–309.

356. TRIMBLE, M. R., and GRANT, I. "Psychiatric Aspects of Multiple Sclerosis," in D. F. Benson and D. Blumer, eds., *Psychiatric Aspects of Neurologic Disease,* vol.

2. New York: Grune & Stratton, pp. 279–300.

357. TYLER, H. R. "Neurological Disorders in Renal Failure," *American Journal of Medicine*, 44 (1968):734–748.

358. VAN PUTTEN, T., and MENKES, J. H. "Huntington's Disease Masquerading as Chronic Schizophrenia," *Diseases of the Nervous System*, 34 (1973):54–56.

359. VARSAMIS, J., ZUCHOWSKI, T., and MAINI, K. K. "Survival Rates and Causes of Death and Geriatric Psychiatric Patients," *Canadian Psychiatric Association Journal*, 17 (1972):17–22.

360. VEITH, R. C., et al. "Cardiovascular Effects of Tricyclic Antidepressants in Depressed Patients with Chronic Heart Disease," *New England Journal of Medicine*, 306 (1982):954–959.

361. VEREKER, R. "The Psychiatric Aspects of Temporal Arteritis," *Journal of Mental Science*, 98 (1952):280–286.

362. VICTOR, M., and HOPE, J. M. "The Phenomenon of Auditory Hallucination in Chronic Alcoholism," *Journal of Nervous and Mental Disease*, 126 (1958):451–481.

363. VICTOR, M., ADAMS, R. D., and COLLINS, G. H. *The Wernicke-Korsakoff Syndrome*. Philadelphia: F. A. Davis, 1971.

364. VINKEN, P. J., and BRUYN, G. W., eds. *Disorders of Higher Nervous Activity*, vol. 3 of *Handbook of Clinical Neurology*. Amsterdam: North Holland Publishing Co., 1969.

365. ———. *Disorders of Speech, Perception and Symbolic Behavior*, vol. 4 of *Handbook of Clinical Neurology*. Amsterdam: North Holland Publishing Co., 1970.

366. ———. *Neurological Manifestations of Systemic Disease*, parts 1 and 2, vols. 38 and 39 of *Handbook of Clinical Neurology*. Amsterdam: North Holland Publishing Co., 1979, 1980.

367. WAGGONER, R. W., and BAEGHI, B. K. "Initial Masking of Organic Brain Changes by Psychic Symptoms: Clinical and Electroencephalographic Studies," *American Journal of Psychiatry*, 110 (1954):904–910.

368. WALKER, S. *Psychiatric Signs and Symptoms Due to Medical Problems*. Springfield, Ill.: Charles C Thomas, 1967.

369. ———. "The Psychiatric Presentation of Wilson's Disease (Hepatolenticular Degeneration) with an Etiological Explanation," *Behavioral Neuropharmacology*, 1 (1969):38–43.

370. WALSHE, J. M. "Wilson's Disease," *Biochemical Journal*, 111:(1969):8–9.

371. WARD, N. G., ROWLETT, H. D. B., and BURKE, P. "Sodium Amylobarbitone in the Differential Diagnosis of Confusion," *American Journal of Psychiatry*, 135 (1978):869–870.

372. WEBB, W. L., Jr., and GEHI, M. "Electrolyte and Fluid Imbalance: Neuropsychiatric Manifestations," *Psychosomatics*, 22 (1981):199–203.

373. WEDDINGTON, W. W., Jr., MUELLING, A. E., and MOOSA, H. H. "Adverse Neuropsychiatric Reaction to Cimetidine," *Psychosomatics*, 23 (1982):49–53.

374. WEINER, H. M. *Psychobiology and Human Disease*. New York: Elsevier, 1977.

375. WEINGARTNER, H., et al. "Cognitive Impairments in Parkinson's Disease," *Psychiatry Research*, 11 (1984):223–235.

376. WELLS, C. E. "Chronic Brain Disease: An Overview," *American Journal of Psychiatry*, 135 (1978):1–12.

377. ———. "Pseudodementia," *American Journal of Psychiatry*, 136 (1979):895–900.

378. ———. "Diagnosis of Dementia: A Reassessment," *Psychosomatics*, 25 (1984):183–190.

379. WELLS, C. E. ed. *Dementia*, 2nd ed. Philadelphia: F. A. Davis, 1977.

380. WELLS, C. E., and DUNCAN, G. W. *Neurology for Psychiatrists*. Philadelphia: F. A. Davis, 1980.

381. WEST, L. J., "A Clinical and Theoretical Overview of Hallucinatory Phenomena," in R. Siegel and L. J. West, eds., *Hallucinations, Behavior, Experience, and Theory*. New York: John Wiley & Sons, 1975, pp. 287–311.

382. WHARTON, R. N. "Atrial Myxoma Masquerade," *American Journal of Psychiatry*, 134 (1977):1441–1442.

383. WHITE, J. C., and COBB, S. "Psychological Changes Associated with Giant Pituitary Neoplasms," *Archives of Neurological Psychiatry*, 74 (1955):383–396.

384. WHITLOCK, F. A. "The Aetiology of Hys-

teria," *Acta Psychiatrica Scandinavica*, 43 (1967):144–162.

385. WHITLOCK, F. A., and EVANS, L. E. "Drugs and Depression," *Drugs*, 15 (1978):53–56.

386. WHITLOCK, F. A., and SISKIND, M. "Depression and Cancer: A Follow-up Study," *Psychological Medicine*, 9 (1979):747–752.

387. ———. "Depression as a Major Symptom of Multiple Sclerosis," *Journal of Neurology, Neurosurgery and Psychiatry*, 43 (1980):861–865.

388. WHYBROW, P. C., PRANGE, A. J., and TREADWAY, C. R. "Mental Changes Accompanying Thyroid Gland Dysfunction," *Archives of General Psychiatry*, 20 (1969):48–63.

389. WIENER, J. S., and HOPE, J. M. "Cerebral Manifestation of Vitamin B_{12} Deficiency," *Journal of the American Medical Association*, 170 (1959):1038–1041.

390. WILLIAMS, S. E., BELL, S. D., and GYE, R. S. "Neurosurgical Disease Encountered in a Psychiatric Service," *Journal of Neurology, Neurosurgery and Psychiatry*, 37 (1974):112–116.

391. WILLNER, A. E., and RABINER, C. J. "Psychopathology and Cognitive Dysfunction Five Years After Open-heart Surgery," *Comprehensive Psychiatry*, 20 (1979):5.

392. WILSON, L. G. "Viral Encephalopathy Mimicking Functional Psychosis," *American Journal of Psychiatry*, 133 (1976): 165–170.

393. WISE, T. N. "The Pitfalls of Diagnosing Depression in Chronic Renal Disease," *Psychosomatics*, 15 (1974):83–84.

394. WOLF, J. K., SANTANA, H. B., and THORPY, M. "Treatment of Emotional Incontinence with Levodopa," *Neurology* 29 (1979):1435–1436.

395. WOLFSON, L. I., and KATZMAN, R. "The Neurologic Consultation at Age 80," in R. Katzman and R. Terry, eds., *The Neurology of Aging*. Philadelphia: F. A. Davis 1983, pp. 221–244.

396. ZARCONE, V. "Narcolepsy," *New England Journal of Medicine*, 288 (1973):1156–1166.

397. ZARIT, S. H. *Aging and Mental Disorders: Psychological Approaches to Assessment and Treatment*. New York: Free Press, 1980.

CHAPTER 32

MEDICAL SIDE EFFECTS OF PSYCHOACTIVE DRUGS

Roger A. Boshes and John M. Davis

¶ **Introduction**

The history of the discovery and development of the major psychotropic agents provides an ideal way of introducing a chapter on side effects. Phenothiazines, tricyclic antidepressants, monoamine oxidase inhibitors, and lithium were all initially investigated for purposes entirely unrelated to their current usage. It was the recognition of a significant clinical side effect by an astute observer that led to their ultimate utilization as psychotropic agents.

One is reminded of the profound observation of Louis Pasteur stated in an address at Lille, France: *"Dans les champs de l'observation, le hasard ne favorise que les ésprits preparés."* Translated literally, this reads, "In the field of observation (research), luck favors only prepared minds." It is worth reiterating that adverse reactions, correctly appreciated by thoughtful observers with prepared minds, have played a major role in the discovery and/or development of most of the psychotropic drugs: antipsychotic, antidepressant, and antimanic agents.

The phenothiazine promethazine hydrochloride, which was known to have antihistaminic properties, was introduced in France in 1952 for the purpose of potentiating anesthetic agents. In the same year, chlorpromazine was noted to produce "artificial hibernation." But it was not until the report of Delay and Deniker that the long-term antipsychotic potential was fully appreciated. These workers recognized that the efficacy of chlorpromazine was not simply the result of sedation but was due to amelioration of the psychotic process itself.[49]

While chlorpromazine was being clinically tested as an antipsychotic agent, it was found to produce an inordinate amount of liver damage (about one in two hundred cases initially). This adverse reaction prompted the development of chemically related compounds, one of which was imipramine hydrochloride. Imipramine demonstrated antidepressant "side effects" when given to schizophrenic patients. This effect was noted and pursued, leading ultimately to a new class of antidepressant compounds. [30,86]

The discovery of monoamine oxidase inhibitors (MAOIs) as antidepressants provides another classical example of the importance of both recognizing and understanding pharmacological side effects. In 1956 iproniazid was clinically tested as an antitubercular agent. A prominent, unanticipated feature of patient response was mood elevation, which led to its trial as an antidepressant. Upon further investigation, it was appreciated that iproniazid also inhibited the enzyme monoamine oxidase (MAO). These clinical and biochemical observations were linked for the first time, suggesting a correlation between mental states and levels of activity of a specific enzyme. This sequence of events, which ironically was entirely serendipitous, represents an early milestone in the history of biological psychiatry. [15] It is reminiscent of the fortuitous observation of Alexander Fleming leading to the discovery of penicillin, which opened the antibiotic era.

The story of lithium differs slightly from the just-mentioned histories, but it too is typical of the pattern of serendipitous events that characterizes the history of psychopharmacology. Cade used lithium to make a soluble uric acid salt from the urine of mental patients, which he injected into guinea pigs in the belief that a toxin, present in the urine, caused mania. What Cade observed was not that the experimental animals became agitated, but that, in fact, after receiving the lithium-containing injection, they became lethargic. He did not merely dismiss the observation as contradictory to his hypothesis but made an inductive leap and treated manic patients with lithium. Yet again, a side effect proved to be a central effect from a historical perspective. [31]

Another point to be made before beginning the substantive material of the chapter concerns ascertainment of data in psychopharmacology—particularly data concerning side effects. Anecdotal reports of side effects caused by psychoactive drugs become myths. These myths permeate the field and become part of the lore of psychopharmacology just as do therapeutic drug effects that cannot be clinically substantiated. Since many side effects may be rare, it is essential to observe large numbers of cases in a carefully controlled fashion in order to substantiate these claims in an accurate and quantitative manner. Even then, a high index of suspicion must be maintained. Psychiatric patients often experience somatic symptoms, believing themselves to be physically ill. They may complain of symptoms identical to drug-induced side effects while on placebo. Therefore, in order to utilize subjective ratings of side effects by patients, one must develop a double-blind, placebo-controlled paradigm that includes the quantitation of side effects. Also, coincidental physical disease may produce signs and symptoms that may be falsely attributed to the drug. Because a patient is on a drug and has a physical symptom or disease does not mean they are causally related; the association may be entirely coincidental.

In addition to myth and subjectivity, evaluation of side effects suffers from lack of agreed-upon, readily defined criteria to identify these untoward reactions. For example, the incidence of chlorpromazine-induced drowsiness reported by different authors ranges from 2 to 92 percent. [43] Authors may disagree on terminology, classification, or even whether certain phenomena are side effects or symptoms of the diathesis itself. [65] This latter point will be reiterated in several sections of the chapter—particularly the discussion on tardive dyskinesia. Since side effects data reflect differences in definition as well as ascertainment, caution should be taken in comparing differential occurrences of side effects.

¶ Antipsychotics

Most peripheral side effects associated with psychotropic agents are mediated via the autonomic nervous system and are manifested primarily in the gastrointestinal tract, cardiovascular system, and genitourinary tract. These autonomic side effects will be discussed, together with the cutaneous manifestation of neuroleptic agents; however, the bulk of the chapter focuses on the central nervous system (CNS), where the side effects are often more troublesome.

Table 32–1 sets out an estimate of the incidence of side effects of phenothiazines based on a number of large, relatively well-controlled studies in which such effects were quantified. This comparison provides an estimate superior to any single study, but it is still a crude approximation owing to widely divergent terminologies and classifications utilized by different workers.

A few generalizations are useful in estimating side effects of antipsychotic drugs. The principal one is stated by Gelenberg: "Molecules with greater milligram potency produce less sedation and hypotension but more acute extrapyramidal reactions" (p. 125).[61] This axiom is roughly quantitated in table 32–2.

There is a high correlation among measurements of anticholinergic activity assayed in several experimental systems, both among the *in vitro* preparations and between the experimental assays and clinical observations of such effects. Affinity for muscarinic receptors can be measured by quinuclindinyl benzilate (QNB) binding, using rat brain or human caudate nucleus, or by the muscarinic acetylcholine (ACh) receptor-mediated cyclic guanosine monophosphate (GMP) formation in cultured mouse-neuroblastoma cells.[120,143] The consensus is that thioridazine hydrochloride has the most anticholinergic properties, followed by mesoridazine and chlorpromazine. It is clear that the so-called high-potency drugs have reduced anticholinergic properties. There is minor disagreement concerning the estimates of the binding as determined by the QNB or the cyclic GMP methods.[119] All were therefore given the equivalent rating of minimal activity.

Autonomic Nervous System Effects

Antipsychotic agents block cholinergic muscarinic receptors. These receptors are located on postganglionic neurons of the parasympathetic chain. The effect of these drugs, therefore, is to antagonize the parasympathetic nervous system; in pharmacological parlance, to produce an atropinelike effect. As can be seen in tables 32–2 and 32–3, thioridazine is the most potently anticholinergic antipsychotic agent, while haloperidol, trifluoperazine hydrochloride, and thiothixene have almost no such properties.

Reduced secretions in the mouth produce the most common anticholinergic side effect. Dry mouth often results in bitter complaints and may lead to noncompliance. The best remedy for this condition is frequent small sips of water to moisten the oral mucosa. Kane and Anderson[79] have reported four cases of oral moniliasis resulting from the use of phenothiazines (three cases with chlorpromazine and one with thioridazine), suggesting that the phenothiazine-caused dry mouth may have predisposed these patients to oral infections. Nasal congestion, mouth breathing, decreased salivation, and the chronic use of sugar-containing candies or gum to alleviate dry mouth discomfort may predispose to oral infection with sucrose-dependent monilia. Pollack, Buck, and Kalnins[112] investigated such lesions and found monilia present in the oral smears of many psychiatric patients.

Autonomic nervous system manifestations of antimuscarinic medication include mydriasis, leading to difficulty in visual accommodation and increased intraocular pressure. This latter complication can occasionally lead to an acute onset of narrow-angle glaucoma. According to Gelenberg, the more common open-angle glaucoma, when properly treated, is not likely to be exacerbated by treatment with antipsychotic medication.[61] Additional peripheral manifestations of the antimuscarinic effect of these medications include drying of secretions in the lungs and nasal congestion.

TABLE 32–1

Differential Incidence of Side Effects (percentages)

Effect	Incidence Caused by										
	Aceto-phena-zine	Chlor-proma-zine	Flu-phena-zine	Mepa-zine	Per-phena-zine	Pheno-bar-bital	Prochlor-pera-zine	Proma-zine	Thio-rida-zine	Trifluo-pera-zine	Triflu-proma-zine
Central nervous system											
Extrapyramidal effects	10.1	11.9	15.4	1.9	21.1	0.0	33.4	26.0	11.8	23.7	6.5
Dystonia	2.9	2.8	8.0	0.97	2.8	1.0	1.8	—	0.88	3.5	1.3
Akathisia	4.3	12.1	21.6	11.6	27.3	10.8	11.5	—	8.9	4.8	10.4
Seizures, convulsions	1.4	1.3	0.0	0.97	0.67	0.0	1.0	16.2	1.2	1.3	0.56
Drowsiness, somnolence	7.2	23.8	19.5	27.2	16.3	31.0	10.1	6.6	36.2	20.8	11.8
Toxic confusion	—	8.6	—	—	—	—	—	20.0	5.2	—	—
Depression	—	13.9	—	14.6	6.2	18.2	5.2	—	0.0	4.3	4.8
Autonomic nervous system											
Dizzy, faint, weak	15.9	6.0	7.0	17.5	12.0	18.6	7.2	6.6	23.3	21.2	11.5
Dry mouth and throat	—	27.8	8.0	23.3	18.8	11.6	20.0	6.6	28.1	2.3	10.0
Disturbed sexual function	—	—	—	—	—	—	—	—	—	3.4	0.0
Urinary disturbance	—	3.0	1.3	—	—	—	—	—	5.5	0.64	0.0
Nasal stuffiness	—	2.5	9.2	—	0.97	—	0.45	—	—	—	3.1
Visual disturbances	2.9	14.4	4.3	23.3	17.8	8.5	14.0	—	16.3	1.8	8.3
Hypotension	1.4	3.4	0.79	—	0.99	—	—	13.3	2.4	0.79	—
Constipation	—	13.9	9.6	22.3	4.6	8.5	1.8	—	16.8	1.1	4.5
Diarrhea	—	1.1	1.1	—	—	—	—	—	3.3	1.1	1.2
Gastrointestinal effects											
Anorexia	—	2.9	—	—	4.2	—	18.8	—	0.0	12.3	0.0
Nausea, vomiting	—	5.0	4.3	4.8	2.9	5.4	3.6	3.3	29.3	2.4	4.5
Blood disturbances											
Agranulocytosis	—	0.32	—	—	0.0	—	—	—	0.0	—	0.0
Eosinophilia	—	—	0.0	—	—	—	—	—	0.0	3.4	—
Leukocytosis	—	—	0.0	—	—	—	—	—	2.4	—	—
Leukopenia	—	0.32	0.0	—	—	—	—	—	1.5	0.0	—
Endocrine effects											
Menstrual changes	—	16.3	4.4	—	—	—	—	—	3.3	—	—
Breast swelling	—	1.1	2.2	—	—	—	—	—	0.60	—	—
Lactation	—	0.72	3.3	—	0.97	—	0.15	—	3.1	—	0.0
Edema	2.9	2.8	0.0	—	0.77	—	2.4	—	2.3	1.4	0.44
Weight gain or loss	—	29.8	—	—	5.9	—	13.6	—	—	1.1	4.5
Allergic reactions	2.9	6.6	2.6	1.9	0.83	3.0	1.6	—	3.2	4.2	3.2
Liver abnormalities											
Abnormal hepatic tests	—	3.7	0.39	—	—	—	—	—	0.51	6.9	—
Jaundice	—	0.64	0.0	—	0.0	0.0	0.0	—	0.0	0.0	0.0

— indicates either that no data were available or the available data were considered extremely unreliable.
SOURCE: J. M. Davis, "Concluding Remarks: Mechanisms of Antidepressants," *Progress in Neuro-Biological Psychiatry*, 7 (1983):365.

TABLE 32–2
Relationship of Potency and Major Side Effects

Drug	Mgm Equivalent	Sedation	Hypotension	Extrapyramidal System	Anticholinergic
Chlorpromazine	100	3	3	2	3
Thioridazine	100	3	3	1	5
Mesoridazine	50	2	2	3	4
Acetophenazine	20	2	2	3	1
Perphenazine	10	2	2	3	1
Loxapine	10	1	1	4	1
Molindone	10	1	1	4	1
Trifluoperazine	3	1	1	4	1
Thiothixene	5	1	1	4	1
Fluphenazine	1.2	1	1	4	1
Haloperidol	1.6	1	1	4	1

Source: C. Salzman, "Introduction to Antipsychotics," lecture given at Massachusetts Mental Health Center, July 15, 1983.

TABLE 32–3
Spectrum of Adverse Effects Caused by Antipsychotic Drugs

Low Potency	High Potency
Fewer extrapyramidal reactions (especially thioridazine)	More frequent extrapyramidal reactions
More sedation, postural hypotension	Less sedation, postural hypotension
Greater effect on the seizure threshold, electrocardiogram (especially thioridazine)	Less effect on the seizure threshold
More likely skin pigmentation and photosensitivity	Fewer anticholinergic effects
Occasional cases of cholestatic jaundice	Occasional cases of neuroleptic malignant syndrome

Source: A. Gelenberg, "Psychoses," in E. L. Bassuck, S. C. Schoonover, and A. J. Gelenberg, eds., *The Practitioner's Guide to Psychiatric Drugs"* (New York: Plenum Press, 1983), p. 125.

Nor is the genitourinary system spared. The sphincter controlling outflow of urine from the bladder is under cholinergic control. Antipsychotic agents may interfere with the function of this sphincter, leading to urinary retention or at least difficulty in voiding. Thioridazine, among the phenothiazines, is most often associated with delayed, inhibited, or retrograde ejaculation without interfering with erectile function. This effect has been utilized therapeutically by some physicians for treating *ejaculatio praecox*.[52] However, any agent with anticholinergic properties may cause delayed or inhibited ejaculation.[133]

Skin and Eye Manifestations

The manifestations of muscarinic blockade are myriad. In the peripheral nervous system, under the control of the parasympathetic ganglian, the effect on the skin is to reduce diaphoresis, producing warmth and dryness. In addition, there is flushing.

A variety of skin eruptions can occur in the first few weeks of therapy with antipsychotics. These include a maculopapular urticaria, edema, and petechiae. Contact dermatitis can also occur in staff who handle chlorpromazine. Patients should be advised that antipsychotics, usually chlorpromazine, cause photosensitivity, so that they will be sunburned much more easily. Sunscreen is useful for those who cannot avoid extended exposure to sunlight.[98]

Skin discoloration has been found to be a long-term manifestation occurring in patients who have been taking chlorpromazine in excess of fifteen years. Skin more often exposed to sunlight—that is, the face, arms, and neck—takes on first a golden-brown color, which gradually fades into a blue-gray metallic discoloration. This can progress to blue or even purple. Skin biopsies show the deposition of pigment granules containing a substance that looks like melanin.[35]

Slit-lamp examination reveals whitish-brown granular deposits in the anterior lens and posterior cornea of some patients on long-term, high-dose chlorpromazine. They are not related to cataracts, which occur in the normal aging population, but tend to occur in patients who also show skin changes. The retina is never affected, and vision is not impaired. The total lifetime dose of chlorpromazine in these patients is estimated to exceed two to three kilograms. The reported incidence of these effects in inpatients at that cumulative dosage ranges from 1 to 30 percent. The variability is probably related to differences in sun and dose exposure in separate inpatient settings. It has been suggested that decreasing the dose or using a different antipsychotic agent can delay or prevent the development of skin and eye signs in patients who must remain on medication.[138]

A much more serious ophthalmological complication can occur when thioridazine is used in high doses. A form of retinitis pigmentosa develops in doses higher than 1,600 mg daily. Visual impairment results that does not always disappear when the drug is discontinued. For this reason, thioridazine dosage should never exceed 800 mg per day.[138]

Endocrine Effects

Pharmacological doses of antipsychotics produce changes in a number of endocrine systems, but the most apparent and therefore important clinical effects for patients concern lactation and sexual dysfunction (in males). Dopamine (DA) exerts an inhibitory effect on the release of prolactin from the pituitary; this inhibitory hypothalamic influence is unique among the pituitary hormones. By blocking these inhibitory DA receptors, antipsychotics cause prolactin to escape its negative control, and elevated blood levels ensue. This effect often leads to impotence secondary to prolactin inhibition of follicle-stimulating hormone (FSH) and luteinizing hormone (LH), which, in turn, reduces testosterone production. Because serum prolactin levels correlate with serum antipsychotic levels, it has been suggested that prolactin levels may be useful as an indirect assay of antipsychotic action. We have reviewed the studies in which both plasma levels and prolactin were measured and have found the average correlation between them to be about 0.5, with most correlations between 0.3 to 0.8. (This correlation is too low to allow prolactin levels to be an effective measure of plasma neuroleptic levels.) Although associated, there is no linear relationship. In addition, since females have normally higher prolactin concentrations than males, one must have separate norms for comparison. A major consequence of elevated serum prolactin level is to induce lactation. The exact incidence of breast engorgement and lactation in women is unknown, but manual pressure on the breast results in milk flow in about 20 to 40 percent of female patients. Nevertheless, only 5 percent will present this complaint to their physician. Similarly, gynecomastia can occur in men, which may be psychologically devastating. Both of these symptoms can usually be dealt with by lowering the dose or switching to another agent. Menstrual irregularities have also been reported by patients using these drugs, probably secondary to elevated serum prolactin levels.[134] False positive pregnancy tests owing to elevation in serum progesterone have also been reported.[106]

Since patients often do not bring their complaints to medical attention, it is important to inquire. If these very disturbing side effects are not dealt with openly, noncompliance often results. It should be noted that many practitioners consider thioridazine a particularly poor choice of medication for paranoid males because of side effects involving sexual dysfunction.

Weight gain is yet another consequence of antipsychotic use, but its cause remains obscure. Molindone hydrochloride reportedly does not have this effect. Remaining minor endocrine changes include occasional shifting of the glucose tolerance curve in a diabetic direction.

Bone Marrow Suppression

Aside from the potentially fatal but exceedingly rare laryngospasm and neuroleptic malignant syndrome, idiosyncratic agranulocytosis is the most serious potential side effect of antipsychotic use, with a mortality rate of about 30 percent.[110] Fortunately it is rare, with an incidence thought to be less that one in 500,000. This side effect is more common in elderly females. It typically develops six to eight weeks after the initiation of therapy, and its onset is heralded by the appearance of fever, sore throat, and ulcerations. The offending agent, again most commonly chlorpromazine, should be withdrawn immediately. Other phenothiazines, including thioridazine, prochlorperazine, promazine hydrochloride, and mepazine have also been implicated. Patients should be transferred directly to a hospital facility that has the capacity for isolation as well as reverse isolation.

Because of the rarity and abrupt onset of the syndrome, monitoring of the hematological profile is not useful. A baseline complete blood count can be obtained for purposes of comparison. Antipsychotics may suppress the bone marrow, leading to a gradual decrease in the leukocyte count by 40 to 80 percent.[61] Unless the absolute granulocyte count drops below 500 cells per mm, this phenomenon is of no clinical significance. Purpura, with and without thrombocytopenia, pancytopenia, and/or hemolytic anemias have all been reported in association with antipsychotic drugs. The best strategy is switching to another antipsychotic agent or stopping antipsychotics if this can be tolerated.

Cardiovascular Effects

Cardiovascular effects include tachycardia, which is a primary anticholinergic effect of decreased vagal tone and a secondary reflex in response to orthostatic hypotension. Phenothiazines, in general, but especially thioridazine, have the effect of prolonging the Q-R interval and flattening the T-wave. These changes have been observed with as little as 300 mg thioridazine and were rapidly reversed after stopping the drug.[48] These electrocardiogram (ECG) effects are of no known clinical importance.

Sudden death has been reported in young individuals on antipsychotic agents, but a causal relationship with medication has not been clearly established; this association may, in fact, be no more than coincidental. Nor is there a greater likelihood with any particular agent despite the different profiles in the balance of autonomic side effects. The suspected cause of death in most cases would be by arrhythmia, in particular ventricular fibrillation.[89] It has been speculated that neuroleptics predispose to a peculiar variety of ventricular tachycardia known as *torsade des pointes*, in which the amplitude of successive beats fluctuates on the ECG in a sine-wave pattern.[82,92] In spite of this observation, there has been no excess of cardiac mortality in the psychotic population since the inception of antipsychotic medication. Moreover, the extreme stress of a psychotic episode may be a relevant variable in evaluating the frequency of sudden death; the disease itself rather than the therapy could be responsible for these rare events.

The more well-known and serious peripheral vascular complication of antipsychotic agents is orthostatic hypotension. Symptoms include weakness and light-headedness. They are most severe during the first week of treatment, since accommodation is rapid. However, among elderly populations, with their attendant osteoporosis, the sequence of dizziness and falling, followed by hip fractures with complications, can evolve into a fatal chain of events ultimately referable to antipsychotic medication. Patients should be educated about the Trendelenburg position (elevating the legs), as well as getting out of bed slowly, particularly in the middle of the night. If the patient is elderly and not reliable, the choice of high-potency versus low-potency medication may be the difference between discomfort and a broken hip. It is useful to remind oneself that patients rarely die from dystonias, akathisias, or other extrapyramidal side effects.

Gastrointestinal Symptoms

Gastrointestinal (GI) complaints are not limited to reduced oral secretions. Acid secretion in the stomach is diminished and motility in the bowel is reduced, often leading to constipation. Nausea and vomiting are occasionally reported with phenothiazines in spite of the proven efficacy of these agents as antiemetics, but these phenomena are not frequent. Finally, weight gain is not uncommon, particularly among females.

An increasingly rare GI symptom is jaundice. Cholestatic jaundice may be a manifestation of an allergic reaction. It is most frequently associated with chlorpromazine, but it has also been known to occur with thioridazine, prochlorperazine, mepazine, promazine, and, rarely, with fluphenazine hydrochloride and triflupromazine hydrochloride. Nonphenothiazines have not been conclusively linked to this phenomenon. Shortly after the introduction of chlorpromazine, the incidence of jaundice was one in two hundred; it is now about one in one thousand, although exact data are lacking. According to Hollister, this drop may be related to improved synthetic methods. It is possible that an impurity resulting from the manufacturing process is responsible.[73]

Jaundice appears one to five weeks after the initiation of antipsychotic therapy. It is typically preceded by a flulike syndrome lasting up to a week, associated with fever, malaise, abdominal pain, nausea, vomiting, and diarrhea. The symptoms and signs are reminiscent of gastroenteritis or mild hepatitis. The liver is neither enlarged nor tender, but laboratory tests reveal elevated bilirubin, with an increased direct fraction, and elevated alkaline phosphatase. If transaminase elevations are present, they are mild. The leukocyte differential shows eosinophilia. A liver biopsy typically will show periportal eo-

sinophilic infiltration and bile plugs in the canaliculi. The latter is characteristic of cholestatic jaundice. Early onset of symptoms, eosinophilia, and recurrence with a repeated challenge, even decades later, support the hypothesis that this is an allergic phenomenon.

It is usually recommended that the offending agent be discontinued, even though the illness has spontaneously resolved in patients who remain on chlorpromazine. The disease is self-limiting and only very rarely progresses to the more persistent exanthematous biliary cirrhosis, which can last from six months to one year.

Miscellaneous Side Effects

In addition, a potpourri of reports on side effects of neuroleptics includes a decrease in antibody synthesis following oral polio virus vaccination. Finally, perphenazine has been reported to increase the level of protein-bound iodine without altering thyroid function, but this observation may be an artifact —the result of traces of iodine in crystalline perphenazine.[37]

Central Nervous System Effects

Antipsychotic drugs affect the CNS either globally or focally. Examples of the latter include the extrapyramidal system (EPS), which will be a primary focus of this section. One of the frequent CNS side effects common to all antipsychotics, but prominently associated with low potency agents, is drowsiness. This symptom is usually most severe during the first weeks of treatment but then abates. Nearly all patients develop a tolerance to this effect; therefore, their drug dosage should not be adjusted downward. Under no circumstances should patients be given amphetamine stimulants to counteract the sedating effect, since stimulants may worsen the psychosis. However, Lehman states that patients may safely increase their coffee consumption.[90]

Seizures may occur in patients on antipsychotic medication. They are seen primarily in those patients with a known seizure disorder as a result of lowering the seizure threshold. But they may also be seen in patients with no known history of epilepsy.[54]

CNS anticholinergic effects can produce memory difficulties, confusion, and, in extreme cases, delirium. Atropinelike delirium, especially in the elderly, is a medical emergency. This is characterized by florid hallucination (tactile, visual), impaired memory, confusion, and loss of orientation. If the clinical picture, which includes agitation and disorientation, is misperceived as psychotic behavior, more treatment with the offending agent will only compound the crisis. Physical symptoms include mydriatic pupils, hot flushed skin, and dry mucous membranes. Tachycardia and reduced bowel sounds complete the picture. Generally, this condition is treated by reducing the dose or by giving a similar antipsychotic with less anticholinergic property, as well as discontinuing unnecessary anticholinergic agents. Intravenous physostigmine, an acetylcholinesterase inhibitor that increases available brain ACh, can reverse the symptoms. But physostigmine can produce many of its own side effects, and it should be used with caution and only under special circumstances. The anticholinergic properties of various psychotropics can potentiate each other.

EXTRAPYRAMIDAL SYSTEM EFFECTS

The EPS is the primary target of the side effects of antipsychotic agents in the CNS. The clinical manifestations may be divided into three sets of reaction, which appear along a temporal vector. The first type of reaction is dystonia, which generally occurs within the first week or so of treatment; indeed, dystonia may present within minutes after treatment. However, dystonia can also occur years after commencement of treatment, but even in this case, it is more likely to occur following an injection of fluphenazine decanoate or after a bolus of oral medication.

The second class of reactions, which may manifest itself after a period of five to twenty days, is the parkinsonianlike syndrome. Another EPS manifestation that may occur at about the same time or a little later than the parkinsonian picture is akathisia, or motor restlessness. The final EPS side effect, which may have an irreversible form and is becoming a very controversial subject among psychopharmacologists and neurologists, is tardive dyskinesia (see chapter 20). This complication appears late in the course of treatment—sometimes only after years of drug therapy or after medication has been discontinued. A discussion of the conventional wisdom as well as more controversial notions about this condition and some innovative speculations will conclude this section.

ACUTE DYSTONIC REACTIONS

Acute dystonic reactions are the most dramatic side effects in both onset and appearance. They are characterized by acute spasms of the muscles of the back, neck, jaw, eyes, and tongue, causing such phenomena as opisthotonos (spasms of the neck and back that arch the back pulling the head backward), trismus (lockjaw), occulogyric crisis (gaze fixed in one position, often upward), and torticollis, or twisted neck. Dystonias appear either as muscle spasms or bizarre involuntary stereotyped movements. Such reactions are not limited to the upper body; they may also affect the muscles of the pelvic girdle or, rarely, the legs. The dystonias may occur hours or days following the commencement of antipsychotic medication or following a marked dosage increase. They may occur after administration of a small dose of phenothiazine given as an antiemetic. The symptoms are episodic, lasting from seconds to hours. They are often painful or uncomfortable but are rarely dangerous. However, rare instances of life-threatening laryngeal spasm have been reported.[97]

Not all antipsychotic medications are equally likely to produce dystonic syndromes. The high-potency drugs are the prime candidates, ranging downward in probability to the low-potency agents. Thioridazine is the least likely phenothiazine to cause dystonia. Young people are said to have a greater risk for having a dystonic reaction than older people, and males are said to be at greater risk than females.[61]

Diagnosing an acute dystonia is not always an easy matter, even when the signs are not subtle. The naive or psychotic patient will often have difficulty communicating the problem, more so if the muscles of the tongue and throat are involved, so the clinician should be alert to signs of unusual motor behavior early in therapy. Dystonias are readily confused with the bizarre posturing seen in some acutely disturbed patients and can be distinguished only by response within minutes to an intramuscular antiparkinsonian agent. If the phenomenon is misdiagnosed as increasingly psychotic behavior, the patient will be needlessly treated with a larger dose of antipsychotic. The dystonias are often painful, always uncomfortable, and frequently embarrassing as well; swift relief is merciful. The differential diagnosis includes many neuropsychiatric syndromes, conversion reactions, tetanus, and atypical seizures, to name a few.

The antiparkinsonian agents in common use for the treatment of EPS side effects include diphenhydramine (Benadryl), benztropine (Cogentin), and procyclidine (Kemadrin). The authors recommend 25 mg diphenhydramine (Benadryl) intramuscularly (IM), which can be repeated, since it has the fewest complicating side effects. Amantadine hydrochloride (Symmetrel) is also used, particularly since it is a relatively weaker anticholinergic agent. However, it has the drawback of sometimes exacerbating psychosis because it is a weak DA agonist. Parenteral treatment is preferred to oral treatment because relief of symptoms is more rapid, and the diagnosis can be quickly confirmed. The intravenous (IV) route is faster than the intramuscular. Some clinicians have used intravenous diazepam (Valium). If these agents fail to relieve the symptoms, one may proceed to methylphenidate, caffeine, diazepam, and, in extreme circumstances, barbiturate-induced

sleep. Hypocalcemia lowers the threshold for the development of EPS side effects, which predictably occur with a greater frequency in hypoparathyroidism.

Following amelioration of the acute dystonic symptoms, one may wish to maintain the patient on an oral dose of the effective antiparkinsonian drug at the lowest possible level for several weeks, after which it may be tapered. The wisdom of prophylactic administration of an agent to prevent an occurrence of dystonia is controversial. Why treat patients with needless drugs? is one argument. However, opponents point out that the benefits of prophylaxis outweigh the costs. It is said that young men may be particularly vulnerable to dystonic reactions and therefore may be candidates for prophylactic treatment.[32]

PARKINSONIAN SYNDROME

Parkinsonian syndrome is defined by a triad of abnormal signs: tremor, rigidity, and bradykinesia. The tremor has a frequency of four to eight oscillations per second and is greater at rest than when the patient is engaged in purposeful activity (the opposite of an intention tremor of the cerebellum). It is particularly exacerbated when the patient is stressed: for example, asked about the tremor. When the thumb rubs against the tip of the index finger, the tremor has a "pill-rolling" appearance. The tremor may affect other parts of the body, including the wrist, elbow, arm, head, tongue, and so forth. It is characteristically bilateral. While often the first of the clinical signs of parkinsonian syndrome to appear naturally, tremor is the least common sign in the iatrogenic form.

Rigidity is defined as an increase in the normal resting tone of muscles. It cannot be seen; it can only be perceived by measuring it or feeling it. The way to do this is to ask the patient to relax and then extend, flex, or rotate various parts of the body. Feeling resistance to such passive movement as well as observing how slowly a raised limb returns by gravity to a resting state denotes the presence of rigidity. When rigidity is combined with tremor, one notices a "ratcheting" movement of an arm or leg moved passively. This "cogwheeling" is very characteristic of parkinsonism.

Bradykinesia, or slowed motion, is the most common of the triad seen in the drug-induced parkinsonian state. Its most striking feature is the expressionless, unblinking, masklike facies of the affected patient. This look is often described as "zombielike." The patients often move or turn as if they had no joints. They do not sequentially rotate, starting with the eyes, then the head, shoulders, hips, and lower extremities; rather, they turn *en bloc.* Patients with parkinsonian symptoms have a very characteristic stance and gait that combines aspects of all of the signs. They are flexed and stooped. They are inclined forward and walk with a festinating gait of small rapid steps *(marche avec petits pas),* which tend to accelerate. Ironically, their bradykinesia often makes stopping as difficult as starting, causing them to career into doors, walls, or pieces of furniture in order to stop.

This clinical picture may appear within a few days or after several months of antipsychotic drug treatment. The pathophysiology of naturally occurring Parkinson's disease results from reduced DA input from the substantia nigra in the midbrain to the caudate nucleus in the basal ganglia. However, instead of destruction of dopaminergic neurons causing the DA deficiency, the iatrogenic syndrome results from blockade of DA receptors—the target of the antipsychotic agents—in the striatum or basal ganglia. Since dopaminergic systems appear to be balanced by ACh and gamma-aminobutyric acid (GABA)–mediated neurons, the amelioration of symptoms is produced either by reducing the DA blockade by lowering the dose of antipsychotic medication or by bringing the other circuits into balance by enhancing the ACh-mediated circuits with antiparkinsonian agents that have primarily anticholinergic properties. The one antiparkinsonian agent that is not primarily an anticholinergic agonist is amantadine, which may be a DA agonist. It is important to keep this agent in mind for those patients suffering from EPS complications who may be particularly sensitive to anticholinergic side effects.[74]

The antipsychotic drugs with the highest potency generally are those that bind to DA receptors with greater avidity. As might be expected, these agents—haloperidol, thiothixene, and fluphenazine—are the most likely to produce the parkinsonian syndrome. Thioridazine, the least potent as well as most anticholinergic of the phenothiazines, has the lowest incidence of EPS complications.[148]

AKATHISIA

A third EPS side effect, which is often mistakenly associated with the parkinsonian syndrome is akathisia. The victim feels restless and compelled to keep his legs in motion—either pacing around, constantly shifting his weight from foot to foot, marching in place while standing, or crossing and uncrossing his legs in a compulsive fashion while sitting. Akathisia, if severe, may lead to sleep disturbance because the patient cannot find a comfortable position, or it may exacerbate psychotic symptoms. In the latter case, the physician may respond by increasing the offending antipsychotic agent, thus compounding the problem. Another common misperception is that akathisia is a manifestation of apparent agitated depression, leading to more medication and more side effects. Akathisia may occur days or months after onset of drug therapy. It is also associated with postencephalitic Parkinson's disease.

Akathisia is, like the dystonic reactions, subjectively very unpleasant and potentially can lead to noncompliance. Unlike the other EPS side effects that respond to the several agents noted earlier, treatment of akathisia with anticholinergics, antiparkinsonian agents, antihistaminics, or benzodiazepines is much less reliable, although all of these are worth trying. Alternatively, lowering the dose of the antipsychotic agent or switching to one of lower potency may be useful.[7]

Several recent reports recommend the use of beta-blockers like propranolol hydrochloride, which may be more effective than the more traditional treatments for akathisia. Lipinski and associates reported that nine of fourteen patients had a complete remission of akathisia, some within twenty-four hours; all fourteen improved. The doses of propranolol were low, ranging from 30 to 80 mg per day, which all patients tolerated. Interestingly, some of these patients were also on lithium carbonate; and their tremors were also ameliorated. However, parkinsonian side effects and tardive dyskinesia were not altered by propranolol. These findings suggest mediation via peripheral beta-2 receptors or central beta-blockade. These authors favor the mechanism of central beta-blockade on the basis of washout studies—the therapeutic effect lingers several days after propranolol is discontinued, suggesting CNS binding.[93]

A syndrome commonly confused with akathisia is the "restless leg" syndrome, as described by Blom and Ekbom (not drug-related). It is characterized by a creeping or crawling sensation in the lower limbs, usually symmetrical, which most commonly comes on prior to sleep. It is apparently sufficiently unpleasant to cause insomnia. It may be associated with poliomyelitis, avitaminosis, cold exposure, diabetes, pregnancy, iron deficiency, anemia, carcinoma, uremia, chronic pulmonary disease, or gastric surgery.[17] A paper reporting that quinine sulfate (650 mg/day) was effective in completely reversing refractory akathisia in a forty-two-year-old woman who reported a twenty-nine-year history of restless legs may have, in fact, been about the restless leg syndrome. This patient had never taken antipsychotic medication but had a generalized anxiety reaction as well as dystonia. She had observed that drinking tonic water before sleep ameliorated the symptoms, and the trial of quinine sulfate confirmed these impressions.[141]

Tardive Dyskinesia

Tardive dyskinesia (TD) is a late-onset complication of antipsychotic medication (see also chapter 20). In fact, it was not recognized as causally linked to such treatment until the early 1970s, in spite of the fact that descriptions of the movement disorder had appeared in the literature. Since these reports were anecdotal, the association between the syndrome and exposure to antipsychotic medication was questioned. Instead, the observations were attributed to senile choreas, stereotyped movements and/or mannerisms of schizophrenia, frontal release signs, or nonspecific brain disorders, or to be secondary to other side effects. Mouth movements were attributed to xerostomia or poor dentition.[61]

However, the persistent association between utilization of antipsychotic agents and TD was finally established as the syndrome became more widely appreciated. Currently, most psychopharmacologists believe that prolonged usage of antipsychotic medication can lead to a dyskinetic disorder that may be transient or persistent.[97] The syndrome most commonly consists of involuntary movements of oral, buccal, lingual, and masticatory muscles, which appear as sucking, lip-smacking, or fly-catching tongue movements. Athetoid writhing of the extremities is also noticeable, as well as sudden, jerky, choreiform movements. Reports of impaired breathing owing to TD have appeared. The movements of TD are more choreoathetoid and less purposeful and voluntary than the stereotypies or mannerisms of schizophrenia. The muscles of the face and neck are more usually involved in older patients, while younger ones show abnormal movements in the limbs and digits as well as abnormal posture.[7] In its most extreme forms, TD may include bizarre grimaces and tongue thrusting, which are very disfiguring, as well as opisthotonic posturing of the body. These symptoms can be very disabling socially. Despite this, the affected individual's subjective distress is surprisingly variable; some patients seem almost oblivious to the bizarre movements. But for the majority, TD is humiliating, further exacerbating problems of social isolation and impaired function for which, ironically, the putative offending drugs are being given. Estimates of the prevalence of TD vary widely—from 1 percent to 50 percent of patients receiving antipsychotic medications.[80] When data from all surveys are combined, the prevalence of TD is around 20 percent.[80,81] A population of chronic patients of a comparable demographic distribution not treated with antipsychotic medication would have a prevalence rate of such movements of 5 percent (the true prevalence rate may thus be 15 percent [5 from 20 percent]).[80]

The causal relationship linking antipsychotic medication to this delayed movement disorder is primarily epidemiological. Most workers agree that longer exposure to larger total amounts of these agents may increase the probability of acquiring TD, but even this generalization is not accepted by all investigators. Older patients and females (possibly because of their longevity relative to males) appear to be at greater risk for acquiring an irreversible form of TD. However, specific predictors of risk—type of drug and dose, appearance of EPS side effects, use of antiparkinsonian agents, or inclusion of drug-free periods or drug holidays—do not contribute to predicting useful risk factors for TD.[9]

It is clear that TD can be unmasked either by lowering the dosage of medication or by stopping it abruptly. Conversely, the syndrome may be ameliorated by increasing the dosage of medication, although this approach ultimately worsens the situation. If the movements are misperceived as an EPS side effect and treated with antiparkinsonian agents, they will worsen. If a patient is on antiparkinsonian medication along with the antipsychotic, discontinuing the former drug will improve the picture. These observations have led to formulating the hypothesis that TD is a manifestation of postsynaptic DA receptor supersensitivity following prolonged DA receptor blockade. The condition is pharmacologically analogous to Huntington's chorea and the opposite of Parkinson's disease.[74]

The hypothesis of supersensitivity of postsynaptic DA receptors as a response to prolonged DA deprivation is currently widely accepted. However, several prominent research groups have proposed alternative theories about TD. Perhaps the most controversial one is promulgated by Timothy Crow and his group in the United Kingdom.[40] These authors maintain that TD is no more than a motoric manifestation of schizophrenia, which was described by Kraepelin long before DA receptor agonists were available. The following description is from Kraepelin's earliest publication on dementia praecox:

> The spasmodic phenomena in the musculature of the face and speech, which often appear, are extremely peculiar disorders. . . . Some of them resemble movements of expression, wrinkling of the forehead, distortion of the corners of the mouth, irregular movements of the tongue and lips. . . . They remind one of the corresponding disorder of chronic patients. . . . Connected with these are further smacking and clicking of the tongue. . . . But besides we observe specially in the lip muscles, fine lightning-like or rhythmical twitchings, which in no way bear the stamp of voluntary movements. The same is the case in the tremor of the muscles of the mouth which appear sometimes in speaking. . . . Several patients continually carried out peculiar sprawling, irregular choreiform outspreading movements which I think I can best characterize by the expression "athetoid ataxia." (p. 181)[85]

Crow and associates[40] cite a study by Brandon, McClellands, and Protheroe, who examined 910 patients in a British institution for signs of TD. They found an incidence of 12 percent in untreated men compared to 17 percent in men treated with phenothiazines. In women, the respective figures were 29 percent and 31 percent. The authors concluded that in some cases, dyskinesia seemed to result from drug treatments, "but in general the association between the two is of theoretical rather than clinical significance"[21] (p. 83). In order to specifically look for increased DA receptor sensitivity, Crow and his collaborators examined DA receptors in postmortem tissue of patients who had been treated with phenothiazines for long periods of time. They expected to find an increase in receptor binding in those patients who had suffered from TD as assessed by the Abnormal Involuntary Movement Scale (AIMS). In fact, they found no difference in either D-1 or D-2 receptors among patients whose AIMS scores varied from 0 to 11. They concluded that abnormal movements are a motoric symptom of schizophrenia. Moreover, whether the occurrence of these movements is caused by, exacerbated by, or unrelated to drug treatment has not been established.

The report of Crow and associates [40] is very intriguing but has not been widely accepted. The consensus remains that there is a causal relationship between neuroleptic medication and TD. Perhaps the most compelling evidence is the emerging recognition that some forms of TD are reversible after long periods of time off medication. It had been known that patients often suffer dyskinesias after cessation of antipsychotic medications, but these frequently remit spontaneously after a short period of time. This transient dyskinesia, referred to as withdrawal dyskinesia, had been thought to be a variant of the classical TD, which was characterized as being irreversible. [7] However, reports are now starting to appear that question whether, in fact, "permanent" TD is reversible after a prolonged period of time—often up to ten years. Klawans, Tanner, and Barr [83] followed six patients for twelve years. All had TD, all were under sixty-one years of age, and all had remissions of their abnormal movements after five years.

Prevention and treatment of TD is complicated by our inability to identify authentic risk factors as well as by the absence of any consistently beneficial drug regimen. The optimum strategy for preventing TD remains the maxim that is the cornerstone of medical therapeutics: *"primum non nosare"* (first do no harm). Medicate psychotic patients for the shortest possible time with the lowest efficacious dose of antipsychotic agent. [7] The American Psychiatric Association Task Force on Tardive Dyskinesia has concluded that antipsychotic medication should not be utilized for over six months in any condition other than schizophrenia.

Even then, medication should be reevaluated with the goal of minimum possible exposure to the patient. [149]

If, after having gone through the extensive differential diagnosis (see table 32–4), the diagnosis of TD is established, treatment options are not extensive. No agent alleviates all of the movements in any patient. Since neuroleptic medication is thought by most workers to cause TD, lowering the dose or stopping the drug entirely may eventually treat the condition but can, in the short term, exacerbate the movements owing to withdrawal dyskinesia. On the other hand, increasing the dosage of medications may mask the dyskinesia but will ultimately exacerbate it.

Medications that have therapeutic value in some patients are presented in table 32–5, along with their presumed mechanisms of action. It should be stressed that most of these agents were evaluated in short-term research protocols and are not practical for clinical use. These drugs may modulate the degree of expression of TD rather than produce a long-term beneficial effect. There is a distinction between a drug that can worsen or suppress the expression of a symptom and a drug that cures the disease. In addition, as stated earlier, none of these drugs has been effective in the majority of patients tested. The best treatment for TD remains the use of the lowest effective dose of antipsychotic agent for the shortest possible time.

Clozapine

Recently a new antipsychotic agent has appeared—clozapine, a dibenzoxazepine with no reported extrapyramidal side effects. Because it is structurally more similar to the anxiolytic family of benzodiazepines than the antipsychotics/phenothiazines, a separate section is devoted to its profile of side effects.

EXTRAPYRAMIDAL SYSTEM EFFECTS

To date, there is no data suggesting that clozapine causes extrapyramidal side effects. [139] We are not able to document un-

TABLE 32–4
Tardive Dyskinesia: Differential Diagnosis

Disorder	Associated Mental Disturbances	Family History	Laboratory Tests
Dyskinesias or withdrawal from neuroleptic medication	Yes	No	None
Schizophrenic stereotypies and mannerisms	Yes	No	None
Spontaneous oral dyskinesias associated with aging (including Meige syndrome)[a]	Yes	No	None
Oral dyskinesias related to dental conditions or prostheses[b]	No	No	None
Torsion dystonia	No	Yes	None
Idiopathic focal dystonia (oral mandibular dystonia, blepharospasm, spasmodic "habit spasms" [tics])	No	No	None
Huntington's disease[c]	Yes	Yes	CT scan
Wilson's disease	Yes	Yes	Serum copper and ceruloplasmin
Magnesium and other heavy metal	Yes	No	Specific for metals
Fahr's syndrome or other disorders with calcification of the basal ganglia	No	Yes	Skull x-rays
Extrapyramidal syndromes following anoxia or encephalitis	Yes	No	None
Rheumatic (Sydenham's) chorea ("St. Vitus' Dance")	No	No	None
Drug intoxications—levodopa, amphetamines, anticholinergics, antidepressants, lithium, phenytoin	Yes	No	For specific agents
CNS complications of systemic metabolic disorders (e.g., hepatic or renal failure, hyperthyroidism, hypoparathyroidism, hypoglycemia, vasculitides)	Yes	Possible	For specific disorders
Brain neoplasms (thalamic, basal ganglia)	Yes	No	CT scan, other brain scans, EEG, etc.
Tetany	No	No	Calcium

NOTE: Reprinted, by permission of the publisher, from A. Gelenberg, "Psychoses," in E. Bassuk, S. C. Schoonover, and A. J. Gelenberg, eds., *The Practitioner's Guide to Psychiatric Drugs*. (New York: Plenum Press, 1983), chap. 4, table 2.
[a]Meige syndrome is a disorder of middle age characterized by progressive oral, lingual, and buccal dystonia together with blepharospasms. The movements are indistinguishable from those of TD, but patients with Meige syndrome need not have had antedating antipsychotic drug exposure, and Meige syndrome is a progressive disorder.
[b]Be sure to ask patients about the state of their mouths and teeth and whether they are chewing gum when you are examining them for TD.
[c]The abnormal movements of Huntington's disease are primarily chorea, with little dystonia or athetosis. The movements are generalized, producing a "fidgety" appearance in the early stages. Although movements of TD are more stereotyped and abnormal, the movements of Huntington's disease appear to be normal movements at an increased frequency. Patients with TD have dyskinesias other than chorea. In general, patients with Huntington's disease have more trouble keeping their tongues out, whereas TD patients may have trouble keeping their tongues in their mouths.

equivocally any report of clozapine-induced dystonias. Moderate to severe parkinsonian rigidity is routinely encountered with the standard antipsychotics but is very rare with clozapine. The incidence of parkinsonian side effects with clozapine, in fact, is near to what would be expected with placebo. In blind studies, an occasional placebo patient has displayed mild parkinsonianlike effects. As noted earlier, akathisia can be difficult to distinguish from psychotic agitation; and parkinsonian hypokinesis may present as apathy or withdrawal.

It is the authors' opinion that these exceptional reports may represent nonspecific placebo side-effect symptoms rather than authentic side effects. If clozapine does, in fact, cause parkinsonian side effects, one would expect to see typical extrapyramidal side effects, such as dystonia, but these have not been reported. At this time, we cannot distinguish between the very-low-incidence hypothesis and the no-extrapyramidal-side-effect hypothesis, although we favor the latter. In order to determine which hypothesis is correct, a large placebo-clozapine com-

TABLE 32–5
Therapeutic Agents in Tardive Dyskinesia

Agents That Partially Suppress TD	Agents with Variable or Negligible Effects
Dopamine antagonists	Amantadine
Phenothiazines	Antihistamines
Haloperidol	Cyproheptadine
Clozapine	Deanol
Pimozide	Lithium salts
Metoclopramide	Naloxone, metenkephalin,
Apomorphine (mixed agonist)	des-tyrosine-γ-endorphin
Papaverine (through	Propranolol
dopamine blockers)	Pyridoxine
Amine-depleting agents	Tryptophan
Reserpine	
Tetrabenazine (also a dopamine	
antagonist)	
Blockers of amine synthesis	
Alpha-methyldopa	
Alpha-methyltyrosine	
Cholinergic agents	
Choline	
Lecithin	
Physostigmine	
GABA agonist	
γ-acetylenic GABA	
γ-vinyl GABA	
Muscimol	
Tetrahydroisoxazolopyridinol	
Clonazepam and other benzodiazepines	
Miscellaneous	
Baclofen (GABA mechanism unproven)	
Sodium valproate (GABA mechanism	
unproven)	

NOTE: Reprinted, by permission of the publisher, from D. Tarsay and R. J. Baldessarini, "Tardive Dyskinesia," *Annual Review of Medicine*, 35 (1984): 619.

parison with double-blind ratings of neurological side effects would be required.

Because there have been no long-term studies of clozapine treatment, there are no conclusive data on whether clozapine will produce TD. In order to establish clozapine's relationship to TD, several thousand patients would need to be treated with clozapine for ten years or more. To date, only about three hundred patients have been treated with clozapine for only a few years, and no clozapine-induced TD has been noted. Eight studies have investigated clozapine treatment in patients with TD induced by other antipsychotics. Although some of these patients did improve after three weeks to six months on clozapine, the finding is difficult to interpret. When patients with TD are switched to placebo, some worsen for a few weeks but may improve later.

AGRANULOCYTOSIS

Although clozapine may not produce significant extrapyramidal symptoms, it is not free from other serious side effects. One of the more alarming of these side effects is agranulocytosis, defined as less than 500 granulocytes per mm.[3] Approximately eighty cases of severe neutropenia among patients taking clozapine have been reported. In all such cases, bone marrow examination revealed normal neutrophilic precursors, as well as normal erythroid and thrombocytic elements.[54] The peripheral smear was entirely normal except for the absence of mature polymorphonuclear lymphocytes or bands. The effect of clozapine appears to be a disturbance in the maturation of white blood cell precursors as opposed to the bone marrow suppression seen with an agent such as chloramphenicol, which either suppresses all of the cell lines in the bone marrow—erythrocytic, lymphocytic, leukocytic, and megakaryocytic— or destroys stem cells, leading to an irreversible aplastic anemia.

Clozapine suppresses granulocytic production but the effect is completely reversible.[139] Moreover, with current techniques such as reverse isolation and white blood cell (WBC) transfusions, the lethal risk of even something as unlikely as this effect is further reduced. Almost half the cases occurred during 1975. In the last few years, there have been only one or two reported cases a year. Many drugs, including mianserin, antipsychotics, and the tricyclic antidepressants, are known to cause bone marrow suppression. In two out of three such cases involving clozapine, the patient was receiving another drug known to cause agranulocytosis. However, there have been enough cases reported where patients did not receive any other drug known to cause agranulocytosis to establish that clozapine is, indeed, responsible. Severe neutropenia can occur in patients of all ages, and agranulocytosis can occur in patients on relatively low doses of clozapine.

There is an important relationship between the onset of agranulocytosis and duration of exposure to clozapine. Agranulocytosis is rare during the first four weeks of treatment; the highest incidence occurs during weeks 5 to 25. This is important clinically, because it means that a four-week therapeutic trial on clozapine can be undertaken without an appreciable risk of agranulocytosis. If clozapine does produce a good clinical response, it may be continued after the clinician weighs the benefits of its observed efficacy versus the long-term risk of agranulocytosis.[71] If the patient fails to respond to clozapine, it can be discontinued before the

time period of maximum risk for agranulocytosis.

When clozapine was first introduced, around 1975, the mortality rate from agranulocytosis was approximately 40 percent. In recent years, this figure has decreased by half, owing to the advances just noted. In patients who have agranulocytosis complicated by infection, the mortality rate has been approximately 40 percent; in patients who have agranulocytosis without infection, the rate is currently 10 percent. It may be that after agranulocytosis was described in the literature as a side effect associated with clozapine, clinicians made earlier diagnoses and discontinued the drug more rapidly, resulting in substantially lower morbidity. Alternatively, reduced mortality may reflect improved management.

Because it is a rare side effect, it is difficult to formulate a precise estimate of the incidence of agranulocytosis. In clinical trials, where the number of patients treated and the number of patients developing agranulocytosis is known, the incidence is about 1.5 per thousand. Other estimates use the ratio of total number of reported cases in countries with good reporting systems to the estimated number of patients taking the drug; this method places the incidence at about 0.5 per one thousand patients. Many cases of severe neutropenia have occurred in Finland—the so-called Finnish epidemic. During this period, fifteen out of sixteen cases occurred in only six of the sixty-two hospitals in Finland in which clozapine was used. Interestingly, some patients who had clozapine-induced agranulocytosis were later treated with phenothiazines but did not acquire agranulocytosis with phenothiazines.[71]

Agranulocytosis has an insidious onset. The first complaints are often fatigue and weakness, followed by frank infection with fever and pharyngitis. When the drug is discontinued, polymorphonuclear bands appear in four to five days, and the WBC count returns to normal values within two or three weeks. Management consists of prophylactic reverse isolation, aggressive treatment of infections with appropriate combinations of antibiotics after obtaining cultures, as well as WBC transfusions if needed. By definition, leukopenia is a reduction of the WBC count to less than 3,500 per mm^3, with a granulocyte count above 1,500 per mm^3. Granulocytopenia is a decrease in granulocyte count to below 1,500 per mm^3, and agranulocytosis is a decrease in granulocyte count to below 500 per mm^3. Fatal complications related to severe neutropenia are generally associated with total granulocyte counts below 500 cells per mm^3.

Conventional antipsychotic drugs may suppress bone marrow production, leading to leukopenia or granulocytopenia in 5 to 15 percent of cases. This phenomenon is thought to be different from agranulocytosis and is of no particular clinical significance. Studies in both the United States and Europe compared the prevalence of leukopenia and granulocytopenia in patients taking clozapine to that in patients taking conventional antipsychotics. These studies established that clozapine causes fewer cases of leukopenia or granulocytopenia than did the conventional antipsychotics. It is not uncommon for patients on antipsychotic drugs to have their WBC count drop below 5,000 and then shortly return to within normal limits. In some patients, the WBC count drops below 5,000 and fluctuates between 3,500 and 5,000 for a period of time. In such cases, this fall in WBC count does not progress to agranulocytosis.

We recommend that patients on clozapine have their WBC count followed at approximately weekly intervals (or even at twice-weekly intervals) during the period of greatest risk—five to twenty-five weeks. If a patient's WBC count drops below 3,500 per mm^3, a WBC count should be done twice a week. If a patient's WBC count falls below 3,500 or the granulocyte count below 1,500, clozapine should be promptly discontinued. Patients whose WBC count is below 1,000 or total granulocyte count is below 500 should be placed in reverse isolation.

MISCELLANEOUS SIDE EFFECTS

An unusual side effect of clozapine is that 10 to 15 percent of patients taking the drug show a slight increase in body temperature (usually 0.5 to 1° C, 1 to 2° F). This generally occurs between the fifth and fifteenth day of treatment, after which temperature returns to normal. The cause of this mild increase in temperature is not known. This temperature virtually never reaches 40° C (104° F), which distinguishes this phenomenon from malignant hyperthermia. In no instance have cases of this mild, transitory elevation in temperature progressed to malignant hyperthermia, which is defined by temperatures that are markedly elevated—often 41 to 42° C (106–108° F).

Clozapine also produces postural hypotension and tachycardia, especially in patients started on moderate-to-large doses of the drug. These side effects can occur after the first dose and be quite severe even on the second or third day of treatment. For this reason, patients should be started on a low dose of clozapine. A therapeutic dose of clozapine is approximately 300 or 450 mg per day. However, it is advisable to start clozapine at 50 mg b.i.d. or t.i.d. for two days, and then gradually increase the dose in 25-mg increments over a week to ten days until the dose is in the range of 300 to 450 mg per day administered in divided doses. Since tachycardia and postural hypotension are dose-related and tolerance does develop, side effects are minimized by titrating the dosage upward from a small starting dose. As far as is known, abrupt discontinuance of clozapine does not produce any adverse cardiovascular side effects, although common sense would dictate gradual discontinuance over the course of a few days. If a gradual-increment dosage schedule is followed, only 3 to 5 percent of patients on clozapine experience significant postural hypotension, although a large number of patients do experience a mild degree of it. Clozapine produces nonspecific inverted T-waves, as do conventional neuroleptics, but this is not known to have any clinical importance.

TABLE 32–6
Selective Neurotransmitter Reuptake Blockade of Currently Available
Antidepressants

Drug	NE Uptake[a]	5HT Uptake	Muscarinic ACh Blockade[b]
Amitriptyline	130	300	50
Imipramine	60	490	280
Doxepin	320	3,400	200
Trimipramine	4,400	5,400	125
Nortriptyline	30	1,400	950
Desipramine	2	2,000	2,200
Protriptyline	2	1,600	115
Amoxapine	23	566	c
Maprotiline	20	24,000	c
Trazodone	100,000	760	c

SOURCES: R. J. Baldessarini, "How Do Antidepressants Work?" in J. M. Davis and J. W. Maas, eds.,
The Affective Disorders (Washington, D.C.: American Psychiatric Association Press, 1983), pp.
243–260; and S. C. Schoonover, "Depression," in E. L. Bassuk, S. C. Schoonover, and A. J.
Gelenberg, eds., *The Practitioner's Guide to Psychiatric Drugs* (New York: Plenum Press, 1983),
pp. 19–78
[a]IC 50.
[b]Nanomoles: greater than IC 50, the less the effect.
[c]No information.

Seizures are a relatively rare side effect with clozapine, but they do occur, especially with doses in the range of 800 to 900 mg per day—which is substantially above the therapeutic dose range of 300 to 450 mg. Seizures also have been known to occur in patients on low doses of clozapine.

Approximately one-third of patients on clozapine experience increased salivation, which occurs during both day and night. Patients will complain about waking up with a wet pillow. The salivation is generally mild to moderate in intensity but can be severe, although it is rarely, if ever, severe enough to warrant discontinuation of the drug. The increased salivation can disappear with time; it can disappear with a dose reduction, or it can persist and constitute a serious problem. Anticholinergics, such as atropine, can be used to decrease excessive salivation.

¶ Tricyclics

The tricyclic antidepressants (TCAs), as chemical congeners of aliphatic phenothiazines, would be expected to have a profile of side effects similar to drugs such as chlorpro-mazine, which have already been discussed. The first-generation agents, imipramine and amitriptyline hydrochloride, do, in fact, resemble chlorpromazine in their spectrum of side effects but have significantly more anticholinergic potency. More recently developed antidepressant ring compounds all have structures that are not truly tricyclic. They will be referred to as "heterocyclic antidepressants" or HCAs, following the nomenclature of Schoonover.[126]

Before undertaking a review of the adverse effects of heterocyclic antidepressants, we shall briefly describe proposed mechanisms of action of these agents. Earlier investigations established that these drugs increased intrasynaptic availability of catecholamines by blocking reuptake by the presynaptic neuron (see table 32–6). Most of these data are obtained from animal studies and may not be strictly applied to the human condition in spite of the apparent clinical correlation of neurotransmitter reuptake with expected clinical consequences.

These experimental findings dovetailed nicely with the hypothesis proposed independently by Schildkraut[125] and Bunney and Davis,[27] that catecholamine deficiency might be the biochemical lesion underlying some kinds of depression. However, the catecholamine hypothesis for explaining the therapeutic efficacy of TCAs was complicated by the observation that reuptake blockade of norepinephrine (NE) and serotonin (5HT) occurred almost immediately and continued on a chronic basis, while symptomatic relief always required several weeks. Moreover, mianserin, a second-generation TCA, has no significant effect on catecholamine uptake but increases NE synthesis and has been shown to be clinically effective.

An alternative hypothesis that accounts for the ten-to-fourteen-day lag between achieving adequate serum levels and seeing clinical effect was promulgated by Sulser and his co-workers.[146] They proposed that an excess of NE was the cause of certain depressions and that the antidepressants worked by reducing the sensitivity of postsynaptic NE receptors. Several groups have now corroborated this theory by demonstrating that reduction or down-regulation of postsynaptic beta-adrenergic receptors and "up-regulation" of presynaptic alpha-adrenergic inhibitory receptors are both cotemporal with the onset of clinical efficacy.[105] The authors believe both hypotheses can be reconciled: Down-regulation is a compensatory effect to NE potentiation; hence, the direction of the effect is consistent with the original hypothesis that depression results from reduced noradrenergic tone. Other findings relevant to the pharmacological action of heterocyclics are summarized in table 32–7.

Many of the side effects discussed in the next sections are now better understood in light of the pleicotropic effects of these compounds.

Therapeutic Use of Side Effects

As is the case with antipsychotic medication, properties of the HCAs other than their major pharmacological effects are often considered in making a choice of which HCA to prescribe for a particular patient. It cannot be stressed too much that there appear to be few, if any, significant differences in general

TABLE 32–7
Pharmacodynamic Actions of Heterocyclic Antidepressants

Immediate actions

Block amine uptake (NE, 5HT)
Reduce firing rate and turnover (NE, 5HT cells)
Block ACh receptors (3′, 2′ amine agents)
Inconsistent effects on 5HT, $alpha_1$, and H_2 receptors
No MAO inhibition (or very weak)

Later actions

Block amine uptake
Increase firing rates
Decrease sensitivity of $alpha_2$- and beta-NE receptors
Increase NE release per impulse
Increase 5HT sensitivity but decrease 5HT binding

SOURCE: R. J. Baldessarini, "How Do Antidepressants Work?" in J. M. Davis and J. W. Maas, eds., *The Affective Disorders* (Washington, D.C.: American Psychiatric Association Press, 1983), pp. 243–260

therapeutic efficacy among the HCAs, in spite of anecdotal reports to the contrary. The choice of HCA is, therefore, primarily based on the tolerance of the patient to the adverse effects, which will be discussed further.

HCAs can be divided into two major groups, based on the presence of activating or sedating side effects. The sedating HCAs are most commonly represented by amitriptyline and the relatively activating HCAs by nortriptyline hydrochloride, protriptyline hydrochloride, and desipramine hydrochloride. Amitriptyline had been considered to be more sedating than most other HCAs, but among the newer agents, trazodone hydrochloride is probably at least equal in such properties. If sedation is not desired, imipramine may be a better choice. If an HCA with specifically activating properties seems indicated, protriptyline may be used. The tricyclic drugs are sometimes classified as to whether they potentiate serotonergic or adrenergic function. The sedating HCAs are thought to be more serotonergic, while the activating HCAs are primarily thought to potentiate noradrenergic function.

The so-called serotonergic antidepressants

also affect NE; a more accurate description, therefore, might refer to these drugs as serotonergic and noradrenergic antidepressants in contradistinction to the many antidepressants that are exclusively noradrenergic. However, correlating pharmacological studies carried out in animal systems with clinical observations may ultimately prove to be naively simplified and therefore more confusing than illuminating.

For example, chlorimipramine, currently available in the United States only on a research basis, is described as having potent serotonergic properties, but its metabolite desmethylchlorimipramine has noradrenergic properties.[47] Amitriptyline is relatively serotonergic, but, like chlorimipramine, its metabolite nortriptyline is noradrenergic. Currently, the drug with the most serotonergic activity is trazodone, but trazodone also down-regulates NE receptors so presumably potentiates NE as well.[123] Chlorimipramine, imipramine, and amitriptyline have been studied in man and found to decrease CSF levels of 5-hydroxyindoleacetic acid (5-HIAA) and 3-methoxy-4-hydroxy-phenylglycol (MHPG). It had been thought that either a serotonergic action or a noradrenergic action respectively would result in a feedback inhibition of one of these compounds, not both simultaneously. These data are consistent with the theory that these drugs are equally noradrenergic and serotonergic. An added caveat is that cerebrospinal fluid (CSF) studies, in many cases, have not been proven to indicate unequivocally what is happening in the human brain and so must be interpreted with a certain degree of skepticism. It is tempting to speculate prematurely about the relationship of one or another pharmacological property of these drugs to a clinical effect in man. We would urge caution before accepting such premature hypotheses as proven.

Side Effects That May Interfere with Treatment

Some of the side effects of the HCAs may be particularly detrimental to an occasional patient's general health or to the success of therapy, and in these cases, special care may be needed in monitoring the treatment response.

INDUCTION OF MANIA

One of the more commonly reported unwanted effects of HCA treatment of depression is the induction of manic or hypomanic states in some patients, particularly those known to be bipolar. This effect has been reported for a large number of the HCAs, including those with only noradrenergic properties and those with serotonergic and noradrenergic properties. In some patients this effect is transitory, but in others it may last longer or induce rapid cycling.[3,26,91,159] The use of HCAs to treat depression in patients with a history of manic or hypomanic symptoms requires caution, and the patient should be observed carefully for the appearance of these symptoms.

CARDIOVASCULAR EFFECTS

The HCAs significantly affect several parameters of cardiovascular activity. These effects are potentially life-threatening and therefore must be attended to. The HCAs generally tend to lower blood pressure, especially systolic blood pressure, and in some patients the hypotensive response to HCA treatment is sufficient to produce syncope on standing. Patients' sensitivity to this side effect may prevent increasing dosage to therapeutic levels. Reflex tachycardia is associated with rapid falls in blood pressure and is a common side effect of HCA use.

An additional complication involves the effects of HCAs on the electrical-mechanical aspects of cardiac function. The specific effects of these compounds on the conduction system include prolongation of the P-R interval, which can lead to atrial-ventricular (A-V) block in toxic dosages. Broadening of the QRS complex, elongation of the QT interval, and flattening of the S-T segment may also occur.[63] Patients with premature ventricular contraction are, in fact, benefited from this quinidinelike effect.[14] Patients with ventricular arrhythmias, therefore, may derive substantial clinical benefit from a well-chosen antidepressant, and imipramine can replace quinidine for these patients.[63] In overdose, however, a wide variety of arrhythmias can occur.[88]

Avery and Winokur[4] have identified a factor that confuses the issue of the actual contribution of HCAs to cardiovascular mortality in depressed patients. They have reported excess mortality from heart disease in patients with affective disorders who have not been adequately treated for depression with HCAs (less than 300 mg/day of imipramine) or electroconvulsive therapy (ECT). Treatment with drugs clearly reduces total mortality in spite of the cardiac toxicity. Reed and associates[118] studied the effects of nortriptyline in geriatric patients and confirmed Avery and Winokur's findings. They found that while these patients, compared with controls, showed mild hypotension (postural drop of 15.2/1.9 mm Hg), mild conduction delay (10 milliseconds), and nonsignificant tachycardia (increase of 3.5 beats/minute), even those patients with preexisting cardiovascular disease showed no evidence of increased cardiovascular morbidity or mortality while using the drug when careful dosing and plasma-level monitoring was maintained.

In a review of more recent studies that focused on cardiovascular effects of HCAs at normal therapeutic levels, Glassman and Bigger[63] concluded that orthostatic hypotension is the single serious adverse reaction. Hypotension does not usually preclude the use of HCAs, but in those instances where it may be troublesome, some physicians advise the use of fluorohydrocortisone (0.025 to 0.05 mg b.i.d.).[42] Since falls due to hypotension and fainting may result in broken bones or head injuries, common-sense precautions are important.[42]

Anticholinergic Effects

The other major pharmacological property of most HCAs that accounts for a spectrum of adverse reactions is anticholinergic blockade—an atropinelike action. The HCAs can cause typical autonomic effects: dry mouth, palpitations, tachycardia, loss of accommodation, postural hypotension, fainting, dizziness, vomiting, constipation, edema, and aggravation of narrow-angle glaucoma. In rare instances, urinary retention and/or paralytic ileus has also been observed, which can lead to serious, or even fatal, complications. These problems can be compounded if the HCA has been combined with other drugs with similar anticholinergic effects—for example, a phenothiazine plus an antiparkinsonian drug.

In general, dry mouth is the most notable of the autonomic side effects, and patients should be alerted to its possible occurrence. Dental caries have been reported in patients receiving anticholinergics when they attempt to relieve dry mouth by ingesting hard candy or soft drinks. Fluoride-containing lozenges may prove preferable for dry mouth. Profuse sweating, especially at night, has also been reported. The precise mechanism responsible for that effect is unknown. The autonomic side effects are usually very mild and tend to become less bothersome after the first few weeks of treatment. In any event, they can usually be controlled by adjusting the dosage of the drug. Bethanechol chloride has been recommended for the treatment of anticholinergic side effects such as urinary retention, although many patients may eventually develop tolerance to atropinic side effects.[126]

The tricyclic drugs differ in spectrum and intensity of anticholinergic properties. In the case of a patient who has had difficulty with anticholinergic effects such as urinary retention and constipation, the clinician may wish to consider a tricyclic with fewer anticholinergic properties. Several *in vitro* techniques have been developed to measure anticholinergic properties. In 1977 Snyder and Yamamura[142] found amitriptyline to have the strongest anticholinergic properties, doxepin to be intermediate in that respect, and desipramine to have the weakest anticholinergic properties. There are assays for measuring the binding of atropinelike agents to the muscarinic receptor of the brain, the intestine, or other tissue.

It is not known for sure to what degree the *in vitro* assays correlate with what patients experience, but it is likely there is a good relationship. In 1978 Blackwell and his group[108] provided results that are confirmatory by using salivation as an index of peripheral cholinergic effects. Amitriptyline reduced saliva far more than did desipramine. Exact comparisons required dose-response information for both drugs. In view of the percentage of difference in anticholinergic effects at a given dose and relative clinical potency, it is reasonable to conclude that desipramine has fewer anticholinergic properties than does amitriptyline. Similarly, doxepin has more anticholinergic properties than does desipramine.[108]

Allergic and Hypersensitivity Effects

Skin reactions may occur early in therapy but often subside with reduced dosage. Jaundice, which can occur early, is of the cholestatic type similar to that attributed to chlorpromazine. Agranulocytosis is a very rare complication. Rare cases of leukocytosis, leukopenia, and eosinophilia have also been observed and are thought to have an autoimmune etiology.

Central Nervous System Effects

All the HCAs produce CNS side effects that are roughly similar, although there are slight quantitative differences. For example, amitriptyline and trazodone are usually more sedating, while nortriptyline, protriptyline, and desipramine are less sedating than imipramine. A general untoward effect, common to all, is psychomotor slowing, not unlike that reported with antipsychotic agents. Some patients complain of difficulty in concentrating or planning a sequential activity. It is difficult to evaluate these so-called side effects, because they are so difficult to differentiate from symptoms of depression. Many depressed patients feel some deterioration of function, be it mental function or bodily function, and may falsely attribute this feeling of deterioration to their body. Such symptoms often remit when the patient recovers from the depression and are better correlated to the patient's psychiatric status than to the plasma level of HCA.

The HCAs may cause a persistent, fine, rapid tremor, particularly in the upper extremities but also in the tongue. The tremor is similar to essential tremor. Twitching, convulsions, dysarthria, paresthesia, peroneal palsies, and ataxia have been reported anecdotally. Disturbances of motor functions are rare but are most likely to occur in elderly patients. Insomnia has also been noted among elderly patients on occasion, but it is transitory and responds well to nightly sedation. Protriptyline and MAOIs are often responsible for this complication. Alternatively, a more serotonergic HCA like amitriptyline can be given at night to take advantage of its sedating property.[114]

From time to time, both amitriptyline and imipramine may cause episodes of schizophrenic excitement (very rare), confusion, or mania. Such episodes usually occur in patients with a predisposition to schizophrenia, chronic brain syndrome, or bipolar manic-depressive disorder. This suggests that a preexisting substratum of disease must be present for the drug to exert its psychotomimetic properties. It is imperative to differentiate which type of CNS toxicity is present, since their treatments may differ radically.

Atropinelike psychosis, the so-called central anticholinergic syndrome, produces a characteristic symptom profile of florid visual or tactile hallucinations (such as hallucinations of lights and/or formication, the tactile sensations of insects crawling on the skin), loss of immediate memory, confusion, and disorientation.[57] When these symptoms are observed after the administration of tricyclics, evidence that the syndrome is a central anticholinergic one is indicated both by its emergence as the typical anticholinergic symptom picture and, more important, by the fact that it is reversible by the administration of physostigmine, an anticholinesterase inhibitor that increases available brain ACh, pharmacologically overcoming the atropine blockade.

Generally, conservative management dictates withdrawal of the anticholinergics, which should result in reversal of the syndrome within a day. In selected cases, physostigmine may be indicated to produce a more rapid reversal. However, an error in diagnosis or the use of too much physostigmine may produce cholinergic toxicity. Since tricyclics may convert a depression to mania, one should be alert to that switch among bipolar patients. Although controlled studies are lacking, some clinicians treat bipolar depressive episodes with lithium-tricyclic combinations.

Mild withdrawal symptoms have been reported with the abrupt termination of imipramine; the reactions include nausea, vomiting, and malaise. Since a gradual reduction in dosage is usually preferred to abrupt cessation, such reactions should not pose a clinical problem. The sedation produced by the antidepressants may add to the sedation produced by other CNS depressants such as ethyl alcohol. Indeed, empirical studies verify the common-sense observation that the sedation caused by different sedative-type drugs and that caused by alcohol can combine to produce a greater effect than either agent alone. This caveat does not necessarily apply to all tricyclics, only to those with significant sedating properties.

Cutaneous Manifestations

Rare reports of maculopapular rashes, petechiae, or urticaria have appeared. In all cases, local treatment or discontinuing the HCA has reversed the problem.

Photosensitivity, similar to that caused by phenothiazines, has also been reported. This reaction can be prevented by the use of topical sunblocks like paraminobenzoic acid (PABA) or by reduced exposure to the sun.

Miscellaneous Reactions

Male and female patients taking HCAs may experience increased or decreased sexual desire. Males, in particular, have reported specific sexual dysfunction, including impotence and delayed ejaculation. Whether all or some of these symptoms are referable to the action of the drugs on the autonomic nervous system or their anticholinergic properties, or are, in fact, a manifestation of the depression itself is virtually impossible to distinguish.

Additional idiosyncratic side effects include tinnitus, weight loss, anorexia, weight gain, increase in appetite, black tongue, alopecia, swelling of the parotid glands, and an allergic reaction characterized by generalized edema or edema localized to the face or periorbital regions.[126] Again, several of these symptoms may be manifestations of the drugs or may represent symptoms of depression—particularly those involving changes in eating patterns.

The safe use of HCAs during pregnancy is an unresolved controversy.[115] There is no empirical evidence that establishes a causal relationship between tricyclic administration and teratological consequences, in spite of occasional reports. Although there is no proof of such an association, it is equally difficult to be certain that this connection can be ruled out. Most authorities believe that prudence dictates giving no medication of any kind during the first trimester and as little as possible during the remainder of pregnancy. Of course, in some cases such advice is impossible to implement. HCAs have, in fact, been given during the first trimester without reports of congenital malformations or developmental sequelae.

Neonates born to mothers receiving HCAs at the time of delivery may have urinary retention, irritability, hyperhidrosis, tachycardia, tachypnea, and/or cyanosis. These symptoms are not life-threatening and remit spontaneously within several days postpartum.[56,135] Nursing mothers should be advised that HCAs are passed into breast milk, and they should be counseled to bottle-feed if medication is essential.[5] For a pregnant woman with morbid depression or suicidal ideation, therefore, a trial of HCAs is not contraindicated. However, both physician and patient should be aware of risks, benefits, and uncertainties when making this decision.

Overdose

The most serious clinically adverse effect of HCAs is toxic overdose. A brief clinical digression vis-à-vis overdose seems appropriate regarding hospital management of depressed patients. When such patients are initially evaluated, they often deny suicidal intentions—perhaps owing to anergia, feelings of powerlessness to control their own destiny, or lack of autonomy. However, it is a well-known clinical observation that these feelings of powerlessness or helplessness often remit before the patient feels less depressed. Therefore, such patients may be more active and therefore at a substantially higher risk for suicide after initiation of treatment than they were when first seen. Clinicians must be aware of this dangerous phase of treatment when prescribing, in terms of number of pills ordered and number of refills permitted. Close supervision is essential during this high-risk period.[46] Even so, it is impossible to anticipate and prevent every foreseeable means of suicide. The dilemma that the threat of suicide presents to the therapist is a "no-win" or "double-blind" situation. Elaborate precautions, "specialing" the patient, placing him or her in a single room, or otherwise treating him like a V.I.P. provides, for many patients, enormous secondary gain. It encourages them as well as others to play the suicide game with escalating suicide threats. It is, in fact, impossible to keep a patient from harming him- or herself. One of the goals of psychotherapy is to encourage such patients to take responsibility for their actions. As outpatients, it is neither feasible nor reliable to rewrite prescriptions every day or two so they will not have enough pills; they can hoard them. If patients cannot or will not make a contract to take responsibility for their behavior, they may require rehospitalization, which may reinitiate escalating self-destructive behavior.

Poisoning by the tricyclic antidepressants through overdose occurs most commonly via the quinidinelike effects of these agents on the heart, which cause conduction failure.

The clinical picture of the toxic patient is that of the central anticholinergic syndrome —atropinelike coma, or easily arousable coma with a tachycardia. But these tricyclic comas can be complicated by cardiac arrhythmias and/or seizures. The tricyclic tachycardia of anticholinergic etiology is almost always benign and rarely requires treatment.[38] The efficacy of physostigmine remains unclear. It can reverse a tachycardia as well as a central anticholinergic coma. If a patient has ingested a number of drugs with potent atropinelike properties, physostigmine can be helpful. Its usefulness for pure tricyclic coma, however, is more controversial. While some advocate its use,[28] others are critical, noting that it may be harmful in cases where junctional or idioventricular arrhythmia exists. Indeed, it has been stated that physostigmine is contraindicated when heart block or bradycardia exists. Its primary indication is for supraventricular rather than ventricular arrhythmias.[38,67] In addition, if too much physostigmine is given, it can produce a cholinergic crisis, including seizures, bradycardia, and excessive salivation.

The care of patients with a tricyclic coma should be left to an emergency physician familiar with the treatment of pharmacological overdose. Nevertheless, the psychiatrist needs to know some of the idiosyncracies of tricyclic coma. An overdose of tricyclics initially produces agitation and confusion, which progress to muscular twitching, delirium, and, finally, coma. Coma is generally an easily arousable condition lasting less than twenty-four hours. Following recovery, disturbed behavior, confusion, and hallucinations may persist for several days. The anticholinergic signs include dilated pupils, dry mouth, warm skin, urinary retention, diminished bowel sounds, and deep coma; respiratory depression is an ominous sign. The most pronounced cardiac effects are the quinidinelike properties of tricyclic drugs, characterized by delayed A-V conduction with the ECG abnormality of prolonged P-R interval. When plasma levels are above 100 ng per ml, there is a moderately good correlation between QRS-complex duration and plasma concentration.

Some workers advocate the use of a small dose of a prophylactic anticonvulsant for the prevention of seizures in tricyclic overdose. The degree to which the coma is deepened by a small dose of such a CNS depressant is negligible. As seizures represent a serious management problem, patients can be treated with intravenous diazepam. If the patient is conscious, induction of vomiting can be useful to minimize further absorption. For the unconscious patient, activated charcoal administered via a naso-gastric tube also is helpful, even many hours after the suspected ingestion.[39] In addition, absorption is delayed due to the atropinelike effect on gastric motility, and the toxic drug is recirculated via the interhepatic circulation. Hypotension will usually respond to elevation of the foot of the bed (the Trendelenburg maneuver). Attention to electrolyte balance, hypoxia, and acidosis is essential; the administration of sodium bicarbonate can be quite helpful to control the latter problem.

The half-life of tricyclics in patients who have overdosed can be several days. Serious cardiac arrhythmias occurring after the patient awakens from a deep coma are not uncommon. Continuous cardiac monitoring for up to a week is required despite the patient's alert mental status. The administration of sodium bicarbonate decreases acidosis, thereby increasing protein binding of the drug and reducing the concentration of unbound drug at critical receptors.[126]

¶ Second-generation Antidepressants

Since many of the "second-generation" antidepressants have been developed with the goal of ameliorating specific side effects, these agents will be reviewed individually. Table 32–8 summarizes the pharmacological profile of many of the newer HCAs.

Alprazolam

Alprazolam is a recently released benzodiazepine that, in dosages higher than required for anxiolytic efficacy, is an effective antidepressant agent. We have found that it down-regulates beta-receptors[105] as well as demonstrating the standard antidepressant pattern of increasing rapid-eye-movement (REM) latency time and decreasing REM density. Its structure defines it as a triazolobenzodiazepine, which is both absorbed and eliminated rapidly. Its potential advantages over traditional HCAs include rapid onset of action, few adverse side effects, virtually no anticholinergic properties, and very minimal risk of death on overdosing, unless it is combined with alcohol.

In direct comparison with imipramine, alprazolam was equally effective in treating depression and significantly better in relieving somatic symptoms, as well as having an earlier onset of action. Imipramine, furthermore, produced more adverse side effects; only drowsiness was reported more frequently by users of alprazolam.[60] This report, as well as more recent data summarized in the review by Davis and Fredman,[45] suggests that this agent will be a useful addition to the psychiatric pharmacopoeia for depression. A current report comparing alprazolam with amitriptyline and doxepin confirms not only its efficacy as an antidepressant but also its superior profile of side effects (fewer than the others).[121] Like HCAs, alprazolam can precipitate a manic attack.[3] It otherwise has a similar side-effect profile to other benzodiazepines, including the liability of potential abuse.

Amoxapine

Released for use in 1982, amoxapine is a dibenzoxazepine derivative similar to phenothiazines as well as to HCAs. However, its pharmacological properties are characteristic of an antidepressant: It potentiates catecholamines and antagonizes reserpine-induced depression. It inhibits the reuptake

TABLE 32–8
Pharmacological Properties of New Antidepressant Drugs

Drug	Central Action	Anticholinergic Effect	Cardiovascular Toxicity
Alprazolam	GABAergic; noradrenergic	None	Very low
Bupropion	Dopaminergic in effect; noradrenergic	None	Less than tricyclics
Fluoxetine	Inhibits 5HT reuptake	None	None
Fluvoxamine	Inhibits 5HT reuptake	None	Low
Maprotiline	Inhibits NE reuptake	Mild–moderate	Less than tricyclics
Mianserin	Presynaptic alpha$_2$-receptor blockade	Slight; less than maprotiline	Low
Nomifensine	Inhibits NE reuptake; potently inhibits DA reuptake	Very mild	Less than tricyclics
Oxaprotiline	Potently inhibits NE reuptake	Mild; less than maprotiline	Less than tricyclics
Trazodone	Blocks 5HT reuptake; potentiates 5-HTP[a]	None	Low
Zimelidine	Inhibits 5HT reuptake; inhibits NE reuptake	None	Low

SOURCE: J. P. Feighner, "Clinical Efficacy of the Newer Antidepressants," *Journal of Clinical Psychopharmacology*, 1 (Supplement) (1981):23–26.
[a] 5-HTP = 5-hydroxytryptophan.

of NE and 5HT. Amoxapine is catabolized to an active metabolite that has DA-blocking properties. Plasma-level studies using the radioreceptor assay demonstrate the same degree of DA blockade in plasma as is found in a patient receiving an antipsychotic. Not unexpectedly, patients have reported extrapyramidal side effects and withdrawal dyskinesia following the use of amoxapine. The side-effect profile is more similar to antipsychotic agents than HCAs; therefore, long-term administration carries the attendant risk of TD.[144] In spite of the fact that amoxapine is pharmacologically similar to phenothiazine and would, therefore, be expected to be less likely to produce cardiac-conduction problems, there have been several reports of overdoses of amoxapine producing bundle-branch block,[19] premature atrial contraction,[64] and atrial flutter.[170] One benefit of amoxapine is its slightly decreased incidence of anticholinergic effect as estimated by xerostomia.[46]

Doxepin

Doxepin hydrochloride was initially touted as an HCA with reduced risk of cardiac toxicity based on the observation that it

rarely altered pulse rate, ECG pattern, or blood pressure.[111] Burrows and coworkers in Australia corroborated these findings in a series of studies[29,163] comparing the effects of doxepin on the cardiovascular system with other HCAs. They found that milligram for milligram, doxepin caused less alteration in the conduction rate, as well as ECG pattern, and had less effect on cardiovascular performance: that is, on pulse rate and maintenance of blood pressure. With the development of reliable methods for measuring plasma levels of HCAs, however, these data have required reevaluation. For the average patient, a therapeutic plasma level of doxepin requires a significantly larger oral dose than is required with amitriptyline or imipramine. When 400 mg orally administered doxepin is compared with 300 mg orally administered imipramine or amitriptyline, all dosages within therapeutic limits, the plasma levels are approximately the same; and the cardiac-sparing effect of doxepin disappears.[62]

Finally, Pitts's observation[111] that doxepin causes less orthostatic hypotension than other HCAs has not been confirmed by subsequent studies. In a carefully controlled animal study, Brown and Leversha[24] found doxepin to be more potent than either amitriptyline or imipramine (least potent) in causing orthostatic changes in dogs. Doxepin offers no other noteworthy advantage in direct comparison with other HCAs in terms of therapeutic efficacy or profile of side effects. However, it should be reemphasized that unlike the other HCAs, which generally require a dose of no more than 300 mg per day, a patient receiving doxepin may require up to 400 mg per day to achieve the same plasma level and clinical effect. In evaluating whether doxepin causes fewer adverse reactions, the dosage effect must be kept in mind.

Maprotiline

Maprotiline is one of several HCAs released for clinical use by the Food and Drug Administration in 1982. It has a tetracyclic structure that was initially thought to account for its decreased anticholinergic side effects. After early publicity about it being tolerable to patients who could not adjust to the anticholinergic properties of other HCAs, reports began to appear that patients on maprotiline had more frequent seizures than patients taking other HCAs.[122] The great majority of such patients were receiving a daily dose exceeding 225 mg per day. At this dose the incidence of seizures ranged between 0.1 and 0.4 percent, in comparison with other HCAs whose incidence of seizures ranged from 0.05 to 0.2 percent.[51,78] Lowering the dose appears to reduce the incidence of seizures, perhaps to a frequency comparable to other HCAs. Ciba-Geigy, the manufacturer of maprotiline, now recommends 225 mg per day as the maximum dose.[132]

In addition, in spite of its tetracyclic structure and early claims to the contrary, maprotiline retains many of the cardiovascular effects observed with other HCAs. It causes a similar pattern of conduction delays in the therapeutic dose range; in toxic overdoses, deaths from heart block and asystole have been reported.[55] Frequent occurrences of orthostatic hypotension among patients using maprotiline have been reported. When maprotiline is taken in overdose, there is a significant lethality. Unlike the tricyclics, whose cardiac effects are noteworthy, maprotiline is relatively free of heart effects, but the occurrence of seizures and other CNS toxicities are notable. Table 32–9 summarizes the clinical profiles of a number of the new antidepressants.

Mianserin

Mianserin hydrochloride is another of the new HCAs that has been widely used in Europe. It is a tetracyclic compound that has similar clinical efficacy in controlled comparisons with older agents. Its primary mode of action is to block alpha-2-adrenergic receptors in the CNS, thereby acting to increase NE synthesis. In addition, it is a potent blocker of H_2-histamine receptors.[59] This latter property may explain its particular pattern of side effects, which includes weight gain, lethargy, and drowsiness. It is reported to have virtually no anticholinergic or cardiovascular side effects.[22] It is clearly more effective than placebo and marginally less effective than the HCAs.[46]

Nomifensine

Unlike maprotiline and mianserin, nomifensine is not structurally related to HCAs. Rather, it is a tetrahydroisoquinoline compound that inhibits both NE and DA reuptake. Since nomifensine is an activating compound, it has been suggested that it might be particularly effective for a depressed patient with prominent psychomotor retardation. Nomifensine is, in fact, not only effective in this condition, but it also works in a clinically broad spectrum of depressive disorders. Its side-effect profile is, not unexpectedly, related to the particular symptoms for which it is targeted. These untoward effects include hyperactivity, insomnia, and tremulousness. In addition, nomifensine has the usual complement of anticholinergic side effects, but these are said to be milder than in the HCAs.[23,59] This drug does not cause convulsions and therefore should be considered in patients with seizure disorders.

TABLE 32–9
Clinical Profiles of New Antidepressant Drugs

Drug	R or E[a]	As Effective as Tricyclics?	Dosage
Alprazolam	R	Yes, in unipolar depression; probably not in bipolar disorders	0.5–4.0 mg/day, single or divided doses
Bicyclic compounds	E	Probably; clinical trials underway	Zimelidine: 100–300 mg/day; fluoxetine: 40–80 mg/day. Toxicity produces Guillain-Barre syndrome
Bupropion	E	Yes	200–600 mg/day, divided doses
Fluoxetine	E	Yes/no	20–80 mg/day, divided doses
Maprotiline	R	Yes	50–225 mg/day, single or divided doses
Mianserin	E	Slightly less effective	30–150 mg/day, given at bedtime
Nomifensine	E	Yes	100–200 mg/day, single or divided doses
Oxaprotiline	E	Yes	50–150 mg/day, single or divided doses
Trazodone	R	Yes	50–800 mg/day, single or divided doses, with largest dose at bedtime
Unicyclic compounds	E	Probably; clinical trials underway	Fluvoxamine and clovoxamine: 50–300 mg/day, single or divided doses

SOURCE: J. P. Feighner, "Clinical Efficacy of the Newer Antidepressants," *Journal of Clinical Psychopharmacology,* 1 (Supplement) (1981): 245.
[a] Released (R) or experimental (E) in United States.

Trazodone

Trazodone is a triazolopyridine compound that is unique; its primary pharmacological action in the CNS is to block 5HT reuptake. It has peripheral and adrenergic blocking action as well. Trazodone down-regulates NE beta-receptors, so it also has noradrenergic activity.

Initially trazodone seemed like a very promising compound because it had unambiguous efficacy in treating a large number of depressive symptoms, and it had virtually no anticholinergic side effects. The early line on side effects mentioned drowsiness and lethargy. Occasionally headaches or GI complaints were reported.

The drowsiness associated with trazodone seems as tenacious as the well-known drowsiness commonly caused by amitriptyline, but it is not transient. Although a fair degree of tolerance develops, patients do not appear to be free of the problem. This lassitude can be so overwhelming as to be incapacitating,

thereby vitiating whatever antidepressant effect the drug provides. Moreover, it can be dangerous for patients who have to drive or operate machinery, particularly when combined with alcohol.[152]

Initial studies established that trazodone does not alter A-V conduction. Dogs given toxic doses of trazodone showed no alteration in cardiac conduction or performance; instead, they died from seizures at very high doses.[66] Neither did orthostatic hypotension seem so severe, although it was reported anecdotally. However, clinical experience has substantiated a newly appreciated cardiac effect of trazodone, the exacerbation of ventricular irritability in patients so predisposed.

Janowsky and associates[76] have shown that among patients with preexisting cardiac problems, trazodone exacerbated ventricular ectopy and, in one patient, precipitated an episode of ventricular tachycardia. After trazodone was discontinued, the frequency of premature ventricular contractions fell to pretrial levels.[76] This report was not a blind, or controlled study, and patients were on the drug for a greater period of time than on no drug. This cardiac effect may therefore have been coincidental.

Lippmann and coworkers[94] reported the occurrence of junctional arrhythmia in a fifty-three-year-old woman receiving 300 mg per day who had several previously normal ECGs. When trazodone was stopped, the arrhythmia disappeared. Their recent review of the literature suggests that trazodone is capable of perturbing A-V conduction, although its mode of action is not well understood.[94] Alternatively, since it does not have the antiarrhythmic quinidinelike properties of other HCAs, it may not protect the heart against ventricular irritability. All of these factors must be considered when using this drug.

The final adverse effect, apparently unique to trazodone, that is currently receiving attention is the occurrence of priapism—defined as prolonged dysfunctional penile erection. According to *Biological Therapeutics in Psychiatry*,[99] Mead Johnson, the manufacturer of trazodone, had received reports as of January 1983 of ten episodes of priapism, some of which required surgery to achieve detumescence. Priapism can lead to permanent impotence or, in its most severe form, ischemia with attendant complications. These adverse reactions, in conjunction with the others noted, have all been reported in consideration of the fact that trazodone is now among the most widely prescribed HCAs. It is therefore difficult to make a firm recommendation for or against the agent. Such side effects as priapism in a second-generation drug must be viewed in the context of agranulocytosis and jaundice in the first-generation tricyclics. The practitioner should weigh all these considerations and carefully monitor patients.

If there are any possible generalizations to be made about the so-called second-generation antidepressants, it is that they share many of the untoward effects of the "first-generation" agents, as well as contributing a few new wrinkles of their own.

¶ Monoamine Oxidase Inhibitors

The history of MAOIs, their discovery and early enthusiastic reception, followed by recognition of unacceptable adverse effects leading to their decline in popularity, and their new popularity, is, in fact, a history of response to their side effects. The subsequent narrative is a replay of this important leitmotif, which runs through this chapter.

Initial enthusiasm for MAOIs flagged when several patients on iproniazid developed cirrhosis and died. However, new chemical congeners structurally related to iproniazid were identified that inhibited MAO activity without hepatic toxicity. The second wave of enthusiasm for MAOIs, which were extensively used in the 1960s, was dampened by reports of hypertensive crises caused by tyramine, a metabolite that accumulated in the GI tracts of patients whose MAOs were inhibited. When absorbed into the general circulation, tyramine, a vasoactive amine in fermented foods can lead to acute elevation of blood pressure with sometimes fatal consequences. Since the early 1960s pharmacological research has been directed toward identifying compounds that selectively inhibit MAO receptors in the CNS while sparing peripheral receptors, particularly in the GI tract. No such compound has been marketed. In fact, no new MAOI has appeared since 1962.[15]

All MAOIs available for clinical use have similar affinities for the two classes of MAOs found throughout the body (gut, liver, CNS, platelets, and blood vessels). Type A MAO accounts for 20 percent of CNS activity but the majority of gastrointestinal activity. This enzyme metabolizes 5HT and NE. Type B MAO accounts for 80 percent of CNS activity and primarily oxidizes DA in human brain and phenylalanine. It contributes 20 percent of MAOI activity in the GI tract. Three partially selective MAOIs are currently under investigation: Clorgyline is selective for MAO-type A, while pargyline hydrochloride is partially selective for MAO-type B. Deprenaline is selective for MAO-type B. Preliminary findings suggest that the more important adverse side effects are associated with MAO-type A inhibition.[109]

The spectrum of side effects of MAOIs is remarkably similar to several other classes of psychotropic agents, with the exception of the tyramine or "cheese" reaction. This most serious complication is the result of either excessive doses of an MAOI or combination of an MAOI with heterocyclic antidepressants or sympathomimetic agents, or, most commonly, by the dietary ingestion of excess tyramine, which is not catabolized in its inactive metabolites by MAOs normally active in the gut.

MAOIs are currently enjoying a resurgence in popularity owing, in part, to the fact that they may be selectively efficacious in particular forms of depression.[41] In addition, panic disorders, which were previously thought to be characterological reactions, have recently been found to be responsive to MAOIs, tricyclics, and alprazolam, and may be particularly sensitive to MAOIs. It is thus particularly timely to review adverse reactions associated with this group of medications that is enjoying a recrudescence of popularity.

Before setting out the particulars of MAOI side effects, a brief comment on a pharmacokinetic issue is pertinent. Therapeutic efficacy is achieved when MAO inhibition of greater than 80 percent of activity is reached. Since MAOIs bind irreversibly to MAOs, discontinuing medication does not reverse inhibition. The patient needs to resynthesize MAOs to replace the permanently inactivated ones, and this process takes up to two weeks. Thus some manifestation of side effects can be expected to linger as long as two weeks.

A sensible approach to thinking about adverse reactions associated with MAOIs is to separate untoward effects into the interaction of MAOIs with foodstuffs and medications and side effects intrinsic to the drug.

We have already described the mechanism of the tyramine reaction, which was one of the cataclysmic side effects recognized early and which nearly took MAOIs out of the pharmacopoeia. It is now known that the vasoactive substances that are released into the circulation, if not catabolized, include sympathomimetic amines as well as tyramine. The earliest symptoms of an impending hypertensive crisis may include some or all of the following: headache—developing rapidly with pain limited to the temporal or occipital region—diaphoresis, pallor, nuchal rigidity, chest pain, or palpitations. An occasional patient may suffer a cerebral hemorrhage, which can be fatal, but this is very rare.

Foods that contain tyramine (or levodopa) are all potentially harmful, but the dangerous ones are those that contain high concentrations of these vasoactive catecholamines. Thus a general principle is the smellier the cheese, the more tyramine it contains and the more dangerous it is. However, cheddar cheese can vary enormously in its tyramine content, depending on its maturity. Figure 32-1, a reprint of a diet and drug warning card prepared by the British Medical Association, is an example of the kind of information a patient on MAOIs should receive.

Table 32-10 contains tyramine content of foods along with recommendations for consumption by patients being treated with MAOIs.

Tyramine content is highly variable even within the same piece of cheese or meat extract. In addition, tyramine content may vary with time of fermentation. Therefore, it is impossible to do large statistical studies on it. Furthermore, some foods are placed on the avoidance lists for unclear reasons. There is agreement on the more dangerous foods, such as cheddar or stilton cheese, pickled herring, Chianti, Bovril, and broad bean pods; more controversy exists on some of the other foods. Additionally, foods containing high concentrations of aged protein, such as smoked salmon (lox), figs, raisins, sauerkraut, snails, and soy sauce, should be consumed in moderation but need not be absolutely forbidden. Coffee, tea, chocolate, and cocoa are on many lists of excluded foods, but most authorities on this subject are skeptical of the genuine risks associated with them.

FIGURE 32–1
Treatment Card

Carry this card with you at all times. Show it to any doctor who may treat you other than the doctor who prescribed this medicine, and to your dentist if you require dental treatment.

INSTRUCTIONS TO PATIENTS

Please read carefully

While taking this medicine and for 10 days after your treatment finishes, you must observe the following simple instructions—

1. Do not eat CHEESE, PICKLED HERRING OR BROAD BEAN PODS.

2. Do not eat or drink BOVRIL, OXO, MARMITE OR ANY SIMILAR MEAT OR YEAST EXTRACT.

3. Do not take any other MEDICINES (including tablets, capsules, nose drops, inhalations, or suppositories) whether purchased by you or previously by your doctor, without first consulting him.

   NB: Cough and cold cures, pain relievers and tonics are medicines.

4. Drink ALCOHOL only in moderation and avoid CHIANTI WINE completely.

Report any severe symptoms to your doctor and follow any other advice given by him.

Note: Reprinted, by permission of the publisher, from P. J. Tyrer, *Drugs in Psychiatric Practice* (London: Butterworth & Co., 1982), p. 262.

Peter Tyrer,[154] in his excellent chapter on MAOIs, dismisses much of the data on forbidden foods. He notes that many items are on the list as the result of unsubstantiated anecdotal reports. In fact, some of these offenders, including bananas, red wine, port sherry, beer, yogurt, chocolate, and avocado pears, all contain very low concentrations of tyramine or DA. He states that commercial preparations are entirely safe. He does caution against homemade wines, beers, and yogurt. He quotes Blackwell, Marley, and Taylor,[16] one of the first groups to associate hypertensive episodes with dietary ingestion of vasoactive amines; they report that prior to the circulation of forbidden food lists, many patients on MAOIs freely ate items on the list without any problem.

The observation that many patients can tolerate the ingestion of vasoactive catecholamines has led some workers to speculate that these individuals have alternative metabolic pathways for inactivating these amines, for example, via sulphate conjugation. These inquiries have, however, produced no measurable differences between patients who do not demonstrate the vascular response and those who do.[20] Tyrer wryly notes that amid these uncertainties, more misinformation has become part of the psychopharmacological lore.[154]

MAOIs interact with indirectly acting medicinal amines as well. Sympathomimetic agents including amphetamine, methylamphetamine, ephedrine, and over-the-counter cold preparations containing sympathomimetic decongestants or asthma medication (e.g., phenylpropanolamine, pseudoephedrine, phenylephrine) are also potentially dangerous and should be avoided scrupulously. Levodopa is also dangerous. This includes agents such as those used in nose or eye drops. Histamine and bee venom may be potentially active.

The possibility of complications such as headache, hypertensive crisis, and intracranial bleeding can be virtually eliminated by careful attention to diet and by avoidance of pressor drugs and related substances. Patients should, therefore, be appropriately educated. Should those side effects occur, they can be treated by the administration of alpha-adrenergic blockers, such as phentolamine: 5 to 10 mg IM administered while

TABLE 32–10
MAOI Dietary Restrictions

Foods with High Tyramine Content—NOT PERMITTED

Unpasteurized cheeses (aromatic): cheddar, emmanthal, stilton, bleu, etc.
Meat extracts: Bovril, Marmite, etc.
Smoked/pickled protein: herring, sausage
Aged/putrifying protein: chopped chicken liver, seasoned game, etc.
Chianti wines and other fortified wine
Italian broad beans (fava) pods (because of high levodopa content)
Caviar

Foods with Limited Tyramine Content—LIMITED AMOUNTS ALLOWED

Meat extract: bouillion, consommé
Pasteurized light and pale beers
White wines: champagne; some red wines; sherry
Ripe avocado, ripe banana
Sour cream, yogurt

Foods with Low Tyramine Content—PERMISSIBLE

Port wine
Distilled spirits (in moderation)
Pasteurized cheeses: cream, cottage
Chocolate
Yeast breads
Fruits: figs, grapes, raisins
Soy sauce, meat tenderizer
Caffeine-containing beverages

SOURCE: A. Nies, "Clinical Application of MAOIs," in G. D. Burrows, T. R. Norman, and B. Davies, eds., *Antidepressants* (Amsterdam: Elsevier, 1983), p. 243.

monitoring blood pressure, or 2 to 5 mg IV, which is effective in minutes or may require a second dose. Blood pressure needs to be carefully monitored and medications adjusted appropriately. Phenoxybenzamine can also be used, as can chlorpromazine, if other drugs are unavailable.

Interactions with Other Drugs

The combination of an MAOI with an imipramine-type drug can lead to a syndrome with restlessness, dizziness, tremulousness, muscle twitching, sweating, convulsions, hyperpyrexia (104° to 109° F), and, sometimes, death. Those reactions can also occur after chronic administration of an MAOI is combined with a bolus of an imipramine-type drug, dextromethorphan, or meperidine, given in high doses or intramuscularly. Con-

sequently, a washout period of at least seven days is recommended to allow the MAO enzyme to regain activity before such medication is given.

Some clinicians have used a combination of tricyclic-MAOI with reasonable safety by closely supervising their patients. By starting the drugs sequentially, adding the MAOIs to a preexisting low-dose tricyclic while cautiously adjusting dosages where indicated, they have obtained good results without adverse effects. However, these drugs should not be used in combination as a routine measure until their safety, efficacy, and appropriate dosage schedules have been worked out by skilled clinical investigators. The danger is most acute when high doses of imipramine-type or amephetaminelike drugs are given in cases in which MAO has been inhibited to a considerable degree. Death, in fact, has been reported after a single IM injection of 25 mg imipramine in a newly hospitalized patient whose prior MAO-inhibiting treatment was not known to the hospital staff.[11,131] The need to obtain a careful history of previous drug treatment in depressed patients before initiating a new course of drug therapy is clearly evident. The earlier caveat of waiting sufficient time for the regeneration of new MAOs after discontinuing MAOI treatment cannot be stressed too often. Table 32–11 lists some of the MAOI incompatabilities.

The MAOIs can interfere with liver microsomal enzyme, leading to potentiation of a great variety of drugs, including alcohol,

TABLE 32–11
MAOI Drug Incompatibilities

Contraindication

Stimulants: amphetamines, cocaine, anorectic drugs
Decongestants: sinus, hay fever, cold tablets
Antihypertensives: methyldopa, guanethidine, reserpine
Antidepressants: imipramine, desipramine, chlorimipramine, trimipramine given in high doses (particularly IM)
MAOIs: Tranylcypromine after other MAOIs
Narcotics: Meperidine (pethidine)

Relatively Contraindicated (marked potentiation)

Amine precursors: levodopa, L-tryptophan

Potentiation

General anesthetics
Sympathomimetics: adrenaline, noradrenaline, dopamine, isoprel
Narcotics: morphine, codeine, etc.
Sedatives: alcohol, barbiturates, benzodiazepines
Local anesthetics containing vasoconstrictors
Hypoglycemic agents: insulin, tolbutamide, chlorpropamide

Insufficient Knowledge

Antidepressants: maprotiline, amoxapine, trazodone, zimelidine
MAOI-MAOI: reversible after irreversible

SOURCE: A. Nies, Clinical Applications of MAOIs," in G. D. Burrows, T. R. Norman, and B. Davies, eds., *Antidepressants* (Amsterdam: Elsevier, 1983), p. 244.

antihistamines, antiparkinsonian agents, barbiturates, hypoglycemic agents, tricyclics, phenothiazines, opiates, methyldopa, ganglionic blocking agents, procaine, anesthetic agents, chloral hydrate, and aspirin.

It is important to recall that psychopharmacological intervention is never benign. Death may also occur in conjunction with ECT and tricyclics as well as with an MAOI. The death rate with ECT is estimated to be in the ratio of 1 in 10,000 cases; the estimated death rate with iproniazid is 1 in 10,000 cases; and with tranylcypromine, 1 in 100,000 cases. For purposes of comparison, death rates from the surgical treatment of peptic ulcer vary from 1 in 100 to 1 in 1,000.

The side effects associated with MAOIs that are attributable to the primary action of the drug, as opposed to their interaction with foods or other drugs, can be conveniently summarized according to physiological systems.

Autonomic Nervous System Effects

The MAOIs cause autonomic side effects such as dry mouth, dizziness, orthostatic hypotension, epigastric distress, constipation, delayed micturition, delayed ejaculation, and impotence. This side-effect profile is very similar to that of other psychotropic agents, and no further description is necessary. Many of these unpleasant side effects are transitory, and patients can be encouraged to push through the discomfort; they may very well develop tachyphylaxis. Alternatively, dosage schedules may be adjusted or another agent from the same group tried.

Hepatic Necrosis

Severe hepatic necrosis has been discussed in conjunction with iproniazid. It occurs very rarely but has a high fatality rate (about 25 percent), as initially reported. This complication led to the drug's withdrawal from clinical use. Similar hepatocellular damage has been reported to occur very rarely in patients treated with other hydrazine MAOI antidepressants—phenelzine, nialamide, and isocarboxazid. Although definitive studies of the incidence of such reactions have not been made, it is believed that they occur much less frequently with phenelzine, niala-mide, and isocarboxazid than with iproniazid and are, in fact, extremely rare. It is reported that a patient placed on a second trial of MAOIs can have a recurrence of hepatocel-lular jaundice, regardless of whether the MAOI is of the same structural family of hy-drazines or not. Jaundice is not reported in association with nonhydrazine MAOIs. Con-sequently, the free hydrazine, rather than the MAO-inhibiting property, is suspected as the causative agent. [107]

Central Nervous System Effects

In general, the most common behavioral toxicity with MAOIs has been the precipita-tion of a hypomanic or manic episode, but restlessness, hyperactivity, agitation, irrita-bility, and confusional states with sensory dis-tortion and disorientation can also occur. [34] Rare cases of paranoid psychosis have been reported. [136] In addition, vertigo, ataxia, dull-ness, drowsiness, memory impairment, tremulousness, hyperreflexia, fasciculations, and seizures have all been associated with the use of MAOIs. [101] These, however, all occur very occasionally. The mechanism of this relationship has not been well estab-lished. [126]

MAOIs suppress REM sleep, [169] and this suppression is associated with restoration of normal mood. [87] Since REM suppression pre-cedes alleviation of depressive symptoms, it is an excellent predictor of treatment re-sponse. Discontinuance of MAOI treatment is accompanied by REM rebound. [151] Para-doxically, some patients experienced insom-nia, while others experienced sedation. The former can be given drug in the morning and at noon and the latter at night.

Miscellaneous Effects

Ankle edema occurs in about 5 percent of patients and can be managed by diuretics if necessary.

MAOI Overdose

An overdose of an MAOI produces adren-ergic hyperactivity, agitation, tachycardia, hyperreflexia, sweating, alternating hypo-tension and hypertension, hyperpyrexia, convulsions, and death. The hyperpyrexia is noteworthy, and the clinician should be pre-pared to treat this condition, which has a lag period of a few hours to twelve or more hours. Patients may initially have only mild symptoms, but the syndrome can proceed to a severe state.

Finally, tranylcypromine in combination with disulfiram (Antabuse) has caused con-vulsion and death in animals.

¶ Lithium

Lithium is the most recent addition to the armamentarium of the American psy-chopharmacologist. Cade's report of the calming effect of lithium on ten agitated patients appeared in 1949[31]; but the drug did not gain approval for use in the United States until 1970, because of the death of several cardiac patients using lithium as a sodium substitute. The paradox of lithium— on the one hand, an apparently benign and effective treatment for bipolar illness and, on the other hand, a potentially lethal drug —is epitomized by the reluctance of the Food and Drug Administration to permit the use of lithium in the United States for over a decade, despite the fact that hun-dreds of thousands of patients elsewhere were enjoying remission from the ravages of manic-depressive illness, which affects up to 0.9 percent of the general population (lifetime incidence). [164]

The problems for the practitioner in assess-ing the risk-benefit ratios for lithium are manifold, but all are referrable to the thera-peutic index, which is the ratio of the toxic serum level to the therapeutic serum level. In the case of lithium, this ratio can be very low (about 2). This means that increasing the dosage of lithium by only 100 percent can lead to serious toxicity. In the field of psychopharmacology, where dosages of medication often range over orders of magnitude, these narrow tolerances are drastically different and can make clinical management complicated. The problem is compounded by the fact that serum-lithium levels, which are used for monitoring, may not accurately reflect intracellular levels or even CSF levels of the ion.

Lithium is one of the more intriguing psychotropic agents—perhaps because it is an ion of low atomic weight rather than a complex, heterocyclic ring-compound of high molecular weight. Its clinical potency has profoundly influenced thinking about the molecular mechanisms underlying emotional disorders. How can a simple ion, so similar to sodium, modulate and affect behavior? Is there any pattern to the side-effect profile, as there is in the antipsychotic preparations, that suggests an understanding of the mechanism of action of lithium? At the time of this writing, the answer to both questions is no; but since we still do not fully understand the side effects themselves, it is not surprising that we do not appreciate their significance.

Sodium balance has important implications for lithium treatment. As the serum-sodium level decreases, it leads to increased reabsorption of sodium and lithium in the proximal tubule, where lithium is handled like sodium. The result is a decrease in lithium clearance and an increase in serum lithium level. This phenomenon is not intrinsically dangerous, because it can be compensated for by alteration of lithium intake if the clinician or patient is aware of the danger—in cases of extreme dehydration or salt depletion, the added burden of obligate fluid and electrolyte loss can lead to rapid hyponatremia and/or dehydration with the attendant concentration of lithium. Diaphoresis in very hot or humid weather or prolonged diarrhea in a patient with previously therapeutic levels of lithium can rapidly become a clinical emergency unless prompt action is taken to adjust lithium intake or rehydrate the patient with appropriate sodium-laden parenteral replacement volume.

In fact, if intervention is not prompt, the phenomenon of obligate sodium loss and lithium sparing, which is a vicious cycle, may have a disastrous outcome. Since there is a change in lithium balance when there is a change in sodium, particular care in management of electrolytes is essential after surgery or acute medical emergency when the patient is critically ill.

Gastrointestinal Effects

GI side effects are commonly associated with initiations of lithium therapy and are generally self-limited. They include gastritis, nausea, vomiting, anorexia, abdominal cramps, and diarrhea. Nausea occurring a few hours after the tablet is taken, when the peak plasma lithium level occurs, is seen early in lithium treatment but often abates spontaneously. If symptoms continue, they can be treated by changing the lithium preparation (some pills are enterically coated) or time of administration to after mealtime, when the stomach is full. Alternatively, dosages may be divided initially to minimize fluctuations in serum levels. Persistent GI complaints may herald impending toxicity and must not be ignored lest they lead to the scenario of diarrhea, dehydration, hyponatremia, and increasing levels of plasma lithium. Similarly, diarrhea can be associated with delivery of lithium to the large intestine, which can occur with certain European depot preparations. This complication can be avoided by using nondepot tablets or capsules or by using other brands of depot formulation.

Endocrine Effects

Schou first observed that lithium inhibited the release of thyroid hormone.[130] The mechanism of action is plieotropic, including suppressing multiple steps in the production of thyroid hormones, reducing iodine uptake by the thyroid gland, reducing iodination of tyrosine, reducing the release of T_3 and T_4, altering the peripheral degradation of thyroid hormone (variable effects), and lowering the sensitivity of the thyroid to thyroid-stimulating hormone (TSH).[58,77]

While most patients are able to compensate for the inhibiting effect of the lithium, approximately 5 to 10 percent of such patients will manifest clinical signs of hypothyroidism and/or diffuse, nontender goiter.[129] Goiter most typically appears in females up to two years after lithium therapy is started. Up to 30 percent of patients treated with lithium may have an elevated TSH as well as decreased T_3 and T_4 levels. In addition, elevated titers of antithyroid hormone antibodies are frequently seen.

Elevated TSH need not be treated if the patient is not manifesting signs of hypothyroidism. However, if the patient is symptomatic, replacement therapy is advisable. All of these abnormalities are generally reversible when lithium is discontinued. The complication of iatrogenic hypothyroidism must be kept in mind by practitioners using lithium, since it can mimic a depressive disorder. Patients on lithium should therefore have thyroid function tests (TFTs) prior to treatment as well as a routine part of their treatment. If TSH is elevated, a complete battery of TFTs is advisable.

Perturbations in the glucose tolerance test are seen in patients taking lithium. The observed effects are small, and the result of the studies are sometimes contradictory. The occasional lithium recipient may develop mild diabetes mellitus,[158] but this may be coincidental and not causatively related to lithium. Conversely, insulin-requiring diabetics who need lithium for control of their affective disorder may require an adjustment in their insulin dosage after their lithium level has been stabilized.[137] Since affectively ill patients have an altered carbohydrate metabolism, it is difficult to specify the exact causal relationships between their illness and the treatment (i.e., lithium).

Hematological Effects

A fascinating side effect of lithium therapy is its effect on bone marrow. Lithium causes a mild to moderate increase in polymorphonuclear leukocyte production. It is well established that this effect is not the result of a mobilization of the marginated pool of leukocytes but is rather an increase in granulocyte production. This leukocytosis has no negative medical import. In fact, lithium has been utilized as a treatment for Felty's syndrome as well as neutropenia secondary to chemotherapy and reportedly has reversed these dangerous conditions.[18,69,96] The efficacy of lithium for the treatment of aplastic anemia remains unclear, since reports are contradictory and erythroid and megakaryocytic precursors are also reported to be stimulated.[10] The mechanism of selective stimulation of the myeloid element of the bone marrow, which is more commonly seen, is entirely unknown.

Cardiovascular Effects

Lithium, like potassium, causes predictable "repolarization" changes in the ECG, including flattening or inversion of T-waves and occasional appearance of U-waves in 20 percent of patients.[50,127] It is recommended that patients with or at risk for cardiac disease or with bradycardia get a baseline ECG before initiation of treatment. Lithium has been associated with impaired sinus node function.[147,168] Adverse cardiac reactions to lithium have been reported, including first-degree A-V block, paroxysmal left-bundle-branch block, irregular or delayed nodal rhythm (particularly in older patients), and finally, increased premature ventricular contractions.

If sinoatrial block occurs, use of digitalis may aggravate the block. However, during lithium toxicity, ventricular tachycardia, atrial fibrillation, and A-V block have been reported. Magnesium has been reported to palliate severe lithium toxicity.[147,153,168] Patients on lithium have allegedly developed severe myocarditis, but the relationship of these conditions to lithium is not firmly established and should be assumed to be coincidental until proven.

Cutaneous Manifestations

A pruritic maculopapular rash occasionally appears in the first month of treatment. It generally remits spontaneously. Rarely it progresses to dermatitis, which may require lithium discontinuance if the lesion does not respond to topical treatment. Lithium is also known to exacerbate preexisting skin lesions like psoriasis, acne, or chronic folliculitis. If lithium treatment must be stopped, it is worth restarting after the skin condition has improved, because a second trial of lithium may not induce a recrudescence of the skin condition.[137]

Renal Manifestations

From the inception of lithium therapy, it was clear that this agent altered the function of the kidney. Lithium causes reduction of water resorption in the distal tubules and collecting ducts by inhibiting the action of antidiuretic hormone (ADH) on adenylate cyclase in the kidney.[2,140,145] This inhibition produces iatrogenic diabetes insipidus (DI), with the attendant inability of the kidney to concentrate urine. The potential risk of DI to patients is that it leaves them unprotected against dehydration if either water intake is restricted or fluid loss is increased by diaphoresis, diarrhea, or vomiting. The serious consequences of obligate fluid and electrolyte loss are further compounded by the selective reabsorption of lithium, which itself is potentially toxic, particularly in the face of volume depletion. While this scenario, which has already been discussed, sounds ominous, it is rarely encountered, particularly if the patient is educated about fluid intake and output as well as the early signs of lithium toxicity, including the need to drink water when thirsty.

Many patients on lithium initially experience polyuria and polydipsia, which persist in a significant minority of patients. This condition may remit spontaneously or respond to adjustment of the lithium dose, or it may persist. Discontinuing lithium does not always reverse the condition, as there are reported cases where this phenomenon has continued for years after lithium was stopped.[113] Use of diuretics, known to help nephrogenic DI, will also help the lithium-induced DI, but particular care needs to be taken, because the diuretic decreases lithium clearance and hence reduces the dose needed to achieve a therapeutic level. Carbamazepine has also been effective as a substitute for lithium.

Lithium is alleged to affect the structure as well as function of the kidney, but the topic remains controversial. Hestbech and associates[72] examined the kidneys of patients who had suffered from lithium intoxication or DI. Renal biopsies revealed a pattern of focal atrophy of nephrons and/or diffuse and focal interstitial nephrosis that was not caused by atherosclerotic disease. A control group matched for age and sex had half as much interstitial fibrosis, one-third of the tubular atrophy, and far fewer sclerotic glomeruli.

The early reports on the morphological changes in the kidney prompted further investigations into lithium's effects on its structure and function. New, Manschreck, and Flodes[102] reported chronic tubulo-interstitial nephropathy associated with long-term lithium treatment six years ago. These workers observed focal glomerular atrophy and interstitial fibrosis with significant impairment of tubular function. The changes appeared in 10 to 20 percent of patients after less than one year of lithium treatment.

Schou and Vestorgaard[129] reviewed the renal histology of approximately 150 patients who had received long-term lithium therapy. While 10 to 20 percent of this group had morphological changes in their kidneys, abnormal renal morphology was also seen in 10 to 20 percent of the kidneys examined in a control group of manic-depressive patients who had never received lithium. And even among those affected, there was no evidence of any decrement in filtering capacity. Filtration rates lower than 50 percent of normal were rarely found. Schou concluded that the risk of progressive renal failure with azotemia is remote.

Thus the first generation of studies failed to determine definitively the role, if any, of lithium as a renal toxin. Table 32–12 is a summary of those studies designed to establish whether or not lithium causes clinical or anatomical evidence of renal pathology. Some of these studies also addressed the question of whether the changes that are putatively induced by lithium therapy are reversed when the medication is discontinued.

While the results from the studies are often disparate, the current consensus is that patients who experience lithium toxicity are more likely to manifest pathological changes in their renal histology than control patients. However, renal function may not appear severely impaired because of the fact that most people have considerable reserve renal capacity. This latter point should not be taken to minimize the significance of lithium toxicity in general, since the syndrome is a potentially fatal complication.

A series of further studies have found similar pathological changes but have not resolved the questions. Interpretation of the data has been clouded by the absence of such variables as valid, age-matched normals as well as control biopsies from nonlithium-treated affectively ill subjects. Experimental designs have not taken into account the effects of other drugs or the effect of lithium overdose, as distinguished from usual lithium dosage. In estimating the incidence of such structural changes, obviously patients who have undergone biopsies following an overdose, toxic-dose exposure, or DI would be expected to demonstrate an increase in abnormal finding, thus biasing the data on the basis of ascertainment. Nevertheless, studies of a more representative sample, such as those of Rafaelsen and associates[116] or Bucht and Whalin,[25] do find a 15 percent incidence of such changes. This finding should be considered in the context that most "long-term" lithium patients have been treated for no longer than five to ten years, with fifteen years as an upper limit, except in rare cases.

We do not know what fifty years of lithium treatment would do to the kidney.

To place these findings in perspective, if lithium clearly damaged structure and function, one would predict the following: (1) there would be a high correlation between biopsy abnormality and consistently impaired renal function; (2) the situation would be observed in lithium-treated patients much more frequently than in controls; (3) there would be a high correlation of renal pathology with dosage; and, finally, (4) a dramatic correlation of renal impairment with duration of lithium therapy would be observed. The data so far have revealed no such picture. Few studies, in fact, find any significant correlation. However, there remains a body of data showing that at least some patients have evidence of impaired tubular function, which persists after lithium is discontinued, in comparison to controls. Renal biopsy studies do show chronic pathological lesions in the tubular regions of the nephron, and there is an association of functional impairment with structural damage. There is a correlation in some studies between dose, time exposure to lithium, and concentrating ability, even after lithium has been discontinued for some time. Sensitivity to vasopressors is decreased after lithium is discontinued as well as during lithium treatment. The situation is further complicated by the possibility that an unanticipated manifestation of the affective illness itself may be to alter the kidney's concentration ability. Frank DI, persisting long after lithium is discontinued, is rare but does occur; amelioration of impaired concentrating ability occurs very slowly after medication is stopped. And finally, there does seem to be a small fraction of lithium-treated patients (5 percent) who have persistently impaired tubular function in the absence of lithium intoxication.

A rare patient may have compromised glomerular function, but it is difficult to prove that lithium reduces glomerular function. Prospective studies have failed to show unequivocally increasing impairment in glomerular function with time; and cross-sec-

TABLE 32–12
Effects of Long-term Lithium Treatment on the Kidney

Authors	No. patients examined (N)	Renal Features Studied				
		Tubular	Glomerular	Morphology # pathological diagnoses per biopsied patients	Function	
					Polyuria	Concentrating Ability
Bucht and Wahlin[25]	20 (?)	X	X	3/20	Lithium and neuroleptics worse than lithium alone	
Coopen et al.[36]	101 (?)	X	X	—	Abnormalities in concentrating abilities same as other affective patients not treated with lithium	
Donker et al.[53]	30 (42)	X	X	—	27%	37%
Grof et al.[68]	50 (?)	X	X	—	Correlates with time on lithium	
Hullin et al.[75]	30 (123)	X	X	No structural changes after mean of 8.3 yrs of low-dose lithium		
Rafaelsen et al.[116]	37 (100)	X	X	6/37, 4 with polyuria	4 l/day among those treated long term	Associated with polyuria
Tyrer et al.[156]	48 (?)	X	—	—	in patients on lithium in comparison with affective patients on other medication	
Vestergaard and Amidsen[160]	184 (272)	X	X	—	33% of all treated	80% of those with polyuria
Vestergaard, Amidsen, and Hansen[161]	237 (272)	X	X	—		33% of all treated who had polyuria
Whalin and Alling[166]	278 (400)	X	X	10–15 years of lithium treatment does not correlate with structural change	Polyuria does not correlate with concentrating ability	

SOURCE: H. Bendz, S. Andersch, and M. Aurell, "Kidney Function in an Unselected Lithium Population," *Acta Psychiatrica Scandinavica*, 68 (1983): 324–334.

tional studies have failed to demonstrate un-equivocally that glomerular function is altered in patients as a function of either dosage of lithium or duration of time treated. Such an association of lithium with these kidney effects has been substantiated by animal studies. One suggestion is that the combina-tion of lithium with neuroleptics increases the risk of kidney damage, but this is doubtful.

It was once thought that a sustained-release lithium preparation that avoided peaks and troughs of the drug would reduce lithium toxicity. Some evidence has suggested that there is, in fact, more renal toxicity associated with sustained-release preparations than in peak-and-trough patterns of administration. The evidence is contradictory, however, so this question remains unresolved.

Since lithium rarely, if ever, leads to reduced glomerular filtration rate (GFR), a finding of reduced GFR in a treated patient should not be automatically attributed to lithium; instead, the patient should be carefully evaluated. Lithium clearly does not have an acutely toxic or rapidly progressive effect on the kidney, so renal disease is in no sense an absolute contraindication to lithium treatment in patients who would derive benefit.

Baseline functional studies before onset of lithium treatment should be done, including an estimate of tubular function (serum creatinine, maximal urine osmolality, and twenty-four-hour urine volume) and a measure of GFR. Plasma lithium should be followed monthly (or at least every three months) and plasma creatinine every six months. Annually repeated kidney function tests (tubular or glomerular) are not clearly indicated in the absence of renal symptoms or changes in plasma lithium with a constant dose. However, renal function should be evaluated every two years.

It is important to try to find the minimal effective maintenance dose, although just how to arrive at this level is problematical. A strong therapeutic alliance with the patient that permits adjusting the dose in order to evaluate the patient without risking a full episode of mania or depression is probably the best approach. This is particularly important in patients with polyuria, although the kidney effect needs to be balanced against the risk of relapse.

In summary, for patients maintained on lithium who do not ever become toxic, the question of the long-term effects of lithium remains unanswered. A minority suffer from irreversible loss of concentrating ability, possibly referable to the inhibiting effect of lithium on ADH. However, these patients have normal glomerular function. The few reports

that include histological studies show an increase in interstitial nephropathy and tubular atrophy in comparison with controls. Whether these findings are a result of lithium therapy or a previously unappreciated aspect of major affective disease remains unclear. Whether these findings are sufficiently worrisome to outweigh the therapeutic efficacy of lithium also remains unresolved. Renal failure among patients on lithium is virtually unreported. [11,155]

Ocular Effects

Lithium occasionally is reported to cause itching, tearing, or burning of the eyes. These symptoms are usually transient, and they can be treated topically with decongestant eye drops. [126]

Weight Gain

Weight gain is a significant problem, little talked about but often resulting in noncompliance. Allegedly 20 to 60 percent of patients gain more than twenty pounds. [162] The cause of this problem is unknown. It may represent an increased fluid intake, which often takes the form of highly caloric soft drinks, or improved appetite secondary to resolution of depression, and it is possible but unproven that lithium's effect on the thyroid or possible effect on carbohydrate or lipid metabolism may play a role. Patients need to be warned of this complication in order to prevent weight gain by a careful dietary management.

Pregnancy and Lactation

Lithium is contraindicated during the first trimester of pregnancy except under extreme circumstances. Congenital malformations associated with lithium include abnormalities of the heart, great vessels, and combinations thereof, such as Ebstein's anomaly. [165] The fact that Ebstein's anomaly is reported more frequently in the fetuses of women taking lithium than among normal gestations suggests a correlation but does not constitute proof; it is difficult to establish a causal association, since there is a greater likelihood of an abnormal baby being reported to a registry than a normal one. Large prospective studies, along with data from animal experiments, are needed to substantiate the alleged relationship.

Lithium may be safely restarted in the third trimester, but these patients should be given the lowest possible dose. Lithium clearance is reduced in the first half of pregnancy. In the second half of pregnancy, lithium clearance is increased, so larger doses may be required. After delivery, lithium clearance returns to normal. Lithium should be discontinued a few days or weeks before delivery; lithium concentrations are in equilibrium in fetal and maternal bloodstreams. Babies born to mothers on lithium often show signs of CNS depression with poor muscular tone and reduced feeding activity. These findings quickly resolve postpartum as the lithium in their system is excreted. These infants have also been noted to develop goiter owing to thyroid suppression. Hypothyroidism generally resolves in two months.[167]

Finally, lithium is present in the milk of lactating mothers in sufficient concentration (10 to 50 percent of plasma levels) to cause CNS toxicity in nursing infants, although some mothers have breast-fed their babies with no obvious problems.[13]

Anesthesia

Lithium has no effect on anesthetics per se, but may prolong the neuromuscular blockade of both depolarizing and nondepolarizing agents. This should be remembered when giving ECT. Increased confusion, disorientation, memory impairment, and restlessness have occurred with lithium and ECT concomitantly. It is wise to discontinue lithium a few days before surgery or ECT.

Central Nervous System Effects

Patients started on lithium therapy sometimes report a vague sense of dysphoria. Specific complaints include lethargy, muscle weakness, headache, fatigue, mental dullness, decrement of memory and mental concentration, and tremulousness. These symptoms usually remit spontaneously after several days or weeks.[154]

Essential tremor manifested by a fine hand tremor is reported in 50 percent of patients started on lithium but is uncommon in maintenance treatment. It generally has a rate of 5 to 10 cycles per second and is worsened by intentional activity, CNS stimulants like caffeine, or anxiety. This side effect is more likely to occur when there is a personal or family history of essential tremor. It generally is time-limited but may persist (4 percent incidence after two years). In the persistent form, propranolol in a dose of 20 to 160 mg per day may relieve the symptom.[126] Tremulousness is generally limited to the extremities but occasionally affects the face, especially the eyelids.

Other occasionally encountered CNS manifestations of lithium that affect the cerebellum—dysarthria, ataxia, nystagmus, as well as the intention tremor just described—may be seen. Vertigo, tinnitus, autonomic slowing of bowel and bladder function, visual distortions, muscle irritability (fasciculations, heightened deep tendon reflexes, twitching), and, finally, an organic brain syndrome have also been described in toxicity. In addition, a parkinsonian picture of extrapyramidal side effects has episodically been observed. Whether lithium can truly cause parkinsonian side effects is in doubt, since such symptoms could be caused by concomitant antipsychotics or tardive dyskinesia, or be misdiagnosed as essential tremor or idiopathic parkinsonian symptoms. The parkinsonian syndrome includes bradykinesia, cogwheeling, masklike facies, and so forth.[70] It is most commonly reported in elderly patients who are concomitantly receiving antipsychotic medication or in those patients whose lithium level exceeds 1.5 mEq per l. There are contradictory reports on whether lithium at more toxic levels may increase or decrease seizure frequency in epileptic patients. CNS and neuromuscular symptoms are the most prominent manifestations of lithium toxicity.

Toxicity and Overdose

The preceding discussions have stressed the need for careful monitoring of lithium levels in patients. The concerns are twofold: On the one hand is the narrow therapeutic range for lithium—from 0.8 mEq per l to 1.2 mEq per l; on the other hand are the severe, albeit rarely irreversible, consequences of lithium toxicity, which can be seen at a level just beyond the therapeutic range. In fact, owing to peculiarities in lithium distribution or the effects of age or unknown factors, a patient may have a serum level well within (or just outside) acceptable limits but have CNS toxicity. Indeed, it is not uncommon for elderly patients to be toxic with normal plasma levels and respond therapeutically at low plasma levels.

Tyrer and Shaw[155] report that individuals in steady-state conditions with acceptable plasma levels of lithium ranging from 0.6 to 1.2 mEq per l may have toxic levels in their brains. These authors set toxic plasma levels at 1.5 mEq per l or greater, but caution that some patients may become toxic at far lower levels—0.5 to 1.0 mEq per l. The population at greatest risk is the elderly. For adults, there is a twofold safety factor, since therapeutic responses occur at 0.8 to 1.0 mEq per l, but toxicity often begins at about double these levels. Indeed, at one time 2 mEq per l was considered the upper limit of normal, with therapeutic level set at 1 to 1.5 mEq per l. Schoonover[126] places toxic limits for lithium at greater than 2.0 mEq per l, although he acknowledges the possibility of the occasional patient being afflicted at a considerably lower level.

The initial symptoms of lithium toxicity include difficulty in concentrating, sluggishness, apathy, dizziness, dysarthria, a coarse hand tremor, ataxia, heaviness of limb, muscular weakness, and slight muscular twitching when dizzy. This progresses to severe apathy, lethargy, sleepiness, truncal and appendicular ataxia, dysarthria, and a more severe irregular tremor with definite myoclonic twitching.

The terminal stage of CNS toxicity progresses to an arousable coma, where the patients react to tactile or verbal stimuli with only movements of head or eyes. Deep tendon reflexes are increased and seizure, opisthotonic posture, severe nystagmus, hyperextension of the extremities, and hyperpyrexia occur. At this stage, cardiovascular collapse with precipitously falling blood pressure, irregular cardiac rhythm, and cardiac conduction irregularities is eminent. Cardiac collapse leads to irregular perfusion, further damaging the kidneys by ischemic insult. The combination of lithium, direct renal toxicity, and ischemia can lead to renal shutdown (ATN) and decreased urine output or anuria. During overdose, one should follow the urine flow and plasma lithium so that the clearance of lithium by the kidney can be monitored. Fifty percent of toxic patients manifest gastrointestinal symptomatology: nausea, vomiting, cramps, and diarrhea.

For severe intoxication, osmotic dialysis, peritoneal dialysis, or hemodialysis may save the patient. Patients with levels greater than 4.0 mEq per l still have a chance of surviving without sequelae if treated aggressively. Patients with plasma levels of 9 mEq per l have reportedly survived. Overdose can result in irreversible neurological damage or death, but most patients (70 to 90 percent) can be expected to recover.[126]

Table 32–13 summarizes the signs and symptoms of toxicity, starting with normal side effects and progressing to those that herald impending death. The time course of recovery from intoxication over days to weeks is substantially slower than the disappearance of lithium from plasma. Sometimes the intoxication can transiently worsen during the first few hours (one to twenty-four hours).

One aspect of lithium toxicity that remains unresolved concerns the allegedly catastrophic interaction of lithium with haloperidol. This combination is frequently employed when a manic patient is particularly disorganized. Anecdotal reports have suggested that neurological damage occurred in

TABLE 32–13
Lithium Side Effects

Degree	Symptoms
Very mild	Nausea (particularly during first few days of treatment)
	Fine tremor of hands
Mild	Polyuria and polydipsia
	Slight muscular weakness, feeling of heaviness in limbs
	Muscle hyperirritability with twitching
	Myoclonic twitching when going to sleep
	Sluggishness, languidness, drowsiness, giddiness
	Slight apathy and reduced ability to concentrate
	Coarse tremor
	Ataxia
	Anorexia
	Vomiting
	Diarrhea
	"Upset stomach" or "abdominal pain"
Moderate	Definite myoclonic twitching
	Definite muscular weakness
	Sedation, dizziness
	Definite ataxia and dysarthria
	Irregular tremor
	More severe GI symptoms
Severe	Hypertonic muscles
	Hyperactive deep tendon reflexes
	Hyperextension of arms and legs with grunts and gasping
	Hyperpyrexia
	Chorea, athetotic movements
	Impairment of consciousness, definite apathy
	Somnolence, confusion, stupor
	Seizures
	Transient focal neurological signs
	Dysarthria
	Cranial nerve signs
Very severe	Coma
	Opisthotonous
	Complications of coma
	Death

NOTE: Reprinted, by permission, from D. F. Klein et al., *Diagnosis and Drug Treatment of Psychiatric Disorders: Adults and Children,* 2nd ed. (Baltimore: Wilkins & Wilkins, 1980), p. 471.

patients receiving both lithium and haloperidol.[6,34,95,150] All of these cases described individuals with slightly elevated serum lithium levels (1.5–2.0 mEq/l), who were also receiving high doses of haloperidol. The victims became hyperpyrexic and comatose and often developed a variety of neurological symptoms, including grand mal seizures. While these are the most frequent neurological manifestations of this condition, other clinical reports have described coma, which may be so profound as to require ventilatory support. Brain-stem findings also included opisthotonous on occasion. Some of these patients died, but many recovered following either hemodialysis or careful parenteral management of their fluids and electrolytes plus intensive neurological support. However, many of the survivors have been left with significant neurological sequelae. One unexplained aspect of this complication is that it has been reported to occur five times more frequently in females than in males.

A recent study has raised the question

whether all patients treated with lithium and haloperidol may be neurologically damaged to some degree. The study compared the discrepancies between verbal scores and performance scores on the Wechsler Adult Intelligence Scale in matched populations of patients who had received either haloperidol or chlorpromazine together with lithium. The report described significantly greater discrepancies in performance in those who had received haloperidol, rather than chlorpromazine, together with lithium, and the authors concluded that this finding indicated nonfocal brain damage that had not been previously appreciated. This conclusion has been disputed, with workers claiming that the sample was too small and also that the single neuropsychological measurement did not warrant a conclusion of nonfocal neurological damage.[157] However, the report adds fuel to the debate about the relationship between these agents.

A proposed mechanism for the suspected toxicity is that the combination of lithium and haloperidol potentiates the entry of lithium into the CNS, either at a greater rate or in greater concentration, leading to lithium toxicity or, alternatively, that the combination synergistically potentiates haloperidol to enter cells more readily, leading to a picture of the neuroleptic-malignant syndrome (NMS). The question of whether the lithium-haloperidol combination is, in fact, a neurotoxic one has not been answered. However, for the practitioner using these drugs in combination, it is imperative that patients be carefully monitored to avoid excessive levels of either drug and that the clinical status of such patients be scrupulously followed.

Many patients have been treated with lithium and haloperidol without any problem. It is quite possible that at least some of the initially reported cases actually suffered from NMS alone, and that what happened to them was entirely the result of NMS, the concomitant lithium treatment being irrelevant. Without case-controlled statistical studies, it is difficult to ascribe cause. We do not feel that we can unequivocally attribute this syndrome to either lithium or haloperidol or a combination of the two. In the absence of knowledge, common sense would dictate that the clinician avoid extremely high plasma levels of either lithium or haloperidol when these drugs are being used in combination. The clinician should be alert to NMS and the treatment that exists, namely, cooling to combat the hyperthermia and administering dantrolene sodium (Dantrolene) and DA agonists, such as bromocriptine mesylate.

Hypothermia has been reported very rarely in patients receiving lithium and diazepam.

Anti-inflammatory drugs and related substances (indomethacin, phenylbutazone, ketoprofen, oxyphenbutazone, dichlofenac, ibuprofen, and glafenine) may decrease lithium clearance, and as a result, plasma lithium level may rise, necessitating a lowering of lithium dose. Ataxia and slurred speech occurred in a patient on methyldopa and lithium. It is possible that these reports have been pure lithium toxicity or a coincidental association.

¶ Acknowledgment

We wish to gratefully acknowledge the support of the MacArthur Foundation.

¶ Bibliography

1. ANANTH, J., and LUCHINS, D. "A Review of Combined Tricyclic and MAOI Therapy," *Comprehensive Psychiatry*, 18 (1977):221–230.

2. ANGRIST, B. M., et al. "Lithium-induced Diabetes Insipidus-like Syndrome," *Comprehensive Psychiatry*, 11 (1970): 141–146.

3. ARANA, G., PEARLMAN, C., and SHADER, R. "Alprazolam-induced Mania," *American Journal of Psychiatry*, 142 (1985):368–369.

4. AVERY, D., and WINOKUR, G. "The Efficacy of Electroconvulsive Therapy and Antidepressants in Depression," *Biological Psychiatry*, 12 (1977):507–523.

5. AYD, F. J. "Excretion of Psychotropic Drugs in Human Breast Milk," *International Drug Therapy Newsletter*, 8 (1973):33–40.

6. BAASTRUP, P. C., et al. "Adverse Reactions in Treatment with Lithium Carbonate and Haloperidol," *Journal of the American Medical Association*, 236 (1976):2645–2646.

7. BALDESSARINI, R. J. *Chemotherapy in Psychiatry*. Cambridge, Mass.: Harvard University Press, 1977.

8. ———. "How Do Antidepressants Work?" in J. M. Davis and J. W. Maas, eds., *The Affective Disorders*. Washington, D.C.: American Psychiatric Association Press, 1983, pp. 243–260.

9. BALDESSARINI, R. J., and TARSAY, D. "Relationship of the Actions of Neuroleptic Drugs to the Pathophysiology of Tardive Dyskinesia," *International Review of Neurobiology*, vol. 21. New York: Academic Press, 1979, pp. 1–40.

10. BARRETT, A. J. "Hematological Effects of Lithium and Its Use in Treatment of Neutropenia," *Blut Journal of Experimental & Clinical Hematology*, 40 (1980):1–6.

11. BENDZ, H. "Kidney Function in Lithium-treated Patients—A Literature Survey," *Acta Psychiatrica Scandinavica*, 68 (1983):303–324.

12. BENDZ, H., ANDERSCH, S., and AURELL, M. "Kidney Function in an Unselected Lithium Population," *Acta Psychiatrica Scandinavica*, 68 (1983):325–334.

13. BERKOWITZ, R. L., CONSTAN, D. R., and MICHIZUKI, T. *Handbook for Prescribing Medication During Pregnancy*. Boston: Little, Brown, 1980.

14. BIGGER, J. T., et al. "Cardiac Antiarrhythmic Effect of Imipramine Hydrochloride," *New England Journal of Medicine*, 296 (1977):206–208.

15. BLACKWELL, B. "Adverse Effect of Antidepressant Drugs. Part I. Monoamine Oxidase Inhibitors and Tricyclics," *Drugs*, 21 (1981):201–219.

16. BLACKWELL, B., MARLEY, E., and TAYLOR, D. "Effects of Yeast Extract After Monoamine Oxidase Inhibition," *Lancet*, 1 (1965):1166.

17. BLOM, S., and EKBOM, K. A. "Comparison Between Akathisia Developing on Treatment with Phenothiazine Derivatives and the Restless Leg Syndrome," *Acta Medica Scandinavica*, 170 (1981): 684–694.

18. BLUM, S. F. "Lithium Therapy of Aplastic Anemia," *New England Journal of Medicine*, 300 (1979):677.

19. BOCK, J. L., Cummings, K. C., and JATLOW, P. I. "Amoxapine Overdose: A Case Report," *American Journal of Psychiatry*, 139 (1982):1619–1620.

20. BONHAM CARTER, S. "Tyramine Conjugation Defect and Its Identification," ——— —*Colloqium on MAOI Therapy*. London: Dataspeed, 1971, pp. 75–81.

21. BRANDON, S., McCLELLANDS, H. A., and PROTHEROE, C. "A Study of Facial Dyskinesia in a Mental Hospital Population," *British Journal of Psychiatry*, 118 (1971):171–184.

22. BRODGON, R., et al. "Mianserin: A Review of Its Pharmacological Properties and Therapeutic Efficacy in Depressive Illness," *Drugs*, 16 (1978):273–301.

23. BRODGON R., et al. "Nomifensine: A Review of Pharmacologic Properties and Therapeutic Efficacy in Depressive Illness," *Evaluation of New Drugs*, 1 (1979): 1–24.

24. BROWN, T.C.K., and LEVERSHA, A. "Comparison of the Cardiovascular Toxicity of Three Tricyclic Antidepressant Drugs: Imipramine, Amitriptyline, and Doxepin," *Clinical Toxicology*, 14 (1979):253–256.

25. BUCHT, G., and WHALIN, A. "Renal Concentrating Capacity in Long-term Lithium Treatment and After Withdrawal of Lithium," *Acta Medica Scandinavica*, 207 (1980):309–314.

26. BUNNEY, W. E., Jr. "Psychopharmacology of the Switch Process in Affective Illness," in M. A. Lipton, A. DiMascio, and K. F. Killam, eds., *Psychopharmacology: A Generation of Progress*. New York: Raven Press, 1978, pp. 1249–1260.

27. BUNNEY, W. E., Jr., and DAVIS, J. M. "Norepinephrine in Depressive Reactions. A Review," *Archives of General Psychiatry*, 13 (1965):483–494.

28. BURKS, J. S., et al. "Tricyclic Antidepressant Poisoning: Reversal of Coma, Choreoathetosis, and Myoclonos by Physostigmine," *Journal of the American*

Medical Association, 230 (1974):1405–1407.

29. BURROWS, J. D., et al. "Tricyclic Antidepressant Drugs and Cardiac Conduction," *Progress in Neuro-Psychopharmacology and Biological Psychiatry,* 1 (1977):329–334.

30. BYCK, R. "Drugs and the Treatment of Psychiatric Disorders," in L. S. Goodman and A. Gilman, eds., *The Pharmacological Basis of Therapeutics,* 5th ed. New York: Macmillan, 1975, pp. 152–200.

31. CADE, J. F. J. "Lithium Salts in the Treatment of Psychotic Excitement," *Medical Journal of Australia,* 2 (1949):349–352.

32. CASEY, D. E., CLAPPISON, V. J., and KEEPERS, G. A. "Anticholinergic Drugs in Neuroleptic Induced Extrapyramidal Symptoms," Paper presented at the American Psychiatry Association Meeting, New Orleans, May 11–15, 1981.

33. COHEN, R., and PICKAR, D. "Implications of Monoamine Oxidase Inhibitor and Induced Hypomania," *Archives of General Psychiatry,* 35 (1978):1393–1394.

34. COHEN, W. J., and COHEN, N. H. "Lithium Carbonate—Haloperidol and Irreversible Brain Damage," *Journal of the American Medical Association,* 230 (1974):1283–1288.

35. COLE, J. O., and DAVIS, J. M. "Antipsychotic Drugs," in L. Bellak and L. Loeb, eds., *The Schizophrenic Syndrome.* New York: Grune & Stratton, 1969, pp. 478–568.

36. COOPEN, A., et al. "Renal Function in Lithium and Non-lithium Treated Patients with Affective Disorders," *Acta Psychiatrica Scandinavica,* 62 (1980):343–355.

37. CRANSWICK, E. H., and SIMPSON, G. M. "Perphenazine and Thyroid Function," *American Journal of Psychiatry,* 120 (1964):1133–1134.

38. CROME, P. "Antidepressant Overdosage," *Drugs,* 23 (1982):431.

39. CROME, P., et al. "Effect of Activated Charcoal on Absorption of Nortriptyline," *Lancet,* 2 (1977):1203–1205.

40. CROW, T. J., et al. "Abnormal Involuntary Movements in Schizophrenia: Are They Related to the Disease Process or Its Treatment? Are They Associated with Changes in Dopamine Receptors?" *Journal of Clinical Psychopharmacology,* 2 (1982):336–340.

41. DAVIDSON, J. R. T., et al. "Atypical Depression," *Archives of General Psychiatry,* 39 (1982):527–534.

42. DAVIES, B., et al. "Pressor Actions of Noradrenalin, Angiotensin II, and Saralasin in Chronic Automatic Failure Treated with Fludrocortisone," *British Journal of Clinical Pharmacology,* 8 (1979):253–260.

43. DAVIS, J. M. "Review of Antispychotic Drug Literature," in D. F. Klein and J. M. Davis, eds., *Diagnosis and Treatment of Psychiatric Disorders.* Baltimore: Waverly Press, 1969, pp. 52–138.

44. ——. "Concluding Remarks: Mechanisms of Antidepressants," *Progress in Neuro-Psychopharmacology and Biological Psychiatry,* 7 (1983):365.

45. DAVIS, J. M., and FREDMAN D. M. "The New Generation of Antidepressants," in J. H. Masserman, ed. *Current Psychiatric Therapies,* vol. 20. New York: Grune & Stratton, 1981, pp. 293–297.

46. DAVIS, J. M., FREDMAN, D. M., and LINDEN, R. D. "A Review of the New Antidepressant Medications," in J. M. Davis, and J. W. Maas, eds., *The Affective Disorders.* Washington, D. C.: American Psychiatric Press, 1983, pp. 1–29.

47. DAVIS, J. M., et al. "Some Conceptual Aspects of Laboratory Tests in Diagnosis," *Journal of Clinical Psychiatry,* 44 (1983):21–26.

48. DEGLIN, S. M., DEGLIN, J. M., and CHENG, E. K. "Drug-induced Cardiovascular Disease," *Drugs,* 14 (1977):29–40.

49. DELAY, J., and DENIKER, P. "Trente-huit cas de psychoses traitées par la cure-prolongée et continué de 4560 RP." Le Congres des AL et Neurologie de Langue Francaise, in *Compte Rendue Congress.* Paris: Masson et Cie, 1952.

50. DEMERS, R. G., and HENINGER, G. R. "Electrocardiographic Changes During Lithium Treatment," *Diseases of the Nervous System,* 31 (1970):674.

51. DESSAM, E. C., et al. "Maprotiline Treatment in Depression—A Perspective on Seizures," Paper presented at the Four-

teenth Annual Congress of the Collegium Internationale Neuro-Psychopharmacologicum, Florence, 1984.

52. DOEPFNER, R. "Der Thioridazin-Aspermatismus (Beitrag zur Behandlung der Ejaculatiopraecox)," *Zietschrift für Haut und Geschlectskrank-heiten*, 36 (1964):265–273.

53. DONKER, A. J., et al. "A Renal Function Study in 30 Patients on Long-term Lithium Therapy," *Clinical Nephrology*, 12 (1979):254–262.

54. EDWARDS, J. G. "Unwanted Effects of Psychotropic Drugs and Their Mechanisms," in H. M. van Praag, et al., eds., *Handbook of Biological Psychiatry*. New York: Marcel Dekker, Inc., 1981, pp. 1–39.

55. EDWARDS, J. G., and GOLDIE, A. "Mianserin, Maprotiline, and Intracardiac Conduction," *British Journal of Pharmacology*, 15 (Supplement) (1983):249s–254s.

56. EGGERMONT, E., et al. "The Adverse Influence of Imipramine on the Adaptation of the Newborn Infant to Extrauterine Life," *Acta Paediatrica Belgica*, 26 (1972):197–204.

57. EL-YOUSEF, M. K., et al. "Reversal by Physostigmine of Antiparkinsonian Drug Toxicity: A Controlled Study," *American Journal of Psychiatry*, 130 (1973):141.

58. EMERSON, C. H., DYSON, W. L., and UNGER, R. P. "Serum Thyrotropin and Thyroxin Concentration in Patients Receiving Lithium Carbonate," *Journal of Clinical Endocrinology & Metabolism*, 36 (1973):338–346.

59. FEIGHNER, J. P. "Clinical Efficacy of the Newer Antidepressants," *Journal of Clinical Psychopharmacology*, I (Supplement) (1981):23s–26s.

60. FEIGHNER, J. P., et al. "Comparison of Alprazolam, Imipramine and Placebo in the Treatment of Depression," *Journal of the American Medical Association*, 249 (1983):3057–3064.

61. GELENBERG, A. "Psychoses," in E. L. Bassuck, S. C. Schoonover, and A. J. Gelenberg, eds., *The Practitioner's Guide to Psychiatric Drugs*. New York: Plenum Press, 1983, pp. 115–166.

62. GLASSMAN, A. H. "Antidepressant Treatment and the Cardiovascular System," Lecture given at Massachusetts Mental Health Center, Boston, March 9, 1984.

63. GLASSMAN, A. H., and BIGGER, T., Jr. "Cardiovascular Effects of Therapeutic Doses of Tricyclic Antidepressants," *Archives of General Psychiatry*, 38 (1981): 815–820.

64. GOLDBERG, M. J., and SPECTOR, R. "Amoxapine Overdose: Reports of Two Patients with Severe Neurologic Damage," *Annals of Internal Medicine*, 96 (1982):463–464.

65. GOLDMAN, D. "The Results of Treatments of Psychotic States with Newer Phenothiazine Compounds Effective in Small Doses," *American Journal of Medical Sciences*, 235 (1958):67–77.

66. GOMON, A. W., and BYRUG, J. E. "Cardiovascular Effects of Trazodone in Animals," *Journal of Clinical Psychopharmacology*, I (Supplement) 6 (1981):70s–75s.

67. GRANACHER, R. D., and BALDESSARINI, R. J. "Physostigmine: Its Use in Acute Anticholinergic Syndrome with Antidepressant and Antiparkinsonian Drugs," *Archives of General Psychiatry*, 32 (1975):375–379.

68. GROF, P., et al. "Long-term Lithium Treatment and the Kidney," *Canadian Journal of Psychiatry*, 25 (1980):535–543.

69. GUPTA, R. C., ROBINSON, W. A., and KURNECK, J. E. "Felty's Syndrome: Effect of Lithium on Granulopoiesis," *American Journal of Medicine*, 61 (1976):29–32.

70. HANSEN, H. E., and AMIDSEN, A. "Lithium Intoxication: Report of 23 Cases and Review of 100 Cases in the Literature," *Quarterly Journal of Medicine*, 47 (1978):123–144.

71. HEIKKILA, J., et al. "Clozapine and Agranulocytosis," *Lancet*, 2 (1975):611.

72. HESTBECH, J., et al. "Chronic Renal Lesions Following Long-term Treatment with Lithium," *Kidney International*, 12 (1977):205–213.

73. HOLLISTER, L. E. "Chlorpromazine Jaundice," *Journal of the American Medical Association*, 169 (1959):1235–1236.

74. ———. *Clinical Pharmacology of Psychotherapeutic Drugs*. New York: Churchill-Livingstone, 1983.

75. HULLIN, R. P., et al. "Renal Function

After Long-term Treatment with Lith-ium," *British Medical Journal,* 1 (1979): 457–459.

76. JANOWSKY, D., et al. "Ventricular Ar-rythmias Possibly Aggravated by Trazo-done," *American Journal of Psychiatry,* 140 (1983):796–797.

77. JEFFERSON, J. W. "Lithium Carbonate-induced Hypothyroidism—Its Many Faces," *Journal of the American Medi-cal Association,* 242 (1979):271–272

78. JUCK, H., et al. "Tricyclic Antidepres-sants and Convulsions," *Journal of Clinical Psychopharmacology,* 3 (1983): 182–185.

79. KANE, F. J., Jr., and ANDERSON, W. B. "A Fourth Occurrence of Oral Moniliasis During Tranquilizer Therapy," *Ameri-can Journal of Psychiatry,* 120 (1964): 1199–1200.

80. KANE, J. M., and SMITH, J. M. "Tardive Dyskinesia Prevalence and Risk Fac-tors, 1959–1979," *Archives of General Psychiatry,* 39 (1982):473–481.

81. KANE, J. M., et al. "Epidemiology of Tar-dive Dyskinesia," *Clinical Neurophar-macology,* 2 (1983):109–115.

82. KEMPER, A. J., DUNLAP, R., and PIETRO, D. A. "Thioridazine-induced Torsade de Pointes: Successful Therapy with Iso-proterenol," *Journal of the American Medical Association,* 49 (1983):2931–2934.

83. KLAWANS, H. L., TANNER, G. M., and BARR, A. "The Reversibility of 'Perma-nent' Tardive Dyskinesia," *Clinical Neuropharmacology,* 7 (1984):153–159.

84. KLEIN, D. F., et al. *Diagnosis and Drug Treatment of Psychiatric Disorders: Adults and Children,* 2nd ed. Balti-more: Williams & Wilkins, 1980.

85. KRAEPELIN, E. *Dementia Praecox and Pa-raphrenias 1919,* trans. R. M. Barclay. New York: Robert E. Krieger, 1971.

86. KUHN, R. "The Treatment of Depressive States with 622355 (Imipramine Hydro-chloride)," *American Journal of Psychi-atry,* 107 (1950):159–174.

87. KUPFER, D. J., and BOWERS, M. B., Jr. "REM Sleep and Central Monoamine Oxidase Inhibition," *Psychopharmaco-logia,* 27 (1972):183–190.

88. LANGOV, R. A., et al. "Cardiovascular Manifestations of Tricyclic Antidepres-sant Overdose," *American Heart Jour-nal,* 100 (1980):458–464.

89. LEESTRIN, J. E., and KOENIG, K. L. "Sud-den Death and Phenothiazine. A Cur-rent Controversy," *Archives of General Psychiatry,* 18 (1968):137–148.

90. LEHMAN, H. E. "Drug Treatment of Schizophrenia," in H. E. Lehman, ed., *Psychopharmacology.* Boston: Little, Brown, 1965, pp. 717–751

91. LERER, B., et al. "48-hour Depressive Cy-cling Induced by Antidepressant," *Brit-ish Journal of Psychiatry,* 137 (1980): 183–185.

92. LIBERATORE, M. A., and ROBINSON, D. S. "Torsade de Pointes: A Mechanism for Sudden Death Associated with Neuro-leptic Drug Therapy," *Journal of Clini-cal Psychopharmacology,* 4 (1984):143–147.

93. LIPINSKI, J. F., et al. "Propranolol in the Treatment of Neuroleptic-induced Aka-thisia," *American Journal of Psychiatry,* 141 (1984):412–415.

94. LIPPMANN, S., et al. "Trazodone Cardio-toxicity," *American Journal of Psychia-try,* 140 (1983):1383.

95. LONDEN, J. B., and WARING, H. "Toxic Reaction in Lithium and Haloperidol," *Lancet,* 2 (1976):1088.

96. LYNNAN, G. H., WILLIAMS, C. C., and PRESTON, D. "The Use of Lithium Car-bonate to Reduce Infection and Leuko-penia During Systemic Chemother-apy," *New England Journal of Medicine,* 302 (1980):257–260.

97. MARSDEN, C. D., TARSAY, D., and BAL-DESSARINI, R. J. "Spontaneous and Drug-Induced Movement Disorders in Psychotic Patients," in D. F. Bensen and D. Blumer, eds., *Psychiatric As-pects of Neurological Diseases.* New York: Grune & Stratton, 1975, pp. 219–256.

98. MASSEY, L. W. C. "Skin Pigmentation, Corneal and Lens Opacities with Pro-longed Chlorpromazine Treatment," *Canadian Medical Association Journal,* 92 (1965):186–187.

99. "More Problems with Trazodone (Desy-rel)," *Biological Therapies in Psychia-try,* 7 (1984):2.

100. MURPHY, D. L. "The Behavioral Toxicity of Monoamine Oxidase Inhibiting An-

tidepressants," *Advances in Pharmacology and Chemotherapy*, 14 (1977):71–105.

101. MURPHY, D. L., SUNDERLAND, T., and COHEN, R. J. "Monoamine Oxidase Inhibiting Antidepressants: A Clinical Update," *Psychiatric Clinics of North America*, 7 (1984):549–562.

102. NEW, C., MANSCHRECK, T. C., and FLODES, J. M. "Renal Damage Associated with Long-term Use of Lithium Carbonate," *Journal of Clinical Psychiatry*, 40 (1979):460–463.

103. NEWTON, R. W. "Computer-assisted Tomography," *Journal of the American Medical Association*, 231 (1975):941–943.

104. NIES, A. "Clinical Applications of MAOI's," in G. D. Burrows, T. R. Norman, and B. Davies, eds., *Antidepressants*. Amsterdam: Elsevier, 1983, p. 244.

105. PANDEY, G. N., and DAVIS, J. M. "Treatment with Antidepressants and Down-regulation of Beta-adrenergic Receptors," *Drug Development Research*, 3 (1983):393–406.

106. PAOLETTI, F., et al. "Positive Pregnancy Test in an 82-Year-Old Woman," *American Journal of Medical Science*, 252 (1966):570–572.

107. PARE, C. M. B. "Toxicity of the Psychotropic Drugs. Side Effects and Toxicity of the Antidepressants." *Proceedings of the Royal Society of Medicine*, 57 (1984):757–778.

108. PETERSON, G., et al. "Anticholinergic Activity of the Tricyclic Antidepressants Desipramine and Doxepin in Nondepressed Volunteers," *Communications in Psychopharmacoloy*, 2 (1975):145.

109. PICKAR, D., et al. "Selective and Nonselective Monoamine Oxidase Inhibitors," *Archives of General Psychiatry*, 39 (1982):535–540.

110. PISCIOTTA, A. V. "Mechanisms of Phenothiazine Induced Agranulocytosis," in D.H.E. Crow ed., *Psychopharmacology, A Review of Progress, 1957–1967*. Washington, D.C.: U.S. Government Printing Office, 1968.

111. PITTS, N. E. "The Clinical Evaluation of Doxepin: A New Psychotropic Agent," *Psychosomatic*, 10 (1969):164–171.

112. POLLACK, B., BUCK, I. F., and KALNINS, L.

"An Oral Syndrome Complicating Psychopharmacotherapy Study II," *American Journal of Psychiatry*, 121 (964):381–386.

113. RABIN, E. Z., et al. "Persistent Nephrogenic Diabetes Insipidus Associated with Long-term Lithium Carbonate Therapy," *Canadian Medical Association Journal*, 121 (1979):194–198.

114. RABKIN, J., KLEIN, D. F., and QUITKIN, F. M. "Somatic Treatment of Acute Depression," in A. Rifkin, ed., *Schizophrenic and Affective Disorders: Biology and Drug Treatment*. Boston: John Wright, 1983, pp. 35–77.

115. RACHELFSKY, G. S., et al. "Possible Teratogeneity of Tricyclic Antidepressants," *Lancet*, 1 (1972):838.

116. RAFAELSEN, O. J., et al. "Kidney Function and Morphology in Long-term Lithium Treatment," Paper presented at International Lithium Congress, New York, 1978.

117. RAMSEY, T. A., and COX, M. "Lithium in the Kidney: A Review," *American Journal of Psychiatry*, 139 (1982):443–449.

118. REED, K., et al. "Cardiovascular Effects of Nortriptyline in Geriatric Patients," *American Journal of Psychiatry*, 137 (1980):986–989.

119. RICHELSON, E. "Antipsychotics Block Muscarinic Acetylcholine Receptor-Mediated Cyclic GMP Formation in Cultured Mouse Blastoma Cells," *Nature*, 266 (1977):371–373.

120. RICHELSON, E., and NELSON, A. "Antagonism by Neuroleptics of Neurotransmitter Receptors of Normal Human Brain *in vitro*," *European Journal of Pharmacology*, 103 (1984):197–204.

121. RICKLES, K., FEIGHNER, J. P., and SMITH, W. T. "Alprazolam, Amitriptyline, Doxepin, and Placebo in the Treatment of Depression," *Archives of General Psychiatry*, 42 (1985):134–141.

122. ROBINSON, T. S. "Adverse Reactions, Toxicities, and Drug Interactions of Newer Antidepressants: Anticholinergic, Sedative, and Other Side Effects," *Pharmacology Bulletin*, 20 (1984):280–290.

123. RUDORFER, M. V., GOLDEN, R. N., and POTTER, W. Z. "Second Generation Antidepressants," *Psychiatric Clinics of North America*, 7 (1984):519–534.

124. SALZMAN, C. "Introduction to Antipsychotics," Lecture given at Massachusetts Mental Health Center, July 15, 1983.

125. SCHILDKRAUT, J. J. "Catecholamine Hypothesis of Affective Disorders," *American Journal of Psychiatry*, 122 (1965): 509–522.

126. SCHOONOVER, S. C. "Depression," in E. L. Bassuk, S. C. Schoonover, and A. J. Gelenberg, eds., *The Practitioner's Guide to Psychiatric Drugs.* New York: Plenum Press, 1983, pp. 19–78.

127. SCHOU, M. "Electrocardiographic Changes During Treatment with Lithium and with Drugs of the Imipramine Type," *Acta Psychiatrica Scandinavica* 169 (Supplement) (1963):258–259.

128. ———. "Long-lasting Neurological Sequelae After Lithium Intoxication," *Acta Psychiatrica Scandinavica,* 70 (1984): 594–602.

129. SCHOU, M., and VESTORGAARD, P. "Lithium Treatment: Problems and Precautions," in G. D. Burrows, T. R. Norman, and B. Davies, eds., *Antidepressants.* Amsterdam: Elsevier, 1983, pp. 269–276.

130. SCHOU, M., et al. "Occurrence of Goiter During Lithium Treatment," *British Medical Journal,* 3 (1968):710–713.

131. SCHUCKIT, M., ROBINS, E., and FEIGHNER, J. "Tricyclic Antidepressants and Monoamine Oxidase Inhibitors," *Archives of General Psychiatry,* 24 (1971):509–514.

132. "Seizures with Maprotiline (Ludiomil)," *Biological Therapies in Psychiatry,* 7 (1984):37–38.

133. SHADER, R. I. "Sexual Dysfunction Associated with Thioridazine Hydrochloride," *Journal of the American Medical Association,* 188 (1964):1007–1009.

134. SHADER, R. I., et al. *Psychotropic Drug Side Effects. Clinical and Theoretical Perspectives.* Baltimore: Williams & Wilkins, 1970.

135. SHEARER, W. T., SHREINER, R. L., and MARSHALL, R. F. "Urinary Retention in a Neonate Secondary to Maternal Ingestion of Nortriptyline," *Journal of Pediatrics,* 81 (1972):570–572.

136. SHEEHY, L. M., and MAXMEN, J. S. "Phenelzine-induced Psychosis," *American Journal of Psychiatry,* 135 (1978):1422–1423.

137. SHOPSIN, B., and GERSHON, S. "Lithium in Psychiatry," *American Journal of Medical Science,* 268 (1974):307–320.

138. SIDDALL, J. R. "Ocular Toxic Changes Associated with Chlorpromazine and Thioridazine," *Canadian Journal of Ophthalmology,* 1 (1966):190–198.

139. SIMPSON, G. M., and VARJA, E. "Clozapine—A New Antipsychotic Agent," *Current Therapeutic Research,* 16 (1974):679–686.

140. SINGER, T., and ROTENBERG, D. "Mechanisms of Lithium Action," *New England Journal of Medicine,* 289 (1973): 254–260.

141. SNYDER, S. "Restless Legs Syndrome Treated with Quinine Sulfate," *Journal of Psychiatric Treatment and Evaluation,* 5 (1983):385–386.

142. SNYDER, S., and YAMAMURA, H. "Antidepressants and the Muscarinic Acetylcholine Receptor," *Archives of General Psychiatry,* 34 (1977):236–238.

143. SNYDER, S., et al. "Antischizophrenic Drugs: Affinity for Muscarinic Cholinergic Receptor Sites in the Brain Predicts Extrapyramidal Effects," *Journal of Psychiatric Research,* 11 (1974):91–95.

144. STEELE, T. E. "Adverse Reactions Suggesting Amoxapine-induced Dopamine Blockade," *American Journal of Psychiatry,* 139 (1982):1500–1501.

145. STERN, S. L. "Update on Lithium Therapy," in J. Z. Yetiv and J. Bianchine, eds., *Recent Advances in Clinical Therapeutics.* New York: Grune & Stratton, 1983, pp. 61–77.

146. SULSER, F. "New Perspectives on the Mode of Action of Antidepressant Drugs," *Trends in Pharmacological Science,* 1 (1979):92–94.

147. TANGEDAHL, T. N., and GAU, G. "Myocardial Irritability Associated with Lithium Carbonate Therapy," *New England Journal of Medicine,* 287 (1972):867.

148. TARSAY, D. "Movement Disorders with Neuroleptic Drug Treatment," *Psychiatric Clinics of North America,* 7 (1984):453–471.

149. TARSAY, D., and BALDESSARINI, R. J. "Tardive Dyskinesia," *Annual Review of Medicine,* 35 (1984):605–623.

150. THOMAS, C., TATHAM, A., and JAKUBOW-SKI, S. "Lithium/haloperidol Combinations and Brain Damage," *Lancet,* 1 (1982):626.

151. TOLLELSON, G. D. "Monoamine Oxidase Inhibition: A Review," *Journal of Clinical Psychiatry,* 44 (1983):280–288.

152. "Trazodone (Desyrel)," *Biological Therapies in Psychiatry,* 5 (1982):17.

153. TUKIAN, A., et al. "The Cardiovascular Effects of Lithium in Man," *American Journal of Medicine,* 61 (1976):665–670.

154. TYRER, P. J. "Monoamine Oxidase Inhibitors and Amine Precursors," in P.J. Tyrer, ed., *Drugs in Psychiatric Practice.* London: Butterworth and Co., 1982, pp. 249–279.

155. TYRER, S., and SHAW, D. M. "Lithium Carbonate," in P. J. Tyrer, ed., *Drugs in Psychiatric Practice.* London: Butterworth and Co., 1982, pp. 280–312.

156. TYRER, S. P., et al. "Lithium and the Kidney," *Lancet,* 1 (1980):94–95.

157. VANDER KOLK, B. "Recent Advances in the Use of Lithium," Lecture given at Massachusetts Mental Health Center, April 20, 1984.

158. VANDER-VELLS, C. D., and GIORDON, M. W. "Manic Depressive Illness, Diabetes Mellitus and Lithium Carbonate Treatment," *Archives of General Psychiatry,* 21 (1969):478–485.

159. VAN SCHEYEN, J. D., and VAN KAMMEN, D. P. "Clomipramine-induced Mania in Unipolar Depression," *Archives of General Psychiatry,* 36 (1979):560–565.

160. VESTERGAARD, P., and AMIDSEN, A. "Lithium Treatment and Kidney Function," *Acta Psychiatrica Scandinavica,* 63 (1981):335–345.

161. VESTERGAARD, P., AMIDSEN, A., and HANSEN, H. E. "Lithium Treatment and Kidney Function," *Acta Psychiatrica Scandinavica,* 60 (1979):504–520.

162. VESTERGAARD, P., AMIDSEN, A., and SCHOU, M. "Clinically Significant Side Effects of Lithium Treatment: A Survey of 237 Patients in Long-term Treatment," *Acta Psychiatrica Scandinavica,* 62 (1980):193–200.

163. VOHRA, J., BURROWS, J. D., and SLOMAN, J. "Assessment of Cardiovascular Side Effects of Therapeutic Doses of Tricyclic Antidepressant Drugs," *Australian and New Zealand Journal of Medicine,* 5 (1975):7–11.

164. WEISSMAN, M., and BOYD, J. H. "The Epidemiology of Affective Disorders—Rates and Risk Factors," in L. Grinspoon, ed., *Psychiatric Update,* vol. 2. Washington, D.C.: American Psychiatric Association Press, 1983, pp. 406–428.

165. WEISTEIN, M., and GOLDFIELD, M. "Cardiovascular Malformations with Lithium Rise During Pregnancy," *American Journal of Psychiatry,* 132 (1975):529–531.

166. WHALIN, L., and ALLING, C. "Effect of Sustained-release Lithium Tablets on Renal Function," *British Medical Journal,* 2 (1979):1332.

167. WILBANKS, J. D., et al. "Toxic Effects of Lithium in a Mother and Newborn Infant," *Journal of the American Medical Association,* 213 (1970):56–57.

168. WORTHEY, L. J. C. "Lithium Toxicity and Refractory Cardiac Arrhythmia Treated with Intravenous Magnesium," *Anesthesia and Intensive Care,* 2 (1974):357–360.

169. WYATT, R. J., et al. "Total Prolonged Drug-induced REM Sleep Suppression in Anxious-depressed Patients," *Archives of General Psychiatry,* 24 (1971): 145–155.

170. ZAVODNICK, S. "Atrial Flutter with Amoxapine: A Case Report," *American Journal of Psychiatry,* 138 (1981):1503–1504.

PART FOUR

Controversies in Biological Psychiatry

CHAPTER 33

ELECTROCONVULSIVE THERAPY

Iver F. Small, Joyce G. Small, and Victor Milstein

¶ Introduction

The first modern physician to induce seizures for therapeutic purposes was Ladislas von Meduna in 1934. In 1938 Ugo Cerletti and Lucio Bini introduced electroconvulsive therapy (ECT) as a more efficient and reliable procedure. Some authors place the origin of convulsive therapy at the time of the medicinal use of electric eels by the Romans. The first therapeutic use of ECT in the United States may have been initiated by Dr. Ben Franklin in 1752.[187] Despite this 200- or 2,000-year history of ECT, this review will, with minor exceptions, concern itself with contemporary literature, emphasizing almost exclusively that of the last decade. The subject matter will be treated in six general areas, namely indications and patterns of use, adverse effects, efficacy, procedure and techniques, ethical issues, and mechanisms of action.

¶ Indications and Patterns of Use

A number of reports have described the role of ECT in psychiatry based on reviews and interpretations of the literature and personal experience.* However, it is important to know how the technique actually is applied in practice, the kinds of patients that receive such treatment, and the observed complications and outcome. In the last decade, there have been a number of surveys involving large numbers of hospitals, psychiatrists, and patients from different nations.† Major depression was the primary indication given for ECT in all reports. However, most of the studies stated that schizophrenia, affective and schizo-affective disorders, and failure to respond to drug therapy also were indications for ECT.

The rate of use of ECT varies considerably. Reports from Europe and North America indicated a range of approximately 2 to 5 percent of hospitalized psychiatric patients. In Canada it was used in 11 percent of such patients, with a wide range between reporting hospitals.[56] Figures of 7 percent[74] in Scotland, 17 percent in Denmark,[94] and 4.1 percent in Sweden[73] have been reported. Surveys from other countries and continents showed higher rates, with 14.3 percent in

---

*See references 63,71,106,163,175, and 201.
†See references 12,15,17,27,53,56,73,74,91,94,97,136,-148,157, and 167.

India[167] and 49 percent[142] to 66 percent[97] in Nigeria. One hospital in Massachusetts[91] treated 70 percent of its patients with ECT.

Usual practice in the United States is to give *three* treatments per week, while in England and Europe treatment is regularly given *twice* a week. Usually one electrical stimulus is provided per treatment session, although occasionally multiple stimuli are given. Bilateral electrode placement and sine wave stimulation is still the most common method employed. The number of treatments given in a series ranges from as low as two or three to more than twenty, although most patients receive six to eight ECTs, with series averaging from 6.1 to 9.4 treatments.[91,97] Schizophrenic patients generally receive more treatments than those with affective disorder.* The American Psychiatric Association (APA) recommends no more than thirty treatments in one year nor more than fifty in a lifetime.[12]

With the exception of reports from India and Nigeria, more women than men are treated with ECT, a fact understandable in light of the greater incidence of affective disorder in females. More females with depression receive ECT, while more males than females with schizophrenia are so treated.[97] Similarly, older patients are more likely to receive ECT than younger persons in Great Britain and the United States.[16,148] However, in India ECT is used mostly with younger patients, 91 percent being less than forty years of age.[167] Most of the surveys indicate that ECT is used only occasionally with adolescents. In one report[15] only one patient less than thirteen years of age received ECT. Recently ECT was used successfully in a twelve-year-old child with mania,[31] although most authorities do not recommend such treatment at this age.

With the exception of the reports from Nigeria[97] and India,[167] the other surveys indicate that almost all treatments are given with premedications of atropine, a short-acting barbiturate, and a muscle relaxant. Some facilities employ an anesthesiologist or

*See references 12,53,73,91,94,136, and 148.

nurse anesthetist some or all of the time for ECT, while others do not.

Apnea commonly occurs with ECT, and prolonged apnea is considered a complication of treatment.[53] Early in the history of ECT apnea resulted in anoxia, which some psychiatrists believed was inevitable and a few thought was necessary for therapeutic benefit.[63] This belief has since been discarded, and some of the negative aftereffects of ECT, especially cognitive impairment and posttreatment headache, have been reduced or eliminated by scrupulous attention to oxygenation. Many of the surveys emphasized the use of 100 percent oxygen and stressed that patients should breathe it before the seizure as well as receive it afterward to assist breathing in the postictal period. Most surveys commented upon the short-term outcome of ECT. Seventy-five percent or more patients with affective disorders were reported to improve or remit. The largest survey[12] found that 88 percent of all patients were moderately improved or better, and a more recent geographically restricted survey using the same questionnaire found the same.[136]

In addition to the official surveys of ECT, there are other more informal reports of consumer attitudes[18,104] and comparisons of public and private hospitals. One survey showed that patients, professionals, and the laity alike had positive attitudes about ECT.[104] The three groups agreed to a remarkable extent upon the indications for ECT and the low probability of memory impairment. Other surveys, however, have expressed negative opinions.[21,80] American studies showed that private patients were more likely to receive ECT than patients in public institutions.[15,68,91] This difference may be based on increased demand for staff and equipment required for ECT in public facilities as opposed to financial incentives that encourage this form of treatment among private patients.[17] Whether this is indeed the explanation, an opposite relation exists in West Germany, where ECT is frequently employed in public clinics and rarely in private hospitals.[157] A similar though not as marked a trend appears to exist in France.[27]

Other issues relating to use of ECT that were important in earlier years appear to have been resolved, some the result of reports of systematic studies and others apparently the product of consensus based on clinical experience. For example, despite reports of favorable results in schizophrenic patients treated with regressive ECT,[59] this procedure is no longer in use. Regressive ECT involves the administration of multiple treatments in a single day over several days, with patients usually manifesting confusion, incontinence, and inability to feed themselves. It has not been demonstrated that the "regression" is necessary for therapeutic effect, and the syndrome described may have contributed to fears and misunderstandings about ECT.

Blachley and Gowing[25] reported a procedure in which several electrically induced seizures were administered in a single session with seizures spaced at two- to three-minute intervals. The electroencephalogram (EEG) and electrocardiogram (EKG) were monitored throughout, resulting in the name multiple monitored ECT, or MMECT. This procedure attracted considerable interest because of its promise of producing more rapid remission. The procedure had the additional advantage of keeping patients sufficiently relaxed through the use of large amounts of succinylcholine chloride, so that they could be ventilated easily during the seizure, thus avoiding any possibility of anoxia. A retrospective study reported that patients who received MMECT had a more rapid course of treatment and fewer sessions of general anesthesia, but there was no difference in efficacy between MMECT and single treatments.[23] However, Maletzky reported more positive results.[130] In addition, he noted the potentially important finding that the degree of improvement was related to the total number of seconds of electrical afterdischarge for the series of ECT. Total seizure times less than 210 seconds were not associated with positive response. His data further indicated that total afterdischarge

duration in excess of 1,000 seconds produced little additional benefit, regardless of diagnostic category. This report of a therapeutic "window" of seizure duration has not been replicated. Anecdotally we have found that total seizure time per ECT series almost always exceeds 210 seconds. However, no significant correlations between seizure time and clinical status have yet been identified with standard three-times-weekly ECT. The APA Task Force Report concluded that data on MMECT were insufficient to evaluate.[12]

Because Blachley and Gowing[25] had their patients completely relaxed, only EEG monitoring could indicate the presence of seizure activity. (EKG monitoring was instituted for safety reasons in their relatively long-lasting general anesthetic procedure.) However, with all forms of ECT, monitoring of the electrical activity of the brain is desirable for a number of reasons, the primary one being to establish that an adequate treatment has been provided.[113,172] The tonic-clonic motor convulsion that accompanies the cerebral afterdischarge is not a necessary part of the treatment[61] (see the section entitled "Procedures and Techniques"), and, given sufficient muscle relaxant, will not occur. Thus, especially in patients in whom large doses of succinylcholine are required, it is necessary to record the electrical activity of the brain. Even neurological signs after treatment are less reliable than the EEG.[111] Fink and Johnson proposed occluding the circulation to the ipsilateral arm (the cuff method) to observe whether or not a bilateral seizure had been induced.[66] However, with this method, the duration of motor activity is shorter than the electrical afterdischarge by several seconds. Even electromyographic (EMG) monitoring is not a reliable indicator of seizure duration,[37,183] for EMG-monitored seizures were 43 to 89 percent as long as the EEG afterdischarge.

The generally accepted requirements for an adequate treatment include a major generalized (grand mal) seizure of duration greater than twenty-five to thirty seconds, as experience indicates that short, partial, focal, or petit mal seizures tend not to be associated with clinical improvement.[204] The only way to identify these events is by EEG monitoring. In this respect, it is likely that early experience with unilateral ECT, in which longer series were needed than with bilateral treatment, occurred mainly for mechanical reasons, because it is more difficult to induce major generalized seizures with unilateral stimulation.[63] Without monitoring the EEG or using the cuff method, it was not possible to discern whether unilateral ECT was associated with a higher number of inadequate or missed seizures than bilateral treatment. Moreover, one study reported that clinical observation alone without EEG monitoring misjudged 43 percent of treatments as unsuccessful and would have resulted in the unnecessary application of a second stimulus.[38] Nevertheless, the one-channel, bipolar recording from frontal electrodes provided by one commercial apparatus is susceptible to eyelid flutter and other artifacts, and is no substitute for multichannel EEG recording.[28]

¶ Adverse Effects

In the early years of its use, ECT was associated with a variety of side effects ranging from chipped teeth through fractures and dislocations to amnesia, prolonged apnea, and even death. Modifications of the procedure involving oxygenation; administration of anticholinergic, sedative, and muscle-relaxing agents; electrode placement; and stimulus parameters have eliminated or drastically reduced most of these adverse effects (see the "Procedures and Techniques" section). However, there remain two related areas of concern, namely whether ECT produces structural changes that may be characterized as brain damage and whether cognitive impairment and especially memory loss is an inevitable consequence of the treatment.

That ECT produces transient neurological dysfunction is generally accepted. In fact, the term acute organic mental syndrome has been used to refer to effects of bilateral ECT.[190] What is disputed is the nature of the dysfunction, its severity, and especially whether it is transient or permanent. In a recent study[190] 48 percent of subjects developed an acute organic syndrome that persisted for less than three weeks (mean of twenty days, range five to forty-three). These patients were treated with bilateral, 60 Hertz (Hz) sine-wave stimulation, and less than 10 percent received oxygen prior to the induction of the seizure. The severity of the organic syndrome was proportional to the number of seizures and the dosages of concomitant psychoactive medications with anticholinergic effects. In another investigation patients were examined before and immediately after dominant and nondominant unilateral ECT.[112] Most treatments were followed by signs of neurological dysfunction that were transitory and referable to the stimulated hemisphere: "All neurological abnormalities tested resolved within 20 minutes of treatment" (p. 1135).[112] However, a review of studies quantitatively examining degrees of disorientation after ECT concluded that various components recovered at different rates, with temporal orientation the slowest to recover.[44]

The issue of whether ECT produces structural and permanent central nervous system (CNS) impairment has been examined from other points of view. One deals with the development of spontaneous seizures during or after a course of ECT. The relationship between seizures-epilepsy and ECT harks back to von Meduna's hypothesis of an inverse relationship between epilepsy and schizophrenia. Fink[63] estimated the occurrence of tardive seizures after ECT as less than one in 500 patients. Although seizure threshold tends to rise after the first few ECTs,[175] in light of his work on kindling, Goddard[86] warned that ECT had many potential hazards. Kindling is a phenomenon in which repeated, low-intensity, subthreshold stimulation of the brains of animals eventually results in spontaneous seizures. Despite early as well as recent case reports of post-ECT spontaneous seizures,[203,207] Blackwood and coworkers[26] and Small and associates[179] found no evidence to suggest that kindling as such was a hazard associated with ECT. (The kindling phenomenon is further discussed in the section entitled "Mechanisms of Action.")

The question of structural change or brain damage is important in evaluating the safety of ECT. Postmortem reports of petechial hemorrhages, gliosis, and neuronal loss appeared soon after the introduction of ECT. Generally, these early treatments were unmodified with anesthesia and muscle relaxants, and were associated with a high incidence of other side effects. Garcia[79] reported on a comprehensive review of the literature related to the neuropathology of ECT. He concluded that ECT causes reversible changes in circulation of the brain parenchyma. This conclusion was supported by Beresford,[24] who stated that most clinical neurologists agree that after the early postictal delirium subsides it is impossible to detect abnormal neurological findings in a patient who has had an uncomplicated generalized seizure (i.e., one that is not for some reason complicated by prolonged hypoxia). He pointed out that several of the older neuropathological studies suggested that inadequate ventilation was responsible for cerebral injury, and he stressed the need to avoid hypoxemia, acidosis, and increased lactate production by the brain.

Using computerized tomography (CT), Weinberger and colleagues[199] reported the presence of enlarged cerebral ventricles in chronic schizophrenic patients, many of whom had received ECT. Ventricular enlargement did not appear to be related to previous treatment modalities. However, cortical atrophy, as determined by measuring the width of sulci and fissures, occurred significantly more frequently in ECT-treated patients. Nevertheless, the authors pointed out that in the majority of chronic patients, CT findings developed independently of treatment with ECT.[200] Further, schizophrenic patients referred for ECT are likely to have more severe forms of illness. Other workers have failed to demonstrate associations between larger ventricles and a history of ECT.[54,69] Another study specifically evaluated the ECT history in forty-one elderly depressive patients who had CT scans.[30] No relationship was found between ventricular atrophy and ECT, but there was a significant association between cortical atrophy and a history of ECT. Lippmann and coworkers[125] found no significant pattern of cerebellar abnormalities associated with a history of ECT in schizophrenic and bipolar affective disorder patients. A case study was reported of a thirty-year-old woman with bipolar depression who was given ten ECTs over forty-five minutes.[135] Three hours later, a repeat CT scan was performed; despite the fact that the patient was amnesic and disoriented, no changes were observed when the scan was compared with that obtained the day before. Similarly, Jacoby and associates,[98] examining brain-tissue density rather than ventricular or sulcal width, found no association with ECT in elderly, depressed patients. Finally, Kendell and Pratt[105] found no CT changes in twelve patients who received a large number of mainly unilateral ECTs.

Following reports of increased ventricular size in schizophrenic patients, which was initially interpreted as cortical atrophy associated with ECT, it was hoped that the relatively precise, noninvasive technique of CT would unequivocally indicate whether ECT does or does not produce structural change. Unfortunately, the technical uncertainties associated with CT (such as whether density or width should be the measure; the use of side-effect-producing, enhancing contrast agents; choice of "slices" to measure; and so on) coupled with problems of selection of appropriate subjects and comparison groups and control of possibly confounding variables have combined to prevent fulfillment of that expectation.

The EEG is a readily available, noninvasive procedure that has been employed with ECT as an indicator of brain damage. Electrically induced seizures are characterized by spiking that begins immediately after the application of the stimulus and persists after its termination.[167,175] The afterdischarge frequently ends abruptly and may be followed by a flat EEG, especially after bilateral ECT early in the course of treatment. Slow-wave activity then typically characterizes the recovery period. With repeated seizures, slowing becomes more persistent in the interictal interval. The EEG may show lateralized changes that are different for bilateral and unilateral ECT. Following the end of the ECT series, the amount of slow-wave activity in the EEG diminishes over time and disappears after a few weeks to a few months.[63,202] The lateralized asymmetry, high-voltage slow waves, and other phenomena in the interictal EEG have been adduced as evidence of the presence of brain damage. However, all of these signs are reversible and do not suggest any persistent structural change. This is confirmed by more specific evoked potential (EP) EEG studies performed after ECT.[111,169,176] Neither visual nor auditory EPs manifested significant hemispheric asymmetries one hour or one day after unilateral ECT. The auditory brain stem EP also is unaffected by ECT,[179] even when recorded during the seizure.[205] Further commentary on these issues is contained in the section "Mechanisms of Action."

Although the illnesses for which ECT primarily is employed, namely the major affective disorders and schizophrenia, are themselves associated with significant cognitive deficits, there is little doubt that ECT produces both short- and long-term intellectual impairment. Retrograde and anterograde amnesia, verbal and nonverbal memory, impaired concentration and attention, markedly slowed reaction time, difficulty abstracting and making complex discriminations, and impaired perception and visuomotor ability are all aspects of cognitive functioning that are affected by ECT. Diffuse, mild, or moderate dysfunction may be noted, and a profound dementia with gross cognitive dysfunction and marked general functional impairment occurs rarely.

Cognitive deficits may, for convenience, be divided into those relating to memory as opposed to all others. The previously described acute neurological impairment associated with ECT as well as orientation difficulties fall into the nonmemory aspect of cognition. However, evaluation of available evidence indicates that ECT does not produce permanent or long-term nonmemory cognitive impairment.[22,155] But there is no doubt that memory impairment is the most troublesome and most widely known side effect associated with ECT.[57,62] There is also general agreement that long-term, enduring memory deficits are not a necessary consequence of ECT. Their occurrence may be influenced by number and frequency of treatments,[154] bilateral as opposed to unilateral stimulation,[197,198] and, to a lesser extent, physical characteristics of the electrical stimulus and the amount of energy employed.[44]

A number of reviews of studies of memory impairment with ECT as well as experimental reports have appeared recently. The reviews show a high level of consensus in their interpretations of the literature and their conclusions. These can be summarized as follows:

- Deficits in memory are maximal immediately after each seizure but recover rapidly so that evaluations done two weeks after a series of treatments fail to show these deficits.[63,71] The amount of impairment appears to be directly related to the frequency and number of seizures, the location of the electrodes, the intensity of the stimulating current, and the time between the last seizure and the evaluation.*
- Memory and recall of events that occurred before the illness tend to recover completely. In a small number of patients, ECT may cause permanent memory impairment, but the significance of this is not clear at this time.[154,192,204]
- Anterograde amnesia recedes gradually after each individual treatment but is cumulative over the series of ECT[45,154,192] and is recovered substantially by six to nine months.[154] Memory for long past events recovers by six to nine months; memory for very recent events occurring just prior to ECT may be lost permanently.†

*See references 12,45,63,71,77, and 154.
†See references 12,154,184,185, and 192.

- Bilateral ECT is associated with greater anterograde and retrograde amnesia than is unilateral treatment.*
- Nondominant unilateral ECT produces less verbal memory impairment[92] and less verbal anterograde and retrograde amnesia than does bilateral ECT.[46,184]
- Nondominant unilateral ECT selectively impairs nonverbal retrograde memory, while dominant unilateral treatment selectively impairs verbal retrograde memory.[77,154]
- Bilateral ECT is associated with more subjective complaints of memory impairment,[12,154] and there may even be an inverse relationship between objective findings of impaired memory function and subjective complaints![103]

The question of whether or not memory impairment induced by ECT is essential to its therapeutic effects has been addressed by many authors. Most investigations show no such relationships,[76,192,204] but there are researchers who still hold opposite views.[118] Some studies have shown that memory deficits are accompanied by EEG slowing.[188] Other work has demonstrated that neuropsychological test performance improves with ECT, particularly unilateral ECT, and that these changes parallel clinical improvement.[170,171] Further studies of these interesting interrelationships may clarify which changes are necessary and sufficient for the therapeutic actions of ECT.

¶ Efficacy

Depression

Convulsive therapy was introduced into clinical medicine before the era of the double-blind study. Evidence of its efficacy was derived from personal experience and observations of dramatic recoveries in patients presumed to be hopelessly ill. Then followed studies of patients randomly assigned to receive ECT or antidepressant medications, as

*See references 12,47,154,184, and 192.

the latter became available. Although these studies were nonblind, the results were remarkably consistent; almost invariably ECT was found superior to antidepressant drug treatment. Reports on the results of double-blind studies that began to appear in the late 1970s were much less enthusiastic. Most still found ECT to be superior to drug treatment, but the differences were not nearly as impressive. Many factors may account for discrepancies between the open and blind trials, not the least of which is observer bias and expectation. However, it is also true that patients referred for ECT have become more treatment resistant, since there are more alternative treatments available and ECT may be used only as a last resort. In most of the studies, group differences were also minimized by the use of concomitant therapies. Some used benzodiazepines and other agents with anticonvulsant effects, which may have interfered with the production of seizures. Moreover, seizure induction is more difficult with the unilateral technique, and missed seizures may have occurred without EEG monitoring. Some of the blind studies were done in very chronically ill patients. Finally, formal studies generally exclude the most extremely suicidal and disturbed patients who often show the most dramatic response to ECT.

Whatever the reason for the lack of outstanding results in recent controlled trials, ECT is still firmly established as an important treatment modality in psychiatry. As indicated by the Task Force position papers,[12] the major indication for ECT is endogenous depression particularly when accompanied by psychosis. Its use in schizophrenia, mania, and other mental disorders is less well established.

Several double-blind controlled trials of ECT in the treatment of depression have been conducted in the past several years. Barton[19] summarized the results from six studies of ECT compared to simulated ECT in 192 hospitalized depressed patients. Taken together, the results of these studies gave overwhelming evidence that ECT was more effective than simulated ECT. Lambourn and Gill[119] compared two groups of sixteen patients with depressive psychosis. One group received six unilateral ECTs, while the second group was given the same procedure without the electrical stimuli and consequent seizures. The outcome of treatment was remarkably positive in both groups, although there was a small trend in favor of ECT. The study raised questions about unilateral brief-pulse ECT and whether partial or missed seizures could have influenced the results, particularly since a report published at about the same time[75] showed that bilateral ECT with sinusoidal stimulus waveform was significantly more effective than simulated ECT. The results in the latter study were all the more outstanding because antidepressant drug treatment was permitted in both treatment groups. In the Northwick Park Electroconvulsive Therapy Trial,[102] seventy patients with endogenous depression were randomly allocated to a course of eight sham ECTs or to eight bilateral treatments. No other antidepressant treatment was given, but benzodiazepine hypnotics were given nightly. Both groups improved, but improvement was greater in the real ECT group after the second week of treatment. Differences between the groups disappeared at one and six months following ECT. The authors concluded that electrically induced seizures enhanced the rate of recovery from an episode of depression but the antidepressant effects are of relatively short duration. This study has been criticized for its fixed, brief duration of treatment and the concomitant use of benzodiazepines.

In a study from India[78] thirty-two patients with primary affective disorder were randomized to treatment with bilateral ECT and placebo or simulated ECT and imipramine hydrochloride. The researchers concluded that improvement with ECT occurred more rapidly when combined with imipramine and that ECT was a superior form of treatment for endogenous depression. West's randomized double-blind controlled study of real and simulated ECT also demonstrated a marked superiority of real ECT.[208] Although

not a controlled trial, a remarkable National Institute of Mental Health report published in 1981 found that eight of nine extremely ill, treatment-resistant depressed patients responded to ECT and were well for at least a year afterward.[146] Most recently Janicak and coworkers[100] combined data from nine studies of 901 patients who were randomly assigned to ECT or sham treatment. They concluded that real ECT was superior to simulated ECT by a margin of 41 percent with a statistical probability of < 0.001. ECT similarly was compared to antidepressant drug treatment by pooling of data from studies of either tricyclic antidepressants (TCAs) or monoamine oxidase inhibitors (MAOIs). Again, ECT was superior with an estimated difference in effectiveness of 45 percent.

ECT has a special place in the treatment of depression accompanied by delusions and other psychotic features and in schizo-affective disorder. In the former, antidepressant drugs alone are usually ineffective and must be combined with neuroleptics for therapeutic efficacy.[85,138] In this situation ECT has been designated as an alternative treatment approach. A retrospective survey comparing the effectiveness of ECT and TCAs combined with neuroleptic therapy in the treatment of psychotic depression revealed a favorable treatment response in 86 percent of ECT-treated patients and 42 percent with the drug combination, suggesting that ECT has therapeutic advantages.[147] Ries and associates[160] prescribed ECT to nine schizo-affective patients who did not respond to pharmacological treatment and observed rapid improvement and remission. These patients were characterized by early-age of onset and first psychiatric treatment, positive family history for mental disorder, and symptomatology of prominent confusion and paranoia.* Prospective evaluations of ECT versus neuroleptic-tricyclic combinations are in

---

*Kupfer and Reynolds[117] suggested that rapid-eye-movement (REM) sleep latencies of less than twenty minutes in depressed patients with low sleep efficiency are predictive of poor antidepressant drug response and better outcome with ECT or antipsychotic-antidepressant combination therapy.

progress at several institutions, but have not been published as far as we are aware.

Schizophrenia

Schizophrenia is the second most common indication stated for the use of ECT in psychiatric patients. There have been a number of controlled, prospective, and later double-blind studies of its usefulness in this context. The older literature contains three studies in which ECT and neuroleptic drug treatment were compared and four reports in which ECT combined with drugs was compared with drug treatment alone. (Only prospective studies in which comparable patients were randomly assigned to treatment groups have been considered in this review.) Langsley, Enterline, and Hickerson[120] compared chlorpromazine to ECT in the treatment of acute schizophrenic and manic reactions in 106 hospitalized patients. The two diagnostic groups were not analyzed separately. Fifteen to twenty bilateral ECTs unmodified by anesthetics or muscle relaxants were given. Drug-treated patients received 200 to 2,000 mg per day of chlorpromazine. Outcome measures indicated equivalent findings with ECT and chlorpromazine at eight and twelve weeks. King[107] obtained similar results with ECT and chlorpromazine. The most definitive work in this area is that of May,[133] who randomly assigned a sample of 228 hospitalized schizophrenic patients to receive neuroleptic drugs, ECT, psychotherapy, or milieu treatment. ECT was given three times a week to limits decided by clinicians, with a mean of nineteen treatments for men and twenty-five for women. Drug-treated patients were given chlorpromazine and/or trifluoperazine hydrochloride in low to moderate doses. Short-term results indicated that the drug-treated patients did better than those who received ECT in terms of most of the outcome measures, which included days in hospital, quality of remission, and cost of treatment. ECT was intermediate in effectiveness compared with drug therapy and psychotherapy, with better results in men than in women. Long-term

follow-up[134] revealed fewer relapses and rehospitalizations in patients who received drugs or ECT, with a trend for better results in the ECT group.

ECT in combination with neuroleptic drugs in the treatment of schizophrenia has been studied with comparisons of drugs plus ECT versus drugs alone. The older literature contains studies with reserpine and chlorpromazine.[35,87,141,182] In the main, equivalent results were obtained in patients treated with drugs or the drug-ECT combination. However, methodological problems prevent firm conclusions because the doses of drugs and the number of ECTs administered were below usual therapeutic levels. Two studies[87,141] showed no advantage to the use of ECT combined with drugs in very chronically ill schizophrenic patients. The other two studies[35,182] found that patients receiving ECT combined with drugs did better than those treated with drugs alone on short-term follow-up. In the Smith and associates study there were no differences between treatment groups six and twelve months later.[182]

More recently, Janakiramaiah, Channabasavanna, and Narasimha Murthy[99] reported a study in schizophrenia of ECT combined with 300 or 500 mg daily of chlorpromazine versus 500 mg of chlorpromazine alone. ECT enhanced therapeutic response at low drug dosages but offered no significant advantages at the higher dosage. Taylor and Fleminger[194] evaluated chronically ill schizophrenic patients receiving regular neuroleptic therapy randomized to receive either real or sham ECT with double-blind evaluation of treatment results. Most groups improved but the ECT group was better after six treatments and at the end of the ECT series. However, the differences between the groups disappeared by sixteen weeks. Small and coworkers[181] studied ECT combined with neuroleptics versus neuroleptics or ECT alone in the treatment of seventy-five chronically ill schizophrenic patients. Comparable therapeutic results were achieved with the ECT-neuroleptic combination and neuroleptic drugs, with less favorable results with unilateral ECT alone. There were suggestions that the course of treatment with the neuroleptic-ECT combination was smoother, with fewer problems with drug compliance; less apathy, withdrawal, indifference, and other negative features of schizophrenia; and fewer movement disorders. There was also better familial adjustment after hospitalization in the ECT-drug combined group.

In general, the outcome studies in chronic schizophrenia indicate that ECT conveys little advantage over neuroleptic drug management. In acute schizophrenia and schizophreniform disorder the situation is probably different[67] because the course of these illnesses is more typical of the affective disorders. Definitive studies of ECT in the treatment of acute psychosis have yet to be accomplished and may not even be feasible in today's climate, given other available effective methods of management.

Some investigators have tried to determine which features of schizophrenia predict improvement with ECT. A retrospective study[108] found that affective features predict improvement, as does an absence of Schneiderian first-rank symptoms. In clinical practice patients are often referred for ECT on the basis of presentation with catatonic features, affective symptomatology, and high risk of aggressive or suicidal behavior. Refusal to eat and drink or intolerance of medications are other common indications.

Formal studies of most of these aspects have not been accomplished and probably will not be done in the future as many of these kinds of patients are not able to give informed consent, cooperate for assessments, or tolerate the delays inherent in a formal research protocol.

Mania

The use of ECT in the treatment of mania has been studied much less than its use in depression or schizophrenia. However, in the past clinicians have relied on ECT for relieving symptoms during acute manic episodes, and maintenance ECT has been used to prevent recurrence.[82] Surveys of practicing psychiatrists in several countries consistently indicate that ECT is widely accepted as a treatment for mania, which is the third most common diagnosis treated with ECT.

The place of ECT in the present-day treatment of mania is uncertain, particularly since prospective studies comparing ECT with lithium carbonate and other methods of management have not yet been accomplished. We made an abortive attempt to perform such a study with prospective randomization of treatment with either lithium or ECT. The study was stopped after intake of only four manic patients because even these cooperating, consenting patients were not able to maintain compliance long enough for either form of treatment to take effect! In a subsequent ongoing study, neuroleptics were permitted in both treatment groups to facilitate compliance and to manage disruptive behavior. Preliminary results from the first twelve patients entering the trial suggest that either form of treatment can bring about remission in four to six weeks with similar needs for neuroleptic therapy in the two groups. This study is continuing with attention to long-range influences on recurrence.

The older literature[166] found that 62 percent of 466 manic patients recovered with ECT and 19 percent improved. This suggests that the efficacy of ECT in mania is less than in severe depression, but better than in schizophrenia, although allowances must be made for changes in diagnosis with current nosologic systems. Other reviews of the subject estimate that ECT leads to therapeutic recovery in mania in 75 percent of cases.[193] In a retrospective survey, McCabe[126] found that 82 percent of manic patients receiving ECT were markedly improved as compared with 36 percent improving without ECT or drug treatment.

The only studies comparing ECT with pharmacological and other treatments of mania have been retrospective in nature.[126,127,195] All reports agreed that ECT was as effective as drug treatment in the management of mania. One study found that patients who received ECT tended to have longer remissions than patients receiving neuroleptics alone.

Clearly, prospective investigations in this area are greatly needed. The major comparison between lithium and ECT is particularly important since, as of this writing, these are the standard methods of management of mania. Such studies must take into account the possible toxic interactions between the two treatments, and a period of lithium withdrawal should be instituted in both treatment groups prior to such an investigation.[178] There has been much recent interest in the usefulness of carbamazepine in the treatment of affective episodes, particularly manic states. (See chapter 15.) It has been suggested that ECT and carbamazepine may share a common therapeutic mechanism, wherein anticonvulsant effects of both treatments may act to stabilize limbic system dysfunctions.[151] In this regard concern has been expressed that ECT may actually worsen patients with rapidly recurring cycles of mania and depression.[116,152] TCAs have also been implicated in aggravating and possibly causing rapid cycling,[143] but carbamazepine in particular has not been examined in this context. The entire subject of the use of ECT in manic and depressed phases of bipolar disorder is worthy of much further investigative attention.

ECT Combination Therapies

Studies of ECT combined with neuroleptic medications in psychotic depression, schizoaffective illness, and schizophrenia have already been described. A number of other drug combinations with ECT have also been investigated. Combinations with antidepressant medications have been shown not to confer any additional therapeutic advantages, and in fact may be associated with more memory loss and confusion in proportion to the anticholinergic effects of the medications.[140,190] ECT should not be combined with MAOIs because of potential interactions with anesthetic agents. ECT combined with lithium has been shown to be associated with neurological complications and possibly reduced therapeutic efficacy.[178] However, lithium or antidepressant medications should be prescribed following ECT to prevent relapse.[41] ECT has also been studied in combination with l-tryptophan, a precursor of central amines possibly deficient in depression.[51,52] Placebo-controlled trials revealed negative findings with no indication of beneficial effects with the combination.[93]

Other studies have focused on combining ECT with different types of drugs in hopes of reducing postictal memory loss and confusion. Based on promising results from animal studies, the ACTH 4–10 fragment was examined in double-blind, placebo-controlled assessments of memory test performance in patients receiving bilateral ECT. Negative findings were consistently reported.[49,50,177] Similarly, piracetam did not exert effects on post-ECT amnesia,[137] providing indirect evidence that such amnesia is not secondary to hypoxia. In other work the long-acting stimulant pemoline was shown to improve scores on the Weschler Memory Scale during ECT.[179] However, long-term follow-up showed these patients had as much if not more objective and subjective memory impairments.[168]

Special Indications

Although most of the formal studies of ECT have been conducted in populations of patients with depression, schizophrenia, or mania, a number of other indications for ECT have gained clinical acceptance. Moreover, ECT has come to be regarded as a safe method of treatment particularly in high-risk situations, as it can be administered under carefully controlled conditions, as in an operating theater. This is a remarkable change from previous attitudes that ECT is dangerous or potentially harmful, and may have evolved because of increasing recognition of the toxicity and limitations of drug treatments as well as the adoption of unilateral ECT as the standard.[174]

An important situation in which ECT may be the preferred method of treatment is in psychotic illnesses or severe depressions that occur during pregnancy. Drug treatment may be associated with congenital malformations and often does not provide rapid enough control of behavior that can be potentially life-threatening to both mother and fetus. This is especially true during the first trimester. Guidelines have been proposed for the use of ECT in pregnancy that include thorough physical and pelvic evaluations, the latter with anesthesia if needed.[158] Obstetrical consultation and monitoring is needed, particularly in the high-risk pregnancy with hazards of induction of premature labor. External fetal monitoring would add to the safety of the procedure and also contribute data about maternal and fetal physiology.

Treatment of the elderly is another area in which drug treatment may be associated with unacceptably high risks because of coexisting medical conditions and the increased vulnerability of the aged to anticholinergic and other toxic effects of drugs. Moreover, the aged are often resistant to drug treatment.[81] At the same time, the aging nervous system is also more sensitive to the unwanted side effects of ECT, particularly confusion and delayed recovery. In this situation unilateral ECT is associated with much less impairment, so much so that it is usually the treatment of choice in the older patient.[77]

ECT is known to be associated with transient elevations in blood pressure, which is of concern in hypertensive patients, particularly the elderly. Intravenous sodium nitroprusside can be effective in counteracting elevated blood pressure during ECT.[40] Patients with cardiac arrhythmias have been successfully treated with ECT, even those patients with a pacemaker.[1] Fixed-rate pacing may be used to avoid ventricular ectopic activity and postconvulsive bradycardia.[156] Ventricular arrhythmias following ECT also can be treated with propranolol hydrochloride,[206] although this would have the potential for interfering with the therapeutic actions of ECT (see the section entitled "Mechanisms of Action").

Convulsive therapy has been given successfully to patients with a number of coexisting neurological disorders accompanied by affective illnesses or psychosis. Improvement in both psychiatric and neurological status has been observed with ECT in Parkinson's disease.[95,121] There are conflicting data about the effects of ECT upon extrapyramidal side effects of medications and tardive dyskinesia.[13,32] Case reports have appeared about the successful use of ECT for the treatment of depression in patients with normal-pressure hydrocephalus with a shunt in place,[196] meningomyelocele and hydrocephalus,[132] acute brain trauma,[164] and severe mental retardation.[20] Modified ECT has even been used successfully in patients who experienced severe delirium or status epilepticus with standard bilateral ECT.[48,203] Some of the most dramatic responses to ECT are seen in the treatment of pseudodementia in which patients present clinically with apparent organic cognitive deficits.[11] Another recognized indication for ECT is the syndrome of delirium acutum or lethal catatonia[174] as well as neuroleptic-induced malignant hyperthermia.[70,101] It has been shown recently that patients on short-acting anticoagulants can receive ECT without the occurrence of CNS bleeding.[7]

ECT has been used in a number of medical conditions complicated by psychotic, depressive, or manic symptomatology. Contradictory findings in control of diabetes mellitus following ECT have been reported.[60,211] In one study sixty patients with adult-onset diabetes mellitus who were not insulin dependent experienced sustained improvement following one or two ECTs.[60] The mechanism may have involved activation of neurons in the ventromedial nucleus of the hypothalamus that are responsive to changes in blood glucose concentration. This unusual finding awaits replication.

ECT has been used in various endocrine disorders, including a case with hypothalamic hypopituitarism that was followed by recovery of endocrinological function.[149] ECT has also been used successfully in the treatment of psychosis following pituitary surgery.[159] Outstanding results in depressed patients with lupus erythematosus and lupus cerebritis have been reported, a situation in which drug treatment is often unsatisfactory.[10,55]

In the past decade the use of unilateral nondominant ECT has been advocated because of its lower incidence of interference with memory and cognitive impairment. Although the literature is consistent on this issue, there is still controversy concerning whether or not unilateral ECT is as effective as bilateral treatment. Most Scandinavian researchers and some American investigators find that the two techniques yield comparable results if sufficient attention is devoted to ensuring the production of generalized major seizures. However, other workers disagree. Abrams and associates[5] found better therapeutic results with bilateral than unilateral ECT in fifty-one endogenously depressed male patients who were assigned randomly to receive bilateral or unilateral ECT. After six treatments, 81 percent were rated as improved in the bilateral group as compared with 55 percent in the unilateral patients. Moreover, clinicians prescribed more treatments in the unilateral group and frequently switched from unilateral to bilateral ECT because of deterioration or lack of response. The authors suggest that electrical stimulation of the diencephalon may be an important aspect of the therapeutic efficacy of bilateral treatment. Janicak and coworkers[100] have pooled data from the literature and compared results with unilateral and bilateral ECT in more than 500 patients. The results of these analyses showed no clear differences favoring bilateral ECT over unilateral nondominant treatment. The authors have preliminary data showing that bilateral ECT is more effective than unilateral ECT in the treatment of mania.

It is possible that differences in stimulus waveform and distances between electrodes with unilateral and bilateral treatment may also influence therapeutic outcome. Daniel and Crovitz[45] found no differences between sine wave and brief pulse stimulation, but Robin and DeTissera[162] showed that low-energy pulse stimulation was less effective than sine wave or high-energy pulse stimuli, despite the production of equally long motor convulsions. This observation led to the conclusion that while generalized seizures are necessary for clinical efficacy, not all such seizures produce a therapeutic response. This is consistent with clinical observations that some patients respond to either unilateral or bilateral ECT, some to bilateral but not unilateral, and some to neither.

¶ Procedures and Techniques

The decision to prescribe ECT begins with a recommendation from the psychiatrist to the patient and family. That recommendation is based on the patient's history, diagnosis, and presenting symptoms, as well as the record of previous therapeutic interventions in the patient and other family members. Other important considerations involve physical condition, the urgency of the presenting illness, and social and occupational needs. Frequently the decision is made in consultation with other professional colleagues. The reasons for recommending ECT must be explained to the patient and relatives, the possible risks and expected benefits discussed, and questions elicited and answered. A consent form is signed by the patient and/or the legal guardian where appropriate, and the form becomes a part of the permanent treatment record.

This section will not detail the various routines and procedures required for administration of ECT as these are readily available from a variety of sources,[2,63,71] perhaps the best of which remains the APA Task Force Report.[12] These volumes as well as others set out standards of performance, qualifications, and procedures that should be thoroughly mastered before undertaking the administration of ECT. However, we will draw attention to several issues that we feel have not been emphasized sufficiently in the literature.

Prior to the prescription of ECT, the patient's history and physical examination should be evaluated with special attention to cardiac and pulmonary functions. In addition, the ocular fundi should be examined, and the condition of the mouth and teeth assessed. Although ECT is unlikely to result in spinal injuries, standard practice dictates that pre- and post-ECT cervical, thoracic, and lumbar spine x-rays should be obtained. It is believed that the very high incidence of compression fractures of the spine in the early days of unmodified ECT has been reduced almost to zero with the present-day use of muscle relaxants. However, this has not been documented in the literature. Until it has been demonstrated that the costs (exposure to irradiation, expense) outweigh the benefits (findings of spurs, old fractures, and demineralization indicating need for a greater than usual degree of relaxation and /or participation of an anesthesiologist), these practices should be continued. In any case, x-rays should be done in elderly patients, postmenopausal women, and medicolegal situations. Normal values on laboratory screening test profiles and results of blood and urine studies should also be documented. In some facilities EEG screening before ECT also has been found to be useful.[177]

Because of its complicating effect on patients treated with ECT, lithium therapy should be discontinued at least one week or longer before starting ECT. Similarly, the MAOIs, reserpine, anticonvulsant medications, and all benzodiazepines should be discontinued.

Even the individual private practitioner should devise a systematic procedure for evaluation of patients to be accomplished before, during, and after ECT. This can be as simple as a listing of the pretreatment target symptoms and assaying their presence during the course of ECT and afterward, along with some overall evaluation of clinical condition and short- and long-term memory, all of which may be scored on a 0- to 4-point rating scale. Orientation in three spheres should be recorded. In larger or academic institutions where facilities are available, more elaborate assessments involving standardized neuropsychological procedures and tests of memory can be applied as well. It is especially important for the patient to be evaluated systematically and repeatedly during the course of ECT. This is most easily accomplished on a weekly basis on a nontreatment day. These procedures will aid in assessing the patient's progress and assist in determining when to discontinue ECT. These very brief assessments also serve as written documentation for decisions made by the clinician.

We stress the *elective* nature of ECT. Only in the most unusual and rare instances should ECT be considered an emergency procedure. The consequence of accepting the elective nature of the procedure is that anything that serves to increase the very small but real risk associated with ECT provides a reason to withhold or discontinue the treatment. Thus upper respiratory infections, elevated temperature, increases in blood pressure, absence of sufficient trained staff, or anything else that might compromise a normal response to the anesthesia or muscle relaxant or the ECT is a sufficient reason to withhold the treatment. (This includes known or suspected violations of the orders of nothing by mouth after midnight.)

As in other areas of medicine, the goal should be to treat with the smallest dosages of modifying medications and electricity consistent with clinical efficacy. Thus the smallest amount of methohexital, which is preferable to thiopental (Pentothal) because of fewer arrhythmias,[11,150] sufficient to render the patient unconscious both behaviorally and electrographically is all that is required. At the first treatment, a bolus of 50 or 60 mg methohexital is injected; if typical high-voltage slow waves do not appear on the EEG, additional 10 to 20 mg amounts are injected. If, during the course of a series of treatments, patients become more anxious and agitated, additional methohexital may be required to ensure a sufficient depth of sleep. On the other hand, if postictal apnea becomes prolonged, the amount of the anesthetic and muscle relaxant should be reduced. Succinylcholine is administered only to relax the patient with minimal alternating tonic-clonic movements remaining. It is critical that patients be asleep before the succinylcholine is injected. In certain cases of severe osteoporosis, unhealed fractures or other injuries, recent surgery, and so on, more complete relaxation, perhaps to the point of paralysis, would be required. In these cases, the presence of an anesthesiologist is necessary. However, we agree with Abrams and Essman[2] that routine ECT should be performed in the psychiatry unit and not in a surgical or anesthesia recovery area.

Two instruments account for most of the ECT given in the United States. The more common is the Medcraft, a 60 Hz, constant voltage, sine-wave machine; the other, the MECTA, is a biphasic square wave, constant-current unit. It is only an accident of history that allowed sine-wave stimulation a preeminent position. Square wave or pulse stimuli permit greater precision and control of the stimulus and, perhaps most important, allow much lower energy stimulation. Our experience has been that the Medcraft at typical settings (140 volts, 0.4 sec) produces 25 to 40 watt-seconds or joules, while the MECTA yields 8 to 15 joules (60 Hz, 0.75 msec, 1.25 sec). At maximum settings these machines may produce 130 and 80 joules respectively. Using the MECTA, we have performed adequate ECT leading to clinical improvement with as little as 2 to 4 joules of energy per treatment. Although there is little research evidence as yet, we and others hypothesize that low-energy treatments are associated with fewer side effects.

The nondominant unilateral placement of electrodes is strongly recommended to minimize cognitive deficits. However, it should be noted that some patients do not respond adequately to unilateral nondominant stimulation and do improve with bilateral treatments. After a trial of several unilateral treatments, repeated evaluations of patients at regular intervals will allow the clinician to determine whether a switch to bilateral treatment is indicated. On the other hand, bilateral ECT may be switched to unilateral treatment if severe amnesic effects appear.

At the time of the initial treatment or any time within the series, a previously effective stimulus may fail to produce a major generalized seizure lasting at least twenty-five seconds. When this occurs, increase the dose of electricity, wait thirty to sixty seconds as there appears to be a refractory period, and repeat the stimulus. If the second stimulus also is ineffective, increase the dose again and repeat for a third time. We do not use more than three stimuli at any session. If the second or third stimulus is successful, the settings that produced the seizure are repeated for following treatments. If the seizure is too short (less than twenty-five seconds) or not a major motor seizure (that is, focal or petit mal), we do not repeat the stimulation that day, but record an inadequate treatment on the chart. The next time the dose is increased, usually by extending the duration of the stimulus, in the hope of entraining a longer afterdischarge. We increase pulse width or voltage if a major or generalized seizure was not produced by the initial stimulus.

Although some ECT facilities report a significant incidence of posttreatment headache, we do not, and we believe this is a consequence of scrupulous attention to oxygenation of the patient. However, such complaints are common with multiple electrical stimuli in a single session. Patients should breathe 100 percent oxygen through a mask for at least sixty seconds as soon as the intravenous (IV) channel has been established. At the end of at least one minute, glycopyrrolate, methohexital, and succinylcholine are injected, each flushed with normal saline. In elderly patients we require three to five minutes of oxygenation. With 100 percent oxygen flowing, the mask is held on the patient's face throughout the induction, stimulus, and ictus until spontaneous respirations are established. We continue EEG/EKG recording throughout this time. The IV channel is maintained until patients are breathing well and are ready to be moved out to a recovery area where they are observed by nursing staff until fully responsive.

¶ Ethical Issues

Ethical issues involving ECT are not specific to that treatment but are identical to ethical issues in general medical practice. These include such matters as determination of the risks of the procedure, who should receive such treatment, the right to refuse treatment, procedures for obtaining informed consent, and the training and preparation of psychiatrists in general and those who administer ECT in particular. Fink[65] has emphasized the risk-benefit analysis with regard to ECT. Such an analysis involves consideration of efficacy, safety, and adverse effects as well as alternative treatments and their risk-benefit ratios and the consequences of not using ECT or any treatment. The latter is known to be associated with increased duration of illness and hospitalization, as well as suicide and death. That is, nontreatment of the psychiatric illnesses for which ECT is indicated carries a high price. Alternative therapies may be contraindicated in medically ill patients because of their physical condition or concomitant medications, while carefully prepared and performed ECT has essentially no contraindications (except perhaps in the presence of a space-occupying lesion with increased intracranial pressure). Thus ECT has been used successfully in patients with a variety of physical illnesses (see the section entitled "Special Indications").

Some have viewed the higher proportion of females to males receiving ECT as proof of a sexist application of an undesirable therapeutic intervention. These individuals, aside from objecting to ECT generally, overlook the fact that more females than males receive a diagnosis of depression—the major indication for ECT—and also occupy more beds in mental health facilities. On the other hand, the finding that the poor and blacks tend to be underrepresented among those receiving ECT[15,191] has resulted in the suggestion that this efficacious treatment is more likely to be applied to white, middle-class patients.[15,16] Whatever the accuracy of these assertions, ECT's clear record of efficacy, especially in the major affective disorders, requires that all patients be considered for and have such therapy available to them.

The issue of refusal of ECT should be considered as part of the larger question of the right of psychiatric patients to refuse treatment of any sort. Patients who are competent may decline ECT or indeed any other treatment regardless of the apparent need for therapy perceived by the patient's family and professionals. Patients who are legally determined to be incompetent to make medical decisions should have such decisions made for them on the basis of best medical judgment. In this instance there must be scrupulous attention to issues of informed consent. Both the risks and the benefits as well as the empirical basis of ECT must be carefully explained to the patient and the legally designated responsible individuals. This serves to protect the patient, the physician, and the interests of society generally.

ECT is a safe and useful treatment in psychiatry and should be part of the armamentarium of psychiatric facilities and treating psychiatrists. From this it follows that all psychiatrists should receive training in ECT. The degree of exposure and training should be sufficient to allow the psychiatrist to perform the treatment and, after more experience, to supervise others in training.

¶ Mechanisms of Action

Mechanisms whereby ECT exerts its therapeutic and other effects are still not fully understood, but important advances in knowledge have been made recently in parallel with studies of the modes of action of antidepressants and other medications. Neurophysiological, biochemical, and neuroendocrinological investigations have contributed to current knowledge on the subject.

Neurophysiological data indicate, but do not absolutely establish, that major, generalized seizures are essential for therapeutic efficacy. Studies have confirmed that tonic-clonic motor movements, specific electrical or chemical agents used for seizure induction, and the occurrence of memory loss and confusion are not essential for therapeutic action. Repeated, not single, seizures are necessary for therapeutic benefit. Serial seizures are associated with increasing interictal EEG slowing, which is more prominent hours after the seizure than immediately postictally, and varies with the number, frequency, and spacing of treatments. [172,175] Recordings of sensory-evoked potentials during and following the ictal phases have shown that not all of the brain is engaged during the generalized seizure. Bilateral ECT is associated with transient suppression of somatosensory and visual evoked responses. [114,115] Similar somatosensory findings occur with unilateral ECT, but ipsilateral visual evoked responses are suppressed for up to thirty minutes postictally with corresponding sensory inattention to the side of stimulation. However, ipsilateral pupillary dilation may contribute to these observations. Recent studies with positron emission tomography (PET) in epilepsy have shown that blood flow is increased during seizures and decreased interictally in patients with focal epileptogenic lesions. Similar PET findings were described in a patient during and following ECT. [161] Visual and automatic EEG analysis of seizures recorded at the scalp during ECT have revealed progressive stages of electrical activity. [29,186] Phase I, at the beginning of the seizure, is characterized by 14 to 22 Hz rhythmic activity. Phase II consists of arrhythmic polyspikes that are of higher amplitude on the stimulated side with unilateral ECT. Phase III appears next with rhythmic 2½ to 3½ Hz spike-polyspike and wave activity, which is occasionally more prominent on the stimulated side. Others have found both ipsilateral and contralateral voltage asymmetries with unilateral ECT in the later part of the seizure. [175] These findings suggest that seizures do not necessarily start with diencephalic activation, as was previously proposed. [3] Diencephalic participation may even be delayed until the transition from Phase II to Phase III. Spectral density analysis confirmed predominance of electrical energy over the stimulated hemisphere early in ECT with differences in energy and seizure duration corresponding to the convulsant and anticonvulsant properties of different anesthetics. [83]

Other interesting investigations have been accomplished with studies of all-night sleep, particularly in patients with primary depressive disorder before, during, and following antidepressant drug treatment. [34,117] Similar studies with ECT have thus far been limited. However, in both humans and animals, ECT or electroconvulsive shock (ECS) reduces time in REM sleep, exerts variable effects on REM latency, increases slow-wave sleep and total sleep time, and abolishes REM rebound. All of these changes can be related to certain biochemical alterations associated with antidepressant drug treatment and ECT.

It has been hypothesized that the mechanisms of therapeutic action and adverse effects of ECT can be understood within the framework of the animal theory of kindling. Kindling is not an analogous situation since it involves repeated stimulation of the brain with stimuli that initially do not produce ictal or behavioral effects. However, when stimuli of fixed intensity are applied to focal brain areas in a spaced sequence, they can eventually lower the seizure threshold and produce behavioral alterations and spontaneous afterdischarges. These mechanisms may apply in the development of complex partial epilepsy and other states of neuronal hyperexcitability in man. ECT, which involves suprathreshold stimulation from the onset, seems to exert opposite effects with increasing seizure thresholds and progressively shorter afterdischarges. ECT is not likely to be associated with an increased incidence of spontaneous seizures, and EEG changes following ECT are not sustained. [26,180]

Some studies have shown that deviant photic excitability is more common in patients who have had ECT. [175] This is likely explained by greater psychopathology and other deviant CNS characteristics in patients referred for such treatment rather than by exposure to convulsive therapy itself. Likewise, neuropsychological tests do not demonstrate persisting impairments after ECT. However, these kinds of evidence are admittedly indirect, and there have been no crucial experiments accomplished to determine if kindling may occur as a consequence of ECT in relation to either its therapeutic or its adverse effects. Studies limited to scalp EEG recordings cannot eliminate the possibility that some of these kinds of changes may occur in strategic cortical or subcortical areas. Adamec and Stark-Adamec[6] suggest that convulsive therapy and kindling may share some common mechanisms wherein both involve an "overwhelming of inhibitory networks," and both may produce long-lasting postsynaptic potentiation that may underlie interictal behavioral changes. They suggest that inhibitory systems may be hypoactive in depressed patients and excitation might be associated with improvement, whereas pathological changes could develop in the biochemically normal brain. It has been demonstrated in animals that ECS can inhibit the kindling sequence. In humans positive results with ECT in the treatment of uncontrolled epileptic seizures were reported in the older literature, as was the effectiveness of ECT in states of toxic delirium and drug withdrawal accompanied by low seizure thresholds.[63]

Numerous and complex neurochemical changes accompany single and repeated seizures, some of which are likely to be essential to the therapeutic effects of ECT. Many of the changes that occur acutely are probably nonspecific and are related more to the stress of the seizure itself. ECS increases brain energy metabolism, oxygen consumption, and protein turnover in animals. Changes in capillary permeability and vascular resistance occur, and the blood-brain barrier becomes more penetrable.[58] Seizures are also accompanied by shifts in electrolyte distribution and alterations in protein synthesis. Hypoxia may develop as a consequence of the muscular convulsion and apnea, but not due to the electrical seizure. Slowly occurring adaptive changes in catecholamine and other neurotransmitter

receptor systems that develop over time and parallel the course of antidepressant response are more likely to be relevant to the therapeutic process of ECT.

Animal studies have shown that repeated daily ECS induces sustained increases in activity of norepinephrine (NE) neurons in various brain areas, but not of dopamine (DA) or serotonin (5-hydroxytryptamine, 5HT) neurons.[139] Repeated ECS in animals also results in increased behavioral sensitivity to chemical agents mimicking the actions of brain monoamines, suggesting increased receptor response.[88] These effects were not particularly long-lasting in the animals studied, which may indicate a difference between disturbing the functions of a normal brain versus restoring an abnormal system to normal equilibrium. Time-dependent, delayed effects of either single or repeated ECS in rats have been observed in which subsensitivity of the DA autoreceptors develops in the substantia nigra.[36] Similar time-dependent effects have been observed with TCAs. These observations with single ECS do not parallel the human experience in which a series of seizures must be induced for therapeutic effects. Chronic ECS produces a reduction in the sensitivity of beta-adrenergic receptors in rat brain as do TCAs.[144] ECS causes increased release and turnover of NE and possibly DA as well, whereas TCAs inhibit the reuptake of biogenic amines. Although antidepressant medications have different actions, all effective therapeutic interventions increase postsynaptic biogenic amine concentrations and reduce the sensitivity of beta-adrenergic receptors.[33] Reduced receptor binding may make more released transmitter available for reuptake, thereby reducing synthesis and demand on the synapse for transmitter. This effect may be biphasic with opposite effects if the system is highly active,[122] which could account for the positive effects of ECT in both depression and mania.

In humans pretreatment 3-methoxy-4-hydroxy-phenylglycol (MHPG) concentrations in urine may predict response to certain TCAs. There have been too few studies conducted with ECT or other drugs to draw conclusions about relationships between pretreatment MHPG concentrations and treatment outcome. McDougle and Milstein[128] did not find significant associations between baseline MHPG level, and ECT response, but they did observe a significant increase in urinary MHPG levels with successive ECTs, with a correspondingly significant decrease in ratings of depressive symptomatology. Considerable evidence has shown that a variety of long-term antidepressant treatments reduce NE and isoproterenol-stimulated cyclic 3',5'-adenosine monophosphate (cAMP) accumulation in the brain.[33] This effect, which has been proposed as a model of antidepressant action, is shared by all major classes of clinically effective antidepressant treatments, including ECT. Repeated ECT enhances adrenergic stimulation of brain cAMP levels, thus causing desensitization of the cyclic response to NE. This observation provides a key model system for studying the molecular basis of antidepressant action and has stimulated studies of antidepressant-induced changes in neurotransmitter receptor binding. Studies of the latter have shown that TCAs reduce the density of beta-adrenergic receptors in brain homogenates as do other antidepressant treatments including MAOIs, ECT, and REM-sleep deprivation. Beta-receptor binding decrements occur with long-term treatment, but not with acute dosing or single seizures.

It has been shown that a variety of antidepressant treatments in humans—including lithium, TCAs, MAOIs, and ECT—yield a reduction in total production and turnover of NE and its metabolites found in peripheral blood.[123,124] This can be attributed to reduced spillover from the synapses and increased presynaptic reuptake. These observations are compatible with animal findings that ECS increases CNS NE turnover, decreases nonadrenergic beta-receptor sensitivity, and produces DA autoreceptor subsensitivity. Antidepressant treatment causes subsensitivity of NE-sensitive adenylate cyclase and/or down-regulation of beta-adrenergic receptors.[189] This may be a compensatory mechanism to offset the increased availability of synaptic NE.

In animal experiments destruction of nonadrenergic pathways in the locus coeruleus abolishes ECS effects.[90] This implies that concurrent treatment with beta-receptor blocking agents such as propranolol hydrochloride might interfere with the therapeutic effects of ECT in humans. We have some retrospective data relating to this issue. Twelve patients who were receiving beta-blocking agents primarily for the treatment of hypertension were treated with ECT. They were compared with controls matched for age, sex, diagnosis, and pre-ECT clinical status. Quantitative ratings of depressive symptomatology before, during, and after ECT showed no significant differences between the groups. However, there was a positive correlation between dosage of beta-blocking drugs and level of psychopathology after ECT. Whether this was a reflection of greater interference of the higher doses on the therapeutic actions of ECT or whether higher doses of drugs were associated with treatment resistance on some other basis is unknown, and worthy of further investigation.

DA turnover is reduced with both lithium and MAOIs but not with TCAs or ECT.[122] Unlike a single ECS, a series of ECT has no effects on central DA synthesis or turnover. However, there are major discrepancies between behavioral and biochemical methods of assessing receptor sensitivity. If ECT did enhance DA-receptor sensitivity, it would likely worsen symptoms of schizophrenia and mania, which is not observed clinically. Nevertheless, there have been suggestions that ECT may aggravate rapid cycling in bipolar disorder.[116,152] Reports of ECT effects on tardive dyskinesia, in which there may be hypersensitive DA receptors, have been inconsistent.[32,174,210] However, ECT has been shown to benefit parkinsonism, a state of DA insufficiency.[95,121] It is possible that pre- and postsynaptic receptor effects may be different with presynaptic subsensitivity and postsynaptic supersensitivity.

Series of seizures do not induce changes in

the content or rate of synthesis of 5HT, although increased behavioral sensitivity to drugs that stimulate central serotonergic receptors has been observed.[88] A newly recognized class of receptors, the $5HT_2$ receptors, are reduced by TCAs.[33] ECT may have opposite effects causing increased ^{3}H-spiperone binding, which suggests increased $5HT_2$ receptors. ECT may increase central 5HT sensitivity, and there are clinical suggestions of 5HT deficiencies in some depressions based on reduced 5-hydroxyindoleacetic acid (5-HIAA) levels in cerebrospinal fluid (CSF) and the possible therapeutic applications of 5HT precursors.[122] However, studies with ECT have not shown consistent correlations between CSF–5-HIAA levels and treatment outcome.[4]

Less attention has been given to effects of repeated ECS on other neurotransmitter systems. Gamma-aminobutyric acid (GABA) concentrations in the caudate nucleus and nucleus accumbens increase with daily ECS, and the synthesis rate of GABA decreases.[122] Also, consistent with diminished inhibitor GABA tone and increased DA sensitivity, chronic ECS attenuates haloperidol-induced cataplexy. Malitz, Sackeim, and Decina[131] and Sackeim and associates[165] hypothesized that the major therapeutic effect of ECT is related to its anticonvulsant effects, which are mediated by increased GABA transmission. Repeated ECS or kindled seizures in animals results in increased numbers of hippocampal benzodiazepine receptors.[129]

It is now well established that many depressed patients have measurable neuroendocrine abnormalities of the hypothalamic-pituitary-adrenal axis, with most data suggesting hypofunction of these systems. Fink,[64] Fink and Ottosson,[67] and others have proposed that the essential action of ECT is to normalize these dysfunctions by increasing the release and diffusion of hypothalamic peptides with behavioral effects. Although this hypothesis is tenable, it is difficult to test, in part because the seizures themselves contribute to nonspecific stress effects that may overwhelm or obscure the essential therapeutic ingredients. In this regard, clinical and animal studies that use "sham ECT" are not adequate, since the stress of the seizure itself is not controlled.

However, some hormonal changes with ECT may be selective, that is, not explained by generalized pituitary or hypothalamic responses to stimulation or stress. Arató and Bagdy[14] concluded that elevation in prolactin with ECT in humans was not a stress reaction because it was not inhibited by pretreatment with diazepam. However, the occurrence of generalized seizures was not validated. Whalley and others[209] concluded that ECT effects on hormone release are selective because there are differential effects upon the so-called stress hormones: prolactin, growth hormone (GH), and cortisol. During ECT they observed prominent elevations of prolactin, no changes in GH, and decreases in the basal output of cortisol. There were also elevations in nicotine and estrogen-stimulated neurophysins, associated with vasopressin and oxytocin respectively. Minimal changes were observed in luteinizing hormone-releasing hormone and thyrotropin-releasing hormone. These data suggest that the therapeutic actions of ECT may be ascribed to release of specific neural hypophyseal hormones into the central circulation.

There is some evidence that neuroendocrine test abnormalities in depressed patients normalize with successful treatment and are predictive of sustained remission.[89,145] However, negative and opposite results have also been reported.[42] The specific neurotransmitter abnormality responsible for the positive dexamethasone suppression test in some depressed patients has not been definitely identified. One possibility is that decreased noradrenergic postsynaptic activity results in diminished tonic inhibitory influence on the neurons of the medial eminence of the hypothalamus.[33] Normalization following recovery may be due to increased sensitivity of NE-hypothalamic postsynaptic receptors. Such normalization could occur secondary to effects on other neurotransmitter systems. It is also possible that increased permeability of the blood-brain barrier and increased cerebral blood flow may increase the availability of peptides for release from the hypothalamus into brain tissue. The intracellular movement of calcium that occurs with ECT is also necessary for hormonal discharge.[63]

The GH response to amphetamine or clonidine hydrochloride is a more specific test of adrenergic receptor function. It has been shown to be reduced in depressed patients and to normalize in patients who respond to antidepressant treatment, but not all studies are congruent. GH response to apomorphine, a DA agonist, was shown to increase following a course of ECT in depressed patients, suggesting that ECT produces an enhancement of DA-mediated responses in the brain.[43] However, Glass and associates[84] observed that GH responses to clonidine in depressed patients who responded to treatment were inhibited by TCAs but not with ECT. Others found no significant changes in responses of GH, prolactin, and cortisol to apomorphine before and after a successful course of ECT.[39]

The hypothalamic-pituitary-thyroid axis is also involved in depression and may normalize with recovery. However, the neurotransmitter regulation of this hormonal system is extremely complex. The prolactin response to thyroid-releasing hormone, which is mediated by a central 5HT mechanism, is potentiated by ECT.[33] This is consistent with results of behavioral and electrophysiological studies showing that long-term antidepressant treatment produces supersensitivity of postsynaptic 5HT receptors. These effects on NE and 5HT postsynaptic receptors may be viewed as a "final common pathway" for antidepressant activity.

There is recent growing awareness of the existence of peptides in the brain, some of which may act as both neurotransmitters and hormones. Studies in rats show that repeated ECS causes a persistent increase of met-enkephalin (met-ENK) content in the hypothalamus and limbic areas such as the nucleus accumbens, septum, and amygdala.[96] The temporal characteristics of this increase resembled the time course of the clinical effects of ECT. Additional controls revealed that subconvulsive shocks and seizures blocked by anesthetic doses of phenobarbital did not affect hypothalamic or septal met-ENK content. Repeated ECS did not change the beta-endorphin content of the hypothalamus. Thus met-ENK changes might participate in the antidepressant action of ECS. Other studies showed that there are transient elevations of immunoreactive plasma beta-endorphin levels after ECT that probably reflect a hypothalamic response to ECT.[8]

It is now known that numerous peptides exist in the central nervous system.[109,110] The hypothalamic-releasing and -inhibitory hormones that regulate anterior pituitary hormone secretion have a wide distribution throughout the CNS. The same is true for the posterior pituitary peptides and a number of other substances originally discovered in the gastrointestinal tract. Although these substances are in much lower concentrations than the classical biogenic amine neurotransmitters, this is not indicative of their likely functional importance. Methods of studying these substances depend on highly complex technological advances involving immunoassay, immunocytochemistry, and single-unit recordings. These methods hold great potential for further elucidation of the effects of ECT in animals and man, which may define the biochemical and electrical alterations necessary for the therapeutic process and the site or sites of such changes in the brain.

In summary, this section has described many changes that occur in different areas of the brain with ECT as reflected by observations of its electrical activity, neurochemistry, and neuroendocrinological, physical, vascular, and membrane characteristics. The therapeutic process of ECT is likely to be related to slowly evolving changes in these systems within the nervous system, many of which also occur with other kinds of antidepressant treatment. Readjustment in the sensitivity of pre- and postsynaptic receptors and a resetting of the dynamic equilibrium between multiple transmitter systems appears to occur, dictated in large part by the preexisting state of the organism. ECT appears to have the facility to up- or down-regulate systems within the brain and to normalize relationships between various neurophysiological, chemical, and endocrinological axes. Various systems that may be implicated are touched upon in this chapter, but knowledge is still fragmentary. Ongoing investigations in this area are on the "cutting edge" of knowledge about functioning of the brain in health and disease states.

¶ Bibliography

1. ABIUSO, P., DUNKELMAN, R., and PROPER, M. "Electroconvulsive Therapy in Patients with Pacemakers," *Journal of the American Medical Association*, 240 (1978):2459–2460.
2. ABRAMS, R., and ESSMAN, W. B., eds. *Electroconvulsive Therapy*. Jamaica, N.Y.: Spectrum, 1982.
3. ABRAMS, R., and TAYLOR, M. A. "Diencephalic Stimulation and the Effects of ECT in Endogenous Depression," *British Journal of Psychiatry*, 129 (1976): 482–485.
4. ABRAMS, R., et al. "Concentration of 5-Hydroxyindoleacetic Acid, Homovanillic Acid, and Tryptophan in the Cerebrospinal Fluid of Depressed Patients Before and After ECT," *Biological Psychiatry*, 11 (1976):85–90.
5. ABRAMS, R., et al. "Bilateral Versus Unilateral Electroconvulsive Therapy; Efficacy in Melancholia," *American Journal of Psychiatry*, 140 (1983): 463–465.
6. ADAMEC, R. E., and STARK-ADAMEC, C. "Limbic Kindling and Animal Behavior —Implications for Human Psychopathology Associated with Complex Partial Seizures," *Biological Psychiatry*, 18 (1983):269–293.
7. ALEXOPOULOS, G. S., et al. "Electroconvulsive Therapy in Patients on Anticoagulants," *Canadian Journal of Psychiatry*, 27 (1982):46–47.
8. ALEXOPOULOS, G. S., et al. "Plasma Immunoreactive β-Endorphin Levels in Depression," *Archives of General Psychiatry*, 40 (1983):181–183.
9. ALLEN, R. M. "Pseudodementia and ECT," *Biological Psychiatry*, 17 (1982): 1435–1443.
10. ALLEN, R. E., and PITTS, F. N. "ECT for Depressed Patients with Lupus Erythematosus," *American Journal of Psychiatry*, 135 (1978):367–368.
11. ———, and SUMMERS, W. K. "Drug Modification of ECT: Methohexital and Diazepam. II," *Biological Psychiatry*, 15 (1980):257–264.
12. AMERICAN PSYCHIATRIC ASSOCIATION. *Electroconvulsive Therapy, Task Force Report 14*. Washington, D.C.: American Psychiatric Association, 1978.
13. ANANTH, J., SAMRA, D., and KOLIVAKIS, T. "Amelioration of Drug-induced Parkinsonism by ECT," *American Journal of Psychiatry*, 136 (1979):1094.
14. ARATO, M., and BAGDY, G. "Neuroendocrine Study of the Mechanism of Action of Electroconvulsive Therapy," *Neuropsychobiology*, 8 (1982):162–168.
15. ASNIS, G. M., FINK, M., and SAFERSTEIN, S. "ECT in Metropolitan New York Hospitals: A Survey of Practice, 1975–1976," *American Journal of Psychiatry*, 135 (1978):479–482.
16. BABIGIAN, H. "Patient Selection for Electroconvulsive Therapy in Monroe County, New York," Conference entitled *ECT: Efficacy and Impact*, New Orleans, February 1978.
17. BAILINE, S. H., and RAU, J. H. "The Decision to Use ECT: A Retrospective Study," *Comprehensive Psychiatry*, 22 (1981):274–281.
18. BARCIA, D., and PARDO, F. M. "Encuesta Acera de las Actitudes de los Psiquiatras Españoles Ante la T.E.C.," *Actas Luso-Españolas de Neurlogia, Psiquiatria y Ciencias Afines*, 6 (1976):117–156.
19. BARTON, J. L. "ECT in Depression; The Evidence of Controlled Studies," *Biological Psychiatry*, 12 (1977):687–695.
20. BATES, W. J., and SMELTZER, D. J. "Electroconvulsive Treatment of Psychotic Self-Injurious Behavior in a Patient with Severe Mental Retardation," *American Journal of Psychiatry*, 139 (1982):1355–1356.
21. BEN-TOVIM, J. M., and BEN-TOVIM, D. I. "ECT in Developing Countries," *British Journal of Psychiatry*, 141 (1982):102.
22. BERENBAUM, S. A., and TAYLOR, M. A.

"Nonmemory Higher Cognitive Function and Electroconvulsive Treatment," *Psychopharmacology Bulletin*, 18 (1982):101–109.

23. BERENS, E. S., YESAVAGE, J. F., and LEIRER, V. O. "A Comparison of Multiple and Single Electroconvulsive Therapy," *Journal of Clinical Psychiatry*, 43 (1982):126–128.

24. BERESFORD, H. R. "Electroconvulsive Therapy: Neurological Side Effects." Conference entitled *ECT: Efficacy and Impact*. New Orleans, February 1978.

25. BLACHLEY, P. H., and GOWING, D. "Multiple Monitored Electroconvulsive Treatment," *Comprehensive Psychiatry*, 7 (1966):100–109.

26. BLACKWOOD, D.H.R., et al. "A Study of the Incidence of Epilepsy Following ECT," *Journal of Neurology, Neurosurgery and Psychiatry*, 43 (1980):1098–1102.

27. BOURGEOIS, M., et al. "Situation Actuelle de L'électroconvulsivethérapie (E.C.T.) I. Aspects Numérigues, Indications, Efficacité, Media, Préjuges et Idéologies," *Annales Medico-Psychologiques*, 139 (1982):1122–1135.

28. BRUMBACK, R. A., "EEG Monitoring of ECT," *British Journal of Psychiatry*, 142 (1983):104–105.

29. BRUMBACK, R. A., and STATON, R. D. "The Electroencephalographic Pattern During Electroconvulsive Therapy," *Clinical Electroencephalography*, 13 (1982):148–153.

30. CALLOWAY, S. P., et al. "ECT and Cerebral Atrophy. A Computed Tomographic Study," *Acta Psychiatrica Scandinavica*, 64 (1981):442–445.

31. CARR, V., et al. "The Use of ECT for Mania in Childhood Bipolar Disorder," *British Journal of Psychiatry*, 143 (1983):411–415.

32. CHACKO, R. C., and ROOT, L. "ECT and Tardive Dyskinesia: Two Cases and a Review," *Journal of Clinical Psychiatry*, 44 (1983):265–266.

33. CHARNEY, D. S., MENKES, D. B., and HENINGER, G. R. "Receptor Sensitivity and the Mechanism of Action of Antidepressant Treatment," *Archives of General Psychiatry*, 38 (1981):1160–1180.

34. CHEN, C. "Sleep Depression and Antidepressants," *British Journal of Psychiatry*, 135 (1979):385–402.

35. CHILDERS, R. T., JR. "Comparison of Four Regimens in Newly Admitted Female Schizophrenics," *Clinical Notes*, (April) (1964):1010–1011.

36. CHIODO, L. A., and ANTELMAN, S. M. "Electroconvulsive Shock: Progressive Dopamine Autoreceptor Subsensitivity Independent of Repeated Treatment," *Science*, 210 (1980):799–801.

37. CHRISTENSEN, P., and HEDEMAND, E. "EEG and EMG Monitored Electroconvulsive Therapy," *Psychopharmacology Bulletin*, 19 (1983):20–22.

38. CHRISTENSEN, P., and KOLDBAEK, I. "EEG Monitored ECT," *British Journal of Psychiatry*, 141 (1982):19–23.

39. CHRISTIE, J. E., et al. "Effect of ECT on the Neuroendocrine Response to Apomorphine in Severely Depressed Patients," *British Journal of Psychiatry*, 140 (1982):268–273.

40. CIRAULO, D., et al. "Sodium Nitroprusside Treatment of ECT-Induced Blood Pressure Elevations," *American Journal of Psychiatry*, 135 (1978):1105–1106.

41. COPPEN, A., et al. "Lithium Continuation Therapy Following Electroconvulsive Therapy," *British Journal of Psychiatry*, 139 (1981):284–287.

42. CORYELL, W., and ZIMMERMAN, M. "The Dexamethasone Suppression Test and ECT Outcome: A Six Month Followup," *Biological Psychiatry*, 18 (1983): 21–27.

43. COSTAIN, D. W., et al. "Electroconvulsive Therapy and the Brain: Evidence for Increased Dopamine-Mediated Responses," *Lancet*, 2 (1982):400–404.

44. DANIEL, W. F., and CROVITZ, H. F. "Recovery of Orientation After Electroconvulsive Therapy," *Acta Psychiatrica Scandinavica*, 66 (1982):421–428.

45. ———. "Acute Memory Impairment Following Electroconvulsive Therapy. I. Effects of Electrical Stimulus Waveforms and Number of Treatments," *Acta Psychiatrica Scandinavica*, 67 (1983):1–7.

46. ———. "Acute Memory Impairment Following Electroconvulsive Therapy. II. Effects of Electrode Placement," *Acta Psychiatrica Scandinavica*, 67 (1983): 57–68.

47. DANIEL, W. F., et al. "The Effects of ECT Modifications on Autobiographical and Verbal Memory," *Biological Psychiatry,* 17 (1982):919–924.

48. DANIEL, W. F., et al. "ECT Induced Delirium and Further ECT: A Case Report," *American Journal of Psychiatry,* 140 (1983):922–924.

49. D'ELIA, G., and FREDERIKSEN, S.O. "ACTH (4-10) and Memory in ECT-Treated and Untreated Patients. I. Effect on Consolidation," *Acta Psychiatrica Scandinavica,* 62 (1980):418–428.

50. ———. "ACTH (4-10) and Memory in ECT-Treated Patients and Untreated Controls. II. Effect on Retrieval," *Acta Psychiatrica Scandinavica,* 62 (1980): 429–435.

51. D'ELIA, G., LEHMANN, J., and RAOTMA, H. "Evaluation of the Combination of Tryptophan and ECT in the Treatment of Depression: I. Clinical Analysis," *Acta Psychiatrica Scandinavica,* 56 (1977): 303–318.

52. ———. "Influence of Tryptophan on Memory Functions in Depressive Patients Treated with Unilateral ECT," *Acta Psychiatrica Scandinavica,* 57 (1978):259–268.

53. D'ELIA, G., OTTOSSON, J. O., and STROMGREN, L. S., "Present Practice of Electroconvulsive Therapy in Scandinavia," *Archives of General Psychiatry,* 40 (1983):577–581.

54. DEMYER, M. K., et al. "Third Ventricle Size and Ventricular/Brain Ratio in Treatment-Resistant Psychiatric Patients," *Journal of Operational Psychiatry,* 15 (1984):2–8.

55. DOUGLAS, C. J., and SCHWARTZ, H. I. "ECT for Depression Caused by Lupus Cerebritis: A Case Report," *American Journal of Psychiatry,* 139 (1982):1631–1632.

56. EASTWOOD, M. R., and STIASNY, S. "The Use of Electroconvulsive Therapy," *Canadian Psychiatric Association Journal,* 23 (1978):29–34.

57. EDITORIAL. "The Present Status of Electroconvulsive Therapy," *New Zealand Medical Journal,* 91 (1980):215–216.

58. ESSMAN, W. B. "Electroconvulsive Shock and Cerebral Chemistry: Changes and Sequelae," in R. Abrams and W. B. Essman, eds., *Electroconvulsive Therapy.* Jamaica, N.Y.: Spectrum, 1982, pp. 199–244.

59. EXNER, J. E., JR., and MURILLO, L. G. "A Long-Term Follow-up of Schizophrenics Treated with Regressive ECT," *Diseases of the Nervous System,* 38 (1977):162–168.

60. FAKHRI, O., FADHLI, A. A., and EIRAWI, R. M. "Effect of Electroconvulsive Therapy on Diabetes Mellitus," *Lancet,* 2 (1980):775–777.

61. FINK, M. "Myths of 'Shock Therapy,'" *American Journal of Psychiatry,* 134 (1977):991–996.

62. ———. "Efficacy and Safety of Induced Seizures (EST) in Man," *Comprehensive Psychiatry,* 19 (1978):1–18.

63. ———. *Convulsive Therapy, Theory and Practice.* New York: Raven Press, 1979.

64. ———. "Neuroendocrinology and ECT: A Review of Recent Developments," *Comprehensive Psychiatry,* 21 (1980): 450–459.

65. ———. "Convulsive Therapy: A Risk-Benefit Analysis," *Psychopharmacology Bulletin,* 18 (1982):110–116.

66. FINK, M., and JOHNSON, L. "Monitoring the Duration of Electroconvulsive Therapy Seizures. Cuff and EEG Methods Compared," *Archives of General Psychiatry,* 39 (1982):1189–1191.

67. FINK, M., and OTTOSSON, J. "A Theory of Convulsive Therapy in Endogenous Depression: Significance of Hypothalamic Functions," *Psychiatry Research,* 2 (1980):49–61.

68. FOWLER, D. R., and MAYFIELD, D. G. "Psychiatric Hospitalization I. Comparison of Public and Private Delivery Systems," *Diseases of the Nervous System,* 38 (1977):314–317.

69. FRANGOS, E., and ATHANASSENAS, G. "Differences in Lateral Brain Ventricular Size Among Various Types of Chronic Schizophrenics," *Acta Psychiatrica Scandinavica,* 66 (1982):459–463.

70. FRANKS, R. D., et al. "ECT Use for a Patient with Malignant Hyperthermia," *American Journal of Psychiatry,* 139 (1982):1065–1066.

71. FRASER, M. *ECT: A Clinical Guide.* New York: John Wiley & Sons, 1982.

72. FRASER, R. M., and GLASS, I. B. "Recovery from ECT in Elderly Patients," *British Journal of Psychiatry,* 133 (1978):524–528.

73. FREDERIKSEN, S.O., and D'ELIA, G. "Electroconvulsive Therapy in Sweden," *British Journal of Psychiatry,* 134 (1979):283–287.

74. FREEMAN, C.P.L., and KENDELL, R. E. "ECT: I. Patient's Experiences and Attitudes," *British Journal of Psychiatry,* 137 (1980):8–16.

75. FREEMAN, C.P.L., BASSON, J. V., and CRIGHTON, A. "Double-Blind Controlled Trial of Electroconvulsive Therapy (ECT) and Simulated ECT in Depressive Illness, *Lancet,* 1 (1978): 738–740.

76. FREEMAN, C.P.L., WEEKS, D., and KENDELL, R. E. "ECT: II: Patients Who Complain," *British Journal of Psychiatry,* 137 (1980):17–25.

77. FROMM-AUCH, D. "Comparison of Unilateral and Bilateral ECT: Evidence for Selective Memory Impairment," *British Journal of Psychiatry,* 141 (1982):608–613.

78. GANGADHAR, B. N., KAPUR, R. L., and KALYANASUNDARAM, S. "Comparison of Electroconvulsive Therapy with Imipramine in Endogenous Depression; a Double-Blind Study," *British Journal of Psychiatry,* 141 (1982):367–371.

79. GARCIA, J. H. "Electroconvulsive Therapy (ECT): Its Effect on the Brain and Other Tissues (A Review)," Conference entitled *ECT: Efficacy and Impact,* New Orleans, February 1978.

80. GARCIA-ESTRADA PEREZ, A. "Doing Without ECT," *British Journal of Psychiatry,* 142 (1983):314.

81. GASPAR, D., and SAMARASINGHE, L. A. "ECT in Psychogeriatric Practice—A Study of Risk Factors, Indications and Outcome," *Comprehensive Psychiatry,* 23 (1982):170–175.

82. GEOGHEGAN, J. J., and STEVENSON, G. H. "Prophylactic Electroshock," *American Journal of Psychiatry,* 105 (1949):494–496.

83. GERST, J. W., et al. "The Electroencephalographic Pattern During Electroconvulsive Therapy. II. Preliminary Analysis of Spectral Energy," *Clinical Electroencephalography,* 13 (1982):251–256.

84. GLASS, I. B., et al. "The Effect of Desipramine Upon Clinical Adrenergic Function in Depressed Patients," *British Journal of Psychiatry,* 141 (1982):372–376.

85. GLASSMAN, A. H., KANTOR, S. J., and SHOSTAK, M. "Depression, Delusions and Drug Response," *American Journal of Psychiatry,* 132 (1975):716–719.

86. GODDARD, G. V. "Development of Epileptic Seizures Through Brain Stimulation at Low Intensity," *Nature,* 214 (1967):1020–1021.

87. GOLLER, E. S. "A Controlled Trial of Reserpine in Chronic Schizophrenia," *Journal of Mental Science,* 106 (1960): 1408–1414.

88. GRAHAME-SMITH, D. G., GREEN, A. R., and COSTAIN, D. W. "Mechanism of the Antidepressant Action of Electroconvulsive Therapy," *Lancet,* 1 (1978):254–256.

89. GREDEN, J. F., et al. "Dexamethasone Suppression Tests in Antidepressant Treatment of Melancholia," *Archives of General Psychiatry,* 40 (1983):493–500.

90. GREEN, A. R., and DEAKIN, J.F.W. "Brain Noradrenaline Depletion Prevents ECS-Induced Enhancement of Serotonin- and Dopamine-Mediated Behavior," *Nature,* 285 (1980):232–233.

91. GROSSER, G. H., et al. "The Regulation of Electroconvulsive Treatment in Massachusetts: A Follow-up," *Massachusetts Mental Health Journal,* 5 (1975):12–25.

92. HARPER, R. G., and WIENS, A. N. "Electroconvulsive Therapy and Memory," *Journal of Nervous and Mental Disease,* 161 (1975):245–254.

93. HERRINGTON, R. N., et al. "Comparative Trial of L-Tryptophan and ECT in Severe Depressive Illness," *Lancet,* 2 (1974):731–734.

94. HESHE, J., and ROEDER, E. "Electroconvulsive Therapy in Denmark," *British Journal of Psychiatry,* 128 (1976):241–245.

95. HOLCOMB, H. H., STERNBER, D. E., and HENINGER, G. R. "Effects of Electroconvulsive Therapy on Mood, Parkinsonism and Tardive Dyskinesia in a Depressed Patient: ECT and Dopamine

Systems," *Biological Psychiatry,* 18 (1983):865–873.

96. HONG, J. S., et al. "Repeated Electroconvulsive Shocks and the Brain Content of Endorphins," *Brain Research,* 177 (1979):273.

97. IHEZUE, H. U., and EBIGBO, P. O. "Present Status and Practice of Electroconvulsive Therapy at the Psychiatric Hospital, Enugu, Nigeria," *Acta Psychiatrica Scandinavica,* 63 (1981):325–332.

98. JACOBY, R. J., et al. "Quantitative Computed Tomography in Elderly Depressed Patients," *British Journal of Psychiatry,* 143 (1983):124–127.

99. JANAKIRAMAIAH, N., CHANNABASAVANNA, S. M., and NARASIMHA MURTHY, N. S. "ECT/Chlorpromazine Combination Versus Chlorpromazine Alone in Acutely Schizophrenic Patients," *Acta Psychiatrica Scandinavica,* 66 (1982): 464–470.

100. JANICAK, P. G., et al. "Efficacy of Electroconvulsive Therapy (ECT): A Meta Analysis," *American Journal of Psychiatry,* in press.

101. JESSEE, S. S., and ANDERSON, G. F. "ECT in the Neuroleptic Malignant Syndrome: Case Report," *Journal of Clinical Psychiatry,* 44 (1983):186–188.

102. JOHNSTONE, E. C., et al. "The Northwick Park Electroconvulsive Therapy Trial," *Lancet,* 2 (1980):1317–1320.

103. KAHN, R. L., et al. "Memory Complaint and Impairment in the Aged," *American Journal of Psychiatry,* 32 (1975): 1569–1573.

104. KALAYAM, B., and STEINHART, M. J. "A Survey of Attitudes on the Use of Electroconvulsive Therapy," *Hospital and Community Psychiatry,* 32 (1981):185–188.

105. KENDELL, B., and PRATT, R.T.C. "Brain Damage and ECT," *British Journal of Psychiatry,* 143 (1983):99–100.

106. KENDELL, R. E. "The Present Status of Electroconvulsive Therapy," *British Journal of Psychiatry,* 139 (1981):265–283.

107. KING, P. D. "Chlorpromazine and Electroconvulsive Therapy in the Treatment of Newly Hospitalized Schizophrenics," *Journal of Clinical and Experimental Psychopathology,* 21 (1960):101–105.

108. KOEHLER, K., and SAUER, H. "First Rank Symptoms as Predictors of ECT Response in Schizophrenia," *British Journal of Psychiatry,* 142 (1983):280–283.

109. KRIEGER, D. T., and MARTIN, J. B. "Brain Peptides I," *New England Journal of Medicine,* 304 (1981):876–885.

110. ———. "Brain Peptides II," *New England Journal of Medicine,* 304 (1981):944–951.

111. KRISS, A., HALLIDAY, A. M., and PRATT, R.T.C. "Transitory Electrophysiological and Neurological Asymmetries Following Unilateral ECT," in R. L. Palmer, ed., *Electroconvulsive Therapy: An Appraisal.* New York: Oxford University Press, 1981, pp. 236–252.

112. KRISS, A., et al. "Neurological Asymmetries Immediately After Unilateral ECT," *Journal of Neurology, Neurosurgery and Psychiatry,* 41 (1978):1135–1144.

113. KRISS, A., et al. "EEG Immediately After Unilateral ECT," *Acta Psychiatrica Scandinavica,* 58 (1978):231–244.

114. KRISS, A., et al. "Evoked Potentials Following Unilateral ECT. I. The Somatosensory Evoked Potential," *Electroencephalography and Clinical Neurophysiology,* 48 (1980):481–489.

115. KRISS, A., et al. "Evoked Potentials Following Unilateral ECT. II. The Flash Evoked Potential," *Electroencephalography and Clinical Neurophysiology,* 48 (1980):490–501.

116. KUKOPULOS, A., et al. "Rapid Cyclers, Temperament and Antidepressants," *Comprehensive Psychiatry,* 24 (1983): 249–258.

117. KUPFER, D. J., and REYNOLDS, C. F. "Electroencephalographic Sleep Changes in Psychiatric Patients," in J. R. Hughes and W. P. Wilson, eds., *EEG and Evoked Potentials in Psychiatry and Behavioral Neurology.* Woburn, Mass. Butterworth Press, 1983, pp. 127–148.

118. LAMBOURN, J. "Is Cognitive Impairment One of the Therapeutic Ingredients of ECT? in R. L. Palmer, ed., *Electroconvulsive Therapy: An Appraisal.* New York: Oxford University Press, 1981, pp. 97–105.

119. LAMBOURN, J., and GILL, D. "A Con-

trolled Comparison of Simulated and Real ECT," *British Journal of Psychiatry*, 133 (1978):514–519.

120. LANGSLEY, D. G., ENTERLINE, J. D., and HICKERSON, G. X. "A Comparison of Chlorpromazine and EST in Treatment of Acute Schizophrenic and Manic Reactions," *Archives of Neurology and Psychiatry*, 81 (1959):384–391.

121. LEBENSOHN, Z. M., and JENKINS, R. B. "Improvement of Parkinsonism in Depressed Patients Treated with ECT," *American Journal of Psychiatry*, 132 (1975):283–285.

122. LERER, B., and BELMAKER, R. H. "Receptors and the Mechanism of Action of ECT," *Biological Psychiatry*, 17 (1982): 497–511.

123. LINNOILA, M., KAROUM, F., and POTTER, W. Z., "Effects of Antidepressant Treatments on Dopamine Turnover in Depressed Patients," *Archives of General Psychiatry*, 40 (1983):1015–1017.

124. LINNOILA, M., et al. "Electroconvulsive Treatment and Lithium Carbonate," *Archives of General Psychiatry*, 40 (1983):677–680.

125. LIPPMANN, S., et al. "Cerebellar Vermis Dimensions on Computerized Tomographic Scans of Schizophrenic and Bipolar Patients," *American Journal of Psychiatry*, 139 (1982):667–668.

126. MCCABE, M. S. "ECT in the Treatment of Mania: A Controlled Study," *American Journal of Psychiatry*, 133 (1976):688–691.

127. MCCABE, M. S., and NORRIS, B. "ECT Versus Chlorpromazine in Mania," *Biological Psychiatry*, 12 (1977):245–254.

128. MCDOUGLE, C. J., and MILSTEIN, V. "MHPG and Depression: A Naturalistic, Clinical Evaluation," submitted for publication.

129. MCNAMARA, J. O., PEPER, A. M., and PATRONE, V. "Kindled and Electroshock Seizures Cause Increased Numbers of Hippocampal Benzodiazepine Receptors," in J. A. Wada, ed., *Kindling 2*. New York: Raven Press, 1981, pp. 289–294.

130. MALETZKY, B. M. "Seizure Duration and Clinical Effect in Electroconvulsive Therapy," *Comprehensive Psychiatry*, 19 (1978):541–550.

131. MALITZ, S., SACKEIM, H. A., and DECINA, P. "ECT in the Treatment of Major Affective Disorders: Clinical and Basic Research Issues," *Psychiatric Journal of University of Ottawa*, 7 (1982):126–133.

132. MANSHEIM, P. "ECT in the Treatment of a Depressed Adolescent with Meningomyelocele, Hydrocephalus, and Seizures," *Journal of Clinical Psychiatry*, 44 (1983):385–386.

133. MAY, P.R.A. *Treatment of Schizophrenia: A Comparative Study of Five Treatment Methods*. New York: Science House, 1968.

134. MAY, P.R.A., et al. "Schizophrenia—A Follow-up Study of Results of Treatment," *Archives of General Psychiatry*, 33 (1976):481–486.

135. MENKEN, M., et al. "Multiple ECT: Morphologic Effects," *American Journal of Psychiatry*, 136 (1979):453.

136. MILSTEIN, V., and SMALL, I. F., "ECT Revisited: Indiana 1982–83," Submitted for publication.

137. MINDUS, P., CRONHOLM, B. and LEVANDER, S. E. "Does Piracetam Counteract the ECT-Induced Memory Dysfunction in Depressed Patients?" *Acta Psychiatrica Scandinavica*, 51 (1975): 319–326.

138. MINTER, R. E., and MANDEL, M. R. "The Treatment of Psychotic Major Depressive Disorder with Drugs and Electroconvulsive Therapy," *Journal of Nervous and Mental Disease*, 167 (1979):726–733.

139. MODIGH, K. "Long-Term Effects of Electroconvulsive Shock Therapy on Synthesis Turnover and Uptake of Brain Monoamines," *Psychopharmacology*, 49 (1976):179–185.

140. MONDIMORE, F. M., et al. "Post-ECT Confusional States Associated with Elevated Serum Anticholinergic Levels," *American Journal of Psychiatry*, 140 (1983): 930–931.

141. NAIDOO, D. "The Effects of Reserpine (Serpasil) on the Chronic Disturbed Schizophrenic: A Comparative Study of Rauwolfia Alkaloids and Electroconvulsive Therapy," *Journal of Nervous and Mental Disease*, 123 (1956):1–13.

142. ODEJIDE, A. O. "A Study of the Inpatient

Service of a Nigerian Psychiatric Hospital," *Comprehensive Psychiatry*, 21 (1980):302–307.

143. OPPENHEIM, G. "Drug-Induced Rapid Cycling: Possible Outcomes and Management," *American Journal of Psychiatry*, 139 (1982):939–941.

144. PANDEY, G. N., et al. "Electroconvulsive Shock Treatment Decreases β-Adrenergic Receptor Sensitivity in Rat Brain," *Nature*, 280 (1979):234–235.

145. PAPAKOSTAS, Y., et al. "Neuroendocrine Measures in Psychiatric Patients: Course and Outcome with ECT," *Psychiatry Research*, 4 (1981):55–64.

146. PAUL, S. M., et al. "Use of ECT with Treatment-Resistant Depressed Patients at the National Institute of Mental Health," *American Journal of Psychiatry*, 138 (1981):486–489.

147. PERRY, P. J., et al. "Treatment of Unipolar Depression Accompanied by Delusions," *Journal of Affective Disorders*, 4 (1982):195–200.

148. PIPPARD, J., and ELLAM, L. "Electroconvulsive Treatment in Great Britain," *British Journal of Psychiatry*, 139 (1981):563–568.

149. PITTS, F. N., JR., and PATTERSON, C. W. "Electroconvulsive Therapy for Iatrogenic Hypothalamic-Hypopituitarism (CRF-ACTH Type)," *American Journal of Psychiatry*, 136 (1979):1074–1076.

150. PITTS, F. N., JR., et al. "Induction of Anesthesia with Methohexital and Thiopental in Electroconvulsive Therapy," *New England Journal of Medicine*, 273 (1965):353–360.

151. POST, R. M., et al. "Kindling and Carbamazepine in Affective Illness," *Journal of Nervous and Mental Disease*, 170 (1982):717–731.

152. POTTER, W. Z., et al. "Clorgyline," *Archives of General Psychiatry*, 39 (1982): 505–510.

153. PRICE, T.R.P. "Unilateral Electroconvulsive Therapy for Depression," *New England Journal of Medicine*, 304 (1981): 53.

154. ———. "Short- and Long-term Cognitive Effects of ECT: Part I—Effects on Memory," *Psychopharmacology Bulletin*, 18 (1982):81–90.

155. ———. Short- and Long-term Cognitive Effects of ECT: Part II—Effects on Nonmemory Associated Cognitive Functions," *Psychopharmacology Bulletin*, 18 (1982):91–101.

156. REGESTEIN, Q. R., and LIND, L. J. "Management of Electroconvulsive Treatment in an Elderly Woman with Severe Hypertension and Cardiac Arrhythmias," *Comprehensive Psychiatry*, 21 (1980):288–290.

157. REIMER, F., and LORENZEN, D. "Die Elektrokonvulsions-Behandlung in Psychiatrischen Kliniken der Bundes-Republik Deutschland und West-Berlin," *Nervenarzt*, 52 (1981):554–556.

158. REMICK, R. A., and MAURICE, W. L. "ECT in Pregnancy," *American Journal of Psychiatry*, 135 (1978):761–762.

159. RIES, R., and BOKAN, J. "Single Case Study: Electroconvulsive Therapy Following Pituitary Surgery," *Journal of Nervous and Mental Disease*, 167 (1979):767–768.

160. RIES, R. K., et al. "ECT in Medication-Resistant Schizoaffective Disorder," *Comprehensive Psychiatry*, 22 (1981): 167–173.

161. RISBERG, J. "Regional Cerebral Blood Flow Measurements by Xe-Inhalation: Methodology and Applications in Neuropsychology and Psychiatry," *Brain and Language*, 9 (1980):9–34.

162. ROBIN, A., and DeTISSERA, S. "A Double-Blind Controlled Comparison of the Therapeutic Effects of Low and High Energy Electroconvulsive Therapies," *British Journal of Psychiatry*, 141 (1982):357–366.

163. ROYAL COLLEGE OF PSYCHIATRISTS. "Memorandum on the Use of Electroconvulsive Therapy," *British Journal of Psychiatry*, 131 (1977):261–272.

164. RUEDRICH, S. L., CHU, C., and MOORE, S. L. "ECT for Major Depression in a Patient with Acute Brain Trauma," *American Journal of Psychiatry*, 140 (1983): 928–929.

165. SACKEIM, H. A., et al. "Anticonvulsant and Antidepressant Properties of Electroconvulsive Therapy: A Proposed Mechanism of Action," *Biological Psychiatry*, 18 (1983):1301–1310.

166. SCHIELE, B. C., and SCHNEIDER, R. A. The Selective Use of Electroconvulsive

Therapy in Manic Patients," *Diseases of the Nervous System*, 10 (1949):291–297.

167. SHUKLA, G. D., "Electroconvulsive Therapy in a Rural Teaching General Hospital in India," *British Journal of Psychiatry*, 139 (1981):569–571.

168. SMALL, I. F. "Inhalant Convulsive Therapy," in M. Fink et al., eds., *Psychobiology of Convulsive Therapy*. Washington, D.C.: V.H. Winston & Sons, 1974, pp. 65–77.

169. SMALL, I. F., and SMALL, J. G. "Electroencephalographic (EEG), Evoked Potential, and Direct Current (DC) Responses with Unilateral Electroconvulsive Treatment (ECT)," *Journal of Nervous and Mental Disease*, 152 (1971):396–404.

170. SMALL, I. F., MILSTEIN, V., and SMALL, J. G. "Relationships Between Clinical and Cognitive Changes with Bilateral and Unilateral ECT," *Biological Psychiatry*, 16 (1981):793–794.

171. SMALL, I. F., et al. "Neuropsychological Observations with Psychosis and Somatic Treatment," *Journal of Nervous and Mental Disease*, 155 (1972):6–13.

172. SMALL, J. G. "EEG and Neurophysiological Studies of Convulsive Therapies," in M. Fink et al., eds., *Psychobiology of Convulsive Therapy*. Washington, D.C.: V.H. Winston & Sons, 1974, pp. 47–63.

173. SMALL, J. G., and SMALL, I. F. "Is EEG Screening Before EST Worthwhile?" *Journal of Nervous and Mental Disease*, 142 (1966):72–77.

174. ———. "Electroconvulsive Therapy Update," *Psychopharmacology Bulletin*, 17 (1981):29–41.

175. SMALL, J. G., SMALL, I. F., and MILSTEIN, V. "Electrophysiology of EST," in M. A. Lipton et al., eds., *Psychopharmacology: A Generation of Progress*. New York: Raven Press, 1978, pp. 759–769.

176. SMALL, J. G., et al. "Electroencephalographic and Neurophysiological Studies of Electrically Induced Seizures," *Journal of Nervous and Mental Disease*, 150 (1970):479–489.

177. SMALL, J. G., et al. "Effects of ACTH-4-10 on ECT-Induced Memory Dysfunctions," *Acta Psychiatrica Scandinavica*, 55 (1977):241–250.

178. SMALL, J. G., et al. "Complications with Electroconvulsive Treatment Combined with Lithium," *Biological Psychiatry*, 15 (1980):103–111.

179. SMALL, J. G., et al. "Auditory Brain Stem Evoked Responses in Hospitalized Patients Undergoing Drug Treatment or ECT," *Biological Psychiatry*, 16 (1981): 287–290.

180. SMALL, J. G., et al. "Does ECT Produce Kindling?" *Biological Psychiatry*, 16 (1981):773–778.

181. SMALL, J. G., et al. "ECT Combined with Neuroleptics in the Treatment of Schizophrenia," *Psychopharmacology Bulletin*, 18 (1982):34–35.

182. SMITH, K. W., et al. "ECT-Chlorpromazine and Chlorpromazine Compared in the Treatment of Schizophrenia," *Journal of Nervous and Mental Disease*, 144 (1967):284–290.

183. SORENSEN, P. S., et al. "Electroconvulsive Therapy: A Comparison of Seizure Duration as Monitored with Electroencephalograph and Electromyograph," *Acta Psychiatrica Scandinavica*, 64 (1981):193–198.

184. SQUIRE, L. R. "ECT and Memory Loss," *American Journal of Psychiatry*, 134 (1977):997–1001.

185. ———. "The Neuropsychology of Human Memory," *Annual Review of Neuroscience*, 5 (1982):241–273.

186. STATON, R. D., HASS, P. J., and BRUMBACK, R. A. "Electroencephalographic Recording During Bitemporal and Unilateral Non-Dominant Hemisphere (Lancaster Position) Electroconvulsive Therapy," *Journal of Clinical Psychiatry*, 42 (1981):264–269.

187. STILLINGS, D. "A Medical Electrical Cure by Benjamin Franklin," *Medical Instrumentation*, 10 (1976):27.

188. STROMGREN, L. S., and JUUL-JENSEN, P. "EEG in Unilateral and Bilateral Electroconvulsive Therapy," *Acta Psychiatrica Scandinavica*, 51 (1975):340–360.

189. SULSER, F. "Deamplification of Noradrenergic Signal Transfer by Antidepressant: A Unified Catecholamine-Serotonin Hypothesis of Affective Disorders," *Psychopharmacology Bulletin*, 19 (1983):300–307.

190. SUMMERS, W. K., ROBINS, E., and REICH, T. "The Natural History of Acute Organic Mental Syndrome Bilateral Elec-

troconvulsive Therapy," *Biological Psychiatry*, 14 (1979):905–912.

191. TAINTOR, Z. "Summary Report of Electroconvulsive Therapy in the Multi-Stable Information System," Conference entitled *ECT: Efficacy and Impact*. New Orleans, February 1978.

192. TAYLOR, J. R., et al. "Electroconvulsive Therapy and Memory Dysfunction: Is There Evidence for Prolonged Defects?" *Biological Psychiatry*, 17 (1982): 1169–1193.

193. TAYLOR, M. A. "Indications for ECT," in A. ABRAMS and W. B. ESSMAN, eds., *Electroconvulsive Therapy, Biological Foundations and Clinical Applications*. New York: SP Medical and Scientific Books, 1982, pp. 7–39.

194. TAYLOR, P., and FLEMINGER, J. J. "ECT for Schizophrenia," *Lancet*, 1 (1980): 1380–1382.

195. THOMAS, J., and REDDY, B. "The Treatment of Mania," *Journal of Affective Disorders*, 4 (1982):85–92.

196. TSUANG, M. T., TIDBALL, J. S., and GELLER, D. "ECT in a Depressed Patient with Shunt in Place for Normal Pressure Hydrocephalus," *American Journal of Psychiatry*, 136 (1979):1205–1206.

197. WEEKS, D., FREEMAN, C.P.L., and KENDELL, R. E. "ECT: III: Enduring Cognitive Deficits?" *British Journal of Psychiatry*, 137 (1980):26–37.

198. ———. "Does ECT Produce Enduring Cognitive Deficits? in R. L. Palmer, ed., *Electroconvulsive Therapy: An Appraisal*, New York: Oxford University Press, 1981, pp. 159–181.

199. WEINBERGER, D. R., et al. "Lateral Cerebral Ventricular Enlargement in Chronic Schizophrenia," *Archives of General Psychiatry*, 36 (1979):735–739.

200. WEINBERGER, D. R., et al. "Structural Abnormalities in the Cerebral Cortex of Chronic Schizophrenic Patients," *Archives of General Psychiatry*, 36 (1979): 935–939.

201. WEINER, R. D. "The Psychiatric Use of Electrically Induced Seizures," *American Journal of Psychiatry*, 136 (1979): 1507–1517.

202. ———. "The Persistence of Electroconvulsive Therapy–Induced Changes in the Electroencephalogram," *Journal of Nervous and Mental Disease*, 168 (1980):224–228.

203. ———. "ECT-Induced Status Epilepticus and Further ECT: A Case Report," *American Journal of Psychiatry*, 138 (1981):1237–1238.

204. ———. "Does Electroconvulsive Therapy Cause Brain Damage?" *Behavioral and Brain Sciences*, 7 (1984):1–54.

205. WEINER, R. D., ERWIN, C. W., and WEBER, B. A. "Acute Effects of Electroconvulsive Therapy on Brain Stem Auditory Evoked Potentials," *Electroencephalography and Clinical Neurophysiology*, 52 (1981):202–204.

206. WEINER, R. D., et al. "Propranolol Treatment of an ECT-Related Ventricular Arrhythmia," *American Journal of Psychiatry*, 136 (1979):1594–1595.

207. WEINER, R. D., et al. "Seizures Terminable and Interminable with ECT," *American Journal of Psychiatry*, 137 (1980):1416–1418.

208. WEST, E. D. "Randomized Double-Blind Controlled Trial of ECT," in R. L. Palmer, ed., *Electroconvulsive Therapy: An Appraisal*. New York: Oxford University Press, 1981, pp. 202–213.

209. WHALLEY, L. J., et al. "Immediate Increases in Plasma Prolactin and Neurophysin but Not Other Hormones After Electroconvulsive Therapy," *Lancet*, 7 (1982):1064–1068.

210. YUDOFSKY, S. C. "Parkinson's Disease, Depression, and Electroconvulsive Therapy: A Clinical and Neurobiologic Synthesis," *Comprehensive Psychiatry*, 20 (1979):579–581.

211. YUDOFSKY, S. C., and ROSENTHAL, N. E. "ECT in a Depressed Patient with Adult-Onset Diabetes Mellitus," *American Journal of Psychiatry*, 137 (1980): 100–101.

CHAPTER 34

A CRITICAL ASSESSMENT OF PSYCHIATRIC SURGERY: PAST, PRESENT, AND FUTURE

H. Thomas Ballantine, Jr.

¶ Introduction

In 1950, the Salmon Lectures were delivered by John Farquahr Fulton, M.D., Sterling Professor of Physiology at Yale University. They were published the following year under the title *Frontal Lobotomy and Affective Behavior.* [18] In the foreword to his monograph, Fulton wrote:

A conservative estimate suggests that in the interval since Egas Moniz first introduced his leucotomy procedure in 1935, at least 20,000 human beings have been subjected to this operation. Many phases of the problem are, however, still obscure both anatomically and physiologically (not to mention psychiatrically), and it has been our purpose in developing these studies, which have been generously supported by a grant from the United States Veteran's Administration, to secure basic information concerning the anatomy and the physiology of the frontal lobes in the belief that the therapeutic benefit which is sometimes seen following a radical lobotomy, can be more effectively secured, and with fewer undesirable side effects, with the use of a more restricted interruption of frontotemporal projections as well as those of the visceral brain—i.e., the cingulate and associated hippocampal structures. (Pp. 12–13) [18]

The final paragraph of the monograph stated:

In conclusion, I think that we can be assured that were Thomas Salmon alive today, he would view with satisfaction and eager interest the new approaches to the problems of mental disease and the possibility which they afford of relieving both mental and physical anguish in our fellow beings. The implications of lobotomy are vast, for the neurosurgeon is in fact dissecting the matrix of the mind with the end in view of correcting faulty structure and interrupting the vicious circles which form the basis of abnormal mental states. . . . Mental disease might, in fact, be looked upon as little more than faulty interpretations of sensory data, and if it is possible to help the mentally ill to interpret their sensations more correctly, it is our duty as physicians to continue to explore every means that might achieve this end. The possibilities inherent in lobotomy for returning the mentally ill to a happier and more useful existence provides one of the most challenging problems in medicine today. (Pp. 128–129)[18]

Thirty-five years have now passed since Fulton voiced these opinions. In this chapter I intend to explore the accomplishments, the difficulties, and the lessons of the past and to give an overview of the present state of psychiatric surgery, which may have been inappropriately called psychosurgery and now, I believe, might be more appropriately described as limbic system surgery. Finally, I shall attempt to look into the future and consider whether there will be a place for this type of neurosurgical intervention and, if so, whether while treating psychiatric illnesses in this way, further information can be adduced that will lead to a better understanding of their causes.

¶ **Historical Background**

In August 1935 Egaz Moniz, Portugal's preeminent neurologist, returned to Lisbon from the Second World Congress of Neurology in London and immediately embarked on an investigation of the effects of frontal lobotomy on intractable psychiatric illness. This innovative study was the impetus for the development of so-called psychosurgery, and in 1949 Moniz was awarded the Nobel Prize for his contributions.

The *force majeure* underlying this new development in psychiatric treatment was, however, the decision of John Fulton and his psychologist colleague, Carlyle Jacobsen, to study frontal lobe function by ablation in two chimpanzees. The investigative approach and the preliminary observations obtained by these two scientists and by others over the next fifteen years deserve to be set down here in some detail, lest limbic system surgery be regarded as devoid of any scientific foundation.

In October 1933 Jacobsen set about training these two animals, named Lucy and Becky. Lucy was described as "crotchety" and not overly friendly, while Becky was said

to be affectionate. The chimpanzees were trained to perform three tasks of increasing complexity in order to gain food. By March 1934 the training was complete and both animals underwent removal of one frontal lobe anterior to the precentral gyrus: the right lobe in Lucy and the left in Becky. During three months of observation no change in skill or behavior was noted in either animal, and in June 1934 similar frontal lobectomies were performed on the opposite sides of the brains of both animals.

Following these bilateral ablations, significant changes in the ability to perform skilled acts and in behavior were noted in both animals. However, the chimpanzees were able to carry out all but the most difficult tasks, and the "intellectual" deficit seemed secondary to an increased distractibility and a lessened attention span as well as diminished memory. On the other hand, the behavioral changes were striking. In Fulton's words:

Following this procedure [the second lobectomies] there was no sign of reflex change in either animal and on superficial inspection their cage behavior did not seem to have altered particularly. On closer scrutiny, however, it was evident that a profound change had occurred, for prior to the second operation both animals showed frustrational behavior, i.e., when unrewarded after having made the wrong choice in the discrimination test or in the delayed-reaction procedure, both animals had temper tantrums and, if unrewarded many times in succession, signs of experimental neurosis became apparent. Following the second operation, the animals seemed devoid of emotional expression. If a wrong choice were made, the animal shrugged its shoulders and went on doing something else—as Jacobsen said picturesquely: "It was as if the animals had joined the happiness cult of the Elder Micheaud* and had placed their burdens on the Lord." Animals with bilateral ablation also failed the double stick-and-platform test. (P. 63)[17]

A remarkable concatenation of interests and events took place in 1935. The Second International Congress of Neurology was held in London in August of that year. At-

---

*Jacobsen was referring to a popular quasireligious radio program of the time.

tending it were Fulton, Jacobsen, Moniz, and Walter J. Freeman, Jr. A graduate of Yale University (1916) and the University of Pennsylvania Medical School (1920), Freeman had, after four years of postgraduate study, been appointed neuropathologist to St. Elizabeth's, the federal psychiatric hospital just outside of Washington, D.C. He was also made Chief of its Laboratory Division and soon thereafter became Associate Professor of Pathology at George Washington University. In 1927 he was named Professor of Neurology at the latter institution in recognition of his brilliance as a teacher, investigator, and clinician.

One of Freeman's interests was the possibility that there might be a biological basis for psychiatric illness, an interest that was stimulated by his neuropathological observations at St. Elizabeth's. As a neurologist, however, he also had been exploring the possible use of Thorotrast for ventriculography and had attended the First International Congress of Neurology in 1931, where he heard Moniz report on the use of this contrast medium for cerebral angiography.

At the Second Congress both Moniz and Freeman had exhibits on the use of Thorotrast, which gave them an opportunity to meet once again and to attend together Fulton's presentation of the postoperative changes in Lucy and Becky.

Again, according to Fulton:

After the paper was read . . . Dr. Moniz arose and asked that, if frontal lobe removal prevents the development of experimental neurosis in animals and eliminates frustration, would it not be feasible to relieve anxiety states in man by surgical means? At the time, we were a little startled by this suggestion for I felt that Dr. Moniz envisaged a bilateral lobectomy which, though possible, would be a very formidable undertaking. (P. 63)[17]

Shutts recounts:

After the Symposium, Freeman and Moniz talked briefly. Moniz was adamant in his belief that surgical destruction of the frontal lobes in humans could be performed with benefit. . . .

The personal dynamism and conviction of

the Portuguese scientist had greatly affected Freeman: "Had I not met him at this time I would not have been ready to accept his second major contribution." [Freeman felt that cerebral angiography was Moniz's first great contribution.] The prospect of following the development of the mind-altering operation excited Freeman. Thus, Moniz and Freeman agreed to communicate with one another throughout Moniz's research and development phase. (P. 41)[43]

After the congress, Moniz returned to Lisbon and sought the collaboration of a young Portuguese neurosurgeon, Almeida Lima, as well as the help of a neurologically oriented clinician, Caucela Abreu, and two psychiatrists, Barahone Fernandez and Sobral Cid. Cid was at that time Professor of Psychiatry at the University of Lisbon; Moniz, Professor of Neurology. Three months after the London congress, Moniz and Lima carried out their first operation by injecting alcohol in the white matter of the frontal lobes. This technique was used in three additional patients before the two men moved to the use of a "leucotome" to sever volumes of white matter about 1 centimeter in diameter, several such lesions being placed in each frontal lobe.

Early in 1936 Moniz began to publish and in June of that year brought forth a monograph on the subject.[34] In it he recounted how he had speculated on the possibility of surgery for psychiatric illness since about 1933 but had his ideas crystallized by the work of Fulton and Jacobsen. He also described the postoperative state of his first twenty patients: Seven were felt to be greatly benefited, another seven were helped, and the psychiatric status of the remaining six was unchanged.

During the next few months Moniz and Lima flooded the scientific and medical communities with reports on lobotomy, publishing no less than ten papers on the subject in French, Portuguese, German, and American journals. This obviously attracted a great deal of attention in the neurosurgical world, but no one was more fascinated than Walter Freeman who, with the assistance of his neurosurgical colleague, James Watts, carried out the first American frontal lobotomy on September 14, 1936.[16]

During the period November 1936 to December 1941, Freeman and Watts operated on 108 patients. There were three deaths in the immediate postoperative period, and a later one in a patient who sustained a right hemiplegia following surgery and succumbed four months later from pneumonia.

Freeman and Watts recorded this experience in the first volume of *Psychosurgery,*[16] in which seventy-four cases were described in great detail. The authors felt that 63 percent of the patients had sustained worthwhile benefit, 23 percent were relatively unchanged, and 14 percent (including the fatalities) were made worse. In this last group, the living patients were described as having a "frontal lobe syndrome" characterized by nonchalance, inability to carry out tasks, and loss of social control.

These complications had been noted by others, and the search began for methods of making more restricted lesions that might still be beneficial but would have fewer undesirable side effects. A detailed review of these various restricted lobotomies can be found in Greenblatt, Arnot, and Solomon's *Studies in Lobotomy.*[20]

In view of the mortality and morbidity resulting from these early operations, one might legitimately ask why such operations continued to be performed. There were two primary reasons.

First, in this early period and particularly prior to 1938, before electroshock therapy was introduced, there was virtually no biological treatment for the psychiatrically ill. Manfred Sakel had, in 1933, introduced insulin shock therapy with modest results and many complications, but in the 1930s psychiatric treatment consisted primarily of rest, sedation with Veronal (a type of liquid barbital), and hydrotherapy for the more disturbed patients. Indeed, "lunatics" were looked upon as the pariahs of society and psychiatric care was just emerging from the dark era of seclusion and incarceration.

Second, it was generally felt by those physicians who had embraced the medical model of psychiatry that the risks, although great, were outweighed by the benefits. Two important reports may serve to corroborate this feeling.

In a collaborative study involving six Veterans Administration hospitals, which was begun in 1950 by Jones and Holsopple and published by Ball, Klett, and Gresock[1] in 1959, 373 patients, all but twelve of whom had been diagnosed as schizophrenic, were divided into two groups. One hundred eighty-five served as controls and 188 had the following operative procedures: radical frontal leucotomy (144), bimedial frontal leucotomy (26), orbital gyrus undercutting (13), and transorbital leucotomy (9).

Of the twenty-six patients who had the bimedial operation, 23 percent were discharged from the hospital, as were 17.8 percent of those having the radical operation. Only 9.7 percent of the 185 matched controls were sufficiently improved to leave the hospital.

In a similar study, Tooth and Newton[46] reviewed for the British Ministry of Health 2,139 leucotomies performed during the years 1942 to 1954. They reported that about 50 percent of the patients had "good results," that 25 percent were improved, and that in 20 percent there was no change or the patients were worse. The operative mortality was given as 6 percent. In view of the almost hopeless prognosis for the patients involved in these two series, one might well understand the enthusiasm for lobotomy despite its risks.

At this point, I wish to review briefly some of the progress in neuroscience in the first half of the twentieth century and present arguments in support of my thesis that current neurosurgical treatment of psychiatric illness should be called limbic system surgery.

Pierre Paul Broca (1824–1880) was a Parisian surgeon with a wide variety of interests. He is best known for his 1861 description of two cases of aphasia (which he called aphemia) from which he deduced the locus of the primary motor speech area (Broca's area) in the left frontal lobes of right-handed individuals. This particular contribution earned him a reputation as a neuroanatomist and neuropathologist, but he was also regarded during his lifetime as an outstanding anthropologist. In 1878 Broca[11] identified and published an account of a volume of brain tissue with a distinct border (or "limbus") made up of the gyrus cinguli and the parahippocampal gyrus. He noted that within this border were the rostral brain stem and the interhemispheric connections and commissurae. This region was termed by Broca *le grande lobe limbique.* Also included within the limbic lobe were the corpus callosum, the subcallosal gyri, the hippocampal formation, and dentate gyrus.

No great attention was given at first to the limbic lobe concept, since that region was felt to be a part of the primitive smell brain —the rhinencephalon. Ramon Cajal[12] however, had concluded in 1901 that the limbic lobe and the primary olfactory apparatus were distinct from one another.

James Wenceslas Papez (1883–1958), whose name is pronounced "Pāpes," spent most of his professional life as a neuroanatomist at Cornell University. According to MacLean,[33] in 1937 Papez read that a large grant had been made in England for the study of the role of the brain in emotional behavior. Irritated because he felt that "the English proposal seemed to ignore what was already known about this subject," Papez quickly wrote his classic paper, "A Proposed Mechanism of Emotion."[37] The introductory paragraph stated: "The following discussion presents some anatomic, clinical and experimental data dealing with the hypothalamus, the gyrus cinguli, the hippocampus and their interconnections. *Taken as a whole, this ensemble of structures is proposed as representing theoretically the anatomic basis of the emotions.*" (p. 725, italics added). In explaining his use of the terms emotional expression and central emotion Papez wrote:

The term "emotion" as commonly used implies two conditions: a way of acting and a way of feeling. The former is designated as emotional expression; the latter, as emotional experience or subjective feeling. The experiments of Bard have demonstrated that emotional expression depends upon the interpretive action of the hypothalamus rather than on that of the dorsal thalamus or cortex, since it may occur when the cerebral hemispheres and the dorsal thalamus are totally removed. For subjective emotional experience, however, the participation of the cortex is essential. Emotional expression and emotional experience may in the human subject be dissociated phenomena, hence, emotion as a subjective state must be referred to the higher psychic level [i.e., the cerebral cortex]. (P. 726)[37]

Papez further theorized that afferent impulses from receptor organs involved in emotion split at the thalamic level into three main pathways. One, conducting information to the corpus striatum via the dorsal thalamus and internal capsule, he called the stream of movement. The second, traveling from the thalamus and internal capsule to the lateral cerebral cortex, represented the stream of thought. Finally, the third pathway, involving impulses conducted through the ventral thalamus to the hypothalamus and also through the mamillary bodies and the anterior thalamic nuclei to the gyrus cinguli, was termed the stream of feeling. This was the basic construct of the now-famous Papez circuit.

His bold, imaginative concept was, however, largely ignored and, for the next ten years, when discussed was usually criticized. The criticisms apparently came from two disparate directions: first, that the theory (as Papez himself admitted) was founded on scant anatomic evidence and, second, that it gave materialistic flavor to those mystical processes which produce the triumphs of intellectual activity in the humanities.

In 1947, however, the Papez circuit was discovered by Paul D. MacLean, a young investigator working at the Massachusetts General Hospital under the direction of Stanley Cobb, Chief of Psychiatry at the hospital and Professor of Neuropathology at Harvard Medical School. MacLean was engaged in recording basal electroencephalograms in cases of temporal lobe epilepsy when he accidentally ran across Papez's 1937 paper. This chance finding and an opportu-

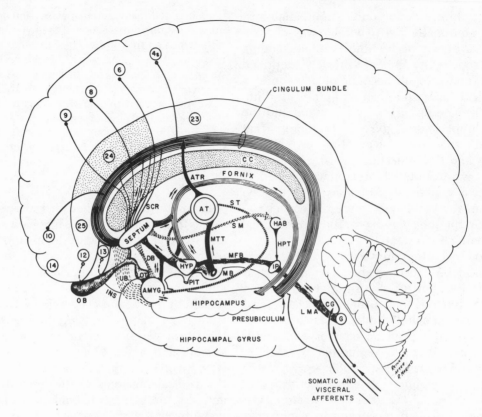

Figure 34–1. Schematic model of the limbic system.

NOTE: Reprinted, by permission of the publisher, from H. T. Ballantine, Jr., et al., "Stereotaxic Anterior Cingulotomy for Neuropsychiatric Illness and Intractable Pain," *Journal of Neurosurgery,* 26 (1967):489.

nity to meet with Papez gave MacLean's research a new direction. In 1949, a year after his visit to Papez, MacLean published "Psychosomatic Disease and the 'Visceral Brain;' Recent Developments Bearing on the Papez Theory of Emotion,"[31] in which he contributed further to the Papez theory. According to MacLean:

I used the expression "visceral brain" as a means of avoiding the narrow implications of the term rhinencephalon that had commonly been applied to the same constellation of structures. . . . I chose the word "visceral" because in its original 16th century sense, it applies to strong, inward feelings. I found, however, that physiologists objected to this term because they interpreted "visceral" in the narrow sense as applying only to glands and hollow organs, including the blood vessels. Consequently, I reverted to Broca's descriptive term "limbic" when referring to the cor-

tex of the limbic lobe and structures of the brain stem with which it has primary connections—hoping that the neutral, descriptive word "limbic" would not give people—especially my colleagues—unpleasant "visceral" feelings! This is how the term "limbic system" crept into the literature in 1952. (P. 6)[33]

MacLean's observations supplied an incentive for a number of other investigations, many of which are recorded in the Proceedings of the Limbic System Symposium held in 1976.[33] Thus we see the progression of our understanding of the "seat of the emotions" over a period of almost one hundred years. According to Nauta:[36]

the term limbic lobe thus came to subsume a great diversity of neural structures ranging in architecture from neocortical (gyrus cinguli) and allocortical (olfactory cortex and most of the remainder of the parahippocampal gyrus) to subcortical (amygdala). Despite this structural heterogenicity, and almost despite the fact that the term, limbic lobe, originally referred merely to a superficially apparent gross-anatomical entity, a need for a collective name for this vast complex in the medial wall of the hemisphere remained even after Broca's term fell into disuse. One such collective designation the long-lived term, rhinencephalon—was based on the widely held assumption that all components of the limbic lobe subserved the sense of smell. When later this functional notion proved untenable, or at least too restrictive, the nomenclature gradually returned to a modification of Broca's original, functionally non-committal term. (P. 303)[36]

A schema to represent current concepts of the anatomy and function of this complex limbic circuit is represented in figure 34–1. Sensory stimuli can be assembled in an area of the midbrain (the "limbic midbrain area of Nauta") consisting of the nucleus of Gudden, the paramedian reticulum, and the central gray matter. From this region, afferent impulses can travel to the hypothalamus and make connections through the medial forebrain bundle with the amygdala and septum, from which fibers radiate to the limbic cortex of the temporal region. From the hypothalamus stimuli can pass into the mamillary bodies, then to the anterior thalamic nuclei and via its radiations to the cingulate region. Radiations from this last structure can be transmitted to the frontal cortex where they would, in the words of Papez, "add emotional coloring to the psychic process."

In similar fashion, the frontal cortex can transmit psychic processes with emotional coloring back to the cingulum, and these efferent impulses can form a reverberant circuit involving the hippocampus, the fornix and mamillary bodies, the tract of Vicq D'Azyr back to the cingulum and finally, again, the hippocampus. After appropriate (or inappropriate?) emotional modification these efferent "emotional experiences" are translated into emotional expression by the same pathways involved in the reception of visceral and extracorporeal stimuli.

Cobb conceptualized this process in his 1949 Salmon Lectures.[13] In explaining his di-

agram of a definition of emotion (see figure 34–2) Cobb wrote:

> From the psychological point of view, emotions may be looked upon as having three main parts. . . . First, there is the private feeling, the affect that is felt by you or me, but that must be interpreted to anyone else by symbols. Second, there is the complex set of physiological changes set up in nerves, viscera, glands and muscles. These make the characteristic stirred-up internal state. Finally, there are the patterns of behavior which overtly express the stirred-up internal state, and back of that, the feeling. All this is shown diagrammatically. . . . Added to them is an arrow, joining the arrows of overt expression with the private feeling. This indicates that overt expression causes various changes in the environment which register via sense organs and change the private feeling. Thus, from the psychological point of view, as well as the neurological, the emotions depend on feedback systems with reverberating circuits. (Pp. 112.)[13]

Cobb also attempted to diagram the primary normal feelings with certain of their pathological counterparts (see figure 34–3). The current mystery of the relationship between a normal emotion, such as a grief reaction, and an abnormal one, such as chronic depression, and the causation in general of disorders of affect is one in urgent need of solution.

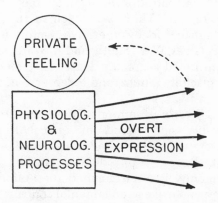

Figure 34–2. Definition of "emotion" (multidimensional referent).

NOTE: Reprinted, by permission of the publisher, from S. Cobb, *Emotions and Clinical Medicine* (New York: W. W. Norton, 1950), p. 112.

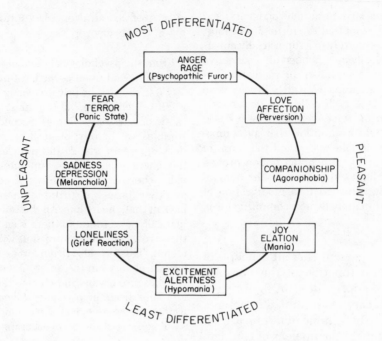

Figure 34–3.   Classification of emotions.

NOTE: Reprinted, by permission of the publisher, from S. Cobb, *Emotions and Clinical Medicine* (New York: W. W. Norton, 1950), p. 108.

The years immediately following World War II produced not only neuroanatomical advances such as those pioneered by Mac-Lean but neurophysiological and clinical progress as well. Fulton and coworkers continued their nonhuman primate investigations, concentrating more upon the cingulate region. They were joined in this nonhuman work by other investigators, notably P. Glees, W. K. Smith, and A. Ward, all of whom noted a greater degree of tameness and placidity (Smith) and a decrease in fear of man (Ward).

J. G. Lyerly attempted to minimize the undesirable side effects of radical frontal lobotomy as early as 1938; this was followed by J. Poppen's introduction of bimedial leucotomy. But it remained for Fulton to once again make a fundamental contribution to limbic system surgery.

At the 1947 meeting of the Society of British Neurological Surgeons there was a general discussion of the benefits and risks of frontal lobotomy. Fulton suggested that, if it

were feasible, cingulectomy might be an appropriate limited operation. He elaborated on this idea the next year in his Withering Lectures at the Birmingham Medical School:

> The question of whether the cingulate gyrus is concerned in the favorable results of lobotomy is also unsettled. In cases which have been deemed favorable therapeutically and have subsequently come to autopsy, the anterior cingulate has been involved almost invariably, and since isolated removal of the cingulate in animals causes profound changes in behavior in the direction of making aggressive animals tamer and more pacific, it is quite conceivable that a lesion restricted to the cingulate might have a beneficial effect even if all the remaining frontal area projections remained intact. This likewise must be kept for further experimental analysis. (Pp. 92–93)[17]

Fulton's hypothesis has been amply confirmed over the years; moreover, a variety of neurosurgical procedures performed in several locations within the brain are currently in use. However, they all involve a portion of the limbic system. Since the term psychosurgery was originally coined by Moniz to describe frontal lobotomy, I believe these modern neurosurgical operations can be more appropriately subsumed under the generic term of limbic system surgery.

Soon after the 1947 neurosurgical meeting Sir Hugh Carins at Oxford and Professor Jacques LeBeau in Paris proceeded promptly to act upon Fulton's suggestion, and in 1961 Lewin[29] reviewed the results of anterior cingulectomies performed by Cairns and his coworkers. Of twenty-six patients with affective illness, twenty-one were said to have benefited from the operation and eleven were classified as greatly improved.

The year 1947 saw a contribution to modern psychiatric surgery that I believe was equal in importance to Fulton's—the introduction by E. A. Spiegel and H. T. Wycis of their stereoencephalatome and the initiation of the stereotactic approach to hitherto inaccessible regions of the human brain. Stereotaxis, the technique of using a probe guidance system and three-dimensional coordinates, had been employed by Sir Victor Horsley four decades earlier in animal brain research but, inexplicably, had not been adapted to humans as a therapeutic tool. Today it is the method preferred by most neurosurgeons who perform intracranial operations for psychiatric illness and chronic pain, since these procedures demand the inactivation of deep-lying cerebral regions.

During this same period Walter Freeman, who had pioneered and popularized frontal lobotomy, was searching for an alternative that would sever primarily the frontal-thalamic connections, thereby, he thought, eliminating or at least reducing the behavioral deficits. In 1946 he introduced transorbital leucotomy. Unfortunately, however, he chose for a surgical instrument a simple ice pick and quickly concluded that there was no need for a neurosurgeon or even an operating room.

Freeman's usual procedure was to administer electric shock to the patient. In the postictal phase of coma he would drive the ice pick through the orbital plates and swing the handle from side to side.[43]

This crude technique was condemned by most psychiatrists and almost all neurosurgeons, but the greater the criticism the more active Freeman became. His behavior was such that eventually he lost his professional appointments at George Washington University and moved to California. He also lost his prestige in the very field in which he had been a leader. Finally the term and procedure of "ice pick lobotomy" caused such revulsion in the medical community that psychosurgery was regarded by many with extreme distaste.

This setback for psychiatric surgery was, however, to be delayed for several years, and in 1948 interest in the field was such that the First International Congress of Psychosurgery was inaugurated at Lisbon in August. Individuals from twenty-eight countries participated and statistics (of varying value) on about 8,000 lobotomies were presented.

Of particular importance was a preliminary report by William B. Scoville on the technique of undercutting the orbital gyrus.[42] This limited leucotomy was also adopted or developed at about the same time by Geoffrey Knight in London, but he eventually replaced it with a procedure that currently is called subcaudate tractotomy. According to Knight,[26] after performing undercuttings on 600 patients he concluded that the operation was of benefit only if the incision was carried far enough posteriorly to reach the zona innominata. As a result, he devised a stereotactic method of implanting Yttrium-90 pellets under x-ray visualization solely in that region.

In Louisville, Kentucky, Grantham developed in 1950 a somewhat similar method for producing electrolytic lesions in the inferomedial quadrants of the frontal lobes for the treatment of intractable chronic pain and psychiatric illness.[19]

Kenneth Livingston reported in 1953 the results of a study begun in 1949 of anterior cingulectomy using the direct approach.[30] Seventy-two patients were operated upon, with one death. A subgroup of twenty-four "psychotic" patients (exact diagnosis not given) had been hospitalized for at least four years preoperatively and followed two years or longer postoperatively. Twelve were able to leave the hospital and another was judged to be markedly improved.

Sixteen of these patients had been placed in four groups of four each. Three patients in each group underwent standard cingulectomy; a sham operation was performed on the fourth. After an observation period of one to three months, the four patients with the sham operations (who had shown no psychiatric improvement) underwent cingulectomy. Although sham operations might not be condoned today, I believe Livingston's contribution weakens the "placebo effect" argument concerning the cause of improvement.

Thus was the stage set for the inauguration of present-day psychiatric surgery, only to be delayed by the introduction of chlorpromazine, the first of the myriad psychopharmacologic agents so familiar to all psychiatrists. Although I believe the psychoanalysts' dogmatic approach had slowed the acceptance of the medical model of psychiatric illness, an increasing number of psychiatrists were coming to believe that psychotropic drugs and electroshock therapy would prove to be the cure for disorders of affect and the amelioration of the manifestations of schizophrenia.

It gradually became apparent, however, that neither of these modalities alone or in combination had proven to be the long-sought-after panacea. Moreover, the side effects of the psychoactive drugs, particularly tardive dyskinesia, became increasingly recognized. Once again, in the 1960s, there was an increase of interest in psychiatric surgery. Foltz and White[15] reported on their experience with stereotaxic anterior cingulumotomy (sic) for the treatment of chronic pain. Refining the procedure described by Grantham a decade earlier for creating lesions in the frontal lobes, they described the beneficial effects of stereotactic anterior cingulotomy in sixteen patients with chronic pain.

I was impressed by two of their findings; first, that the more emotionally "involved" their patients were with their pain syndromes, the better the postoperative status seemed to be, and second, that in a group of patients with pain of uncertain or unknown etiology, the results were impressive. I concluded from this account that bilateral anterior stereotactic cingulotomy might be an appropriate procedure for testing Fulton's hypothesis that were it feasible, the cingulum might be an appropriate locus for psychiatric surgery. In 1962 I began a study of this operation with two psychiatrists, Norris B. Flanagan and Walter Cassidy.[12]

¶ Modern Psychiatric Surgery

The present era began in 1970 with the inauguration in Copenhagen of the Second International Congress on Psychosurgery. Fifty-one papers were contributed by seventy-seven authors from eleven countries. The effects of ablations in regions of the frontal lobes, temporal lobes, cingulum, thalamus, and hypothalamus were presented and discussed.

One of the most important reports was given by Knight[26] regarding 450 patients who had undergone bilateral Yttrium-90 implantation in the subcaudate regions. Sadao Hirose from Japan described a modification of Scoville's orbital undercutting in which the incision was restricted to the medial portion of the white matter of the orbital gyri.

My colleagues and I documented our experiences with bilateral stereotactic anterior cingulotomy.[4] During the previous eight years, 160 patients had undergone the procedure; 121 were suffering from intractable disorders of affect and thirty-nine from chronic pain.

The Third International Congress of Psychosurgery was held two years later in Cambridge, England, and emphasized the current state of knowledge concerning the neurophysiology of the limbic system and its connections. There were also, however, additional clinical reports supplementing those of 1970 and two preliminary accounts of different approaches to limbic system surgery: the limbic leucotomy of Kelly and Richardson in London[24] and stereotactic anterior capsulotomy as performed in Sweden by Bingley and Leksel.[8] Both of these procedures will be discussed subsequently.

It would appear from this account that psychiatric surgery had finally been accepted as a therapeutic tool, but countervailing forces were also at work. The international counterculture revolt was having its greatest impact during the period 1965 to 1975. Its likely effect on medicine in general and psychiatric surgery in particular had been aptly described by Oliver Wendell Holmes, Senior, in an invited oration to the Massachusetts Medical Society in 1860.[21] Dr. Holmes spoke in part as follows:

. . . The truth is that Medicine, professedly founded on observation, is as sensitive to outside influences, political, religious, philosophical and imaginative as is the barometer to the changes of atmospheric density. Theoretically it ought to go on its own straightforward inductive path, without regard to changes of government or to fluctuations of public opinion. But look a moment while I clash a few facts together, and see if some sparks do not reveal by their light a closer relation between the Medical Sciences and the conditions of Society and the general thought of the time, than would at first be suspected. (P. 9)[21]

The profundity of this observation was illustrated to me over the next several years by the vicious and hysterical attacks on psychosurgery and electroconvulsive therapy that led to legislation limiting these potentially therapeutic procedures. In 1973 the state of Oregon passed a law creating a Psychosurgery Review Board that essentially made it impossible for a patient to be operated on no matter how much the patient and his or her psychiatrist wished to have the procedure carried out. That same year the Honorable

Louis Stokes, a representative from Ohio, introduced a bill in Congress that would have banned all psychosurgery in the United States. In 1974 California passed a law similar to that of Oregon and, again, psychiatric surgery was for all intents and purposes impossible to obtain in that state.

Perhaps the most devastating blow to psychiatric surgery occurred in Michigan when, in 1973, a lawyer named Gabe Kaimowitz of Michigan Legal Services intervened on behalf of a mental patient who had been involuntarily confined to a state mental hospital because he had murdered and then raped a young nursing student. After eighteen years of incarceration it was proposed that he undergo stereotactic hypothalamotomy in order to reduce any tendency toward sexual aggression. It was clearly explained that the operation was experimental/investigational and the patient had consented to it. Kaimowitz intervened on the grounds that it was impossible for this man to give informed consent for the procedure.[22]

A three-judge Michigan court prohibited the performance of the operation on the grounds (among others) that it was "clearly experimental." Unfortunately, however, the judges also stated: "Throughout this opinion the Court will use the term psychosurgery to describe the proposed innovative or experimental surgical procedure defined in the questions for consideration by the Court." Thus these judges set down as a legal precedent what I believe to be the erroneous conclusion that all limbic system surgery was "clearly experimental." This failure to distinguish between various psychosurgical procedures has continued to hamper psychiatric surgery to this day.

Following these legal actions, however, an action more favorable to psychosurgery was taken. In September 1973, Congress created the National Commission for the Protection of Human Subjects of Biomedical and Behavioral Research. The commission undertook to study psychiatric surgery in the United States as it had been performed during the period 1965 to 1975 and issued its report in 1977.

To the surprise of many objective observers and the consternation of those opponents of psychiatric surgery, the report was somewhat favorable. In his letter of transmittal to the President and the Congress on March 14, 1977, Kenneth J. Ryan, M.D., the chairman of the commission, stated in part, "On the basis of data from pilot studies that were conducted under contract to assess the effects of psychosurgery, the Commission has determined unanimously that there are circumstances under which psychosurgical procedures may appropriately be performed."[11]

The commission also developed a set of requirements "to protect the access of individuals to a potential therapy, while recognizing the responsibility of the state to protect individual rights and safety." The "safeguards" recommended by the commission were essentially those that had been followed for more than seven years by Massachusetts General Hospital. Unfortunately, however, the commission also said that "the safety and efficacy of specific psychosurgical procedures for the treatment of particular disorders . . . have not been demonstrated to the degree that would permit such procedures to be considered 'an accepted practice.' "

To resolve these doubts, the commission further called upon the Department of Health and Human Services to set up a Psychosurgery Review Board to be certain that psychiatric surgery was carried out only in approved hospitals with an Institutional Review Board that could certify that the patient was in need of the operation, that all generally accepted nonoperative methods of treatment had been tried without success, that the surgeon was competent, and that the patient had given informed consent. These recommendations have not been acted upon as of this date and, as a consequence, there is no official body that can certify that such procedures as stereotactic cingulotomy or subcaudate tractotomy can be considered "accepted practice."

¶ The Current Status of Limbic System Surgery

Despite the obstacles that have just been described, successful symposia on psychiatric surgery were held at the 1982 International Congress of Biological Psychiatry in Stockholm and in 1983 at The World Congress of Psychiatry in Vienna. The following data have been compiled from those meetings and other communications presented since 1970.

Psychiatric surgery is still being performed on a limited international basis but more frequently in the United Kingdom and the United States than elsewhere. Although open bilateral medial leucotomies and bilateral orbital undercuttings are still done in small numbers, as of this writing four stereotactic approaches—subcaudate tractotomy, bilateral anterior cingulotomy, a combination of these two termed limbic leucotomy, and anterior capsulotomy—appear to be the most frequently carried out procedures.

Two important questions must be answered in reference to these operations: What are the risks and what benefits can be expected? If the surgery is carried out with reasonable expertise, the answer to the former can be stated with confidence.

Subcaudate tractotomy has been performed by Knight, Bridges, and Bartlett on about 1,000 patients. A review of 580 of the earlier cases disclosed that there had been one death and a 1 percent incidence of postoperative epilepsy. A detailed psychiatric review of 150 of these patients disclosed that twenty-one of them "had developed some post-operative behavioral and psychological changes which were lasting and troublesome in four, but minor and trivial in seventeen."[44]

In the United States it has been possible to collect a series of 923 patients who have been subjected to 1109 cingulotomies from 1962 to 1984. Since each such procedure puts the patient at risk for complications, the following statistics seem reliable. There has been one death, which gives an operative mortality of

0.09 percent; and four patients have been rendered hemiplegic as a result of intracerebral hematoma, an incidence of 0.36 percent.

A consecutive subgroup of 179 of my patients are being followed independently by the Department of Psychology at the Massachusetts Institute of Technology (MIT), a study first commissioned in 1974 by the National Commission for the Protection of Human Subjects of Biomedical and Behavioral Research and continued by the National Institute of Mental Health. In 1980 the MIT group stated that

on the basis of six years of research, in which 137 patients who underwent bilateral cingulotomy [by my group] have been examined, it can be concluded first of all that no patient (except possibly one who experienced a subdural hemorrhage during a recent operation) showed the severe adverse effects that had been associated with prefrontal lobotomy during the 1940's and 1950's. In fact, there is so far no evidence of any lasting neurological abnormality attributable to the cingulate lesions and only one test in which there are lasting behavioral deficits after cingulotomy. This test requires the patient to copy a complex drawing from a model. . . .[14]

In the early 1950s, Lars Leksell in Sweden introduced the operation of stereotactic anterior capsulotomy, a procedure designed to interrupt the fibers connecting the anterior frontal lobe cortex and the thalamus at their convergence in the internal capsule. Thirty-five patients with severe obsessive-compulsive neurosis were operated on, and their postoperative status was reported in 1975 at the Fourth World Congress of Psychiatric Surgery in Madrid.[9] Twenty-five patients were symptom-free or "much improved" and ten were unchanged, a success rate of 71 percent. Although the numbers are relatively small, the results are impressive in view of the acknowledged difficulty in treating this illness by other methods.

In a series of 148 patients subjected to limbic leucotomy and the thirty-five patients who underwent anterior capsulotomy, there was one lasting memory deficit in the former and no mention of complications in the latter. Thus it can be safely concluded that, although stereotactic limbic system surgery is not entirely free from risk, it is as safe, or safer, than any other intracranial neurosurgical procedure.

Assessment of the effectiveness of present-day limbic system surgery presents a much more difficult problem. A uniform standard of judgment from observer to observer is lacking, as is any objective attempt at categorization of degrees of improvement. Everyone understands, for example, the categories of "well," "unimproved," and "worse," but almost all analyses of the results include a category of "useful improvement," which must invariably be subjective. It is of some interest, however, that when Moniz reported the results of frontal lobotomy in his first twenty patients, he and his colleagues felt that useful improvement had been obtained in 70 percent.[34] This remains the average figure for postoperative benefit even today. It is with these caveats in mind that the following reports from the literature are presented.

In 1981 Bartlett, Bridges, and Kelly[7] reported that 68 percent of patients with depression made a complete or nearly complete recovery after subcaudate tractotomy. Those with a diagnosis of anxiety showed 63 percent useful improvement, and in the patients with obsessional illness it was 53 percent.

In 1975 my associates and I presented the postoperative status of 154 patients who had undergone stereotactic bilateral anterior cingulotomy for disorders of affect.[5] Seventeen percent were said to be "well" and an additional 58 percent were categorized as having been "significantly improved."

Kelly[23] documented the postoperative status of 148 patients subjected to stereotactic limbic leucotomy. Ninety-nine (67 percent) were categorized as "clinically improved" twenty months postoperatively. He stated that the results were best in those with obsessional neurosis, 84 percent of forty-nine patients with that diagnosis being placed in the improved category. Patients with a primary diagnosis of anxiety and/or depression did not improve quite so strikingly, good results being obtained in only 60 percent.

Although limbic system surgery is generally thought to be helpful only for the treatment of intractable affective illness, Kelly presented a surprisingly different view. Nineteen of the patients in his series were said to be schizophrenic and 63 percent were classified as clinically improved. It was stated, however, that these patients had been chosen for operation because of "very distressing psychotic symptoms, or high levels of anxiety, depression or obsessions. . . . Postoperatively there was not only a reduction of anxiety and depression but also a decrease in the number of psychotic episodes (pp. 229–30)."[23] This raises an interesting question as to the accuracy of diagnostic classification when dealing with psychiatric illness; it varies from country to country and within a country may differ markedly from psychiatrist to psychiatrist. The patient diagnosed by an American psychiatrist as suffering from paranoid schizophrenia may be diagnosed by his British colleagues as suffering from a primary disorder of affect with secondary cognitive problems bordering on the delusional. This brings up the matter of selection of patients for limbic system surgery.

It is my belief and the belief of many who support the concept of surgical intervention for intractable psychiatric illness that all generally accepted methods of nonoperative treatment should have been tried unsuccessfully before any patient is considered for operation. In 1981 Bartlett, Bridges, and Kelly[7] published a statement on this subject in the *British Journal of Psychiatry.* It was their opinion that patients suffering from long-term illness with inadequate or absent response to "routine therapies" should be assessed for surgery even if the symptoms were not especially severe but did cause disability and emotional suffering. Patients who were severely ill with a high risk of suicide should, they stated, be referred early after the onset of the illness.

In 1962 my colleagues at Massachusetts General Hospital and I began a study of stereotactic anterior cingulotomy, and for the next eight years thereafter patients were referred primarily from a very small group of psychiatrists in the Boston area. Because of the wide range of diagnoses, it was decided early on (since this was a clinical study) to accept any patient for assessment who had chronic, disabling psychiatric illness that had failed to respond to nonoperative treatment and in whom emotional suffering was either the sole or the most prominent psychiatric symptom. In 1970, when patients were being referred from all sections of the United States, additional criteria were added, and at the present time the following preoperative conditions must be met.

First, the patient must be under psychiatric treatment and referred for evaluation by the treating psychiatrist accompanied by a written statement that all reasonable methods of nonoperative treatment had been tried without success and that the psychiatrist would continue to treat the patient after surgery for as long as seemed necessary.

Second, the patient must agree to return to psychiatric care and, almost without exception, have the emotional support of a family member or close friend, both before and after surgery.

Third, an institutional review board, consisting of the operating neurosurgeon and also a psychiatrist and neurologist appointed by the governing board of the hospital as independent evaluators, must assess the patient from the standpoint of diagnosis and prior treatment. Only if all three of these individuals agree that surgical intervention is appropriate will it be carried out.

The need for psychiatric follow-up care cannot be overemphasized. Most observers agree that maximum benefit may not occur for one to two years postoperatively and that surgical intervention should be considered an adjunct to, not a substitute for, continued psychiatric care for as long as the patient is symptomatic.

The selection of the site or sites for operative intervention in the limbic system remains somewhat controversial. In London it has been agreed that patients diagnosed as suffering from depression, anxiety, obsessional neurosis (with associated depression), or schizo-affective illness should undergo subcaudate tractotomy. Limbic leucotomy—that is, the production of multiple small cingulate and subcaudate lesions—is reserved for those patients with obsessional neurosis alone and for carefully selected cases of schizophrenia in whom symptoms of depression, anxiety, or obsessional behavior are very prominent.

Our experiences at Massachusetts General Hospital have been confined, almost without exception, to stereotactic anterior cingulotomy. The absence of undesirable personality changes or postoperative intellectual deficits has been gratifying, but in about 40 percent of our patients a good result has not been obtained until a second, or even a third, region in the anterior cingulum has undergone ablation. In a few very sick patients, whose personalities were already damaged by their illnesses, we have interrupted larger volumes during one operation. Invariably these patients have shown postoperative confusion and other transient disorders of cortical function. These findings create quite a dilemma since each cingulotomy procedure puts the patient at risk for a complication. Moreover, our results in obsessional neurosis and germ phobia have not been as satisfactory as with depression. It is quite possible that those patients should be subject to limbic leucotomy as described by Kelly and Richardson. To date we have been reluctant to perform this operation because of the very slight but definite risk of undesirable alterations of personality following subcaudate tractotomy. In Great Britain this risk is apparently acceptable in view of the potential benefit. In the United States it might not be tolerated at this time.

¶ **The Future of Psychiatric Surgery**

Modern neurosurgical techniques, particularly the stereotactic procedures, for the treatment of otherwise intractable disorders of affect were considered so favorably in 1968 that planning was begun for the 1970 Second World Congress of Psychosurgery. Five years later there were state statutes so restrictive that from 1973 to the present psychiatric surgery has virtually disappeared from view in Oregon and California.

As a result of these legal actions, psychiatrists and neurosurgeons became reluctant to recommend the surgical approach, and those who did wrote very little about their experiences. Only in England and a few centers in the United States and Europe did clinicians continue to perform limbic system surgery at about the same rate as prior to 1970.

In the early 1980s, however, there were signs that society was taking what I believe to be a more rational view. The media, particularly television, produced documentaries that introduced the public to the benefits of psychiatric surgery, and the shrill voices of the critics became more subdued. Two of the largest neurosurgical societies in North America issued statements that were supportive, and an increasing number of psychiatrists began referring patients for surgery after other treatment modalities had failed.

What then of the future? In the words of John Fulton, quoted earlier, "Many phases of the problem [of psychiatric surgery] are, however, still obscure both anatomically and physiologically (not to mention psychiatrically). . . ." Due to the progress in the neurosciences, we now have many more questions that need answers than were considered when Fulton wrote those words thirty-four years ago. Nevertheless, we have more tools than he had. Some of these problems follow.

Although the relative risks of certain types of limbic system surgery seem to have been established firmly, and the efficacy of such surgery has been reasonably well documented, the basic reasons for success or failure are conjectural. Two theories (or, perhaps, hypotheses) are currently in vogue, the anatomical and the neurochemical.

The first, and older, of these is based on Papez's theory of emotion and its three "streams" of movement, thought, and feeling. Since each of these may follow divergent pathways, it might seem logical to devise different operations for different psychiatric illnesses. For example, an interruption of the fibers in the "stream of movement" might be helpful for obsessive-compulsive behavior, while a lesion in the "stream of feeling" might benefit unipolar depression. This could be the basis for the recommendations of the British school mentioned earlier.

On the other hand, if the Papez circuit is a truly reverberant one, then it may be that it is the volume of interruption rather than the exact locus that is the operant factor. If so, what is fundamentally accomplished by a given operation? Could it be that the surgery alters brain chemistry as much or more than it alters pathways? Some credence is lent to this view by the fact that it is more common for improvement in psychiatric status (when it occurs) to take place slowly. One would expect, if anatomic disruption were the only factor, that the result would be almost immediately apparent. Moreover, we have evidence that neurotransmitter concentration is altered in some patients who are to be subjected to anterior cingulotomy.

Ventricular cerebrospinal fluid (CSF) was assayed from twenty-one patients with severe depressive disorders.[10] Ventricular CSF from fourteen patients with hydrocephalus and lumbar CSF from twelve patients with no known neurosurgical or psychiatric disease were used as controls. Immunoassayable beta-endorphin levels were similar in all groups: 24.4 ± 11.8 pg per ml for normal controls, 17.11 ± 7.8 pg per ml in the patients with hydrocephalus, and 17.2 ± 8.8 pg per ml for patients with depression.

Somatostatin was significantly less in the depressed patients, who had a value of 25.2 ± 18.5 pg per ml. Control values were 62.8 ± 28.2 pg per ml for patients without known neurological disease and 70.4 ± 54.3 pg per ml for hydrocephalic patients.

Although these data suggest that depressive disease may be associated with a derangement in CSF somatostatin, the significance of these findings, particularly the pathophysiological relationship, is currently unclear. It should be possible in the future to obtain tissue for microneurochemical analysis from the region selected for ablation prior to carrying out the procedure. Careful and detailed clinical and neuroscience studies must be done to solve the problem of anatomy versus neurochemistry.

A problem of immediate concern, however, is the climate of public and psychiatric opinion regarding limbic system surgery. It would appear that psychiatric patients and their relatives are currently more cognizant of these procedures than the psychiatrists. It is not uncommon for us to accept patients for evaluation after they or their families have read about "psychosurgery" and have then persuaded the treating psychiatrist to make a referral.

Another issue concerns the belief that modern pharmacotherapy has obviated the need for psychiatric surgery, and in England it is true that there has been some reduction in operations since 1982. On the other hand, in the United States there has been a steady increase both in the number of disabled psychiatric patients and in the suicide rate. The National Centers for Disease Control, for example, has recently published statistics on premature deaths (defined as death occurring before the age of sixty-five) for the year 1982.

The leading cause of premature death was cancer followed by heart disease, suicides, and homicides (which alone accounted for 43,999 deaths) and then cerebrovascular disease. While the suicide rate in our operated series is 9 percent, the rate for a similar group of unoperated patients has been variously estimated at between 15 percent and 30 percent. Moreover, it has been estimated that on any one day in the United States there are about 45,000 individuals disabled by emotional illnesses refractory to treatment and a burden to themselves, their families, and society. These are the patients who are included in the grim statistics on suicide and homicide. If these statistics are even approximately correct and if they were more widely known, I believe there would be a marked increase in the use of psychiatric surgery in the near future.

Contributing greatly to the current lack of

use is the fact that information on modern psychiatric surgery is scarce and published in obscure journals. However, the major obstacle seems to be the reluctance of many psychiatrists to become informed and involved, and it has been the neurosurgeons rather than the psychiatrists who have taken the lead in assuring the viability of this treatment in the United States. I believe this state of affairs should be reversed in the future. One step in that direction might be the implementation of a prospective controlled study such as that first proposed by the Research Committee of the British Royal College of Psychiatrists and published in 1977.[40] This is a most important paper and should be read by all interested psychiatrists because of its assessment of psychiatric surgery in Great Britain as well as the detailed description of the method proposed.

Briefly, after referral by the treating psychiatrist and acceptance for surgery by the evaluating team (to include a neurosurgeon), the patient would then be randomly chosen for operation or further nonoperative treatment by an independent research psychiatrist. At the end of a suitable period of observation, the nonoperated patient would be offered surgery if his or her clinical state had not improved. Such a study could be carried out in the United States at selected sites chosen by the National Institute of Mental Health, which should fund the study as well.

In the opening paragraph, describing the clinical trial, the Research Committee observed, "because of the National Health Service, freedom from political influence, and the availability of suitable research workers, Britain is one of a few countries in which a trial of psychosurgery might be achieved" (p. 175).[40] It is ironic that the study was never funded because of political opposition from the same groups that stultified progress in psychiatric surgery in the United States.

¶ Epilogue

Papez, in his famous paper, posed this question: "Is emotion a magic product or is it a physiologic process which depends on an anatomic mechanism?" (p. 743)[37] I have recently addressed this question in this way:

Advances in neurochemistry have revealed to mankind a much greater miracle than magic. We are beginning to understand and wonder at the disclosure of another of the beauties of nature— the probability that atoms of which all things are made can combine into billions of molecules which build and run the human brain and that it in turn can produce great music, writing, painting and even greater opportunities for Man to know himself. (Pp. 2535–36)[2]

In the future there will be more advances in psychopharmacological therapy, but for the near term it seems apparent to me that there is a place for psychiatric surgery. Moreover, as the public comes increasingly to understand the almost miraculous transmutation of matter into mind and emotion, neuroscientists will be given greater opportunities and responsibilities. Psychiatrists and neurosurgeons will cooperate in greater numbers, and psychiatric surgery may then come to be regarded as casually as heart surgery. This will increase the obligation of neurosurgeons and neuroscientists, neurologists and psychiatrists in their quest toward a better understanding of the neurophysiological basis of mental health and mental illness.

It is essential, however, to be ever mindful that these neurosurgical attempts to benefit the psychiatrically disabled have the potential to alter human behavior in the general population. For this reason, neurosurgeons have a special ethical responsibility to be certain that their skills are employed only to benefit the health and welfare of suffering patients and never for "scientific" or social or political ends.

¶ Bibliography

1. BALL J., KLETT C. J., and GRESOCK C. J. "The Veteran's Administration Study of Prefrontal Lobotomy," *Journal of Clinical and Experimental Psychopathology,* 20 (1959):205–217.
2. BALLANTINE, H. T., JR. "Neurosurgery for

Behavioral Disorders," in Wilkins and Rengachary, eds., *Neurosurgery*. New York: McGraw-Hill (in press).

3. BALLANTINE, H. T., JR., et al. "Stereotaxic Anterior Cingulotomy for Neuropsychiatric Illness and Intractable Pain," *Journal of Neurosurgery*, 26 (1967): 488–495.

4. BALLANTINE, H. T., JR., et al. "Frontal Cingulotomy for Mood Disturbance," in H. Hitchcock, L. Laitinen, and K. Vaernet, eds., *Psychosurgery*. Springfield, Il.: Charles C Thomas, 1972, pp. 221–229.

5. BALLANTINE, H. T., JR., et al. "Cingulotomy for Psychiatric Illness: Report of 13 Years' Experience," in W. H. Sweet, S. Obrador, and J. G. Martin-Rodriguez, eds., *Neurosurgical Treatment in Psychiatry, Pain and Epilepsy*. Baltimore, Md.: University Park Press, 1977, pp. 333–353.

6. BARTLETT, J. R., and BRIDGES, P. K. "The Extended Subcaudate Tractotomy Lesion," in W. H. Sweet, S. Obrador, and J. G. Martin-Rodriguez, eds., *Neurosurgical Treatment in Psychiatry, Pain and Epilepsy*. Baltimore, Md.: University Park Press, 1977, pp. 387–398.

7. BARTLETT, J. R., BRIDGES, P., and KELLY, D. "Contemporary Indications for Psychosurgery," *British Journal of Psychiatry*, 138 (1981):507–511.

8. BINGLEY, T., et al. "Stereotactic Anterior Capsulotomy in Anxiety and Obsessive-compulsive States," in L. Laitinen and K. Livingston, eds., *Surgical Approaches in Psychiatry*. Baltimore, Md.: University Park Press, 1973, pp. 165–173.

9. BINGLEY, T., et al. "Capsulotomy in Chronic Obsessive-compulsive Neurosis," in W. H. Sweet, S. Obrador, and J. G. Martin-Rodriguez, eds., *Neurosurgical Treatment in Psychiatry, Pain and Epilepsy*. Baltimore, Md.: University Park Press, 1977, pp. 287–299.

10. BLACK, P. McL., et al. "Beta-endorphin and Somatostatin Concentrations in the Cerebrospinal Fluid of Patients with Depressive Disorder (Abstract)," Society of Biological Psychiatry, Los Angeles, 1984.

11. BROCA, P. "Anatomie Comparee Circonvolutions Cerebrales: Le Grand Lobe Limbique et La Scissure Limbique dans la Serie des Mammiferes," *Revue Anthropologie* (Paris) 1 (1878):385–498.

12. CASSIDY, W. L., BALLANTINE, H. T., JR., and FLANAGAN, N. B.: "Frontal Cingulotomy for Affective Disorders," *Recent Advances in Biology and Psychiatry*, 8 (1965):269–275.

13. COBB, S. *Emotions and Clinical Medicine*. New York: W. W. Norton, 1950.

14. CORKIN, S. Personal communication, 1984.

15. FOLTZ, E. L., and WHITE L. E., JR. "Pain 'relief' by Frontal Cingulotomy," *Journal of Neurosurgery*, 19 (1962):89–100.

16. FREEMAN, W. L., and WATTS, J. W. *Psychosurgery*. Springfield, Ill.: Charles C Thomas, 1942.

17. FULTON, J. F. *Functional Localization in Relation to Frontal Lobotomy*. New York: Oxford University Press, 1949.

18. ———. *Frontal Lobotomy and Affective Behavior*. New York: W.W. Norton, 1951.

19. GRANTHAM, E. G. "Prefrontal Lobotomy for Relief of Pain with a Report of a New Operative Technique," *Journal of Neurosurgery*, 8 (1951):405–410.

20. GREENBLATT, M., ARNOT, R., and SOLOMON, H. C., eds. *Studies in Lobotomy*. New York: Grune and Stratton, 1950.

21. HOLMES, O. W. "Currents and Counter-Currents in Medical Science," Address delivered to the Massachusetts Medical Society, May 30, 1860.

22. KAIMOWITZ v. Department of Mental Health, Civil no. 73-19434-AW (Cir. Ct., Wayne County, Mich., July 10, 1973).

23. KELLY, D. *Anxiety and Emotions: Physiological Basis and Treatment*. Springfield, Ill.: Charles C Thomas, 1980.

24. KELLY, W., RICHARDSON, A., and MITCHELL-HEGGS, N. "Technique and Assessment of Limbic Leucotomy," in W. Laitinen and K. Livingston, eds., *Surgical Approaches in Psychiatry*. Baltimore, Md.: University Park Press, 1973, pp. 165–173.

25. KNIGHT, G. "Stereotactic Tractotomy in the Surgical Treatment of Mental Illness," *Journal of Neurology, Neurosurgery, and Psychiatry*, 28 (1965):304–310.

26. ———. "Bifrontal Stereotaxic Tractotomy in the Substantia Innominata: An Experience of 450 Cases," in E. Hitchcock, L.

Laitinen, and K. Vaernet, eds., *Psychosurgery.* Springfield, Ill: Charles C Thomas, 1972.

27. ———. "Psychosurgery Today," *Proceedings of the Royal Society of Medicine,* 65 (1972):1099–1108.

28. KULLBERG, G. "Differences in Effect of Capsulotomy and Cingulotomy," in W. H. Sweet, S. Obrador, and J. G. Martin-Rodriguez, eds., *Neurosurgical Treatment in Psychiatry, Pain and Epilepsy.* Baltimore, Md.: University Park Press, 1977, pp. 301–308.

29. LEWIN, W. "Observations on Selective Leucotomy." *Journal of Neurology Neurosurgery, and Psychiatry,* 24 (1961):37–44.

30. LIVINGSTON, K. E. "Cingulate Cortex Isolation for the Treatment of Psychoses and Psychoneuroses," *Proceedings, Association for Research in Nervous and Mental Disease,* 21 (1951):374–378.

31. MACLEAN, P. D. "Psychosomatic Disease and the 'Visceral Brain'; Recent Developments Bearing on the Papez Theory of Emotion," *Psychosomatic Medicine,* 11 (1949):338–353.

32. ———. "Some Psychiatric Implications of Physiological Studies on Frontotemporal Portion of Limbic System (Visceral Brain)," *Electroencephalography and Clinical Neurophysiology* 4 (1952): 407–418.

33. ———. "Challenges of the Papez Heritage," in K. E. Livingston and D. Hornykiewicz, eds., *Limbic Mechanisms.* New York: Plenum Press, 1978, pp. 1–15.

34. MONIZ, E. *Tentatives Operatoires Dans le Traitement de Certaines Psychoses.* Paris: Masson & Cie, 1936.

35. NAUTA, W. J. H. "Hippocampal Projections and Related Neural Pathways to the Midbrain in the Cat," *Brain,* 81 (1958):319–340.

36. ———. "Connections of the Frontal Lobe with the Limbic System," in L. V. Laitinen and K. E. Livingston, eds., *Surgical Approaches in Psychiatry,* Baltimore, MD.: University Park Press, 1973, p. 303.

37. PAPEZ, J. W. "A Proposed Mechanism of Emotion," *Archives of Neurology and Psychiatry,* 38 (1937):725–743.

38. PRIBRAM, K. H., and FULTON, J. F. "An Experimental Critique of the Effects of Anterior Cingulate Ablations in the Monkey, *Brain,* 77 (1954):34–44.

39. RAMON Y CAJAL, S. *Studies on the Cerebral Cortex (Limbic Structures),* L. M. Kraft, transl. London: Lloyd-Luke Ltd., 1955.

40. RESEARCH COMMITTEE, ROYAL COLLEGE OF PSYCHIATRISTS. "Evaluation of the Surgical Treatment of Functional Mental Illness: Proposal for a Prospective Controlled Trial," in W. H. Sweet, S. Obrador, and J. G. Martin-Rodriguez, eds., *Neurosurgical Treatment in Psychiatry, Pain and Epilepsy.* Baltimore, Md.: University Park Press, 1977, pp. 175–188.

41. RICHARDSON, A. "Stereotactic Limbic Leucotomy: Surgical Technique," *Postgraduate Medical Journal,* 49 (1973): 860–864.

42. SCOVILLE, W. B., and BETTIS, D. B. "Results of Orbital Undercutting Today: A Personal Series," in W. H. Sweet, S. Obrador, and J. G. Martin-Rodriguez, eds., *Neurosurgical Treatment in Psychiatry, Pain and Epilepsy.* Baltimore, Md.: University Park Press, 1977, pp. 189–202.

43. SHUTTS, D. *Lobotomy: Resort to the Knife.* New York: Van Nostrand Reinhold, 1982.

44. STROM-OLSEN, R., and CARLISLE, S. "Bifrontal Stereotactic Tractotomy: A Follow-up Study of Its Effect on 210 Patients," *British Journal of Psychiatry,* 118 (1971):141–154.

45. SYKES, M. K., and TREDGOLD, R. F. "Restricted Orbital Undercutting: A Study of Its Effects on 350 Patients Over Ten Years, 1951–1960," *British Journal of Psychiatry,* 110 (1964): 609–640.

46. TOOTH, G. C., and NEWTON, M. P. *Leucotomy in England and Wales 1942–1954.* Reports on Public Health and Medical Subjects No. 104, Ministry of Health, London: Her Majesty's Stationery Office, 1961.

CHAPTER 35

A CRITICAL REVIEW OF THE USE OF LABORATORY TESTS IN PSYCHIATRIC DISORDERS

Stephen M. Stahl and Kerry D. Kravitz

¶ **Introduction and Overview of Diagnostic Tests in Psychiatry**

Introductory Comments

The purposes of this chapter are several-fold: to provide a conceptual framework within which to define the clinical usefulness of diagnostic laboratory tests in psychiatric practice; to clarify the common statistical concepts used in the literature; and to summarize briefly the literature with respect to the current state of the art for several specific diagnostic tests. We are not attempting to comprehensively review the literature for each diagnostic test under investigation in psychiatry.

We preface our remarks with the caveat that we remain largely ignorant of the mol-ecular basis for neurobiological dysfunction in mental illness. Currently, laboratory tests in psychiatry are predominantly exploratory, hypothesis-generating research tools. Pragmatic, empirical applications of research tools as clinical laboratory tests are, in fact, just beginning to emerge in the practice of psychiatry. This chapter attempts to review laboratory parameters that link neurobiology and mental illness and to critique these parameters from the perspective of their potential application as clinical laboratory tests in psychiatry. As of 1985, the state of the art in this field is still quite primitive, and future advances will require enhanced knowledge of the neurobiological basis of mental illness. Nevertheless, it may be timely to assess the status of contemporary laboratory research tools, since their implementation as clinical laboratory tests would be expected to dramatically alter the practice of modern clinical psychiatry.

Clinical Applications of Laboratory Tests

A laboratory test may be used to: (1) clarify a diagnosis; (2) rule out certain disorders; (3) make decisions about the need to embark upon further work-up; (4) aid in treatment decisions; (5) predict prognosis; (6) screen for disease in a given population; (7) monitor the effects of treatment; and (8) predict increased risk of developing a disease at some future time.[115,142] While these uses are not mutually exclusive, it is clear that a laboratory test may be appropriate for one use but lack utility for another. For example, the oral glucose tolerance test has been used to detect occult diabetes but has no practical use in the management of patients with overt diabetes.

Prior to ordering a laboratory test, clinicians should have some idea of the cost of the test, both in terms of money and, more important, in terms of risk to the patient, and the context in which they plan to use the test. For example, a test used for screening purposes should have a relatively low cost, low risk, and high sensitivity. Clinicians should also have an estimate of the probability of a false negative and false positive test; know the *a priori* probability that the disease is present in a given patient (e.g., see the discussion on the exercise electrocardiogram in the next section and in the DST general considerations section); and know the risk to the patient of making a decision based on a false negative or a false positive test.

Statistical Concepts for Laboratory Tests

In addition to these considerations, there are statistical concepts that help to determine the usefulness of a diagnostic test.[20,115] These are the sensitivity, specificity, and predictive value of a given test. *Sensitivity* is defined as the probability of a positive test result in an individual with a given disease.

Specificity is the probability of a negative test result in an individual who does not have the disease. *Positive predictive value* is defined as the percentage of all positive results that are true positives. The predictive value is a function of sensitivity, specificity, and prevalence of the disease.

Some warnings about these useful concepts are in order. First, these concepts are defined in certain populations, whereas clinicians deal with decisions regarding individuals. It may be problematic to use probabilistic data to make clinical decisions in individual patients. While probabilistic concepts lend themselves well to populations, they are more difficult to use when a decision must be made for an individual patient. Furthermore, even if the sensitivity and specificity of a diagnostic test is known with certainty, some important clinical variables that are difficult to quantify must be considered in the decision-making process. For example, what is the risk to the patient of a false positive or a false negative test? What is the added cost versus benefit of additional increments of certainty in making a diagnosis?

Second, the estimates of sensitivity, specificity, and predictive value will vary depending on the population studied. Therefore, in examining research studies that attempt to estimate these parameters, it is essential that clinicians pay attention to the criteria defining the population that was studied, in order to assess whether those estimates are appropriate for an individual patient being seen in clinical practice. For example, the exercise electrocardiogram (ECG) has been shown to have the highest rate of false positives in the population of patients who have the lowest *a priori* probability of having coronary artery disease.[289] To rephrase this observation in terms of the population of high-risk individuals, the conclusions seem obvious: namely, those at greatest risk for coronary artery disease have the lowest rate of false positive results on the exercise ECG. Thus a positive exercise ECG is most informative in that population of patients whose diagnosis is the most certain.

Third, in most statistical studies, populations are defined by one or, at most, several parameters. Clinicians, on the other hand, must take into account many variables. Hence the estimates of sensitivity, specificity, and predictive value cannot be the only considerations in assessing the utility of a clinical test as applied at the bedside.

Fourth, sensitivity and specificity refer to tests that are dichotomous—that is, yes/no or positive/negative—rather than continuous. Frequently clinicians must make decisions based on the use of a continuous variable. An example is blood glucose. Although patients with glucose of 175 and 1,075 both have "abnormal" values, these two abnormal values have quite different implications for diagnosis, treatment, and prognosis.

Finally, in order to have meaning, the measure of sensitivity of a test must be compared with a measure that is more sensitive. To return to the example of the exercise ECG, the sensitivity and specificity can be estimated only because there is a more sensitive and specific test, namely, coronary angiography. Such is not the case when psychiatric diagnoses are considered. There are widely divergent theories about the etiology and treatment of various psychiatric disorders. For the most part, our diagnostic categories are simply syndromes, since we lack precise knowledge of the pathophysiology of most disorders.

Psychiatric Nosology and Laboratory Tests

In considering the clinical utility of any test, we must unfortunately touch upon the thorny problem of nosology in psychiatry. The advantages and disadvantages of DSM-III have been debated elsewhere,[165] and we are not attempting to add further considerations to the controversy. However, several comments are in order. In order to put this question in perspective, it may be helpful to consider the manner in which clinical knowledge has evolved in branches of medicine other than psychiatry. We acknowledge that there are those involved in the treatment of the mentally ill who sense the limitations of the medical model as applied to psychiatry. We are not attempting to argue that point here. In general, however, clinicians in other specialties of medicine have begun with an observation that several symptoms and/or signs are frequently associated as a syndrome. Examples in clinical medicine are abundant: symptoms of diabetes include polyuria, polydipsia, and polyphagia; symptoms of pneumonitis include fever, cough, sputum, and pleuritic chest pain. Research leads to the subdivision of the syndrome into various etiologies. In general, then, syndromes represent a heterogeneous collection of diseases leading to a given symptom cluster. Returning to the pneumonitis example, the aforementioned symptoms may have been caused by a variety of etiologies, each of which has very different treatment implications. Furthermore, even if a specific diagnosis of pneumonia is made, which is reaffirmed by diagnostic tests, the clinician will ask why the patient contracted the pneumonia. Is the patient already debilitated from some chronic disease such as congestive heart failure? Or perhaps the development of pneumonia in an otherwise apparently healthy individual is the first sign of obstruction of the airway from an occult carcinoma. Hence the process of diagnosis is an iterative one, and there is no ultimate "diagnosis." In other words, when one arrives at a diagnosis, one may still ask why and how the pathological process started.

Thus the process of research in medicine has been one that begins with an association of symptoms and signs (a syndrome) and moves toward more specific understanding of etiology, treatment, and prognosis. Similarly, biological tests in psychiatry may eventually lead to a subtyping of depression, psychoses, and other disorders that have specific etiologic and treatment implications, in an analogous manner to the specificity of sputum culture in pneumonia. At present, however, our diagnostic categories reflect syndromes and lack that specificity. As a result, there is frequently confusion about whether diagnoses reflect transient states or enduring traits.[189]

There is likely to be heterogeneity in many of the psychiatric diagnostic categories as well as overlap between diagnoses. In addition, there is frequently confusion about the precise meaning of certain terms. Current psychiatric diagnoses are full of examples. One example is the term endogenous, which has been used in at least two different ways to describe depression. The first is defined as a lack of precipitating factors. This corresponds to the standard English usage of the term, meaning that the depression developed from within. This is contrasted with neurotic or secondary depressions, which are attributed to characterological problems or to other diagnoses that may precede or cause the depression. The term endogenous is also used to denote the lack of reactivity of depressive symptoms once they are established. The first usage implies an etiology; the second denotes a certain clinical picture or set of symptoms. It is important to distinguish between these two meanings and to avoid the assumption that all those patients who have a clinical picture of depression with pervasive loss of pleasure and lack of reactivity to normally pleasurable activities also lack characterological, environmental, or other precipitants to their depression. In such cases, the term endogenomorphic has been suggested[164] in order to avoid that confusion. Nosology and terminology will probably continue to create confusion until etiologies are known and are capable of being validated by laboratory tests.

Types of Laboratory Tests in Psychiatry

In this chapter we confine our comments to biochemical laboratory tests in three general categories: neuroendocrine tests, biochemical tests of biogenic amines and their metabolites, and biochemical tests of enzymes and receptors for neurotransmitters. Neuroendocrine studies (see table 35–1) are based on the ability to assay serum hormones whose concentrations are regulated by central nervous system (CNS) neurons. Thus changes in the concentrations of serum hormones in response to diseases or to provocation with drugs can be an index of the functioning of their CNS regulatory neurons. The neurotransmitter biogenic amines and their metabolites (see table 35–2) can be assayed in a number of body fluids (blood, urine, and cerebrospinal fluid [CSF]) from patients. These studies attempt to demonstrate abnormalities in the production of a number of CNS neurotransmitters in patients with psychiatric disorders by directly sampling the neurotransmitters or their metabolites in body fluids. Neurotransmitter enzymes and receptors (see table 35–3) are present in peripheral tissues that can be sampled in psychiatric patients. In those cases in which platelets, lymphocytes, red blood cells, or fibroblasts contain the same neurotransmitter enzyme or receptor as CNS neurons, the peripheral tissue can serve as a potential model for the same enzyme or receptor in the CNS. Other potential laboratory tests such as sleep physiology, structural and metabolic brain imaging, serum drug levels, and others are reviewed elsewhere in this volume.

¶ Neuroendocrine Tests

Dexamethasone Suppression Test— General Considerations

The dexamethasone suppression test (DST) is one of the most thoroughly investigated diagnostic laboratory tests in psychiatry. Yet its utility in clinical psychiatry is hotly debated.[19,66,146,153]

The evidence linking depression and neuroendocrine abnormalities dates back to Thomas Addison, who was the first to describe an association of adrenal insufficiency and depressive symptoms. In the late 1950s a number of investigators began to measure serum and urinary cortisol in depressed patients.* Initial studies regarded cortisol elevations as a nonspecific response to stress.[181,236,242] Sachar and associates mea-

*See references 39,40,121,236,239, and 240.

TABLE 35–1
Proposed Neuroendocrine Laboratory Tests in Clinical Psychiatry

Proposed Test	Proposed Clinical Application
Dexamethasone suppression test (DST)	Depression, (diagnosis, prognosis, treatment)
Thyrotropin-releasing hormone (TRH) stimulation test	Depression (diagnosis)
Growth hormone	Depression (diagnosis, treatment responses)
Prolactin	Depression, schizophrenia (diagnosis, treatment responses)

TABLE 35–2
Proposed Biochemical Laboratory Tests of Neurotransmitters and Their Metabolites in Clinical Psychiatry

Neurotransmitter/Metabolite	Body Fluid	Proposed Clinical Application
NE (norepinephrine)	CSF	Depression (diagnosis)
MHPG (3-methoxy-4-hydroxy-phenylethyleneglycol)	CSF, serum, urine	Depression (diagnosis, treatment response)
5HT (serotonin)	CSF, platelet	Schizophrenia, infantile autism, mental retardation
5-HIAA (5-hydroxyindoleacetic acid)	CSF	Depression (diagnosis, suicidal behavior, treatment response); schizophrenia (diagnosis)
Epinephrine	CSF	Schizophrenia (diagnosis)
Endorphins	CSF	Schizophrenia (diagnosis)
HVA (homovanillic acid)	CSF, serum	Schizophrenia (diagnosis, treatment response)

TABLE 35–3
Proposed Laboratory Tests of Neurotransmitter Enzymes and Receptors from Peripheral Models in Clinical Psychiatry

Neurotransmitter Enzyme Receptor	Peripheral Tissue	Proposed Clinical Application
MAO (monoamine oxidase)	Platelet, fibroblast	Schizophrenia (diagnosis); depression (monitoring MAO inhibition)
5HT (serotonin) uptake	Platelet	Depression (diagnosis, genetics, treatment response)
^{3}H-IMI (^{3}H-imipramine) binding sites	Platelet	Depression (diagnosis, suicide behavior)
Alpha-2 adrenergic receptors	Platelet	Depression (diagnosis, treatment response)
Beta-adrenergic receptors	Lymphocyte, fibroblast	Depression (diagnosis, treatment response)
NE-stimulated adenylate cyclase	Lymphocyte fibroblast	Depression (diagnosis, treatment response)
Na^+/K^+-ATPase (Sodium-potassium adenosine triphosphatase)	Red blood cells	Mania, depression, obesity
COMT (catechol-O-methyl-transferase)	Red blood cells, fibroblast	Depression
Muscarinic cholinergic receptors	Red blood cells, fibroblast	Depression (diagnosis, genetics)

sured serum cortisol every twenty minutes for twenty-four hours and found that depressed patients tended to have higher cortisol spikes than controls, along with blunting of the normal diurnal pattern.[243] Meanwhile, the search was underway for less cumbersome tests to use as a biologic marker for depression.

The overnight DST was initially used as a screening test to rule out the diagnosis of Cushing's syndrome.[89,210,221] Nearly two decades ago, several independent investigators applied it to depression.* Since these preliminary studies with the DST, there has been a proliferation of investigations into its utility in assessing diagnosis, treatment, course of illness, and prognosis in depressed patients.

Detailed reviews of the literature on the DST in depression may be found elsewhere.† We shall briefly summarize the literature with respect to considerations of clinical utility, and we shall avoid speculation about pathophysiological implications. The pathophysiology of dexamethasone nonsuppression in endogenous depression has not yet been clarified.[146]

Carroll and associates have suggested a standardization of the DST.[72] On day one 1.0 mg dexamethasone is given orally at 11 or 11:30 P.M. On day two plasma samples are collected at 4 P.M. and 11 P.M. A cortisol value greater than 5 μg per dl in either sample is defined as a positive or abnormal result. A variation of this standardization consists of one sample obtained at 4 P.M. or two samples obtained at 8 A.M. and 4 P.M. Some investigators have used doses of 2 mg or, less commonly, 0.5 mg dexamethasone. Abnormal DST means nonsuppression. Since abnormal DST is also referred to as "positive DST," confusion has resulted about the terms nonsuppression and positive DST; both have come to mean an abnormal DST.

Differing laboratory assays are available for determination of cortisol. Colorimetric and fluorometric methods are not recommended because they generally yield higher cortisol values than competitive protein binding (CPB) or radioimmunoassay (RIA). The accuracy of the CPB and RIA is decreased in the lower range of cortisol values (0–5 μg/dl). Therefore, post-dexamethasone cortisol values in the 3 to 7 μg per dl range need to be interpreted with caution.[66,185]

The DST is generally considered to be a specific test (92 to 100 percent) for the diagnosis of endogenous depression or melancholia.[65,132,136] Table 35–4 shows the average rate of DST nonsuppression in normal controls to be 7 percent. This confirms a high specificity in that population. Recent reports, however, have begun to question its specificity in populations of patients with other psychiatric diagnoses.[86,275]

The sensitivity has been estimated to be only about 45 percent.[65,132,136] The predictive value has varied depending on the population studied (see discussion in the next section).[252] Recall that the positive predictive value depends not only on the specificity, which may vary with the population studied, but also on the prevalence of the disease in the population studied.

The DST is a state-dependent variable.* In other words, the DST tends to normalize before or concurrent with clinical improvement. Other variables that are known to affect the DST are given in table 35–5. Age was initially not considered to affect the DST[72,250,284]; however, more recent studies suggest otherwise.[9,95,215,261] The increase in DST nonsuppression in elderly patients may be a factor in the high incidence of positive DST in demented patients (see table 35–14).[132] Any drugs that stimulate the hepatic microsomal enzyme system, such as barbiturates or anticonvulsants, may cause a positive DST because of an acceleration in the rate of degradation of dexamethasone.[66] Severe illness, infection, pregnancy, Cushing's disease, uncontrolled diabetes, alcohol withdrawal, or recent heavy alcohol intake may cause a positive DST in the absence of depression.[66]

*See references 59,69,120,273, and 274.
†See references 19,65,66,77,132,136,146,153,235,252, and 283.

*See references 6,55,67,101,131,211,217,278, and 301.

TABLE 35–4
Rates of Dexamethasone Nonsuppression in Normal Controls

Study	N^{+a}	N^b	$\%^{+c}$
Amsterdam, Winokur, and Caroff [10]	2	22	9
Amsterdam et al.[11]	8	53	15
Carroll et al.[72]	3	70	4
Charles et al.[77]	0	11	0
Coppen et al.[86]	9	79	11
Holsboer, Doerr, and Sippell[148]	0	10	0
Nuller and Ostroumova[211]	8	85	9
Peselow et al.[222]	2	49	4
Raskind et al.[228]	0	15	0
Rothschild et al.[234]	1	31	3
Schatzberg et al.[246]	1	31	3
Schlesser, Winokur, and Sherman[249]	0	80	0
Stokes et al.[275]	8	77	10
Winokur et al.[292]	4	24	17
TOTAL	46	637	7

[a] The number of normal controls in each study who showed positive DST (nonsuppression).
[b] The total number of normal controls in each study.
[c] The percentage of positive DST in normal controls in each study.

TABLE 35–5
Conditions Affecting the Dexamethasone Suppression Test

False Positive	False Negative
Pregnancy	Pituitary, adrenal disease
Cushing's syndrome	Steroids
Alcohol withdrawal	High-dose benzodiazepine treatment
Severe weight loss	High-dose cyproheptadine treatment
Severe illness:	Indomethacin
advanced carcinoma	
congestive heart failure	
traumas	
infection	
dehydration	
uncontrolled diabetes	
cerebrovascular accident	
Obesity	
Temporal lobe epilepsy	
Anorexia nervosa	
Neuroleptic withdrawal	
Dementia	
Medications:	
high-dose estrogens	
narcotics	
sedative hypnotics	
anticonvulsants	
spironolactone	

An abnormal DST has been reported in 52 percent of a sample of twenty-five stroke patients.[110] All of the DST nonsuppressors in that study had some depressive symptoms of mood, sleep, and/or appetite disturbance.

Weight loss[30,66,102,165] and obesity also predispose toward DST nonsuppression.[89] Recent reports suggest the possibility that neuroleptic withdrawal may cause DST nonsuppression.[97,98] False negative results may be caused by high-dose benzodiazepine therapy, steroids, and high-dose cyproheptadine treatment, as well as by pituitary or adrenal disease.[66] Indomethacin has also been reported to cause a false negative DST.[182]

Most of the studies of the DST have involved inpatients. The sensitivity of the DST in an outpatient population has been found to be lower than that found in inpatients. This finding may be an artifact of the sampling procedure, since inpatient protocols have generally sampled post-dexamethasone cortisol at 4 P.M. and 11 P.M., while outpatient studies have generally sampled only at 4 P.M.[72] Incidence of DST nonsuppression has not been found to correlate with severity of depression.[132]

It is clear that the DST is not a useful screening test for identification of patients with endogenous depression in the general population. Because of the low sensitivity, many endogenously depressed individuals have a false negative DST. Furthermore, in a general population in which the incidence of depression is relatively low, the predictive value of the DST would be low in spite of a high specificity. Because of the high probability of a false negative, the DST cannot be used to rule out major depression. Approximately one-half of those with the diagnosis of major depressive episode have a negative DST. That percentage of false negatives is higher in an outpatient sample. Nonetheless, a positive DST increases the diagnostic certainty. Exactly what that means from a clinical point of view remains open to question, because endogenous depression is a syndrome, not a disease with a known etiology, and the relationship of the DST to clinical response is not clear (i.e., do DST nonsuppressors respond differently to treatment than suppressors?).

In order to explicate these issues, we return now to a common example in clinical practice in internal medicine, the exercise ECG. By comparing and contrasting the exercise ECG to the DST, we may shed some light upon the crucial questions regarding the clinical utility of the DST, as well as illuminate the directions in which the DST may go in the future.

Endogenous depression (Research Diagnostic Criteria)[263] or melancholia (DSM-III)[8] is a syndrome, analogous to the syndrome of angina pectoris. As mentioned previously, the exercise ECG has been used to increase the diagnostic certainty of the diagnosis of coronary artery disease as an etiology of the anginal chest pain. The diagnosis of coronary artery disease may also be confirmed by coronary angiography, which essentially provides a "picture" of the coronary artery lesions that may account for the symptom of chest pain. Hence angiography is a more sensitive and specific test for coronary artery disease than is the exercise ECG. Furthermore, the estimates of sensitivity and specificity of the exercise ECG are based on results of angiography, which either confirm or rule out that diagnosis.

This is not the case with regard to the DST, for which estimates of sensitivity and specificity are only based on the presence of a syndrome. This would be equivalent to estimating sensitivity of the exercise ECG by counting how many individuals with angina pectoris have a positive exercise ECG. Those with classical angina pectoris have a greater frequency of positive exercise ECGs than those with atypical chest pain,[289] and so a positive exercise ECG may confirm the "diagnosis" of angina pectoris. If so, is there any clinical utility to that observation? It is clear that coronary artery disease is one cause of anginal chest pain and that those with classical angina are more likely to have coronary artery disease than those with atypical chest pain. In spite of this clear relationship, it would create confusion to equate angina pec-

TABLE 35-6

Rates of Dexamethasone Nonsuppression in Bipolar Versus Unipolar Depression

Study	Bipolar			Unipolar		
	$N+^a$	N^b	$\%+^c$	$N+^a$	N^b	$\%+^c$
Amsterdam et al.[11]	5	17	29	10	41	24
Berger et al.[29]	2	8	25	3	12	25
Carroll[66]	24	42	57	36	61	59
Charles et al.[78]	2	3	67	7	9	78
Kasper and Beckman[161]	5	11	45	17	31	55
Mendlewicz, Charles, and Franckson[191]	19	25	76	24	29	82
Papakostas et al.[217]	0	4	0	14	20	70
Rothschild et al.[234]	1	8	13	10	14	71
Schatzberg et al.[246]	7	20	35	28	45	62
Schlesser, Winokur, and Sherman[250]	28	33	85	65	146	45
Sternbach, Gwirtsman, and Gerner[272]	1	3	33	7	11	64
Stokes et al.[275]	10	37	27	25	74	34
TOTAL	104	211	49	246	493	50

[a]The number of unipolar and bipolar depressed patients in each study who showed positive DST (nonsuppression).
[b]The total number of unipolar and bipolar depressed patients in each study.
[c]The percentage of positive DST in normal controls in each study.

toris and coronary artery disease or to use the two terms synonymously.

Endogenous depression, unlike coronary artery disease, is not a specific diagnosis. Further research may lead to more precise understanding of pathophysiology of depression and revision of nosology, but at present it is not clearly understood. Therefore, the practical applicability of increased diagnostic certainty remains questionable. The applicability of the DST in differential diagnosis is explored further in the next section.

Dexamethasone Suppression Test as an Aid in Differential Diagnosis, Prognosis, and Therapy of Depression

The rate of positive DST has been examined in various subtypes of depression: unipolar versus bipolar (see table 35–6); endogenous versus nonendogenous (see table 35–7); primary versus secondary (see table 35–8); and familial versus sporadic (see table 35–9). These tables should be interpreted with caution, because many variables were not uniform across these studies. These include: (1) the dose of dexamethasone administered; (2) the number of post-dexamethasone blood samples obtained; (3) the time(s) at which the

samples were obtained; (4) the criteria defining a positive (abnormal) DST; (5) the type of laboratory assay used (colorimetric, fluorometric, competitive protein binding, or RIA); (6) the diagnostic criteria used to define the patient population; (7) the criteria used to exclude subjects from the study; and (8) the population studied.

The tables are thus provided to give an overview of the research in this area rather than to give precise and valid estimates of sensitivity and specificity. The rate of DST nonsuppression is similar in unipolar and bipolar endogenous depression (see table 35–6). Thus the DST cannot be used to distinguish between these two diagnostic categories. Furthermore, the validity of differentiating these two diagnostic categories has been questioned on the basis of the DST findings and the fact that the most prevalent psychiatric disorder found in probands of bipolar depressives is unipolar depression.[66] Most studies have found a low rate of nonsuppression in patients with mania. Patients with mixed mania and depression have a high rate of DST nonsuppression. These findings are in accord with the notion that DST is a state variable.

The results of the studies of DST have lent

TABLE 35-7

Rates of Dexamethasone Nonsuppression in Endogenous Versus Nonendogenous Depression

Study	Endogenous			Nonendogenous		
	$N+^a$	N^b	$\%+^c$	$N+^a$	N^b	$\%+^c$
Alexopoulous et al.[7]	41	73	56	—	—	—
Ames et al.[9,d]	11	28	39	19	62	31
Arana et al.[12]	6	15	40	8	14	57
Beeber et al.[26]	9	15	60	6	8	75
Berger et al.[29]	5	20	25	4	19	21
Brown and Shuey[55]	4	6	67	7	43	16
Brown, Johnston, and Mayfield[56]	8	20	40	—	—	—
Caroff et al.[62]	19	29	66	—	—	—
Carroll et al.[72,e]	92	215	43	1	100	1
Coppen et al.[86]	63	78	81	20	41	49
Dotti, Bersani, and Nocera[100]	0	10	100	10	10	100
Evans and Nemeroff[106]	4	4	100	7	12	58
Greden et al.[131]	21	31	68	—	—	—
Holsboer, Lieble, and Hofschuster[146]	5	10	50	2	10	20
Holsboer et al.[151,f]	14	59	24	5	34	15
Jaffe, Barnshaw, and Kennedy[156]	3	7	43	0	15	0
Kasper and Beckman[161]	21	41	51	6	26	23
Meltzer et al.[187,g]	6	20	30	4	6	67
Nasr et al.[200]	6	14	39	5	26	19
Nelson et al.[205]	5	28	18	—	—	—
Nuller and Ostroumova[211]	36	52	69	—	—	—
Papakostas et al.[217]	14	24	58	—	—	—
Peselow et al.[222]	13	52	25	7	36	19
Reus[230]	20	42	48	—	—	—
Rudorfer, Hwu, and Clayton[237,h]	13	31	42	—	—	—
Rush et al.[238]	13	32	41	2	38	5
Sherman, Pfohl, and Winokur[254]	5	15	33	3	10	30
Soloff, George, and Nathan[259,i]	3	8	38	0	6	0
Stokes et al.[275]	9	37	24	26	74	35
Targum, Rosen, and Capodanno[280]	23	49	47	—	—	—
Targum, Sullivan, and Byrnes[281]	23	54	43	—	—	—
TOTAL	515	1119	46	142	590	24

[a]The number of normal controls in each study who showed positive DST (nonsuppression).
[b]The total number of normal controls in each study.
[c]The percentage of positive DST in normal controls in each study.
[d]Diagnostic criteria unspecified.
[e]Endogenous depression defined by one of four sets of criteria: Research Diagnostic Criteria,[261] *International Classification of Diseases,* Newcastle Scale,[60] or DSM-III melancholia.[8]
[f]DST dose: 2 mg.
[g]Includes schizo-affective depressed.
[h]Criterion for +DST: cortisol > 3 µg per dl.
[i]Includes patients with borderline personality disorder.

support to the notion of differentiating between endogenous and nonendogenous depression.[66,132] "Endogenous" is used here to denote a pervasive lack of pleasure and lack of reactivity, as in the DSM-III subtype of melancholia. Carroll reports a 43 percent rate of DST nonsuppression in melancholic (endogenous) depressed patients, while only 1 percent of nonendogenously depressed patients had a positive DST.[66] Table 35-7 shows that across studies the sensitivity is 48 percent, close to that reported by Carroll. However, the average rate of DST nonsuppression in nonendogenously depressed patients is higher (25 percent) than that reported by Carroll.

TABLE 35–8

Rates of Dexamethasone Nonsuppression in Primary Versus Secondary Depression

Study	Endogenous			Nonendogenous		
	$N+^a$	N^b	$\%+^c$	$N+^a$	N^b	$\%+^c$
Berger et al.[29]	8	36	22	1	9	11
Brawley[44]	32	49	65	—	—	—
Brown and Qualls[54]	18	39	46	—	—	—
Brown and Shuey[55]	9	18	50	2	31	6
Brown, Johnston, and Mayfield[56]	8	16	50	1	4	25
Charles et al.[77]	8	14	57	2	15	13
Charles et al.[78]	9	12	75	1	7	14
Coryell, Gaffney, and Burkhardt[88]	19	69	28	1	24	4
Davis et al.[94]	25	42	60	—	—	—
Evans and Nemeroff[106]	15	21	71	1	7	14
Extein, Pottash, and Gold[107]	25	50	50	—	—	—
Greden et al.[131]	21	31	68	—	—	—
Meltzer et al.[187]	6	17	35	—	—	—
Mendlewicz, Charles, and Franckson[191,d]	43	54	79	9	41	21
Nasrallah and Coryell[201]	7	17	41	0	5	0
Papakostas et al.[217]	14	24	58	0	16	0
Rudorfer, Hwu, and Clayton[237]	13	31	41	—	—	—
Rush et al.[238]	10	58	17	5	12	42
Schlesser, Winokur, and Sherman[250]	93	179	52	0	42	0
Sherman, Pfohl, and Winokur[252]	8	25	32	—	—	—
Targum, Rosen, and Capodanno[280]	23	49	47	—	—	—
Winokur et al.[292]	4	26	15	—	—	—
TOTAL	418	877	48	23	213	11

[a]The number of normal controls in each study who showed positive DST (nonsuppression).
[b]The total number of normal controls in each study.
[c]The percentage of positive DST in normal controls in each study.
[d]Does not include those with schizo-affective disorder.

Table 35–8 summarizes the data for DST in primary versus secondary depression. Those with primary depression are much more likely (58 percent) to be DST nonsuppressors than those with secondary depression (11 percent).

There is disagreement about whether the DST differentiates between familial depressive disease and sporadic depression (see table 35–9). Two studies have shown that in those with familial pure depressive disease,[291] there is a higher incidence of DST nonsuppression than in those with depressive spectrum disease or sporadic depressive disease.[88,250] However, other reports have failed to confirm that observation.

The DST has been studied in patients with various psychiatric disorders other than endogenous depression. Carroll notes that the rate of positive DST in syndromes related to depression (e.g., schizo-affective disorder, catatonia, and depressed patients with borderline personality disorder) is similar to that seen in depressed inpatients.[38,65,126] Table 35–10 shows the rate of DST nonsuppression in patients with borderline personality disorder. Sixty-three percent of depressed borderline patients have positive DST (nonsuppression), as compared with only 18 percent of nondepressed borderline patients.

There have also been reports of DST nonsuppression in schizophrenia (see table 35–11), mania (see table 35–12), alcoholism (see table 35–13), dementia (see table 35–14), anorexia nervosa,[99,119] bulimia,[137] obsessive compulsive disorder,[154] and agoraphobia with panic attacks.[90,253] Thus the specificity of the DST in these populations may differ from that found in populations of normal controls.

TABLE 35–9

Rates of Dexamethasone Nonsuppression in Familial Pure Depressive Disease (FPDD),
Depressive Spectrum Disease (DSD), and Sporadic Depressive Disease (SDD)

Study	FPDD			DSD			SDD		
	$N+$[a]	N[b]	$\%+$[c]	$N+$[a]	N[b]	$\%+$[c]	$N+$[a]	N[b]	$\%+$[c]
Amsterdam, et al.[11]	2	16	13	1	7	14	6	24	25
Carroll et al.[70]	1	2	50	5	6	83	4	5	80
Coryell, Gaffney, and Burkhardt[88]	8	11	73	4	15	27	8	21	38
Fleming et al.[112]	13	28	46	8	17	47	12	32	38
Kasper and Beckman[161]	2	6	33	0	3	0	12	22	55
Mendlewicz, Charles, and Franckson[191]	6	7	85	2	3	67	16	19	84
Rudorfer, Hwu, and Clayton[237]	1	6	17	5	15	33	6	9	67
Rush et al.[238]	7	23	30	2	14	14	1	22	5
Schlesser, Winokur, and Sherman[250]	38	50	76	3	41	7	24	55	44
TOTAL	78	149	52	30	121	25	89	209	43

[a] The number of normal controls in each study who showed positive DST (nonsuppression).
[b] The total number of normal controls in each study.
[c] The percentage of positive DST in normal controls in each study.

The question of specificity becomes further clouded when considering the fact that depression may coexist with other psychiatric disorders. In addition, it is often difficult to distinguish between syndromes with similar symptoms, for example, schizo-affective depressed versus psychotic depression versus schizophrenia with negative symptoms. Table 35–11 shows similar rates of DST nonsuppression in depressed schizophrenic patients ($^7/_{23}$ = 30 percent), schizo-affective depressed patients ($^8/_{21}$ = 38 percent), and schizophrenic patients with negative symptoms ($^8/_{25}$ = 32 percent). In contrast, in those schizophrenic patients without symptoms of depression, the rate of DST nonsuppression is 13 percent. This includes some studies that did not specify whether depressive or negative symptoms were absent. Preliminary reports[97,98] suggest that neuroleptic withdrawal may cause DST nonsuppression. The extent to which neuroleptic withdrawal accounts for DST nonsuppression in this population deserves further study.

The rate of DST nonsuppression in patients with mania shows considerable variability, ranging from zero percent to 88 percent (see table 35–12). This variability may in part be due to some methodological differences noted earlier (e.g., different dexamethasone dose and criteria for positive DST). Another factor is that DST nonsuppression may precede or follow the onset of depressive symptoms by about one week.[130] Therefore, DST nonsuppression in this population may represent an imminent switch to depression.[66]

Interpretation of DST nonsuppression in alcoholics (see table 35–13) may be complicated by several factors. Depression, alcohol withdrawal, and abnormal liver function, all of which predispose to DST nonsuppression, are common in this population. Table 35–13 shows little difference in rate of positive DST between alcoholic patients abstinent less than three weeks (21 percent) and those abstinent longer than three weeks (15 percent). However, one study[86] did not specify whether the patients were free of depressive symptoms or whether their liver function tests were normal. Excluding that study, only three of eighty-three (4 percent) alcoholic patients who were abstinent at least three weeks had an abnormal DST.

The high rate of DST nonsuppression in demented patients (see table 35–14) is difficult to interpret for several reasons: (1) depression and dementia may coexist; (2) depression may present with cognitive deficits that remit along with depressive symptoms;

TABLE 35–10

Rates of Dexamethasone Nonsuppression in Borderline Personality Disorder

Study	With Depression			Without Depression		
	$N+^a$	N^b	$\%+^c$	$N+^a$	N^b	$\%+^c$
Baxter et al.[25,d]	18	19	95	1	20	5
Beeber et al.[26]	8	13	62	—	—	—
Carroll et al.[71]	8	13	62	5	8	63
Soloff, George, and Nathan[259]	3	14	21	0	5	0
TOTAL	37	59	63	6	33	18

[a]The number of normal controls in each study who showed positive DST (nonsuppression).
[b]The total number of normal controls in each study.
[c]The percentage of positive DST in normal controls in each study.
[d]Depressed group includes those with diagnosis of schizo-affective disorder.

TABLE 35–11

Rates of Dexamethasone Nonsuppression in Schizophrenia

Study	Without Depression[a]			With Depression[b]		
	$N+^c$	N^d	$\%+^e$	$N+^c$	N^d	$\%+^e$
Abou-Saleh, Miller, and Coppen[3]	—	—	9	—	—	32
Arana et al.[12]	1	9	11			
Brown, Johnston, and Mayfield[56]	0	8	0			
Carman et al.[60]			46			
Castro et al.[75]	7	23	30			
Charles et al.[77]	0	4	0			
Coppen et al.[86]	2	21	10	8	25	32
Dewan et al.[98]	6	20	30			
Holsboer et al.[151]	1	9	11			
Meltzer et al.[187]	2	5	40	6	16	38
Munro, Hardiker, and Leonard[195]	0	23	0	7	23	30
Myers[198,f]	11	55	20			
Papakostas et al.[217]	0	6	0			
Rothschild et al.[234]	2	14	14			
Schlesser, Winokur, and Sherman[250]	0	48	0			
Sternbach, Gwirtsman, and Gerner[272]				2	5	40
Stokes et al.[275]	2	12	17			
TOTAL	34	257	13	23	69	33

[a]Includes studies that did not specify whether the patients had any depressive or negative symptoms.
[b]Includes studies of schizo-affective depressed patients,[187,272] depressed schizophrenic patients,[195] and schizophrenic patients with negative symptoms, flat affect, impoverished speech, diminished drive.[86]
[c]The number of normal controls in each study who showed positive DST (nonsuppression).
[d]The total number of normal controls in each study.
[e]The percentage of positive DST in normal controls in each study.
[f]Five nondepressed schizophrenic patients underwent eleven serial DSTs over a twelve-week period.

TABLE 35–12
Rates of Dexamethasone Nonsuppression in Mania

Study	$N+$[a]	N[b]	$\%+$[c]
Amsterdam et al.[11,d]	1	6	17
Arana et al.[12]	14	16	88
Carroll, Curtis, and Mendels[67,d]	0	1	0
Charles et al.[77]	0	7	0
Graham et al.[124,e]	23	50	46
Meltzer et al.[187]	0	3	0
Schlesser, Winokur, and Sherman[250]	0	61	0
Stokes et al.[275]	8	16	50
TOTAL	46	160	29

[a]The number of normal controls in each study who showed positive DST (nonsuppression).
[b]The total number of normal controls in each study.
[c]The percentage of positive DST in normal controls in each study.
[d]Bipolar, Hypomania Criterion for +DST: cortisol > 7.6 μg per dl.
[e]+DST based on post-dexamethasone cortisol > 3.6 μg per dl; dexamethasone dose: 2 mg.

TABLE 35–13
Rates of Dexamethasone Nonsuppression in Alcoholism

Study	Abstinent > 3 Weeks			Abstinent < 3 Weeks		
	$N+$[a]	N[b]	$\%+$[c]	$N+$[a]	N[b]	$\%+$[c]
Abou-Saleh, Miller, and Coppen[3,d]	—	—	9			
Brown, Johnston, and Mayfield[56]	0	10	0			
Coppen et al.[86,e]	20	72	28	—	—	—
Dackis et al.[91]	0	32	0			
Kroll, Palmer, and Greden[169,f]	1	22	5			
Newsom and Murray[207]	0	13	0	17	75	23
Swartz and Dunner[276,g]				6	28	21
Targum et al.[282]	2	6	33	16	83	19
TOTAL	23	155	15	39	186	21

[a]The number of normal controls in each study who showed positive DST (nonsuppression).
[b]The total number of normal controls in each study.
[c]The percentage of positive DST in normal controls in each study.
[d]Length of abstinence was not specified. Those with elevated LFTs were excluded, 53 percent of whom had +DST.
[e]Not specified whether depressive symptoms were present or whether liver function tests (LFTs) were normal.
[f]Three patients with DST nonsuppression were excluded because of elevated LFTs.
[g]Fifteen patients with elevated LFTs were excluded from the table, eight of whom had positive DST (nonsuppression).

TABLE 35–14
Rates of Dexamethasone Nonsuppression in Dementia

Study	$N+$[a]	N[b]	$\%+$[c]	Mean Age
Abou-Saleh, Millar, and Coppen[3]	21	45	47	—
Coppen et al.[86,d]	20	45	44	78
Raskind et al.[228,e]	7	15	47	64
Spar and Gerner[260,f]	9	17	53	72
TOTAL	57	122	47	

[a]The number of normal controls in each study who showed positive DST (nonsuppression).
[b]The total number of normal controls in each study.
[c]The percentage of positive DST in normal controls in each study.
[d]Not specified whether these patients were free of depressive symptoms.
[e]Zero of fifteen controls (mean age sixty-eight) had +DST.
[f]None met DSM-III[8] criteria for major depressive episode.

and (3) DST nonsuppression may increase as a function of age. Thus the utility of the DST in distinguishing depressive pseudodementia from dementia remains controversial.[141,228,260]

Now that the results of studies pertaining to differential diagnosis of an abnormal DST have been presented, let us consider the general state of the art of differential diagnosis in psychiatry. We do not argue that we must dispense with the medical model in psychiatry, but we do believe its limitations need to be stressed in order to clarify where we are and where we might eventually be in terms of making specific diagnoses. In clinical medicine, a differential diagnosis is a set of hypotheses regarding possible causes of a set of subjective complaints and objective findings in a given patient. Each of the possibilities in the differential has its own etiological and treatment implications. In depression, precise etiologies of various disorders have not been agreed upon in the same way as, for instance, pneumococcus has been as a cause of pneumonia. Thus, in assessing the clinical utility of the DST, the primary focus at this point must be upon treatment implications. Let us now turn to studies that consider the utility of the DST in the prediction of response to specific treatments and the prediction of prognosis, and for decisions about the long-term management of depressed patients.

Results are inconclusive regarding the use of DST to predict response to specific treatments. One study found nonsuppressors responded to imipramine hydrochloride and desipramine hydrochloride, but not to amitriptyline hydrochloride and clomipramine hydrochloride.[54] Another found nonsuppressors had better response to amitriptyline than to imipramine or desipramine.[44] Results are also conflicting about whether DST nonsuppressors are more likely[55,56,127,205] or less likely[179] to respond to treatment in general. Several studies show no difference in response rates between DST suppressors and nonsuppressors.[9,54,129,153,261] Nonsuppressors who subsequently revert to normal suppression have been shown to have a greater degree of clinical improvement than those who remain nonsuppressors.[131,132] Those patients whose depressive symptoms remit but whose DST remains abnormal may be at higher risk for relapse within six months.* However, it should be noted that occurrence of clinical improvement with continued DST nonsuppression is infrequent. Finally, preliminary studies suggest that DST may be useful in prediction of increased risk of suicide.†

In conclusion, the following guidelines may be offered regarding the DST. At present, it is easier to define inappropriate than appropriate uses. To begin with the former, the low sensitivity of the DST precludes its use as a means of ruling out endogenous depression. Because of the high rate of false negatives, it would be a mistake to withhold antidepressant medication solely on the basis of a negative DST. Furthermore, the DST is not useful as a screening test for depression in the general population for two reasons. The first is its low sensitivity, as previously mentioned. The second is that even with a high specificity, the predictive value of the test will be low because of the low prevalence of endogenous depression in the general population. Even if we estimate the population prevalence of depression to be 5 percent, with a specificity of 95 percent and a sensitivity of 60 percent, the positive predictive value would be 39 percent. In other words, nearly two-thirds of the positive tests would be false positives. This contrasts markedly to a psychiatric inpatient population, in which the positive predictive value would be 92 percent (assuming a prevalence of 50 percent for endogenous depression).

Although a positive DST is additional (and perhaps confirmatory) evidence for a diagnosis of endogenous depression (melancholia), it is unclear how that result should affect the initial treatment decision. There have been no consistent indications that a patient with endogenous depression and a positive DST is likely to respond better to one specific treat-

---

*See references 6, 122, 128, 131, 149, 150, 217, 233, and 279.
†See references 21, 65, 87, 98, 129, 280, and 300.

ment than another. Nor is it clear that a positive DST forecasts positive response to somatic treatments in general. Two preliminary studies do suggest, however, that patients with major depressive disorder and negative DSTs have a 50 percent response rate to placebo, while those with positive DSTs have a zero percent response rate to placebo.[54,118]

There is also evidence that DST normalization in a patient who initially was a nonsuppressor may be indicative of good prognosis and early remission. Furthermore, even in those patients who improve clinically, persistence of DST nonsuppression may signal poor prognosis, including a higher rate of suicide. Thus the DST continues to hold great promise for utility in clinical psychiatry. Current and future research must clarify several issues discussed in this section so that the transition from "interesting biological correlate" to "practical clinical laboratory test" may be accomplished. As such, the DST is the one laboratory test in psychiatry that is the farthest along in that transition process.

Thyrotropin-releasing Hormone Stimulation Test

Thyrotropin-releasing hormone (TRH) is a tripeptide found in the CNS and other tissues.[41,58,176] It is secreted by hypothalamic neurons into the portal venous system of the pituitary, where it stimulates the release of thyroid-stimulating hormone (TSH),[144,245] as well as prolactin[43] and growth hormone.[180] Norepinephrine (NE) stimulates and serotonin (5HT) inhibits release of TRH.

The TRH test consists of an injection of TRH followed by measurement of TSH. Standardization has been suggested as follows.[176] The patient should be drug-free for at least seven days and not malnourished. After fasting the night prior to the test, the patient, in a recumbent position, is administered 0.5 mg of TRH intravenously over one minute. TSH is measured prior to and thirty minutes after the TRH is given. A positive test is defined as a change in TSH of less than 5.0 µIU per ml.

Variables that affect the TRH test are age, renal function, nutritional status, repetitive administration of TRH,[176] and administration of any of the following: somatostatin, neurotensin, dopamine (DA), thyroid hormones, or glucocorticoids. Individuals with Klinefelter's syndrome have been noted to have blunted TSH response to TRH.

Clinical studies reviewed elsewhere[176] have shown blunting of response to TRH in depressed patients. However, this blunting is not specific to depression but is also found in alcoholism, mania, and anorexia nervosa. Schizophrenic patients do not show blunting of the TSH response to TRH. Further research in this area holds promise in elucidating a specific neuroendocrine defect in a subpopulation of depressed individuals. However, at present this test has no proven clinical utility. In fact, it is still unclear whether blunted response represents a state or a trait variable.[176]

Other Neuroendocrine Tests

DA and NE have been implicated in the control of human growth hormone (hGH) secretion.[81] hGH has been investigated as a neuroendocrine marker of a hypothesized noradrenergic abnormality in depression.[52,157]

Factors that influence hGH secretion include stress, sleep, prolonged fasting, arginine infusion, alteration of protein intake, excessive fatty acids, and changes in plasma glucose.[104] hGH release is also influenced by sex,[105,113] age,[140,223] oral contraception medication,[105] and phase of menstrual cycle.[104]

The hGH response to various stimuli has been studied in depressed patients. Depressed patients have been found to have a blunted hGH response to methylamphetamine,[80,82] clonidine,[83,183] 5-hydroxytryptophan,[277] and insulin-induced hypoglycemia.* Further research is needed to establish the clinical utility of these hGH stimulation tests and to clarify the complex interrelationships

*See references 63,64,73,103,133,134,194,225,241, and 244.

between psychiatric symptoms, neurotransmitter function, and endocrine parameters.

Prolactin has been studied in relation to schizophrenia, depression, and neuroleptic medication.[157] It is released from the anterior pituitary in response to sleep, stress, and estrogens. DA agonists and 5HT antagonists inhibit its release, while 5HT agonists, DA antagonists, and TRH stimulate secretion. Prolactin may eventually be used as an index of DA blockade to assess neuroleptic compliance and adequacy of a therapeutic trial. However, at present the clinical utility of prolactin has yet to be established. Neuroendocrine tests as research tools are reviewed elsewhere in this volume.

¶ Biogenic Amines and Their Metabolites in Blood, Urine, and Cerebrospinal Fluid

The biogenic amines are neurotransmitters in the central and peripheral nervous systems. Several decades of research have elucidated the synthesis, storage, release, and metabolism of these neurotransmitters (see chapter 2). The biogenic amines are known to have important roles as mediators of neuronal communication in discrete pathways in the brain (see chapter 1). Numerous hypotheses also link the biogenic amines to the pathophysiology of mental illness, notably depression and schizophrenia. These hypotheses are explained in detail in chapter 12 and chapter 17. More recently, anxiety disorders (see chapter 21) and Alzheimer's disease (see chapter 25) have also been linked to abnormalities in the functional activity of biogenic amines.

Research on the relationship of biogenic amines to various mental disorders has led to attempts to develop diagnostic laboratory tests for specific disorders (see table 35–2). This pursuit continues today in the form of measuring biogenic amines and their metabolites in body fluids that can be sampled clinically: blood, urine, and CSF. The goals of this research are to find clinically identifiable abnormalities in biogenic amine

metabolites that: (1) distinguish patients with clinical syndromes (e.g., depression) from normal controls; (2) permit biological subtyping of syndromes that can be identified clinically (e.g., endogenous versus nonendogenous depression); (3) enable the clinician to predict good or bad outcomes; and (4) enable the clinician to predict treatment response to different drugs and/or psychotherapies.

Unfortunately, in 1985 these goals remain largely unfulfilled, and the utility of laboratory tests of biogenic amines and their metabolites to the practicing clinician is very limited. On the other hand, research in this area is progressing rapidly, and it is likely that psychiatric practitioners will someday be able to apply these tests in their practices to aid their understanding of a given patient's disorder as well as how best to treat it. Thus it may be valuable for clinicians to have an overview of the state of the art in 1985, so that they will understand the historical scientific content from which numerous diagnostic tests will likely emerge.

Catecholamines and Affective Disorders

The catecholamine NE and its principal CNS metabolite 3-methoxy-4-hydroxyphenylglycol (MHPG) have had a hypothesized link to affective disorders for over twenty years.[57,247] The attempt to identify a deficiency in CNS noradrenergic functioning led to assaying NE and its metabolites in blood, urine, and CSF from patients with major depressive disorder. Early evidence suggested decreased urinary or CSF MHPG concentrations.[57,178,247] However, the status of this work is currently unclear; not all investigators find this abnormality in depressed patients, and those who do are unable to show clinical differences in the subtypes of depressed patients with differing MHPG concentrations.[79] Furthermore, there appears to be no consistent correlation between the changes in MHPG concentrations and the treatment response of patients on long-term antidepressants.[79,85,262] As research progresses in this field and as the debate continues over the clinical utility of catecholamine measurements, it will become clearer as to how the practicing clinician will apply them in clinical practice.

Indoleamines and Affective Disorders

The indoleamine 5HT and its metabolite 5-hydroxyindoleacetic acid (5-HIAA) have also been hypothesized to be related to major depressive disorders. These investigations, performed over the past twenty years, have reached two tentative conclusions.[16,189,197,224] The first is that CSF 5-HIAA concentrations are distributed bimodally in patients with depression. That is, there is one subgroup of depressed patients with low 5-HIAA. The second conclusion, first suggested by Asberg and colleagues, is that the patients with low CSF 5-HIAA are more likely to commit suicide and are more likely to use violent methods for their suicide attempts. In Asberg's original study of sixty-eight depressed patients,[14] more of the patients who had attempted suicide (including two who later did commit suicide) were in the low CSF 5-HIAA group. More recently, Asberg's group has shown a 20 percent mortality by suicide within a year of lumbar puncture in depressed patients with low CSF 5-HIAA concentrations.[285]

Many studies by several groups of investigators have now documented a potential relationship between CSF 5-HIAA concentrations and suicidal behavior.* However, CSF 5-HIAA does not yet have a role in clinical practice as a reliable, valid predictor of suicidal behavior. Continuing studies may bring this tool to bear on the very important clinical need to be able to help predict suicide.

CSF 5-HIAA concentrations appear to decrease in depressed patients given virtually any tricyclic antidepressant medication.[79] However, this change occurs whether or not the patient's depression improves and is therefore unable to assist the clinician in choosing an antidepressant or in predicting its clinical usefulness in a given patient.[15,36,79]

Neurotransmitters in Schizophrenia

Pharmacological evidence supports an association between increased DA activity and schizophrenic symptoms (see chapter 17). However, no striking abnormalities have been identified in the CSF DA metabolite homovanillic acid in schizophrenic patients.[33,34] CSF NE has been reported to be elevated[123,162,170] in some schizophrenic patients, as has CSF epinephrine.[31] CSF 5-HIAA in schizophrenics may be correlated with "mannerisms and posturing," one of the items of the Brief Psychiatric Rating Scale.[163] Blood platelet 5HT levels may also correlate with mannerisms and posturing and with CSF 5-HIAA concentrations.[163] Furthermore, blood platelet 5HT levels are increased in schizophrenic patients as a group.[268] Another group of neurotransmitters are the endorphins, morphinelike peptides that serve as neuromodulators in the brain. They appear to be normal in biological fluids of schizophrenic patients.[32,288]

In summary, a number of interesting leads relate a variety of neurotransmitters and metabolites to schizophrenia, but clinical applications of these laboratory tests are not yet apparent.

¶ Peripheral Models for Studying Neurotransmitter Receptors and Enzymes in Psychiatric Illness

Introduction

Increasing attention is being paid to the role of enzymes and receptors of biogenic amines in mental illness (see chapters 2, 12, 17, 20, 21, 23, 24, and 25). Since direct measurement of enzymes and receptors in brain is possible only in postmortem autopsy tissues, new strategies are being developed to

---

*See references 4, 14, 17, 21, 22, 23, 49, 50, 51, 68, 209, 213, 285, and 287.

study these same neurotransmitter enzymes and receptors from other tissues, such as blood cells or fibroblasts, that can be obtained ethically from living patients. These strategies are based on scientific evidence that allows one to draw analogies between a peripheral tissue and the brain.

Human platelets contain monoamine oxidase (MAO), alpha-2 adrenergic receptors, 5HT reputake sites, ^{3}H-imipramine (^{3}H-IMI) binding sites, and 5HT membrane receptors (5HT$_2$ sites and shape-change receptors).[266] Human lymphocytes contain beta-adrenergic receptors[171] linked to a NE-stimulated adenylate cyclase.[42] Human red blood cells contain the enzymes catechol-O-methyl-transferase (COMT)[290] and sodium-potassium adenosine triphosphate (Na$^+$/K$^+$ ATPase),[208] as well as a transport mechanism for lithium[138,216] and cholinergic receptors (^{3}H-QNB [^{3}H-quinuclidinyl benzicate] binding sites).[13] Human fibroblasts contain MAO, COMT,[155] and a number of membrane receptors, including cholinergic receptors.[199] Each of these enzymes and receptors in the peripheral tissue is a model for the same enzyme or receptor in brain (see table 35-3). Each has been studied in various psychiatric populations and proposed as an aid in diagnosis. The tests in general are highly technical, expensive, and suitable at this time only for relatively sophisticated research laboratories, as opposed to routine clinical laboratories. Although a number of leads are quite promising, none of these tests is ready for routine clinical use. Here we will review a few of these studies in peripheral tissues and suggest how they might come to be employed in clinical practice as a laboratory test in psychiatry.

Rationale for Using Peripheral Models of CNS Neurotransmitter Enzymes and Receptors to Study Psychiatric Disorders in Man

Recent years have witnessed a rapid proliferation in the number of biological substances that are candidate neurotransmitters in the CNS. Similarly, the number of known enzymes and receptors relating to each neurotransmitter has also greatly increased. Neurotransmitters are frequently employed by the body in multiple sites by multiple receptors for multiple functions.[266] One example of this is the dual use of "gut" peptides by the brain and "brain" peptides by the gut. Brain neurotransmitters are frequently used as well by the hypothalamus and pituitary for secretion into the systemic circulation. Brain transmitters are found in the peripheral nervous system, in the adrenals, in other endocrine organs, and in platelets. Brain neurotransmitter enzymes and receptors are not only found in the tissues just listed, but also in lymphocytes, red blood cells, and fibroblasts. Thus nature appears to have been parsimonious by applying neurotransmitter molecules for several purposes in several tissues and with multiple receptors.

These observations may create an opportunity for the psychiatrist who wishes to understand diseases and drug effects in terms of modern molecular neurobiology. That is, there are certain analogies between the neurotransmitter pharmacology of the brain and that of the peripheral tissues that may link the similar processes in the different tissues, especially when they are both controlled by genetic factors. Since it is often not practical or ethical to study the brain directly in CNS disorders, the best window to the CNS may be the study of these same neurotransmitters and receptors in peripheral tissues whenever the latter behave analogously to the CNS. The development of platelets, lymphocytes, red blood cells, and fibroblasts as models for some of these CNS neurotransmitter functions depends on rigorous studies documenting exactly which peripheral tissues and their receptors and enzymes accurately model the CNS and which do not. The following sections give a brief overview of the state of the art for several applications of peripheral models to the study of neurotransmitter enzymes and receptors in psychiatric disorders.

Platelets as Models

Platelets are perhaps the best developed peripheral model and the most extensively studied.[258,265,266] Platelets and neurons both possess a limiting membrane rich in receptors, mitochondria, and storage vesicles for neurotransmitter. Differences between platelets and neurons include the fact that platelets contain alpha granules, which store glycogen, whereas neurons do not; on the other hand, neurons contain a cell nucleus, but platelets do not.[258,266]

Specific enzymes and receptors that are shared by platelets and neurons include mitochondrial MAO, 5HT reuptake sites, ^{3}H-IMI binding sites, alpha-2 adrenergic receptors, and possibly $5HT_2$ receptors.[258,266] Each enzyme and receptor has been studied in both brain and platelet and the results are reviewed in detail elsewhere[266]; brief overviews follow.

PLATELET MONOAMINE OXIDASE

It is known that platelet MAO is of the B type and is analogous to the B type found in brain (i.e., inhibited with greater specificity by deprenyl and pargyline and having phenylethylamine and benzylamine as preferred substrates).* Thus platelet MAO B is a good model for brain MAO B.

Beginning in the 1970s, large-scale investigations of platelet MAO in numerous psychiatric disorders (especially schizophrenia)[296] have been conducted to determine the potential utility of this laboratory test as an aid to diagnosis and a clue to pathophysiology. Although early studies suggested that platelet MAO B may be reduced in schizophrenia, numerous problems have limited its application in clinical practice.[186,248,293,297] These problems include: (1) technical difficulties with the assays; (2) disputes about the methods used to isolate platelets and platelet subpopulations; (3) a wide overlap of individual values for platelet MAO activity when comparing the schizophrenic population to the

*See references 141, 158, 167, 196, 264, 298, and 299.

normal control population; (4) the possibility of a confounding medication (neuroleptic) effect on platelet MAO activity; and (5) lack of diagnostic specificity, since other disorders such as depression may also be associated with reduced platelet MAO activity.

A newer potential use of platelet MAO activity under active investigation is to monitor the pharmacological and therapeutic effects of MAO inhibitors administered to patients. That is, therapeutic effects (e.g., antidepressant, antipanic, etc.) may be associated with a high degree (greater than 80 to 90 percent) of inhibition of platelet MAO activity.[174,229,232] It is possible that determining percentage of platelet MAO inhibition in patients receiving MAO inhibitors may be useful in three situations: to monitor compliance, to determine if a dosage increase is necessary (low platelet MAO inhibition), and to determine true therapeutic failure (no clinical response despite adequate MAO inhibition). This promising potential application may serve a clinical role in the near future.

PLATELET SEROTONIN UPTAKE AND ^{3}H-IMIPRAMINE SITES

Recent investigations have demonstrated remarkable analogies between the platelet and the CNS serotonergic neuron in the mechanism by which both tissues transport 5HT.[266] It appears that both tissues possess a macromolecular complex for transporting 5HT that is composed of several components located in the outer cellular membrane. These include a 5HT reuptake binding site,[256,257,258,267] a sodium binding site,[256,257] a ^{3}H-IMI binding site,[46,218,220] and NA^+/K^+ ATPase.[258] When sodium binds to its membrane site, the affinity of the 5HT binding site for 5HT is increased, thereby facilitating the intracellular transport of both sodium and 5HT. Once inside the cell, Na^+/K^+ ATPase extrudes the sodium, and the storage granule binds the 5HT. A ^{3}H-IMI binding site also appears to be closely linked to the 5HT reuptake site, but not identical with it. When tricyclic antidepressants bind this ^{3}H-IMI binding site, the membrane binding site for 5HT itself is inhibited, and the transport of 5HT ceases. Exciting and provocative new evidence suggests that the brain may synthesize its own endogenous imipraminelike substance (a naturally occurring antidepressant? or depressant?) that binds to the ^{3}H-IMI binding site.[24,172]

Numerous clinical studies now suggest that the 5HT transporter complex is abnormal in patients with affective disorders.* Not only is the capacity (i.e., Vmax) of the 5HT reuptake mechanism decreased in platelets from patients with major depressive disorder, but so is the number (i.e., Bmax) of platelet ^{3}H-IMI binding sites. Furthermore, ^{3}H-IMI binding sites are reduced in the cortex from brains of patients who committed suicide.[271] Reductions in platelet ^{3}H-IMI binding may also correlate with reductions in CSF 5-HIAA concentrations in depressed patients and thus be a potential additional biological link to depression and/or suicidal behavior[18] (see also the section entitled "Indoleamines and Affective Disorders"). First-degree relatives of depressed patients with reduced platelet 5HT uptake may express this same abnormality, and this biological parameter may label a disease trait that is present in the patient regardless of clinical state (i.e., depressed or euthymic).[268]

These preliminary findings are currently the subject of intense investigation and debate. Further research may well bring platelet 5HT uptake and platelet ^{3}H-IMI binding studies into the realm of laboratory tests for practicing clinicians in the near future.

PLATELET ALPHA-2 ADRENERGIC RECEPTORS

Physiological and pharmacological studies indicate that the actions of catecholamines involve both alpha- and beta-adrenergic receptors in several tissues. Both alpha- and beta-adrenergic receptors are further classified into subtypes (alpha-1, alpha-2, beta-1, beta-2).[147,192] Human platelets apparently do not contain beta-adrenergic receptors or al-

pha-1 adrenergic receptors in their outer membranes. However, the platelet does contain alpha-2 adrenergic receptors, which have similar kinetic and pharmacological properties to those in the brain.* This suggests that the alpha-2 adrenergic receptor in platelets may constitute an adequate model for the same receptor in the brain.

The platelet alpha-2 adrenergic receptor has been investigated in patients with major depressive disorder, both before and after treatment with antidepressant medications.† No clear abnormalities have yet been identified that would allow application to clinical practice. Future research in patients with disorders that possibly are linked to alpha-2 adrenergic receptors (such as depression, obsessive-compulsive disorder, anxiety, and Tourette syndrome) may lead to a useful clinical application for platelet alpha-2 adrenergic receptor assays.

Lymphocytes as Models

Compared to the human platelet, the human lymphocyte has been less well studied as a model system for brain neurotransmitter receptors and enzymes. The most interesting potential application is that of beta-adrenergic membrane receptors, which are linked to an adenylate cyclase system in a receptor-enzyme complex very similar to that in the brain.‡ Other lymphocyte receptors for steroid hormones such as dexamethasone[255] and for various neuropeptides will require further basic research comparing their properties in the lymphocyte and in the brain before we will know whether analogies can be appropriately made.

Although the kinetic and pharmacological properties of lymphocyte beta-adrenergic receptors and their linked enzyme (NE-stimulated adenylate cyclase) do share model characteristics for the same receptor and enzyme in the CNS, little application of this concept has yet been made in psychiatric dis-

---

*See references 35, 47, 184, 219, 268, and 269.

*See references 93, 139, 159, 206, and 286.
†See references 92, 116, 117, 160, 196, 270, 294, and 295.
‡See references 1, 2, 37, 48, 109, 168, 171, and 193.

orders. Preliminary investigations suggest possible abnormalities in major depressive disorder,[27,28,108,173] but much more study will be required to develop these assays as clinical laboratory tests.

Red Blood Cells as Models

Although several enzymes and receptors relating to neurotransmitters in the CNS exist in human red blood cells (see the section entitled "Introduction"), the status of current investigations does not allow immediate application of these laboratory tests to the practice of clinical psychiatry. In the future, red blood cell Na^+/K^+ ATPase may help clarify our understanding of major depressive disorder, mania, obesity, and the mechanism of action of lithium.* Red blood cell cholinergic receptors could potentially render insight into diseases of CNS cholinergic receptors.[13]

Fibroblasts as Models

Cultured human skin fibroblasts hold considerable promise for characterizing molecular abnormalities in psychiatric disorders.[45] These cells are relatively easily accessible by simple skin biopsy and they can be cultured without transformation, grown in large enough quantities so that numerous biochemical assays can be performed, and frozen for later use. Most significant from a theoretical point of view is the fact that fibroblasts contain receptors and enzymes for neurotransmitters that are analogous to those in neurons. These include (among others) adenylate cyclase,[143] glutamic acid decarboxylase,[125] nerve growth factor,[251] high-affinity choline uptake,[231] MAO,[155] COMT,[155] and muscarinic cholinergic receptors.[199] Psychiatric disorders with a genetic basis that were related to molecular abnormality in any one of these parameters could potentially be diagnosed by assaying cultured skin fibroblasts instead of the brain,

*See references 5, 74, 76, 84, 96, 111, 114, 145, 152, 175, 177, 188, 190, 202, 203, 204, 214, 226, and 227.

just as several metabolic abnormalities causing mental retardation are currently diagnosed (e.g., fibroblasts from amniocentesis assayed for hexosaminidase to diagnose Tay-Sachs disease).[45,212]

Perhaps the most elegant clinical application of peripheral models for the CNS has been the use of the fibroblast as a model of the brain's enzymatic machinery for the disposition of lipids. For example, Tay described the clinical picture of Tay-Sachs disease in 1881, and Sachs expanded the clinical picture and presented the pathological findings in 1886. However, it was not until 1969 that the basic enzymatic defect was described, when Okada and O'Brien[212] found that hexosaminidase A was markedly diminished in skin fibroblasts grown *in vitro* for many cellular generations from patients with Tay-Sachs disease, as well as in the liver, brain, skin, kidney, leukocytes, and serum. Since this discovery, the diagnosis of several of the cerebral lipidoses has been made possible on the basis of assaying enzymes in cultured fibroblasts.

Although no psychiatric disorder is currently known to be related to a specific molecular abnormality of an enzyme or receptor present in fibroblasts, this area is the subject of intense investigation, and the day may not be too far away when patients with psychiatric disorders can have a diagnosis made or verified by a skin biopsy for these assays. In fact, one preliminary study suggests that an increase in muscarinic cholinergic receptors from cultured skin fibroblasts may be present in patients and their affected relatives with major affective illness (unipolar or bipolar).[199] These and similar investigations may finally begin the long-sought-after process of linking psychiatric illnesses and molecular neurobiology.

¶ Conclusion

Clinical psychiatry in 1985 is just beginning to inherit the benefits of the past two decades of explosive research and new knowledge of fundamental neurobiology. As this research has begun to clarify molecular mechanisms of mental illness, new laboratory tests have begun to trickle into clinical psychiatric practice. This chapter reviews only three of the areas of new laboratory testing in clinical psychiatry: neuroendocrine tests, biochemical tests of neurotransmitters and their metabolites, and biochemical tests of neurotransmitter enzymes and receptors in peripheral tissues.

We attempt to provide the reader not only with an up-to-date status report on the use of these laboratory tests from the perspective of the practicing clinician, but also a strategy whereby clinicians will be able to evaluate the literature as new advances unfold in the future. We do not touch upon the fiscal issue of where research ends (i.e., payment by research grants) and where clinical standard of care begins (i.e., payment by patients and third parties). While we are purposely conservative in promoting widespread or indiscriminate use of these laboratory tests, we do not wish to imply that some of these tests are not justifiably "standard of care," particularly by more innovative practitioners. It would be a great tragedy in the current era of cost containment if third-party payers shut the door to applications of laboratory tests in psychiatry just as our specialty is on the verge of entering the field of modern molecular medicine.

¶ Bibliography

1. AARONS, R. D., and MOLINOFF, P. B. "Changes in the Density of Beta-Adrenergic Receptors in Rat Lymphocytes, Heart and Lung After Chronic Treatment with Propranolol," *Journal of Pharmacology and Experimental Therapeutics*, 221 (1982):439–443.

2. AARONS, R. D., et al. "Decreased Beta-adrenergic Receptor Density on Human Lymphocytes After Chronic Treatment with Agonists," *Journal of Pharmacology and Experimental Therapeutics*, 224 (1983):1–6.

3. ABOU-SALEH, M. T., MILLER, R., and COPPEN A. "Dexamethasone Suppression Test in Depression," *Neuropharmacology*, 22 (1983):549–550.

4. AGREN, H. "Symptom Patterns in Unipolar and Bipolar Depression Correlating with Monoamine Metabolites in Cerebrospinal Fluid, II: Suicide," *Psychiatry Research*, 193 (1980):225–236.

5. AKAGAWA, K., WATANABE, M., and TSUKADA, Y., "Activity of Erythrocyte Na, K-ATPase in Manic Patients," *Journal of Neurochemistry*, 35 (1980):258–260.

6. ALBALA, A. A., et al. "Changes in Serial Dexamethasone Suppression Tests Among Unipolar Depressives Receiving Electroconvulsive Treatment," *Biological Psychiatry*, 16 (1981):551–60.

7. ALEXOPOULOUS, G. S., et al. "Dexamethasone Suppression Test in Geriatric Depression," Paper presented at the 135th Annual Meeting of the American Psychiatric Association, Toronto, Canada, 1982.

8. American Psychiatric Association Committee on Nomenclature: *Diagnostic and Statistical Manual of Mental Disorders*, (DSM-III). Washington, D.C.: American Psychiatric Association, 1980.

9. AMES, D., et al. "A Study of the Dexamethasone Suppression Test in Hospitalized Depressed Patients," *British Journal of Psychiatry*, 144 (1984):311–313.

10. AMSTERDAM, J. D., WINOKUR, A., and CAROFF, S. N. "The Dexamethasone Suppression Test in Outpatients with Primary Affective Disorder and Healthy Control Subjects," *American Journal of Psychiatry*, 139 (1982):287–291.

11. AMSTERDAM, J. D., et al. "A Neuroendocrine Test Battery in Bipolar and Healthy Subjects," *Archives of General Psychiatry*, 40 (1983):515–521.

12. ARANA, G. W., et al. "The Dexamethasone Suppression Test in Psychotic Disorders," *American Journal of Psychiatry*, 140 (1983):1521–1523.

13. ARONSTAM, R. L., ABOOD, L. G., and MACNEIL, M. K. "Muscarinic Cholinergic Binding in Human Erythrocyte Membranes," *Life Sciences*, 20 (1977):1175–1180.

14. ASBERG, M., TRASBERG, L., and THOREN, P. "5-HIAA in the Cerebrospinal Fluid.

A Biochemical Suicide Predictor," *Archives of General Psychiatry*, 338 (1976):1193–1197.

15. ASBERG, M., et al. "Monoamine Metabolites in Cerebrospinal Fluid and Serotonin Uptake Inhibition During Treatment with Chlorimipramine," *Clinical Pharmacologic Therapy*, 21 (1975):201–207.

16. ASBERG, M., et al. "Serotonin Depression: A Biochemical Subgroup within Affective Disorders," *Science*, 191 (1976):478–480.

17. ASBERG, M., et al. "Monoamine Metabolites in Cerebrospinal Fluid in Relation to Depressive Illness, Suicidal Behavior and Personality," in B. Angrist, ed., *Recent Advances in Neuropharmacology*. New York: Pergamon Press, 1981, pp. 271–275.

18. ASBERG, M., et al. "Serotonin and Suicidal Behavior," *Clinical Neuropharmacology*, 7 (Supplement 1) (1984):570–571.

19. BALDESSARINI, R. J. *Biomedical Aspects of Depression and Its Treatment*. Washington, D.C.: American Psychiatric Press, 1983.

20. BALDESSARINI, R. J., FINKLESTEIN, S., and ARANA, G. W. "The Predictive Power of Diagnostic Tests and the Effect of Prevalence of Illness," *Archives of General Psychiatry*, 40 (1983):569–573.

21. BANKI, C. M., and ARATO, M. "Amine Metabolites and Neuroendocrine Responses Related to Depression and Suicide," *Journal of Affective Disorders*, 5 (1983):223–232.

22. ———. "Amine Metabolites, Neuroendocrine Findings and Personality Dimensions as Correlates of Suicidal Behavior," *Psychiatry Research*, 10 (1983): 253–261.

23. BANKI, C. M., VOJNIK, M., and MOLNAR, G. "Cerebrospinal Fluid Amine Metabolites, Tryptophan and Clinical Parameters in Depression," *Journal of Affective Disorders*, 3 (1981):81–89.

24. BARBACCIA, M. L., et al. "Putative Endogenous Ligands for Antidepressant Recognition Sites," *Clinical Neuropharmacology*, 7 (Supplement 1) (1984):308–309.

25. BAXTER, L., et al. "Dexamethasone Suppression Test and Axis I Diagnoses of Inpatients with DSM-III Borderline Personality Disorder," *Journal of Clinical Psychiatry*, 45 (1984):150–153.

26. BEEBER, A. R., et al. "Dexamethasone Suppression Test in Hospitalized Depressed Patients with Borderline Personality Disorder," *Journal of Nervous and Mental Disease*, 172 (1984):301–303.

27. BELMAKER, R. H. "Receptors, Adenylate Cyclase, Depression and Lithium," *Biological Psychiatry*, 16 (1981):333–350.

28. BELMAKER, R. H., ZOHAR, J., and EBSTEIN, R. P. "Cyclic Nucleotides in Mental Disorder," in P. Hament and H. Sands, eds., *Advances in Cyclic Nucleotide Research*, vol. 12. New York: Raven Press, 1980, pp. 187–197.

29. BERGER, M., et al. "Neuroendocrinological and Neurophysiological Studies in Major Depressive Disorders: Are There Biological Markers for the Endogenous Subtype?" *Biological Psychiatry*, 17 (1982):1217–1242.

30. BERGER, M., et al. "Influence of Weight Loss on the Dexamethasone Suppression Test," *Archives of General Psychiatry*, 40 (1983):585–586.

31. BERGER, P. A., "Epinephrine in Schizophrenia." Abstracted at the American College of Neuropsychopharmacology, 1983.

32. BERGER, P. A., and BARCHAS, J. D. "Pharmacological Studies of a β-endorphin in Psychopathology," *Psychiatric Clinics of North America*, 6 (1983):377–391.

33. BERGER, P. A., ELLIOTT, G. R., and BARCHAS, J. D. "Neuroregulators and Schizophrenia," in M. A. Lipton, A. DiMascio, and K. F. Killam, eds., *Psychopharmacology: A Generation of Progress*. New York: Raven Press, 1978, pp. 1071–1095.

34. BERGER, P. A., et al. "CSF Monoamine Metabolites in Depression and Schizophrenia," *American Journal of Psychiatry*, 137 (1980):174–180.

35. BERRETTINI, W. H., et al. "Platelet ^{3}H-imipramine Binding in Euthymic Bipolar Patients," *Psychiatry Research*, 7 (1982):215–219.

36. BERTILSSON, L., ASBERG, M., and THOREN, P. "Differential Effect of Chlorimipramine and Nortriptyline on Cerebrospinal Fluid Metabolites of

Serotonin and Noradrenaline in Depression," *European Journal of Clinical Pharmacology,* 21 (1976):194–200.

37. BISHOPRIC, N. H., COHEN, H. J., and LEFKOWITZ, R. J. "Beta Adrenergic Receptors in Lymphocyte Subpopulations," *Journal of Allergy and Clinical Immunology,* 65 (1980):29–33.

38. BLOODWORTH, R. C. "The Use of the Dexamethasone Suppression Test in the Differential Diagnosis of Catatonic Stupor," *International Journal of Psychiatry in Medicine,* 12 (1982):93–101.

39. BOARD, F., PERSKY, H., and HAMBURG, D. A. "Psychological Stress and Endocrine Function: Blood Levels of Adreno-Cortical and Thyroid Hormones in Acutely Disturbed Patients," *Psychosomatic Medicine,* 18 (1956):324–333.

40. BOARD, F., WADESON, R., and PERSKY, H. "Depressive Affect and Endocrine Function," *Archives of Neurology and Psychiatry,* 78 (1957):612.

41. BOLER, J., et al. "The Identity of Chemical and Hormone Properties of the Thyrotropin Releasing Hormone and Pyroglutamyl-histadyl-proline-amide," *Biochemical and Biophysical Research Communications,* 37 (1969):705–710.

42. BOURNE, H. R., and MELMON, K. L. "Adenyl Cyclase in Human Leukocytes: Evidence for Activation by Separate Beta Adrenergic and Prostaglandin Receptors," *Journal of Pharmacologic Experimental Therapy,* 178 (1971):1–10.

43. BOWERS, C. Y., et al., "Prolactin and Thyrotropin Release in Man by Synthetic Pyroglutamyl-histadyl-prolinamide," *Biochemical and Biophysical Research Communications,* 45 (1971):1033–1041.

44. BRAWLEY, P. "Dexamethasone, Methylphenidate and Depression." Abstracted in *American Psychiatric Association Scientific Procedures,* 161 (1979):352.

45. BREAKEFIELD, X. O., and PINTAR, J. E. "The Use of Cell Culture to Analyze the Genetic Basis of Human Neurologic Disease," in E. S. Gershon, et al., eds., *Genetic Research Strategies in Psychobiology and Psychiatry.* Pacific Grove, Calif: Boxwood Press, 1981, pp. 407–414.

46. BRILEY, M. S., RAISMAN, R., and LANGER, S. Z. "Human Platelets Possess High-affinity Binding Sites for ^{3}H-imipra-mine," *European Journal of Pharmacology,* 58 (1979):347–348.

47. BRILEY, M. S., et al. "Tritiated Imipramine Binding Sites Are Decreased in Platelets of Untreated Depressed Patients," *Science,* 209 (1980):303–305.

48. BRODDE, O. E., et al. "The Beta Adrenergic Receptor in Human Lymphocytes: Subclassification by the Use of a New Radio-ligand, ^{125}Iodocyanopindolol," *Life Sciences,* 29 (1981):2189–2198.

49. BROWN, G. L., GOODWIN, F. K., and BUNNEY, W. E. "Human Aggression and Suicide: Their Relationship to Neuropsychiatric Diagnoses and Serotonin Metabolism," in B. T. Ho, J. C. Schoolar, and E. Usdin, eds., *Serotonin in Biological Psychiatry,* vol. 34. New York: Raven Press, 1982, pp. 287–307.

50. BROWN, G. L., et al. "Aggression in Humans Correlates with Cerebrospinal Fluid Amine Metabolites," *Psychiatry Research,* 1 (1979):131–139.

51. BROWN, G. L., et al. "Aggression, Suicide and Serotonin: Relationships to Cerebrospinal Fluid Amine Metabolites," *American Journal of Psychiatry,* 139 (1982):741–746.

52. BROWN, G. M., et al. "Psychoendocrinology and Growth Hormone: A Review," *Psychoneuroendocrinology,* 3 (1978):131–153.

53. BROWN, W. A. Dexamethasone Suppression Test. Unpublished presentation, American College of Neuropsychopharmacology Meeting Abstracts, 1984.

54. BROWN, W. A., and QUALLS, C. B. "Pituitary-adrenal Disinhibition in Depression: Marker of a Subtype with Characteristic Clinical Features and Response to Treatment," *Psychiatry Research,* 4 (1981):115–128.

55. BROWN, W. A., and SHUEY, I. "Response to Dexamethasone and Subtype of Depression," *Archives of General Psychiatry,* 37 (1980):747–751.

56. BROWN, W. A., JOHNSTON, R., and MAYFIELD, D. "The 24-hour Dexamethasone Suppression Test in a Clinical Setting: Relationship to Diagnosis, Symptoms, and Response to Treatment," *American Journal of Psychiatry,* 136 (1979):543–547.

57. BUNNEY, W. E., and DAVIS, J. M. "Norepi-

nephrine in Depressive Reactions: A Review," *Archives of General Psychiatry,* 13 (1965):483–494.

58. BURGUS, R., et al., "Structure Moleculaire du Facteu Hypothalamique Hypophysitrope TRF d'Origine Ovine: Mise En Evidence Spectrometric de Masse de la Sequence, PCA-His-Pro-NH2," *Compte Rendus of the Academy of Science* (Paris), 269 (1969):1870–1873.

59. BUTLER, P.W.P., and BESSER, G. M. "Pituitary Adrenal Function in Severe Depressive Illness," *Lancet,* 2 (1968):1234–1236.

60. CARMAN, J. S., et al. "Dexamethasone Non-suppression: Predictor of Thymoleptic Response in Catatonic and Schizo-affective Patients," Abstracted in *Society of Biological Psychiatry,* 4 (1980):36.

61. CARNEY, M.W.P., ROTH, M., and GARSIDE, R. F. "The Diagnosis of Depressive Syndromes and the Prediction of ECT Response," *British Journal of Psychiatry,* 111 (1965):659–674.

62. CAROFF, S., et al. "Response to Dexamethasone in Psychotic Depression," Paper presented at the 135th Annual Meeting of the American Psychiatric Association, Toronto, Canada, 1982.

63. CARROLL, B. J. "Hypothalamic-pituitary Function in Depressive Illness: Insensitivity to Hypoglycaemia," *British Medical Journal,* 3 (1969):27–28.

64. ———. "The Hypothalamic-pituitary-adrenal Axis in Depression," in B. Davies, B. J. Carroll, R. M. Mobray, eds., *Depressive Illness: Some Research Studies.* Springfield, Ill.: Charles C Thomas, 1972, pp. 23–201.

65. ———. "The Dexamethasone Test for Melancholia," *British Journal of Psychiatry,* 140 (1982):292–304.

66. ———. "Biologic Markers and Treatment Response," *Journal of Clinical Psychiatry,* 44 (1983):30–40.

67. CARROLL, B. J., CURTIS, G. C., and MENDELS, J. "Neuroendocrine Regulation in Depression. I. Limbic System—Adrenocortical Dysfunction," *Archives of General Psychiatry,* 33 (1976):1039–1044.

68. CARROLL, B.J., GREDEN, J.F., and FEINBERG, M. "Suicide, Neuroendocrine Dysfunction and CSF 5HIAA Concentrations in Depression," in B. Angrist and A. Betal, eds., *Recent Advances in Neuropsychopharmacology: Advances in the Bio-Science,* vol. 31. Elmsford, N.Y.: Pergamon Press, 1981, pp. 307–313.

69. CARROLL, B. J., MARTIN, F.I.R., and DAVIES, B. M. "Resistance to Suppression by Dexamethasone of Plasma 11-OHCS Levels in Severe Depressive Illness," *British Medical Journal,* 3 (1968):285–287.

70. CARROLL, B. J., et al. "Neuroendocrine Dysfunction in Genetic Subtypes of Primary Unipolar Depression," *Psychiatry Research,* 2 (1980):251–258.

71. CARROLL, B. J., et al. "Neuroendocrine Evaluation of Depression in Borderline Patients," *Psychiatric Clinics of North America,* 5 (1981):650–653.

72. CARROLL, B. J., et al. "A Specific Laboratory Test for the Diagnosis of Melancholia," *Archives of General Psychiatry,* 38 (1981):15–22.

73. CASPER, R. C., and DAVIS, J. "Neuroendocrine and Amine Studies in Affective Illness," *Psychoneuroendocrinology,* 2 (1977):105–115.

74. CASPER, R. C., et al. "Intracellular Lithium and Clinical Response," *Lancet,* 2 (1976):418–419.

75. CASTRO, P., et al. "Abnormal DST Results in Patients with Chronic Schizophrenia," *American Journal of Psychiatry,* 140 (1983):1261.

76. CAZULLO, C. L., et al. "Intracellular Lithium Concentration and Clinical Response," *British Journal of Psychiatry,* 126 (1975):298–300.

77. CHARLES, G., et al. "Plasma and Urinary Cortisol Levels After Dexamethasone in Affective Disorders," *Journal of Affective Disorders,* 3 (1981):397–406.

78. CHARLES, G., et al. "Reproducibility of the Dexamethasone Suppression Test in Depression," *Biological Psychiatry,* 17 (1982):845–848.

79. CHARNEY, D. S., MENKES, D. B., and HENINGER, G. R. "Receptor Sensitivity and the Mechanism of Action of Antidepressant Treatment: Implications for the Etiology and Therapy of Depression," *Archives of General Psychiatry,* 38 (1981):1160–1180.

80. CHECKLEY, S. A. "Corticosteroid and Growth Hormone Responses to Methylamphetamine in Depressive Illness," *Psychological Medicine,* 9 (1979):107–116.

81. ——. "Neuroendocrine Studies of Monoamine Function in Man: A Review of Basic Theory and Its Application to the Study of Depressive Illness," *Psychological Medicine,* 10 (1980):35–53.

82. CHECKLEY, S. A., and CRAMMER, J. L. "Hormonal Responses to Methylamphetamine in Depression: A New Approach to the Noradrenaline Depletion Hypothesis," *British Journal of Psychiatry,* 131 (1977):582–586.

83. CHECKLEY, S. A., SLADE, A. P., and SHUR, E. "Growth Hormone and Other Responses to Clonidine in Patients with Endogenous Depression," *British Journal of Psychiatry,* 138 (1981):51–55.

84. CHOI, S. J., TAYLOR, M. A., and ABRAMS, R. "Depression, ECT and Erythrocyte Adenosinetriphosphatase Activity," *Biological Psychiatry,* 12 (1977):75–81.

85. COPPEN, A., et al. "Urinary 4-hydroxy-3-methoxy-phenylglycol Is Not a Predictor for Clinical Response to Amitriptyline in Depressive Illness," *Psychopharmacology,* 64 (1979):95–97.

86. COPPEN, A., et al. "DST in Depression and Other Psychiatric Illness," *British Journal of Psychiatry,* 142 (1983):498–504.

87. CORYELL, W., and SCHLESSER, M. A. "Suicide and the Dexamethasone Suppression Test in Unipolar Depression," *American Journal of Psychiatry,* 138 (1981):1120–1121.

88. CORYELL, W., GAFFNEY, G., and BURKHARDT, P. W. "The Dexamethasone and Familial Subtypes of Depression—A Naturalistic Replication," *Biological Psychiatry,* 17 (1982):33–40.

89. CRAPO, L. "Cushing's Syndrome: A Review of Diagnostic Tests," *Metabolism,* 28 (1979):955–977.

90. CURTIS, G. C., CAMERON, O. G., and NEESE, R. M. "The Dexamethasone Suppression Test in Panic Disorder and Agoraphobia," *American Journal of Psychiatry,* 139 (1982):1043–1046.

91. DACKIS, C. A., et al. "Specificity of the DST and the TRH Test for Major Depression in Alcoholics," *American Journal of Psychiatry,* 141 (1984):680–683.

92. DAIGUJI, M., MELTZER, H. Y., and U'PRICHARD, D. C. "Human Platelet Alpha-2-Adrenergic Receptors: Labelling with ^{3}H-Yohimbine, a Selective Antagonist Ligand," *Life Sciences,* 28 (1981):2705–2709.

93. DAIGUJI, M., et al. "Alpha-2-adrenergic Receptors in Platelet Membranes of Depressed Patients: No Change in Number or ^{3}H-Yohimbine Affinity," *Life Sciences,* 29 (1981):2059–2064.

94. DAVIS, K. L., et al. "Neuroendocrine and Neurochemical Measurements in Depression," *American Journal of Psychiatry,* 138 (1981):1555–1562.

95. DAVIS, K. L., et al. "Age and the Dexamethasone Suppression Test in Depression," *American Journal of Psychiatry,* 141 (1984):872–874.

96. DELVECCHIO, M., et al. "Cell Membrane Predictors of Response to Lithium Prophylaxis of Affective Disorders," *Neuropsychobiology,* 7 (1981):243–247.

97. DEVANAND, D. P., PANDURANGI, A. K., and DEWAN, M. J. "False-positive Dexamethasone Suppression Test Results Related to Antipsychotic Drug Withdrawal: Case Report," *Journal of Clinical Psychiatry,* 45 (1984):275–276.

98. DEWAN, M., et al. "Abnormal Dexamethasone Suppression Test Results in Chronic Schizophrenics," *American Journal of Psychiatry,* 139 (1982):1501–1503.

99. DOERR, P., et al. "Relationship Between Weight Gain and Hypothalamic Pituitary Adrenal Function in Patients with Anorexia Nervosa," *Journal of Steroid Biochemistry,* 12 (1980):529–537.

100. DOTTI, A., BERSANI, G., and NOCERA, F. "Dexamethasone Suppression Test as a Factor of Differential Diagnosis in Endogenous Depression." Abstracted in *Proceedings of the International Society of Psychoneuroendocrinology,* 11th International Congress, Florence, Italy, 1980.

101. DYSKEN, M. W., et al. "Serial Postdexamethasone Cortisol Levels in a Patient Undergoing ECT," *American Journal of Psychiatry,* 136 (1979):1328–1329.

102. EDELSTEIN, C. K., et al. "Effects of Weight

Loss on the Dexamethasone Suppression Test," *American Journal of Psychiatry,* 140 (1983):338–341.

103. ENDO, M., et al. "Endocrine Studies in Depression," in N. Hatotani, ed., *Psychoneuroendocrinology.* New York: S. Karger, 1974, pp. 23–31.

104. ETTIGI, P. G., and BROWN, G. M. "Psychoneuroendocrinology of Affective Disorder: An Overview," *American Journal of Psychiatry,* 134 (1977):493–501.

105. ETTIGI, P. G., et al. "Effect of Sex, Oral Contraceptives and Glucose Loading on Apomorphine Induced Growth Hormone Secretion," *Journal of Clinical Endocrinology and Metabolism,* 40 (1975):1094–1098.

106. EVANS, D. L., and NEMEROFF, C. B. "Use of the Dexamethasone Suppression Test Using DSM-III Criteria on an Inpatient Psychiatric Unit," *Biological Psychiatry,* 18 (1983):505–511.

107. EXTEIN, I., POTTASH, A.L.C., and GOLD, M. S. "Relationship of Thyrotropin-Releasing Hormone Test and Dexamethasone Suppression Test Abnormalities in Unipolar Depression," *Psychiatry Research,* 4 (1981):49–53.

108. EXTEIN, I., et al. "Changes in Lymphocyte Beta-Adrenergic Receptors in Depression and Mania," *Psychiatry Research,* 1 (1979):191–197.

109. FELDMAN, R. D., et al. "Alterations in Leukocyte Beta Receptor Affinity with Aging: A Potential Explanation for Altered Beta Adrenergic Sensitivity in the Elderly," *New England Journal of Medicine,* 310 (1984):815–819.

110. FINKLESTEIN, S., et al. "Mood, Vegetative Disturbance, and the Dexamethasone Suppression Test After Stroke," *Annals of Neurology,* 12 (1982):463–468.

111. FLEMENBAUM, A., WEDDIGE, R., and MILLER, J. "Lithium Erythrocyte/Plasma Ratio as a Predictor of Response," *American Journal of Psychiatry,* 135 (1978):336–338.

112. FLEMING, J. E., et al. "The Thyrotropin-releasing Hormone and Dexamethasone Suppression Tests in the Familial Classification of Depression," *Psychiatry Research,* 9 (1983):53–58.

113. FRANTZ, A. G., and RABKIN, M. T. "Effect of Estrogen and Sex Difference on Secretion of Human GH," *Journal of Clinical Endocrinology and Metabolism,* 25 (1965):1470–1480.

114. FRAZER, A., GOTTLIEB, J., and MENDELS, J. "Lithium Ratio and Clinical Response in Manic-depressive Illness," *Lancet,* 1 (1977):41–42.

115. GALEN, R. S., and GAMBINO, S. R. *Beyond Normality: The Predictive Values and Efficiency of Medical Diagnoses.* New York: John Wiley & Sons, 1975.

116. GARCIA-SEVILLA, J. A., et al. "Platelet Alpha-2-adrenergic Receptors in Major Depressive Disorder: Binding of Titrated Clonidine Before and After Tricyclic Antidepressant Drug Treatment," *Archives of General Psychiatry* 38 (1981):1327–1330.

117. GARCIA-SEVILLA, J. A., et al. "Tricyclic Antidepressant Drug Treatment Decreases Alpha 2-Adrenoreceptors on Human Platelet Membranes," *European Journal of Pharmacology,* 69 (1981):121–122.

118. GEORGOTAS, A. Dexamethasone Suppression Test. Unpublished presentation, American College of Neuropsychopharmacology Meeting Abstracts, 1984.

119. GERNER, R. H., and GWIRTSMAN, J. W. "Abnormalities of Dexamethasone Suppression Test and Urinary MHPG in Anorexia Nervosa," *American Journal of Psychiatry,* 138 (1981):650–653.

120. GIBBONS, J. L., and FAHY, T. J. "Effect of Dexamethasone on Plasma Corticosteroids in Depressive Illness," *Neuroendocrinology,* 1 (1966):358–363.

121. GIBBONS, J. L., and McHUGH, P. R. "Plasma Cortisol in Depressive Illness," *Psychiatry Research,* 1 (1962):162–171.

122. GOLDBERG, I. K. "Dexamethasone Suppression Test as Indicator of Safe Withdrawal of Antidepressant Therapy," *Lancet,* 1 (1980):376.

123. GOMES, U.C.R., et al. "Noradrenergic Overactivity in Chronic Schizophrenia: Evidence Based on Cerebrospinal Fluid Noradrenaline and Cyclic Nucleotide Concentrations," *British Journal of Psychiatry,* 137 (1980):346–351.

124. GRAHAM, P. M., et al. "The Dexamethasone Suppression Test in Mania," *Jour-*

nal of Affective Disorders, 4 (1980):201–211.

125. GRAY, P. N., and DANA, S. L. "GABA Synthesis by Cultured Fibroblasts Obtained from Persons with Huntington's Disease," *Journal of Neurochemistry,* 33 (1978):985–992.

126. GREDEN, J. F., and CARROLL, B. J. "The Dexamethasone Suppression Test as a Diagnostic Aid in Catatonia," *American Journal of Psychiatry,* 136 (1979):1199–1200.

127. GREDEN, J. F., et al. "Dexamethasone Test Predicts Treatment Response," Abstracted in *Scientific Proceedings of the American Psychiatric Association,* No. NR36, New Research Abstracts, 1980.

128. GREDEN, J. F., et al. "Normalization of Dexamethasone Suppression Tests: A Probable Index of Recovery Among Endogenous Depressives," *Biological Psychiatry,* 15 (1980):449–458.

129. GREDEN, J. F., et al. "Dexamethasone Suppression Test and Selection of Antidepressant Medications," *Journal of Affective Disorders,* 3 (1981):389–396.

130. GREDEN, J. F., et al. "Serial Dexamethasone Suppression Tests Among Rapidly Cycling Bipolar Patients," *Biological Psychiatry,* 17 (1982):455–462.

131. GREDEN, J. F., et al. "Dexamethasone Suppression Tests in Antidepressant Treatment of Melancholia: The Process of Normalization and Test-Retest Reproducibility," *Archives of General Psychiatry,* 40 (1983):493–500.

132. GREEN, H. S., and KANE, J. M. "The Dexamethasone Suppression Test in Depression," *Clinical Neuropharmacology,* 6 (1983):7–24.

133. GREGOIRE, F., et al. "Hormone Release in Depressed Patients Before and After Recovery," *Psychoneuroendocrinology,* 2 (1977):303–312.

134. GRUEN, P. H., et al. "Growth Hormone Responses to Hypoglycemia in Postmenopausal Depressed Women," *Archives of General Psychiatry,* 32 (1975): 31–33.

135. GRUNHAUS, L., et al. "Depressive Pseudodementia: A Suggestive Diagnostic Profile," *Biological Psychiatry,* 18 (1983): 215–225.

136. GWIRTSMAN, H. E., GERNER, R. H., and

STERNBACH, H. "The Overnight Dexamethasone Suppression Test: Clinical and Theoretical Reviews," *Journal of Clinical Psychiatry,* 43 (1982):321–327.

137. GWIRTSMAN, H. E., et al. "Neuroendocrine Abnormalities in Bulimia," *American Journal of Psychiatry,* 140 (1983): 559–563.

138. HAAS, M., SCHOOLER, J., and TOSTESON, D. C. "Coupling of Lithium to Sodium Transport in Human Red Cells," *Nature,* 258 (1975):425–427.

139. HAGA, T., and HAGA, K. "Characterization of Alpha-Adrenergic Receptor Subtypes in Rat Brain: Estimation of Ability of Adrenergic Ligands to Displace ^{3}H-Dihydroergocryptine from the Receptor Subtypes," *Life Sciences,* 26 (1980): 211–214.

140. HALBREICH, U., et al. "Growth Hormone Response to Dextroamphetamine in Depressed Patients and Normal Subjects," *Archives of General Psychiatry,* 39 (1982):189–192.

141. HALL, D.W.E., LOGAN, B. W., and PARSONS, G. H. "Further Studies on the Inhibition of Monoamine Oxidase by M and B 9302 (Clorgyline). I. Substrate Specificity in Various Mammalian Species," *Biochemical Pharmacology,* 18 (1969):1447–1454.

142. HARVEY, A. M., et al. *The Principles and Practice of Medicine,* 12th ed., New York: Appleton-Century Crofts, 1980.

143. HASLAM, R. J., and GOLDSTEIN, S. "Adenosine 3':5'-cyclic monophosphate in Young and Senescent Human Fibroblasts During Growth and Stationary Phases *in vitro,*" *Biochemistry Journal,* 144 (1974):253–263.

144. HERSHMAN, J. M. "Clinical Application of Thyrotropin-releasing Hormone," *New England Journal of Medicine,* 290 (1974):886–890.

145. HESKETH, J. E., GLEN, A.I.M., and READING, H. W. "Membrane ATPase Activities in Depressive Illness," *Journal of Neurochemistry,* 28 (1977):1401–1402.

146. HIRSCHFELD, R.M.A., KOSLOW, S. H., and KUPFER, D. J. "The Clinical Utility of the Dexamethasone Suppression Test in Psychiatry: Summary of an NIMH Workshop," *Journal of the American*

Medical Association, 250 (1983):2172–2174.

147. HOFFMAN, B. B., and LEFKOWITZ, R. J. "Alpha-adrenergic Receptor Subtypes," *New England Journal of Medicine*, 302 (1980):1390–1396.

148. HOLSBOER, F., DOERR, H. G., and SIPPEL, W. G. "Dexamethasone Suppression of 11-deoxycorticosterone, Corticosterone and Cortisol in Depressed Female Patients and Normal Controls," *Acta Psychiatrica Scandinavica*, 66 (1982):18–25.

149. HOLSBOER, F., LIEBLE, R., and HOFSCHUSTER, E. "Repeated Dexamethasone Suppression Test During Depressive Illness: Normalization of Test Result Compared with Clinical Improvement," *Journal of Affective Disorders*, 4 (1982):93–101.

150. HOLSBOER, F., STEIGER, A., and MAIER, W. "Four Cases of Reversion to Abnormal Dexamethasone Suppression Test Response as Indicator of Clinical Relapse: A Preliminary Report," *Biological Psychiatry*, 18 (1983):911–916.

151. HOLSBOER, F., et al. "Diagnostic Values of the Dexamethasone Suppression Test in Dopamine," *Lancet*, 2 (1980):706.

152. HOPKIN-NAEVERSON, M., SPIEGEL, D. A., and LEWIS, W. C. "Deficiency of Erythrocyte Sodium Pump Activity in Bipolar Manic-depressives," *Life Sciences*, 15 (1974):1739–1748.

153. INSEL, T. R., and GOODWIN, F. K. "The Dexamethasone Suppression Test: Promises and Problems of Diagnostic Laboratory Tests in Psychiatry," *Hospital and Community Psychiatry*, 34 (1983):1131–1138.

154. INSEL, T. R., et al. "The Dexamethasone Suppression Test in Patients with Primary Obsessive-Compulsive Disorder," *Psychiatry Research*, 6 (1982):153–160.

155. JACOBOWITZ, D. M. "Localization of Catechol-O-methyltransferase and Monoamine Oxidase in Fibroblasts in Tissue Culture," *Life Sciences*, 11 (1972):965–974.

156. JAFFE, K., BARNSHAW, H. D., and KENNEDY, M. E. "The Dexamethasone Suppression Test in Depressed Outpatients With and Without Melancholia," *American Journal of Psychiatry*, 140 (1983):492–493.

157. JOHNSON, G.F.S. "Endocrine Dysfunction in Depression," in P.J.V. Beumont and G. D. Burrows, eds., *Handbook of Psychiatry and Endocrinology*. New York: Elsevier Biomedical Press, 1982, pp. 239–266.

158. JOHNSTON, J. P. "Some Observations Upon a New Inhibitor of Monoamine Oxidase in Brain Tissue," *Biochemical Pharmacology*, 17 (1968):1285–1298.

159. KAFKA, M. S., et al. "Alpha-adrenergic Receptors on Human Platelets," *Life Sciences*, 21 (1977):1429–1432.

160. KAFKA, M. S., et al. "Alpha-adrenergic Receptor Function in Schizophrenia, Affective Disorders and Some Neurological Diseases," *Communications in Psychopharmacology*, 4 (1980):477–480.

161. KASPER, S., and BECKMAN, H. "Dexamethasone Suppression Test in a Pluridiagnostic Approach: Its Relationship to Psychopathological and Clinical Variables," *Acta Psychiatrica Scandinavica*, 68 (1983):31–37.

162. KEMALI, D., DEL VECCHIO, M., and MAJ, M. "Increased Noradrenaline Levels in CSF and Plasma of Schizophrenic Patients," *Biological Psychiatry*, 17 (1982): 711–717.

163. KING, R., et al. "Serotonin and Schizophrenia: Correlations Between Serotonergic Activity and Schizophrenic Motor Behavior." Abstracted at the American College of Neuropsychopharmacology, 1983.

164. KLEIN, D. F. "Endogenomorphic Depression: A Conceptual and Terminological Revision," *Archives of General Psychiatry*, 31 (1974):447–454.

165. KLERMAN, G. L., et al. "A Debate on DSM-III," *American Journal of Psychiatry*, 141 (1984):539–553.

166. KLINE, M. D., and BEEBER, A. R. "Weight Loss and the Dexamethasone Suppression Test," *Archives of General Psychiatry*, 40 (1983):1034–1035.

167. KNOLL, J., and MAGYAR, K. "Some Puzzling Pharmacological Effects of Monoamine Oxidase Inhibitors," *Advances in Biochemical Psychopharmacology*, 5 (1972):393–407.

168. KRAWIETZ, W., et al. "Different Numbers of Beta-receptors in Human Lympho-

cyte Subpopulations," *Biochemical Pharmacology*, 31 (1982):133–136.

169. KROLL, P., PALMER, C., and GREDEN, J. F. "The Dexamethasone Suppression Test in Patients with Alcoholism," *Biological Psychiatry*, 18 (1983):441–450.

170. LAKE, C. R., et al. "Schizophrenia: Elevated Cerebrospinal Fluid Norepinephrine," *Science*, 207 (1980):331–333.

171. LANDMANN, R. BURGIESSER, E., and BUKLER, F. R. "Human Lymphocytes as a Model for Beta-Adrenergic Receptors in Clinical Investigation," *Journal of Receptor Research*, 3 (1983):71–88.

172. LANGER, S. Z., et al. "Molecular Mechanisms in Imipramine and Desipramine Binding to Synaptic Membranes," *Clinical Neuropharmacology*, 7 (Supplement 1) (1984):302–303.

173. LERER, B., EBSTEIN, R. P., and BELMAKER, R. H. "Subsensitivity of Human Beta-adrenergic Adenylate Cyclase after Salbutamol Treatment of Depression," *Psychopharmacology*, 75 (1981): 169–172.

174. LIEBOWITZ, M. R. et al. "Phenelzine Versus Imipramine in Atypical Depression: A Preliminary Report," *Archives of General Psychiatry*, 41 (1984):669–677.

175. LINNOILA, M., et al. "RBC Membrane Adenosine Triphosphatase Activities in Patients with Major Affective Disorders," *Archives of General Psychiatry*, 40 (1983):1021–1026.

176. LOOSEN, P. T., and PRANGE, A. J. "Serum Thyrotropin Release to Thyrotropin-Releasing Hormone in Psychiatric Patients: A Review," *American Journal of Psychiatry*, 139 (1982):405–416.

177. LYTTKENS, L., SODERBERG, U., and WETTERBERG, L. "Relationship Between Erythrocyte and Plasma Lithium Concentrations as an Index of Psychiatric Disease," *Uppsala Journal of Medical Sciences*, 81 (1976):123–128.

178. MAAS, J. W. "Biogenic Amines and Depression: Biochemical and Pharmacological Separation of Two Types of Depression," *Archives of General Psychiatry*, 32 (1975):1357–1361.

179. McLEOD, W. "Poor Response to Antidepressants and Dexamethasone Nonsuppression," in B. Davies, B. J. Carroll, and R. M. Mowbray, eds., *Depressive Ill-*

ness: Some Research Studies. Springfield, Ill.: Charles C Thomas, 1972, pp. 202–206.

180. MAEDA, K., et al. "Growth Hormone and Prolactin Release After Injection of Thyrotropin Releasing Hormone in Patients with Depression," *Journal of Clinical Endocrinology and Metabolism*, 40 (1975):501–505.

181. MASON, J. W. "A Review of Psychoendocrine Research on the Pituitary-Adrenal Cortical System," *Psychosomatic Medicine*, 30 (1968):576–607.

182. MATHE, A. A. "False Normal Dexamethasone Suppression Test and Indomethacin," *Lancet*, 2 (1982):714.

183. MATUSSEK, N. "Neuroendokrinologische Untersuchungen bei Depressiven Syndrome," *Der Nervenarzt*, 49 (1978):569–575.

184. MELLERUP, E. T., PLENGE, P., and ROSENBERG, R. "^{3}H-imipramine Binding Sites in Platelets from Psychiatric Patients," *Psychiatry Research*, 7 (1982):221–227.

185. MELTZER, H. Y., and FANG, V. S. "Cortisol Determination and the Dexamethasone Suppression Test," *Archives of General Psychiatry*, 40 (1983):501–505.

186. MELTZER, H. Y., et al. "Platelet Monoamine Oxidase and Plasma Amine Oxidase in Psychiatric Patients," *Schizophrenia Bulletin*, 6 (1980):213–219.

187. MELTZER, H. Y., et al. "Effect of Dexamethasone on Plasma Prolactin and Cortisol Levels in Psychiatric Patients," *American Journal of Psychiatry*, 139 (1982):763–768.

188. MENDELS, J., and FRAZER, A. "Intracellular Lithium Concentration and Clinical Response: Toward a Membrane Theory of Depression," *Journal of Psychiatric Research*, 10 (1973):9–18.

189. MENDELS, J., et al. "Biogenic Amine Metabolites in the Cerebrospinal Fluid of Depressed and Manic Patients," *Science*, 175 (1972):1380–1382.

190. MENDLEWICZ, J., and VERBANEK, P. "Lithium Ratio and Clinical Response in Manic-depressive Illness," *Lancet*, 1 (1977):41.

191. MENDLEWICZ, J., CHARLES, G., and FRANCKSON, J. M. "The Dexamethasone Suppression Test in Affective Disorder: Relationship to Clinical and Ge-

netic Subgroups," *British Journal of Psychiatry,* 141 (1982):464–470.

192. MINNEMAN, K. P., PITTMAN, R. N., and MOLINOFF, P. B. "Beta-adrenergic Receptor Subtypes: Properties, Distribution and Regulation," *Annual Review of Neuroscience,* 4 (1981):419–461.

193. MOLINOFF, P. B., and AARONS, R. D. "Effects of Drugs on Beta-adrenergic Receptors on Human Lymphocytes," *Journal of Cardiovascular Pharmacology,* 5 (Supplement 1) (1983):S63–S67.

194. MUELLER, P. S., HENINGER, G. B., and MACDONALD, R. K. "Studies on Glucose Utilization and Insulin Sensitivity in Affective Disorders," in T. A. Williams, M. M. Katz, and J. A. Shield, eds., *Recent Advances in Psychobiology of Depressive Illnesses.* Washington, D.C.: U.S. Department of Health, Education and Welfare, 1972, pp. 235–248.

195. MUNRO, J. G., HARDIKER, T. M., and LEONARD, D. P. "The Dexamethasone Suppression Test in Residual Schizophrenia with Depression," *American Journal of Psychiatry,* 141 (1984):250–252.

196. MURPHY, D. L., and DONNELLY, C. H. "Monoamine Oxidase in Man: Enzyme Characteristics in Platelets, Plasma and Other Human Tissues," *Advances in Biochemical Psychopharmacology,* 12 (1974):71–85.

197. MURPHY, D. L., CAMPBELL, I., and COSTA, J. L. "Current Status of the Indoleamine Hypothesis of Affective Disorders," in M. A. Lipton, A. DiMascio, and K. F. Killam, eds., *Psychopharmacology: A Generation of Progress.* New York: Raven Press, 1978, pp. 1235–1248.

198. MYERS, E. D. "Serial Dexamethasone Suppression Tests in Male Chronic Schizophrenic Patients," *American Journal of Psychiatry,* 141 (1984):904–905.

199. NADI, N. S., NURNBERGER, J. I., and GERSHON, E. S. "Muscarinic Cholinergic Receptors on Skin Fibroblasts in Familial Affective Disorder," *New England Journal of Medicine,* 211 (1984):225–230.

200. NASR, S. J., et al. "Symptoms Profile of Patients with Positive DST: A Pilot Study," *Biological Psychiatry,* 18 (1983):571–574.

201. NASRALLAH, H., and CORYELL, W. H. "Dexamethasone Nonsuppression Predicts the Antidepressant Effects of Sleep Deprivation," *Psychiatry Research,* 6 (1982):61–64.

202. NAYLOR, G. J., and SMITH, A.H.W. "Defective Genetic Control of Sodium-Pump Density in Manic-Depressive Psychosis," *Psychological Medicine,* 11 (1981):257–263.

203. NAYLOR, G. J., et al. "Erythrocyte Membrane Cation Carrier in Depressive Illness," *Psychological Medicine,* 3 (1973): 502–508.

204. NAYLOR, G. J., et al. "A Biochemical Study of Short-cycle Manic-depressive Psychosis in Mental Defectives," *British Journal of Psychiatry,* 128 (1976):169–180.

205. NELSON, W., et al. "Hypothalamic-pituitary Axis Activity and Tricyclic Response in Major Depression," *Archives of General Psychiatry,* 49 (1982):1033–1036.

206. NEWMAN, K. D., et al. "Identification of Alpha-Adrenergic Receptors in Human Platelets by ^{3}H-dihydroergocriptine binding," *Journal of Clinical Investigations,* 612 (1978):395–402.

207. NEWSOM, G., and MURRAY, N. "Reversal of Dexamethasone Suppression Test Non-suppression in Alcohol Abusers," *American Journal of Psychiatry,* 140 (1983):353–354.

208. NIGGLI, V., et al. "Purified $(Ca^{2+}-Mg^{2})$-ATPase of the Erythrocyte Membrane," *Journal of Biological Chemistry,* 256 (1981):395–401.

209. NINAN, P. T., et al. "CSF 5-hydroxyindole Acetic Acid Levels in Suicidal Schizophrenic Patients," *American Journal of Psychiatry,* 141 (1984):566–569.

210. NUGENT, C. A., NICHOLS, T., and TYLER, F. H. "Diagnosis of Cushing's Syndrome. Single Dose Dexamethasone Suppression Tests," *Archives of Internal Medicine,* 116 (1965):172–176.

211. NULLER, J. L., and OSTROUMOVA, M. N. "Resistance to Inhibiting Effect of Dexamethasone in Patients with Endogenous Depression," *Acta Psychiatrica Scandinavica,* 61 (1980):169–177.

212. OKADA, S., and O'BRIEN, J. S. "Tay-Sachs Disease: Generalized Absence of a Beta-D-N-Acetylhexosaminidase Component," *Science,* 165 (1969):698–701.

213. ORELAND, L., et al. "Platelet Monoamine Oxidase Activity and Monoamine Metabolites in Cerebrospinal Fluid in Depressed and Suicidal Patients and in Healthy Controls," *Psychiatry Research,* 4 (1981):21–29.

214. OSTROW, D. G., et al. "Ion Transport and Adrenergic Function in Major Affective Disorders," *Biological Psychiatry,* 17 (1982):971–980.

215. OXENKRUG, G. F., et al. "Aging and Cortisol Resistance to Suppression by Dexamethasone: A Positive Correlation," *Psychiatry Research,* 10 (1983): 125–130.

216. PANDEY, G. N., SARKADI, R., and GUNN, R. B. "Lithium Transport Pathways in Human Red Cells," *Psychopharmacology Bulletin,* 14 (1978):16–19.

217. PAPAKOSTAS, Y., et al. "Neuroendocrine Measures in Psychiatric Patients: Course and Outcome with ECT," *Psychiatry Research,* 4 (1981):55–64.

218. PAUL, S. M., et al. "Demonstration of Specific 'High Affinity' Binding Sites for ³H-imipramine on Human Platelets," *Life Sciences,* 26 (1980):953–959.

219. PAUL, S. M., et al. "Depressed Patients Have Decreased Binding of Tritiated Imipramine to Platelet Serotonin 'Transporter,'" *Archives of General Psychiatry,* 38 (1981):1315–1320.

220. PAUL, S. M., et al. "Does High Affinity ³H-imipramine Binding Label Serotonin Reuptake Sites in Brain and Platelet?" *Life Sciences,* 28 (1981):2753–2760.

221. PAVLATOS, F. C., SMILO, R. P., and FORSHAM, P. H. "A Rapid Screening Test for Cushing's Syndrome," *Journal of the American Medical Association,* 193 (1965):720–723.

222. PESELOW, E. D., et al. "The Dexamethasone Suppression Test in Depressed Outpatients and Normal Control Subjects," *American Journal of Psychiatry,* 140 (1983):245–247.

223. PLOTNICK, L. P., et al. "Integrated Concentration of Growth Hormone Correlated with Stage of Puberty and Estrogen Levels in Girls," *Journal of Clinical Endocrinology and Metabolism,* 38 (1974):436–439.

224. POST, R. M., BALLENGER, J. C., and GOODWIN, F. K. "Cerebrospinal Fluid Studies of Neurotransmitter Function in Manic and Depressive Illness," in J. H. Wood, ed., *Neurobiology of Cerebrospinal Fluid,* vol. 1. New York: Plenum Press, 1980, pp. 685–717.

225. PUIG-ANTICH, J., et al. "Growth Hormone Secretion in Prepubertal Children with Major Depression. I. Final Report on Insulin-induced Hypoglycemia During a Depressive Episode," *Archives of General Psychiatry,* 41 (1984):455–460.

226. RAMSEY, T., et al. "Intracellular Lithium and Clinical Response," *British Journal of Psychiatry,* 128 (1976):103–104.

227. RAMSEY, T. A., et al. "The Erythrocyte Lithium-Plasma Lithium Ratio in Patients with Primary Affective Disorder," *Archives of General Psychiatry,* 36 (1979):457–461.

228. RASKIND, M., et al. "Dexamethasone Suppression Test and Cortisol Circadian Rhythm in Primary Degenerative Dementia," *American Journal of Psychiatry,* 139 (1982):1468–1471.

229. RAVARIS, C. L., et al. "A Multiple-dose Controlled Study of Phenelzine in Depression-Anxiety States," *Archives of General Psychiatry,* 33 (1976):347–350.

230. REUS, V. I. "Pituitary-adrenal Disinhibition as the Independent Variable in the Assessment of Behavioral Symptoms," *Biological Psychiatry,* 17 (1982):317–326.

231. RIKER, D. K., ROTH, R. M., and BREAKEFIELD, X. O. "High-affinity [³H]choline Accumulation in Cultured Human Skin Fibroblasts," *Journal of Neurochemistry,* 36 (1981):746–752.

232. ROBINSON, D. S., et al. "The Monoamine Oxidase Inhibitor Phenelzine in the Treatment of Depressive-Anxiety States," *Archives of General Psychiatry,* 29 (1973):407–413.

233. ROTHSCHILD, A. J., and SCHATZBERG, A. F. "Fluctuating Postdexamethasone Cortisol Levels in a Patient with Melancholia," *American Journal of Psychiatry,* 139 (1982):129–130.

234. ROTHSCHILD, A. J., et al. "The Dexamethasone Suppression Test as a Discriminator Among Subtypes of Psychotic Pa-

tients," *British Journal of Psychiatry*, 141 (1982):471–474.

235. ROY, A., PICKAR, D., and PAUL, S. "Biologic Tests in Depression," *Psychosomatics*, 10 (1983):125–130.

236. RUBIN, R. T., and MANDELL, A. J. "Adrenal Cortical Activity in Pathological Emotional States: A Review," *American Journal of Psychiatry*, 123 (1966):347–400.

237. RUDORFER, M. F., HWU, H., and CLAYTON, P. J. "Dexamethasone Suppression Test in Primary Depression: Significance of Family History and Psychosis," *Biological Psychiatry*, 17 (1982):41–48.

238. RUSH, A. J., et al. "Sleep EEG and Dexamethasone Suppression Test Findings in Unipolar Major Depression," *Biological Psychiatry*, 17 (1982):327–341.

239. SACHAR, E. J. "Corticosteroids in Depressive Illness. I. A Re-evaluation of Control Issues and of the Literature," *Archives of General Psychiatry*, 17 (1967):544–553.

240. ———. "Corticosteroids in Depressive Illness. II. A Longitudinal Psychoendocrine Study," *Archives of General Psychiatry*, 17 (1967):554–557.

241. SACHAR, E. J., FINKELSTEIN, J., and HELLMAN, L. "Growth Hormone Responses in Depressive Illness: Response to Insulin Tolerance Test," *Archives of General Psychiatry*, 25 (1971):263–269.

242. SACHAR, E. J., HELLMAN, L., and FUKUSHIMA, D. K. "Cortisol Production in Depressive Illness: A Clinical and Biochemical Clarification," *Archives of General Psychiatry*, 23 (1970):289–298.

243. SACHAR, E. J., et al. "Disrupted 24-hour Patterns of Cortisol Secretion in Psychotic Depression," *Archives of General Psychiatry*, 28 (1973):19–24.

244. SACHAR, E. J., et al. "Growth Hormone and Prolactin in Unipolar and Bipolar Depressed Patients: Responses to Hypoglycemia and L-Dopa," *American Journal of Psychiatry*, 130 (1973):1362–1367.

245. SAWIN, C. T., and HERSHMAN, J. M. "Clinical Use of Thyrotropin-Releasing Hormone," *Pharmacology and Therapeutics Part C*, 1 (1976):351–366.

246. SCHATZBERG, A. F., et al. "The Dexamethasone Suppression Test: Identification of Subtypes of Depression," *American Journal of Psychiatry*, 140 (1983):88–91.

247. SCHILDKRAUT, J. J. "The Catecholamine Hypothesis of Affective Disorders: A Review of Supporting Evidence," *American Journal of Psychiatry*, 122 (1965):509–522.

248. SCHILDKRAUT, J. J., et al. "Platelet Monoamine Oxidase Activity in Subgroups of Schizophrenic Disorders," *Schizophrenia Bulletin*, 6 (1980):220–225.

249. SCHLESSER, M. A., WINOKUR, G., and SHERMAN, B. M. "Genetic Subtypes of Unipolar Primary Depressive Illness Distinguished by Hypothalamic-pituitary-adrenal Axis Activity," *Lancet*, 1 (1979):739–741.

250. ———. "Hypothalamic-pituitary-adrenal Axis Activity in Depressive Illness," *Archives of General Psychiatry*, 37 (1980): 737–743.

251. SCHWARTZ, J. P., and BREAKEFIELD, X. O. "Altered Nerve Growth Factor in Fibroblasts from Patients with Familial Dysautonomia," *Proceedings of the National Academy of Sciences*, 77 (1980): 1154–1158.

252. SHAPIRO, M. F., and LEHMAN, A. F. "The Diagnosis of Depression in Different Clinical Settings: An Analysis of the Literature on the Dexamethasone Suppression Test," *Journal of Nervous and Mental Disease*, 171 (1983):714–720.

253. SHEEHAN, D. V., et al. "Panic Attacks and the Dexamethasone Suppression Test," *American Journal of Psychiatry*, 140 (1983):1063–1064.

254. SHERMAN, B., PFOHL, B., and WINOKUR, G. "Circadian Analysis of Plasma Cortisol Levels Before and After Dexamethasone Administration in Depressed Patients," *Archives of General Psychiatry*, 41 (1984):271–275.

255. SMITH, E. M., MEYER, W. J., and BLALOCK, J. E. "Virus-induced Corticosterone in Hypophysectomized Mice: A Possible Lymphoid Adrenal Axis," *Science*, 218 (1982):1311–1313.

256. SNEDDON, J. M. "Sodium-dependent Accumulation of 5-hydroxytryptamine by Rat Blood Platelets," *British Journal of Pharmacology*, 37 (1969):680–688.

257. ———. "Relationship Between Internal Na^+/K^+ and the Accumulation of

^{14}C-5-hydroxytryptamine by Rat Platelets," *British Journal of Pharmacology,* 43 (1971):834–844.

258. ——. "Blood Platelets as a Model for Monoamine-containing Neurones," *Progress in Neurobiology,* 1 (1973):151–198.

259. SOLOFF, P. H., GEORGE, A., and NATHAN, R. S. "The Dexamethasone Suppression Test in Patients with Borderline Personality Disorders," *American Journal of Psychiatry,* 139 (1982):1621–1623.

260. SPAR, J. E., and GERNER, R. "Does the Dexamethasone Suppression Test Distinguish Dementia from Depression?" *American Journal of Psychiatry,* 139 (1982):238–240.

261. SPAR, J. E., and LaRUE, A. "Major Depression in the Elderly: DSM-III Criteria and the Dexamethasone Suppression Test as Predictors of the Treatment Response," *American Journal of Psychiatry,* 140 (1983):844–847.

262. SPIKER, D. G., et al. "Urinary MHPG and Clinical Response to Amitriptyline in Depressed Patients," *American Journal of Psychiatry,* 137 (1980):1183–1187.

263. SPITZER, R. L., ENDICOTT, J., and ROBINS, E. *Research Diagnostic Criteria (RDC) for a Selected Group of Functional Disorders,* 3rd ed. New York: New York State Psychiatric Institute, Biometrics Research, 1977.

264. SQUIRES, R. F. "Multiple Forms of Monoamine Oxidase in Intact Mitochondria as Characterized by Selective Inhibitors and Thermal Stability: A Comparison of Eight Mammalian Species," *Advances in Biochemical Psychopharmacology,* 5 (1972):355–370.

265. STAHL, S. M. "The Human Platelet: A Diagnostic and Research Tool for the Study of Biogenic Amines in Psychiatric and Neurologic Disorders," *Archives of General Psychiatry,* 34 (1977):509–516.

266. ——. "Platelets as Pharmacologic Models for the Receptors and Biochemistry of Monoaminergic Neurons," in G. Longenecker, ed., *The Platelets: Physiology and Pharmacology.* New York: Academic Press, 1985, pp. 307–340.

267. STAHL, S. M., and MELTZER, H. Y. "A Kinetic and Pharmacologic Analysis of 5-hydroxytryptamine Transport by

Human Platelets and Platelet Storage Granules: Comparision with Central Serotonergic Neurons," *Journal of Pharmacological Experimental Therapy,* 205 (1978):118–132.

268. STAHL, S. M., CIARANELLO, R. D., and BERGER, P. A. "Platelet Serotonin in Schizophrenia and Depression," in B. T. Ho, E. Usdin, and E. Costa, eds., *Serotonin in Biological Psychiatry.* New York: Raven Press, 1982, pp. 183–198.

269. STAHL, S. M., et al. "Hyperserotonemia and Platelet Serotonin Uptake in Schizophrenia and Affective Disorders," *American Journal of Psychiatry,* 140 (1983):26–30.

270. STAHL, S. M., et al., "Platelet Alpha-2 Adrenergic Receptor Sensitivity in Major Depressive Disorders," *Psychiatry Research,* 10 (1983):157–164.

271. STANLEY, M., VIRGILIO, J., and GERSHON, S. "Tritiated Imipramine Sites Are Decreased in the Frontal Cortex of Suicides," *Science,* 216 (1982):1337–1339.

272. STERNBACH, H., GWIRTSMAN, H., and GERNER, R. H. "The Dexamethasone Suppression Test and Response to Methylphenidate in Depression," *American Journal of Psychiatry,* 138 (1981): 1629–1631.

273. STOKES, P. E. "Pituitary Suppression in Psychiatric Patients." Abstracted in *The Endocrine Society (USA),* 49th meeting abstracts, 1966.

274. ——. "Studies on the Control of Adrenocortical Function in Depression," in T. A. Williams, M. M. Katz., and J. A. Shield, eds., *Recent Advances in the Psychobiology of the Depressive Illnesses.* Washington, D.C.: U.S. Government Printing Office, 1972, pp. 199–220.

275. STOKES, P. E., et al. "Pretreatment Dexamethasone Suppression Test and Hypothalamic - pituitary - adrenocortical Function in Depressed Patients and Comparison Groups," *Archives of General Psychiatry,* 41 (1984):257–267.

276. SWARTZ, C. M., and DUNNER, F. J. "Dexamethasone Suppression Testing of Alcoholics," *Archives of General Psychiatry,* 39 (1982):1309–1312.

277. TAKAHASHI, S., et al. "Growth Hormone Responses to Administration of L-5-hydroxytryptophan (L-5-HTP) in Manic

Depressive Psychosis," in H. N. Tsum, ed., *Psychoneuroendocrinology*. Basel: S. Karger, 1974, pp. 32–38.

278. TARGUM, S. D. "The Application of Serial Neuroendocrine Challenge Studies in the Management of Depressive Disorder," *Biological Psychiatry*, 18 (1983): 3–19.

279. ———. "Persistent Neuroendocrine Dysregulation in Major Depressive Disorder: A Marker for Early Relapse," *Biological Psychiatry*, 19 (1984):305–310.

280. TARGUM, S. D., ROSEN, L., and CAPODANNO, A. E. "The Dexamethasone Suppression Test in Suicidal Patients with Unipolar Depression," *American Journal of Psychiatry*, 140 (1983):877–879.

281. TARGUM, S. D., SULLIVAN, A. C., and BYRNES, S. M. "Neuroendocrine Interrelationships in Major Depressive Disorder," *American Journal of Psychiatry*, 139 (1982):282–286.

282. TARGUM, S. D., et al. "Abnormal Dexamethasone Suppression Tests in Withdrawing Alcoholic Patients," *Biological Psychiatry*, 19 (1984):401–405.

283. TASKA, R., and BRODIE, K. H. "New Trends in the Diagnosis and Treatment of Depression," *Journal of Clinical Psychiatry*, 44 (1983):11–13.

284. TOURIGNY-RIVARD, M. F., RASKIND, M., and RIVARD, D. "The Dexamethasone Suppression Test in an Elderly Population," *Biological Psychiatry*, 16 (1981): 1177–1184.

285. TRASKMAN, L., et al. "Monoamine Metabolites in Cerebrospinal Fluid and Suicidal Behavior," *Archives of General Psychiatry*, 38 (1981):631–636.

286. U'PRICHARD, D. C., GREENBERG, D. A., and SNYDER, S. H. "Binding Characteristics of a Radiolabeled Agonist and Antagonist at Central Nervous System Alpha Noradrenergic Receptors," *Molecular Pharmacology*, 13 (1977):454–459.

287. VAN PRAAG, H. M., and DE HAAN, S. "Depression Vulnerability and 5-hydroxytryptophan Prophylaxis," *Psychiatry Research*, 3 (1980):75–83.

288. WAHLSTROM, A., JOHANSSON, L., and TERENIUS, L. "Characterization of Endorphins (Endogenous Morphine-like Factors) in Human CSF and Brain Extracts," in H. Kosterlitz, ed., *Opiates and Endogenous Opioid Peptides*. Amsterdam: Elsevier Press, 1976, pp. 49–56.

289. WEINER, D. A., et al. "Correlations Among History of Angina, ST Segment Response, and Prevalence of CAD in the Coronary Artery Surgery Study," *New England Journal of Medicine*, 301 (1979):230–235.

290. WEINSHILBOUM, R. M. "Human Erythrocyte Catechol-O-methyl Transferase: Correlation with Lung and Kidney Activity," *Life Sciences*, 22 (1978):625–630.

291. WINOKUR, G., et al. "Is a Familial Definition of Depression Both Feasible and Valid?" *Journal of Nervous and Mental Diseases*, 166 (1978):764–768.

292. WINOKUR, G., et al. "Variability of Hormonal Responses to a Series of Neuroendocrine Challenges in Depressed Patients," *American Journal of Psychiatry*, 139 (1982):39–44.

293. WISE, C. D., et al. "Sources of Error in the Determination of Platelet Monoamine Oxidase: A Review of Methods," *Schizophrenia Bulletin*, 6 (1980):245–253.

294. WOOD, K., and COPPEN, A. "Platelet Alpha-Adrenoreceptor Sensitivity in Depressive Illness," *Advances in Biological Psychiatry*, 7 (1981):85–89.

295. ———. "Prophylactic Lithium Treatment of Patients with Affective Disorders Is Associated with Decreased Platelet ^{3}H-dihydroergocriptine Binding," *Journal of Affective Disorders*, 5 (1983):253–256.

296. WYATT, R. J., POTKIN, S. G., and MURPHY, D. L. "Platelet Monoamine Oxidase Activity in Schizophrenia: A Review of the Data," *American Journal of Psychiatry*, 136 (1979):377–385.

297. WYATT, R. J., et al. "Monoamine Oxidase in Schizophrenia: An Overview," *Schizophrenia Bulletin*, 6 (1980):199–207.

298. YANG, H.Y.T., and NEFF, N. H. "Beta-phenylethylamine: A Specific Substrate for Type B Monoamine Oxidase of Brain," *Journal of Pharmacology and Experimental Therapeutics*, 187 (1973): 365–371.

299. ———. "The Monoamine Oxidase of Brain: Selective Inhibition with Drugs and the Consequences for the Metabo-

lism of the Biogenic Amines," *Journal of Pharmacology and Experimental Therapeutics*, 189 (1974):733–740.

300. YEREVANIAN, B. I., et al. "Normalization of the Dexamethasone Suppression Test at Discharge from Hospital (Its Prognos-

tic Value)," *Journal of Affective Disorders*, 5 (1983):191–197.

301. YEREVANIAN, B. I., et al. "The Dexamethasone Suppression Test During Major Depressive Episodes," *Biological Psychiatry*, 19 (1984):407–412.

CHAPTER 36

ETHICS IN BIOLOGICAL PSYCHIATRY

Alan A. Stone

¶ Introduction

It is useful in thinking about medical ethics to make a basic distinction. The important locus of ethical inquiry involves questions that arguably have two or more conflicting or contradictory answers. For example, is it proper to give an efficacious treatment to a psychotic patient who refuses that treatment? The medical benefits arguably make this ethically proper, but respect for the patient's privacy and autonomy arguably make it improper. And these arguments will be further complicated by the question of competency versus incompetency.

In contrast, there are actions taken by psychiatrists and other physicians without any ethical justification that directly violate principles of professional ethics.[2] Although these violations are the province of "ethics committees," they essentially deal with unethical conduct. For example, selling prescriptions to drug addicts, sexually exploiting patients, billing for treatments that never took place, gossiping about patients, and prescribing drugs without adequate knowledge of psychopharmacology or side effects are professional transgressions that have no ethical justification. They are simply wrong and present no ethical question; the only ethical issue is how such offenses should properly be dealt with by the profession and by the law.[73] Should there be punishment or rehabilitation or some combination of both? The medical profession in recent years has recognized that unethical and incompetent physicians are often impaired physicians—frequently substance abusers.[79] A concerted effort has been made to deal with these impaired physicians and to rehabilitate and discipline them. But despite these efforts, critics believe and statistics indicate that the medical profession has not responsibly dealt with either impaired or unimpaired ethical transgressors.[43] "Professional etiquette," covering up for a colleague's failings,[30] is said to be more important than professional responsibility, which in theory requires exposing incompetent and unethical colleagues. These criticisms have led to state laws mandating the reporting of impaired physicians[4]; and the task of disciplining unethical physicians increasingly is given by legislatures to "licensing" and "quality assurance" boards no longer dominated by the medical profession or by "professional etiquette."[43] This chapter will not deal with these extensive legal developments or the obviously unethical practices of psychiatrists, psychotherapists, and other physicians.

The important ethical questions arise when the well-meaning physician faces a choice between two or more contradictory actions, both of which can be ethically justified—the dilemma is in deciding which ethical justification should prevail. Here we confront the hard choices at the core of medical ethics, and these choices become even more difficult when the patient is unable to express a preference. This is the typical situation for the biological psychiatrist; hard choices are compounded by the fact that patients are often marginally incompetent and unable to participate in the choices in terms of their own values or self-interests.

The dichotomy between simple unethical behavior and the conflict between two ethically justified actions is not as fixed as this presentation might suggest. For example, a major reason for loss of medical licensure in this century was illegal and "unethical" abortion. Judged by contemporary values and standards, and excluding those who did it "for the money," these unethical physicians now appear to have made a choice between two actions with conflicting ethical justifications. In fact, the changes in law and medical ethics around the legalization of abortion marked an important turning point for modern medicine, medical ethics, and morality. It made the subject of medical ethics an ongoing concern to the mass media, to politics, and to organized religion. Indeed, it would be fair to say that the Supreme Court's abortion decision[22,62] was one of the most important events to transform medical ethics and move it, perhaps irrevocably, into the public domain.

"Medical ethics has come of age once again," says one well-known commentator. Judging by sheer volume, he is certainly correct. As books, monographs, collections of essays, and articles on medical ethics cross one's desk in increasing numbers, and with many of them dealing with psychiatry, certain common themes begin to emerge.* This chapter discusses seven that are relevant to medicine generally and are particularly pertinent to the ethics of biological pyschiatry.

The Good Old Days

First, there is the historical view, which is universally shared, that physicians and medical researchers in the "good old days" accepted as standard practice procedures that are today ethically quite unacceptable. Vulnerable populations were used for research, and improper inducements were offered. Patients were unwittingly subjected to research and treatments of dubious value and with significant risks. Race and class considerations influenced the selection of experimental subjects.

It is impossible not to conclude that patients were exploited—both by today's standards and even by the ethical standards already articulated in the 1947 Nuremberg Agreement,[41] which was developed in response to Nazi concentration camp experiments by physicians. Yet it was not until 1966 that Professor Henry Beecher,[10] of Harvard Medical School, "blew the whistle" on ethically dubious biomedical research being carried out in the most respected medical institutions in the United States—including his own medical school. Beecher courageously discussed and listed "ethically dubious" biomedical research in an article that was published by the prestigious and equally courageous *New England Journal of Medicine*.

Professor Jay Katz, a psychiatrist, subsequently published an encyclopedic edited

*See references 9, 12, 17, 20, 34, 36, 56, 59, 67, 84, and 85.

collection, *Experimentation with Human Beings,*[41] which included notable abuses, controversial examples, and a broad spectrum of critical, psychological, and analytic perspectives on the ethics of such human experimentation. More recently, a Presidential Commission for the Study of Ethical Problems in Medicine and Biomedical and Behavioral Research was convened to deal with these questions. The chairman of the commission has described the process of public involvement that produced twelve volumes of reports including much that is relevant to psychiatry.[1]

A great deal that was done in the name of medical research on human subjects, even after World War II, is in retrospect horrifying, and much of it had little or no scientific value. We look back with the wisdom of hindsight, although some will argue that medical science would not have progressed as much as it has if at an earlier time it had been forced to meet our present-day ethical standards. Historians who judge the medical practices of the past will have to decide how much weight to give this consideration. Whatever their verdict, it seems clear that Beecher's publication marked the end of the "good old days" and the beginning of a new era of sensitivity about medical ethics.

It is in this historical context that biological psychiatrists should consider three notorious examples of research and innovation that occurred during the post–World War II era. First, there was the widespread introduction of prefrontal and transorbital lobotomy for a variety of mental disorders. This brain surgery was often performed by psychiatrists without neurosurgical training and often without even the pretense of obtaining consent. Readily available electroconvulsive therapy (ECT) was used as anesthesia for the procedure of transorbital lobotomy. Only in 1959 did the chief proponent of this approach acknowledge significant side effects.[29]

Second was the Tuskegee syphilis study, in which, to determine the natural course of tertiary syphilis, black patients went untreated despite the availability of pencillin.[39] Third, the Willowbrook hepatitis study,[41] though not performed by psychiatrists, illustrates the practice of using helpless and noncomprehending patients in mental "institutions" for medical research. This Willowbrook research in fact produced an immunization procedure for type-B hepatitis and was heralded by the editors of the *Journal of the American Medical Association;* but was it ethically justified? Willowbrook, an institution for the mentally retarded, was plagued by endemic infectious hepatitis. Nonetheless, parents were so eager to institutionalize their retarded children that they consented to allow their children, who would very likely contract the disease, to be inoculated experimentally with hepatitis. The parents who thus consented obtained priority for their children's admission to a facility that could not meet even minimal standards of care or provide basic hygiene.

The grim details and the pros and cons of this "good old days" practice and research need not be rehearsed here. (Later I describe the introduction of ECT.) However, these examples illustrate the legacy of ethical criticisms that modern biological psychiatry has inherited.

A Priori *Ethical Solutions*

A second theme in the literature of medical ethics is the attempt to apply a variety of ethical approaches to solve problems of medical ethics—deontological, Kantian, neo-Kantian, Rawlsian, act utilitarian, rule utilitarian, situational ethics, religious, contractarian, and so on. Although some of these efforts have been made by physicians, most are the work of philosophers, ethicists, theologians, and lawyers. Although it would be impossible to discuss all of these attempts (of which the main outlines are described in the following text), it is worth emphasizing that these efforts have achieved no compelling victories. No one application of an ethical approach has captured the field and convinced the medical profession that it has the answers to ethical questions. Indeed, there has been some sentiment that no *a priori* set of ethical rules or casuistry can be expected to solve the problems of medical ethics.[84,85] This belief has led to the development of what has been called situational ethics.[26] Moral rules are considered, but can be rejected under the special circumstances of the case.

A review of the burgeoning biomedical ethics literature produces only two inescapable conclusions: Medical ethics is clearly in disarray, and medical ethics is now clearly in the public domain and no longer the private preserve of physicians. Even the physicians' claim to priority as the actual providers of care is being challenged by nurses who claim, not without some justification, that they deserve the title of caretakers and the right to be heard on ethical questions of clinical care, a right that goes with the responsibility of giving and withholding the actual care.[37]

The Medical Establishment's Principles of Ethics

A third and related theme is the almost complete lack of weight and importance given to the "official" principles of medical ethics generated by the medical establishment itself. These include the American Medical Association's *Principles of Medical Ethics,* which includes a preamble and seven sections. The American Psychiatric Association has appended to this *Annotations Especially Applicable to Psychiatry.*[2] As already noted, these principles indicate what actions are unethical and set forth minimum standards of conduct.

Earlier versions of the AMA's Principles of Ethics nonetheless were attacked by economists and lawyers as protectionistic. It was argued that certain ethical prohibitions merely protected the status and economic interests of the profession, rather than serving the interests of patients. The most often cited instance is the AMA's reliance on its Principles of Ethics to oppose the development of health maintenance organizations (HMOs); but the medical establishment has also opposed in this century Blue Cross, Medicare and Medicaid, nurse practitioners, advertising, and so forth.

Beyond these criticisms, it is striking how little weight or importance is given to the profession's own promulgated ethics by serious writings on ethical problems in medicine. This seems not to be a matter of mere oversight but rather a justified recognition that establishment medical ethics provide precious little guidance in dealing with true ethical problems—specifically, conflicts between ethically justifiable actions. Thus even such basic ethical problems confronting psychiatrists as their ethical responsibilities in dealing with patients who exercise the right to refuse treatment are not considered; nor do the Principles of Ethics instruct the physician as to how to resolve conflicts in specific provisions of the code. Perhaps the most glaring examples are conflicts between the requirement of confidentiality and the requirement to expose the unethical conduct of colleagues whose misconduct is often reported to psychiatrists in a therapeutic context.[73]

Veatch has suggested we "abandon the idea that an ethic for medicine can be based on a professionally articulated code" (p. 6).[85] In reality, the essential AMA "principles" on which the annotations for psychiatrists are based seem to have been reformulated over the years to pacify the Federal Trade Commission and others who have attacked medicine's "protectionistic ethics" and to minimize legal liabilities, rather than to instruct the practitioner. Most physicians and psychiatrists are nonetheless highly ethical. I shall argue that if medicine and psychiatry lack a useful code of ethics or an organized theory of ethics, we do have a traditional and meaningful ethical praxis.

The "Rights" of Patients

A fourth theme found in much of the ethical writing is the new emphasis on the "rights" of the patient, particularly the right to participate in, if not control, decisions affecting one's bodily and mental integrity. A central focus of this concern is the legal doctrine of informed consent. Putting to one side all of the very real problems inherent in truly informed consent, there can be no doubt that it offers at least a partial solution to many troubling ethical questions. Although a psychiatrist cannot abandon ethical responsibility for his or her actions, an important ethical boundary is crossed when the patient shares that responsibility by giving informed consent.

Informed consent has therefore been proposed as the panacea for a broad range of practical and ethical problems in medicine,[49] and it is regularly invoked in a variety of legal contexts. Informed consent is relevant to malpractice law and to state statutes that have addressed particular treatments of public concern. Statutes governing the administering of ECT, for example, have required detailed procedures for obtaining informed consent.[70]

Informed consent also plays a significant role in many government agency regulations, including regulations governing psychiatric research involving human subjects.[19] Even routine but controversial treatments are regulated in this way; guidelines mandate informed consent (as well as a minimum thirty-day waiting period) before a Medicaid-financed sterilization may be performed.[24] Informed consent is also prominent in regulations imposed by nongovernmental groups,[38] as well as in the body of constitutional law that has developed surrounding the right to refuse treatment.[64]

The doctrine of informed consent, and its importance to writers on ethics, is deeply rooted in the basic philosophical values of individual autonomy, self-determination, and personal freedom, central tenets of liberal philosophy.[50] The legal presumption derived from liberal philosophy is that any constraint on individual autonomy or freedom must have a compelling justification. Such constraints, when imposed by the state without sufficient justification, are viewed in legal terms as violations of constitutional guarantees of liberty, privacy, and the "right to be left alone." Many problems of medical ethics in biological psychiatry, as we shall see, have become legal questions and have been recast in the language of constitutional law, dealing with the "rights of patients."

The Bottomless Pit

A fifth theme in ethical writings that has achieved particular importance in the past decade is the so-called bottomless pit problem.[88] Assume that the medically correct thing to do in a given situation is to provide a given patient with a given treatment. For example, some biological psychiatrists suggest that every patient thought to have schizophrenic disorder should have a computerized tomographic (CT) scan. However, if every such patient were given a CT scan, the cost and resources required would open a bottomless pit, creating serious limitations on other social obligations that also have ethical standing. The artificial heart is an often-cited example of a medical innovation that would create a bottomless pit. As the health care industry exceeds 10 percent of the gross national product, health care itself is viewed as a bottomless pit, and this is now discussed as a justification for some form of rationing of health care.

The significance of the bottomless pit in discussions of medical ethics is multifold. It makes economics and future aggregate cost count as relevant and appropriate ethical considerations in research, and it raises the question of the criteria to be used in selecting the patients who obtain a resource that others are denied. But accepting the relevance of the bottomless pit in an ethical dialogue about the treatment of patients and deciding how much weight to give it and who should do the weighting is one of the great questions in contemporary medical ethics and public policy.

There has been little discussion of the bottomless pit problem in psychiatry; yet one wonders if the history of institutional psychiatry in this century does not suggest an implicit judgment by society, explicitly adopted by its elected officials, that quality care of the mentally disabled is a bottomless pit and a waste of social resources that should be devoted to higher priorities. State governors objecting to court-ordered right to treatment have made arguments that come close to openly stating this.[73] What other explanation can there be for the ways in which the richest country in the world has allocated resources to its most vulnerable citizens?

The Committee Solution

A sixth theme that emerges from the literature of medical ethics is the ubiquitous committee approach to all ethical problems. Lawyers have often suggested that in order to deal with ethical problems, medicine needed to incorporate some of the notions of due process that are basic to law. The ubiquitous committee is the most compelling evidence that "due process" of a sort exists in medicine and in psychiatry. Due process in law does not require a single specific procedure for making decisions, but the essence of due process is to ensure that the various interests at stake are heard. Above all, due process is meant to promote fairness among competing interests.

The use of committees in medicine to deal with ethical questions involved in treatment and research approximates some of the goals of due process, depending, of course, on the membership of the committee and the rules by which it functions. However, solving or resolving ethical questions by hearing the various interests and then deciding by vote of a committee composed of diverse members is not the same as deciding ethical problems by applying ethical principles or reaching a decision by moral reasoning. Due process is meant to ensure that a decision is approached in a fair manner, but committee voting by representatives of interest groups can be closer to political decision making than moral reasoning.

More Questions Than Answers

A final striking aspect of the medical ethics literature is that it seems to raise many more compelling questions than it provides compelling answers. Physicians and psychiatrists have had their ethical sensibilities raised, but they have been given very little guidance as to practical resolutions. The ethical literature is in a certain sense muckraking. Problems that were formerly dealt with in private are now exposed to public airing, promoting distrust of physicians and of psychiatry. For example, there has been much legal and ethical attention given to the side effects of the administration of antipsychotic drugs, emphasizing arrant abuses and incompetent practice, and little attention paid to the great benefits of competent practice. This muckraking approach has given rise to the expression of a constitutional right of involuntarily confined and psychotic patients to refuse antipsychotic drug treatment. In the process, with the attendant media hoopla, public confidence in the benefits of these drugs when properly prescribed by competent psychiatrists has been undermined. Nor have the courts or the ethicists established clear guidelines to help psychiatrists decide when these beneficial drugs are legally and ethically appropriate. There is ongoing legal confusion about who should make the decisions and by what criteria.

A similarly confusing scenario has grown up in medicine around the treatment of the dying patient and the defective newborn. Thus, in these and many other important areas, there is a heightened ethical awareness in the medical profession and a sense of greater public concern, but no clearer legal or ethical directives. The result is a growing distrust of the medical establishment and the psychiatric profession, a distrust that feeds on itself and that neither the law nor the ethicists have resolved through their interventions.

The seven themes that I have extracted from the recent literature on medical ethics are not meant to be inclusive or definitive, but they should give some sense of the terrain. The terrain has been shaped not just by intellectual debate and scholarly reflection. Medical ethics has in a certain sense also become the final common pathway for a variety of social, political, economic, and legal forces now influencing the medical profession in the United States.

For example, medical ethics is one of the battlegrounds for the rise of consumerism, for the regulation of medical practice by courts and legislatures, for rationing of health care to control the cost of health care, for death with dignity in an aging population, for egalitarianism between physicians and related professions, for holistic medicine and against dehumanizing medical care, for patients' rights against medical authority, for the increasing antipathy against medical paternalism on both the political right and left, and for the growing public concern about iatrogenesis. The legalization of abortion has brought powerful religious interests to bear on medical ethics. Medical ethics, particularly in psychiatry, has even become an important battleground for international politics. Progress in medical science and psychiatry is no longer viewed as a certain social beneficence. The fearful possibilities of recombinant deoxyribonucleic acid and of more sophisticated "mind-altering" drugs suggest to many critics that the future of medical and psychiatric research is too important to be left to those doing the research.

These powerful social, political, religious, and economic forces are now played out in medical ethics and in the ethics of biological psychiatry. Indeed, it may well be that future medical historians will describe the second half of the twentieth century as the period when medical ethics, previously the dominion of the profession, became part of the public domain. In no way is this phenomenon more obvious than when we consider the ethics of biological psychiatry. Indeed the attacks on the ethics of biological psychiatry foreshadowed the attacks on the ethics of the rest of medicine. The contrast between the introduction of electroshock treatment, which I shall now detail, and the current regulation of psychobiological research on human subjects and the formulation of the right to refuse treatment as a basic constitutional right makes clear what an extraordinary transformation has taken place. There are still important and interesting ethical problems unique to biological psychiatry, which I discuss later. These problems deserve our careful attention. Even though the ultimate power to establish policy may no longer be left to the psychiatric profession, its voice should be heard.

¶ The Good Old Days

The pre–World War II era in biological psychiatry provides many examples of the "good old days" mentality in research and treatment. Of the various "innovations" of that era, only "electroshock" remains as a widely accepted treatment. Therefore, I shall focus on the ethical questions that in retrospect seem applicable to the method of its introduction into psychiatric practice.

Describing the development of "electroshock" in the *American Journal of Psychiatry*, Ugo Cerletti[16] conveyed a sense of the ethical context in which the founding fathers of biological psychiatry worked. (All of the following quotations are from his 1950 article.[16]) Cerletti had used both Sakel's method of treating schizophrenia by means of insulin coma and Meduna's method of pentylenetetrazol (Cardiazol, Metrazol)–induced convulsions. Cerletti believed, as did Meduna, that the grand mal convulsion was the essential curative factor. He wrote:

[i]t was natural that the idea should occur to me, and perhaps to others also, that electricity could be applied to men as a convulsive stimulus . . . but this idea then, and for a long time to come, appeared utopian, because of the terror with which the notion of subjecting a man to high tension currents was regarded. (P.89)

Cerletti was able to overcome this terror by fortunate happenstance, when he learned of a slaughterhouse where pigs were supposedly killed by electrocution. Investigating, he found instead that the electricity produced convulsions and unconsciousness, allowing the butchers to cut the pigs' throats. The pigs were not being killed by electricity; they were in fact being slaughtered. Cerletti secured permission to experiment at the slaughterhouse and learned that pigs survived even after five to six minutes of electric current across the head. Only current across the pigs' chests had fatal consequences.

These clear proofs, certain and often repeated, caused all my doubts to vanish, and without more ado I gave instructions in the clinic to undertake, next day, the experiment upon men. . . . A schizophrenic of about 40, whose condition was organically sound was chosen for the first test. He expressed himself exclusively in an incomprehensible gibberish made up of odd neologisms, and, since his arrival from Milan by train without a ticket, not a thing had been ascertainable about his identity. (P. 90)

The first treatment was given at a reduced tension, 70 volts with a duration of 0.2 seconds. The voltage proved inadequate to produce a convulsion, and the assembled doctors began to whisper about whether to give a second treatment at a higher voltage. The patient, hearing the

low toned conversation around him, exclaimed— no longer in his incomprehensible jargon, but in so many clear words and in a solemn tone—"Not a second. Deadly!" . . . This *warning* explicit and unequivocal, shook the persons present to the extent that some began to insist upon the suspension of the proceedings. (P. 90)

But, Cerletti continued, "[a]nxiety lest something that amounted to superstition should interfere with my decision urged me on to action." The electrodes were reapplied "and a 110 volt discharge was sent through for 0.5 seconds" producing the first "electroshock treatments . . . such was the name I forthwith gave it." (p. 91)

The patient gradually awakened and when Cerletti asked " 'What has been happening to you?' he answered, with no more gibberish, 'I don't know, perhaps I have been asleep.' . . . So electroshock was born."

Cerletti reports a complete remission and "[i]t may be of interest to note that 'the patient' was well satisfied because a very tiresome whistling in his ears that had also troubled him for years had also disappeared."

Cerletti was much concerned about "unexpected surprises" (negative side effects) that might be encountered with electroshock therapy. He specifically mentioned

casualties associated with other contemporary medical innovations: myxedema, which followed the "brilliant" operation of goiter ablation by Kocher and Reverdin; the hopeless blindness produced by Atoxil, a proposed cure for sleeping sickness; the "incidents" caused by blood transfusions before the discovery of blood groups; and the disastrous paraplegias consequent to endorachidian injections of sulfonamides. He particularly worried that inducing repeated convulsions would make his patients into epileptics, but neither this nor other unwarranted side effects occurred in his experience. Reporting on his subsequent research to identify "acroagonine," the specific chemical substance he believed was produced by a shocked brain, Cerletti recounted ideas and theories that in retrospect seem quite bizarre. So too does the application of electroshock to certain other diagnostic disorders. Soon physicians in Italy applied electroshock to "progressive paralysis, Parkinsonism, disseminated sclerosis, psoriasis, prurigo, and alopecia areata."

Cerletti, explaining why his patients were afraid of his beneficial therapy, hypothesized that the "terror defense" expressed the biological significance of epileptic fits, and he ended his report of the development of electroshock therapy with a quote from "Padre Dante":

Qaul e colui che sommiando vede, E dope il sogno la passione impressa, Rimane, e l'altro alla mente non riede . . . (Para. XXXIII, 58–61) (As he who while dreaming sees, and after the dream is over, the emotion remains while the picture has faded away . . .)

We now know that Meduna's original theory and his statistics about the low incidence of schizophrenia among epileptics, which led Cerletti to introduce electroshock, were wrong. We know too that although Cerletti introduced electroshock as a treatment for all forms of schizophrenia, its primary indication is now for certain patients with depression and patients with catatonic schizophrenia. And we certainly know that Cerletti's clinical research would today never get past the required committees that supervise research. Not only did Cerletti select as his first subject a patient who had no known identity and who was incompetent to consent, but the patient also had no relatives or friends to represent his interests or to consent on his behalf. Nor did Cerletti stop when the patient clearly said "Not a second. Deadly!" This may have been considered an incompetent refusal of treatment, but these were the first comprehensible words the man had spoken. Cerletti himself described it as a "warning, explicit and unequivocal." Cerletti simply ignored these words and suggested that the patient's warning evoked "superstitions" among the assembled doctors. Perhaps, but how would one today describe the theories that inspired this innovative treatment, or Cerletti's subsequent attempts to treat schizophrenia by injecting pig "acroagonine" into humans?

The selection of Cerletti's first experimental subject, which he described in the *American Journal of Psychiatry* in 1950 without the slightest hint of any ethical concern, exemplifies the "old days" mentality that continued at least until 1966. In making an ethical judgment about Cerletti's method of selecting his first subject, we should remember that his method was identical to that used by most medical schools for selecting cadavers for anatomical dissection. The corpses with no identity and no known relatives were dispatched to the anatomy laboratory for student instruction. Legislatures reflecting the social ethics of that era passed statutes providing for this practice. The point is that Cerletti's ethical mentality in selecting his experimental subjects was not unique to psychiatry.

During my own medical training in the 1950s, when surgical procedures on the heart became common, Down's syndrome children were brought from institutions for repair of their congenital heart disorders and, perhaps more important, to provide surgeons with the necessary experience and training in cardiac surgery. The use of the mentally disabled and the probable class and race discrimination inherent in biomedical research did not then seem relevant or important to doctors, lawmakers, or society. The legal and ethical presumptions that seem so correct today—that the more helpless the person, the greater is the obligation of society to safeguard that person's rights and interests—had not yet emerged. Indeed, one could describe the "old days" mentality as favoring the opposite presumption. If a person was socially, economically, politically, and psychologically powerless, then he was more apt to be a suitable subject for medical experimentation. A kind of social Darwinism governed the selection of subjects in this ethics. This is the red thread that seems to run through what now seems to be the dubious ethical practices of the "good old days." Social Darwinism, as it was then interpreted, was elastic enough to include not only mental disability but also racial, ethnic, and class biases. It is perhaps the only common thread that runs from Nazi concentration camps to Willowbrook, to Tuskegee, and on through the annals of research in medicine and psychiatry.

Cerletti's work took place almost a half century ago, and it led to the development of a treatment method considered by many experts in biological psychiatry to be invaluable even today. This kind of history is more typical of early advances in biological psychiatry than it is exceptional. Bold innovators experimented on sick, helpless patients, often basing their experiments on false theories and incomplete or incorrect scientific knowledge, with little or no consideration of the patients' rights. Cerletti did not receive the Nobel Prize, but his Portuguese contemporary Egon Moniz did, for the clinical development of prefrontal lobotomy, a procedure Moniz performed on violent mental patients after he learned about preliminary research by Fulton and Jacobsen on two chimpanzees. [83]

Psychosurgery, electroshock, Metrazol convulsions, and insulin coma ushered in the practice of biological psychiatry in the midtwentieth century. Probably none of these developments would have been possible if researchers had been required to obtain the informed consent of their subjects. One does not have to look back very far to find authoritarian physicians and psychiatrists who, when confronted with serious and seemingly incurable disorders, took drastic measures. These grandfathers of modern biomedical research knew far less than they imagined, and their failures have generally been forgotten. What this history can teach us is to have greater humility about the wisdom of our current knowledge and to remember that professional ethics becomes morally suspect when scientific progress is achieved on the backs of the helpless.

It is, in part, because of the "good old days" that we now confront the question of whether the advancement of medical science provides a substantial ethical justification for research on human subjects. Most ethicists would agree that it does, but the record of past abuses makes clear that this is a justification that must be carefully limited and qualified. It is also qualified by concerns on the one hand that the advancement of medical science opens a bottomless pit and on the other that supposed beneficences often turn out to be iatrogenic harms. The problem for clinical research in the future in the United States is that the pendulum has swung so far that the advancement of medical science, though valued ethically and socially in the abstract, may be given little weight in the consideration of concrete research proposals. Clinical research, particularly in psychiatry, has been severely restricted.

The irony of these ethical and legal constraints is that they have led to the exporting of clinical research, particularly drug research, to third world countries.[69] Colonialism and the "good old days" continue as these vulnerable populations assume the risks of biomedical research considered inappropriate for American citizens. Indeed, in the United States, the ethical dispute has moved on from human to animal experimentation.[65] The protections afforded American animals may yet exceed those provided some third world citizens who are the subjects of our exported biomedical research.

¶ *A Priori* Ethical Solutions

Five years ago *Psychiatric Annals*,[32] a "throw-away journal," published an issue that dealt with the ethical conflicts in psychiatry. The striking feature of the issue was that all of the articles were authored by psychiatrists who were ordained Catholic priests. There are many reactions one could have to the logic of such an enterprise, but one might well suppose that the editors hoped that psychiatrists trained to the priesthood might have a special contribution to make to the disorganized enterprise of medical ethics.

George Murray began his article,[53] "Ethics at the Crossroad," with a quote: "To begin with, medical ethics is no big deal—K. Danner Clouser." Although it is difficult to know exactly what Murray intended by the quote, presumably he meant that the "big deal" is moral philosophy and that medical ethics is only one of many areas to which moral principles are applied. Murray made the further point that the substance, if there is any, of medical ethics cannot come from mere medical knowledge, but must come from moral philosophy. He identified the basic problem that confounds medical ethics as Hume's is-ought dilemma. This is a version of the fact-value distinction: Physicians know about facts, which are objective—the *is*—but they do not know about values—the *ought*—which cannot objectively be proved true or false by medical science.

This is a theme echoed increasingly by medical writers: Medical ethics has to do with values and medical science has to do with facts. Thus the physician has no priority or claim of authority in medical ethics. For example, Komaroff, writing for the President's Commission for the Study of Ethical Problems in Medicine and Biomedical and Behavioral Research about the ethics of rationing health care, concluded that the advance of the science of clinical practice will only allow "the inescapable ethical problems to be posed more clearly" (p. 251).[42] The more medicine discovers the *is*, the clearer will be the question of the *ought*, which is a separate matter, the province of experts in values.

The is-ought, fact-value dilemma makes psychiatry a particularly vulnerable target. Since even some distinguished biological psychiatrists agree that the diagnosis of mental disorder is partly fact and partly value, the ethics of the act of diagnosing a patient can be criticized as labeling or as imposing the psychiatrist's value judgments. The new *Diagnostic and Statistical Manual* may improve diagnostic reliability but it does not eliminate value judgments. The debate over the diagnosis of homosexuality demonstrates the confusion about facts and values in psychiatry.[7]

Murray conceded that there are philosophers who claim to have solved the is-ought dilemma and overcome the fact-value distinction, but he concluded that their reasoning is so difficult and complicated that it will not convince the "ordinary person" or the ordinary physician. Thus a useful, shared, and principled medical ethics drawn from a moral philosophy that has overcome the is-ought dilemma does not exist. Philosophical principles applied to medical ethics are still too complicated, abstract, or conflicting to be convincing. One might assume that an ordained Catholic priest would then suggest that his religion, with its long tradition of applying theological-moral values to human problems, including medical ethics, has answers to medical ethical questions. But he did not; instead he invoked Wilson's sociobiology and imagined a similar evolution of ethics.

Murray's evolutionary approach is not only highly speculative and scientistic; it also has nothing to do with traditional Catholic morality. Indeed, none of the priest-psychiatrists in this journal offered theological moral solutions to medical-ethical problems. Any of the articles could have been written by agnostics. However, these priest-psychiatrists did convey in their articles a sense of their own personal integrity and their common desire to reach good ethical decisions. But good, as they presented it, had no relation to God or any clearly stated transcendent moral values. At their best, they offered themselves as role models of compassionate physicians.

Although it is not explicit, one can read between the lines of Cassem's excellent article[15] what I shall discuss as the practical dialectic of do no harm and do all you can to help the patient. Cassem, a distinguished liaison psychiatrist, applied this dialectic to the dying patient, where it can be paraphrased as: Do no harm by futile recourse to life-support systems that prolong futile suffering and do all you can to ease the inevitable suffering attendant on a protracted death.

Because of what they leave out, these articles by priest-psychiatrists exemplify what I believe is the most important obstacle to the development of a coherent theory of medical ethics. We live in a diverse society in which diverse and conflicting values proliferate. The conflicting values have strong constituencies: Consider the right to life versus the freedom of choice in the context of abortion. Given these diverse and conflicting values, there is no agreed-upon moral dogma that can be applied to ethical dilemmas in medicine. This great obstacle apparently confronts even psychiatrists trained to the priesthood, whom one might expect to share a strong, consistent religious and moral code. This is not to deny the additional problem that even when such dogma exists, there may be no simple casuistry in applying such dogma to contemporary problems of medical ethics. Thus we see the Catholic Church struggling over the years to reinterpret its dogma so as to apply it to the new problems created by advances in biomedical technology.

Although applied medical ethics may be considered "no big deal," the literature of medical ethics is certainly complicated, compendious, and even arcane when approached by the average physician. Yet despite the density and volume of this literature, one eventually learns that philosophers, within their own hierarchy of intellectual status, look down on medical ethicists, as Murray suggested. Their work is viewed as an attempt to apply standard philosophical ideas to the biomedical area rather than to do original or creative moral philosophy. Be that as it may, I shall here briefly summarize in broad outline some of the contemporary approaches to biomedical ethics. This outline is drawn in the main from the excellent *Principles of Biomedical Ethics* by Beauchamp and Childress. [9]

The two central schools of moral philosophy relied upon by professional ethicists are the utilitarian and the deontological. The utilitarian looks in essence to the consequences of alternative choices and asks which choice will result in the greatest good for the greatest number. Jeremy Bentham and John Stuart Mill are the philosophical fathers of utilitarianism. The deontologists (deontology is the study of moral obligations) reject the idea that morality can be based entirely on consequences. They argue that there are moral values to be served even when the consequences of serving them do not result in promoting the greatest good. For example, preserving the autonomy of the individual may be a more important value than treating a person's manic-depressive disorder.

Both the utilitarian and the deontological schools are subdivided into many sects. The earliest utilitarians, for example, had difficulty defining the desired consequence or utility. Bentham and Mill are described as hedonistic utilitarians because they defined utility—the greatest good—as happiness, pleasure, or the avoidance of unhappiness. Later utilitarians took a more pluralistic view of utility, and today many utilitarians have given up the attempt to define the "good." Instead they look to actual preferences: What is useful is what individuals prefer to obtain. This modern version may have greater analytic clarity and allow for methodological precision; but in accepting any and all preferences, including preferences that we customarily think of as bad or evil, "preference utilitarianism" seems to have lost its connection with our moral traditions. It seems more like a survey of public opinion than a search for higher moral ground. Per-

haps these utilitarians believe there is no higher moral ground.

Beyond disputes about what counts as "utility" in utilitarianism, there is also a major distinction made between act and rule utilitarianism. The question is whether the principle of maximizing utility is to be applied to particular acts or to rules of conduct that determine the right or wrong of particular acts. The rule utilitarian establishes rules of conduct that are justified by the appeal to their utility. These rules then govern specific acts. The act utilitarian applies the principles of utility directly to a particular act. The important difference is that the rule utilitarian must consider the general consequences of everyone's observing a rule. For example, an act utilitarian might accept a particular paternalistic intervention, such as involuntary psychiatric treatment, without having to ask (as the rule utilitarian would) what will be the consequences of a rule in which all such acts of paternalism are justified. Rule utilitarians, going back to David Hume, are further divided into those who suggest that the utility of the whole code of rules must be considered and those who would consider only the utility of a particular rule. If, in the utilitarian school of morality, the right is a function of the good then it turns out that there are many definitions of the good and many conflicting theories about how to think about attaining the greatest good for the greatest number.

Just as there are subdivisions of utilitarianism, there are different deontological theories. Immanuel Kant is the deontological equivalent of Bentham and Mill, the father of modern deontological theory. He specifically rejected the notion that morality could be based on any empirical theory of human good or happiness or utility. The "veil of self love" obscured all such efforts, in his view. Instead he sought to construct a moral theory on *a priori* moral grounds and proposed the categorical imperative. [40]

The categorical imperative has been stated in many ways. Its essence is universalizability. Any moral maxim that a rational person would assert would have to hold for every other rational being in the universe. Kant's attempt to found morality on a single fundamental *a priori* principle has been much admired by philosophers, but it seems so lofty and abstract that it lacks practical value as a program for human affairs, including application to particular moral or ethical problems in medicine.

Perhaps the most notable deontological theorist of modern times is John Rawls. His ideas are set out in his highly influential work, *A Theory of Justice.*[58] The key to his moral theory is to imagine rational persons who are agreeing to a social contract but with a "veil of ignorance" about their personal interests, because they cannot know how they, as individuals, will be subsequently situated. Thus, for example, in deciding what might be just policies for the mentally ill or mentally retarded, one cannot know whether or not one will be so handicapped. Rawls argues that behind "the veil of ignorance," the parties to a social contract would agree to certain principles of justice. Rawls is considered a deontological pluralist, in contrast to Kant's monistic categorical imperative. Rawls's work should be of interest to psychiatrists, because he considers psychological issues of great importance in constructing a just society. It is an interesting propaedeutic experiment to imagine how one would like psychiatrists to behave if one could not know whether one was to be a patient or a psychiatrist, or to consider what mental health laws should exist or what medical ethics should require. Rawls, however, is not a medical ethicist; he is a moral-political philosopher whose work medical ethicists and lawyers have attempted to apply to medical ethics.

Again, just as with utilitarians, deontologists are further divided into act and rule deontologists. Act deontologists have little academic standing. Presumably they have some *a priori* value to guide every ethical decision. Each case is decided by an intuition about what is good or just. God or their conscience speaks to them. The rule deontolo-gist, in contrast, adheres to a set of binding moral rules that classifies acts as right and wrong, obligatory or prohibited. The rule deontologists have a strong foothold in contemporary biomedical ethics. Prolific writers such as Ramsey[57] and Veatch[85] are considered rule deontologists. (Veatch describes his approach as "contractarian.") Hare[33] and Brandt[11] are the leading Anglo-American utilitarians, but as with Rawls, biomedical ethics is not their primary interest. Beauchamp and Childress, authors of the text that informs the summary just given, picture the rule utilitarians and the rule deontologists as the principal players in the contemporary biomedical ethics debate. Their *Principles of Biomedical Ethics,*[9] is an invaluable source for those with a serious interest in the basics of the subject.

There are, however, useful books on biomedical ethics directed to psychiatrists that make no mention of these ethical theories and make no explicit use of them. Culver and Gert's book,[20] *Philosophy in Medicine: Conceptual and Ethical Issues in Medicine and Psychiatry,* does not even include the term deontological (not to mention rule deontologists and rule utilitarians) in its index. Eschewing any analytic discussion of controlling moral and ethical theories, the authors attempt an "ordinary language" approach to medical ethics. Although in their conceptual analysis the authors refer to controlling moral rules, the theoretical source of those rules is left unspecified and, some might say, unjustified. Their approach to dealing with typical ethical problems in medicine and, particularly, in psychiatry is to provide analysis of the concepts and precise definitions of the words used, such as rationality, irrationality, competence, incompetence, paternalism, and "malady." Malady is a term they use in an attempt to clarify the concept of mental illness as a sickness. They believe that after their kind of verbal and conceptual clarification, ordinary moral convictions can provide the rules that decide particular cases.

The reader of the literature of medical ethics will also encounter what is called situational ethics. There are, as might be expected, a variety of interpretations of situational ethics. Beauchamp and Childress[9] describe act utilitarianism and act deontologism as situational ethics. The basic approach of the situational ethicist is to discount any fixed ethical rule that might, in a particular situation, produce what is in their view a wrong result. They recognize ethical rules, but these "intermediate" rules can be set aside in a particular situation to achieve beneficence, the greatest good, the most loving act, or some religious ideal. Beauchamp and Childress argue that situational ethics faces "insurmountable problems of coordination, cooperation, and trust" (p. 43).[9] They quote a rather amusing dialogue involving a patient who is attempting to determine how his doctor will take care of him. It turns out, of course, that the patient can get no trustworthy promise from the physician, because the course of action depends on the "situation." The dialogue, though humorous, is real enough to suggest that perhaps there is a great deal of situational ethics in traditional medical practice and medical paternalism.

This brief outline should give some sense of the broad contours of the intellectual dialogue in contemporary medical ethics. There are surely significant omissions in this capsule summary. There are also significant questions about the real-world importance of this intellectual debate on biomedical ethics. At the level of theory, one is often struck by the ease with which the same ethical proposition can be recast in utilitarian, deontological, or contractarian terms. For example, treating a patient against his will can be seen as a utilitarian proposal, but it can be recast as a deontological proposal to promote beneficence.

At the level of practice, one wonders if these debates alter the behavior of physicians and psychiatrists; or has medical ethics become yet another lifeless intellectual subspecialty, removed from the real world of health care: the emergency room and the ward? Surely over the past three decades it has been law, economics, and politics, not ethics, that have altered the behavior of psychiatrists and changed psychiatric practice

and research. Arguably, the law is influenced by the ongoing ethical dialogue. Ethicists are certainly cited in some important decisions. But it is probably fair to say that the ordinary judge is as removed from this ethical discourse as is the ordinary physician. One can certainly find more politics than ethics in the important constitutional reforms that have changed the practice of psychiatry. However, if one considers Thomas Szasz an ethicist (he could be categorized as a rule deontologist), then the ethical dialogue he initiated has had a profound influence on the legal reforms of psychiatry.

Szasz, one of the apostles of "autonomy," is at the extreme of libertarian positions. By arguing that mental illness was a myth,[77] he challenged every instance in which the law left open the possibility that individual autonomy, when compromised by mental illness, could be discounted. Unlike other "ethicists," Szasz had a practical program for systematic reform, a program that could be translated into legal arguments and could be embraced by civil libertarians of the left and libertarians of the right. Both groups share his emphasis on individual antonomy and his distrust of paternalism. He set out his practical program in his book *Law, Liberty and Psychiatry*,[75] and much of his program has come to pass as the law of the land.

Szasz's theories about the myth of mental illness required him to take a position on the mind-body problem. He adopted the most radical mind-brain dichotomy. He considered mental events to be entirely separate from brain events. He accepted the fact that there were diseases of the brain that were the province of medicine and neurology, not psychiatry. But he asserted that diseases of the mind were invented by psychiatrists. Schizophrenia was his most important example. What he did not anticipate, or chose to ignore, were the developing advances in biological psychiatry that have demonstrated the biological aspect of schizophrenia and other major mental disorders. That diseases of the brain are significantly associated with diseases of the mind can no longer be doubted. To assert that brain events have no bearing on mental events is absurd. Szasz's theory, reported in the *Myth of Mental Illness*,[77] because it is based on this radical mind-brain dichotomy, is without logical or scientific foundation; it is, in fact, a myth. But myth or not, it shaped the views of a generation of legal activists who attacked the traditional practices of psychiatry and, particularly, biological psychiatry.

¶ The Medical Establishment's Principles of Ethics

It would be no exaggeration, based on my own informal surveys, to suggest that the vast majority of physicians and psychiatrists have never even read, not to mention studied, the AMA's *Principles of Medical Ethics with Annotations Especially Applicable to Psychiatry*. This, I think, demonstrates both how unimportant the principles have become in actually disciplining the profession and how little of value they provide when a doctor confronts a genuine ethical dilemma.

It is quite reasonable to suggest that medicine and psychiatry have neither enforced ethical norms nor developed a coherent theory of medical ethics. As Veatch, an ethicist, has written, "[i]t makes no more sense to depend on a health professional to provide knowledge of what is morally appropriate behavior in medicine than to trust a friend who is a rabbi to help select a good ham for Sunday dinner" (p. 8).[85] Business is good for medical ethicists these days, and Veatch is condescending about the physician's confusing and conflicting practical guidelines: Do what will benefit the patient and do no harm. He calls these "slogans" and scoffs at physicians who do not even recognize that they conflict.

Viewed in a less condescending way, this approach presents a dialectic and derives from medical traditions that no longer appear in the AMA's Principles of Ethics. The first is the ancient Hippocratic injunction, *primum non nocere,* first of all do no harm. The second maxim derives from the physician's calling and obligation as caretaker of the sick: Do everything you can to help the patient. Obviously, as Veatch points out, these two maxims will sometimes conflict. Every psychiatrist with clinical experience recognizes this conflict. Does one discontinue neuroleptics in a severely psychotic patient showing early signs of tardive dyskinesia?

There is, as yet, no synthesis of this practical dialectic of do no harm and do what you can to help. The physician must struggle within this dialectic, but the dialectic defines a praxis to be pursued. The lack of synthesis does not explain why these maxims and the praxis they convey have disappeared from the accepted principles of medical ethics. Unfortunately, even this practical approach has been undermined by recent legal regulations intended to control the rising cost of health care. The physician is no longer free to do everything he or she can to help the patient. We will return to the praxis of medical ethics in the discussion of the bottomless pit.

¶ The "Rights" of Patients

Whether it is on deontological or utilitarian grounds, privacy, autonomy, and self-determination have been the key concepts in arguments about the rights of patients. What appears to be an ethical problem because of a particular moral or religious value can, it is argued, be obviated by the patient's exercise of personal autonomy.

An example that sharply defines the implications of autonomy is the ethical dispute over sex-change surgery, a dispute in which psychiatrists have played an active role on both sides.[78] (For the sake of simplifying this discussion, it is limited to male-to-female sex changes.) Obviously, to perform a sex-change operation against the patient's wishes would be unethical, and I know of no modern legal system that would permit such a procedure to be done involuntarily. Some countries have permitted sterilization and castration, but the idea of involuntarily transforming a man into a woman goes beyond what is legally, ethically, and "naturally" acceptable. But if it is too horrible to contemplate such a procedure as an involuntary treatment, it is apparently not horrible—indeed proponents of the procedure now consider it humane—to provide it to a man who feels he is a woman and wants a sex-change operation. His autonomous choice, tested by cross-dressing, feminizing hormones, careful psychiatric evaluation, and continuing informed consent, outweighs any opposing ethical reservations that the procedure violates some principle of "natural law" or the physician's ethical norm of nonmaleficence, or involves the legal crime of maiming. The legal argument of maiming has been invoked by opponents of voluntary stereotaxic psychosurgery,[3] which is arguably less an act of maiming (mutilation) than sex-change surgery. The autonomy of the person is sufficient, by contemporary ethical standards, to trump any social values or religious convictions of the community that might deem medical participation in such "unnatural" surgery immoral, unethical, and perverse.

Arguably, the exercise of personal autonomy in such a case has no impact on society and therefore the state has no interest or responsibility. However, if the same man wanted his physically healthy arm amputated, it is unlikely that such an autonomous choice would meet contemporary ethical standards, or that informed consent would protect the surgeon from civil or criminal liability. The autonomous choice must meet some other unstated criterion. The reason for the choice must be acceptable to a substantial minority, or at least there must be no organized political opposition. The choice to have a sex-change operation meets this other criterion in part because the psychiatric profession has declared that transsexualism is a disease or disorder that can be treated. This is yet another example of the fact-value problem in psychiatry. Is transsexualism a fact or is it the result of changing societal values about sex and sexual identity? Labeling the desire of a man to be a woman a disease—in this instance, contrary to tradi-

tional psychiatric approaches—does not mean that it is the desire that should be cured. Rather the psychiatric cure, unique to this disorder, is to make the "pathological" desire come true. Indeed, one might note that before the development of the relevant surgical methods, the disorder of transsexualism was not included in the psychiatric nosology.

It is nonetheless remarkable to consider the fact that no American city or state has attempted to prohibit sex-change operations, nor are there any legally imposed requirements that involve judicial scrutiny or mandate formal legal review. However, there have been just such legal requirements levied against patients who would voluntarily undergo ECT and psychosurgery.[60] The striking disparity in legal and ethical opinion between voluntary sex-change surgery and voluntary psychosurgery is exemplified in a federal court opinion. The court does not even question the moral or ethical justifications for an "irreversible" sex-change operation; instead it holds that given the doctor's diagnosis and recommendation, sex-change surgery is "necessary medical care," which must be paid for by Medicaid.[55] In contrast, courts have had the gravest reservations about "irreversible" psychosurgery and even the side effects of neuroleptic drugs,[63] and federal courts have ruled that abortion is not "necessary medical care."[8]

If sex-change surgery illustrates the apparent power of personal autonomy in resolving ethical questions, the comparison to *voluntary* ECT and *voluntary* psychosurgery emphasizes the point already made that there are still values that can trump personal autonomy. Vigorous legal and ethical opponents of voluntary psychosurgery and ECT have expressed no such opposition to voluntary sex-change surgery. Yet on further analysis we may see that the values invoked against psychosurgery and ECT are also rooted in autonomy. There is a widespread popular perception that these treatments destroy or alter the individual will, making people into "zombies." Whether opponents of these psychiatric procedures are factually correct or not, they may nonetheless believe that these psychiatric treatments impair a person's autonomy.

Thus the principle behind their opposition might be that autonomy is so precious that one cannot, even with informed consent, make an autonomous choice to sacrifice the capacity to make future autonomous choices, just as the law would not permit a person to choose to be a slave and sign a contract to that end. The objections to neuroleptic drugs have piggybacked on these arguments, labeling these drugs as "mind altering,"[63] thus interfering with the will and autonomy of the person. Nonetheless, the different ways in which the law and medical ethicists respond to sex-change surgery and to biological psychiatric treatment suggest a certain inconsistency. This inconsistency in turn suggests a special public animus and distrust of biological psychiatry.

The personal autonomy of the patient is protected legally and ethically through informed consent. Historically, the legal concept of informed consent was a response to nonconsensual intrusions by physicians upon their patients. These intrusions were deemed batteries and were conceptualized within the realm of tort law. Thus a surgeon who performed an operation without his or her patient's consent was guilty of an illegal touching.[66] Over the past three decades the focus of the courts has shifted to the kind of information given to the patient who is to give consent. Although physicians continue to be sued for battery, the dominant legal approach has become that of negligence (inherent in physicians' failure to provide the kind of information necessary to obtain adequately informed consent).

The modern law of informed consent relevant to malpractice has taken two directions. Some states—still the majority—require a physician to provide to the patient that information which other physicians would provide. Other states take a more consumer-oriented view, requiring the physician to provide to the patient the information he or she needs in order to make an informed decision. The latter is considered the progressive approach. Its rationale of patient autonomy is typified in one court decision:

True consent to what happens to one's self is the informed exercise of a choice, and that entails an opportunity to evaluate knowledgeably the options available and the risks attendant upon each. The average patient has little or no understanding of the medical arts, and ordinarily has only his physician to whom he can look for enlightenment with which to reach an intelligent decision. (P. 780)[14]

Informed consent in psychiatry raises the fundamental and practical problem of competency to consent. This problem is based on the assumption that the autonomy of a person who is irrational, insane, or unable to comprehend his or her available choices is not an autonomy that should be given the same weight as the choice of a competent person should be given. This assumption has been subjected to much critical scrutiny, particularly from radical psychiatrists and civil libertarians. The definition of incompetency to make medical decisions is still quite unclear, both in law and in psychiatry.[28] However, even where there is legal consensus that incompetency exists and negates autonomy, there remains considerable disagreement about the methods for defining and determining incompetency and the appropriate consequences that follow a determination of incompetency.[63] Analyzing these issues is central to understanding many of the ethical problems of biological psychiatry.

The "rights" of psychiatric patients are to a large extent an outgrowth of constitutional litigation in the federal courts, where informed consent has not been the central issue.[86] Rather, the focus has been on the involuntary patient who has not consented to psychiatric intervention. This litigation has attacked every aspect of the discretionary authority exercised by psychiatrists under color of law.

The exact legal interpretation of the

phrase "under color of law" is complicated. It is a reasonable rule of thumb, however, to assume that anything done to a patient in a public mental health facility is done under color of law. Furthermore, anything done to a civilly committed patient, including the decision to commit, is done under color of law whether in a private or public facility. Acting under color of law means acting as an agent of the state. The state mental health statute, for example, establishes provisions for civil commitment and in most states authorizes any psychiatrist to initiate emergency commitment. Thus a private practitioner who initiates commitment acts under color of law.

It is because the psychiatrist acts under color of law that his or her actions can be challenged as violations of constitutional rights under the Civil Rights Act, in what is legally known as a 1983 action.[82] A "1983 litigation" can challenge the constitutionality of the laws that authorize the psychiatrist's actions and can claim that the psychiatrist is personally liable for monetary damages for violating the patient's constitutional rights. Rarely have courts actually awarded monetary damages, and the awards have been minimal.[23] The principal result of such litigation has been for courts to redefine or create rights applicable to the entire class of similarly situated psychiatric patients under the jurisdiction of the court.

The right to treatment, the right to refuse treatment, and the right to the least restrictive alternative are the most important developments affecting the practice and the ethics of psychiatry.[71] This is not the place to examine and explain these judge-made rights. The different federal courts have reached different conclusions about these rights, and the Supreme Court has not as yet held that psychiatric patients have any of these rights.[73] Legal advocates nonetheless can be expected to assert that these rights exist, and that they are relevant to the claims of advocacy groups in the mental health system.

Although the law has taken a broader per-spective, for the purposes of this discussion, patients' rights can be thought of as the obverse of the psychiatrist's discretionary authority. Where the psychiatrist examines, evaluates, and in his or her discretion decides to hospitalize, medicate, seclude, restrain, or restrict the patient, there is a corresponding right that "protects" the patient and challenges the psychiatrist's discretion.[73] What is the relevance of the psychiatrist's professional ethics, when so much of the doctor-patient relationship is now constrained by law?

Before attempting to answer this question, one might do well to ask another question as a propaedeutic. What was the relevance of the psychiatrists' professional ethics when we confined and cared for patients under conditions that were degrading, overcrowded, unsanitary, and countertherapeutic? The psychiatrist had nearly absolute discretionary authority, but to what end, and how were professional ethics squared with the shamefully inadequate resources and conditions? Professional ethics did not mitigate the systemic abuses of the past, and they are unlikely to solve the systemic problems of the present. The ethical psychiatrist will nonetheless find that on occasion, the patients' newfound rights interfere with an ethically responsible effort to provide good care. What should a psychiatrist do when ethics come into conflict with law?

The most important instance of such conflict arises as a result of the right to refuse treatment, particularly "antipsychotic" medication. It merits detailed discussion. Since Massachusetts law is the most extreme example, let us consider the conflict as it occurs in that jurisdiction. Massachusetts law allows patients who meet the legal criteria for involuntary hospitalization to be hospitalized but to refuse antipsychotic medication.[73] The patient's refusal can only be overturned by a judge, who must first decide that the patient is incompetent and then decide whether to permit drug treatment. The latter decision is based on legal criteria that emphasize autonomy. The judge who must decide whether to permit antipsychotic drug treatment is asked not to do what is in the best interest of the patient or to follow the best medical advice. Rather, the judge must attempt to enter the mind of the patient and choose what the patient, if he were in his right mind, would choose. This is an example of the overwhelming importance of individual autonomy in the law's approach to these issues. The law rejects a "reasonable person" test or a "best interest" test, and instead attempts through "substituted judgment" to replicate the particular patient's autonomous will.

Now assume that a competent and ethical psychiatrist has evaluated the patient and made a good-faith effort to explain the "antipsychotic" treatment to the patient and the patient's family. Assume that the patient nonetheless refuses. Assume further that as required by Massachusetts law, the ethical and responsible psychiatrist explains the diagnosis and proposed treatment to a judge, but the judge, after finding the patient incompetent, in a substituted judgment upholds the incompetent patient's refusal of treatment based on the legal criteria of proxy consent. Further assume that the ethical and responsible psychiatrist in good faith believes that antipsychotic drugs are the *essential* element of the treatment. What should the ethical psychiatrist then do? Should the psychiatrist simply accede to the law and continue to take professional responsibility for a patient who refuses the *essential* aspect of treatment? Here there are a number of competing ethical and legal considerations.

The law, no matter how inanely, in the psychiatrist's opinion, has spoken and deserves respect. However, the law now requires the psychiatrist to provide care in a manner that the psychiatrist, by his or her own standards, considers negligent.[72] Should the psychiatrist ignore his or her best medical judgment in deference to the law? Note further that the law claims to speak for the patient. What should any doctor do when a patient asks for treatment but refuses to consent to the *essential* element of the treatment? For example, should an ethical and competent doctor continue to treat a forty-five-year-old man with fulminating pneumonia who refuses antibiotics? We are assuming that an ethical doctor in all of these situations would try to accommodate the patient's wishes with alternative treatment whenever feasible, but in this example, no accommodation can be made that the doctor believes will allow effective treatment. Under these circumstances, at the behest of a court or a patient, should a doctor continue to take responsibility for a negligent treatment? The doctor is being prevented from pursuing either of the practical ethical mandates of the profession. The doctor cannot help the patient, and the inadequate treatment harms the deteriorating patient.

Doctors are sometimes placed in a similar situation as a result of a patient's religious objection to blood transfusions that are necessary for survival. These are instances when the law subjugates medical imperatives not just to the competent patient's autonomy, but also to religious convictions recognized by constitutional precedents. Is the incompetent patient's autonomy sufficient by itself? Is the incompetent patient's judicial proxy sufficient? Whatever answer the law may give to such questions, does the physician have a right based on traditional medical ethics to object to the law's answer and refuse to cooperate?

A psychiatrist cannot impose a treatment barred by the court—a course of action that is illegal and can only be defended as a type of civil disobedience. But is it ethically and legally justifiable for the psychiatrist to ask in these circumstances to be relieved of responsibility for the patient? It is ethically justified, in my view, to attempt to withdraw from treatment responsibility when in good faith a psychiatrist believes he or she cannot help the patient and that the court-ordered withholding of treatment harms the patient. Lawyers routinely ask courts to relieve them of responsibility for an "uncooperative" client. And if a judge interfered with the lawyer's ethical obligation to be a zealous advocate, the legal profession would certainly be up in arms.

If psychiatrists looked to the legal profession as an example, they would, I believe, be sustained in the conviction that their professional ethics justified some action in the specific circumstances I have detailed. What should that action be? They should first notify the patient and the court that they cannot in good conscience continue to be responsible for the patient's care.

Doctors cannot "abandon" patients without risking a suit for malpractice. However, the cases of malpractice arising from abandonment typically involve doctors who abandon patients in an emergency when the patients wanted and needed treatment.[45] The psychiatrist should in any event refer the patient to other professionals. This protects the psychiatrist against a claim of abandonment.

But now the question arises, to whom should a psychiatrist refer such a patient? In the public mental hospital where these situations typically arise, there are now many nonphysician mental health practitioners who are given primary responsibility for patient or "client" care. Since the patient under the law can refuse "biological treatment" but not other treatments, it is perhaps reasonable to look to these practitioners to take responsibility for the refusal of treatment.

What will all this accomplish, even if it is legal and ethical? To some psychiatrists, it seems improper to refer a patient to a psychologist or social worker whose treatments they in good faith believe will not help the patient. They see this as dumping a problem, but it is not a problem of the psychiatrist's making. It is a problem created by the law's regulation of psychiatric practice without regard for the ethical obligations of the psychiatrist.

Such referral is therefore the only available way for the psychiatrist to assert ethical obligations and perhaps at least to force the courts to recognize that there is an ethical problem at issue.

¶ The Bottomless Pit*

Although, as noted earlier, the analogy of the bottomless pit is usually applied to technological advances such as the artificial heart, to many critics the American health care system is itself a "bottomless pit." The health care industry is now estimated to be in excess of 10 percent of the gross national product. The federal government's expenditures for health care have been increasing steeply. Health care insurance is a growing burden to employers and employees alike. There has, therefore, been considerable political pressure to control health care costs.

During the Carter administration, national health insurance became a misnomer for what was in reality an attempt to control health care costs. No coherent legislation has passed the Congress, but there have been a series of makeshift attempts at cost control enacted into federal legislation over the past two decades. These federal regulations, typically augmented by state law, now cast a lengthening shadow over the clinical practice of medicine and psychiatry. PSRO (Professional Standards Review Organization), PRO (peer review organization), DRG (diagnosis-related group), and CON (certificate of need) are acronyms that have entered the physician's consciousness, along with malpractice liability, antitrust actions, and new federal and state regulation.

The health insurance industry, increasingly the target of legal regulation, is itself a powerful regulatory influence and often acts in a quasi-legal capacity, extending the lengthening shadow of legal constraints. Psychiatric care has been a principal victim of the health insurance industry. Psychiatric benefits, which have always been inequitably underinsured, are often the first to be curtailed, and although some states have mandatory minimums on mental health care, these

*Material in this section has been adapted, with permission, from my article "Law's Influence on Medicine and Medical Ethics," *New England Journal of Medicine*, 312 (1985):309–312.

provisions are now being challenged in the courts.[5]

The medical profession is increasingly viewed as a vested-interest group, opposing reforms that are needed to control the bottomless pit of health care. The characterization may be accurate, but I want to consider a narrower question: Is the concern that medical responsibility and medical ethics are being overrun by these legal reforms an intelligible concern deserving of public attention, or is it merely a red herring? One should acknowledge at the outset that there is real confusion and perplexity among physicians because the import of legal constraints seems to be so contradictory. Much of the recent legal regulation has in fact been aimed at creating incentives to lower aggregate health care costs and put a bottom on the bottomless pit. On the other hand, litigation establishing the rights of patients, the "judges at the bedside" *Saikewicz* [74] and *Rogers* decisions,[63] Baby Doe regulations,[25] malpractice rulings,[80] and the threat of loss of Joint Commission on Accreditation of Hospitals accreditation are legal developments that ignore cost and effectiveness considerations.

The right to refuse "antipsychotic" treatment can transform a three-week hospital stay into endless months. Fear that a discharged patient will harm third parties, resulting in malpractice litigation, can also prolong hospitalization and increase the cost of care. And courts addressing the right to treatment of the mentally ill and mentally retarded have said that costs must be ignored when constitutional rights are at stake.[90]

The former legal constraints suggest that the aggregate cost of health care is to be considered an explicit factor in deciding what is ethically and clinically appropriate treatment in particular cases. The latter suggest, explicitly in the case of the proposed Baby Doe regulations and in the *Rogers* right-to-refuse-treatment case, that cost cannot be an ethically, clinically, or legally relevant consideration. How is an ethical physician to react to these mixed legal messages?

Even when legal policy is aimed solely at reducing or containing the bottomless pit of aggregate health care costs, contradictory methods have been applied, with conflicting clinical and ethical implications. Most important, legal health policy experts disagree about whether costs are better contained by command and control regulation or by deregulation and competition.[89] The former policy treats the health care system as an industry to be regulated: It imposes five-year plans, hospital rate setting, price fixing, CON, and other controls on capital expansion. The latter favors the end of centralized control, believing that competition, entrepreneurial ingenuity, the "for profit" sector, and a freer market will lower costs and enhance efficiency.

These contradictory legal policies have attracted different political constituencies. As a result, legislation affecting health care is sometimes an uneasy compromise between these contradictory policies. Federal health planning legislation, for example, embodies such contradictory provisions. Federal guidelines ask state planning agencies to consolidate and regionalize health care services, but they also ask them to promote competition and innovation among health care providers. How these contradictory policies of consolidation and competition are to be reconciled is unclear.[18] Many other recent developments in law reflect these contradictory policies. Some right-to-treatment lawsuits have required massive expenditures to upgrade public inpatient facilities despite mental health planners' preference for innovative partial care facilities.[90]

Legal constraints acceptable to politicians on both sides of the regulation-competition struggle are perhaps even more important for their clinical and ethical implications. DRGs are the most recent example. Although not yet applied to psychiatric patients, they eventually will be. DRGs appeal to politicians on both sides of the regulation-deregulation aisle. DRGs appeal to the regulatory supporters because they allow regulators to set the categories and fix the price tag of hospital treatment. The pro-competition supporters are appeased by the fact that at least there is an incentive for efficiency, and more efficient hospitals will benefit financially from the fixed prices. However, it is probably safe to say that one other good reason politicians endorse DRGs as they did HMOs, PSROs, and PROs is that all of the painful ethical decisions inherent in balancing cost control and quality of health care are passed on to the health care providers and taken off the backs of government officials. If the time comes when patients are deprived of needed services, it will be the providers who will be held accountable for their decisions by angry consumers.

It is, I think, a useful practice to examine each new cost-saving proposal in terms of where politicians seek to place the major burden for the "tragic choices."[13] Congress and the state and federal agencies can bear the burden themselves, as when they limit Medicare or Medicaid coverage. Congress has done this repeatedly by limiting psychiatric coverage. However, confronted with "tragic choices" and a vocal lobby, Congress usually makes resources available, as they did for patients with renal failure by adding the costs to Medicare.

The "tragic choices" of the mental health system have not produced the same kind of federal generosity. The mental patient evokes neither the same kind of human sympathy nor the same kind of political pressure. It is fair to say that Congress prefers to pass the burden of painful political and ethical decisions to others. PSRO and PRO legislation put the burden on the doctor's peer group, as did all forms of utilization review. Limiting tax deductions for health care, cost-sharing, deductible health insurance policies, and limits on psychiatric coverage put the burden on the patient. Rate setting, DRGs, and HMOs put the burden on the health care providers' administrative hierarchy. Health-planning regulation, as originally conceived, put the burden on citizens' groups that were to be representative of the community. Systems have been devised to make the primary care physician shoulder the burden.[52] Finally, there are legal reformers who try to place the burden on group purchasers of health care insurance, such as unions and employers, who presumably can make informed decisions to accept a smaller package of health and mental health care benefits.[35]

The cost-effectiveness of targeting the burden in these different ways is not fully known as yet, and the social justice of these different measures is still being argued. However, it is clear that wherever the burden is placed, there will eventually be an encounter between a doctor and a patient where the issue will be joined, where patients will be turned away or the quality of treatment will be affected by cost-saving considerations. This kind of encounter is an everyday occurrence in the mental health care system. Indeed, responsible quality care is the exception rather than the rule in the public mental health system.

Certain consequences of this burden are already apparent in psychiatry and elsewhere in the practice of medicine. The need to establish cost-control decision-making processes promotes the bureaucratization of care; empowers administrators, be they physicians or not; and favors the proliferation of decision making by committee and by standardized protocols.[67] Even where such measures seem to be effective in containing costs, these developments are changing the practice of medicine, diffusing ethical responsibility, challenging the physician's professional identity and autonomy, and affecting the doctor-patient relationship.[54]

Although there are many physicians who welcome standardized care and the diffused committee approach to ethical problems, some physicians have become increasingly concerned about their own personal responsibilities to their patients. The ethical questions attendant on standardizing and rationing health care to control cost have been frequently discussed. Many prominent physicians seem to feel there is a need to draw firm ethical lines against these threatening legal intrusions, and even highly interventionist courts have expressed a willingness to consider medical ethics in their law making.[74] But is it clear that there exist in medical ethics sufficiently clear principles to permit us or the law givers to draw bright lines?

For example, consider the growing problems of providing quality care for the aged population, a population of great concern to psychiatrists. A recent article denounced discrimination against the elderly as an emerging and dubious national policy of cost-benefit analysis for controlling the bottomless pit of health care costs.[6] The views expressed were in sharp contrast to a paper published only weeks before in the same journal, which argued that it was ethical under appropriate circumstances to "sparingly" provide resuscitation and intensive care to "pleasantly senile" patients. Although the thrust of the latter article was patient autonomy and death with dignity, cost-saving, cost-benefit analysis, and the bottomless pit hovered in the background as a legitimate ethical consideration, for "as society tries to contain the soaring cost of health care, the physician is subject to insistent demands for restraint, which cannot be ignored" (p. 956).[87] These contrasting papers, both written by distinguished physicians, are indicative of the medical profession's current confusion and uncertainty about where, in the face of the bottomless pit, we stand on our own ethical principles. What is the ethical principle that will send physicians or psychiatrists to the barricades to resist cost-saving legal reform?

Cost-saving legal interventions are especially threatening to practical medical ethics because I believe that, to a large extent, physicians learn whatever practical ethics they possess primarily by identifying with the role models they encountered during their training in teaching hospitals. These were conscientious and compassionate physicians who demonstrated a dedication to high-quality care, including mastery of all available technological resources. Our ethical role models were physicians who in the pursuit of excellence pressed for certainty of diagnosis and helpful treatment, even at what is now described as the flattening end of the curve. Their diligence and their continuing mastery of developments in their field, together with their caring for patients, is what distinguished them. Their ethics and their quest for professional excellence were *combined,* not separate, virtues. Do whatever you can to help your patient and first of all do no harm. These contradictory demands constitute the ethical dialectic of the exemplary physician's ethical practice. There is as yet no synthesis. But the praxis is real, and physicians judge themselves and others on these terms as decent and caring healers.

We will have difficulty upholding this praxis of ethical probity and professional excellence when cost-conscious administrators empowered by legal constraints mount their attack on flat-of-the-curve medicine. It is this traditional praxis that now seems threatened both by regulatory constraints and the pro-competition emphasis on entrepreneurial ingenuity and by competitive efficiency. In fact, one of the leading legal proponents of the pro-competitive approach has specifically attacked the "Tyranny of Professional Norms and Standards" as the basic obstacle to market reform.[35] Even Fuchs, an economist sympathetic to the "caring physician," worries that physicians are counterproductively "imprinted" with the "best medical practice" in medical school.[31] There seems to be insufficient appreciation of the crucial link between what makes for practical medical ethics and the best medical practice.

If I am correct in suggesting that the "best medical practice" is half of what is basic to practical medical ethics, then the current concern among practitioners is intelligible. This is not to say that partial solutions cannot be found, or that there is no iatrogenic harm or waste in the "best medical practice," or that the bottomless pit can be ignored. Perhaps the role models of the future will be practitioners who have, as Komaroff suggested, mastered the "science of clinical practice"—including "cost effectiveness analysis." But Komaroff, as earlier noted, frankly acknowledges that the advance of the science of clinical practice will only allow "the inescapable ethical problems to be posed more clearly" (p. 251).[42] His conclusion implies that the ethical questions in medicine cannot be answered by the practice of the new scientific physician. That conclusion is an invitation to further legal intervention in the decades ahead. With the pressure to control aggregate cost in the foreground of political concern, *caveat emptor* may be more relevant than *primum non nocere* in medical practice.

I have described the bottomless pit problem as it applies to the entire health care sector. It seems clear that if mental illness continues to have low political priority, it will bear a disproportionate burden in the face of rationing. The ethics of the individual psychiatrist and the traditional praxis will be no solution to these large-scale problems. The greatest problem facing psychiatry and biological psychiatry is continuity of care. This is a therapeutic and an ethical failure demonstrating a lack of responsibility for patients. Regulation, rationing, and related systemic changes seem to increase fragmentation of care and increase the psychiatrist's sense that the obligation of the profession is to deliver a specific, limited treatment of disorders rather than responsible care of patients.

For psychiatry to stand on a firm ethical foundation in the future, solutions must be found to overcome political, systemic, and economic problems—subjects that are rarely taught in medical schools, residency training programs, or courses on medical or psychiatric ethics. The failure of the great experiment of the community mental health centers gives one pause to wonder whether psychiatry has the will, the power, or the imagination to find solutions to problems that touch directly on the ethical standing of our profession. The most obvious example is the homeless mentally ill.

¶ The Committee Solution

As I have already suggested, the use of committees to resolve ethical questions may not be the way to find ethical solutions. The result of committee decision making may be to obscure the ethical question or to substitute a political decision instead of resolving

the ethical question on the basis of a specific ethical principle. These comments are applicable to the recent legal and ethical controversy over withholding treatment from mentally disabled newborns, the so-called Baby Doe regulations.[25] The government asserted as a legal and ethical principle that quality of future life (profound mental retardation) was not an acceptable consideration in withholding treatment. This was proffered as a substantive ethical and legal position that was intended to govern any decision, no matter what procedure or committee was used in making that decision. The American Academy of Pediatrics, speaking for a divided medical profession, offered no alternative substantive ethical position. The Principles of Ethics in fact provide no real alternative. However, the academy opposed government regulation, emphasizing instead the importance of local hospital committees representing different "interest groups" as the better procedural mechanism to deal with these ethical problems.[25] If the hospital committee were free not to adopt the substantive principle proposed by the government, and if the members followed their own moral intuitions and voted on a case-by-case basis, in what sense could we describe such a committee as engaged in moral reasoning or as applying an ethical principle? Due process may ensure that a decision is approached in a fair manner, but committee voting by representatives of interest groups is closer to political decision making than moral reasoning.

Viewed from this perspective, the proliferation of ethics committees might be seen as serving to bureaucratize, politicize, and obscure medical ethics, rather than serving to forge new and clearer ethical principles. How would a hospital committee confront the alternative ethical principle, contrary to the government view, in the Baby Doe regulations: namely, that a newborn who is so brain-impaired as to never be able to experience sentient existence is not a person?[46] No interest group suggested by the American Academy of Pediatrics to be represented in the hospital committee explicitly holds that view; yet it may be the most compelling ethical argument for withholding treatment. If the view were presented, how would a committee resolve the ethical controversy?

There are, however, many different kinds of committees and layers of committees utilizing a variety of procedures to review the ethics of research and practice; the one constant is the creation of a committee to deal with the problem. Committees have a certain cost whatever their benefits; ethical responsibility is removed from the primary physician, and there is a sacrifice of patient privacy. This alters the doctor-patient relationship and limits the physician's autonomy.

A recent study was done of surgeons who were collaborating in a randomized clinical trial of surgery for breast cancer.[81] Although they had agreed to collaborate, they failed to involve their own patients. The study indicated that some surgeons do not even accept being bound by protocols they collaborate in producing. Their chief objection was the effect of the research protocol's informed consent provisions on the doctor-patient relationship. The committee solution, whatever its benefits—and this is not to say they are not considerable—inevitably contributes to the further depersonalization and bureaucratization of medicine and clinical research. Professional ethicists who do not realize that bureaucracy can be the mortal enemy of the patient's autonomy, privacy, and self-determination have lost contact with the realities of modern medicine. Thus to the extent they promote bureaucracy, ethical reforms may be self-defeating.

This is not to suggest that committees serve no useful ethical function. The committee model that is most familiar is the institutional review boards for research (IRBs), which were begun in 1966. These boards have given special emphasis to informed consent, to adequate safeguards and surveillance for potential hazards, and for the protection of minors and prisoners. The basic test of the IRBs, as suggested by Fost, is whether they have "a better track record of making ethically defensible decisions than physicians acting on their own" (p. 49).[27] He

believes that they do. No doubt he is correct, since IRBs were mandated after widespread media attention to the abuses in medical research. Beecher published his article in 1966[10], and IRBs were a response to the scandal. Fost cogently argues that the creation of IRBs helped the research community to develop a consensus about ethical standards for research. Similarly, he argues that equivalent committees could help to develop a consensus about the treatment of defective newborns. He notes that despite strong opposition from the research community, the standards applied by IRBs are now widely accepted by medical investigators.

I have no doubt that IRBs served a useful function in prohibiting certain abuses that once were common, and in that sense, their track record is ethically defensible. However, ethical decisions involve more than preventing abuses. Consider the special protections now given to prisoners. These protections were the result of a report in 1976 by the National Commission for the Protection of Human Subjects of Biomedical and Behavioral Research.[61] A commission study had found that most prisoners did not regard their consent to research as obtained under coercion or undue influence; the prisoners believed they were making autonomous choices. However, the commission concluded that conditions in prison were potentially coercive and, therefore, invited exploitation and made the prisoners vulnerable.

According to Beauchamp and Childress, the ethically factual, claim-justifying ground was that prison environments were coercive and could not be made free of coercion.[9] Thus the ethical justification rests on a factual claim and the ethical principle is avoiding harm, not a paternalistic overriding of the prisoners' choice. However, the supposed factual claim involves a psychological hypothesis about the nature of coercion and the individual's susceptibility to it. It is a psychological hypothesis that, taken seriously, raises questions about the ability of prisoners to freely consent to anything, and it ignores any consideration of whether prisoners convicted of crimes ought to pay their debt to society in part by accepting the risks of reasonable medical experimentation that may prove beneficial to the members of society. Both the factual conclusion and the ethical principle seem debatable. In fact, the report on research involving prisoners, viewed in this light, is not so much an ethical decision as a political bone thrown to the political activists concerned about prison conditions. It is useful politics, not utilitarian or deontological ethics. I do not claim that the political argument I have made is compelling, only that it raises questions about whether the prohibition of all research on prisoners (no matter how scientifically valuable and no matter how strongly prisoners assert that they feel no coercion), in fact, demonstrates substantial ethical progress.

¶ More Problems Than Solutions

Although I believe that psychiatrists no longer have the power to establish the ethical principles of their profession and have them accepted by the public and respected by the law, psychiatry remains the most crucial ethical force in the mental health system. Constrained by law and regulation, accountable to advocates and ombudsmen, well-trained psychiatrists remain the most qualified decision makers and providers of care to those with serious mental illness. They cannot abandon their ethical responsibilities and they should be aware of what seems to be their special ethical problems. These problems, it can be argued, begin with the mind-brain problem already touched on in the discussion of Szasz.

Szasz's approach to the mind-body problem is the antithesis of the approach taken by biological psychiatrists of the nineteenth century, who assumed that every mental "disease" was the product of a brain "disease." They reduced mind to brain. Even Sigmund Freud, as late as 1893, was attributing nocturnal enuresis to brain lesions and persistent headache to chronic, localized meningitis. As Moore[51] has pointed out, Isaac Ray's influential treatise on legal insan-

ity relied on that reductionistic assumption and asserted that since mental diseases were diseases of the brain, the aberrant behavior of such persons could not possibly be accounted for by such legal and mental terms as will and intention. Ray's treatise demonstrates what is still the most interesting moral and ethical question in biological psychiatry: Where mental illness is explained in biological discourse, does the person as a moral agent disappear? Do the issues of autonomy and responsibility become meaningless?

Using Szasz and Ray as counterexamples, we can outline some of the simplest aspects of the mind-brain problem as they are relevant to the special ethical problems of biological psychiatry. Szasz and Ray, though taking contradictory positions, share certain assumptions. Both would agree that there are persons with diseases of the brain (e.g., general paresis of the insane) whose behavior cannot be fully explicated in a discourse about minds—a self that chooses, intends, and acts on those intentions. There is, therefore, a class of persons whose disturbed behavior is, in some sense, only to be understood in terms of manifestations of a diseased brain. Now one must ask which psychiatric patients actually have brain disease.

The history of biological psychiatry is a convoluted trail of premature attempts to answer this question and to specify the brain disease or other biological disturbance. Even though in recent years the evidence of brain abnormality has been convincingly demonstrated in many psychiatric disorders, it is fair to say that there is still overreaching in the attempts to specify the nature of the abnormal brain event and its relation to complex behavior. Attempts to do this have been and remain premature and reductionistic.

Despite these limitations, once a patient is labeled as having a brain dysfunction, there is often a tendency to attribute all socially unacceptable, immoral, and unethical behaviors to the dysfunction. A decade ago violence was said to be an ictal event in temporal lobe epilepsy.[47] The scientific evidence subsequently proved this assertion to be dubious; but at the time, there was a tendency to assume that violence by temporal lobe epileptics had this specific biological explanation, the activation of the trigger of violence in the amygdala. Once patients were labeled temporal lobe epileptics, they were presumed to be incapable of intentional violence, at least to the extent that the "experts" tended to label all the violent acts of such patients as symptomatic. Furthermore, there was a tendency to assume that episodic violence, even in the absence of electroencephalogram evidence of temporal lobe epilepsy, was caused by temporal lobe dysfunction. Thus the overreaching biological approach tended to negate moral responsibility for violence.

Ray, without any of the neurophysiological or neurochemical evidence available today and apparently as a matter of faith, asserted that the criminal behavior of a schizophrenic was a manifestation of brain disorder. Szasz, in contrast, asserted that the person with schizophrenic disorder is as much a moral agent as any other person.[76] Completely ignoring the biological evidence, Szasz polemically asserted that schizophrenia was "created by psychiatry." Thus he engaged in the opposite kind of reductionistic fallacy. Where Ray reduced mind to brain, Szasz seems to have reduced brain to mind.

The dispute between Szasz and Ray is, however, more complicated. Szasz concedes that there are brain disorders, such as general paresis, that lead to mental disorders. But even in the case of paresis, can it be said that the brain disease explains the content of a particular patient's delusions of grandeur? Does it even explain why delusions of grandeur are typical of the condition? Surely the content of the delusion is based on the life experience of the patient, and perhaps the tendency of these patients to have grandiose delusions is cultural and experiential rather than a function of specific lesions in the brain. Even in the case of a paretic, there is a person experiencing a biological disorder.

Biological psychiatry does not yet have a coherent understanding of the brain in all its complexity, and there is no accepted theory about the relation between brain events and mental events; yet much of the debate in psychiatry has been carried out at a level that ignores these basic problems. If there is evidence of brain abnormality, the behavior of the affected person is cast by many biological psychiatrists in the discourse of diseased organisms. Such persons are not responsible, not competent, and not autonomous. Self, choice, intention, purpose, and will are not terms applicable to a diseased brain. So Isaac Ray advised the law, assuming that psychoses were brain disorders. Conversely, in the absence of brain disease, the person is understood in a discourse of self, choice, intention, purpose, and even free will. So Thomas Szasz advised the law assuming that psychoses or, as he preferred to describe them, "problems in living," had no significant relationship to biological disorders.

This is by no means an antiquated debate, and it is central to the ethical and moral questions in biological psychiatry. A biological psychiatrist testifying on behalf of John Hinckley (attempted assassin of President Reagan) argued that the diazepam Hinckley had taken had released the inhibitory brain, allowing a paroxysm of violence in a person with schizophrenic disorder.[73] All this, of course, was highly speculative, particularly since this explanation was based on a reconstruction of the events weeks after they happened. Hinckley's brain, he said, was demonstrably abnormal (atrophy on a CT scan), and this was sufficient for the biological psychiatrist to cast Hinckley's behavior in the discourse of brain disease: altered thresholds, chemical release of inhibitory brain, and paroxysm of violence. This is a discourse of the caused behavior of an organism, not the intended behavior of a choosing person. Thus the biological psychiatrist excused Hinckley from legal and moral responsibility for his actions in the same form of argument used by Isaac Ray more than a century ago. John Hinckley was not a moral agent.

Conversely, a psychiatrist testifying against Hinckley described a person without schizophrenia and without a brain disorder, who, made anxious by his decision to shoot the President, took diazepam to calm himself down, the better to achieve his purpose.[73] Hinckley, in this description, did not have a paroxysm of violence. He was described as a moral agent, a person purposefully assuming a firing position, intending to carry out his chosen plan to kill the President. It could have been said that the atrophy was, in fact, "garden variety" and within normal limits. This contradictory testimony exemplifies the practical importance of the mind-brain problem in psychiatry.

Understanding mind in terms of brain leads to a discourse about causation in organisms, as opposed to a discourse about the intended actions of persons with choice. The biological discourse excludes free will and moral responsibility. It is a discourse based on an implicit assumption that the presence of a demonstrable brain disorder cancels the self that intends, chooses, and acts on those intentions and choices. But would it not be peculiar if all diseases of the brain cancelled the self? People with brain tumors often recognize their symptoms and decide to seek medical assistance. The self that plans and the self that reflects on the self is apparently still functioning in some persons with serious brain disorders.

There are, of course, patients with such extensive brain disease that it becomes impossible to argue that they have the ability to choose, or to will, or to intend. However, the autonomy and moral responsibility of such cases are not apt to be the subject of ethical or legal dispute. Dispute begins when the brain disorder is more limited and the question arises, In what way is this behavior a product of the brain disorder? Is the presence of a particular brain disorder sufficient to reduce the person and the mind to the mechanistic brain discourse? How can this be possible when we do not yet understand the complexities of the brain? How can the attempt be more than speculative? Is such speculation a sufficient basis to rule out moral responsibility?

The attempt to reduce mind to brain and eliminate the self has, as already noted, been played out in the literature of temporal lobe epilepsy. Violence was once thought to be an ictal event in that disorder, an automatic act and not willed behavior. Thus such violence was thought to carry no moral or legal responsibility. The most notorious example of this overreaching was the suggestion that the violence attendant on the urban race riots of the 1960s could be attributed in some measure to brain disease and particularly disorders of the amygdala.[48] Today's experts believe that the evidence now indicates that among patients with temporal lobe epilepsy, violence is an interictal event and not an epileptic equivalent. However, attributing interictal violence to a kindling disturbance of the limbic brain, the current hypothesis, requires highly speculative accounts of the brain mechanisms at work.[21] These accounts typically omit any reference to how the person, the self, experiences the brain disorder and how the person adapts or reacts to these significant disruptions.

Brain disorder as a direct explanation of violent behavior remains inadequate and highly speculative. The exact nature of the association between the supposed neuronal disorder and violence is by no means fully elucidated without taking into account the person, the context, the cultural mores, and so on. For example, one current speculative theory has it that limbic disorders alter the affective salience of perceptions.[21] Thus one can hypothesize that a chance perception might produce intense hostile affect, but whether the person then hits, stabs, howls insults, or becomes apologetic and ashamed is not explained biologically, nor is it even clear that such theories are based on a complete understanding of relevant brain function in all its complexity. How inadequate, then, must be the accounts in which the various complex schizophrenic symptoms and all other behaviors of such persons are reduced to the discourse of biological causation.

I have described these speculative theories as overreaching. They are not overreaching to the extent that they are hypotheses to be further pursued in research. Biological psychiatrists overreach when they claim to explain complex human actions: violence, sexual preference, or religious conversions, all complex human actions that have been attributed to limbic disorders. What is more, it is this overreaching that backfires and leads the legal critics of biological psychiatry to claim that biological treatment is mind-altering, interfering with mentation, free thought, and even religious belief. These criticisms are in some respects a mirror response to these overreaching claims.

It is important to recognize that in the first simple distinction presented here, brain disease was the crucial distinguishing criterion. Brain disease made the person into an organism. But the brain without disease is no less a brain and no less explicable in terms of brain chemistry, brain physiology, and biological causation. The brain is material, though highly complicated material, and there is a normal organism as well as a diseased organism. The presence or absence of brain disease does not change the underlying biological theory or discourse, nor does it obviate the mind-brain problem.

Making the presence of brain disease the critical criterion, the point at which the person becomes an organism is an arbitrary convention. This is a critical conceptual flaw in Ray's approach to the mind-brain problem. Ray had no basis to assert that the language of intention, will, and action cannot explain brain-disordered persons but can explain nonbrain-disordered persons. It is a conceptual flaw that has not yet been solved by biological psychiatry. One common approach to this problem, once it has been clearly recognized, is to suggest that the person with a brain disorder has less choice or autonomy than a person without such a brain disorder. The notion is of a limited repertoire of responses or a lowered threshold of a given response. This approach, though intuitively appealing, has no real explanatory power. It is a way of saying that there must be a relationship between brain and mind but that the relationship cannot be specified. That, however, is a compromise and not a theory.

Konrad Lorenz, in his popular work on aggression, faced up to the theoretical problem I am emphasizing. He admitted that free will and the self that chooses were the obstacle to acceptance of his mechanistic biological explanations of aggressive behavior. He suggested that when we understood that free will was the will of the "Creator," the dispute would end.[44] Presumably because free will was to Lorenz a religious concept, it could be relinquished if it took on a different religious meaning. Surely it can be argued that free will is a premise about what it means to be a person and a moral agent, even to an atheist. These comments emphasize that the moral and ethical crux of biological psychiatry is its implicit determinism, which excludes the autonomous person, the moral agent, capable of free will. The elimination of the autonomous person is by no means a failing limited to biological psychiatry. It is a failing of all forms of modern-day psychiatry and behavioral science founded on deterministic premises. Like its sister disciplines, biological psychiatry has constructed a theory in which ethics and morality are extraneous matters. This, in turn, suggests that the practice of biological psychiatry is morally neutral. To believe that is to deny the lessons of history in the twentieth century.

¶ Conclusions

What lessons are there to be learned from this overview of themes in medical and psychiatric ethics? First, a definition has been presented: Medical ethics involves conflicts between two or more arguably correct actions. This is not a subject elaborated in the medical professional's Principles of Ethics. Second, the historical record suggests that the medical and psychiatric professions have been insensitive to values other than therapeutic values and the advancement of science through research; thus important ethical values were ignored. Third, psychiatry must now accept the reality that where professional ethics involves conflicts between two arguably correct choices, there must be a dialogue with patients, the public, and the law (e.g., the dying patient, the defective newborn, the right to refuse "antipsychotic" drugs).

Fourth, there seems to be no acceptable system of *a priori* ethical solutions to the many ethical problems the psychiatrist confronts. This does not mean the psychiatrist should ignore such systematic attempts; the study of ethics should be as important to psychiatrists as the study of any other relevant professional subject. There is as yet no definitive theory of the genetics of schizophrenia, but that is not a reason for psychiatrists to ignore that literature. The same ought to be true of ethics.

Fifth, the psychiatrist cannot expect to get much practical guidance from the profession's Principles of Ethics. They do define unethical behavior, and the evidence that many psychiatrists have never even seen a copy is unacceptable; but one can get a great deal from the traditional praxis of doing all you can to help and first of all do no harm. These maxims constitute a dialectical framework, and the framework offers guidance in thinking about one's personal ethical responsibilities as a physician and in making judgments about one's peers.

Sixth, informed consent is not an enemy of good care in psychiatry. For many psychiatric patients, the drug they are taking and its effects on them is the most important consideration. The cooperative patient is an informed patient who understands the purpose of treatment, the risks and benefits, and the alternatives. The patient who knows about side effects will be alert to the need to inform the psychiatrist. Informed consent is a process, a continuing dialogue, and the goal of good psychiatric care includes that dialogue, not only as a matter of ethics but as a matter of good treatment.

The rights of patients as defined by law in some jurisdictions may in fact interfere with treatment. I suggest that the psychiatrist under certain specified conditions can refuse on ethical grounds to be responsible for a patient whose legal rights interfere with essential treatment. Psychiatrists must continue to participate in legal decisions and legislation that shape the rights of patients to ensure that potential legal conflicts between the rights and the needs of patients are fully considered.

Seventh, no psychiatrist can single-handedly address the problems of the bottomless pit. The psychiatrist should be an advocate for his or her own patients' needs. The psychiatric profession as a whole must be alert to regulatory attempts to control the bottomless pit that ignore the needs of the mentally ill or give them short shrift. The individual psychiatrist and the profession must be alert to regulatory constraints that impinge on ethical responsibilities. These questions should be directly confronted, lest the provision of mental health services be designed to meet the demands of regulation and economic incentives rather than the needs of the mentally ill.

The most common ethical failing of medicine and psychiatry is the failure to provide continuity of care, yet rarely is this identified as an ethical failing. Perhaps this is because the provision of health care *is* designed to meet the demands of regulation and therefore seems forced upon us, and rarely does the profession consider the ethical implications of its economic incentives and constraints.

Eighth, the committee solution to ethical problems provides a process of review; it does not guarantee wise or correct substantive ethical decisions. It may be that physicians will fall into the same fallacy as those lawyers who are satisfied that the process was good even though the result may be bad. Such a procedural approach may be enough for a just legal system, but it may not be enough for ethical medical or psychiatric care.

Ninth, this chapter, like the literature on ethics, raises more questions than it provides answers, but that is not a reason for skepticism or cynicism. The medical profession, in the end, depends on the ethical praxis of its individual practitioners, not on laws, committees, or *a priori* theories. A psychiatrist dedicated to high standards of practice and personal responsibility can contribute much to the ethics of the profession, even in these times of ethical uncertainty.

Finally, there are special ethical issues for the biological psychiatrist. The biological psychiatrists (and I would suggest all psychiatrists) have a tendency to treat those problems with ethical implications as part of the patient's illness. This is not some vague theoretical point; rather, it is a matter of everyday practice. Often a liaison psychiatrist is asked to consult on matters that involve ethical as well as psychiatric questions. The patient refuses treatment, the patient is uncooperative, or the patient's family is angry, perhaps with the doctor or the nurses or the hospital.

If the biological psychiatrist thinks in the discourse of brain and ignores the discourse of mind and meaning, he or she may fail to discover that the patient has not been properly informed about his condition and treatment or that he has a legitimate complaint to be angry about. The psychiatrist will fail to discover that medical and surgical colleagues have been derelict in their ethical responsibilities. The temptation to ignore all this is great, as one avoids conflict with colleagues and one is consistent to the discourse of biological causation.

A psychiatrist who is concerned about ethics and about high standards of care will find that life is more difficult, but being a good psychiatrist is not an easy profession. Life is a moral adventure, and a psychiatrist who ignores ethics has no moral direction to guide his or her professional life.

¶ Bibliography

1. ABRAM, M. B., and WOLF, S. M. "Public Involvement in Medical Ethics," *New England Journal of Medicine*, 310 (1984):627–632.

2. AMERICAN PSYCHIATRIC ASSOCIATION. *The Principles of Medical Ethics with Annotations Especially Applicable to Psychiatry.* Washington, D.C.: American Psychiatric Association, 1984.

3. ANNAS, G. J., and GLANTZ, L. H. "Psychosurgery: The Law's Response," *Boston University Law Review*, 54 (1974):249–267.

4. Arizona Revised Statutes §32-1451 (1975 Comm. Supp.).

5. Attorney General v. Travellers Insurance Co., 385 Mass. 598, 1982, 391 Mass. 730 (1984).

6. AVORN, J. "Benefit and Cost Analysis in Geriatric Care: Turning Age Discrimination into Health Policy," *New England Journal of Medicine*, 310 (1984): 1294–1301.

7. BAYER, R. *Homosexuality and American Psychiatry: The Politics of Diagnosis.* New York: Basic Books, 1980.

8. Beal v. Doe, 432 U.S. 438 (1977).

9. BEAUCHAMP, T. L., and CHILDRESS, J. F. *Principles of Biomedical Ethics*, 2nd ed. New York: Oxford University Press, 1983.

10. BEECHER, H. K. "Ethics and Clinical Research," *New England Journal of Medicine*, 274 (1966):1354–1360.

11. BRANDT, R. B. *Ethical Theory.* Englewood Cliffs, N. J.: Prentice-Hall, 1959.

12. BURT, R. A. *Taking Care of Strangers.* New York: Free Press, 1979.

13. CALABRESI, G., and BOBBIT, P. *Tragic Choices.* New York: W.W. Norton, 1978.

14. Canterbury v. Spence, 464 F.2d 772 (1972).

15. CASSEM, E. "When to Disconnect the Respirator," *Psychiatric Annals*, 9 (1979): 38–53.

16. CERLETTI, U. "Old and New Information About Electroshock," *American Journal of Psychiatry*, 107 (1950):87–94.

17. CHILDRESS, J. F. *Who Should Decide: Paternalism in Health Care.* New York: Oxford University Press, 1982.

18. Code of Federal Regulations, National Health Planning and Resources Development Act 42. U.S.C. § 300 N-1(c)(11)(12) 1982.

19. Combined Federal Regulations, 45 C.F.R. § 46 (1982).

20. CULVER, C. M., and GERT, B. *Philosophy in Medicine: Conceptual and Ethical Issues in Medicine and Psychiatry.* New York: Oxford University Press, 1982.

21. DEVINSKY, O., and BEAR, D. "Varieties of Aggressive Behavior in Temporal Lobe Epilepsy," *American Journal of Psychiatry*, 141 (1984):651–656.

22. Doe v. Bolton, 410 U.S. 179 (1973).

23. Donaldson v. O'Connor, 493 F.2d 507 (1974).

24. Federal Register, 43 Fed. Reg. 52146, 52171, 52173 (Nov. 8, 1978).

25. Federal Register, vol. 49, No. 1. (Jan. 12, 1984), p. 1622.

26. FLETCHER, J. *Situation Ethics: The New Morality.* Philadelphia: Westminster Press, 1966.

27. FOST, N. "Letter," *Hastings Center Report,* 13 (1983):49.

28. FREEDMAN, B. "Competence, Marginal and Otherwise," *International Journal of Law and Psychiatry,* 4 (1981):53–72.

29. FREEMAN, W. "Psychosurgery," in S. Arieti, ed., *American Handbook of Psychiatry,* vol. 2. New York: Basic Books, 1959, pp. 1521–1541.

30. FRIEDSON, E. *Professional Dominance: The Social Structure of Medical Care.* New York: Atherton Press, 1970.

31. FUCHS, V. *Who Shall Live.* New York: Basic Books, 1974.

32. GILLS, J. J., ed. "Professional Conflicts: Ethics and Society," *Psychiatric Annals,* 9 (1979):1–74.

33. HARE, R. M. *Applications of Moral Philosophy.* Berkeley: University of California Press, 1973.

34. HARRON, F., BURNSIDE, J., and BEAUCHAMP, T. L. *Health and Human Values, A Guide to Making Your Own Decisions.* New Haven, Conn.: Yale University Press, 1983.

35. HAVIGHURST, C. C. "Decentralizing Decision-Making: Private Contract vs. Professional Norms," in J. A. Meyer, ed., *Market Reforms in Health Care.* Washington D.C.: American Enterprise Institute, 1983, pp. 22–45.

36. HILLER, M. D. *Medical Ethics and the Law.* Cambridge, Mass.: Ballinger Publishing Company, 1981.

37. JAMETON, A. *Nursing Practice: The Ethical Issues.* Englewood Cliffs, N.J.: Prentice-Hall, 1983.

38. Joint Commission on Accreditation of Hospitals, *Standards for Hospital Accreditation.* Chicago: Joint Committee on Accreditation of Hospitals, 1964, 1971.

39. JONES, J. *Bad Blood.* New York: Free Press, 1981.

40. KANT, I. *Foundations of the Metaphysics of Morals.* New York: Bobbs-Merrill, 1969. (Originally published in 1785.)

41. KATZ, J. *Experimentation with Human Beings.* New York: Russell Sage Foundation, 1972.

42. KOMAROFF, A. L. "Securing Access to Health Care," in *President's Commission for the Study of Ethical Problems in Medicine and Biomedical and Behavioral Research,* vol. 3. Washington, D.C.: Government Printing Office, 1979–1983, pp. 225–251.

43. LAW, S. "Can Doctors Police Doctors?" Health Law Project, *Library Bulletin,* 3 (1978): 1–6.

44. LORENZ, K. *On Agression.* New York: Harcourt, Brace and World, 1966.

45. LOUISELL, D. W., and WILLIAMS, H. *Medical Malpractice,* rev. ed. New York: Matthew Bender, 1983.

46. McCORMICK, R. "To Save or Let Die, The Dilemma of Modern Medicine," *Journal of the American Medical Association,* 229 (1974):172–176.

47. MARK, V., and ERVIN, F. *Violence and the Brain.* New York: Harper & Row, 1970.

48. MARK, V., SWEET, R., and ERVIN, F. "Role of Brain Disease in Riots and Urban Violence," *Journal of the American Medical Association,* 201 (1967):895.

49. MEISEL, A. "Informed Consent," in E. D. Hiller, ed., *Medical Ethics and the Law.* Cambridge, Mass.: Ballinger, 1981, pp. 197–217.

50. MILL, J. S. *Utilitarianism, On Liberty and Essay on Bentham,* edited by M. Warnock, New York: New American Library, 1974.

51. MOORE, M. S. *Law and Psychiatry: Rethinking the Relationship.* Cambridge: Cambridge University Press, 1984.

52. MOORE, S. H., MARTIN, D. Q., and RICHARDSON, W. C. "Does the Primary-Care Gatekeeper Control the Cost of Health Care." *New England Journal of Medicine,* 309 (1983):1400–1404.

53. MURRAY, G. "Ethics at the Crossroads," *Psychiatric Annals,* 9 (1979):21–25.

54. PELLEGRINO, E. D. "Competition: New Moral Dilemmas for Physicians and Hospitals," *Hospital Progress,* 64 (1983):8–25.

55. Pinneke v. Preisser, 623 F.2d 546 (1980).

56. PRESIDENT'S COMMISSION FOR THE STUDY OF ETHICAL PROBLEMS IN MEDICINE AND BIOMEDICAL AND BEHAVIORAL RESEARCH. *Summing Up.* Washington, D.C.: Government Printing Office, 1979–1983.

57. RAMSEY, P. *The Patient as Person.* New Haven, Conn.: Yale University Press, 1970.

58. RAWLS, J. *A Theory of Justice.* Cambridge, Mass.: Harvard University Press, 1971.

59. REDLICH, F., and MOLLICA, R. F. "Ethical Issues in Psychiatry," *American Journal of Psychiatry,* 133 (1976):125–136.

60. "Referendum Against ECT," *Mental Disability Law Reporter,* 6 (1982):366–367.

61. *Report and Recommendations: Research Involving Prisoners.* Washington, D.C.: DHEW Publication No. (05)76-131, 1976.

62. Roe v. Wade, 410 U.S. 113 (1973).

63. Rogers v. Commissioner of Mental Health, 390 Mass. 459 (1983).

64. Rogers v. Okin, 478 F. Supp. 1342, 1364–65 (1979), aff'd in part and rev'd in part, 634 F.2d 650 (1980), vacated and remanded sub. nom. Mills v. Rogers, 102 S. Ct. 2442 (1982).

65. RYDER, R. *Victims of Science: The Use of Animals in Research.* London: Davis-Poynter, 1975.

66. Schloendorff v. Society of New York Hospitals, 105 N.E. 92 (1914).

67. SHANNON, T. A., and MANFRA, J. A. *Law and Bioethics.* Ramsey, N.J.: Paulist Press, 1982.

68. SPIVEY, B. E. "The Relation Between Hospital Management and Medical Staff Under a Prospective Payment System," *New England Journal of Medicine,* 310 (1984):984–986.

69. STONE, A. A. "The History and Future of Litigation," in D. M. Gallant, and R. Force, eds., *Legal and Ethical Issues in Human Research and Treatment.* New York: SP Medical and Scientific Books, 1978, pp. 19–69.

70. ———. "Informed Consent: Special Problems for Psychiatry," *Hospital and Community Psychiatry,* 321 (1979):324–325.

71. ———. "Preceptor, Law and Psychiatry," in L. Grinspoon, ed., *Psychiatry 1982 Annual Review.* Washington, D.C.: American Psychiatry Press, 1982, pp. 321–327.

72. ———. "The New Paradox of Psychiatric Malpractice," *New England Journal of Medicine,* 311 (1984):1384–1387.

73. ———. *Law, Psychiatry and Morality; Essays and Analysis.* Washington, D.C.: American Psychiatric Press, 1984.

74. Superintendent of Belchertown State School v. Saikewicz, 373 Mass. 278 (1977).

75. SZASZ, T. *Law, Liberty and Psychiatry.* New York: Macmillan, 1963.

76. ———. *The Manufacture of Madness.* New York: Harper & Row, 1970.

77. ———. *The Myth of Mental Illness,* rev. ed. New York: Harper & Row, 1974.

78. ———. *Sex by Prescription.* Garden City, N.Y.: Anchor Press, 1980, pp. 70–96.

79. TALBOTT, G. D., and BENSON, E. B. "Impaired Physicians: The Dilemma of Identification," *Postgraduate Medicine,* 68 (1980):56–64.

80. Tarasoff v. Regents of University of California, 118 Cal. Rptr. 129 (1974).

81. TAYLOR, K. M., MARGOLESE, R. G., and SOSKOLNE, C. L. "Physician's Reasons for Not Entering Eligible Patients in a Randomized Clinical Trial of Breast Cancer," *New England Journal of Medicine,* 310 (1983):1363–1367.

82. U.S.C. 42 § 1983 (1979).

83. VALENSTEIN, E. *Brain Control.* New York: John Wiley & Sons, 1973.

84. VEATCH, R. M. *Case Studies in Medical Ethics.* Cambridge, Mass.: Harvard University Press, 1977.

85. ———. *A Theory of Medical Ethics.* New York: Basic Books, 1981.

86. WALD, P., and FRIEDMAN, P. R. "The Politics of Mental Health Advocacy in the United States," *International Journal of Law and Psychiatry,* 1 (1978):137–152.

87. WANZER, S. H., et al. "The Physician's Responsibility Toward Hopelessly Ill Patients," *New England Journal of Medicine,* 310 (1984):955–960.

88. WIKLER, D. "Philosophical Perspectives on Access to Health Care: An Introduc-

tion," in *President's Commission for the Study of Ethical Problems in Medicine and Biomedical and Behavioral Research*, vol. 2. Washington, D.C.: Government Printing Office, 1979–1983, pp. 109–151.

89. WING, K. R., and CRAIGE, B. "Health Care Regulation: Dilemma of a Partially Developed Policy," *North Carolina Law Review*, 57 (1979):1165–1195.
90. Wyatt v. Stickney, 325 F. Supp. 781 (1971).

NAME INDEX

SUBJECT INDEX

Extrapyramidal side effects, 13, 16, 76, 438, 481, 482, 560, 926, 951–955; of amoxapine, 309; in children, 629; clozapine and, 957–959; of doxapine, 970; electroconvulsive therapy and, 1010; of lithium, 985; neuroendocrine system and, 130; tricyclics and, 520; *see also* Tardive dyskinesia

Eye disorders, *see* Ocular side effects

Eye movement in schizophrenia, 436

Facial motor nucleus, 14

Factitious mental disorder, 912

Family studies: of affective disorders, 161, 162; of alcoholism, 879; of anorexia nervosa, 775–776; of attention deficit disorder, 630–631; computed tomography in, 219; of obesity, 793; of schizophrenia, 160–161, 429–430

Family therapy, 482; for schizophrenia, 483–486

Fasciculus retroflexus, 6

Fatigue, 905–906

Fear, 597–599

Federal Trade Commission, 1088

Felty's syndrome, 980

Fenfluramine, 389; for bulimia, 780; for childhood disorders, 629; for obesity, 801; prolactin and, 118; serotonin and, 272

Fentanyl, 814

Fibrillary gliosis, 153, 213, 432, 448

Fibroblast studies, 1069

Fisher's Exact Test, 325, 340

FK-33-824, 557

Flagyl, 891

Flooding, 604, 605

Fluorohydrocortisone, 965

Fluoxetine, 314, 316, 317

Flupenthixol, 69, 174, 499; side effects of, 540–541

Fluphenazine, 473, 496; for childhood disorders, 629; depot form of, 480; electroencephalography and, 193; plasma levels of, 492, 494; side effects of, 540, 951, 954

Folate deficiency, 912, 917

Follicle-stimulating hormone (FSH), 114; in alcoholism, 134; in anorexia nervosa and bulimia, 131, 132, 771; in depression, 119–120; drug effects on, 949; in schizophrenia, 128, 130

Folstein Mini Mental State Examination, 906

Food and Drug Administration (FDA), 310, 395, 610, 635, 971, 978

Forced immersion, 602, 604

Fornix, 6, 7

Fourier transformations, 190

Friedrich's ataxia, 691

Frontal cortex: atrophy of, 239; innervation of, 12; magnetic resonance imaging of, 254; neuropeptides in, 74; in positron emission tomography, 239, 240, 242, 245

Frontal horn enlargement, 221, 222

Frontal lobe: decreased activity of, 196; hypothesis perseveration and, 183; in schizophrenia, 439

Frontal lobe syndrome, 921

Frontal lobotomy, *see* Lobotomy

Frontal Lobotomy and Affective Behavior (Fulton), 1029

Frustration-aggression theory, 652, 657

Functional brain imaging, *see* Positron emission tomography

Fusaric acid, 275, 387, 545, 555

GABA-oc-ketoglutarate transaminase (GABA-T), 277–279

Gamma-aminobutyric acid (GABA), 15–17, 37, 45, 412; affective disorders and, 277–279; aggression and, 656; in Alzheimer's disease, 681–682; in anorexia nervosa, 773; anticonvulsants and, 395; anxiety and, 586–592, 919; benzodiazepines and, 851; electroconvulsive therapy and, 1018; growth hormone and, 121; in magnetic resonance spectroscopy, 257; parkinsonism and, 954; in postmortem brain tissue, 154; in schizophrenia, 73, 445–446; somatostatin and, 282; in tardive dyskinesia, 545, 556, 558, 560

Gamma-endorphins, 75–76, 447

Gamma-MSH, 22

Gas chromatography, 42, 378, 379

Gastrin, 20

Gastrointestinal peptides, 19

Gastrointestinal system: alcoholism and, 884; in anorexia nervosa and bulimia, 765–766, 780; antipsychotics and, 951; lithium and, 979; stimulants and, 632; in tardive dyskinesia, 541; tricyclics and, 965

Genain quadruplets, 242

Gene transfer, 178–179

General paresis, 910, 911

Generalized anxiety disorder, 601; behavioral therapy for, 603; pharmacotherapy for, 607–612

Genetic factors, 160–167; in affective disorders, 265–266, 272, 274, 275, 281; in aggression, 653–654; in alcoholism, 879–880; in Alzheimer's disease, 87, 679–680; in anorexia nervosa, 775–776; in attention deficit disorder, 630–631; in autism, 627, 628; in behavioral neurochemistry, 46–47; computed tomography abnormalities and,

219–220; in drug metabolism, 381; in enuresis, 633; family data and, 152; isolation of major genes, 164–166; laboratory tests and, 1069; linkage analysis for, 163; Mendelian, 163–164; molecular neurobiologic studies of, 51; in obesity, 793–795; pathoanatomy and pathophysiology and, 166–167; in schizophrenia, 429–433; in tic disorders, 634; types of inheritance, 162–163

Genitourinary side effects, 948, 965

Germ phobia, surgical treatment of, 1043

Gestalt therapy, 863

Gilles de la Tourette's syndrome, 555, 559, 563, 634–635, 691

Glafenine, 988

Glaucoma, 946, 965

Global Assessment Scale, 127

Global Hamilton Depression Scale, 333

Globus pallidus, 16, 18; neuropeptides in, 74

Glucagon: in Alzheimer's disease, 89; pain and, 716

Glucocorticoids, 41, 1063; in affective disorders, 115; dexamethasone suppression test and, 117; immune function and, 123; in schizophrenia, 129; suicidal behavior and, 123

Glucose metabolic rate, 238–239

Glucose tolerance test, 980

Glue sniffing, 830

Glutamate, 15, 16, 277

Glutamic acid decarboxylase (GAD), 154, 277, 681

Gluten, abnormal reaction to, 449

Glutethimide, 605; abuse of, 814, 847–848

Glycine, 15, 16

Glycopyrrolate, 1013

Goiter, 980

Gonadal steroid hormones: in affective disorders, 119–120; in alcoholism, 134; in anorexia nervosa, 131–132; in schizophrenia, 128; stress and, 125; *see also specific hormones*

Gonadotropin, 114; in affective disorders, 119–120; in alcoholism, 134; in anorexia nervosa, 771, 772; neuroleptics and, 130; premenstrual syndrome and, 421

Gonadotropin-releasing hormone (GnRH), 112, 113; in alcoholism, 134; in anorexia nervosa, 132, 771; in depression, 119, 120; in schizophrenia, 130

Granulocytopenia, 961

Granulovacuolar degeneration, 680

Group for the Advancement of Psychiatry, Committee on Child Psychiatry of, 621

Group therapy, 482; for alcoholism, 890, 891; for anorexia nervosa and